D1587419

Meyler's Side Effects of Drugs

The International Encyclopedia of Adverse Drug Reactions and Interactions

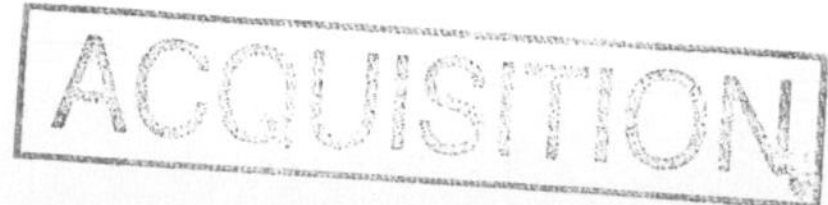

Complementary to this volume
Side Effects of Drugs Annuals 24–29 (1999–2006)
Edited by Jeffrey K. Aronson (Earlier annuals are no longer available in print)

Drugs During Pregnancy and Lactation, Second edition (2006)
Edited by Christof Schaefer et al.

The Law and Ethics of the Pharmaceutical Industry (2005)
By Graham Dukes

Introduction to Clinical Pharmacology, Fifth edition (2006)
By Marilyn Edmunds

Principles of Clinical Pharmacology, Second edition (2006)
Edited by Arthur Atkinson et al.

Writing Clinical Research Protocols (2006)
By E. De Renzo

A Pharmacology Primer (2003)
By Terry Kenakin

Publishing history of *Meyler's Side Effects of Drugs*

*Volume**	*Date of publication*	*Editors*
First published in Dutch	1951	L Meyler
First published in English	1952	L Meyler
First updating volume	1957	L Meyler
Second volume	1958	L Meyler
Third volume	1960	L Meyler
Fourth volume	1964	L Meyler
Fifth volume	1966	L Meyler, C Dalderup, W Van Dijl, and HGG Bouma
Sixth volume	1968	L Meyler and A Herxheimer
Seventh volume	1972	L Meyler and A Herxheimer
Eighth volume	1975	MNG Dukes
Ninth edition	1980	MNG Dukes
Tenth edition	1984	MNG Dukes
Eleventh edition	1988	MNG Dukes
Twelfth edition	1992	MNG Dukes
Thirteenth edition	1996	MNG Dukes
Fourteenth edition	2000	MNG Dukes & JK Aronson
Fifteenth edition	2006	JK Aronson

*The first eight volumes were updates; the ninth edition was the first encyclopedic version and updating continued with the Side Effects of Drugs Annual (SEDA) series.

At various times, full or shortened editions of volumes in the Side Effects series have appeared in French, Russian, Dutch, German, and Japanese.
The website of *Meyler's Side Effects of Drugs* can be viewed at:
http://www.elsevier.com/locate/Meyler.

Meyler's Side Effects of Drugs

The International Encyclopedia of Adverse Drug Reactions and Interactions

Fifteenth edition

Editor

JK Aronson, MA, DPhil, MBChB, FRCP, FBPharmacol S
Oxford, United Kingdom

Honorary Editor

MNG Dukes, MA, DPhil, MB, FRCP
Oslo, Norway

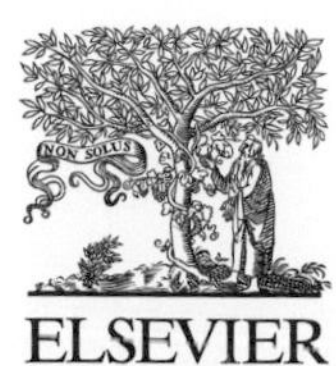

ELSEVIER

AMSTERDAM • BOSTON • HEIDELBERG • LONDON • NEW YORK • OXFORD
PARIS • SAN DIEGO • SAN FRANCISCO • SINGAPORE • SYDNEY • TOKYO

Elsevier
Radarweg 29, PO Box 211, 1000 AE Amsterdam, The Netherlands

Fifteenth edition 2006
Reprinted 2007

British Library Cataloguing in Publication Data
A catalogue record for this book is available from the British Library

Library of Congress Cataloging-in-Publication Data
A catalog record for this book is available from the Library of Congress

ISBN: 978-0-444-50998-7 (Set)
ISBN: 978-0-444-52251-1 (Volume 1)
ISBN: 978-0-444-52252-8 (Volume 2)
ISBN: 978-0-444-52253-5 (Volume 3)
ISBN: 978-0-444-52254-2 (Volume 4)
ISBN: 978-0-444-52255-9 (Volume 5)
ISBN: 978-0-444-52256-6 (Volume 6)

For information on all Elsevier publications
visit our website at books.elsevier.com

Printed and bound in *Great Britain*

07 08 09 10 10 9 8 7 6 5 4 3 2

Contents

Contributors

In this list the main contributors to the Encyclopedia are identified according to the original chapter material to which they made the most contribution. Most have contributed the relevant chapters in one or more editions of the *Side Effects of Drugs Annuals* 23-27 and/or the 14th edition of *Meyler's Side Effects of Drugs*. A few have contributed individual monographs to this edition.

M. Allwood
Derby, United Kingdom
Intravenous infusions—solutions and emulsions

M. Andersen
Odense, Denmark
Antihistamines

M. Andrejak
Amiens, France
Drugs affecting blood coagulation, fibrinolysis, and hemostasis

J.K. Aronson
Oxford, United Kingdom
Antiepileptic drugs
Antiviral drugs
Positive inotropic drugs and drugs used in dysrhythmias

S. Arroyo
Milwaukee, Wisconsin, USA
Antiepileptic drugs

I. Aursnes
Oslo, Norway
Drugs that affect lipid metabolism

H. Bagheri
Toulouse, France
Radiological contrast agents

A.M. Baldacchino
London, United Kingdom
Opioid analgesics and narcotic antagonists

D. Battino
Milan, Italy
Antiepileptic drugs

Z. Baudoin
Zagreb, Croatia
General anesthetics and therapeutic gases

A.G.C. Bauer
Rotterdam, The Netherlands
Antihelminthic drugs
Dermatological drugs, topical agents, and cosmetics

M. Behrend
Deggendorf, Germany
Drugs acting on the immune system

T. Bicanic
London, United Kingdom
Antiprotozoal drugs

L. Biscarini
Perugia, Italy
Anti-inflammatory and antipyretic analgesics and drugs used in gout

J. Blaser
Zurich, Switzerland
Various antibacterial drugs

C. Bokemeyer
Tübingen, Germany
Cytostatic drugs

S. Borg
Stockholm, Sweden
Antidepressant drugs

J. Bousquet
Montpellier, France
Antihistamines

P.J. Bown
Redhill, Surrey, United Kingdom
Opioid analgesics and narcotic antagonists

C.N. Bradfield
Auckland, New Zealand
General anesthetics and therapeutic gases

C.C.E. Brodie-Meijer
Amstelveen, The Netherlands
Metal antagonists

P.W.G. Brown
Sheffield, United Kingdom
Radiological contrast agents

A. Buitenhuis
Amsterdam, The Netherlands
Sex hormones and related compounds, including hormonal contraceptives

H. Cardwell
Auckland, New Zealand
Local anesthetics

A. Carvajal
Valladolid, Spain
Antipsychotic drugs

R. Cathomas
Zurich, Switzerland
Drugs acting on the respiratory tract

A. Cerny
Zurich, Switzerland
Various antibacterial drugs

G. Chevrel
Lyon, France
Drugs acting on the immune system

C.C. Chiou
Bethesda, Maryland, USA
Antifungal drugs

N.H. Choulis
Attika, Greece
Metals
Miscellaneous drugs and materials, medical devices, and techniques not dealt with in other chapters

L.G. Cleland
Adelaide, Australia
Corticotrophins, corticosteroids, and prostaglandins

P. Coates
Adelaide, Australia
Miscellaneous hormones

J. Costa
Badalona, Spain
Corticotrophins, corticosteroids, and prostaglandins

P. Cottagnoud
Bern, Switzerland
Various antibacterial drugs

P.C. Cowen
Oxford, United Kingdom
Antidepressant drugs

S. Curran
Huddersfield, United Kingdom
Hypnosedatives and anxiolytics

H.C.S. Daly
Perth, Western Australia
Local anesthetics

A.C. De Groot
Hertogenbosch, The Netherlands
Dermatological drugs, topical agents, and cosmetics

M.D. De Jong
Amsterdam, The Netherlands
Antiviral drugs

A. Del Favero
Perugia, Italy
Anti-inflammatory and antipyretic analgesics and drugs used in gout

P. Demoly
Montpellier, France
Antihistamines

J. Descotes
Lyon, France
Drugs acting on the immune system

A.J. De Silva
Ragama, Sri Lanka
Snakebite antivenom

H.J. De Silva
Ragama, Sri Lanka
Gastrointestinal drugs

F.A. De Wolff
Leiden, The Netherlands
Metals

S. Dittmann
Berlin, Germany
Vaccines

M.N.G. Dukes
Oslo, Norway
Antiepileptic drugs
Antiviral drugs
Metals
Sex hormones and related compounds, including hormonal contraceptives

H.W. Eijkhout
Amsterdam, The Netherlands
Blood, blood components, plasma, and plasma products

E.H. Ellinwood
Durham, North Carolina, USA
Central nervous system stimulants and drugs that suppress appetite

C.J. Ellis
Birmingham, United Kingdom
Drugs used in tuberculosis and leprosy

P. Elsner
Jena, Germany
Dermatological drugs, topical agents, and cosmetics

T. Erikkson
Lund, Sweden
Thalidomide

E. Ernst
Exeter, United Kingdom
Treatments used in complementary and alternative medicine

M. Farré
Barcelona, Spain
Corticotrophins, corticosteroids, and prostaglandins

P.I. Folb
Cape Town, South Africa
Cytostatic drugs
Intravenous infusions—solutions and emulsions

J.A. Franklyn
Birmingham, United Kingdom
Thyroid hormones and antithyroid drugs

M.G. Franzosi
Milan, Italy
Beta-adrenoceptor antagonists and antianginal drugs

J. Fraser
Glasgow, Scotland
Cytostatic drugs

H.M.P. Freie
Maastricht, The Netherlands
Antipyretic analgesics

C. Fux
Bern, Switzerland
Various antibacterial drugs

P.J. Geerlings
Amsterdam, The Netherlands
Drugs of abuse

A.H. Ghodse
London, United Kingdom
Opioid analgesics and narcotic antagonists

P.L.F. Giangrande
Oxford, United Kingdom
Drugs affecting blood coagulation, fibrinolysis, and hemostasis

G. Gillespie
Perth, Australia
Local anaesthetics

G. Girish
Sheffield, United Kingdom
Radiological contrast agents

V. Gras-Champel
Amiens, France
Drugs affecting blood coagulation, fibrinolysis, and hemostasis

A.I. Green
Boston, Massachusetts, USA
Drugs of abuse

A.H. Groll
Münster, Germany
Antifungal drugs

H. Haak
Leiden, The Netherlands
Miscellaneous drugs and materials, medical devices, and techniques not dealt with in other chapters

F. Hackenberger
Bonn, Germany
Antiseptic drugs and disinfectants

J.T. Hartmann
Tübingen, Germany
Cytostatic drugs

K. Hartmann
Bern, Switzerland
Drugs acting on the respiratory tract

A. Havryk
Sydney, Australia
Drugs acting on the respiratory tract

E. Hedayati
Auckland, New Zealand
General anesthetics and therapeutic gases

E. Helsing
Oslo, Norway
Vitamins

R. Hoigné
Wabern, Switzerland
Various antibacterial drugs

A. Imhof
Seattle, Washington, USA
Various antibacterial drugs

L.L. Iversen
Oxford, United Kingdom
Cannbinoids

J. W. Jefferson
Madison, Wisconsin, USA
Lithium

D.J. Jeffries
London, United Kingdom
Antiviral drugs

M. Joerger
St Gallen, Switzerland
Drugs acting on the respiratory tract

G.D. Johnston
Belfast, Northern Ireland
Positive inotropic drugs and drugs used in dysrhythmias

P. Joubert
Pretoria, South Africa
Antihypertensive drugs

A.A.M. Kaddu
Entebbe, Uganda
Antihelminthic drugs

C. Koch
Copenhagen, Denmark
Blood, blood components, plasma, and plasma products

H. Kolve
Münster, Germany
Antifungal drugs

H.M.J. Krans
Hoogmade, The Netherlands
Insulin, glucagon, and oral hypoglycemic drugs

M. Krause
Scherzingen, Switzerland
Various antibacterial drugs

S. Krishna
London, United Kingdom
Antiprotozoal drugs

M. Kuhn
Chur, Switzerland
Drugs acting on the respiratory tract

R. Latini
Milan, Italy
Beta-adrenoceptor antagonists and antianginal drugs

T.H. Lee
Durham, North Carolina, USA
Central nervous system stimulants and drugs that suppress appetite

P. Leuenberger
Lausanne, Switzerland
Drugs used in tuberculosis and leprosy

M. Leuwer
Liverpool, United Kingdom
Neuromuscular blocking agents and skeletal muscle relaxants

G. Liceaga Cundin
Guipuzcoa, Spain
Drugs that affect autonomic functions or the extrapyramidal system

P.O. Lim
Dundee, Scotland
Beta-adrenoceptor antagonists and antianginal drugs

H.-P. Lipp
Tübingen, Germany
Cytostatic drugs

C. Ludwig
Freiburg, Germany
Drugs acting on the immune system

T.M. MacDonald
Dundee, Scotland
Beta-adrenoceptor antagonists and antianginal drugs

G.T. McInnes
Glasgow, Scotland
Diuretics

I.R. McNicholl
San Francisco, California, USA
Antiviral drugs

P. Magee
Coventry, United Kingdom
Antiseptic drugs and disinfectants

A.P. Maggioni
Firenze, Italy
Beta-adrenoceptor antagonists and antianginal drugs

J.F. Martí Massó
Guipuzcoa, Spain
Drugs that affect autonomic functions or the extrapyramidal system

L.H. Martín Arias
Valladolid, Spain
Antipsychotic drugs

M.M.H.M. Meinardi
Amsterdam, The Netherlands
Dermatological drugs, topical agents, and cosmetics

D.B. Menkes
Wrexham, United Kingdom
Hypnosedatives and anxiolytics

R.H.B. Meyboom
Utrecht, The Netherlands
Metal antagonists

T. Midtvedt
Stockholm, Sweden
Various antibacterial drugs

G. Mignot
Saint Paul, France
Gastrointestinal drugs

S.K. Morcos
Sheffield, United Kingdom
Radiological contrast agents

W.M.C. Mulder
Amsterdam, The Netherlands
Dermatological drugs, topical agents, and cosmetics

S. Musa
Wakefield, United Kingdom
Hypnosedatives and anxiolytics

K.A. Neftel
Bern, Switzerland
Various antibacterial drugs

A.N. Nicholson
Petersfield, United Kingdom
Antihistamines

L. Nicholson
Auckland, New Zealand
General anesthetics and therapeutic gases

I. Öhman
Stockholm, Sweden
Antidepressant drugs

H. Olsen
Oslo, Norway
Opioid analgesics and narcotic antagonists

I. Palmlund
London, United Kingdom
Diethylstilbestrol

J.N. Pande
New Delhi, India
Drugs used in tuberculosis and leprosy

J.K. Patel
Boston, Massachusetts, USA
Drugs of abuse

J.W. Paterson
Perth, Australia
Drugs acting on the respiratory tract

K. Peerlinck
Leuven, Belgium
Drugs affection blood coagulation, fibrinolysis, and hemostasis

E. Perucca
Pavia, Italy
Antiepileptic drugs

E.H. Pi
Los Angeles, California, USA
Antipsychotic drugs

T. Planche
London, United Kingdom
Antiprotozoal drugs

B.C.P. Polak
Amsterdam, The Netherlands
Drugs used in ocular treatment

T.E. Ralston
Worcester, Massachusetts, USA
Drugs of abuse

P. Reiss
Amsterdam, The Netherlands
Antiviral drugs

H.D. Reuter
Köln, Germany
Vitamins

I. Ribeiro
London, United Kingdom
Antiprotozoal drugs

T.D. Robinson
Sydney, Australia
Drugs acting on the respiratory tract

Ch. Ruef
Zurich, Switzerland
Various antibacterial drugs

M. Schachter
London, United Kingdom
Drugs that affect autonomic functions or the extrapyramidal system

A. Schaffner
Zurich, Switzerland
Various antibacterial drugs
Antifungal drugs

S. Schliemann-Willers
Jena, Germany
Dermatological drugs, topical agents, and cosmetics

M. Schneemann
Zürich, Switzerland
Antiprotozoal drugs

S.A. Schug
Perth, Australia
Local anesthetics

G. Screaton
Oxford, United Kingdom
Drugs acting on the immune system

J.P. Seale
Sydney, Australia
Drugs acting on the respiratory tract

R.P. Sequeira
Manama, Bahrain
Central nervous system stimulants and drugs that suppress appetite

T.G. Short
Auckland, New Zealand
General anesthetics and therapeutic gases

D.A. Sica
Richmond, Virginia, USA
Diuretics

G.M. Simpson
Los Angeles, California, USA
Antipsychotic drugs

J.J. Sramek
Beverly Hills, California, USA
Antipsychotic drugs

A. Stanley
Birmingham, United Kingdom
Cytostatic drugs

K.J.D. Stannard
Perth, Australia
Local anesthetics

B. Sundaram
Sheffield, United Kingdom
Radiological contrast agents

J.A.M. Tafani
Toulouse, France
Radiological contrast agents

M.C. Thornton
Auckland, New Zealand
Local anesthetics

B.S. True
Campbelltown, South Australia
Corticotrophins, corticosteroids, and prostaglandins

C. Twelves
Glasgow, Scotland
Cytostatic drugs

W.G. Van Aken
Amsterdam, The Netherlands
Blood, blood components, plasma, and plasma products

C.J. Van Boxtel
Amsterdam, The Netherlands
Sex hormones and related compounds, including hormonal contraceptives

G.B. Van der Voet
Leiden, The Netherlands
Metals

P.J.J. Van Genderen
Rotterdam, The Netherlands
Antihelminthic drugs

R. Verhaeghe
Leuven, Belgium
Drugs acting on the cerebral and peripheral circulations

J. Vermylen
Leuven, Belgium
Drugs affecting blood coagulation, fibrinolysis, and hemostasis

P. Vernazza
St Gallen, Switzerland
Antiviral drugs

T. Vial
Lyon, France
Drugs acting on the immune system

P. Vossebeld
Amsterdam, The Netherlands
Blood, blood components, plasma, and plasma products

G.M. Walsh
Aberdeen, United Kingdom
Antihistamines

T.J. Walsh
Bethesda, Maryland, USA
Antifungal drugs

R. Walter
Zurich, Switzerland
Antifungal drugs

D. Watson
Auckland, New Zealand
Local anesthetics

J. Weeke
Aarhus, Denmark
Thyroid hormones and antithyroid drugs

C.J.M. Whitty
London, United Kingdom
Antiprotozoal drugs

E.J. Wong
Boston, Massachusetts, USA
Drugs of abuse

C. Woodrow
London, United Kingdom
Antiprotozoal drugs

Y. Young
Auckland, New Zealand
General anesthetics and therapeutic gases

F. Zannad
Nancy, France
Antihypertensive drugs

J.-P. Zellweger
Lausanne, Switzerland
Drugs used in tuberculosis and leprosy

A. Zinkernagel
Zürich, Switzerland
Antiprotozoal drugs

M. Zoppi
Bern, Switzerland
Various antibacterial drugs

O. Zuzan
Hannover, Germany
Neuromuscular blocking agents and skeletal muscle relaxants

Foreword

My doctor is
A good doctor
He made me no
Iller than I was

Willem Hussem (The Netherlands) 1900–1974
Translation: Peter Raven

"*Primum non nocere*"—in the first place, do no harm—is often cited as one of the foundation stones of sound medical care, yet its origin is uncertain. Hippocrates? There are some who will tell you so;[1] but the phrase is not a part of the Hippocratic Oath, and the Father of Medicine wrote in any case in his native Greek.[2] It could be that the Latin phrase is from the Roman physician Galenius, while others attribute it to Scribonius Largus, physician to one of the later Caesars,[3] and there is a lot of reason to believe that it actually originated in 19th century England.[4] Hippocrates himself, in the first volume of his *Epidemics*, put it at all events better in context: "When dealing with diseases have two precepts in mind: to procure benefit and not to harm."[5] One must not become overly obsessed by the safety issue, but it is a necessary element in good medical care.

The ability to do good with the help of medicines has developed immensely within the last century, but with it has come the need to keep a watchful eye on the possibility of inflicting harm on the way. The challenge is to recognize at the earliest possible stage the adverse effects that a valuable drug may induce, and to find ways of containing them, so that risk never becomes disproportionate to benefit. The process of drug development will sometimes result in methods of treatment that are more specific to their purpose than were their predecessors and hence less likely to produce unwanted complications; yet the more novel a therapeutic advance the greater the possibility of its eliciting adverse effects of a type so unfamiliar that they are not specifically looked for and long remained unrecognized when they do occur. The entire process of keeping medicines safe today involves all those concerned with them, whether as researchers, manufacturers, regulators, prescribers, dispensers, or users, and it demands an effective and honest flow of information and thought between them.

For several decennia, concerned by its own errors in the past, the science of therapeutics put unbounded faith in the ability of well-planned clinical trials to arrive at the truth about the properties of medicines. Insofar as efficacy was concerned that was and remains a sound move, closing the door to charlatanism as well as to well-meant amateurism. Therapeutic trials with a new medicine were also able to delineate those adverse effects that occurred in a fair proportion of users. If serious, they would bar the drug from entry to the market altogether, while if transient and reasonably tolerable they would form the basis for warnings and precautions as well as the occasional contraindication. The problem lay with those adverse drug reactions that occurred rather less commonly or not at all in populations recruited for therapeutic trials, yet which could soon arise in the much broader spectrum of patients exposed to the drug once it was marketed across the world. The influence of race or climate might explain some of them; others might reflect interactions with foods, alcohol, or other drugs; yet others could only be explained, if at all, in terms of the particular susceptibility of certain individuals. Scattered across the globe, these effects might readily be overlooked, regarded as coincidental, or at worst dismissed contemptuously as "merely anecdotal".

The seriousness of the adverse effects issue became very apparent even as the reputation of controlled trials deservedly grew, and it touched on both newer and older drugs. The thalidomide calamity, involving several thousand cases of drug-induced phocomelia, was fortunately recognized by Widukind Lenz and others in the light of individual case reports within two years of the introduction of the product. On the other hand, generations elapsed between the patenting of aspirin in 1899 and the realization in 1965 that it might induce Reye's syndrome when used to treat fever in children. Such events, and many less spectacular, showed that, however vital well-controlled studies had become, there was good reason to remain alert for signals emerging from individual cases. Unanticipated events occurring during drug treatment might indeed reflect mere coincidence, but again they might not; and for many of the patients who suffered in consequence there was nothing in the least anecdotal about them.

Fortunately, the 1950s and 1960s of the 20th century saw the first positive reactions to the adverse reaction issue. Effective drug regulation emerged in one country after another. In 1952, Prof. Leo Meyler of The Netherlands produced his first "Side Effect of Drugs" to pull together data from the world literature. A number of national adverse reaction monitoring bureaux were established to gather data from the field and examine carefully reports of suspected side effects of medicines, creating the basis for the World Health Organization to establish its global reporting system. The pharmaceutical industry has increasingly realized its duty to collect and pass on the information that comes into its possession through its wide contacts with the health professions. Later years have seen the emergence, notably in Sweden and in Britain, of systems through which patients themselves can report possible adverse effects to the medicines they have taken. All these processes fit together in what the French language so appropriately terms "pharmacovigilance", with vigilance as the watchword for all concerned.

In this continuing development, the medical literature provides a resource with vast potential. The world is believed to have some 20 000 medical journals, of which a nuclear group of a thousand or so can be relied upon to publish reports and analyses of adverse effects—not only in the framework of formal investigations but also in letters, editorials, and reports of meetings large and small. Much of that information comprises not so much firm facts as emergent knowledge, based directly on experience in the field and calling urgently for attention. The book that Leo Meyler created has, in the course of fifteen editions and with the support of an ever-larger team of professionals, provided the means by which that attention can be mobilized. It has become the world's principal tool in bringing together, encyclopedically but critically, the evidence on the basis of which adverse drug effects and interactions can be recognized, discussed, and accommodated into medical practice. Together with its massive database and its complementary *Side Effects of Drugs Annuals*, it has evolved into a vital instrument in ensuring that drugs are used wisely and well and with due caution, in the light of all that is known about them. There is nothing else like it, nor need there be; across the world, *Meyler* has become a pillar of responsible medical care.

M.N. Graham Dukes
Honorary Editor, *Meyler's Side Effects of Drugs*
Oslo, Norway

Notes

1. Lichtenhaeler C. Histoire de la Médicine, Fayard, Paris, 1978:117.
2. Smith CM. Origin and uses of *Primum non nocere*. J Clin Pharmacol 2005;45:371–7.
3. Albrecht H. Primum nil nocere. Die Zeit, 6 April, 2005.
4. Notably in a book by Inman T. *Foundation for a New Theory and Practice of Medicine*. London, 1860.
5. I am indebted to Jeffrey Aronson for his own translation of the Greek original from Hippocrates *Epidemics*, Book I, Section XI, which seems to convey the meaning of the original [ἀσκεῖν περὶ τὰ νοσημάτα δῦο, ὠφελειν ἤ μὴ βλάπτειν] rather better than the published translations of his work.

Preface

This is a completely new edition of what has become the standard reference text in the field of adverse drug reactions and interactions since Leopold Meyler published his first review of the subject 55 years ago. Although we have retained the old title, *Meyler's Side Effects of Drugs*, the subtitle of this edition, *The Encyclopedia of Adverse Drug Reactions and Interactions*, reflects both modern terminology and the scope of the review. The structure of the book may have changed, but the *Encyclopedia* remains the most comprehensive reference source on adverse drug reactions and interactions and a major source of informed discussion about them.

Scope

The scope of the *Encyclopedia* remains wide. It covers not only the vast majority of prescription drugs, old and new, but also non-prescribed substances (such as anesthetics, antiseptics, lifestyle compounds, and drugs of abuse), herbal medicines, devices (such as blood glucose meters), and methods in alternative and complementary medicine. For this edition, entries on some substances that were regarded as obsolete, such as thalidomide and smallpox vaccine, have been rewritten and restored. Other compounds, such as diethylstilbestrol, although no longer in use, continue to cast their shadow and are included. Yet others, currently regarded as obsolete, have been retained, both for historical reasons and because one can never be sure when an old compound may once more become relevant or provide useful information in relation to another compound. Some drugs have been withdrawn from the market in some countries since the last edition of *Meyler* was published; rofecoxib, cisapride, phenylpropanolamine, and kava (see Piperaceae) are examples. Nevertheless, detailed monographs have been included on these substances because of the lessons that they can teach us and in some cases because of their relevance to other compounds in their classes that are still available; it is also not possible to predict whether these compounds will eventually reappear in some other form or for some new indication.

In the last 15 years there has been increasing emphasis on the use of high-quality evidence in therapeutic practice, principally as obtained from large, randomized clinical trials and from systematic reviews of the results of many such trials. However, while it has been possible to obtain useful information about the beneficial effects of interventions in this way, evidence about harms, including adverse drug reactions, has been more difficult to obtain. Even trials that yield good estimates of benefits are poor at providing evidence about harms for several reasons:

- benefits are usually single, whereas harms are usually multiple;
- the chance of any single form of harm is usually smaller than the chance of benefit and therefore more difficult to detect; however, multiple harms can accumulate and affect the benefit-to-harm balance;
- benefits are identifiable in advance, whereas harms are not or not always;
- the likely time-course of benefits can generally be predicted, while the time-course of harms often cannot and may be much delayed by comparison with the duration of a trial.

For all these reasons, larger and sometimes longer studies are needed to detect harms. In recent years attempts have been made to conduct systematic reviews of adverse reactions, but these have also been limited by several problems:

- harms are in general poorly collected in randomized trials and trials may not last long enough to detect them all;
- even when they are well collected, as is increasingly happening, they are often poorly reported;
- even when they are well reported in the body of a report, they may not be mentioned in titles and abstracts;
- even when they are well reported in the body of a report, they may be poorly indexed in large databases.

All this means that it is difficult to collect information on adverse drug reactions from randomized, controlled trials for systematic review. This can be seen from the evidence provided in Table 1, which shows the proportion of different types of information that have been used in the preparation of two volumes of the *Side Effects of Drugs Annual*, proportions that are likely be the same in this *Encyclopedia*.

Wherever possible, emphasis in this *Encyclopedia* has been placed on information that has come from systematic reviews and clinical trials of all kinds; this is reflected in new headings under which trial results are reported (observational studies, randomized studies, placebo-controlled studies). However, because many reports of adverse drug reactions (about 30%) are anecdotal, with evidence from one or just a few cases, many individual case studies (see below) have also been included. We need better methods to make use of the information that this large body of anecdotes provides.

Structure

The first major change that readers will notice is that the chapter structure of previous editions has given way to a monographic structure. That is because some of the information about individual drugs has previously been scattered over different chapters in the book; for example ciclosporin was previously covered in Chapter 37 and in scattered sections throughout Chapter 45; it is now dealt with in a single monograph. The monographs are arranged in alphabetical order, with cross-referencing as required. For example, if you turn to the monograph on cetirizine, you will be referred to the complementary general monograph on antihistamines, where much information that is relevant to cetirizine is given; the monograph on cetirizine itself contains information that is relevant only to cetirizine and not to other antihistamines. Within each monograph the material is arranged in the same way as in the *Side Effects of Drugs Annuals* (see "How to use this book").

Case Reports

A new feature, recognizable from the Annuals, but not incorporated into previous editions, is the inclusion of case reports of adverse effects. This feature reflects the fact that about 30% of all the literature that is reported and discussed in the Annuals derives from such reports (see Table 1). In some cases the only information about an adverse effect is contained in an anecdotal report; in other cases the report illustrates a variant form of the reaction. A case report also gives more immediacy to an adverse reaction, allowing the reader to appreciate more precisely the exact nature of the reported event.

Classification of Adverse Drug Reactions

Another new feature of this edition is the introduction of the DoTS method of classifying adverse drug reactions, based on the **Dose** at which they occur relative to the beneficial dose, the **Time-course** of the reaction, and individual **Susceptibility factors** (see "How to use this book"). This has been done for selected adverse effects, and I hope that as volumes of SEDA continue to be published and the *Encyclopedia's* electronic database is expanded, it will be possible to classify increasing numbers of adverse reactions in this way.

References

Because all the primary and secondary literature is thoroughly surveyed in the Annuals, the *Encyclopedia* has become increasingly compact relative to the amount of information available (even though it has increased in absolute size), with many unreferenced statements and cross-references to the Annuals, on the assumption that all the information would be readily available to the reader, although that may not always be the case. To restore all the reference material on which the *Encyclopedia* has been based as it has evolved over so many years would be a gargantuan task, but in this edition a major start has been made. Many references to original material have been restored, and there is now hardly a statement that is not backed up by at least one reference to primary literature. In addition, almost all of the material that was published in Annuals 23 to 27 (SEDA-23 to SEDA-27) has been included, complete with citations. This has resulted in the inclusion of more than 40 000 references in this edition. Readers will still have to refer to earlier editions of the Annual (SEDA-1 to SEDA-22) and occasionally to earlier editions of *Meyler's Side Effects of Drugs* for more detailed descriptions, but now that the *Encyclopedia* is available electronically this will be repaired in future editions.

Methods and Contributors

I initially prepared the text of the *Encyclopedia* by combining text from the 14th edition of *Meyler's Side Effects of Drugs* and the five most recent annuals (SEDA-23 to SEDA-27). [Later literature is covered in SEDA-28 and the forthcoming SEDA-29.] I next restored missing references to the material and extended it where important information had not been included. The resulting monographs were then sent to experts for review, and their comments were incorporated into the finished monographs. I am grateful to all those, both authors of chapters in previous editions and Annuals and those who have reviewed the monographs for this edition, for their hard work and for making their expertise available.

Acknowledgements

This 15th edition of *Meyler's Side Effects of Drugs* was initiated and carefully planned with Joke Jaarsma at Elsevier, who has provided unstinting support during the production of several previous editions of *Meyler's Side Effects of Drugs* and the *Side Effects of Drugs Annuals*. Early discussions with Dieke van Wijnen at Elsevier about the structure of the text were invaluable. Professor Leufkens from the Faculty of Pharmacy at the University of Utrecht was instrumental in helping us to assemble the preliminary content for this edition; pharmacy students in his department entered the text

Table 1 Types of articles on adverse drug reactions published in 6576 papers in the world literature during 1999 and 2003 (as reviewed in SEDA-24 and SEDA-28)

Type of article	Number of descriptions* (%)
An anecdote or set of anecdotes (that is reported case histories)	2084 (29.9)
A major, randomized, controlled trial or observational study	1956 (28.1)
A minor, randomized, controlled trial or observational study or a non-randomized study (including case series)	1099 (15.8)
A major review, including non-systematic statistical analyses of published studies	951 (13.7)
A brief commentary (for example an editorial or a letter)	362 (5.19)
An experimental study (animal or in vitro)	263 (3.77)
A meta-analysis or other form of systematic review	172 (2.47)
Official statements (for example by Governmental organizations, the WHO, or manufacturers)	75 (1.07)
Total no. of descriptions*	6962
Total no. of articles	6576

* Some articles are described in more than one way

electronically into templates under the guidance of Joke Zwetsloot from Elsevier. Christine Ayorinde provided excellent assistance while I expanded and edited the material. The International Non-proprietary Names were checked by Renée Aronson. At Elsevier the references were then checked and collated by Liz Perill, who also copyedited the material, with Ed Stolting, and shepherded it through conversion to different electronic formats. Bill Todd created the indexes. Stephanie Diment oversaw the project and coordinated everyone's efforts.

The History of Meyler

The history of *Meyler's Side Effects of Drugs* goes back 55 years; a full account can be found at http://www.elsevier.com/locate/Meyler and the various volumes are listed before the title page of this set. When Leopold Meyler, a physician, experienced unwanted effects of drugs that were used to treat his tuberculosis, he discovered that there was no single text to which medical practitioners could turn for information about the adverse effects of drug therapy; Louis Lewin's text *Die Nebenwirkungen der Arzneimittel* ("The Untoward Effects of Drugs") of 1881 had long been out of print (SEDA-27, xxv–xxix). Meyler therefore surveyed the current literature, initially in Dutch as *Schadelijke Nevenwerkingen van Geneesmiddelen* (Van Gorcum, 1951), and then in English as *Side Effects of Drugs* (Elsevier, 1952). He followed up with what he called surveys of unwanted effects of drugs. Each survey covered a period of two to four years and culminated in Volume VIII (1976), edited by Graham Dukes (SEDA-23, xxiii-xxvi), Meyler having died in 1973. By then the published literature was too extensive to be comfortably encompassed in a four-yearly cycle, and an annual cycle was started instead; the first *Side Effects of Drugs Annual* (SEDA-1) was published in 1977. The four-yearly review was replaced by a complementary critical encyclopaedic survey of the entire field; the first encyclopaedic edition of *Meyler's Side Effects of Drugs*, which appeared in 1980, was labeled the ninth edition.

Since then, *Meyler's Side Effects of Drugs* has been published every four years, providing an encyclopaedic survey of the entire field. Had the cycle been adhered to, the 15th edition would have been published in 2004, but over successive editions the quantity and nature of the information available in the text has changed. In the new millennium it was clear that for this edition a revolutionary approach was needed, and that has taken a little longer to achieve, with a great deal of effort from many different individuals.

We have come a long way since Meyler published his first account in a book of 192 pages. I think that he would have approved of this new *Encyclopedia*.

J. K. Aronson
Oxford, October 2005

How to use this book

In a departure from its previous structure, this edition of *Meyler's Side Effects of Drugs* is presented as individual drug monographs in alphabetical order. In many cases a general monograph (for example Antihistamines) is complemented by monographs about specific drugs (for example acrivastine, antazoline, etc.); in that case a cross-reference is given from the latter to the former.

Monograph Structure

Within each monograph the information is presented in sections as follows:

GENERAL INFORMATION
Includes, when necessary, notes on nomenclature, information about the results of observational studies, comparative studies, and placebo-controlled studies in relation to reports of adverse drug reactions, and a general summary of the major adverse effects.

ORGANS AND SYSTEMS
Cardiovascular (includes heart and blood vessels)
Respiratory
Ear, nose, throat
Nervous system (includes central and peripheral nervous systems)
Neuromuscular function
Sensory systems (includes eyes, ears, taste)
Psychological, psychiatric
Endocrine (includes hypothalamus, pituitary, thyroid, parathyroid, adrenal, pancreas, sex hormones)
Metabolism
Nutrition (includes effects on amino acids, essential fatty acids, vitamins, micronutrients)
Electrolyte balance (includes sodium, potassium)
Mineral balance (includes calcium, phosphate)
Metal metabolism (includes copper, iron, magnesium, zinc)
Acid–base balance
Fluid balance
Hematologic (includes blood, spleen, and lymphatics)
Mouth and teeth
Salivary glands
Gastrointestinal (includes esophagus, stomach, small bowel, large bowel)
Liver
Biliary tract
Pancreas
Urinary tract (includes kidneys, ureters, bladder, urethra)
Skin
Hair
Nails
Sweat glands
Serosae (includes pleura, pericardium, peritoneum)
Musculoskeletal (includes muscles, bones, joints)
Sexual function
Reproductive system (includes uterus, ovaries, breasts)
Immunologic (includes effects on the immune system and hypersensitivity reactions)
Autacoids
Infection risk
Body temperature
Multiorgan failure
Trauma
Death

LONG-TERM EFFECTS
Drug abuse
Drug misuse
Drug tolerance
Drug resistance
Drug dependence
Drug withdrawal
Genotoxicity
Mutagenicity
Tumorigenicity

SECOND-GENERATION EFFECTS
Fertility
Pregnancy
Teratogenicity
Fetotoxicity
Lactation

SUSCEPTIBILITY FACTORS (relates to features of the patient)
Genetic factors
Age
Sex
Physiological factors
Cardiac disease
Renal disease
Hepatic disease
Thyroid disease
Other features of the patient

DRUG ADMINISTRATION
Drug formulations
Drug additives
Drug contamination (includes infective agents)
Drug adulteration
Drug dosage regimens (includes frequency and duration of administration)
Drug administration route
Drug overdose

DRUG–DRUG INTERACTIONS
FOOD–DRUG INTERACTIONS
SMOKING
OTHER ENVIRONMENTAL INTERACTIONS
INTERFERENCE WITH DIAGNOSTIC TESTS
DIAGNOSIS OF ADVERSE DRUG REACTIONS
MANAGEMENT OF ADVERSE DRUG REACTIONS
MONITORING THERAPY

Classification of Adverse Drug Reactions

Selected major reactions are classified according to the DoTS system (BMJ 2003;327:1222–5). In this system adverse reactions are classified according to the **Dose** at which they usually occur relative to the beneficial dose, the **Time-course** over which they occur, and the **Susceptibility factors** that make them more likely, as follows:

1 **Relation to dose**
- *Toxic reactions* (reactions that occur at supratherapeutic doses)
- *Collateral reactions* (reactions that occur at standard therapeutic doses)
- *Hypersusceptibility reactions* (reactions that occur at subtherapeutic doses in susceptible patients)

2 **Time-course**
- *Time-independent reactions* (reactions that occur at any time during a course of therapy)
- *Time-dependent reactions*
  - Immediate reactions (reactions that occur only when a drug is administered too rapidly)
  - First-dose reactions (reactions that occur after the first dose of a course of treatment and not necessarily thereafter)
  - Early reactions (reactions that occur early in treatment then abate with continuing treatment)
  - Intermediate reactions (reactions that occur after some delay but with less risk during longer- term therapy, owing to the "healthy survivor" effect)
  - Late reactions (reactions the risk of which increases with continued or repeated exposure), including withdrawal reactions (reactions that occur when, after prolonged treatment, a drug is withdrawn or its effective dose is reduced)
  - Delayed reactions (reactions that occur some time after exposure, even if the drug is withdrawn before the reaction appears)

3 **Susceptibility factors**
- *Genetic*
- *Age*
- *Sex*
- *Physiological variation*
- *Exogenous factors* (for example drug–drug or food–drug interactions, smoking)
- *Diseases*

Drug Names And Spelling

Drugs are usually designated by their recommended or proposed International Non-proprietary Names (rINN or pINN); when these are not available, chemical names have been used. If a fixed combination has a generic combination name (for example co-trimoxazole for trimethoprim + sulfamethoxazole) that name has been used; in some cases brand names have been used.

Spelling

Where necessary, for indexing purposes, American spelling has been used, for example anemia rather than anaemia, estrogen rather than oestrogen.

Cross-references

The various editions of *Meyler's Side Effects of Drugs* are cited in the text as SED-13, SED-14, etc.; the *Side Effects of Drugs Annuals* 1-22 are cited as SEDA-1, SEDA-2, etc. This edition includes most of the contents of SEDA-23 to SEDA-27. SEDA-28 and SEDA-29 are separate publications, which were prepared in parallel with the preparation of this edition.

Indexes

Index of drug names
An index of drug names provides a complete listing of all references to a drug for which adverse effects and/or drug interactions are described. The monograph on herbal medicines contains tabulated cross-indexes to the plants that are covered in separate monographs.

Index of adverse effects
This index is necessarily selective, since a particular adverse effect may be caused by very large numbers of compounds; the index is therefore mainly directed to adverse effects that are particularly serious or frequent, or are discussed in special detail; before assuming that a given drug does not have a particular adverse effect, consult the relevant monograph.

Alphabetical list of drug monographs

The number in parentheses after each heading is the number of the corresponding chapter in the Side Effects of Drug Annuals (SEDA-28 and later) in which the item is usually covered.

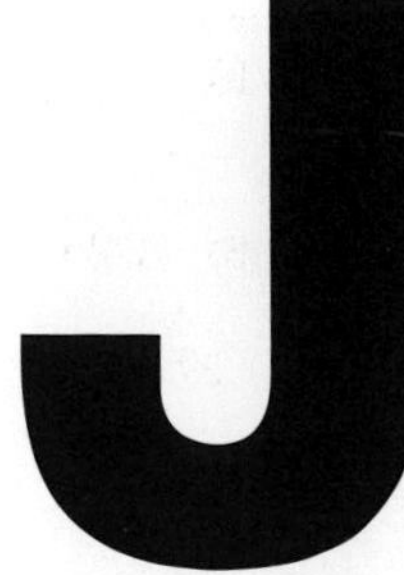

Japanese encephalitis vaccine

See also Vaccines

General Information

During the last half century, Japanese encephalitis has been recognized as an important arboviral disease in man in Japan, China, Korea, Thailand, India, Nepal, Sri Lanka, and Vietnam. In 1954, Japanese encephalitis vaccine of the mouse brain type for human use was licensed in Japan. However, there was strong criticism of mouse brain vaccine, which has continued for many years. Therefore, in 1965, the Nippon Institute of Biological Products and the Biken Foundation implemented more advanced purification procedures, such as alcohol precipitation and ultracentrifugation.

Three types of Japanese encephalitis vaccine are currently produced:

1. mouse brain-derived inactivated vaccine, commercially available;
2. cell culture-derived inactivated vaccine;
3. cell culture-derived attenuated vaccine, produced and used exclusively in China.

The Chinese cell culture-derived inactivated vaccine is produced in primary hamster kidney cells; a highly purified Vero cell culture-derived inactivated vaccine is under clinical development in France. A Chinese live-attenuated vaccine is also produced in primary hamster kidney cells. The efficacy of one dose is 80%, and the efficacy of two doses, given 1 year apart, is 97.5%; this vaccine was evaluated in a randomized trial in 26 239 children, half of whom received the vaccine and half served as controls, and its adverse effects have been reviewed (SEDA-22, 350).

In 1965, a special surveillance team was formed by the Japanese Ministry of Health and Welfare to investigate adverse events following the administration of Japanese encephalitis vaccine. No severe adverse event was reported among 21 396 vaccinees of whom 18 401 were adolescents and children under 18 years of age. Some mild reactions (fever, malaise, abdominal symptoms) were noted in 1.2% of the vaccinees. Using a countrywide hospital network, the surveillance team studied any severe neurological disease occurring within 1 month after receipt of the vaccine. During 1957–66, 26 cases (nine cases of meningitis, ten cases of convulsions, five cases of polyneuropathy, and two cases of demyelinization) were analysed. No evidence was provided showing a causative relation between these clinical syndromes and Japanese encephalitis immunization. The incidence of neurological disease was considered minor compared with the millions of doses distributed annually in Japan (1).

Since 1989, urticaria and/or angioedema of the extremities, face, and oropharynx, and respiratory distress have been reported from Europe, North America, and Australia as a new pattern of adverse effects. Collapse due to hypotension has required hospitalization in several cases, and erythema multiforme and erythema nodosum have also occurred; the reported rates of such adverse effects varied markedly in different countries (respective ranges 0.7–12 per 10 000 and 50–104 per 10 000). The vaccine constituents responsible for the adverse effects have not yet been identified.

Japanese encephalitis vaccine has been reviewed (2). A supplementary volume of the journal Vaccine has dealt with results presented at a WHO meeting held in Bangkok, Thailand, in 1998 (3–6). Comprehensive data were provided on the epidemiological and virological situation in southeast Asia and Australia, control measures, vaccine production capacities, and different vaccines against Japanese encephalitis. Adverse events after the use of inactivated mouse brain vaccine (the only vaccine that is currently licensed for international use) have been reviewed in detail (3).

Organs and Systems

Nervous system

Postmarketing surveillance data of adverse events after Japanese encephalitis immunization in Japan and the USA have been compared (7). The rates of total reported adverse events were 2.8 per 100 000 doses in Japan and 15.0 per 100 000 doses in the USA. In Japan, 17 neurological disorders were reported from April 1996 to October 1998 (0.2 per 100 000 doses), whereas in the USA there were no serious neurological adverse events temporally associated with Japanese encephalitis vaccine from January 1993 to June 1999. Rates for systemic hypersensitivity reactions were 0.8 and 6.3 per 100 000 doses in Japan and the USA respectively.

Acute disseminated encephalomyelitis after Japanese encephalitis immunization has been reported from Japan.

- A 6-year-old girl and a 5-year-old boy had drowsiness, paresthesia, and gait disturbance 14 and 17 days respectively after immunization with Japanese encephalitis vaccine. Treatment with prednisolone improved the clinical findings (8,9).

Another report included seven cases of acute disseminated encephalomyelitis after administration of Japanese encephalitis vaccine between 1968 and 1990 (10). Three other cases of neurological complications after the use of Japanese encephalitis vaccine have been reported in Denmark. In two cases the clinical picture was consistent with acute demyelinating encephalomyelitis (SEDA-21, 334).

The rate of neurological complications seen in Japan in 1965–73 was of the order of 1 per 2.3 million vaccinees, and in Denmark the rate was 3 per 175 000 immunized individuals (one of them with a predisposition to multiple sclerosis) (11).

Two deaths from acute anaphylaxis and four cases of acute encephalopathy or acute disseminated encephalomyelitis (two fatal), temporally related to Japanese encephalitis immunization, have been reported from the Republic of Korea (3). The live-attenuated vaccine developed and used in China had 98% efficacy in a two-dose schedule. Concern that a live vaccine derived from an encephalitogenic virus might lead to vaccine-associated encephalitis could not be addressed satisfactorily, even in a study of 26 000 children. During efficacy studies in different geographic areas of China and in different years, the observations were combinable: the average encephalitis risk after live-attenuated Japanese encephalitis vaccine was 1.59 per 100 000 vaccinees.

Immunologic

Hypersensitivity reactions (generalized urticaria or angioedema) after the use of Japanese encephalitis vaccine have been reported from some countries (see Table 1); the vaccine constituents responsible for these events have not been identified (12). There has been a detailed report of the adverse effects, mainly allergic mucocutaneous reactions, of Biken vaccine in Danish travellers and US Marine Corps personnel (SEDA-22, 351).

The Advisory Committee on Immunization Practices (ACIP) has recommended that vaccinees should be observed for 30 minutes after immunization and that medications to treat anaphylaxis should be available (12) [http://www.cdc.gov/mmwr/PDF/rr/rr4201.pdf]. A personal history of allergic disorders should be considered when weighing the risks and benefits of the vaccine for an individual. Japanese encephalitis vaccine should not be given to persons who had a previous adverse reaction after receiving Japanese encephalitis vaccine or a previous hypersensitivity reaction to other vaccines of neural origin.

In Japan, children who had immediate-type allergic reactions to Japanese encephalitis vaccine had antigelatin IgE in their sera. However, the immunological mechanism of non-immediate-type allergic reactions that consist of cutaneous signs developing several hours or more after Japanese encephalitis immunization is not yet clear. Serum samples taken from 28 children who had non-immediate-type allergic skin reactions have been compared with serum samples taken from 10 children who had immediate-type reactions (13). All the children who had had immediate-type reactions had antigelatin IgE and IgG. Of 28 children who had had non-immediate-type reactions, one had antigelatin IgE and nine had antigelatin IgG. These results suggest that some children who develop non-immediate-type allergic reactions have also been sensitized to gelatin.

Table 1 Allergic reactions after Japanese encephalitis immunization

Country	Estimated number of vaccines	Number of reactions	Estimated rate per 100 000 vaccines
Denmark	42 000	21	50
Sweden	15 000	1	7
UK	1950	1	51
Australia			
Nationwide	3400	4	118
Fairfield Hospital	601	3	499
Canada			
University of Calgary	96	1	1042
USA			
Travellers	1328	2	151
Army	526	1	190
Army and dependents (Okinawa)	35 253	220	624
Total	100 154	254	254

Susceptibility Factors

An association between reactions to Japanese encephalitis vaccine and a history of urticaria or allergic rhinitis has been identified (14).

References

1. Oya A. Japanese encephalitis vaccine. Acta Paediatr Jpn 1988;30(2):175–84.
2. Sabchareon A, Yoksan S. Japanese encephalitis. Ann Trop Paediatr 1998;18(Suppl):S67–71.
3. Tsai TF. New initiatives for the control of Japanese encephalitis by vaccination: minutes of a WHO/CVI meeting, Bangkok, Thailand, 13–15 October 1998. Vaccine 2000;18(Suppl 2):1–25.
4. Markoff L. Points to consider in the development of a surrogate for efficacy of novel Japanese encephalitis virus vaccines. Vaccine 2000;18(Suppl 2):26–32.
5. Kurane I, Takasaki T. Immunogenicity and protective efficacy of the current inactivated Japanese encephalitis vaccine against different Japanese encephalitis virus strains. Vaccine 2000;18(Suppl 2):33–5.
6. Tsarev SA, Sanders ML, Vaughn DW, Innis BL. Phylogenetic analysis suggests only one serotype of Japanese encephalitis virus. Vaccine 2000;18(Suppl 2):36–43.
7. Takahashi H, Pool V, Tsai TF, Chen RT. Adverse events after Japanese encephalitis vaccination: review of post-marketing surveillance data from Japan and the United States. The VAERS Working Group. Vaccine 2000;18(26):2963–9.
8. Demmler M, Heidel G. Trigeminus-Affektion nach Influenza-Schutzimpfung. [Trigeminal involvement following preventive influenza vaccination.] Psychiatr Neurol Med Psychol (Leipz) 1985;37(7):428–33.
9. Ohtaki E, Murakami Y, Komori H, Yamashita Y, Matsuishi T. Acute disseminated encephalomyelitis after Japanese B encephalitis vaccination. Pediatr Neurol 1992;8(2):137–9.
10. Ohtaki E, Matsuishi T, Hirano Y, Maekawa K. Acute disseminated encephalomyelitis after treatment with Japanese B encephalitis vaccine (Nakayama–Yoken and Beijing strains). J Neurol Neurosurg Psychiatry 1995;59(3):316–17.
11. Anonymous. Vaccination against Japanese encephalitis for all travellers not currently recommended. Drugs Ther Perspect 1997;10:11–13.
12. Advisory Committee on Immunization Practices (ACIP). Inactivated Japanese encephalitis virus vaccine. MMWR Recomm Rep 1993;42(RR-1):1–15.
13. Sakaguchi M, Miyazawa H, Inouye S. Specific IgE and IgG to gelatin in children with systemic cutaneous reactions to Japanese encephalitis vaccines. Allergy 2001;56(6):536–9.
14. Sakaguchi M, Yoshida M, Kuroda W, Harayama O, Matsunaga Y, Inouye S. Systemic immediate-type reactions to gelatin included in Japanese encephalitis vaccines. Vaccine 1997;15(2):121–2.

Josamycin

See also Macrolide antibiotics

General Information

In a randomized open study, 325 children aged 2–15 years with acute tonsillitis and a positive test for *Streptococcus pyogenes* antigen were treated with josamycin 25 mg/kg bd for 5 days, or penicillin 50 000–100 000 IU/day for 10 days; in five patients taking josamycin treatment was withdrawn because of gastrointestinal adverse events (nausea/vomiting) (1).

Organs and Systems

Liver

Cholestatic hepatitis has been attributed to josamycin (2).

Biliary tract

In female rats josamycin caused bile duct proliferation at a high dose of 1460 mg/kg (3).

References

1. Portier H, Bourrillon A, Lucht F, Choutet P, Gehanno P, Meziane L, Bingen E. Groupe d'etude de pathologie infectieuse pediatrique. [Treatment of acute group A beta-hemolytic streptococcal tonsillitis in children with a 5-day course of josamycin.] Arch Pediatr 2001;8(7):700–6.
2. Lavin I, Mundi JL, Trillo C, Trapero A, Fernandez R, Lopez MA, Cervilla E, Quintero D, Palacios A. [Cholestatic hepatitis by josamycin.] Gastroenterol Hepatol 1999;22(3):160.
3. Kasahara K, Nishikawa A, Furukawa F, Ikezaki S, Tanakamaru Z, Lee IS, Imazawa T, Hirose M. A chronic toxicity study of josamycin in F344 rats. Food Chem Toxicol 2002;40(7):1017–22.

Juglandaceae

See also Herbal medicines

General Information

The family of Juglandaceae contains three genera:

1. *Carya* (hickory)
2. *Juglans* (walnut)
3. *Pterocarya* (pterocarya).

Juglans regia

The fresh fruit-shell of *Juglans regia* (English walnut) contains the naphthoquinone constituent juglone, which is mutagenic and possibly carcinogenic. The juglone content of dried shells has not yet been studied adequately.

In a placebo-controlled study in 60 Persian hyperlipidemic subjects, walnut oil encapsulated in 500 mg capsules reduced plasma triglyceride concentrations by 19–33% of baseline (1).

Adverse effects

Hyperpigmentation and contact dermatitis have been attributed to *J. regia* (2) as has dermatitis bullosa (3).

A brown orange pigmentation occurred in a patient who used the bark of *J. regia* for cleaning teeth (4).

References

1. Zibaeenezhad MJ, Rezaiezadeh M, Mowla A, Ayatollahi SM, Panjehshahin MR. Antihypertriglyceridemic effect of walnut oil. Angiology 2003;54(4):411–14.
2. Bonamonte D, Foti C, Angelini G. Hyperpigmentation and contact dermatitis due to *Juglans regia*. Contact Dermatitis 2001;44(2):101–12.
3. Barniske R. Dermatitis bullosa, ausgelost durch den Saft gruner Walnussfruchtschalen (*Juglans regia*). [Dermatitis bullosa, caused by the juice of green walnut shells (*Juglans regia*).] Dermatol Wochenschr 1957;135(8):189–92.
4. Ashri N, Gazi M. More unusual pigmentations of the gingiva. Oral Surg Oral Med Oral Pathol 1990;70(4):445–9.

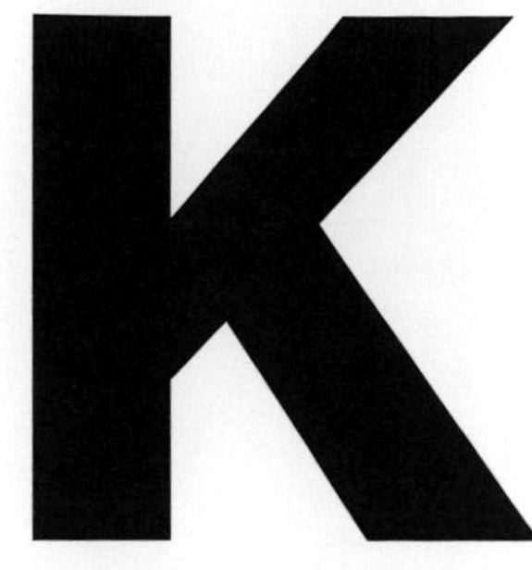

Kanamycin

See also Aminoglycoside antibiotics

General Information

Kanamycin can be used for short-term treatment of severe infections caused by susceptible strains (for example *Escherichia coli*, *Proteus* species, *Enterobacter aerogenes*, *Klebsiella pneumoniae*, *Serratia marcescens*, and *Mima-Herellea*) that are resistant to other less ototoxic aminoglycosides. It is not indicated for long-term therapy, for example in tuberculosis.

Organs and Systems

Neuromuscular function

Like the other aminoglycosides, kanamycin has neuromuscular blocking properties, particularly if given directly into the peritoneum (1). However, it seems to be less dangerous in this respect than neomycin or streptomycin.

Sensory systems

Kanamycin causes mainly cochlear damage (2). After prolonged administration (for example 1 g for periods of 30–180 days) the frequency of this adverse reaction is higher than 40%. Vestibular toxicity occurs in less than 10% of cases treated with usual doses and is generally reversible soon after withdrawal.

Gastrointestinal

Presurgical bowel preparation with oral kanamycin is seldom practiced and can be followed by an intestinal malabsorption syndrome (3). Only negligible amounts of kanamycin are absorbed through an intact intestinal mucosa, but increased systemic availability and potential toxicity can result from the presence of ulcerated or denuded areas.

Urinary tract

Kanamycin causes very little nephrotoxicity after short courses of treatment with daily doses of less than 15 mg/kg; if total doses of 30 g or more are given, the incidence of renal damage can be 50% or higher (1).

Immunologic

Sensitization (rash, drug fever) after parenteral administration of kanamycin is less frequent than with streptomycin. Anaphylaxis has only rarely been described. Cross-allergy with the other aminoglycosides is frequent (4).

References

1. Finegold SM. Toxicity of kanamycin in adults. Ann NY Acad Sci 1966;132(2):942–56.
2. Hinojosa R, Nelson EG, Lerner SA, Redleaf MI, Schramm DR. Aminoglycoside ototoxicity: a human temporal bone study. Laryngoscope 2001;111(10):1797–805.
3. Lees GM, Percy WH. Antibiotic-associated colitis: an in vitro investigation of the effects of antibiotics on intestinal motility. Br J Pharmacol 1981;73(2):535–47.
4. Chung CW, Carson TR. Cross-sensitivity of common aminoglycoside antibiotics. Arch Dermatol 1976;112(8):1101–7.

Kaolin

General Information

Kaolin, commonly given together with pectin in the treatment of diarrhea, is generally regarded as safe.

The absorbent properties of kaolin could result in the binding of other drugs that are given at about the same time. For example, kaolin adsorbs mefenamic acid and flufenamic acid, phenylbutazone, indometacin, and methiazinic acid (1). One should not therefore be surprised if it reduces the effect of any non-steroidal anti-inflammatory agent, requiring an increase in dosage by 50–100% to maintain efficacy. The reduction of lincomycin absorption is quite drastic, perhaps amounting to 90% of the dose given (2).

Organs and Systems

Respiratory

Industrial exposure to kaolin can cause lung damage. In more than 2000 kaolin workers from east central Georgia the presence of ventilatory impairment was related to the presence of complicated pneumoconiosis, employment in clay calcining, and cigarette smoking (3). In those who worked with calcined clay, there was an increased prevalence of abnormal FEV_1, but not FVC, compared to both wet and dry processors, which could not be explained by either cigarette smoking or the presence of pneumoconiosis. However, the magnitude of abnormality in the calcined clay workers was unlikely to lead to disabling impairment. Of those who had been exposed for more than 3 years, 90 had simple pneumoconiosis and 18 had complicated pneumoconiosis, adjusted prevalences of 3.2 and 0.63% respectively. Dry processing was associated with a greater risk of pneumoconiosis than wet processing.

In one case, multiple pulmonary kaolin granulomata developed secondary to the use of a liquid kaolin suspension for pleural poudrage to treat recurrent spontaneous pneumothoraces, presumably because the kaolin entered the lung through pleuro-alveolar or pleuro-bronchial openings (4).

References

1. Naggar VF, Khalil SA, Daabis NA. The in-vitro adsorption of some antirheumatics on antacids. Pharmazie 1976;31(7):461–5.
2. Wagner JG. Design and data analysis of biopharmceutical studies in man. Can J Pharm Sci 1966;1:55.
3. Morgan WK, Donner A, Higgins IT, Pearson MG, Rawlings W Jr. The effects of kaolin on the lung. Am Rev Respir Dis 1988;138(4):813–20.

4. Herman SJ, Olscamp GC, Weisbrod GL. Pulmonary kaolin granulomas. J Can Assoc Radiol 1982;33(4):279–80.

Kebuzone

See also Non-steroidal anti-inflammatory drugs

General Information

Kebuzone is an NSAID that is related to phenylbutazone. Allergic reactions, gastrotoxicity, nephrotoxicity, local reactions with necrosis (1), and liver damage have been reported (SED-11, 176) (2). The Japanese authorities have asked that the package insert should indicate that this drug must be used only as a last resort when other anti-inflammatory agents and uricosuric drugs are ineffective (SEDA-12, 83).

Organs and Systems

Liver

In 20 cases of kebuzone-induced liver damage, biopsy showed hepatocellular damage with or without cholestasis, reactive hepatitis, or cholangiolitis (3). There was hepatitis with central lobular necrosis in one case. In five patients, a lymphocyte proliferation test was positive.

Skin

Nicolau syndrome (embolia cutis medicamentosa) is a very rare complication of intramuscular injections, in which there is extensive necrosis of the injected skin area, perhaps due to accidental intra-arterial and/or para-arterial injection; it usually occurs in children (4). Nicolau syndrome has been reported in three patients who had received intramuscular injections of kebuzone (5).

References

1. Capusan I, Moise IG, Maier N. Nicolaus syndrome following intramuscular injections of ketophenylbutazone (Ketazon). Dermatol Venereol 1976;21:205.
2. Porst H, Roschlau G, Schentke U, Weise L. Leberschäden durch Ketophenylbutazone (Ketazon). Dtsch Gesundheitsw 1978;33:1181.
3. Kunze KD, Porst H, Tschopel L. Morphologie und Pathogenese von Leberschäden durch Dihydralazin, Propranolol und Ketophenylbutazon. [Morphology and pathogenesis of liver injury produced by dihydralazine, propranolol and ketophenylbutazone.] Zentralbl Allg Pathol 1985;130(6):509–18.
4. Saputo V, Bruni G. La sindrome di Nicolau da preparati di penicillina: analisi della letteratura alla ricerca di potenziali fattori di rischio. [Nicolau syndrome caused by penicillin preparations: review of the literature in search for potential risk factors.] Pediatr Med Chir 1998;20(2):105–23.
5. Varga L, Asztalos L. Nicolau-szindroma ketazon injekcio utan. [Nicolau syndrome after ketazon injection.] Orv Hetil 1990;131(21):1143–6.

Ketamine

See also General anesthetics

General Information

Ketamine is a short-acting anesthetic that is widely used by emergency physicians (1) and can be given intravenously, intramuscularly, orally, and even nasally (2). Multiple ketamine anesthetics may be safe (3).

Subanesthetic low-dose ketamine is being used increasingly often for acute pain therapy, day-case surgery, and chronic pain management. Ketamine is now available in chiral (*S*+ and *R*–) forms as well as the standard racemic form. *S*-ketamine has twice the analgesic potency of racemic ketamine and four times that of *R*-ketamine. Thus, low dose *S*-ketamine may avoid adverse effects while providing high-quality analgesia.

The pharmacology of ketamine, including its adverse effects, has been reviewed (4), as has the use and adverse effects of *S*-ketamine in the intensive care unit (5).

Ketamine relaxes smooth muscles in the airways and may therefore be a useful induction agent in children with asthma (6). If endotracheal intubation is required, lidocaine 1–2 mg/kg intravenously before intubation has been recommended, although the use of a laryngeal mask airway may be more appropriate. When used in combination with midazolam by infusion, ketamine provides analgesia and prevents and relieves bronchospasm (7).

The addition of ketamine to bupivacaine for spinal anesthesia has been studied in 60 patients undergoing spinal anesthesia for insertion of intracavitary brachytherapy implants for cervical carcinoma (8). They were randomly assigned to receive either bupivacaine 10 mg or bupivacaine 7.5 mg plus ketamine 25 mg. Motor recovery was significantly quicker in the ketamine group. Blood pressure was significantly lower in the bupivacaine group 5 minutes after administration, and perioperative intravenous fluid requirements were significantly higher. Patients given ketamine reported more sedation and dizziness, both intraoperatively and postoperatively. There were no nightmares or dissociative features. Overall satisfaction was better with bupivacaine. The study was abandoned after 30 patients, because of the high rate of adverse effects with ketamine. Although ketamine had local anesthetic-sparing properties, its adverse effects made it unsuitable for intrathecal administration.

When added to standard doses of morphine and a non- steroidal analgesic, *S*-ketamine 0.5 mg/kg had no additional benefit in a randomized, double-blind study in 30 patients undergoing anterior cruciate ligament repair (9).

Organs and Systems

Cardiovascular

Tachycardia and hypertension are common after anesthetic induction with ketamine, although the hypertension can be limited by the addition of diazepam (10). Nodal dysrhythmias can also occur (11). Because of possible reduced cardiac and pulmonary performance, ketamine should be avoided in critically ill patients (12). Pulmonary vasoconstriction and increased ventricular preload secondary to ketamine can be deleterious (13).

The effects of intramuscular premedication with either clonidine 2 micrograms/kg or midazolam 70 micrograms/kg on perioperative responses to ketamine anesthesia have been assessed in a placebo-controlled study in 30 patients (14). Clonidine significantly reduced intraoperative oxygen consumption, mean arterial pressure, and heart rate compared with midazolam and placebo. Thus, clonidine was as effective as midazolam, the standard drug used for this purpose, in reducing the undesirable sympathetic stimulation of ketamine.

Oral clonidine, 2.5 or 5.0 micrograms/kg, 90 minutes before ketamine 2 mg/kg has been compared with placebo in 39 patients (15). In those given clonidine 2.5 micrograms/kg, heart rate responses were reduced compared with placebo (maximum heart rate 97 versus 76 beats/minute). In those given clonidine 5 micrograms/kg, heart rate responses were less (maximum heart rate 97 versus 77 beats/minute) and mean arterial pressure was lower (121 versus 141 mmHg), and there were fewer nightmares and less drooling.

Respiratory

Apnea occurred after the intramuscular injection of ketamine 4 mg/kg to sedate a healthy 4-year-old boy (16). This case illustrates the need for adequate monitoring and preparation for emergency airway management when using ketamine for sedation.

Nervous system

Ketamine causes a significant rise in cerebrospinal fluid pressure, increased electroencephalographic activity, and possibly epileptiform discharges (17).

Delayed acute intracranial hypertension has been described after ketamine anesthesia (18).

Oral ketamine is an effective analgesic in patients with chronic pain. In 21 patients with central and peripheral chronic neuropathic pain treated with oral ketamine, the starting dose was ketamine 100 mg/day, titrated upward by 40 mg/day increments every 2 days until a satisfactory effect was achieved, or until adverse effects became limiting (19). Nine patients discontinued ketamine because of intolerable adverse effects, including psychotomimetic symptoms, such as "elevator" effect or dissociative feelings, somnolence or insomnia, and sensory changes such as taste disturbance and somatic sensations.

In a study of 21 outpatients with refractory neuropathic pain treated with oral ketamine, 17 reported adverse events (20). The most common were light-headedness, dizziness, tiredness, headache, a nervous floating feeling, and bad dreams. The adverse effects were sufficiently important to prevent ten patients from continuing with the trial.

Neurotoxicity due to focal lymphocytic vasculitis has been reported close to the catheter injection site in a patient who received intrathecal ketamine infusion for chronic cancer pain (21).

- A 72-year-old woman with abdominal pain due to peritoneal malignant mesothelioma was given patient-controlled analgesia with morphine and then a thoracic epidural infusion of bupivacaine 0.125% and morphine 0.04 mg/ml at a rate of 6–12 ml/hour, with minor success. A thoracic intrathecal catheter was inserted for infusion of bupivacaine 0.25% plus morphine 0.12 mg/ml at a rate of up to 3.5 ml/hour. The morphine concentration was increased to 0.3 mg/ml and then clonidine 3 micrograms/ml was added. Satisfactory pain relief was finally achieved by adding ketamine 1 mg/ml, containing benzethonium chloride as a preservative. The mean daily intrathecal dose of ketamine was 67 mg. After 7 days she had an acute psychotic reaction and the ketamine was withdrawn. There were no neurological deficits. She died 10 days later. There was focal lymphocytic vasculitis in the spinal medullary tissue, in the nerves, and in the leptomeninges of the thoracolumbar spinal cord.

This neurotoxicity could have been due to the preservative benzethonium chloride or the ketamine. However, several other agents, including bupivacaine, morphine, and clonidine, were also given intrathecally, so causality was not proven, even though the other agents have not been associated with this problem.

There have been several attempts to understand the pathophysiology of schizophrenia using subanesthetic doses of ketamine to probe glutaminergic function in healthy and schizophrenic volunteers; no long-term adverse consequences were attributable to ketamine (22).

Psychological, psychiatric

In a randomized, double-blind, crossover study of cognitive impairment in 24 volunteers who received *S*-ketamine 0.25 mg/kg, racemic ketamine 0.5 mg/kg, or *R*-ketamine 1.0 mg/kg, the ketamine isomers caused less tiredness and cognitive impairment than equianalgesic doses of racemic ketamine (23). In addition, *S*-ketamine caused less reduction in concentration capacity and primary memory.

A placebo-controlled study of low-dose ketamine infusion in ten volunteers showed formal thought disorder and impairments in working and semantic memory (24). The degree of thought disorder correlated with the impairment in working memory.

Psychotomimetic effects

The psychotomimetic effects of ketamine, apart from encouraging illicit use, can lead to distressing psychic disturbances, particularly in children (13); there can be nightmares, delirium, and hallucinations (25). Oral ketamine is an effective analgesic in patients with chronic pain. In 21 patients with central and peripheral chronic neuropathic pain treated with oral ketamine, the starting dose was ketamine 100 mg/day, titrated upward by 40 mg/day increments every 2 days until a satisfactory effect was achieved, or until adverse effects became limiting (19). Nine patients discontinued ketamine because of intolerable adverse effects, including psychotomimetic symptoms, such as "elevator" effect or dissociative feelings, somnolence or insomnia, and sensory changes such as taste disturbance and somatic sensations.

The pharmacological effects of the *R*- and *S*-enantiomers of ketamine have been compared in 11 subjects who received *R*-ketamine 0.5 mg and then *S*-ketamine 0.15 mg, separated by 1 week (26). Before and after each drug administration they were subjected to a painful stimulus using a nerve stimulator applied to the right central incisor tooth. Pain suppression was equal with the two drugs. The subjects reported more unpleasant psychotomimetic effects with *S*-ketamine and more pleasant effects with *R*-ketamine. Seven of eleven subjects preferred *R*-ketamine, while none preferred *S*-ketamine. These results suggest that the neuropsychiatric effect of ketamine may be predominantly due to the *S*-enantiomer, and that *R*-ketamine may be a better alternative. This study is in direct distinction to earlier work suggesting that *R*-ketamine is responsible for most of the undesirable neuropsychiatric side effects of ketamine.

A placebo-controlled study in 10 healthy young men showed a linear relation between ketamine plasma concentrations of 50–200 ng/ml and the severity of psychotomimetic effects (27). The psychedelic effects were also similar to those observed in a previous study of dimethyltryptamine, an illicit LSD-25 type of drug, and were a function of plasma concentration rather than simply an emergence phenomenon. Clinically useful analgesia was obtained at plasma concentrations of 100–200 ng/ml. At plasma concentrations of 200 ng/ml, all subjects had lateral nystagmus. When ketamine is given in large doses, patients rapidly become unresponsive, and so the effects described in this study are usually only observed during the recovery phase.

There have been several attempts to understand the pathophysiology of schizophrenia using subanesthetic doses of ketamine to probe glutaminergic function in healthy and schizophrenic volunteers; no long-term adverse consequences were attributable to ketamine (22).

Prevention

There have been several attempts to attenuate the unpleasant psychological adverse effects that occur after sedation with ketamine.

Prior use of benzodiazepines or opiates limits the psychotomimetic effects of ketamine. There has been a double-blind, placebo-controlled study of the role of lorazepam in reducing these effects after subanesthetic doses of ketamine in 23 volunteers who received lorazepam 2 mg or placebo, 2 hours before either a bolus dose of ketamine 0.26 mg/kg followed by an infusion of 0.65 mg/kg/hour or a placebo infusion (28). The ability of lorazepam to block the undesirable effects of ketamine was limited to just some effects. It reduced the ketamine-associated emotional distress and perceptual alterations, but exacerbated the sedative, attention-impairing, and amnesic effects of ketamine. However, it failed to reduce many of the cognitive and behavioral effects of ketamine. There were no pharmacokinetic interactions between subanesthetic doses of ketamine and lorazepam.

The effect of intravenous midazolam 0.05 mg/kg on emergence phenomena after ketamine 1.5 mg/kg intravenously for painful procedures has been assessed in a randomized, double-blind, placebo-controlled study in 104 children (29). Midazolam was given 2 minutes after the ketamine. There was no significant difference between the two groups in levels of agitation. The overall rate of agitation was low, but probably high enough to detect any significant differences between the groups.

The neuropsychiatric effects of ketamine were modulated by lamotrigine, a glutamate release inhibitor, in 16 healthy volunteers (30). Lamotrigine 300 mg was given 2 hours before ketamine 0.26 and 0.65 mg/kg on two separate days. There were fewer ketamine-induced perceptual abnormalities, fewer schizophreniform symptoms, and less learning and memory impairments. Mood-elevating effects were increased with lamotrigine. The authors commented that the results were experimental and that further studies are needed to confirm the potential benefits in a larger group of patients.

The hypothesis that the unpleasant emergence phenomena that often accompany the use of ketamine, including odd behavior, vacant stare, and abnormal affect, would be reduced by the use of a selected recorded tape played during the perioperative period has been tested in 28 adults (31). The incidence of dreams was higher when the recorded tape was connected. This report emphasizes the current recommendations that a quiet room with minimal stimuli is best for reducing emergence phenomena after ketamine sedation.

Endocrine

In a double-blind, randomized, placebo-controlled crossover comparison of the effects of ketamine and memantine in 15 male volunteers, ketamine increased serum prolactin and cortisol concentrations, whereas memantine and placebo did not (32).

Liver

Serum enzyme activities (alkaline phosphatase, aspartate transaminase, alanine transaminase, and gamma-glutamyl transpeptidase) were raised in 14 of 34 patients anesthetized with ketamine; the significance of this is unknown (33).

Long-Term Effects

Drug abuse

Media reports suggest that in some countries the non-medical (illicit) use of ketamine has greatly increased (34).

Drug Administration

Drug administration route

The addition of ketamine to bupivacaine for spinal anesthesia has been studied in 60 patients undergoing spinal anesthesia for insertion of intracavitary brachytherapy implants for cervical carcinoma (8). They were randomly assigned to receive either bupivacaine 10 mg or bupivacaine 7.5 mg plus ketamine 25 mg. Motor recovery was significantly quicker in the ketamine group. Blood pressure was significantly lower in the bupivacaine group 5 minutes after administration, and perioperative intravenous fluid requirements were significantly higher. Patients given ketamine reported more sedation and dizziness, both intraoperatively and postoperatively. There were no nightmares or dissociative features. Overall satisfaction was better with bupivacaine. The study was abandoned after 30 patients, because of the high rate of adverse effects with ketamine. Although ketamine had local anesthetic-sparing properties, its adverse effects made it unsuitable for intrathecal administration.

Drug–Drug Interactions

Alfentanil

The interaction of ketamine with the respiratory depressant effect of alfentanil has been studied in eight healthy men, who received alfentanil as a continuous computer-controlled infusion aiming at a plasma concentration of 50 ng/ml and either an infusion of racemic ketamine increasing step-wise through 50, 100, and 200 ng/ml or placebo (35). Alfentanil caused hypoventilation by reducing respiratory rate, and this was antagonized by ketamine in a concentration-dependent manner. This combination may be effective in overcoming the adverse effects of either agent individually.

Haloperidol

The interaction of the dopamine antagonist haloperidol 5 mg orally with subanesthetic doses of ketamine has been studied in a placebo-controlled study in 20 healthy volunteers over 4 days (36). Haloperidol pretreatment reduced impairment of executive cognitive functions produced by ketamine and reduced the anxiogenic effects of ketamine. However, it failed to block the ability of ketamine to produce psychosis, perceptual changes, negative symptoms, or euphoria, and it increased the sedative and prolactin responses to ketamine. These results imply that ketamine may impair executive cognitive functions via dopamine receptor activation in the frontal cortex, but that the psychoactive effects of ketamine are not mediated via dopamine receptors, but rather via NMDA receptor antagonism.

References

1. Epstein FB. Ketamine dissociative sedation in pediatric emergency medical practice. Am J Emerg Med 1993;11(2):180–2.
2. Weksler N, Ovadia L, Muati G, Stav A. Nasal ketamine for paediatric premedication. Can J Anaesth 1993;40(2):119–21.
3. Murray Wilson A. Multiple ketamine anaesthesia. Saudi Med J 1979;1:19.
4. Kohrs R, Durieux ME. Ketamine: teaching an old drug new tricks. Anesth Analg 1998;87(5):1186–93.
5. Adams HA. The use of (S)-ketamine in intensive care medicine. Acta Anaesthesiol Scand 1998;42:S212–13.
6. Kremer M. What's new with reactive airways and anesthesia? CRNA 1995;6(3):118–24.
7. Jahangir SM, Islam F, Aziz L. Ketamine infusion for postoperative analgesia in asthmatics: a comparison with intermittent meperidine. Anesth Analg 1993;76(1):45–9.
8. Kathirvel S, Sadhasivam S, Saxena A, Kannan TR, Ganjoo P. Effects of intrathecal ketamine added to bupivacaine for spinal anaesthesia. Anaesthesia 2000;55(9):899–904.
9. Jaksch W, Lang S, Reichhalter R, Raab G, Dann K, Fitzal S. Perioperative small-dose S(+)-ketamine has no incremental beneficial effects on postoperative pain when standard-practice opioid infusions are used Anesth Analg 2002;94(4):981–6.
10. Zsigmond EK, Kothary SP, Kumar SM, Kelsch RC. Counteraction of circulatory side effects of ketamine by pretreatment with diazepam. Clin Ther 1980;3(1):28–32.
11. Cabbabe EB, Behbahani PM. Cardiovascular reactions associated with the use of ketamine and epinephrine in plastic surgery. Ann Plast Surg 1985;15(1):50–6.
12. Waxman K, Shoemaker WC, Lippmann M. Cardiovascular effects of anesthetic induction with ketamine. Anesth Analg 1980;59(5):355–8.
13. Tarnow J, Hess W. Pulmonale Hypertonie und Lungenödem nach Ketamin. [Pulmonary hypertension and pulmonary edema caused by intravenous ketamine.] Anaesthesist 1978;27(10):486–7.
14. Taittonen MT, Kirvela OA, Aantaa R, Kanto JH. The effect of clonidine or midazolam premedication on perioperative responses during ketamine anesthesia. Anesth Analg 1998;87(1):161–7.
15. Handa F, Tanaka M, Nishikawa T, Toyooka H. Effects of oral clonidine premedication on side effects of intravenous ketamine anesthesia: a randomized, double-blind, placebo-controlled study. J Clin Anesth 2000;12(1):19–24.
16. Smith JA, Santer LJ. Respiratory arrest following intramuscular ketamine injection in a 4-year-old child. Ann Emerg Med 1993;22(3):613–15.
17. Gardner AE, Dannemiller FJ, Dean D. Intracranial cerebrospinal fluid pressure in man during ketamine anesthesia. Anesth Analg 1972;51(5):741–5.
18. Fontana M, Mastrostefano R, Pietrangeli A, Madonna V. Acute intracranial hypertension syndrome due to ketamine in a patient with delayed radionecrosis simulating an expansive process. J Neurosurg Sci 1980;24(2):93–8.
19. Enarson MC, Hays H, Woodroffe MA. Clinical experience with oral ketamine. J Pain Symptom Manage 1999;17(5):384–6.
20. Haines DR, Gaines SP. N of 1 randomised controlled trials of oral ketamine in patients with chronic pain. Pain 1999;83(2):283–7.
21. Stotz M, Oehen HP, Gerber H. Histological findings after long-term infusion of intrathecal ketamine for chronic pain: a case report. J Pain Symptom Manage 1999;18(3):223–8.
22. Lahti AC, Warfel D, Michaelidis T, Weiler MA, Frey K, Tamminga CA. Long-term outcome of patients who receive ketamine during research. Biol Psychiatry 2001;49(10):869–75.
23. Pfenninger EG, Durieux ME, Himmelseher S. Cognitive impairment after small-dose ketamine isomers in comparison to equianalgesic racemic ketamine in human volunteers. Anesthesiology 2002;96(2):357–66.
24. Adler CM, Goldberg TE, Malhotra AK, Pickar D, Breier A. Effects of ketamine on thought disorder, working memory, and semantic memory in healthy volunteers. Biol Psychiatry 1998;43(11):811–16.
25. Klausen NO, Wiberg-Jorgensen F, Chraemmer-Jorgensen B. Psychomimetic reactions after low-dose ketamine infusion. Comparison with neuroleptanaesthesia. Br J Anaesth 1983;55(4):297–301.
26. Rabben T. Effects of the NMDA receptor antagonist ketamine in electrically induced A delta-fiber pain. Methods Find Exp Clin Pharmacol 2000;22(3):185–9.
27. Bowdle TA, Radant AD, Cowley DS, Kharasch ED, Strassman RJ, Roy-Byrne PP. Psychedelic effects of ketamine in healthy volunteers: relationship to steady-state plasma concentrations. Anesthesiology 1998;88(1):82–8.
28. Krystal JH, Karper LP, Bennett A, D'Souza DC, Abi-Dargham A, Morrissey K, Abi-Saab D, Bremner JD, Bowers MB Jr, Suckow RF, Stetson P, Heninger GR, Charney DS. Interactive effects of subanesthetic ketamine and subhypnotic lorazepam in humans Psychopharmacology (Berl) 1998;135(3):213–29.

29. Sherwin TS, Green SM, Khan A, Chapman DS, Dannenberg B. Does adjunctive midazolam reduce recovery agitation after ketamine sedation for pediatric procedures? A randomized, double-blind, placebo-controlled trial. Ann Emerg Med 2000;35(3):229–38.
30. Anand A, Charney DS, Oren DA, Berman RM, Hu XS, Cappiello A, Krystal JH. Attenuation of the neuropsychiatric effects of ketamine with lamotrigine: support for hyperglutamatergic effects of N-methyl-D-aspartate receptor antagonists. Arch Gen Psychiatry 2000; 57(3):270–6.
31. Lauretti GR, Ramos MBP, De Mattos AL, De Oliveira AC. Emergence phenomena after ketamine anesthesia: influence of a selected recorded tape and midazolam. Rev Bras Anesthesiol 1996;46:329–34.
32. Hergovich N, Singer E, Agneter E, Eichler HG, Graselli U, Simhandl C, Jilma B. Comparison of the effects of ketamine and memantine on prolactin and cortisol release in men. a randomized, double-blind, placebo-controlled trial. Neuropsychopharmacology 2001;24(5):590–3.
33. Dundee JW, Fee JP, Moore J, McIlroy PD, Wilson DB. Changes in serum enzyme levels following ketamine infusions. Anaesthesia 1980;35(1):12–16.
34. Hall CH, Cassidy J. Young drug users adopt "bad trip" anesthetic. Independent 1992;2:1.
35. Persson J, Scheinin H, Hellstrom G, Bjorkman S, Gotharson E, Gustafsson LL. Ketamine antagonises alfentanil-induced hypoventilation in healthy male volunteers. Acta Anaesthesiol Scand 1999;43(7):744–52.
36. Krystal JH, D'Souza DC, Karper LP, Bennett A, Abi-Dargham A, Abi-Saab D, Cassello K, Bowers MB Jr, Vegso S, Heninger GR, Charney DS. Interactive effects of subanesthetic ketamine and haloperidol in healthy humans. Psychopharmacology (Berl) 1999;145(2):193–204.

Ketanserin

General Information

Ketanserin is a selective 5-HT_2 receptor antagonist with antihypertensive action. Because it antagonizes the vasoconstriction and platelet aggregation induced by 5-HT and increases erythrocyte deformability, its potential usefulness in peripheral vascular disease has been extensively investigated, although never convincingly demonstrated. It has been reported to be beneficial in pre-eclampsia (1).

Most of the adverse effects attributable to ketanserin seem, not surprisingly, to be on the central nervous system. They include drowsiness, fatigue, headache, sleep disturbances, and dry mouth. Other complaints include dizziness, light-headedness, lack of concentration, and dyspepsia. A gradual increase in dosage is therefore recommended. These adverse effects occur in about 10% of patients and lead to withdrawal of the drug in 3–4% (SEDA-17, 243).

Organs and Systems

Cardiovascular

Dose-related prolongation of the QT interval on the electrocardiogram occurs in roughly one-third of patients taking ketanserin (2). Several cases of ventricular dysrhythmias with QT prolongation, leading to syncope, have been reported (SED-11, 392) (SED-12, 473), but the exact incidence of significant ventricular dysrhythmias on the basis of QT prolongation during ketanserin therapy is unknown.

Drug–Drug Interactions

Ecstasy

In 14 healthy subjects, ketanserin attenuated the perceptual changes, emotional excitation, and acute adverse responses induced by ecstasy, but had little effect on positive mood, well-being, extroversion, and short-term sequelae (3). Body temperature was lower with ecstasy plus ketanserin than with ecstasy alone.

Potassium-wasting diuretics

Prolongation of the QT interval by ketanserin is more pronounced when it used in combination with potassium-wasting diuretics (4). This combination must therefore be avoided.

References

1. Bolte AC, van Eyck J, Gaffar SF, van Geijn HP, Dekker GA. Ketanserin for the treatment of preeclampsia. J Perinat Med 2001;29(1):14–22.
2. Zehender M, Meinertz T, Hohnloser S, Geibel A, Hartung J, Seiler KU, Just H. Incidence and clinical relevance of QT prolongation caused by the new selective serotonin antagonist ketanserin. Am J Cardiol 1989; 63(12):826–32.
3. Liechti ME, Saur MR, Gamma A, Hell D, Vollenweider FX. Psychological and physiological effects of MDMA ("Ecstasy") after pretreatment with the 5-HT(2) antagonist ketanserin in healthy humans. Neuropsychopharmacology 2000;23(4):396–404.
4. Prevention of Atherosclerotic Complications with Ketanserin Trial Group. Prevention of atherosclerotic complications: controlled trial of ketanserin. BMJ 1989; 298(6671):424–30. Erratum in: BMJ 1989;298(6674):644.

Ketobemidone

General Information

Ketobemidone is an opioid receptor agonist, with pharmacokinetics and potency similar to morphine. Combined with the antispasmodic drug, *N*,*N*-dimethyl-3,3-diphenyl-1-methylallylamine chloride, ketobemidone is often used in Scandinavia.

In a study of postoperative pain relief, ketobemidone equalled morphine and pethidine with respect to efficacy of analgesia and adverse effects, such as shivering, nausea, and vomiting (SEDA-16, 81).

Organs and Systems

Respiratory

Early cough in 40 of 121 patients given ketobemidone for postoperative analgesia has been reported. Four of the patients found it severe and distressing. The lower frequency of cough in patients previously exposed to ketobemidone in the premedication may reflect tachyphylaxis (SEDA-17, 81).

Ketoconazole

See also Antifungal azoles

General Information

Ketoconazole was the first azole available for oral administration. However, it has been supplanted by newer azoles with fewer adverse effects and more reliable absorption from the gastrointestinal tract. Even after years of use, new adverse effects (often related to high doses and/or newer indications) continue to be reported.

Ketoconazole is water-soluble at a pH of below 3. Its oral absorption is influenced by the acidity of the stomach contents, and the concomitant administration of histamine H_2 receptor antagonists, proton pump inhibitors, antacids, or food affects its absorption. A high carbohy drate meal ingested with ketoconazole reduces total drug absorption, while a high lipid meal increases it. Erratic absorption is particularly apparent in patients with AIDS. Peak serum concentrations are seen within 2–3 hours. The half-life is about 8 hours. CSF penetration is less than 10% (1). Ketoconazole is extensively metabolized in the liver and excreted in the bile in an inactive form; less than 1% of the active drug is excreted in the urine. Clearance is not significantly altered by renal dialysis (1).

In man, higher doses of ketoconazole affect cortisol/cortisone and androgen/testosterone substrates. This finding has led to the use of ketoconazole in Cushing's disease and prostate cancer, but the phenomenon is also responsible for some of the adverse effects, especially those associated with higher doses and prolonged use (SED-12, 677). The potency of ketoconazole in inhibiting P450 isozymes (such as CYP3A4) is a cause of interactions with several other drugs.

Use in non-infective conditions

The efficacy of ketoconazole 400 mg qds in the early treatment of acute lung injury and acute respiratory distress syndrome has been investigated in a randomized, double-blind, placebo-controlled trial in 234 patients (2). Ketoconazole was safe but had no effects on mortality, lung function, or the duration of mechanical ventilation.

Because of its potent inhibitory effects on adrenal steroidogenesis by interference with cytochrome CYP450, ketoconazole controls hypercortisolism when surgery is contraindicated or unsuccessful. The effects of oral ketoconazole 200–1200 mg qds for 65–83 months in three patients who had residual or recurrent Cushing's disease after surgical treatment have been reported (3). The dosage of ketoconazole was adjusted according to the clinical response and 24-hour urinary excretion of free cortisol. All three patients had good clinical and biochemical responses to therapy with ketoconazole and had no adverse effects.

General adverse effects

Gastrointestinal complaints, including anorexia, nausea, gastralgia, and constipation are the most frequent adverse effects of ketoconazole. Hepatotoxicity, varying in degree from mild disturbances of liver function tests to hepatitis and rare cases of fulminating hepatic necrosis, has been reported. Some cases have been reported in the first weeks of treatment, but duration of treatment is of importance and in prolonged courses of treatment, monitoring is advisable. With the use of high doses, especially for longer periods of time, the effects of interference with hormonal balance should be watched for. Adrenal insufficiency has been reported even with low-dose treatment. Pruritus and skin reactions have been reported, but do not in general cause major problems. Hypersensitivity reactions are rare. Tumor-inducing effects have not been reported.

Organs and Systems

Respiratory

Patients undergoing esophagectomy are at increased risk of acute lung injury, perhaps related to increased concentrations of thromboxane in the postpulmonary circulation. In 38 consecutive patients undergoing esophagectomy, perioperative ketoconazole, which inhibits thromboxane synthesis, reduced the incidence of acute lung injury (4).

Nervous system

Headache, dizziness, nervousness, and somnolence have been reported (SED-11, 573). The incidences are low. Encephalopathy can occur as a result of severe liver damage.

Sensory systems

Eyes

Papilledema has been reported in one patient taking ketoconazole. The condition cleared on withdrawal of ketoconazole and recurred on resumption 2 months later (SEDA-18, 284).

Psychological, psychiatric

In one patient taking a high dosage for prostate cancer, weakness was associated with mental disturbances, notably confabulation and disorientation in time and space (SEDA-13, 233).

Endocrine

Gynecomastia was occasionally observed in men when ketoconazole first became available. Ketoconazole has a marked effect on steroid concentrations, including a change in the testosterone/estradiol ratio, and this is most likely to be the basis of the gynecomastia. A lowering of testosterone serum concentrations and a reduced response of testosterone concentrations to human gonadotropin have been shown (SED-11, 573) (5). Various studies have shown suppression of testosterone, androstenedione, and dehydroepiandrosterone, with reciprocal increases in gonadotrophins.

Reductions in serum and urinary cortisol concentrations have been reported in patients taking ketoconazole and signs of hypoadrenalism have been seen during high-dose treatment. However, it is not clear whether the asthenia syndrome described in the past (severe muscle weakness, most pronounced in the legs, fatigue, apathy, and anorexia) is related to hypoadrenalism. In some cases, hypoadrenalism has been described shortly after the start of low-dose treatment. Substitution therapy may be required, since simple withdrawal of ketoconazole may not redress hormonal balance quickly enough.

Various studies have shown that ketoconazole interferes with 17- and 20-hydroxylases and inhibits mitochondrial 11-α-hydroxylase and cytochrome P450-dependent steroid hydroxylase enzymes (SED-12, 677) (6) (SEDA-12, 228) (SEDA-14, 234).

Because of its effects on the pituitary/adrenal system, ketoconazole has been used in the long-term control of hypercortisolism of either pituitary or adrenal origin (SED-12, 677). In seven patients with Cushing's disease and one with an adrenal adenoma, ketoconazole 600–800 mg/day for 3–13 months produced rapid persistent clinical improvement (7). Plasma dehydroepiandrosterone sulfate concentrations and urinary 17-ketosteroid and cortisol excretion fell soon after the start of treatment, and remained normal or nearly so throughout treatment. Urinary tetrahydro-11-deoxycortisol excretion rose significantly. Plasma cortisol concentrations fell. Plasma ACTH concentrations did not change and individual plasma ACTH and cortisol increments in response to CRH were comparable before and during treatment. The cortisol response to insulin-induced hypoglycemia improved in one patient and was restored to normal in another. The patients recovered normal adrenal suppressibility in response to a low dose of dexamethasone during ketoconazole treatment.

The effect of ketoconazole appears to be mediated by inhibition of adrenal 11-β-hydroxylase and 17,20-lyase, and in some unknown way it prevents the expected rise in ACTH secretion in patients with Cushing's disease (SEDA-12, 228) (SEDA-17, 323). It may, however, cause such a rapid reduction in serum cortisol concentrations that a crisis is precipitated, and patients' adrenal function should be carefully monitored. While ketoconazole (400–800 mg/day) may be a good alternative to other adrenal steroid inhibitors, patients should be observed for signs of hepatotoxicity. Acute adrenal crisis occasionally occurs (8).

Because ketoconazole has antiandrogenic properties, it is particularly suitable for women, in whom it has few effects on menstruation and does not cause hirsutism. In men, however, long-term inhibition of androgen production can be disruptive, especially if it leads to gynecomastia and hypogonadism. Combination with aminoglutethimide and metyrapone has been advocated in order to avoid these effects (SEDA-17, 323).

Ketoconazole (400 mg/day) has been used for the treatment of hirsutism and acne in women, but adverse effects, such as headache, nausea, loss of scalp hair, hepatitis, and biochemical changes, were impressive (9–11).

Hematologic

Fatal aplastic anemia has been reported during ketoconazole therapy (12).

Gastrointestinal

Nausea, mild gastrointestinal symptoms, and vomiting can occur in patients taking ketoconazole; diarrhea has been reported, but the incidence is low (SED-12, 678). The incidence of gastrointestinal complaints is higher with the use of daily doses above 800 mg (13).

Liver

Mild and often transient rises in serum liver enzyme activities are not uncommon in patients taking ketoconazole; the incidence is reported to be about 10–15% (SEDA-12, 229). This figure is higher than originally thought (SED-11, 573) (14), the newer figures probably representing a greater awareness of the risk rather than a true increase; it is possible, however, that the use of higher doses plays a role (SED-12, 678).

The incidence of symptomatic hepatic injury associated with ketoconazole is estimated to be about one in 10 000 treated cases (SEDA-18, 284). Biochemically, the pattern was hepatocellular in 54%, cholestatic in 16%, and mixed cholestatic-hepatocellular in 30%. Histology (14 cases) showed a predominantly hepatocellular pattern in 57%, with extensive centrilobular necrosis and mild to moderate bridging (14,15). Lethal cases of toxic hepatitis and a case necessitating transplantation have been reported (14,16,17).

- A girl developed fatal liver failure while taking ketoconazole for Cushing's syndrome (18). The authors proposed using metyrapone when temporary control of hypercortisolism is required in childhood and adolescence.

A cohort study of the risk of acute liver injury among users of oral antifungal drugs has been performed in the general population of the General Practice Research Database in the UK (19). The cohort included 69 830 patients, free from liver and systemic diseases, who had received at least one prescription for oral griseofulvin, fluconazole, itraconazole, ketoconazole, or terbinafine between 1991 and 1996. Five cases of acute liver injury occurred during the use of oral antifungal drugs. Two of the patients were taking ketoconazole, another two itraconazole, and one terbinafine. The incidence rates of acute liver injury were 134 (CI = 37, 488) per 100 000 person-months for ketoconazole, 10 (CI = 2.9, 38) for itraconazole, and 2.5 (CI = 0.4, 14) for terbinafine. One case was associated with past use of fluconazole. Ketoconazole was the antifungal drug that was associated with the highest relative risk, 228 (CI = 34, 933) compared with the risk among non-users, followed by itraconazole and terbinafine, with relative risks of 18 (CI = 2.6, 73) and 4.2 (CI = 0.2, 25) respectively.

Skin

The risk of serious skin disorders has been estimated in 61 858 users, aged 20–79 years, of oral antifungal drugs identified in the UK General Practice Research Database

(20). They had received at least one prescription for oral fluconazole, griseofulvin, itraconazole, ketoconazole, or terbinafine. The background rate of serious cutaneous adverse reactions (corresponding to non-use of oral antifungal drugs) was 3.9 per 10 000 person-years (95% CI = 2.9, 5.2). Incidence rates for current use were 15 per 10 000 person-years (1.9, 56) for itraconazole, 11.1 (3.0, 29) for terbinafine, 10 (1.3, 38) for fluconazole, and 4.6 (0.1, 26) for griseofulvin. Cutaneous disorders associated with the use of oral antifungal drugs in this study were all mild.

Pruritus and occasional rashes can occur in patients taking ketoconazole (21). Rare cases of a fixed drug eruption have been reported (SED-12, 678) (22) (SEDA-17, 323).

Musculoskeletal

- Muscle weakness and diffuse myalgia were reported in a 17-year-old man with multiple endocrine neoplasia syndrome type 1 taking ketoconazole for oral candidiasis. The electromyogram showed a distinct myopathic pattern. Withdrawal of the ketoconazole was followed by rapid improvement (SEDA-17, 323).

In rats, high doses (80 mg/kg) caused syndactyly in one experiment (SED-11, 574). There are insufficient data to determine whether there might be a harmful effect in humans.

Second-Generation Effects

Lactation

Ketoconazole can be found in the milk of lactating dogs receiving ketoconazole; there are insufficient data to decide whether harm might ensue to the breast-fed child.

Susceptibility Factors

Age

Because ketoconazole interferes with steroid synthesis and vitamin D metabolism, ketoconazole should not be used in children. It is not approved for use in children and there is no pediatric dosage range based on pharmacokinetic information in this population.

Sex

Liver complications may be more common in elderly people, in women, or in subjects in whom liver function is already compromised for other reasons.

Other features of the patient

Ketoconazole interferes with steroidogenesis, and those who are critically ill (23) or HIV-positive (24) are particularly susceptible to adrenal insufficiency from the use of ketoconazole.

Drug–Drug Interactions

Aciclovir

Ketoconazole seems to have a synergistic antiviral effect when it is taken with aciclovir (25).

Alcohol

A disulfiram-type reaction of ketoconazole with alcohol has been reported (SEDA-12, 231).

Amphotericin

Combination of ketoconazole with amphotericin reportedly leads to antagonism, particularly if ketoconazole therapy precedes amphotericin (26).

Antacids

Co-administration of antacids reduces the absorption of ketoconazole (13).

Antihistamines

Ketoconazole can increase the concentrations of astemizole and terfenadine by inhibition of CYP3A4. High concentrations of terfenadine can cause cardiac toxicity. Increased plasma concentrations of unmetabolized terfenadine prolong the QT interval and carry the risk of torsade de pointes and other fatal ventricular arrhythmias (13).

Ebastine (10 and 20 mg/day) had no clinically important effect on QT_c interval in adults, including elderly people, children, and patients with hepatic or renal impairment, and co-administration with ketoconazole or erythromycin did not lead to significant changes in the QT_c interval (27,28).

The pharmacokinetic and pharmacodynamic interactions of emedastine difumarate and ketoconazole have been investigated in 12 healthy volunteers (29). Emedastine difumarate 4 mg was given orally for 10 consecutive days, and on days 6–10 ketoconazole 200 mg bd was co-administered. Emedastine steady-state pharmacokinetics were slightly altered by ketoconazole: the AUC rose by about 33% and total clearance fell by about 30%, with no change in the half-life, suggesting that the volume of distribution also changed; this pattern could have arisen from protein binding displacement. However, there was no change in the QT_c interval after 5 days of co-treatment. The authors concluded that concomitant treatment with emedastine and ketoconazole in subjects with normal QT intervals could therefore be undertaken without special precautions.

When single doses of erythromycin (333 mg) or ketoconazole (200 mg) were given to healthy men who used levocabastine, two sprays per nostril (0.05 mg/spray) bd for 6 days, there were no changes in the pharmacokinetics of levocabastine or in the QT_c interval (30).

Ketoconazole affects plasma concentrations of loratadine, a non-sedating antihistamine, but appears to be devoid of any electrocardiographic effects (31). In a randomized, single-blind, multiple-dose, three-way, crossover study, concomitant administration of loratadine 10 mg qds and ketoconazole 200 mg bd resulted in significantly increased mean loratadine plasma concentration by 307% and desloratadine plasma concentrations by 73%; ketoconazole plasma concentrations were unaffected by loratadine. Despite increased concentrations of loratadine and its metabolite, there were no statistically significant differences in the electrocardiographic QT_c interval.

Benzodiazepines

In a double-blind, crossover kinetic and dynamic study of the interaction of ketoconazole with alprazolam and triazolam, two CYP3A4 substrate drugs with different kinetic profiles, impaired clearance by ketoconazole had more profound clinical consequences for triazolam than for alprazolam (32). By the same mechanism ketoconazole also inhibits the metabolism of midazolam (33).

Calcium channel blockers

The effects of ketoconazole 200 mg on the pharmacokinetics of nisoldipine 5 mg have been investigated in a randomized, cross-over trial (34). Pretreatment with and concomitant administration of ketoconazole resulted in 24-fold and 11-fold increases in the AUC and C_{max} of nisoldipine, respectively. The ketoconazole-induced increase in plasma concentrations of the metabolite M9 was of similar magnitude. Thus, ketoconazole and other potent inhibitors of CYP3A should not be used concomitantly with nisoldipine.

In an intestinal perfusion study of the effect of ketoconazole 40 μg/ml on the jejunal permeability and first-pass metabolism of (*R*)- and (*S*)-verapamil 120 μg/ml in six healthy volunteers, ketoconazole did not alter the jejunal permeability of the isomers, suggesting that it had no effect on the P-glycoprotein mediated efflux. However, the rate of absorption increased, suggesting inhibition by ketoconazole of the gut wall metabolism of (*R/S*)-verapamil by CYP3A4 (35).

Carbamazepine

Serum concentrations of ketoconazole are reduced by concomitant use of drugs that induce hepatic microsomal enzymes, such as carbamazepine. There may at the same time be a change in serum carbamazepine concentration (13,25).

Ciclosporin

The fact that ketoconazole inhibits cytochrome P450 accounts for some of its interactions. Ketoconazole increases ciclosporin concentrations, enhancing the risk of renal impairment, as shown by a fall in creatinine clearance (SED-12, 678) (6,13,25,36).

The effect of ketoconazole in ciclosporin-treated kidney transplant recipients has been the subject of a prospective randomized study (37). In 51 ketoconazole-treated patients and 49 controls there was a similar frequency of acute rejection episodes. However, in the control group, rejection episodes were more recurrent, with a poorer response to treatment. Acute ciclosporin nephrotoxicity was more common in the ketoconazole group, but this was encountered more at induction and rapidly reversed on further reduction of the dose of ciclosporin. Chronic graft dysfunction was significantly less in the ketoconazole group during the first year, but by the end of the study the difference was not statistically significant. Hepatotoxicity was similar in the two groups. Serum concentrations of cholesterol, low-density lipoprotein, and triglycerides were lower in the ketoconazole group. The authors concluded that long-term low-dose ketoconazole in ciclosporin-treated kidney transplant recipients is safe and cost-saving.

Citalopram

The effect of ketoconazole on the pharmacokinetics of citalopram has been studied in a double-blind, three-way, crossover trial in 18 men and women (38). The subjects received three treatments with a 14-day washout period: a single dose of ketoconazole 200 mg plus placebo, a single dose of citalopram 40 mg plus placebo, and a single dose of ketoconazole 200 mg plus a single dose of citalopram 40 mg. There were no changes in the pharmacokinetics of citalopram after co-administration of ketoconazole, suggesting that ketoconazole and other CYP3A4 inhibitors can be safely co-administered with citalopram.

Clozapine

The interaction of ketoconazole (400 mg/day for 7 days) with clozapine has been evaluated in five patients with schizophrenia given a single dose of clozapine 50 mg at the end of ketoconazole therapy (39). Ketoconazole did not significantly change the disposition of clozapine or its metabolism to its principal metabolites, desmethylclozapine and clozapine-*N*-oxide.

Donepezil

Donepezil 5 mg produced no change in plasma concentrations of ketoconazole 200 mg (40).

Erythromycin

If erythromycin and ketoconazole, both CYP3A4 inhibitors, are taken in combination, there will be an even more dramatic effect on the metabolism of other drugs, such as terfenadine and astemizole, midazolam and triazolam, and ciclosporin.

Halofantrine

Halofantrine, a highly lipophilic antimalarial drug with poor and erratic absorption, is metabolized to its equipotent metabolite desbutylhalofantrine and this is inhibited by oral ketoconazole (41).

Histamine H_2 receptor antagonists

Co-administration of histamine H_2 receptor antagonists reduces the absorption of ketoconazole (13).

HIV protease inhibitors

The effects of co-administration of ketoconazole 400 mg and amprenavir 1200 mg, which is mostly metabolized by CYP3A4, have been studied in an open, randomized, balanced, single-dose, three-period, crossover study in 12 healthy men (42). Co-administration of the two drugs increased the amprenavir AUC by 31% and reduced its C_{max} by 16%. Amprenavir increased the AUC of ketoconazole by 44% and increased its half-life and C_{max} by 23% and 16% respectively. Thus, co-administration of amprenavir and ketoconazole result in statistically significant increases in the AUCs of both agents, but the clinical significance of these changes remains to be investigated.

The pharmacokinetic interaction of fluconazole 400 mg od and indinavir 1000 mg tds has been evaluated in a placebo-controlled, crossover study for 8 days; there was no significant interaction (43).

The effect of ketoconazole (200 and 400 mg qds) on plasma and cerebrospinal fluid concentrations of ritonavir (400 mg bd) and saquinavir (400 mg bd) have been investigated in a two-period, two-group, longitudinal pharmacokinetic study in 12 HIV-infected patients (44). Ketoconazole significantly increased the AUC and trough concentrations of ritonavir and prolonged its half-life (by 29%, 62%, and 31% respectively). It produced similar changes (37%, 94%, and 38% respectively) in the kinetics of saquinavir. Ketoconazole significantly increased the ritonavir CSF concentration at 4–5 hours after the dose by 178% (from 2.4 to 6.6 ng/ml), with no change in the paired unbound plasma concentration (26 ng/ml). The changes were not related to ketoconazole dose or plasma exposure. The corresponding changes in saquinavir CSF concentrations were not significant. The authors concluded that ketoconazole inhibited the systemic clearance of ritonavir and, because of the disproportionate increase in CSF concentrations compared with the increase in plasma concentrations, that there was greater inhibition of drug efflux from the CSF.

A study in seven HIV-infected men who took saquinavir 600 mg tds in addition to two other antiretroviral drugs and concomitant ketoconazole (200 mg qds for 7 days, followed by 400 mg qds for another 7 days) showed no significant differences in peak and trough concentrations of saquinavir after the addition of ketoconazole (45). There was substantial inter-subject variability in the study, and the authors concluded that saquinavir concentrations may be unpredictable in individual patients and that drug monitoring may be required for optimizing saquinavir treatment.

Ifosfamide

The effect of ketoconazole on the CYP-mediated metabolism of ifosfamide to 4-hydroxyifosfamide and the ultimate cytotoxic ifosforamide mustard, and its deactivation to 2- and 3-dechloroethylifosfamide has been studied in a randomized, crossover study in 16 patients, who received intravenous ifosfamide 3 g/m^2/day, either alone or in combination with ketoconazole 200 mg bd 1 day before treatment and during 3 days of concomitant administration (46). Ketoconazole did not affect the fraction metabolized or exposure to the dechloroethylated metabolites and thus did not alter the pharmacokinetics of ifosfamide or its metabolism.

Isoniazid

Combined administration of ketoconazole with isoniazid can lead to increased concentrations of the latter, and there are possibly also alterations in ketoconazole concentrations (SED-12, 678) (25).

Methylprednisolone

The effect of ketoconazole on steroid metabolism is reflected in other interactions. Ketoconazole increases the total amount of methylprednisolone in the body (SED-12, 678) (47).

Oral contraceptives

The reported reduction in the effect of oral contraceptives (SEDA-12, 231) concurs with the effect of ketoconazole on steroid metabolism; the effect seems to be mild and may be mainly of importance during the use of formulations with low estrogen content (SED-12, 678) (48).

Phenazone

Ketoconazole reduces the clearance of phenazone (antipyrine) (SED-11, 574) (49).

Phenytoin

Serum concentrations of ketoconazole are reduced by concomitant use of drugs that induce hepatic microsomal enzymes, such as phenytoin. There may at the same time be a change in serum phenytoin concentration (SED-12, 678) (13,25,50).

Proton pump inhibitors

Co-administration of proton pump blockers reduces the absorption of ketoconazole (13).

Reboxetine

Reboxetine is metabolized by CYP3A4. In 11 healthy volunteers, ketoconazole increased the AUC of reboxetine by about 50% and increased its half-life (51). The adverse effects profile of reboxetine was not altered by ketoconazole.

Rifamycins

Serum concentrations of ketoconazole are reduced by concomitant use of drugs that induce hepatic microsomal enzymes, such as rifampicin. There may at the same time be a change in rifampicin serum concentration (SED-12, 678) (13,25,36).

Ropivacaine

Ketoconazole 400 mg caused a minor reduction in the clearance of ropivacaine, which is mostly metabolized by CYP1A2 (52).

Statins

In two cases, rhabdomyolysis occurred after co-administration of simvastatin 20 mg/day and ketoconazole (53).

Theophylline

The combination of ketoconazole with theophylline was reported to have reduced theophylline concentrations, suggesting increased metabolism of theophylline (SEDA-13, 234). This is surprising, since one would have expected ketoconazole to have inhibited the metabolism of theophylline, if at all. However, in 10 healthy, non-smoking men aged 18–40 years aminophylline 6 mg/kg intravenously before and after they had taken oral ketoconazole 200 mg/day for 7 days caused no change in the half-life or clearance of theophylline (54), so there is probably no important interaction between these two drugs.

Tolterodine

Tolterodine is eliminated by two different oxidative metabolic pathways: hydroxylation, catalysed by CYP2D6, and *D*-alkylation, catalysed by CYP3A. The pharmacokinetics and safety of tolterodine and its metabolites in the absence and presence of ketoconazole have been investigated in healthy volunteers with deficient CYP2D6 activity (poor metabolizers) (55). Clearance of tolterodine fell by 60% during co-administration of ketoconazole, resulting in a 2.1-fold increase in AUC. Thus, caution is needed when ketoconazole and other potent inhibitors of CYP3A are used concomitantly with tolterodine.

Tretinoin

A potential interaction of ketoconazole with tretinoin (all-trans retinoic acid), resulting in slowed metabolism, is probably not of importance (56).

Warfarin

Potentiation of the effects of warfarin has been reported in one case (SED-12, 678) (57), but absence of interference with anticoagulants was also claimed.

Ziprasidone

Ziprasidone is oxidatively metabolized by CYP3A4, but it does not inhibit CYP3A4 or other isoenzymes at clinically relevant concentrations. The effect of ketoconazole 400 mg qds for 6 days on the single-dose pharmacokinetics of ziprasidone 40 mg has been evaluated in an open, placebo-controlled, crossover study in healthy volunteers (58). Ketoconazole caused a modest increase in the mean AUC (33%) and the mean C_{max} (34%) of ziprasidone. This effect was not considered clinically relevant and suggests that other inhibitors of CYP3A4 are unlikely to affect the pharmacokinetics of ziprasidone significantly. Most of the reported adverse events were mild. The adverse events that were most commonly reported in subjects who took the drugs concomitantly were dizziness, weakness, and somnolence. There were no treatment-related laboratory abnormalities or abnormal vital signs during the study and at the 6-day follow-up evaluation.

Zolpidem

Zolpidem is metabolized by CYP3A. Ketoconazole 200 mg bd impaired the clearance of zolpidem 5 mg and enhanced its benzodiazepine-like pharmacodynamic effects. In contrast, itraconazole 100 mg bd and fluconazole 100 mg bd had small effects on zolpidem kinetics and dynamics (59).

References

1. Lyman CA, Walsh TJ. Systemically administered antifungal agents. A review of their clinical pharmacology and therapeutic applications. Drugs 1992;44(1):9–35.
2. The ARDS Network. Ketoconazole for early treatment of acute lung injury and acute respiratory distress syndrome: a randomized controlled trial. JAMA 2000;283(15):1995–2002.
3. Chou SC, Lin JD. Long-term effects of ketoconazole in the treatment of residual or recurrent Cushing's disease. Endocr J 2000;47(4):401–6.
4. Schilling MK, Eichenberger M, Maurer CA, Sigurdsson G, Buchler MW. Ketoconazole and pulmonary failure after esophagectomy: a prospective clinical trial. Dis Esophagus 2001;14(1):37–40.
5. Krause W, Effendy I. Wie wirkt Ketoconazol auf den Testosteron-Stoffwechsel? [How does ketoconazole affect testosterone metabolism?] Z Hautkr 1985;60(14):1147–55.
6. Drouhet E, Dupont B. Evolution of antifungal agents: past, present, and future. Rev Infect Dis 1987;9(Suppl 1):S4–S14.
7. Loli P, Berselli ME, Tagliaferri M. Use of ketoconazole in the treatment of Cushing's syndrome. J Clin Endocrinol Metab 1986;63(6):1365–71.
8. Khosla S, Wolfson JS, Demerjian Z, Godine JE. Adrenal crisis in the setting of high-dose ketoconazole therapy. Arch Intern Med 1989;149(4):802–4.
9. Venturoli S, Fabbri R, Dal Prato L, Mantovani B, Capelli M, Magrini O, Flamigni C. Ketoconazole therapy for women with acne and/or hirsutism. J Clin Endocrinol Metab 1990;71(2):335–9.
10. De Pedrini P, Tommaselli A, Spano G, Montemurro G. Clinical and hormonal effects of ketoconazole on hirsutism in women. Int J Tissue React 1988;10(3):193–8.
11. Akalin S. Effects of ketoconazole in hirsute women. Acta Endocrinol (Copenh) 1991;124(1):19–22.
12. Duman D, Turhal NS, Duman DG. Fatal aplastic anemia during treatment with ketoconazole. Am J Med 2001;111(9):737.
13. Francis P, Walsh TJ. Evolving role of flucytosine in immunocompromised patients: new insights into safety, pharmacokinetics, and antifungal therapy. Clin Infect Dis 1992;15(6):1003–18.
14. Lewis JH, Zimmerman HJ, Benson GD, Ishak KG. Hepatic injury associated with ketoconazole therapy. Analysis of 33 cases. Gastroenterology 1984;86(3):503–13.
15. Stricker BH, Blok AP, Bronkhorst FB, Van Parys GE, Desmet VJ. Ketoconazole-associated hepatic injury. A clinicopathological study of 55 cases. J Hepatol 1986;3(3):399–406.
16. Knight TE, Shikuma CY, Knight J. Ketoconazole-induced fulminant hepatitis necessitating liver transplantation. J Am Acad Dermatol 1991;25(2 Pt 2):398–400.
17. Duarte PA, Chow CC, Simmons F, Ruskin J. Fatal hepatitis associated with ketoconazole therapy. Arch Intern Med 1984;144(5):1069–70.
18. Zollner E, Delport S, Bonnici F. Fatal liver failure due to ketoconazole treatment of a girl with Cushing's syndrome. J Pediatr Endocrinol Metab 2001;14(3):335–8.
19. Garcia Rodriguez LA, Duque A, Castellsague J, Perez-Gutthann S, Stricker BH. A cohort study on the risk of acute liver injury among users of ketoconazole and other antifungal drugs. Br J Clin Pharmacol 1999;48(6):847–52.
20. Castellsague J, Garcia-Rodriguez LA, Duque A, Perez S. Risk of serious skin disorders among users of oral antifungals: a population-based study. BMC Dermatol 2002;2(1):14.
21. Smith EB, Henry JC. Ketoconazole: an orally effective antifungal agent. Mechanism of action, pharmacology,

clinical efficacy and adverse effects. Pharmacotherapy 1984;4(4):199–204.
22. Cox FW, Stiller RL, South DA, Stevens DA. Oral ketoconazole for dermatophyte infections. J Am Acad Dermatol 1982;6(4 Pt 1):455–62.
23. Albert SG, DeLeon MJ, Silverberg AB. Possible association between high-dose fluconazole and adrenal insufficiency in critically ill patients. Crit Care Med 2001;29(3):668–70.
24. Etzel JV, Brocavich JM, Torre M. Endocrine complications associated with human immunodeficiency virus infection. Clin Pharm 1992;11(8):705–13.
25. Bickers DR. Antifungal therapy: potential interactions with other classes of drugs. J Am Acad Dermatol 1994;31(3 Pt 2):S87 90.
26. Schaffner A, Frick PG. The effect of ketoconazole on amphotericin B in a model of disseminated aspergillosis. J Infect Dis 1985;151(5):902–10.
27. Moss AJ, Chaikin P, Garcia JD, Gillen M, Roberts DJ, Morganroth J. A review of the cardiac systemic side-effects of antihistamines: ebastine. Clin Exp Allergy 1999;29(Suppl 3):200–5.
28. Moss AJ, Morganroth J. Cardiac effects of ebastine and other antihistamines in humans. Drug Saf 1999;21(Suppl 1):69–80.
29. Herranz U, Rusca A, Assandri A. Emedastine–ketoconazole: pharmacokinetic and pharmacodynamic interactions in healthy volunteers. Int J Clin Pharmacol Ther 2001;39(3):102–9.
30. Pesco-Koplowitz L, Hassell A, Lee P, Zhou H, Hall N, Wiesinger B, Mechlinski W, Grover M, Hunt T, Smith R, Travers S. Lack of effect of erythromycin and ketoconazole on the pharmacokinetics and pharmacodynamics of steady-state intranasal levocabastine. J Clin Pharmacol 1999;39(1):76–85.
31. Kosoglou T, Salfi M, Lim JM, Batra VK, Cayen MN, Affrime MB. Evaluation of the pharmacokinetics and electrocardiographic pharmacodynamics of loratadine with concomitant administration of ketoconazole or cimetidine. Br J Clin Pharmacol 2000;50(6):581–9.
32. Greenblatt DJ, Wright CE, von Moltke LL, Harmatz JS, Ehrenberg BL, Harrel LM, Corbett K, Counihan M, Tobias S, Shader RI. Ketoconazole inhibition of triazolam and alprazolam clearance: differential kinetic and dynamic consequences. Clin Pharmacol Ther 1998;64(3):237–47.
33. Lam YW, Alfaro CL, Ereshefsky L, Miller M. Pharmacokinetic and pharmacodynamic interactions of oral midazolam with ketoconazole, fluoxetine, fluvoxamine, and nefazodone. J Clin Pharmacol 2003;43(11):1274–82.
34. Heinig R, Adelmann HG, Ahr G. The effect of ketoconazole on the pharmacokinetics, pharmacodynamics and safety of nisoldipine. Eur J Clin Pharmacol 1999;55(1):57–60.
35. Sandstrom R, Knutson TW, Knutson L, Jansson B, Lennernas H. The effect of ketoconazole on the jejunal permeability and CYP3A metabolism of (R/S)-verapamil in humans. Br J Clin Pharmacol 1999;48(2):180–9.
36. Sugar AM, Stern JJ, Dupont B. Overview: treatment of cryptococcal meningitis. Rev Infect Dis 1990;12(Suppl 3):S338–48.
37. Sobh MA, Hamdy AF, El Agroudy AE, El Sayed K, El-Diasty T, Bakr MA, Ghoneim MA. Coadministration of ketoconazole and cyclosporine for kidney transplant recipients: long-term follow-up and study of metabolic consequences. Am J Kidney Dis 2001;37(3):510–17.
38. Gutierrez M, Abramowitz W. Lack of effect of a single dose of ketoconazole on the pharmacokinetics of citalopram. Pharmacotherapy 2001;21(2):163–8.
39. Lane HY, Chiu CC, Kazmi Y, Desai H, Lam YW, Jann MW, Chang WH. Lack of CYP3A4 inhibition by grapefruit juice and ketoconazole upon clozapine administration in vivo. Drug Metabol Drug Interact 2001;18(3–4):263–78.
40. Tiseo PJ, Perdomo CA, Friedhoff LT. Concurrent administration of donepezil HCl and ketoconazole: assessment of pharmacokinetic changes following single and multiple doses. Br J Clin Pharmacol 1998;46(Suppl 1):30–4.
41. Khoo SM, Porter JH, Edwards GA, Charman WN. Metabolism of halofantrine to its equipotent metabolite, desbutylhalofantrine, is decreased when orally administered with ketoconazole. J Pharm Sci 1998;87(12):1538–41.
42. Polk RE, Crouch MA, Israel DS, Pastor A, Sadler BM, Chittick GE, Symonds WT, Gouldin W, Lou Y. Pharmacokinetic interaction between ketoconazole and amprenavir after single doses in healthy men. Pharmacotherapy 1999;19(12):1378–84.
43. De Wit S, Debier M, De Smet M, McCrea J, Stone J, Carides A, Matthews C, Deutsch P, Clumeck N. Effect of fluconazole on indinavir pharmacokinetics in human immunodeficiency virus-infected patients. Antimicrob Agents Chemother 1998;42(2):223–7.
44. Khaliq Y, Gallicano K, Venance S, Kravcik S, Cameron DW. Effect of ketoconazole on ritonavir and saquinavir concentrations in plasma and cerebrospinal fluid from patients infected with human immunodeficiency virus. Clin Pharmacol Ther 2000;68(6):637–46.
45. Collazos J, Martinez E, Mayo J, Blanco MS. Effect of ketoconazole on plasma concentrations of saquinavir. J Antimicrob Chemother 2000;46(1):151–2.
46. Kerbusch T, Jansen RL, Mathot RA, Huitema AD, Jansen M, van Rijswijk RE, Beijnen JH. Modulation of the cytochrome P450-mediated metabolism of ifosfamide by ketoconazole and rifampin. Clin Pharmacol Ther 2001;70(2):132–41.
47. Glynn AM, Slaughter RL, Brass C, D'Ambrosio R, Jusko WJ. Effects of ketoconazole on methylprednisolone pharmacokinetics and cortisol secretion. Clin Pharmacol Ther 1986;39(6):654–9.
48. Kovacs L, Somos P, Hamori M. Examination of the potential interaction between ketoconazole (Nizoral) and oral contraceptives with special regard to products of low hormone content (Rigevidon, Anteovin). Ther Hung 1986;34;167.
49. D'Mello AP, D'Souza MJ, Bates TR. Pharmacokinetics of ketoconazole–antipyrine interaction. Lancet 1985;2(8448):209–10.
50. Food and Drug Administration. Ketoconazole labeling revised. FDA Drug Bull 1984;14(2):17–18.
51. Herman BD, Fleishaker JC, Brown MT. Ketoconazole inhibits the clearance of the enantiomers of the antidepressant reboxetine in humans. Clin Pharmacol Ther 1999;66(4):374–9.
52. Arlander E, Ekstrom G, Alm C, Carrillo JA, Bielenstein M, Bottiger Y, Bertilsson L, Gustafsson LL. Metabolism of ropivacaine in humans is mediated by CYP1A2 and to a minor extent by CYP3A4: an interaction study with fluvoxamine and ketoconazole as in vivo inhibitors. Clin Pharmacol Ther 1998;64(5):484–91.
53. Gilad R, Lampl Y. Rhabdomyolysis induced by simvastatin and ketoconazole treatment. Clin Neuropharmacol 1999;22(5):295–7.
54. Heusner JJ, Dukes GE, Rollins DE, Tolman KG, Galinsky RE. Effect of chronically administered ketoconazole on the elimination of theophylline in man. Drug Intell Clin Pharm 1987;21(6):514–17.
55. Brynne N, Forslund C, Hallen B, Gustafsson LL, Bertilsson L. Ketoconazole inhibits the metabolism of tolterodine in subjects with deficient CYP2D6 activity. Br J Clin Pharmacol 1999;48(4):564–72.

56. Lee JS, Newman RA, Lippman SM, Fossella FV, Calayag M, Raber MN, Krakoff IH, Hong WK. Phase I evaluation of all-trans retinoic acid with and without ketoconazole in adults with solid tumors. J Clin Oncol 1995;13(6):1501–8.
57. Smith AG. Potentiation of oral anticoagulants by ketoconazole. BMJ (Clin Res Ed) 1984;288(6412):188–9.
58. Miceli JJ, Smith M, Robarge L, Morse T, Laurent A. The effects of ketoconazole on ziprasidone pharmacokinetics—a placebo-controlled crossover study in healthy volunteers. Br J Clin Pharmacol 2000;49(Suppl 1):S71–6.
59. Greenblatt DJ, von Moltke LL, Harmatz JS, Mertzanis P, Graf JA, Durol AL, Counihan M, Roth-Schechter B, Shader RI. Kinetic and dynamic interaction study of zolpidem with ketoconazole, itraconazole, and fluconazole. Clin Pharmacol Ther 1998;64(6):661–71.

Ketolides

General Information

The ketolides cethromycin (ABT-773) and telithromycin are semisynthetic derivatives of 14-membered-ring macrolide antibiotics, members of the macrolide-lincosamide-streptogramin-B, MLS(B), class of antimicrobials, but they differ from macrolides by having a 3-keto group instead of an L-cladinose group on the erythronolide A ring (1–3). In a study of the efficacy of the ketolides HMR 3004 (previously RU 004) and telithromycin (HMR 3647, previously 66 647) against beta-lactamase-producing *Haemophilus influenzae*, the in vitro activity of both ketolides against 30 clinical isolates was comparable to that of azithromycin and superior to clarithromycin and erythromycin A. Furthermore, HMR 3004 and HMR 3647 were both active in a murine model of experimental pneumonia, as assessed by pulmonary clearance of beta-lactamase producing *H. influenzae* (4).

Telithromycin has a good spectrum of activity against respiratory pathogens, including penicillin-resistant and erythromycin-resistant pneumococci, intracellular bacteria, and atypical bacteria. It has an absolute oral availability of 57% in young and elderly subjects (5), and the rate and extent of absorption is unaffected by food (6). It penetrates rapidly into bronchopulmonary, tonsillar, sinus, and middle ear tissues/fluids, achieves high concentrations at sites of infection, and concentrates within polymorphonuclear neutrophils. In a dosage of 800 mg/day it is well tolerated across all patient populations, and adverse events, most commonly diarrhea, nausea, dizziness, and vomiting, are generally mild to moderate in intensity and seldom lead to treatment withdrawal (7–9).

Organs and Systems

Cardiovascular

Telithromycin causes prolongation of the QT interval, especially in elderly patients with predisposing conditions (2).

Long-Term Effects

Drug tolerance

In subjects receiving oral telithromycin (800 mg/day for 10 days), high drug concentrations were detected in the saliva indicating a good therapeutic profile for throat infections. Quantitative ecological disturbances in the normal microflora during administration of telithromycin were moderate, and no overgrowth of yeasts or *Clostridium difficile* occurred. However, resistant bacterial strains emerged (10).

The in vitro activity of cethromycin was very similar to that of telithromycin, with an MIC_{90} of 0.5 mg/l or less for all bacteria examined, except methicillin-resistant *Staphylococcus aureus*, *Enterococcus faecalis*, *Enterococcus faecium*, *H. influenzae*, and *Bacteroides* species. However, the antichlamydial activity of cethromycin was greater than that of telithromycin (11).

Drug–Drug Interactions

Cytokines

Cytokines modify phagocyte activity and may interfere with the immunomodulating properties of antibacterial agents. In an in vitro study, TNF-α and GM-CSF reduced the inhibitory effect of telithromycin on oxidant production by polymorphonuclear neutrophils, suggesting an effect of telithromycin downstream of the priming effect of cytokines. In addition, TNF-α and GM-CSF moderately impaired the uptake of telithromycin by polymorphonuclear neutrophils; the inhibitory effect of these two cytokines seemed to be related to the activation of the p38 mitogen-activated protein kinase (12).

References

1. Nilius AM, Ma Z. Ketolides: the future of the macrolides? Curr Opin Pharmacol 2002;2(5):493–500.
2. Shain CS, Amsden GW. Telithromycin: the first of the ketolides. Ann Pharmacother 2002;36(3):452–64.
3. Van Rensburg DJ, Matthews PA, Leroy B. Efficacy and safety of telithromycin in community-acquired pneumonia. Curr Med Res Opin 2002;18(7):397–400.
4. Piper KE, Rouse MS, Steckelberg JM, Wilson WR, Patel R. Ketolide treatment of *Haemophilus influenzae* experimental pneumonia. Antimicrob Agents Chemother 1999;43(3):708–10.
5. Perret C, Lenfant B, Weinling E, Wessels DH, Scholtz HE, Montay G, Sultan E. Pharmacokinetics and absolute oral bioavailability of an 800-mg oral dose of telithromycin in healthy young and elderly volunteers. Chemotherapy 2002;48(5):217–23.
6. Bhargava V, Lenfant B, Perret C, Pascual MH, Sultan E, Montay G. Lack of effect of food on the bioavailability of a new ketolide antibacterial, telithromycin. Scand J Infect Dis 2002;34(11):823–6.
7. Balfour JA, Figgitt DP. Telithromycin. Drugs 2001;61(6):815–29.
8. Baltch AL, Smith RP, Ritz WJ, Franke MA, Michelsen PB. Antibacterial effect of telithromycin (HMR 3647) and comparative antibiotics against intracellular *Legionella pneumophila*. J Antimicrob Chemother 2000;46(1):51–5.

9. Bearden DT, Neuhauser MM, Garey KW. Telithromycin: an oral ketolide for respiratory infections. Pharmacotherapy 2001;21(10):1204–22.
10. Edlund C, Alvan G, Barkholt L, Vacheron F, Nord CE. Pharmacokinetics and comparative effects of telithromycin (HMR 3647) and clarithromycin on the oropharyngeal and intestinal microflora. J Antimicrob Chemother 2000;46(5):741–9.
11. Andrews JM, Weller TM, Ashby JP, Walker RM, Wise R. The in vitro activity of ABT773, a new ketolide antimicrobial agent. J Antimicrob Chemother 2000;46(6):1017–22.
12. Vazifeh D, Bryskier A, Labro MT. Effect of proinflammatory cytokines on the interplay between roxithromycin, HMR 3647, or HMR 3004 and human polymorphonuclear neutrophils. Antimicrob Agents Chemother 2000;44(3):511–21.

Ketoprofen

See also Non-steroidal anti-inflammatory drugs

General Information

The spectrum of adverse effects of ketoprofen is similar to that of ibuprofen.

Ketoprofen was originally approved for over-the-counter sales in the USA by the FDA, but in the same year, in Italy, the Ministry of Health transferred two ketoprofen-containing products from non-prescription to prescription status (SEDA-20, 93). The reasons for this difference are not clear.

Organs and Systems

Respiratory

A fatal asthmatic reaction has been described (1), and severe bronchospasm with respiratory and cardiac arrest has been reported in a young man with a history of mild asthma after he took ketoprofen (2). Topical application can provoke asthma in predisposed subjects (3).

Even topical formulations of NSAIDs should be avoided in patients with a history of analgesic-induced asthma (4).

- A 74-year-old woman with a history of sinusitis, nasal polyps, and analgesic-induced asthma had a sudden life-threatening attack of asthma 2 hours after the application of a 2% ketoprofen adhesive tape. Asthma had not previously occurred when she had used a 0.3% ketoprofen adhesive patch.

Nervous system

Retention of salt and water, sometimes with reversible pseudotumor cerebri, can occur with ketoprofen (5).

Gastrointestinal

The overall frequency of adverse reactions was 15–50% in different trials; gastrotoxicity predominated, at a frequency of 6.5–42% (6–8), even after rectal administration. In some epidemiological studies, ketoprofen in prescription doses was more gastrotoxic than other NSAIDs (SEDA-18, 99).

There are very few data on the gastrointestinal toxicity of over-the-counter doses of ketoprofen. In an endoscopic short-term study in healthy subjects ketoprofen was associated with significant gastrointestinal toxicity (9). Another endoscopic study showed that the *R*-enantiomer of ketoprofen has less gastrointestinal toxicity than the racemic mixture or the *S*-enantiomer while retaining good analgesic activity (SEDA-22, 116).

Local symptoms, including rectal bleeding, can accompany treatment with ketoprofen suppositories (8.3% of patients) (6).

Liver

Hepatotoxicity has rarely been reported with ketoprofen (SEDA-17, 110).

Urinary tract

Like many other NSAIDs, ketoprofen can cause acute interstitial nephritis (10). Renal insufficiency and the nephrotic syndrome due to membranous glomerulonephritis (an unusual cause of NSAID-induced nephrotic syndrome) have been described in an elderly patient taking long-term ketoprofen (SEDA-12, 86).

As topical NSAIDs can be absorbed via the skin, they cannot be considered safe in high-risk patients, in whom all NSAIDs are contraindicated.

- A 62-year-old woman developed acute renal insufficiency after using topical ketoprofen for 5 days (11). She had several predisposing factors to NSAID-induced acute renal insufficiency, such as advanced age, chronic renal impairment due to polycystic kidney disease, and treatment with an ACE inhibitor and furosemide.

Ketoprofen use has been followed by red discoloration of urine (SEDA-16, 110).

Skin

Topical ketoprofen can cause contact dermatitis and photodermatitis, like other NSAIDs (SEDA-18, 104) (SEDA-22, 116). Data from Sweden have confirmed the photosensitizing potential of topical gel formulations of ketoprofen and have included a number of reports of contact dermatitis (12). In some cases ketoprofen can be responsible for very prolonged photosensitivity after only a single application (13).

Toxic epidermal necrolysis has been described with ketoprofen (SEDA-21, 105).

Drug Administration

Drug administration route

Studies on a modified-release formulation of ketoprofen showed a similar pattern of adverse effects to the usual formulations (SEDA-12, 86).

An injectable form of ketoprofen has acceptable tolerability (6,7), but about 4.5% of patients have local reactions.

Drug overdose

A 64-year-old woman had auditory and visual hallucinations, persecutory delusions, and slurred speech after she took an overdose of ketoprofen; her psychiatric symptoms resolved within 48 hours (14).

Drug–Drug Interactions

Aspirin

Concurrent administration of aspirin reduces ketoprofen protein binding and increases its clearance. Salicylate also reduces the metabolic conversion of ketoprofen to its conjugates and their renal elimination, and enhances its conversion to non-conjugated metabolites (15).

Co-triamterzide

Irreversible renal insufficiency has been reported in an elderly patient who took ketoprofen in combination with co-triamterzide (triamterene + hydrochlorothiazide) (16). The interaction with triamterene is well documented (SEDA-12, 80) and co-administration with ketoprofen has proved dangerous.

Warfarin

Although data from healthy subjects indicate no interaction of ketoprofen with warfarin, severe gastrointestinal bleeding and a prolonged prothrombin time have been attributed to this combination (SEDA-13, 81).

References

1. Egede F. Fatal asthmatic reaction following ketoprofen (Orudis) (Alreumat). Fatalt forlobende astmatisk reaction efter ketoprofen (Alreumat), (Orudis). [A fatal asthmatic reaction following ketoprofen (Alreumat), (Orudis).] Ugeskr Laeger 1979;141(17):1151–2.
2. Schreuder G. Ketoprofen: possible idiosyncratic acute bronchospasm. Med J Aust 1990;152(6):332–3.
3. Miyairi A, Ohori K. Aspirin-induced asthma due to rubbing ketoprofen ointment. Kokyu 1990;9:110.
4. Kashiwabara K, Nakamura H. Analgesic-induced asthma caused by 2.0% ketoprofen adhesive agents, but not by 0.3% agents. Intern Med 2001;40(2):124–6.
5. Larizza D, Colombo A, Lorini R, Severi F. Ketoprofen causing pseudotumor cerebri in Bartter's syndrome. N Engl J Med 1979;300(14):796.
6. Tamisier JN. Ketoprofen. Clin Rheum Dis 1979;5:381.
7. Gougeon J, Mireau-Hottin J, Gaillard F. Clinical trial of the injectable form of ketoprofen. Rheumatol Rehabil 1976;(Suppl):75–8.
8. Willans MJ, Digby JW, Topp JR, et al. Long term treatment of arthritis disease with ketoprofen (Orudis): a Canadian multicentre evaluation. Curr Ther Res 1979;25:35.
9. Lanza FL, Codispoti JR, Nelson EB. An endoscopic comparison of gastroduodenal injury with over-the-counter doses of ketoprofen and acetaminophen. Am J Gastroenterol 1998;93(7):1051–4.
10. Ducret F, Pointet P, Martin D, Villermet B. Insuffisance rénale aigueë réversible induite par le kétoprofene. [Acute reversible renal insufficiency induced by ketoprofen.] Nephrologie 1982;3(2):105–6.
11. Krummel T, Dimitrov Y, Moulin B, Hannedouche T. Drug points: Acute renal failure induced by topical ketoprofen. BMJ 2000;320(7227):93.
12. Swedish Adverse Drug Reactions Advisory Committee. Ketoprofen gel—contact dermatitis and photosensitivity. SADRAC Bull 1998;67:2.
13. Offidani A, Cellini A, Amerio P, Simonetti O, Bossi G. A case of persistent light reaction phenomenon to ketoprofen? Eur J Dermatol 2000;10(2):153–4.
14. Tavcar R, Dernovsek MZ, Brosch S. Ketoprofen intoxication delirium. J Clin Psychopharmacol 1999;19(1):95–6.
15. Williams RL, Upton RA, Buskin JN, Jones RM. Ketoprofen–aspirin interactions. Clin Pharmacol Ther 1981;30(2):226–31.
16. Pazmino PA, Pazmino PB. Ketoprofen-induced irreversible renal failure. Nephron 1988;50(1):70–1.

Ketorolac

See also Non-steroidal anti-inflammatory drugs

General Information

Ketorolac is, like several other NSAIDs, promoted as a non-narcotic analgesic. This is merely a marketing ploy, which does not reflect any special characteristics, except that it is one of many NSAIDs that can be given parenterally. A pyrrolizine carboxylic acid derivative, it is structurally and pharmacologically related to tolmetin, zomepirac, and indometacin. The trometamol salt of ketorolac enhances its solubility and allows parenteral administration; single intramuscular injections are better tolerated than morphine.

Opinions on the safety of ketorolac in EC drug regulatory authorities are conflicting (SEDA-18, 104) (1). However, the risk of adverse effects is higher when ketorolac is used in higher doses, in elderly subjects, and for more than 5 days (SEDA-21, 105).

Other information on the benefit-to-harm balance of parenteral ketorolac tromethamine as a postoperative analgesic has been provided by three studies (SEDA-21, 105). The overall risk of gastrointestinal and operative site bleeding and acute renal insufficiency associated with parenteral ketorolac and a parenteral opiate were relatively small.

The most commonly reported symptoms are somnolence, headache, dizziness, nausea, dyspepsia, and abdominal pain. Edema, hyperkalemia, diarrhea, sweating, self-limiting wheezing, and itching have also been reported occasionally (SEDA-12, 86) (SEDA-16, 110) (SEDA-17, 111).

There are contrasting data on the benefit-to-harm balance of parenteral ketorolac as an analgesic (SEDA-21, 105). This prompted regulatory review of ketorolac in many countries, leading to revision of labelling, dosage recommendations, and prescribing practices. The use of ketorolac should be limited in dosage and duration; in elderly patients it should probably not be used at all. It is important for prescribers to understand that increasing the dosage of ketorolac beyond the label recommendations (60–120 mg/day for a maximum of 2–5 days) will not provide better efficacy, but will increase the risk of serious adverse reactions (2).

Organs and Systems

Sensory systems

Reversible hearing loss with tinnitus and headache were described in a woman with a predisposition to ototoxicity in end-stage renal disease (SEDA-21, 106).

Hematologic

Ketorolac prolongs bleeding time reversibly. The clinical significance of the effect of ketorolac on hemostasis in perioperative use is still imperfectly understood. Serious bleeding, either at the operative site or in the gastrointestinal tract after perioperative administration of ketorolac, has been documented in several reports (SEDA-18, 105) and in controlled studies (SEDA-20, 93). Concomitant use of anticoagulants increases the risk of bleeding (SEDA-18, 105).

Gastrointestinal

Gastric lesions (endoscopically demonstrated erosions, ulcers, and giant duodenal or gastric ulcers) have been described in healthy volunteers (SEDA-14, 94) and patients (SEDA-18, 105) treated with parenteral ketorolac (SEDA-14, 94); gastric damage is dose-related (SEDA-17, 112). A case-control study on hospitalization for upper gastrointestinal tract bleeding and/or perforation provided further evidence of the unfavorable benefit-to-harm balance of ketorolac compared with other NSAIDs. Ketorolac was five times more gastrotoxic than all other NSAIDs. The relative risk with intramuscular ketorolac was higher than with oral ketorolac (SEDA-22, 117).

Further evidence of the unfavorable benefit-to-harm balance of ketorolac compared with other NSAIDs has been provided by another case-control study on first-time hospitalization for gastroduodenal ulcer (documented by endoscopy, radiology, surgery, or autopsy), with or without bleeding or perforation. Of all the NSAIDs used in outpatients the highest rate ratio for lesions of any degree of severity was seen with piroxicam (4.6; 95% CI = 1.4, 8.3); ketorolac ranked second highest (3.4; 95% CI = 1.4, 8.3). For patients who suffered hemorrhage or perforation, the highest rate ratio observed was for ketorolac (5.9; 95% CI = 2.1, 16) (3).

Colonic ulceration with massive bleeding has been reported in a woman who received ketorolac intramuscularly (SEDA-21, 106).

Urinary tract

There have been several reports of impaired renal function in patients taking ketorolac (SEDA-17, 112) (SEDA-18, 105) (SEDA-22, 117). The severity varies from slight to severe forms of renal insufficiency, which may even occur after a single dose of 30 mg. Because recent major surgery is considered a risk factor for renal insufficiency, particularly in elderly patients, the use of ketorolac, or other NSAIDs, for postoperative pain management is warranted only in carefully selected patients. Furthermore, a case report confirmed that oral ketorolac can cause acute renal insufficiency in young subjects without any predisposing factors (SEDA-21, 106).

Immunologic

Anaphylaxis and anaphylactoid reactions have been reported (SEDA-17, 112).

Second-Generation Effects

Pregnancy

As ketorolac crosses the placental barrier, it should not be used in pregnant women. When it is given to mothers during labor, it significantly inhibits platelet aggregation in the neonate (SEDA-14, 94).

Susceptibility Factors

Other features of the patient

Children undergoing tonsillectomy had a significant increase in the risk of major postoperative hemorrhage without beneficial effects, compared with opioid analgesics (SEDA-21, 106).

Several reports have documented the high risk of ketorolac in patients with a history of asthma, nasal polyposis, and sensitivity to aspirin or any other NSAID (SEDA-18, 105). Exacerbation of chronic asthma has been reported after the use of ketorolac eye-drops (SEDA-21, 106).

Drug–Drug Interactions

Lithium

Reports of lithium neurotoxicity resulting from an interaction with ketorolac have been published (SEDA-22, 117) (4).

In a pharmacokinetic study in healthy volunteers ketorolac increased the concentration of lithium in both serum and erythrocytes, which may reflect concentration of the drug in the nervous system more accurately. Ketorolac can therefore increase the risk of adverse reactions of lithium (5), as do many other NSAIDs.

References

1. Lewis S. Ketorolac in Europe. Lancet 1994;343:784.
2. Reinhart DI. Minimising the adverse effects of ketorolac. Drug Saf 2000;22(6):487–97.
3. Menniti-Ippolito F, Maggini M, Raschetti R, Da Cas R, Traversa G, Walker AM. Ketorolac use in outpatients and gastrointestinal hospitalization: a comparison with other non-steroidal anti-inflammatory drugs in Italy. Eur J Clin Pharmacol 1998;54(5):393–7.
4. Iyer V. Ketorolac (Toradol) induced lithium toxicity. Headache 1994;34(7):442–4.
5. Cold JA, ZumBrunnen TL, Simpson MA, Augustin BG, Awad E, Jann MW. Increased lithium serum and red blood cell concentrations during ketorolac coadministration. J Clin Psychopharmacol 1998;18(1):33–7.

Ketotifen

See also Antihistamines

General Information

Ketotifen was originally developed as a drug that would inhibit the release of vasoactive substances from mast cells, as an oral alternative to cromoglicate, but its actions in asthma are probably attributable to its antihistaminic effect (SED-13, 423) (SEDA-22, 194), which occurs within minutes after administration and lasts for up to 12 hours. It also stabilizes mast cells, preventing histamine release, inhibits eosinophil accumulation in the lungs of animals exposed to platelet-activating factor, and reverses beta-adrenoceptor tachyphylaxis (1). It is classified as an antiallergic drug and is used as a prophylactic medicine.

Some trials have suggested that ketotifen has similar efficacy to cromoglicate in asthma (2) and also a small steroid-sparing effect (3). It is more effective than placebo in the treatment of atopic dermatitis (4). The normal therapeutic dose is 1–2 mg/day.

Conjunctival injection, headache, and rhinitis are common. Allergic reactions, stinging, discharge, eye pain, and photophobia occurred in less than 5% of patients. The most common adverse effects noted in long-term clinical trials are sedation and weight gain (SEDA-7, 1).

In young children (with an average age 16 months) effective doses of ketotifen produced adverse effects similar to those seen in adults, including dry mouth (28%) and sometimes increased appetite (5). In a series of 257 older children, increased weight was reported in 17, sedation in 13, and nausea in 3 (6). An evaluation of postmarketing surveillance of ketotifen in the UK showed, however, that the percentage of adverse effects reported in children was rather lower than in adults, sedation occurring in only 6% at the beginning of treatment. The corresponding figure in adults was 14.2% (7).

Organs and Systems

Nervous system

There is considerable controversy about the frequency and severity of sedation. Although it is commonly reported when ketotifen is started (23% in one study), its incidence falls during the first 2 months to about 6%. Only 2–3% of patients discontinue therapy for this reason (8). In a study involving 1791 patients, with allergic paroxysmal asthma, somnolence occurred in 13%. This effect started early in treatment and wore off in more than one-third of the patients (2).

Ketotifen produced seizures in a 5-year-old epileptic boy with allergic rhinitis. This was not specific to ketotifen but the result of H_1 receptor blockade. Administration of D-chlorphenamine increased the number of epileptic discharges seen on the electroencephalograph. It is recommended that centrally acting H_1 receptor antagonists should be avoided in epileptic patients, especially children (9).

Two cases of seizures in children induced by ketotifen have been reported (10).

- A 3-month-old boy was given ketotifen (0.1 mg/kg/day) for atopic dermatitis and after 8 days developed tonic spasms of a mixed flexor extensor type, consisting of flexion of the neck and arms with extension of the legs more than 10 times a day. Each seizure lasted for 5–15 minutes. An electroencephalogram showed a hypsarrhythmic trace. Ketotifen was withdrawn and the seizures were successfully controlled with ACTH and valproic acid. An MRI scan was normal.
- A 3-month-old boy was given ketotifen, 0.1 mg/kg/day, for asthmatic bronchitis. After 10 days his facial movements altered and 1 month after ketotifen was started tonic spasms began. His seizures consisted of a sudden contraction, usually bilateral and symmetrical involving the muscles of the neck, trunk, and limbs. An electroencephalogram showed a hypsarrhythmic trace. He was treated with ACTH and clonazepam without benefit. Ketotifen was withdrawn and ACTH and clonazepam were replaced with valproic acid. This resulted in seizure control, after which the electroencephalogram showed no abnormal discharges. Blood tests and an MRI scan were normal.

There is evidence that the central histaminergic neurons play an important role in inhibiting convulsions in the immature brain, where the GABA system is less effective than in the adult brain. Histamine acts via an H_1 receptor and other H_1 receptor antagonists can cause seizures. The authors proposed that ketotifen induces infantile spasms by antagonizing H_1 receptors.

Urinary tract

A single case of drug-induced cystitis has been reported. The patient had never taken tranilast, and the symptoms resolved on stopping ketotifen and recurred when the drug was restarted. Aseptic pyuria was found and cystoscopy revealed significant reddening over the urinary bladder (11).

Drug Administration

Drug overdose

Eight cases of overdose have been reported in which the patients took doses ranging from 10 to 120 mg (12). The plasma concentrations were considerably higher than those after therapeutic doses. The symptoms of overdose were drowsiness, confusion, coma, dyspnea, bradycardia and tachycardia, hyperexcitability, convulsions, and nystagmus. Six patients were treated with gastric lavage and after supportive treatment all eight patients made a full recovery within 12 hours of admission.

References

1. Garland LG. Pharmacology of prophylactic anti-asthma drugs. In: Page CP, Barnes PJ, editors. Pharmacology of Asthma. Berlin: Springer-Verlag; 1991:261–90.
2. Lebeau B, Gence B, Bourdain M, Loria Y. Le Kétotitine dans le traitement preventif de l'asthme. Analyse

synthetique de 1791 observations de medicine praticienne. [Preventive treatment of asthma with ketotifen: an analysis of 1791 cases treated in general practice.] Poumon Coeur 1982;38(2):125–9.
3. Lane DJ. A steroid sparing effect of ketotifen in steroid-dependent asthmatics. Clin Allergy 1980;10(5):519–25.
4. Falk ES. Ketotifen in the treatment of atopic dermatitis. Results of a double blind study. Riv Eur Sci Med Farmacol 1993;15(2):63–6.
5. El-Hefny A. Treatment of wheezy infants and children with ketotifen. Pharmatherapeutica 1983;3(6):388–92.
6. Sainmont C, Duprat P, Bourdain M, Loria Y. Etudeclinique du kétotifène solution buvable chez l'enfant. Résultats préliminaires sur 257 observations. [Clinical study of an oral solution of ketotifen in children. Preliminary results of 257 cases.] Ann Pediatr (Paris) 1984;31(1):81–4.
7. Craps L. Prophylaxis of asthma with ketotifen in children and adolescents: a review. Pharmatherapeutica 1983;3(5):314–26.
8. Tinkelman DG, Moss BA, Bukantz SC, Sheffer AL, Dobken JH, Chodosh S, Cohen BM, Rosenthal RR, Rappaport I, Buckley CE 3rd, et al. A multicenter trial of the prophylactic effect of ketotifen, theophylline, and placebo in atopic asthma. J Allergy Clin Immunol 1985;76(3):487–97.
9. Yokoyama H, Iinuma K, Yanai K, Watanabe T, Sakurai E, Onodera K. Proconvulsant effect of ketotifen, a histamine H1 antagonist, confirmed by the use of d-chlorpheniramine with monitoring electroencephalography. Methods Find Exp Clin Pharmacol 1993;15(3):183–8.
10. Yasuhara A, Ochi A, Harada Y, Kobayashi Y. Infantile spasms associated with a histamine H_1 antagonist. Neuropediatrics 1998;29(6):320–1.
11. Hara H, Kurita M, Morioka H, Kuwabara T, Kuroda K, Matsuhashi M, Ishii N, Miura K, Shirai M. [Drug induced cystitis due to ketotifen fumarate—a case report.] Nippon Hinyokika Gakkai Zasshi 1992;83(11):1906–9.
12. Jeffreys DB, Volans GN. Ketotifen overdose: surveillance of the toxicity of a new drug. BMJ (Clin Res Ed) 1981;282(6278):1755–6.

Krameriaceae

See also Herbal medicines

General Information

The family of Krameriaceae contains the single genus *Krameria* (ratany). Contact dermatitis has been reported in a patient using an extract of *Krameria triandra* (1).

Reference

1. Goday Bujan JJ, Oleaga Morante JM, Yanguas Bayona I, Gonzalez Guemes M, Soloeta Arechavala R. Allergic contact dermatitis from *Krameria triandra* extract. Contact Dermatitis 1998;38(2):120–1.

Labetalol

See also Beta-adrenoceptor antagonists

General Information

Labetalol is a non-selective alpha- and beta-adrenoceptor antagonist; these actions reside in four different enantiomers.

Labetalol is less likely to increase airways resistance in patients with bronchial asthma or to reduce peripheral blood flow. However, it can produce postural hypotension (SEDA-3, 166–7), and paresthesia of the scalp (1,2) and perioral numbness (3) have been described.

Organs and Systems

Cardiovascular

Labetalol is generally used effectively as an antihypertensive drug without reports of high vascular resistance, even in patients with pheochromocytoma. However, a case of pheochromocytoma with increased systemic vascular resistance and reduced cardiac index has been described (4).

- A 36-year-old man with a pheochromocytoma underwent adrenalectomy. After induction of anesthesia he was given intravenous labetalol 30 mg, and after intubation his blood pressure rose from 147/85 to 247/150 mmHg, his systemic vascular resistance index rose from 1958 to 3458 dyn·sec^{-1} m^2 cm^5, and his cardiac index fell to 3.6 l min^{-1} m^2. During tumor resection, he was given sodium nitroprusside to reduce his blood pressure. After tumor resection, his blood pressure fell to 77/52 mmHg and his systemic vascular resistance index to 1635 dyn·sec^{-1} m^2 cm^5. His blood pressure was effectively controlled with dobutamine.

This case affords a reminder that intravenous labetalol can increase the systemic vascular resistance and cause a hypertensive crisis. In these cases, labetalol should be replaced with a pure alpha-blocker or another vasodilator, to prevent the possibility of cardiovascular complications.

Neonatal cardiac arrest was precipitated in one case by labetalol (5).

Electrolyte balance

Three cases of severe hyperkalemia have been reported in renal transplant recipients taking labetalol for acute hypertension (6) and life-threatening hyperkalemia has been reported after intravenous labetalol (7).

- A 28-year-old man with severe hypertension and end-stage renal disease was given two intravenous doses of labetalol 20 mg 1 hour apart for malignant hypertension. The serum potassium concentration before treatment was 6.2 mmol/l, but 8 hours after labetalol it rose to 9.9 mmol/l and he developed left bundle branch block, ventricular tachycardia, and hypotension. He was given intravenous calcium gluconate, sodium bicarbonate, and lidocaine and reverted to sinus rhythm. The potassium concentration after 2 hours was 8.0 mmol/l. After hemodialysis the potassium concentration fell to 6.1 mmol/l.

In a retrospective chart review in 103 transplanted patients from January to November 1994, hypertension requiring perioperative treatment was observed in 51 cases (8). Treatment for hyperkalemia was necessary in 13 of the 38 patients who were treated with labetalol, compared with 11 of the 65 who were treated with another antihypertensive treatment.

Patients with end-stage renal disease on dialysis can have an enhanced hyperkalemic response to labetalol, which is partly attributable to electrochemical disturbances in the cells, characterized by an increase in intracellular sodium and chloride and a fall in intracellular potassium.

Liver

Eleven cases of hepatotoxicity have been reported with labetalol (9). Acute hepatitis has been described in an East-Asian man (10).

- A 50-year-old man with chronic hepatitis B infection, a hemiparesis due to a hemorrhage in the left basal ganglia, and a high systolic blood pressure was given intermittent intravenous labetalol followed by oral therapy (200 mg bd). After 1 week, his aspartate transaminase, alanine transaminase, and bilirubin started to rise. Ultrasonography of the liver and gallbladder was normal. Labetalol was withdrawn, and all the liver function tests normalized within a few days.

Prior hepatitis B infection may have predisposed this patient to labetalol-induced liver toxicity.

Musculoskeletal

Two children developed a proximal myopathy and rhabdomyolysis, which resolved on withdrawal of labetalol (11).

Immunologic

Antinuclear and antimitochondrial antibodies develop not uncommonly during long-term administration of labetalol (12).

Second-Generation Effects

Fetotoxicity

Labetalol has a high transplacental transfer rate.

- A single intravenous dose of labetalol 30 mg given to a woman with severe pregnancy-related hypertension 20 minutes before cesarean section was associated with significant neonatal beta-adrenoceptor blockade (hypoglycemia, bradycardia, and hypotension), and there were high labetalol concentrations in the umbilical cord blood (150–180 ng/ml) (13).
- An infant was born dead to a woman given intravenous labetalol 50 mg, which lowered her blood pressure from 170/110 to 115/85 mmHg before surgery (14).

Oral labetalol is well tolerated in pre-eclampsia, but if intravenous treatment is necessary, a small dose (5–10 mg) should be used initially and titrated up as necessary.

References

1. Scowen E. Scalp tingling on labetalol. Lancet 1978;1:98.
2. Hua AS, Thomas GW, Kincaid-Smith P. Scalp tingling in patients on labetalol. Lancet 1977;2(8032):295.
3. Gabriel R. Circumoral paraesthesiae and labetalol. BMJ 1978;1(6112):580.
4. Chung PC, Li AH, Lin CC, Yang MW. Elevated vascular resistance after labetalol during resection of a pheochromocytoma (brief report). Can J Anaesth 2002;49(2):148–50.
5. Sala X, Monsalve C, Comas C, Botet F, Nalda MA. Paro cardiaco en neonato de madre tratada con labetalol. [Cardiac arrest in newborn of mother treated with labetalol.] Rev Esp Anestesiol Reanim 1993;40(3):146–7.
6. Arthur S, Greenberg A. Hyperkalemia associated with intravenous labetalol therapy for acute hypertension in renal transplant recipients. Clin Nephrol 1990;33(6):269–71.
7. Hamad A, Salameh M, Zihlif M, Feinfeld DA, Carvounis CP. Life-threatening hyperkalemia after intravenous labetolol injection for hypertensive emergency in a hemodialysis patient. Am J Nephrol 2001;21(3):241–4.
8. McCauley J, Murray J, Jordan M, Scantlebury V, Vivas C, Shapiro R. Labetalol-induced hyperkalemia in renal transplant recipients. Am J Nephrol 2002;22(4):347–51.
9. Clark JA, Zimmerman HJ, Tanner LA. Labetalol hepatotoxicity. Ann Intern Med 1990;113(3):210–13.
10. Marinella MA. Labetalol-induced hepatitis in a patient with chronic hepatitis B infection. J Clin Hypertens (Greenwich) 2002;4(2):120–1.
11. Willis JK, Tilton AH, Harkin JC, Boineau FG. Reversible myopathy due to labetalol. Pediatr Neurol 1990;6(4):275–6.
12. Kanto JH. Current status of labetalol, the first alpha- and beta-blocking agent. Int J Clin Pharmacol Ther Toxicol 1985;23(11):617–28.
13. Klarr JM, Bhatt-Mehta V, Donn SM. Neonatal adrenergic blockade following single dose maternal labetalol administration. Am J Perinatol 1994;11(2):91–3.
14. Olsen KS, Beier-Holgersen R. Fetal death following labetalol administration in pre-eclampsia. Acta Obstet Gynecol Scand 1992;71(2):145–7.

Lamiaceae

See also Herbal medicines

General Information

The genera in the family of Lamiaceae (Table 1) include basil, catnip, germander, lavender, mints, origanum, rosemary, sage, skullcap, and thyme.

Hedeoma pulegoides and *Mentha pulegium*

The volatile oil of pennyroyal (prepared from *Hedeoma pulegoides* or *Mentha pulegium*) is a folk medicine used as an abortifacient. The doses that are required for this effect can cause serious symptoms, including vomiting, seizures, hallucinations, renal damage, hepatotoxicity and shock; deaths have also occurred (1,2).

Adverse effects

The hepatotoxicity of pulegone, the principal constituent of pennyroyal oil, has been demonstrated in animal studies and reported in humans (3).

Two cases of serious or fatal toxicity have been described in two infants who had been treated with herbal tea containing pennyroyal oil (4). One infant developed fulminant liver failure with cerebral edema and necrosis; the other infant developed hepatic dysfunction and a severe epileptic encephalopathy.

Lavandula angustifolia

The volatile oil of *Lavandula angustifolia* (lavender) contains linrayl acetate and linalool, and lavender also contains coumarins. It has been used in aromatherapy to treat insomnia and headaches, and may have small beneficial effects (5).

Adverse effects

Patch tests with lavender oil from 1990 to 1998 in Japan were positive in 3.7% of cases (6). In five of 11 positive cases in 1997 and eight of 15 positive cases in 1998, the patients had used dried lavender flowers in pillows, drawers, cabinets, or rooms.

- A 53-year-old patient with relapsing eczema had contact allergy to various essential oils used in aromatherapy (7). Sensitization was due to previous exposure to lavender, jasmine, and rosewood. Laurel, eucalyptus, and pomerance also produced positive tests, without previous exposure.

Contact dermatitis has been attributed to a lavender oil pillow (8), and to lavender in an analgesic gel (9).

Mentha piperita

The oil of *Mentha piperita* (peppermint) contains cineol, limonene, menthofuran, menthol, and menthone. It has been used as a carminative and antispasmodic for esophageal spasm and irritable bowel syndrome (10).

Adverse effects

Contact dermatitis has been attributed to menthol in peppermint (11).

Salvia species

In China, the root of *Salvia miltiorrhiza* (danshen) has been used traditionally for the treatment of coronary diseases.

The leaf of *Salvia officinalis* (sage) contains 1.0–2.5% of essential oil, consisting of 35–60% of thujone.

Adverse effects

A patient taking warfarin and who had taken a decoction of *S. miltiorrhiza* presented with a prolonged bleeding time and melena (12) and other cases have been reported (13). Pharmacodynamic and pharmacokinetic studies in rats have shown that danshen increases the absorption rate constant, AUC, C_{max}, and half-lives of both *R*- and *S*-warfarin, and reduces their clearances and apparent volumes of distribution (14,15).

Thujone can cause toxicity when the herb is taken in overdose (more than 15 g per dose) or for a prolonged period. Pregnancy is listed as a contraindication to the use of the essential oil or alcoholic extracts of *S. officinalis*.

Table 1 The genera of Lamiaceae

Acanthomintha (thorn-mint)
Acinos (acinos)
Agastach (giant hyssop)
Ajuga (bugle)
Ballota (horehound)
Blephilia (pagoda-plant)
Brazoria (brazos-mint)
Calamintha (calamint)
Cedronella (cedronella)
Chaiturus (lion's tail)
Clinopodium (clinopodium)
Coleus (coleus)
Collinsonia (horsebalm)
Conradina (false rosemary)
Cunila (cunila)
Dicerandra (balm)
Dracocephalum (dragonhead)
Elsholtzia (elsholtzia)
Erythrochlamys (erythrochlamys)
Galeopsis (hemp nettle)
Glechoma (glechoma)
Haplostachys (haplostachys)
Hedeoma (false pennyroyal)
Hyptis (bushmint)
Hyssopus (hyssop)
Isanthus (fluxweed)
Lallemantia (lallemantia)
Lamiastrum (lamiastrum)
Lamium (dead nettle)
Lavandula (lavender)
Leonotis (lion's ear)
Leonurus (motherwort)
Lepechinia (pitchersage)
Leucas (leucas)
Lycopus (waterhorehound)
Macbridea (macridea)
Marrubium (horehound)
Marsypianthes (marsypianthes)
Meehania (meehania)
Melissa (balm)
Mentha (mint)
Moluccella (moluccella)
Monarda (beebalm)
Monardella (monardella)
Mosla (mosla)
Nepeta (catnip)
Ocimum (basil)
Origanum (origanum)
Orthosiphon (orthosiphon)
Perilla (perilla)
Perovskia (perovskia)
Phlomis (Jerusalem sage)
Phyllostegia (phyllostegia)
Physostegia (lion's heart)
Piloblephis (piloblephis)
Plectranthus (plectranthus)
Pogogyne (mesamint)
Pogostemon (pogostemon)
Poliomintha (rosemary mint)
Prunella (self heal)
Pycnanthemum (mountain mint)
Rhododon (sand mint)
Rosmarinus (rosemary)
Salazaria (bladder sage)
Salvia (sage)
Satureja (savory)
Scutellaria (skullcap)
Sideritis (ironwort)
Solenostemon (solenostemon)
Stachys (hedge nettle)
Stachydeoma (mock pennyroyal)
Stenogyne (stenogyne)
Synandra (synandra)
Teucrium (germander)
Thymus (thyme)
Trichostema (bluecurls)
Warnockia (brazos mint)

Scutellaria species

The *Scutellaria* species (skullcap) include over 40 members, which contain a variety of flavonoids and terpenoids, the latter including scutellariosides and smithiandienol. Some also contain pyrrolizidine alkaloids (see separate monograph), which have repeatedly been implicated in veno-occlusive disease of the liver.

Adverse effects

Although Western skullcap formulations are supposed to come from *Scutellaria lateriflora*, it is unclear whether it is responsible for the liver damage that has been associated with skullcap. In the UK, the American germander (*Teucrium canadense*) has been widely used to replace *S. lateriflora* in commercial skullcap materials and products. In one UK case of skullcap-associated hepatotoxicity, the material was found to come from *T. canadense*. This raises the possibility that other cases of skullcap toxicity may also have involved *Teucrium* rather than *Scutellaria* (16).

Respiratory

- A 53-year-old Japanese man, who had taken skullcap intermittently for hemorrhoids, developed recurrent interstitial pneumonitis (17). Re-challenge, after he had stopped taking the herbal remedy and had become symptom free, resulted in a high fever and signs and symptoms of interstitial pneumonitis. Transbronchial lung biopsy showed lymphocytic alveolitis with eosinophilic infiltration. The symptoms subsided again after withdrawal.

Liver

Skullcap has repeatedly been associated with hepatotoxicity, and veno-occlusive disease has been reported (18).

- A 28-year-old man presented with jaundice after taking six tablets of skullcap (together with zinc and pau d'arco) daily for the previous 6 months to help his multiple sclerosis. His liver enzymes were raised and hepatitis A, B, and C serologies were negative. He developed progressive liver failure and received a transplant but died shortly after. His explanted liver showed fibrous stenosis and obliteration of most of the terminal venules with extensive perivenular fibrosis, indicative of veno-occlusive disease.

Teucrium species

Teucrium species (germander) contain a variety of iridoids, monoterpenoids, diterpenoids, and sesquiterpenoids.

Adverse effects

The hepatotoxicity of germander has been well documented. An animal study suggests that the hepatotoxicity resides in one or more reactive metabolites of its furanoditerpenoids (19).

In France, many cases of hepatitis have been associated with the normal use of *Teucrium chamaedrys* (wall germander). The frequency of this adverse effect has been estimated at one case in about 4000 months of treatment (20). Two cases of hepatitis in women who had been taking germander daily for 6 months have been reported from Canada (21). Although most cases are not serious, deaths have been reported (22), and progression to liver cirrhosis has also been described (23).

Seven patients developed hepatitis after taking *T. chamaedrys* and had no other cause of liver damage (24). The hepatitis was characterized by jaundice and a marked increase in serum transaminases 3–18 weeks after taking germander. Liver biopsies in three patients showed hepatic necrosis. After withdrawal of germander the jaundice disappeared within 8 weeks and recovery was complete in 1.5–6 months. In three cases, germander was followed by prompt recurrence of hepatitis.

- A 62-year-old man had taken a tea made from *T. capitatum* for 4 months when he developed anorexia, nausea, and malaise (25). He also noted dark urine and jaundice. He was admitted to hospital with acute icteric hepatitis. A liver biopsy showed bridging necrosis, inflammatory infiltration, and bile emboli. After withdrawal of the herbal tea he made a full recovery within 3 months.

Several other cases have been reported (26–30).

References

1. Ciganda C, Laborde A. Herbal infusions used for induced abortion. J Toxicol Clin Toxicol 2003;41(3):235–9.
2. Anderson IB, Mullen WH, Meeker JE, Khojasteh-Bakht SC, Oishi S, Nelson SD, Blanc PD. Pennyroyal toxicity: measurement of toxic metabolite levels in two cases and review of the literature. Ann Intern Med 1996;124(8):726–34.
3. Sullivan JB Jr, Rumack BH, Thomas H Jr, Peterson RG, Bryson P. Pennyroyal oil poisoning and hepatotoxicity. JAMA 1979;242(26):2873–4.
4. Bakerink JA, Gospe SM Jr, Dimand RJ, Eldridge MW. Multiple organ failure after ingestion of pennyroyal oil from herbal tea in two infants. Pediatrics 1996;98(5):944–7.
5. Hardy M, Kirk-Smith MD, Stretch DD. Replacement of drug treatment for insomnia by ambient odour. Lancet 1995;346(8976):701.
6. Sugiura M, Hayakawa R, Kato Y, Sugiura K, Hashimoto R. Results of patch testing with lavender oil in Japan. Contact Dermatitis 2000;43(3):157–60.
7. Schaller M, Korting HC. Allergic airborne contact dermatitis from essential oils used in aromatherapy. Clin Exp Dermatol 1995;20(2):143–5.
8. Coulson IH, Khan AS. Facial "pillow" dermatitis due to lavender oil allergy. Contact Dermatitis 1999;41(2):111.
9. Rademaker M. Allergic contact dermatitis from lavender fragrance in Difflam gel. Contact Dermatitis 1994;31(1):58–9.
10. Pittler MH, Ernst E. Peppermint oil for irritable bowel syndrome: a critical review and metaanalysis. Am J Gastroenterol 1998;93(7):1131–5.
11. Wilkinson SM, Beck MH. Allergic contact dermatitis from menthol in peppermint. Contact Dermatitis 1994;30(1):42–3.
12. Tam LS, Chan TY, Leung WK, Critchley JA. Warfarin interactions with Chinese traditional medicines: danshen and methyl salicylate medicated oil. Aust NZ J Med 1995;25(3):258.
13. Chan TY. Interaction between warfarin and danshen (*Salvia miltiorrhiza*). Ann Pharmacother 2001;35(4):501–4.
14. Chan K, Lo AC, Yeung JH, Woo KS. The effects of Danshen (*Salvia miltiorrhiza*) on warfarin pharmacodynamics and pharmacokinetics of warfarin enantiomers in rats. J Pharm Pharmacol 1995;47(5):402–6.
15. Lo AC, Chan K, Yeung JH, Woo KS. The effects of danshen (*Salvia miltiorrhiza*) on pharmacokinetics and pharmacodynamics of warfarin in rats. Eur J Drug Metab Pharmacokinet 1992;17(4):257–62.
16. De Smet PA. Health risks of herbal remedies. Drug Saf 1995;13(2):81–93.
17. Takeshita K, Saisho Y, Kitamura K, Kaburagi N, Funabiki T, Inamura T, Oyamada Y, Asano K, Yamaguchi K. Pneumonitis induced by ou-gon (scullcap). Intern Med 2001;40(8):764–8.
18. Akatsu T, Santo RM, Nakayasu K, Kanai A. Oriental herbal medicine induced epithelial keratopathy. Br J Ophthalmol 2000;84(8):934.
19. Loeper J, Descatoire V, Letteron P, Moulis C, Degott C, Dansette P, Fau D, Pessayre D. Hepatotoxicity of germander in mice. Gastroenterology 1994;106(2):464–72.
20. Castot A, Larrey D. Hépatites observées au cours d'un traitement par un médicament ou une tisane contenant de la germandrée petit-chêne. Bilan des 26 cas rapportés aux Centres Régionaux de Pharmacovigilance. [Hepatitis observed during a treatment with a drug or tea containing wild germander. Evaluation of 26 cases reported to the Regional Centers of Pharmacovigilance.] Gastroenterol Clin Biol 1992;16(12):916–22.
21. Laliberte L, Villeneuve JP. Hepatitis after the use of germander, a herbal remedy. CMAJ 1996;154(11):1689–92.
22. Mostefa-Kara N, Pauwels A, Pines E, Biour M, Levy VG. Fatal hepatitis after herbal tea. Lancet 1992;340(8820):674.
23. Dao T, Peytier A, Galateau F, Valla A. Hépatite chronique cirrhogène à la germandrée petit-chêne. [Chronic cirrhogenic hepatitis induced by germander.] Gastroenterol Clin Biol 1993;17(8–9):609–10.
24. Larrey D, Vial T, Pauwels A, Castot A, Biour M, David M, Michel H. Hepatitis after germander (*Teucrium chamaedrys*) administration: another instance of herbal medicine hepatotoxicity. Ann Intern Med 1992;117(2):129–32.
25. Dourakis SP, Papanikolaou IS, Tzemanakis EN, Hadziyannis SJ. Acute hepatitis associated with herb (*Teucrium capitatum L.*) administration. Eur J Gastroenterol Hepatol 2002;14(6):693–5.
26. Mazokopakis E, Lazaridou S, Tzardi M, Mixaki J, Diamantis I, Ganotakis E. Acute cholestatic hepatitis caused by *Teucrium polium* L. Phytomedicine 2004;11(1):83–4.
27. Polymeros D, Kamberoglou D, Tzias V. Acute cholestatic hepatitis caused by *Teucrium polium* (golden germander) with transient appearance of antimitochondrial antibody. J Clin Gastroenterol 2002;34(1):100–1.
28. Perez Alvarez J, Saez-Royuela F, Gento Pena E, Lopez Morante A, Velasco Oses A, Martin Lorente J. Hepatitis aguda por ingestion de infusiones con *Teucrium chamaedrys*. [Acute hepatitis due to ingestion of

Teucrium chamaedrys infusions.] Gastroenterol Hepatol 2001;24(5):240–3.
29. Mattei A, Rucay P, Samuel D, Feray C, Reynes M, Bismuth H. Liver transplantation for severe acute liver failure after herbal medicine (*Teucrium polium*) administration. J Hepatol 1995;22(5):597.
30. Pauwels A, Thierman-Duffaud D, Azanowsky JM, Loiseau D, Biour M, Levy VG. Hépatite aiguë a la germandrée petit-chêne. Hepatotoxicite d'une plante medicinale. Deux observations. [Acute hepatitis caused by wild germander. Hepatotoxicity of herbal remedies. Two cases.] Gastroenterol Clin Biol 1992;16(1):92–5.

Lamivudine

See also Nucleoside analogue reverse transcriptase inhibitors (NRTIs)

General Information

Lamivudine (3TC) is a nucleoside analogue reverse transcriptase inhibitor that has been widely used against HIV infection which also has antiviral effects against hepatitis B (1).

Observational studies

In a 24-week phase I/II study, 89 children aged 3 months to 17 years (median 7.3 years) were treated with lamivudine for 24 weeks in dosages of 1–20 mg/kg/day (2). Dosages over 20 mg/kg/day were not tested because of reported neutropenia in adults at this dosage (3). Lamivudine was generally well tolerated in these children. Ten children were withdrawn because of presumed adverse effects: three because of increased serum transaminase activities, three because of neutropenia, and two because of hyperactivity. One child became ataxic shortly after the start of therapy, and one developed pancreatitis during hospitalization for acute cryptosporidiosis. All of these events resolved with supportive care on withdrawal of lamivudine, except one case of hepatitis, which persisted up to 10 months after withdrawal. Treatment was discontinued temporarily in other patients because of pancreatitis ($n = 2$), rashes ($n = 2$), neutropenia ($n = 1$), anemia ($n = 1$), and increased serum transaminase activities ($n = 1$). On resolution of the presumed adverse reaction, the drug was reintroduced in all of these cases without further problems. There were no significant hematological or biochemical changes. Neither the incidence nor the severity of the observed adverse events was dose-related. The assignment of causality to lamivudine of most of the adverse events was complicated by intercurrent conditions and concomitant medications.

In a study of the efficacy of lamivudine (25, 100, or 300 mg/day for 12 weeks) in the treatment of chronic hepatitis B virus infections, lamivudine was similarly well tolerated in 32 patients (4). Only minor non-specific non-dose-related adverse reactions were observed. In addition, there were mild asymptomatic increases in serum activities of amylase, lipase, and creatine kinase, which in most cases resolved despite continued therapy.

Comparative studies

The safety and efficacy of lamivudine (300–600 mg/day) in combination with zidovudine (600 mg/day) in the treatment of antiretroviral-naive and zidovudine-experienced HIV-infected persons has been compared with zidovudine monotherapy in two placebo-controlled studies of 129 and 223 patients (5,6). There were no significant differences in the incidence or severity of adverse effects between patients taking zidovudine alone or in combination with lamivudine. In both studies gastrointestinal symptoms, notably nausea, were the most commonly observed adverse reactions, occurring in 5–11% of zidovudine-experienced patients and 23–29% of antiretroviral drug-naive individuals. Although one antiretroviral drug-naive patient taking combined therapy had an asymptomatic rise in pancreatic amylase activity, acute pancreatitis was not observed in either study. Grade 1 peripheral neuropathy was reported in one zidovudine-experienced patient taking low-dosage lamivudine (150 mg bd) and zidovudine.

Organs and Systems

Hematologic

A case report has provided strong evidence that lamivudine can on rare occasions cause severe anemia; the mechanism is unclear (7).

Gastrointestinal

In a 1-year trial of lamivudine in 10 children with vertically acquired chronic hepatitis B, lamivudine made serum hepatitis B viral DNA undetectable in all the patients within 24 weeks (8). Serum alanine transaminase activity returned to the reference range within 36 weeks. Although nausea and vomiting were reported in one child, it was not necessary to withhold treatment.

Liver

Lamivudine is used orally to treat chronic hepatitis B in adults and children (9). It increases the rate of loss of hepatitis B e antigen and seroconversion in compensated chronic carriers, with improvement of histology at a similar rate to interferon alfa. However, the tyrosine-methionine-aspartate-aspartate (YMDD) mutation prevents efficacy and can cause flares of hepatitis. The indications for treatment must therefore be established with care and only by those who have expert knowledge of the disease, the drug, and the YMDD mutation.

Nails

Paronychia has been reported in 12 HIV-infected patients who had taken lamivudine only for 3 months before the onset of symptoms (10). Microbiological investigations for fungi or bacteria were negative. All were treated with topical antiseptics; surgical procedures were performed in four. Five patients healed without recurrence, while the paronychia recurred in six. There was no mention of withdrawal of lamivudine. The causative role of lamivudine in the development of paronychia in these patients remains obscure.

Long-Term Effects

Drug tolerance

The incidence of viral resistance to lamivudine increases with the duration of therapy in patients with chronic hepatitis B (11). However, the effect of viral resistance on hepatic synthetic function has not been well defined. In 38 patients (26 with cirrhosis) in an open study there was an initial antiviral response in all patients (hepatitis B virus DNA became undetectable by a hybridization assay), and nine of 22 (41%) hepatitis B e antigen-positive patients underwent hepatitis B e antigen seroconversion. In 29 patients with undetectable serum hepatitis B viral DNA at the end of the study, the mean serum albumin concentration rose from 40 to 43 g/l, corresponding to a yearly increase of 1.85 g/l; this was largely attributable to an increase in the cirrhotic patients. Resistance to lamivudine developed in nine patients. Suppression of viral replication by lamivudine improves hepatic synthetic function in chronic hepatitis B patients, but emergence of drug resistance is associated with a rapid fall in serum albumin.

References

1. Jarvis B, Faulds D. Lamivudine. A review of its therapeutic potential in chronic hepatitis B. Drugs 1999;58(1):101–41.
2. Lewis LL, Venzon D, Church J, Farley M, Wheeler S, Keller A, Rubin M, Yuen G, Mueller B, Sloas M, Wood L, Balis F, Shearer GM, Brouwers P, Goldsmith J, Pizzo PA. Lamivudine in children with human immunodeficiency virus infection: a phase I/II study. The National Cancer Institute Pediatric Branch–Human Immunodeficiency Virus Working Group. J Infect Dis 1996;174(1):16–25.
3. McLean TW, Kurth S, Gee B. Pelvic osteomyelitis in a sickle-cell patient receiving deferoxamine. Am J Hematol 1996;53(4):284–5.
4. Dienstag JL, Perrillo RP, Schiff ER, Bartholomew M, Vicary C, Rubin M. A preliminary trial of lamivudine for chronic hepatitis B infection. N Engl J Med 1995;333(25):1657–61.
5. Katlama C, Ingrand D, Loveday C, Clumeck N, Mallolas J, Staszewski S, Johnson M, Hill AM, Pearce G, McDade H. Safety and efficacy of lamivudine–zidovudine combination therapy in antiretroviral-naive patients. A randomized controlled comparison with zidovudine monotherapy. Lamivudine European HIV Working Group. JAMA 1996;276(2):118–25.
6. Staszewski S, Loveday C, Picazo JJ, Dellarnonica P, Skinhoj P, Johnson MA, Danner SA, Harrigan PR, Hill AM, Verity L, McDade H. Safety and efficacy of lamivudine–zidovudine combination therapy in zidovudine-experienced patients. A randomized controlled comparison with zidovudine monotherapy. Lamivudine European HIV Working Group. JAMA 1996;276(2):111–17.
7. Weitzel T, Plettenberg A, Albrecht D, Lorenzen T, Stoehr A. Severe anemia as a newly recognized side-effect caused by lamivudine. AIDS 1999;13(16):2309–11.
8. Zuccotti GV, Cucchi C, Gracchi V, D'Auria E, Riva E, Tagger A. A 1-year trial of lamivudine for chronic hepatitis B in children. J Int Med Res 2002;30(2):200–2.
9. Sokal E. Lamivudine for the treatment of chronic hepatitis B. Expert Opin Pharmacother 2002;3(3):329–39.
10. Zerboni R, Angius AG, Cusini M, Tarantini G, Carminati G. Lamivudine-induced paronychia. Lancet 1998;351(9111):1256.
11. Hui JM, George J, Liddle C, Lin R, Samarasinghe D, Crewe E, Farrell GC. Changes in serum albumin during treatment of chronic hepatitis B with lamivudine: effects of response and emergence of drug resistance. Am J Gastroenterol 2002;97(4):1003–9.

Lamotrigine

See also Antiepileptic drugs

General Information

Lamotrigine is widely used in the management of partial and generalized seizures. It has a favorable tolerability profile, even though neurological adverse effects and hypersensitivity reactions are sometimes troublesome. Its pharmacology, clinical pharmacology, adverse effects, and interactions have been reviewed (1). Its adverse events are primarily neurological, gastrointestinal, and dermatological and are typically mild or moderate and transient, with the exception of a potentially serious rash. Maculopapular or erythematous skin rashes occur in about 12% of children and are the most common reason for withdrawal. More severe forms of rash, including Stevens–Johnson syndrome, occur occasionally, with a three-fold higher incidence in children (about 1%) than adults (about 0.3).

Observational studies

Among 11 316 patients in a postmarketing surveillance study that included 3994 patients followed for 6 months or longer, the main events leading to drug withdrawal were rash ($n = 210$), drowsiness ($n = 74$), nausea ($n = 66$), dizziness ($n = 63$), headache ($n = 61$), vomiting ($n = 33$), ataxia ($n = 32$), malaise ($n = 29$), and aggression ($n = 26$). Rare serious adverse events included Stevens–Johnson syndrome in 12 cases, neutropenia in 4, thrombocytopenia in 3, and disseminated intravascular coagulation in 2. Leukopenia, a meningitic reaction, acute renal insufficiency, hepatotoxicity, and a lupus-like reaction occurred in one patient each (2).

In an open study, there were adverse events (details not given) in two of 30 patients with serum lamotrigine concentrations between 16 and 39 μmol/l, and in 5 of 11 patients with serum concentrations between 39 and 86 μmol/l (3). This is one of the few studies to have provided preliminary evidence for a relation between serum lamotrigine concentrations and the risk of adverse effects.

The efficacy of lamotrigine as monotherapy has been studied retrospectively in 83 children (mean age 8.7 years) with focal epilepsy ($n = 43$), generalized epilepsy ($n = 32$), or not classified ($n = 8$) (4). The median follow-up period was

8 months (mean = 8.5). Rash was the most common adverse effect, in five patients; two patients discontinued treatment. There were no cases of Stevens–Johnson syndrome.

Lamotrigine has been used as maintenance monotherapy for rapid-cycling bipolar disorder in 324 patients (open label) and 182 patients (double-blind) with rapid-cycling bipolar disorder (5). In all, 265 patients reported adverse events during the open phase. The most common adverse events (over 10%) were headache, infection, influenza, nausea, abnormal dreams, dizziness, and rash. During the double-blind phase 122 patients reported adverse events, equally with lamotrigine and placebo.

In 44 patients with profound mental retardation a retrospective assessment of adjunctive lamotrigine (272 mg/day) showed a significant reduction in seizure frequency from 10.1 to 5.8 seizures per month (6). There were no treatment-related changes in laboratory parameters, vital signs, or body weight, and no serious rashes. In three of five patients there was worsened self-injurious behavior, requiring drug withdrawal.

Lamotrigine has been studied in 32 children with epilepsy refractory for at least 1 year to other antiepileptic drugs (7). Adverse effects were uncommon, and there were no skin rashes.

The efficacy and safety of lamotrigine have been prospectively evaluated in 41 children and young adults (aged 3–25 years) with drug-resistant partial epilepsies (8). Lamotrigine withdrawal was mainly due to lack of efficacy (46%); only two patients developed a transient skin rash, which did not require withdrawal.

The adverse effects of lamotrigine have been surveyed retrospectively in 2701 patients in five tertiary referral epilepsy centers in the UK; 1326 were excluded because lamotrigine and/or comparators had been begun outside the study centers (9). The most common adverse events were rash (10%), dizziness, ataxia, and diplopia. There were four cases of life-threatening adverse events: one case each of hepatic insufficiency, acute exacerbation of ulcerative colitis, disseminated intravascular coagulation, and renal insufficiency caused by rhabdomyolysis and myoglobinuria. The mortality rate was 1.7 per 100 patient-years and the standard mortality ratio was 10.4, similar to other antiepileptic drugs (gabapentin and vigabatrin). No deaths were directly attributable to lamotrigine.

In an open randomized study in 417 patients over 2 years old who took lamotrigine or carbamazepine monotherapy for new-onset epilepsy there was similar efficacy (65% were free of seizures with lamotrigine and 73% with carbamazepine) (10). Although the patients taking lamotrigine tended to have fewer adverse events than those taking carbamazepine (52 versus 60%), the difference was not significant. Somnolence was the only adverse event reported at an incidence of over 5% and it was more frequent in patients taking carbamazepine (11 versus 4% with lamotrigine).

Comparative studies

In a 48-week, double-blind, monotherapy trial of 260 patients with newly diagnosed epilepsy, the proportion withdrawn because of adverse events was 11% in the lamotrigine group (9% with rash) and 21% in the carbamazepine group (13% with rash). Somnolence was more frequent with carbamazepine (22 versus 12%), but the incidence of other common complaints (headache, weakness, rash, nausea, dizziness) did not differ between groups (11). Although it was concluded that lamotrigine is tolerated better than carbamazepine, in this and other trials a design that involved twice-daily dosing may have placed carbamazepine at a disadvantage in the comparison.

In a multicenter, double-blind comparison of lamotrigine and phenytoin (titrated over 6 weeks from starting dosages of 100 and 200 mg/day respectively) in 181 patients with newly diagnosed epilepsy there were comparable seizure freedom rates and comparable trial discontinuation rates with the two drugs (12). Skin rashes leading to withdrawal occurred in 12% of patients assigned to lamotrigine and in 5% of those assigned to phenytoin, but the risk associated with lamotrigine might have been overestimated, owing to an excessively high starting dose. Central nervous system adverse effects were more common with phenytoin, the difference being statistically significant for weakness (29 versus 16%), somnolence (28 versus 7%), and ataxia (12 versus 0%).

A review of the manufacturer's safety database from the adult clinical trial program has been published (13). In placebo-controlled add-on trials involving a total of 1555 patients, the most common adverse events were dizziness (35 versus 15% on placebo), headache (26 versus 21%), diplopia (25 versus 6%), ataxia (20 versus 6%), nausea (19 versus 9%), blurred vision (14 versus 4%), rhinitis (11 versus 8%), somnolence (10 versus 7%), rashes (10 versus 5%), and vomiting (10 versus 5%). Dizziness and rashes led to withdrawal most commonly, each in 2% of patients. Dizziness, diplopia, nausea, blurred vision, and headache occurred more commonly in patients co-medicated with carbamazepine than in those co-medicated with other drugs. In randomized comparative monotherapy studies, somnolence, weakness, dizziness, and ataxia occurred less often with lamotrigine than with carbamazepine or phenytoin, whereas insomnia was slightly more frequent with lamotrigine. Withdrawals due to adverse events were fewer with lamotrigine than with the other drugs. Rash associated with lamotrigine typically occurred within the first 8 weeks. Exceeding the currently recommended slow dosage escalation guidelines and co-administration of valproate are risk factors for rashes. In adults, the incidence of Stevens–Johnson syndrome was approximately 1:1000, but higher rates (1 in 50 to 1 in 300) have been reported in children (SEDA-22, 89).

In a multicenter, double-blind, monotherapy trial in 150 elderly patients with newly diagnosed epilepsy (mean age 77 years) lamotrigine (median dosage 100 mg/day) was better tolerated than carbamazepine (400 mg/day) (14). The drop-out rate for adverse events was 18% with lamotrigine compared with 42% with carbamazepine. Patients taking lamotrigine had a lower incidence of skin rashes (3 versus 19%), somnolence (12 versus 29%), and dizziness (10 versus 17%). Lamotrigine may be a better choice for initial treatment in elderly people, although the toxicity of carbamazepine might have been overestimated by giving a non-modified-release formulation twice daily. Seizure control was comparable with the two drugs, but statistical power was insufficient to demonstrate equal efficacy.

In 126 patients with carbamazepine-resistant or valproate-resistant epilepsy given lamotrigine, 50% during add-on therapy and 53% during lamotrigine monotherapy had at least 50% reduction in total seizures (15). There were adverse events in 49 patients, including respiratory tract infections ($n = 11$), dizziness ($n = 8$), headache ($n = 7$), diplopia ($n = 5$), tremor ($n = 5$), somnolence ($n = 4$), insomnia ($n = 4$), nausea ($n = 4$), and weakness ($n = 3$). Treatment was discontinued in nine patients because of adverse events, in five cases because of rash.

Cognitive adverse effects of lamotrigine and valproate have been compared in a double-blind, randomized, placebo-controlled study in 30 healthy volunteers who took lamotrigine 50 mg, valproic acid 900 mg, or placebo for 12 days (16). Lamotrigine had a relatively good cognitive profile but no different from that of valproic acid at the doses tested. Lamotrigine was associated with a selective general psychostimulant effect. As this study was performed in healthy volunteers taking a low dose, and conducted over a very short time, its conclusions are not generalizable to patients with epilepsy taking long-term treatment.

In a double-blind comparison of gabapentin and lamotrigine in 309 patients with new-onset partial or generalized seizures, the target doses were gabapentin 1800 mg/day and lamotrigine 150 mg/day (17). Severe adverse events were reported in 11% of patients taking gabapentin and 9.3% of patients taking lamotrigine. Two patients had serious adverse events thought to be related to the study drug; one took an overdose of gabapentin and the other had convulsions with lamotrigine. The most frequent treatment-related adverse events in both treatment groups were dizziness, weakness, and headache; 11% of patients taking gabapentin and 15% of those taking lamotrigine withdrew because of adverse events. There was an increase of over 7% in body weight from baseline in 14% of the patients taking gabapentin and 6.6% of those taking lamotrigine. There were benign skin rashes in 4.4% of those taking gabapentin and 11% of those taking lamotrigine.

Placebo-controlled studies

Lamotrigine has been used as maintenance monotherapy for rapid-cycling bipolar disorder in 324 patients (open label) and 182 patients (double-blind) with rapid-cycling bipolar disorder (5). In all, 265 patients reported adverse events during the open phase. The most common adverse events (over 10%) were headache, infection, influenza, nausea, abnormal dreams, dizziness, and rash. During the double-blind phase 122 patients reported adverse events, equally with lamotrigine and placebo.

The analgesic efficacy of lamotrigine in painful HIV-associated distal sensory polyneuropathy has been studied, given anecdotal reports of its efficacy, in a randomized, double-blind, placebo-controlled study (18). Of 42 subjects, 13 did not complete the 14-week study. Of those who took lamotrigine five dropped out because of rashes and one because of a gastrointestinal infection. The rashes were mild or moderate morbilliform rashes and resolved after withdrawal.

Organs and Systems

Nervous system

The most common adverse effects of lamotrigine include dizziness, weakness, headache, diplopia, ataxia, blurred vision, and somnolence (SEDA-18, 65) (SEDA-20, 63) (19). These effects resemble those seen with carbamazepine and can result from an adverse pharmacodynamic interaction. Tolerability is better when lamotrigine is given as monotherapy or with drugs other than carbamazepine; however, tremor develops in some patients taking valproate in combinations (SEDA-18, 66). During monotherapy, serum lamotrigine concentrations associated with intolerable adverse effects (mostly headache, dizziness, and ataxia) were 0.4–18.5 μg/ml and overlapped widely with those tolerated in other patients (20).

Irritability and aggressive behavior occur occasionally, and mentally retarded patients are possibly at greater risk (SEDA-22, 88). Rare central nervous system effects include insomnia, psychosis (SEDA-20, 63), downbeat nystagmus (SEDA-22, 89), movement disorders (SEDA-21, 72), and a Tourette-like syndrome. Lamotrigine can increase seizure frequency and severity in children with severe myoclonic epilepsy (SEDA-21, 72).

- A 47-year-old man developed a rash, fever, and rigors after taking lamotrigine (50 mg/day at maintenance) for 1 month (21). The reaction subsided after withdrawal, but 3 days later he complained of left shoulder pain and numbness in the left arm. The pain worsened over the next 3 weeks and then subsided. Thereafter, he developed weakness of the left arm with muscle wasting and signs of denervation in the biceps, infraspinatus, and supraspinatus. The condition was diagnosed as neuralgic amyotrophy. Almost complete recovery occurred over 8 months.

It is possible that the initial hypersensitivity reaction in this case determined focal neuronal involvement at the brachial plexus.

Worsening seizures

In a multicenter study, lamotrigine aggravated seizures in children with severe myoclonic epilepsy (22). Of 21 patients with severe myoclonic epilepsy given lamotrigine in dosages of 2.5–12.5 mg/kg/day, seizures were worsened in 17. The frequency of convulsive seizures increased by more than 50% in eight of 20 patients and myoclonic seizures worsened in six of 18. Of five patients who improved in at least one seizure type, four had concomitant worsening of more incapacitating seizures. The drug was withdrawn in 19 patients, with consequent improvement in 18. These findings suggest that lamotrigine is inappropriate in severe myoclonic epilepsy.

Paradoxical seizure aggravation may occur in other types of epilepsy.

- In a 5-year-old girl with benign rolandic epilepsy, the addition of lamotrigine (0.5–5 mg/kg/day) to valproate resulted in a temporary reduction in seizure frequency (23). However, her school performance deteriorated insidiously, with poor memory and concentration, clumsiness, stuttering, and emotional lability. After 4 months she developed new daily brief absence-like episodes, with staring, dropping of the head and jaw, and flickering of the eyelids, without loss of consciousness. Ictal electroencephalography showed anterior-predominant 3 Hz sharp slow wave complexes. Withdrawal of lamotrigine resulted in rapid improvement of cognitive function and gradual remission of the new attacks.

- A 9-year-old girl with Lennox–Gastaut syndrome, who had initially had an improvement in seizure frequency, insidiously developed myoclonic status epilepticus after the lamotrigine dosage was increased from 15 to 20 mg/kg (24). Withdrawal of lamotrigine resulted in rapid disappearance of status.
- Two patients (age unspecified) with severe epileptic encephalopathy who had improved on lamotrigine in combination with valproate developed continuous myoclonic jerks after 2–3 years; these were ascribed to high serum concentrations of lamotrigine (65 and 69 μmol/l) (25).

In the last report, the causative role of the drug is difficult to assess, because no mention was made of whether myoclonus regressed after reducing the dosage.

Sleep disorders

Insomnia is a recognized adverse effect of lamotrigine. Among 109 patients treated with lamotrigine in an adult tertiary referral center, 7 had insomnia of sufficient severity to require a change of therapy (26). The symptom occurred shortly after the start of treatment, was dose-dependent, and resolved after withdrawal or dosage reduction. Unlike previous reports, in which insomnia occurred in patients with impaired cognition, no predisposing factor could be identified.

In another report, two boys aged 6 and 8 years developed severe difficulties in falling asleep and fragmented sleep (in one case associated with scary dreams) after being stabilized on lamotrigine, 8 mg/kg (27). These disturbances improved when the dosage was reduced.

Tics

Tics are a rare adverse effect of lamotrigine.

- Three boys and two girls (mean age 7 years) developed simple motor tics (associated with verbal tics in two cases) within 10 months of starting lamotrigine (maintenance dosage 4–18 mg/kg) (28). When lamotrigine was withdrawn, the tics resolved within 3 months in three cases (with recurrence after rechallenge in one child) and improved in one. In the fifth child, improvement occurred despite continuation of treatment. Two of the affected patients had acquired epileptic aphasia syndrome, one had expressive and receptive language dysfunction, one had a static encephalopathy, and one had no mental or neurological impairment.

These data suggest that children with severe language dysfunction may be at increased risk of developing lamotrigine-induced tics.

- A 51-year-old man developed blepharospasm 4 months after starting lamotrigine, while taking a maintenance dosage of 500 mg/day (29). The condition cleared 4 weeks after withdrawal.
- Lamotrigine (250–324 mg/day) caused Tourette syndrome in three children aged 7, 8, and 12 years; in the 12-year-old boy, the syndrome was accompanied by behavioral abnormalities suggestive of obsessive-compulsive disorder (30). All the symptoms disappeared when the dosage was reduced to 175–225 mg/day and recurred on rechallenge with higher dosages.
- Two young men (aged 18 and 22 years) with epilepsy had disabling myoclonic jerks after taking lamotrigine after 2–3 years of therapy when their plasma lamotrigine concentrations rose to about 70 μmol/l (31).
- A retrospective survey yielded five cases of tics in three men and two women aged 2.5–12 years) within the first 10 months of therapy (4–17 mg/kg/day) (32). Four had simple motor tics and one had mostly vocal tics (gasping sounds) with normal laryngoscopic evaluation. In three cases the tics resolved completely within 1 month of drug withdrawal and recurred in two after reintroduction. A fourth had gradual improvement over 4 months after withdrawal; in the fifth, simple motor tics improved spontaneously with a reduction in dose.

Psychological, psychiatric

The cognitive and behavioral effects of lamotrigine 150 mg/day have been compared with those of carbamazepine 696 mg/day in 25 healthy adults in a double-blind, crossover, randomized study with two 10-week treatment periods (33). Lamotrigine had significantly fewer cognitive and behavioral adverse effects than carbamazepine, and 48% of the variables favored lamotrigine. The differences encompassed cognitive speed, memory, graphomotor coding, neurotoxic symptoms, mood, sedation, perception of cognitive performance, and other quality-of-life perceptions. The cognitive and behavioral changes favored lamotrigine over carbamazepine, but the magnitude of the observed effects was modest, although it could be relevant in some patients.

Endocrine

In two children with cranial diabetes insipidus, desmopressin requirements fell while they were taking lamotrigine (34). Lamotrigine may act at voltage-sensitive sodium channels and reduce calcium conductance. Both of these mechanisms of action are shared by carbamazepine, which can cause hyponatremia secondary to inappropriate secretion of antidiuretic hormone.

Metabolism

In a prospective evaluation of the effect of lamotrigine 3.5–14.2 mg/kg on growth in 103 children and adolescents aged 1.6–16 years with epilepsy treated with lamotrigine monotherapy for 6–71 months, the children had normal growth, although the study had several methodological shortcomings (35).

Hematologic

Aplastic anemia occurred in one patient who had recovered 7 years earlier from bone-marrow aplasia ascribed to carbamazepine (SEDA-20, 63). Severe pure red cell aplasia in a patient with heterozygous beta-thalassemia reversed rapidly after lamotrigine withdrawal; however, lamotrigine did not affect hematology parameters in another patient with the same condition (SEDA-20, 64). In two other cases of anemia associated with increased platelet counts the role of lamotrigine could not be ascertained (SEDA-22, 89).

There have been a few reports of leukopenia or neutropenia, and one case of septic shock secondary to leukopenia possibly due to lamotrigine (SEDA-20, 64).

- An 11-year-old girl with congenital left renal agenesis, epilepsy from cortical dysgenesis, and chronic hepatitis B and C, developed a skin rash and agranulocytosis (white cell count 3.1×10^9/l, lymphocytes 92%, and monocytes 8%) 15–20 days after starting to take lamotrigine (36). She recovered rapidly after drug withdrawal.

An inappropriately high starting dose (50 mg/day) may have contributed to this reaction.

Lamotrigine has been associated with agranulocytosis (37).

- A 59-year-old woman, with seizures after resection of a low-grade glioma, chemotherapy, and radiotherapy 2 years before, took lamotrigine 300 mg/day for 9 weeks and developed an agranulocytosis. The lamotrigine serum concentration was 2.2 μg/ml (usual target range 1–15 μg/ml). A bone marrow biopsy showed a hypocellular marrow with reduced myelopoiesis, a shift to the left, and normal cytogenetics. Over the next few days she developed a fever but no infection. She recovered after 10 days, having been given granulocyte-colony-stimulating factor and prophylactic antibiotics for 7 days.
- A 29-year-old woman with Blackfan–Diamond anemia developed an erythroblastopenic crisis after taking phenytoin on two separate occasions and then again after taking lamotrigine (38). The proposed mechanism was inhibition of dihydrofolate reductase, and the crisis responded to treatment with folinic acid. Lamotrigine was then continued without ill effect.
- Reversible agranulocytosis developed in a 30-year-old woman who had taken lamotrigine 100 mg/day for 6 weeks and valproate 250 mg/day for 2 weeks (39). Her white cell count fell from 6.7×10^9/l at 4 weeks to 2.6×10^9/l at 6 weeks and the absolute neutrophil count was 580×10^6/l. The white cell count recovered after withdrawal of lamotrigine; the valproate was continued.

Liver

Liver toxicity from lamotrigine is extremely rare. Acute hepatic necrosis occurred in the context of a hypersensitivity reaction that also involved the skin (SEDA-20, 64).

Four children developed reversible lamotrigine-associated hepatotoxicity (40). One had pre-existing encephalitis and the other three had multiple medical and neurological problems, fever and infections, were taking many other drugs, and had very frequent seizures; two had epilepsia partialis continua. The information given was insufficient to assess the role of lamotrigine in the pathogenesis of the hepatic dysfunction.

Reversible hepatotoxicity occurred in three children taking lamotrigine (41). In one there was severe hepatic failure. The liver abnormalities resolved after withdrawal.

Pancreas

Pancreatitis was reported in a 26-year-old man who had taken lamotrigine for 5 months, but cause and effect was dubious (SEDA-19, 61).

Skin

The rates of lamotrigine-related rash have been analysed from 12 multicenter studies of bipolar depression in 1955 patients taking open-label lamotrigine, 1198 taking lamotrigine in controlled studies, and 1056 taking placebo (42). In controlled studies, the rates of benign rash were 8.3% for lamotrigine and 6.4% for placebo. There were no serious rashes. In the open studies 13% ($n = 257$) had rashes with lamotrigine and one was reported as a mild form of Stevens–Johnson syndrome that did not require hospitalization. Thus, the risk of severe allergic rashes with lamotrigine is low, provided that there is a low initial dose and slow upward titration.

A rash, usually urticarial or maculopapular, is the most common event leading to early withdrawal of lamotrigine. In add-on trials, rashes occurred in up to 15% of patients and led to withdrawal in 2%. Six patients who developed a rash with lamotrigine later had similar rashes after exposure to structurally unrelated anticonvulsants, such as phenytoin and barbiturates (SEDA-22, 89). In 12 patients with probable Alzheimer's disease and seizures and 16 with other neurological disorders, lamotrigine caused three cases of mild rashes (43).

Published and unpublished cases of Stevens–Johnson syndrome ($n = 43$) and toxic epidermal necrolysis ($n = 14$) associated with lamotrigine have been reviewed (44). The patients with Stevens–Johnson syndrome were younger than those with toxic epidermal necrolysis (21 versus 31 years); the median time to onset for both reactions was 17 days; the median dosage at onset (50 mg for Stevens–Johnson syndrome, 87.5 mg for toxic epidermal necrolysis) did not differ significantly. Valproate co-medication was present in 74% and 64% of patients with Stevens–Johnson syndrome and toxic epidermal necrolysis respectively. In three patients, toxic epidermal necrolysis occurred in the context of the anticonvulsant hypersensitivity syndrome.

An expert panel has reviewed published and unpublished data on the incidence and risk factors for lamotrigine-induced rash (45). An allergic skin rash occurs in about 10% of patients, usually in the first 8 weeks. In clinical trials, the incidence of rashes leading to hospitalization, including those associated with hypersensitivity syndrome, was about 1:300 in adults (one third as Stevens–Johnson syndrome) and 1:100 in children (50% as Stevens–Johnson syndrome). The risk increased with excessively rapid dosage titration and in patients co-medicated with valproate. Up to March 1997, the manufacturer had received a total of 150 postmarketing reports of possible cases of Stevens–Johnson syndrome or toxic epidermal necrolysis, and 46 of these were in children aged 12 years or under. Of the 46 children, three were reported as having toxic epidermal necrolysis, 40 as

Stevens–Johnson syndrome, and 3 as suggestive of Stevens–Johnson syndrome; two deaths were reported. Rashes associated with one or more symptoms of hypersensitivity reactions occurred in 19 children. Of 29 patients with Stevens–Johnson syndrome, toxic epidermal necrolysis, or hypersensitivity reactions, for whom precise details were available, 83% were taking lamotrigine with concomitant valproate and 85% were taking lamotrigine dosages higher than recommended.

- A 33-year-old woman, who had taken valproate for 3 years, developed Stevens–Johnson syndrome soon after starting to take lamotrigine 150 mg/day (46). Lamotrigine was withdrawn and prednisolone given; the signs and symptoms progressively resolved over 10 days.

Although serious skin rashes have been reported with traditional anticonvulsants, the risk of Stevens–Johnson syndrome and toxic epidermal necrolysis with these drugs appears to be lower than with lamotrigine. Data from the Saskatchewan Health Plan suggest that the risk of serious rashes is in the order of 0.9:1000 (1.4:1000 in children) for phenytoin, 0.6:1000 (1.4:1000 in children) for carbamazepine, and 0:1000 for valproate, but Stevens–Johnson syndrome constituted only a small minority of these cases (47).

The panel agreed on the following conclusions

(1) most skin rashes from lamotrigine are benign and resolve on withdrawal;
(2) serious skin rashes occur almost entirely during the first 8 weeks and increased vigilance is recommended during this period;
(3) death from skin rashes is extremely rare (under 10 known cases);
(4) a mild rash can progress to a severe rash or to systemic involvement; fever, lymphadenopathy, facial edema, vomiting, or raised liver enzymes may indicate a hypersensitivity reaction and can precede the appearance of a rash;
(5) the following features suggest the development of a serious rash: mucous membrane lesions, blistering or peeling, facial edema, lymphadenopathy, raised liver enzymes, and leukopenia or thrombocytopenia;
(6) the risk of a rash, and possibly also serious rashes, is increased with excessive initial dosages or too fast rates of titration, combination with valproic acid (particularly in the absence of enzyme-inducing drugs), and possibly a history of skin or allergic reactions to another anticonvulsant; physicians should follow dosing instructions carefully, and be aware that dosing varies according to whether lamotrigine is added to valproate, an enzyme-inducing antiepileptic drug (such as phenytoin), or both, or is used as monotherapy;
(7) potential risks and benefits should be discussed with the patient, who should be informed about symptoms suggestive of hypersensitivity;
(8) if a rash appears, the patient should be seen by a physician within 24 hours and, if necessary, a specialist opinion should be sought; suspected cases of Stevens–Johnson syndrome and toxic epidermal necrolysis should be hospitalized for specialist care;
(9) blood chemistry and hematology may be useful to detect systemic involvement;
(10) if no alternative explanation exists, the rash should be presumed to be due to lamotrigine and the drug should be withdrawn; in patients with a rash non-typical of drug-induced rashes, lamotrigine can be continued cautiously under close monitoring if its use is deemed essential.

Fast dose escalation rate and co-administration of valproate are the most important risk factors for skin reactions. Patients should be warned to report immediately any sign of hypersensitivity, such as rash, fever, or lymphadenopathy. In selected patients who have experienced a mild rash, rechallenge with lower initial doses and slower escalation can be attempted under close supervision (48), but this should be done only when the drug is absolutely necessary, owing to the risk of serious reactions. For adults taking valproate (with or without other anticonvulsants), the dose escalation rate currently recommended by the manufacturer is 25 mg on alternate days during weeks 1 and 2, followed by 25 mg daily during weeks 3 and 4, with further increments by 25–50 mg every 1–2 weeks up to the usual maintenance dose of 100–200 mg/day (Europe) or 100–400 mg/day (USA) (49). For adults taking enzyme inducers without valproate, the escalation rate is 50 mg/day during weeks 1 and 2 followed by 50 mg bd during weeks 3 and 4, with further increments by 100 mg daily every 1–2 weeks up to the usual maintenance dose of 200–400 mg/day (Europe) or 300–500 mg/day (USA). For children aged 2–12 years, starting dosages are 0.15 mg/kg/day in the presence of valproate and 0.3 mg/kg bd in the presence of enzyme inducers without valproate (50).

Data on skin reactions from the German registry have confirmed that the risk of serious rashes is reduced by slower dose escalation (51). In 1993 there were five cases of Stevens–Johnson syndrome or toxic epidermal necrolysis, all in patients who were also taking valproate, among 1270 new patients taking lamotrigine, that is one per 254 recipients. After the recommended starting dose with valproate was reduced by a factor of four, the rates of Stevens–Johnson syndrome or toxic epidermal necrolysis fell to two of 15 500 recipients in 1994 and two of 34 700 recipients in 1995. However, this apparent change in incidence could have been explained in part by additional factors, such as greater risk awareness and consequent more cautious use of the drug, prompter withdrawal at first appearance of a rash and possibly changes in ascertainment rates.

Safe reintroduction of lamotrigine proved possible in seven young people (aged 5–19 years) who had previously had a mild rash associated with a first course (52). The lamotrigine was withdrawn immediately when the rash was identified and was subsequently reintroduced after 47–236 days using a slow escalation regimen, starting with 0.1 mg/day. Lamotrigine was successfully reintroduced without recurrence of persistent rash and without any adverse effects in all seven cases.

Hair, nails, sweat glands

Hair loss and hirsutism have been reported rarely with lamotrigine (SEDA-18, 66) (SEDA-19, 71).

Sexual function

- A 37-year-old schizoaffective woman taking lamotrigine monotherapy developed loss of libido and an unpleasant feeling when her erogenous zones were touched when the dosage of lamotrigine was increased from 200 to 400 mg/day (53). Surprisingly, no attempt was made to determine whether the condition could be reversed by lowering the dosage.

The authors speculated that this effect could have been related to inhibition of serotonin reuptake by lamotrigine.

Immunologic

A phenytoin-like hypersensitivity syndrome with skin rash, leukocytosis, and laboratory evidence of liver and kidney dysfunction has been attributed to lamotrigine (SEDA-22, 89).

Twenty-six lamotrigine-associated reactions consistent with the features of the anticonvulsant hypersensitivity syndrome have been reviewed, including nine previously published (54). The patients were aged 3.5–74 (mean 28) years and 14 were female. Valproate was used as co-medication in 60%. Fever was present in all patients, a skin rash in 77% (with Stevens–Johnson syndrome or toxic epidermal necrolysis in five cases), hematological abnormalities in 69% (including eosinophilia in 19%), liver abnormalities in 65%, renal involvement in 23%, disseminated intravascular coagulation in 15%, and musculoskeletal disorders in 8%. Multiorgan involvement was present in 46%. One patient died. Overall, the characteristics of the syndrome were comparable to that induced by aromatic anticonvulsants, except for a somewhat higher incidence of severe skin rashes and a lower frequency of eosinophilia and lymphadenopathy.

- A 35-year-old man with Lennox–Gastaut syndrome developed tender cervical lymphadenopathy 14 weeks after lamotrigine was introduced, when the dosage was increased to 200 mg/day (55). Frozen section examination of a biopsy specimen 10 weeks later suggested lymphoma, but further histopathological investigations documented lymphoid hyperplasia consistent with a diagnosis of pseudolymphoma, which resolved 1 month after withdrawal.

This seems to have been the first report of pseudolymphoma associated with lamotrigine.

Systemic hypersensitivity reactions to lamotrigine can be severe.

- A 27-year-old woman developed disseminated intravascular coagulation, fever, rash, and hepatic dysfunction 11 days after starting lamotrigine (56). The drug dosage was not stated.
- A 17-year-old girl with a history of bipolar disorder developed fever, lymphadenopathy, skin rash, diarrhea, and acute renal insufficiency requiring dialysis after taking lamotrigine for 4 weeks (57). Renal biopsy showed acute interstitial nephritis with focal granulomas; colonic biopsy showed colitis and ileitis with non-necrotizing epithelioid granulomas.
- Severe hypersensitivity affecting the skin, lymph nodes, and liver has been reported with lamotrigine in a 36-year-old man, who had taken high doses of sodium valproate and lamotrigine for about a month (58). Skin tests were negative with both drugs, but lymphocyte stimulation tests were twice positive with lamotrigine. Later re-exposure to sodium valproate was tolerated.

Drug-induced lupus-like syndrome has been associated with lamotrigine (59).

- A 57-year-old woman, who had taken lamotrigine 2 mg/kg/day for about 2 years developed arthralgia affecting the small joints of the hands, wrists, and knees, an erythematous skin rash, myalgia, and Raynaud's phenomenon. Serum antinuclear antibodies were positive (1:320, speckled pattern), as was anti-Ro/SSA. Rheumatoid factor and anticardiolipin antibodies were negative and serum complement was normal. Lamotrigine was withdrawn and the symptoms and abnormal tests gradually normalized.

Multiorgan failure

Multiorgan failure and disseminated intravascular coagulation have been described occasionally with lamotrigine. Although these were originally considered to be secondary to seizure activity and not to lamotrigine itself (SED-13, 154), in at least three recent cases the drug was probably implicated (SEDA-20, 64) (60). In two affected children the presentation included fever, rash, hepatic and renal dysfunction, hypoalbuminemia, intravascular coagulation, and changes in alertness.

Death

Sudden unexplained death in epileptic patients taking lamotrigine has been considered to be related to the underlying disease and not to its treatment (SEDA-21, 72).

Long-Term Effects

Drug withdrawal

Psychomotor inhibition after rapid withdrawal of lamotrigine has been reported (61).

- A 26-year-old man with refractory generalized seizures had taken lamotrigine since the age of 22. At age 26, during presurgical evaluation with video-electroencephalography, lamotrigine was withdrawn and valproic acid 1200 mg/day and levetiracetam 1000 mg/day were continued. After 5 days he became anhedonic and had hyperhidrosis of the hands. He claimed that he had the impression that he was floating or that he was drunk. He had visual hallucinations, with stars in both visual fields, but no diplopia. He had a tremor and a slight tachycardia. Biological and toxicological results were unremarkable. An electroencephalogram ruled out status epilepticus.

The interpretation of this case is confounded by the use of levetiracetam at the onset of the symptoms. In addition, his symptoms appeared just after an admission for video-electroencephalography, during which he suffered at least one generalized tonic-clonic seizure. Thus, his symptoms could have been a mild form of postictal psychosis.

Second-Generation Effects

Pregnancy

Plasma lamotrigine concentrations in one woman fell during pregnancy and increased about six-fold after delivery; such changes could affect the clinical outcome (62).

Changes in lamotrigine clearance before, during, and after pregnancy were retrospectively analysed in 12 pregnancies (63). There was a significant (over 65%) increase in apparent clearance between preconception and the second and third trimesters. In 11 pregnancies higher doses of lamotrigine were required to maintain therapeutic concentrations. In the postpartum period, apparent clearance returned to the preconception baseline, and lamotrigine doses had to be reduced.

Teratogenicity

There were birth defects in eight of 123 offspring exposed to lamotrigine polypharmacy during the first trimester of pregnancy (95% CI = 3, 13%) and in none of 40 exposed to monotherapy (CI = 0, 11%) (64). The wide confidence intervals indicate that sample size was not sufficiently large to determine whether lamotrigine has a lower teratogenic risk than other anticonvulsants.

The results of a prospective study on the outcomes in pregnant women exposed to lamotrigine have been published (65). The report included 168 outcomes in women exposed to lamotrigine monotherapy and 166 after pregnancies exposed to lamotrigine polytherapy during the first trimester. Three of 168 neonates (1.8%) exposed to lamotrigine monotherapy had major birth defects (95% CI = 0.5, 5.5%). There were five major birth defects in 50 neonates (10%) after lamotrigine polytherapy with valproic acid during the first trimester (95% CI = 3.7, 23%). The proportion of major defects on exposure to lamotrigine polytherapy without valproate during the first trimester was 5 of 116 (4.3%) (95% CI = 1.6, 10%). There were no specific patterns of major birth defects in any subgroup or within the register as a whole. Thus, it appears that lamotrigine-exposed women have a relatively low frequency of major birth defects and that the combination of lamotrigine and valproic acid could potentially be especially detrimental in this respect. However, the wide confidence intervals preclude a firm conclusion. Moreover, there were several methodological limitations to this study, such as lack of standardization in outcome ascertainment and other potential sources of bias.

Fetotoxicity

The outcomes of pregnancy in 53 women exposed to lamotrigine included 4 spontaneous abortions, 13 induced abortions (none because of a prenatally detected defect), 34 newborns without birth defects, and 2 newborns with unspecified defects (66). No information on co-medication was given, and more data are required for risk assessment.

Lactation

The breast milk to plasma lamotrigine concentration ratio is about 0.6, and in breast-fed infants serum drug concentrations reach about 30% of maternal concentrations. Although no toxicity has been reported in these infants, close observation is warranted (SEDA-22, 88) (62).

Susceptibility Factors

Age

In adults, the incidence of Stevens–Johnson syndrome was approximately 1:1000, but higher rates (1 in 50 to 1 in 300) have been reported in children (SEDA-22, 89).

The effects of lamotrigine in children have been reviewed (67). Its efficacy has been demonstrated in 13 studies in 1096 children with a variety of seizure types. Generally, lamotrigine treatment in these trials was at higher initial doses and faster dose escalations than are currently recommended. Most adverse events associated with lamotrigine were mild to moderate and did not result in withdrawal. In placebo-controlled, add-on trials 85% of those who took lamotrigine had an adverse event compared with 83% of those who took placebo. Lamotrigine was associated with an increased risk of adverse events in the nervous system (dizziness, tremor, ataxia, and diplopia), gastrointestinal tract (nausea), and urinary tract (infection). Skin rash was reported more often with lamotrigine than placebo and more often by children than by adults.

Other features of the patient

Exceeding the currently recommended slow dosage escalation guidelines and co-administration of valproate are risk factors for rashes.

Drug Administration

Drug overdose

The effects of overdosage of lamotrigine include sedation, ataxia, diplopia, nausea, vomiting, hypertonia, nystagmus, and prolongation of the QRS complex (SEDA-18, 66). Cardiac rhythm should be monitored. Multiple oral dosing with activated charcoal enhances lamotrigine elimination, but its value in overdose is unknown.

The manifestations of acute lamotrigine overdose can mimic the anticonvulsant hypersensitivity syndrome (68).

- A 49-year-old man with bipolar disorder inadvertently took four daily doses of lamotrigine 2700 mg each. He developed a low-grade fever, a skin rash, and periorbital edema. He had a leukocytosis, raised liver enzymes, and acute renal insufficiency. He recovered fully after lamotrigine withdrawal and steroid therapy.

Postmortem blood and tissue concentrations of lamotrigine have been reported in a case of suicide attributed to "mixed drug toxicity" with carbamazepine, lamotrigine, paroxetine, and thioridazine (69). The blood lamotrigine concentration was 155 μmol/l. Two other individuals with high postmortem blood lamotrigine concentrations, who did not die of an overdose, were also taking valproate.

Severe encephalopathy due to lamotrigine overdose has been reported (70).

- A 55-year-old woman taking lamotrigine and valproate for partial epilepsy took an overdose of lamotrigine and became stuporose. A CT scan was unremarkable and the cerebrospinal fluid was normal. Electroencephalography showed generalized slowing without epileptiform activity. The serum valproate concentration was 65 μg/ml and the lamotrigine concentration 32 μg/ml. A toxicology screen was negative. Lamotrigine was withheld and she remained unresponsive for 3 days, when she awoke disoriented. On day 5 she was alert and fully oriented (serum lamotrigine 15 μg/ml).

Drug–Drug Interactions

Carbamazepine

The effects of other antiepileptic drugs on the pharmacokinetics of lamotrigine have been studied in 62 patients with epilepsy (71). Carbamazepine, phenytoin, and phenobarbital, all enzyme inducers, increased the oral clearance of lamotrigine, individually by 58% and in combination by nearly 200%.

The time-course of de-induction following the step-wise withdrawal of carbamazepine in patients treated concomitantly with lamotrigine has been analysed (72). This study was part of an active-control, monotherapy trial. Patients taking carbamazepine were given lamotrigine to attain a target dose of 500 mg/day, while carbamazepine was withdrawn in weekly 20% decrements. After withdrawal, lamotrigine was continued as monotherapy for a further 12 weeks. Of 156 patients, 76 were assigned to lamotrigine, 43 of them completed the withdrawal to monotherapy, and 28 of these 43 successfully completed the study. In a subset analysis of completers, lamotrigine concentration increased by 62% in those who had taken carbamazepine. These differences were significantly different and occurred when carbamazepine plasma concentrations were very low or undetectable.

Cimetidine

The effect of cimetidine on the pharmacokinetics of lamotrigine has been studied in 10 healthy men (73). Cimetidine had no effect on the pharmacokinetics of lamotrigine.

Ketamine

Because some of the cognitive effects of ketamine may be mediated through increased glutamate release, lamotrigine, which inhibits glutamate release, has been used to reduce the neuropsychiatric effects of ketamine in 16 healthy subjects (74). Lamotrigine significantly reduced ketamine-induced perceptual abnormalities and increased its immediate mood-elevating effects.

Lithium

The effect of lamotrigine on steady-state lithium pharmacokinetics has been studied in 20 healthy adult men (75). Lamotrigine did not significantly change the pharmacokinetics of lithium.

Methsuximide

The interaction of methsuximide with lamotrigine has been studied in 16 patients aged 9–19 years with a variety of seizure types and syndromes (76). The mean lamotrigine serum concentration before starting or after stopping methsuximide was 54 μmol/l and the mean concentration while taking methsuximide was 25 μmol/l. Methsuximide lowered the serum lamotrigine concentration in every case, with a mean fall of 53% (range 36–72%). In some patients this led to a deterioration in seizure control when methsuximide was added or an improvement in seizure control after methsuximide was withdrawn. The mechanism is thought to be induction of metabolism.

Oral contraceptives

Plasma concentrations of lamotrigine were reduced in seven women taking an oral contraceptive (mean reduction 49%, range 41–64%), probably through induction of glucuronide conjugating enzymes (77).

Phenobarbital

The effects of other antiepileptic drugs on the pharmacokinetics of lamotrigine have been studied in 62 patients with epilepsy (71). Carbamazepine, phenytoin, and phenobarbital, all enzyme inducers, increased the oral clearance of lamotrigine, individually by 58% and in combination by nearly 200%.

Phenytoin

The effects of other antiepileptic drugs on the pharmacokinetics of lamotrigine have been studied in 62 patients with epilepsy (71). Carbamazepine, phenytoin, and phenobarbital, all enzyme inducers, increased the total oral clearance of lamotrigine, individually by 58% and in combination by nearly 200%.

Choreoathetosis is a rare adverse effect of some anticonvulsants, but has especially been associated with phenytoin. In a retrospective survey, three of 39 adults and one of 38 children developed choreoathetosis acutely when lamotrigine was added to phenytoin or vice versa (78). The effect was reversible by withdrawing one of the drugs. It was calculated that the risk of choreoathetosis is increased more than 50-fold when these drugs are combined, possibly owing to a pharmacodynamic interaction.

The time-course of de-induction following the step-wise withdrawal of phenytoin in patients treated concomitantly with lamotrigine has been analysed (72). This study was part of an active-control, monotherapy trial. Patients taking phenytoin were given lamotrigine to attain a target dose of 500 mg/day, while phenytoin was withdrawn in weekly 20% decrements. After withdrawal, lamotrigine was continued as monotherapy for a further 12 weeks. Of 156 patients, 76 were assigned to lamotrigine, 43 of them completed the withdrawal to monotherapy, and 28 of these 43 successfully completed the study. In a subset analysis of completers, lamotrigine concentration increased by 160% in patients who had previously taken phenytoin. These differences were significantly different and occurred when phenytoin plasma concentrations were very low or undetectable.

Rifampicin

The effects of rifampicin on the pharmacokinetics of lamotrigine have been studied in 10 healthy men (73).

Rifampicin induced the glucuronidation of lamotrigine, increasing total clearance about two-fold.

Valproate

Effects of valproate on lamotrigine

Co-administration of valproate is one of the most important risk factors for skin reactions to lamotrigine; valproate co-medication was present in 74 and 64% of patients with Stevens–Johnson syndrome and toxic epidermal necrolysis respectively (44).

Valproate reduced the oral clearance of lamotrigine by about 70%, but the effect was not related to the concentration of valproate (hence the rather misleading title of the paper, that is there was an effect but it did not appear to be concentration-related) (71). There was no effect on lamotrigine clearance when a single enzyme inducer was combined with valproate, but combinations of enzyme inducers had almost the same effect in the presence or absence of valproate. Consistent with this result, it has also been shown that the effect of valproate on the clearance of lamotrigine is independent of valproate dose and steady-state concentration in 28 patients with intractable epilepsy (79). However, in contrast to these findings, there were good relations between the dose of valproate 200–1000 mg/day and the increase in lamotrigine AUC and the prolongation of half-life in eight patients with epilepsy (80).

Twenty-six lamotrigine-associated reactions consistent with the features of the anticonvulsant hypersensitivity syndrome have been reviewed, including nine previously published (54). The patients were aged 3.5–74 years (mean 28) and 14 were female. Valproate was used as co-medication in 60%.

Effects of lamotrigine on valproate

In a study of 400 serum concentrations from 372 patients taking lamotrigine and valproic acid, lamotrigine was associated with a slight reduction in valproate serum concentrations (81). However, the size of the effect was probably of no clinical significance.

Effects of the combination of lamotrigine with valproate

The tolerability of lamotrigine added to valproate has been assessed in 108 mostly adult patients (82). The median starting dose was 21 mg/day and upward titrations were usually made at 2-week intervals; although these were more cautious than in earlier studies, in many patients the initial dose or titration rate still exceeded those currently recommended by the manufacturer. Adverse events led to withdrawal in 14 patients, including seven of 14 who had a rash. Other adverse events included fatigue (12%), gastrointestinal symptoms (9%), dizziness, headache, and insomnia (3% each). Serious events were hallucinations (two patients), increased liver enzymes (two patients), irritability, and leukopenia (one patient each). These results suggest that, with cautious dosage escalation, lamotrigine can be added to valproate with acceptable safety. In this study, the incidence of rash was not higher than that seen among 310 patients in whom lamotrigine was added to other drug regimens not including valproate (13 versus 14%).

In an open prospective trial, patients with partial seizures who had not responded to lamotrigine or valproate given separately responded well to the combination; this was not due to an effect of valproate on serum lamotrigine concentrations, because after adjusting dosages based on clinical response the serum concentrations of both drugs were lower during combination therapy (83). Hand tremor developed in all 13 patients who took the combination, compared with three of 20 who took valproate without lamotrigine and none of 17 who took lamotrigine without valproate. These findings confirm that valproate plus lamotrigine is a valuable combination in patients unresponsive to either drug alone, partly because of a pharmacodynamic interaction. Patients co-medicated with valproate should be treated with a lower starting dose of lamotrigine and with slower dosage escalation to minimize the risk of a skin rash. Maintenance lamotrigine dosage requirements are also reduced by valproate co-medication. Although tremor is common, it can be maintained within acceptable limits by adjusting the dosage of either drug.

Diagnosis of Adverse Drug Reactions

The usual target range for plasma lamotrigine concentrations is 4–16 μmol/l (1–4 μg/ml).

References

1. Culy CR, Goa KL. Lamotrigine. A review of its use in childhood epilepsy. Paediatr Drugs 2000;2(4):299–330.
2. Mackay FJ, Wilton LV, Pearce GL, Freemantle SN, Mann RD. Safety of long-term lamotrigine in epilepsy. Epilepsia 1997;38(8):881–6.
3. Froscher W, Keller F, Kraemer G, Vogt H. Serum level monitoring in assessing lamotrigine efficacy and toxicity. Epilepsia 1999;40(Suppl 2):252.
4. Barron TF, Hunt SL, Hoban TF, Price ML. Lamotrigine monotherapy in children. Pediatr Neurol 2000;23(2):160–3.
5. Calabrese JR, Suppes T, Bowden CL, Sachs GS, Swann AC, McElroy SL, Kusumakar V, Ascher JA, Earl NL, Greene PL, Monaghan ET. A double-blind, placebo-controlled, prophylaxis study of lamotrigine in rapid-cycling bipolar disorder. Lamictal 614 Study Group. J Clin Psychiatry 2000;61(11):841–50.
6. Gidal BE, Walker JK, Lott RS, Shaw R, Speth J, Marty KJ, Rutecki P. Efficacy of lamotrigine in institutionalized, developmentally disabled patients with epilepsy: a retrospective evaluation. Seizure 2000;9(2):131–6.
7. Lethel V, Chabrol B, Livet MO, Mancini J. Intérêt de la lamotrigine therapy en pédiatrie. Étude rétrospective chez 32 enfants. [Lamotrigine therapy in children. Retrospective study of 32 children.] Arch Pediatr 2000;7(3):234–42.
8. Parmeggiani L, Belmonte A, Ferrari AR, Perucca E, Guerrini R. Add-on lamotrigine treatment in children and young adults with severe partial epilepsy: an open, prospective, long-term study. J Child Neurol 2000;15(10):671–4.
9. Wong IC, Mawer GE, Sander JW. Adverse event monitoring in lamotrigine patients: a pharmacoepidemiologic study in the United Kingdom. Epilepsia 2001;42(2):237–44.
10. Nieto-Barrera M, Brozmanova M, Capovilla G, Christe W, Pedersen B, Kane K, O'Neill F; Lamictal vs. Carbamazepine Study Group. A comparison of monotherapy with lamotrigine or carbamazepine in patients with

newly diagnosed partial epilepsy. Epilepsy Res 2001;46(2):145–55.
11. Brodie MJ, Richens A, Yuen AW. Double-blind comparison of lamotrigine and carbamazepine in newly diagnosed epilepsy. UK Lamotrigine/Carbamazepine Monotherapy Trial Group. Lancet 1995;345(8948):476–9.
12. Steiner TJ, Dellaportas CI, Findley LJ, Gross M, Gibberd FB, Perkin GD, Park DM, Abbott R. Lamotrigine monotherapy in newly diagnosed untreated epilepsy: a double-blind comparison with phenytoin. Epilepsia 1999;40(5):601–7.
13. Messenheimer J, Mullens EL, Giorgi L, Young F. Safety review of adult clinical trial experience with lamotrigine. Drug Saf 1998;18(4):281–96.
14. Brodie MJ, Overstall PW, Giorgi L. Multicentre, double-blind, randomised comparison between lamotrigine and carbamazepine in elderly patients with newly diagnosed epilepsy. The UK Lamotrigine Elderly Study Group. Epilepsy Res 1999;37(1):81–7.
15. Jozwiak S, Terczynski A. Open study evaluating lamotrigine efficacy and safety in add-on treatment and consecutive monotherapy in patients with carbamazepine- or valproate-resistant epilepsy. Seizure 2000;9(7): 486–92.
16. Aldenkamp AP, Arends J, Bootsma HP, Diepman L, Hulsman J, Lambrechts D, Leenen L, Majoie M, Schellekens A, de Vocht J. Randomized double-blind parallel-group study comparing cognitive effects of a low-dose lamotrigine with valproate and placebo in healthy volunteers. Epilepsia 2002;43(1):19–26.
17. Brodie MJ, Chadwick DW, Anhut H, Otte A, Messmer SL, Maton S, Sauermann W, Murray G, Garofalo EA; Gabapentin Study Group 945-212. Gabapentin versus lamotrigine monotherapy: a double-blind comparison in newly diagnosed epilepsy. Epilepsia 2002;43(9):993–1000.
18. Simpson DM, Olney R, McArthur JC, Khan A, Godbold J, Ebel-Frommer K. A placebo-controlled trial of lamotrigine for painful HIV-associated neuropathy. Neurology 2000;54(11):2115–19.
19. Richens A. Safety of lamotrigine. Epilepsia 1994;35(Suppl 5):S37–40.
20. Kilpatrick ES, Forrest G, Brodie MJ. Concentration–effect and concentration–toxicity relations with lamotrigine: a prospective study. Epilepsia 1996;37(6):534–8.
21. Hennessy MJ, Koutroumanidis M, Elwes RD. Neuralgic amyotrophy associated with hypersensitivity to lamotrigine. Neurology 1998;51(4):1224.
22. Guerrini R, Dravet C, Genton P, Belmonte A, Kaminska A, Dulac O. Lamotrigine and seizure aggravation in severe myoclonic epilepsy. Epilepsia 1998;39(5):508–12.
23. Catania S, Cross H, de Sousa C, Boyd S. Paradoxic reaction to lamotrigine in a child with benign focal epilepsy of childhood with centrotemporal spikes. Epilepsia 1999;40(11):1657–60.
24. Guerrini R, Belmonte A, Parmeggiani L, Perucca E. Myoclonic status epilepticus following high-dosage lamotrigine therapy. Brain Dev 1999;21(6):420–4.
25. Jansky J, Rasonyi G, Halasz P, Olajos S, Szucs A. Continuous myoclonus during lamotrigine therapy with high serum level. Epilepsia 1999;40(Suppl 2):282.
26. Sadler M. Lamotrigine associated with insomnia. Epilepsia 1999;40(3):322–5.
27. Champagne J, Whiting SE. Sleep disturbance on lamotrigine. Epilepsia 1999;40(Suppl 7):118–19.
28. Sotero M, Patti M, Cheyette S, Rho JM. Lamotrigine-induced tic disorder: Report of five pediatric cases. Epilepsia 1999;40(Suppl 7):123.
29. Verma A, St Clair EW, Radtke RA. A case of sustained massive gabapentin overdose without serious side effects. Ther Drug Monit 1999;21(6):615–17.
30. Lombroso CT. Lamotrigine-induced tourettism. Neurology 1999;52(6):1191–4.
31. Janszky J, Rasonyi G, Halasz P, Olajos S, Perenyi J, Szucs A, Debreczeni T. Disabling erratic myoclonus during lamotrigine therapy with high serum level—report of two cases. Clin Neuropharmacol 2000;23(2):86–9.
32. Sotero de Menezes MA, Rho JM, Murphy P, Cheyette S. Lamotrigine-induced tic disorder: report of five pediatric cases. Epilepsia 2000;41(7):862–7.
33. Meador KJ, Loring DW, Ray PG, Murro AM, King DW, Perrine KR, Vazquez BR, Kiolbasa T. Differential cognitive and behavioral effects of carbamazepine and lamotrigine. Neurology 2001;56(9):1177–82.
34. Mewasingh L, Aylett S, Kirkham F, Stanhope R. Hyponatraemia associated with lamotrigine in cranial diabetes insipidus. Lancet 2000;356(9230):656.
35. Ueberall MA. Normal growth during lamotrigine monotherapy in pediatric epilepsy patients—a prospective evaluation of 103 children and adolescents. Epilepsy Res 2001;46(1):63–7.
36. de Camargo OA, Bode H. Agranulocytosis associated with lamotrigine. BMJ 1999;318(7192):1179.
37. Fadul CE, Meyer LP, Jobst BC, Cornell CJ, Lewis LD. Agranulocytosis associated with lamotrigine in a patient with low-grade glioma. Epilepsia 2002;43(2):199–200.
38. Pulik M, Lionnet F, Genet P. Successful treatment of lamotrigine-induced erythroblastopenic crisis with folinic acid. Neurology 2000;55(8):1235–6.
39. Solvason HB. Agranulocytosis associated with lamotrigine. Am J Psychiatry 2000;157(10):1704.
40. Mikati M, Fayad M, Choueiri R, Jbeilie D. Potential hepatotoxicity of lamotrigine in children. Epilepsia 1999;40(Suppl 2):233.
41. Fayad M, Choueiri R, Mikati M. Potential hepatotoxicity of lamotrigine. Pediatr Neurol 2000;22(1):49–52.
42. Calabrese JR, Sullivan JR, Bowden CL, Suppes T, Goldberg JF, Sachs GS, Shelton MD, Goodwin FK, Frye MA, Kusumakar V. Rash in multicenter trials of lamotrigine in mood disorders: clinical relevance and management. J Clin Psychiatry 2002;63(11):1012–9.
43. Tsolaki M, Kourtis A, Divanoglou D, Bostanzopoulou M, Kazis A. Monotherapy with lamotrigine in patients with Alzheimer's disease and seizures. Am J Alzheimer's Dis 2000;15:74–9.
44. Schlienger RG, Shapiro LE, Shear NH. Lamotrigine-induced severe cutaneous adverse reactions. Epilepsia 1998;39(Suppl 7):S22–6.
45. Guberman AH, Besag FM, Brodie MJ, Dooley JM, Duchowny MS, Pellock JM, Richens A, Stern RS, Trevathan E. Lamotrigine-associated rash: risk/benefit considerations in adults and children. Epilepsia 1999;40(7):985–91.
46. Yalcin B, Karaduman A. Stevens–Johnson syndrome associated with concomitant use of lamotrigine and valproic acid. J Am Acad Dermatol 2000;43(5 Pt 2):898–9.
47. Tennis P, Stern RS. Risk of serious cutaneous disorders after initiation of use of phenytoin, carbamazepine, or sodium valproate: a record linkage study. Neurology 1997;49(2):542–6.
48. Tavernor SJ, Wong IC, Newton R, Brown SW. Rechallenge with lamotrigine after initial rash. Seizure 1995;4(1):67–71.
49. Besag FMC. Approaches to reducing the incidence of lamotrigine-induced rash. CNS Drugs 2000;13:21–3.
50. Messenheimer JA, Guberman AH. Rash with lamotrigine: dosing guidelines. Epilepsia 2000;41(4):488.
51. Rzany B, Mockenhaupt M, Baur S, Schroder W, Stocker U, Mueller J, Hollander N, Bruppacher R, Schopf E. Epidemiology of erythema exsudativum multiforme majus, Stevens-Johnson syndrome, and toxic epidermal necrolysis in Germany (1990–1992): structure and results

of a population-based registry. J Clin Epidemiol 1996;49(7):769–73.
52. Besag FM, Ng GY, Pool F. Successful re-introduction of lamotrigine after initial rash. Seizure 2000;9(4):282–6.
53. Erfurth A, Amann B, Grunze H. Female genital disorder as adverse symptom of lamotrigine treatment. A serotoninergic effect? Neuropsychobiology 1998;38(3):200–1.
54. Schlienger RG, Knowles SR, Shear NH. Lamotrigine-associated anticonvulsant hypersensitivity syndrome. Neurology 1998;51(4):1172–5.
55. Pathak P, McLachlan RS. Drug-induced pseudolymphoma secondary to lamotrigine. Neurology 1998;50(5):1509–10.
56. Sarris BM, Wong JG. Multisystem hypersensitivity reaction to lamotrigine. Neurology 1999;53(6):1367.
57. Fervenza FC, Kanakiriya S, Kunau RT, Gibney R, Lager DJ. Acute granulomatous interstitial nephritis and colitis in anticonvulsant hypersensitivity syndrome associated with lamotrigine treatment. Am J Kidney Dis 2000;36(5):1034–40.
58. Schaub N, Bircher AJ. Severe hypersensitivity syndrome to lamotrigine confirmed by lymphocyte stimulation in vitro. Allergy 2000;55(2):191–3.
59. Sarzi-Puttini P, Panni B, Cazzola M, Muzzupappa S, Turiel M. Lamotrigine-induced lupus. Lupus 2000;9(7):555–7.
60. Chattergoon DS, McGuigan MA, Koren G, Hwang P, Ito S. Multiorgan dysfunction and disseminated intravascular coagulation in children receiving lamotrigine and valproic acid. Neurology 1997;49(5):1442–4.
61. Gelisse P, Kissani N, Crespel A, Jafari H, Baldy-Moulinier M. Is there a lamotrigine withdrawal syndrome? Acta Neurol Scand 2002;105(3):232–4.
62. Tomson T, Ohman I, Vitols S. Lamotrigine in pregnancy and lactation: a case report. Epilepsia 1997;38(9):1039–41.
63. Tran TA, Leppik IE, Blesi K, Sathanandan ST, Remmel R. Lamotrigine clearance during pregnancy. Neurology 2002;59(2):251–5.
64. Tennis P, Eldridge R. Six-year interim results of the lamotrigine pregnancy registry. Epilepsia 1999;40(Suppl 2):196.
65. Tennis P, Eldridge RR; International Lamotrigine Pregnancy Registry Scientific Advisory Committee. Preliminary results on pregnancy outcomes in women using lamotrigine. Epilepsia 2002;43(10):1161–7.
66. Eldridge RR, Tennis P; The Lamotrigine Pregnancy Registry Advisory Committee. Monitoring birth outcomes in the Lamotrigine Pregnancy Registry. Epilepsia 1995;36(Suppl 4):90.
67. Messenheimer JA, Giorgi L, Risner ME. The tolerability of lamotrigine in children. Drug Saf 2000;22(4):303–12.
68. Mylonakis E, Vittorio CC, Hollik DA, Rounds S. Lamotrigine overdose presenting as anticonvulsant hypersensitivity syndrome. Ann Pharmacother 1999;33(5):557–9.
69. Pricone MG, King CV, Drummer OH, Opeskin K, McIntyre IM. Postmortem investigation of lamotrigine concentrations. J Forensic Sci 2000;45(1):11–15.
70. Shei M, Campellone JV. Stupor from lamotrigine toxicity. Epilepsia 2001;42(8):1082–3.
71. Gidal BE, Anderson GD, Rutecki PR, Shaw R, Lanning A. Lack of an effect of valproate concentration on lamotrigine pharmacokinetics in developmentally disabled patients with epilepsy. Epilepsy Res 2000;42(1):23–31.
72. Anderson GD, Gidal BE, Messenheimer JA, Gilliam FG. Time course of lamotrigine de-induction: impact of step-wise withdrawal of carbamazepine or phenytoin. Epilepsy Res 2002;49(3):211–17.
73. Ebert U, Thong NQ, Oertel R, Kirch W. Effects of rifampicin and cimetidine on pharmacokinetics and pharmacodynamics of lamotrigine in healthy subjects. Eur J Clin Pharmacol 2000;56(4):299–304.
74. Anand A, Charney DS, Oren DA, Berman RM, Hu XS, Cappiello A, Krystal JH. Attenuation of the neuropsychiatric effects of ketamine with lamotrigine: support for hyperglutamatergic effects of N-methyl-D-aspartate receptor antagonists. Arch Gen Psychiatry 2000;57(3):270–6.
75. Chen C, Veronese L, Yin Y. The effects of lamotrigine on the pharmacokinetics of lithium. Br J Clin Pharmacol 2000;50(3):193–5.
76. Besag FM, Berry DJ, Pool F. Methsuximide lowers lamotrigine blood levels: a pharmacokinetic antiepileptic drug interaction. Epilepsia 2000;41(5):624–7.
77. Sabers A, Buchholt JM, Uldall P, Hansen EL. Lamotrigine plasma levels reduced by oral contraceptives. Epilepsy Res 2001;47(1–2):151–4.
78. Beach RL, Zaatreh M, Tennison M, D'Cruz ON. Apparent pharmacodynamic interaction between lamotrigine and phenytoin causing chorea. Epilepsia 1999;40(Suppl 7):145.
79. Kanner AM, Frey M. Adding valproate to lamotrigine: a study of their pharmacokinetic interaction. Neurology 2000;55(4):588–91.
80. Morris RG, Black AB, Lam E, Westley IS. Clinical study of lamotrigine and valproic acid in patients with epilepsy: using a drug interaction to advantage? Ther Drug Monit 2000;22(6):656–60.
81. Mataringa MI, May TW, Rambeck B. Does lamotrigine influence valproate concentrations? Ther Drug Monit 2002;24(5):631–6.
82. Faught E, Morris G, Jacobson M, French J, Harden C, Montouris G, Rosenfeld W. Adding lamotrigine to valproate: incidence of rash and other adverse effects. Postmarketing Antiepileptic Drug Survey (PADS) Group. Epilepsia 1999;40(8):1135–40.
83. Pisani F, Oteri G, Russo MF, Di Perri R, Perucca E, Richens A. The efficacy of valproate–lamotrigine comedication in refractory complex partial seizures: evidence for a pharmacodynamic interaction. Epilepsia 1999;40(8): 1141–6.

Lansoprazole

See also Proton pump inhibitors

General Information

Lansoprazole is a proton pump inhibitor. Its safety profile has been reviewed based on premarketing clinical studies, and has to be regarded with the reservations appropriate to this type of material. In 4749 patients the most frequent adverse effects were headache (4.7%), diarrhea (3.2%), abdominal pain (2.2%), pharyngitis (1.8%), and nausea (1.4%); some patients had upper respiratory complaints or suffered anxiety or depression, or myalgia (1). The adverse reaction profile appears to be closely similar to that of omeprazole.

Lansoprazole 15 and 30 mg/day were more effective than placebo, but not misoprostol 200 micrograms qds, for the prevention of NSAID-induced gastric ulcers in a multicenter, double-blind, placebo-controlled trial in 537 patients without *Helicobacter pylori* infection who were long-term users of NSAIDs (2). However, adverse effects were significantly more frequent (31% versus less than 20%) and treatment adherence significantly less (71% versus more than 90%) in patients taking misoprostol. The most commonly reported adverse effects in all groups were diarrhea, abdominal pain, and nausea.

Drug–Drug Interactions

Roxithromycin

The effect of lansoprazole on roxithromycin concentrations in plasma and gastric tissue have been investigated in 12 healthy volunteers who took lansoprazole 30 mg bd with or without roxithromycin 300 mg bd over 6 days (3). The medications were well tolerated, with only mild adverse events. The more frequent adverse events were nausea, bloating, and diarrhea. Lansoprazole and roxithromycin did not alter the systemic availability of each other. However, lansoprazole increased the local concentration of the antibiotic in the stomach.

References

1. Colin-Jones DG. Safety of lansoprazole. Aliment Pharmacol Ther 1993;7(Suppl 1):56–60.
2. Graham DY, Agrawal NM, Campbell DR, Haber MM, Collis C, Lukasik NL, Huang B; NSAID-Associated Gastric Ulcer Prevention Study Group. Ulcer prevention in long-term users of nonsteroidal anti-inflammatory drugs: results of a double-blind, randomized, multicenter, active- and placebo-controlled study of misoprostol vs lansoprazole. Arch Intern Med 2002;162(2):169–75.
3. Kees F, Holstege A, Ittner KP, Zimmermann M, Lock G, Scholmerich J, Grobecker H. Pharmacokinetic interaction between proton pump inhibitors and roxithromycin in volunteers. Aliment Pharmacol Ther 2000;14(4):407–12.

Latanoprost

See also Prostaglandins

General Information

Latanoprost is an analogue of $PGF_{2\alpha}$, used to treat glaucoma. The use of latanoprost and unoprostone in the treatment of open-angle glaucoma and ocular hypertension has been reviewed (1). More data on safety are needed to calculate its benefit-to-harm balance.

Latanoprost caused reduced intraocular pressure by 20–40% in adults with open-angle glaucoma or ocular hypertension, but its efficacy and safety in children have not been widely reported. Most children reported so far gained little benefit on intraocular pressure from latanoprost, but older children and those with juvenile-onset open-angle glaucoma do gain a significant ocular hypotensive effect. Systemic and ocular adverse effects in children using latanoprost are infrequent (2).

Organs and Systems

Cardiovascular

Two patients in their seventies developed hypertension during treatment with topical latanoprost (dosage not stated) for open-angle glaucoma; both were also taking tocopherol (vitamin E) supplements. Neither had a previous history of hypertension (3). The authors commented that it is likely that systemic absorption of topical latanoprost could cause hypertension. Self-medication with vitamin E has been reported to aggravate or precipitate hypertension.

Respiratory

Latanoprost rarely causes systemic effects. However, it aggravated respiratory symptoms in a patient with chronic bronchitis and emphysema, with improvement after latanoprost was withdrawn (4).

Nervous system

Three cases of headache after latanoprost have been described (5).

- A 65-year-old man with primary open-angle glaucoma intolerant of dipivefrin and beta-blockers used latanoprost in both eyes at bedtime. He had no prior history of migraine, but he began to have headaches, the frequency and severity of which increased until they were occurring daily. The pain was not relieved by over-the-counter or narcotic analgesics, and he was virtually incapacitated. Latanoprost was discontinued and he had almost immediate relief, with only one migraine during the following week, and he was headache-free for the next 10 months. He then agreed to rechallenge. After the second night of latanoprost therapy his headache recurred, and therapy was withdrawn 2 days later when he had incapacitating pain. Headache did not recur within 4 months of follow-up.
- A 65-year-old man with primary open-angle glaucoma, using levobunolol hydrochloride 0.5%, was given a nighttime dose of latanoprost. The next morning he awoke with a severe bifrontal throbbing headache, photophobia, and slight blurring of vision. The headache intensified, and 4 days later a CT scan was normal. On the sixth day he stopped using latanoprost. His headache disappeared within 24 hours and did not recur during follow-up for 1 year.
- A 54-year-old woman with primary open-angle glaucoma, using betaxolol hydrochloride 0.5%, had mild progression of visual field loss in her left eye. Latanoprost was added nightly to her left eye. A few hours after the first dose she was awakened by a severe unilateral pounding headache extending from the left eye and brow to the left cranium. There were no associated neurological symptoms. The headache resolved spontaneously the next day, but recurred on three nights after instillation of latanoprost. On the fourth night the headache did not occur. She continued to use latanoprost, and the headache did not return.

Sensory systems

Corneal damage

Four patients treated with latanoprost developed dendritiform epitheliopathy, a sign of corneal toxicity; the lesions reversed in 1–4 weeks after latanoprost withdrawal (6).

Three cases of *Herpes simplex* keratitis developed during latanoprost therapy (7).

- One patient, with a history of *H. simplex* keratitis, had recurrence with latanoprost (4 months); the infection resolved on withdrawal but recurred on rechallenge.

- The second patient, with a history of *H. simplex* keratitis, had bilateral recurrence with latanoprost (1 month); antiviral therapy did not eradicate the infection until latanoprost was withdrawn.
- The third patient developed the infection after 1 month; the keratitis cleared on withdrawal of latanoprost and antiviral therapy; reinstitution of latanoprost with prophylactic antiviral medication (valaciclovir) kept the cornea clear, but as soon as the antiviral drug was discontinued, *H. simplex* virus keratitis reappeared.

Although the mechanism is unclear, it is known that inhibitors of prostaglandin synthesis reduce recurrence of epithelial *H. simplex* infections and prostaglandins may stimulate their occurrence.

Iris pigmentation

Latanoprost can produce darkening of the iris in 10–25% of patients treated for 0.5–2 years. The incidence of iris pigmentation differs between eyes with differently colored irises: green–brown, yellow–brown, and blue–brown eyes, in that order, have the highest incidences, whereas eyes with uniformly blue, grey, or green irises are much less affected, even after 2 years of treatment. About 60% of eyes with an initial green–brown iris will have increased pigmentation within 1 year. The corresponding figure for initially blue–brown eyes is about 20%. All patients who have developed increased pigmentation of the iris have been withdrawn from studies, and during follow-up for up to almost 3 years the change in iris pigmentation has been stable without signs of reversibility or further increase. Nevi and freckles have not changed color or size. Apart from the change in color the iris looks normal and pigmentation dispersion has not been observed. No cell proliferation is involved and the change in color is due to melanogenesis. It has been concluded that the change in iris pigmentation is unlikely to cause any long-term consequence besides the cosmetic one. The possibility of late loss of pigment and induction of a pigmentary glaucoma also seems unlikely; melanocytes in the iris are continent and do not release melanin (8). In an observational cohort study of 43 patients, 30 had a definite acquired iris anisochromia (9).

The time of onset of the changes in iris pigmentation can be as early as 3 months. The earliest reported change in iris color occurred in a 78-year-old woman, whose iris color changed from blue–green to brown–green within 4 weeks (10). The pigmentation is irreversible. In a 50-year-old man with peripheral iris darkening after latanoprost treatment, the darkening did not change appreciably for several years after withdrawal (11).

The fine structure of an iridectomy specimen from a 65-year-old woman treated with latanoprost has been reported (12). She received latanoprost for 13.5 months and the drug was withdrawn because of iris color change. She underwent cataract surgery 16 months after stopping the drug and a sector iridectomy was obtained. The authors found some melanocytes with atypical features, including nuclear chromatin margination, prominent nucleoli, and invagination of the nucleoli. These characteristics are also seen in precancerous lesions, in the normal ageing iris, and in patients with glaucoma.

The mechanism of iris pigmentation due to latanoprost is unknown. In an in vitro experiment using uveal melanocytes, the addition of latanoprost increased melanin content, melanin production, and tyrosinase activity (13). Alpha-methyl-para-tyrosine, an inhibitor of tyrosinase (the enzyme that transforms tyrosine to levodopa), completely prevented the latanoprost-induced stimulation of melanogenesis.

Of 17 patients requiring filtering surgery for primary open-angle glaucoma randomized to receive latanoprost ($n = 8$) or alternative medications ($n = 9$) for 3 months before surgery, all had peripheral iridectomy specimens, and there were color changes in one case (14). No morphological changes or cellular proliferation were found in any specimen.

Iris cyst associated with latanoprost has been described in a 76-year-old woman (15). Latanoprost was given for 5 weeks, and during a re-examination a large iris cyst was observed in her right eye. The cyst disappeared 3 weeks after latanoprost withdrawal.

Uveitis

In four patients with complicated open-angle glaucoma, in whom anterior uveitis appeared to be associated with latanoprost, the uveitis was unilateral and occurred only in the eye receiving latanoprost in three patients. In one patient, latanoprost was used in both eyes, and the uveitis was bilateral (16). Four of five eyes had a history of prior inflammation and/or prior incisional surgery. All patients were rechallenged. The uveitis improved after withdrawal and recurred after rechallenge in all eyes. The authors concluded that topical prostaglandin analogues may be relatively contraindicated in patients with a history of uveitis or prior ocular surgery. There may also be a risk in eyes that have not had previous uveitis or incisional surgery.

Optic disc and macular edema

A case of bilateral optic disc edema has been described (17).

- A 64-year-old woman was included in a randomized, double-blind trial of drugs used in the treatment of ocular hypertension. After 3 months, examination of the optic nerve showed bilateral edema. She had been using latanoprost 0.0005% eye-drops at night to both eyes. Latanoprost was withdrawn and the disc edema resolved at 1 week.

Cystoid macular edema developed in two patients treated with topical latanoprost for glaucoma (18). Latanoprost was withdrawn, and the cystoid macular edema was treated with topical corticosteroids and ketorolac, with improvement in visual acuity. The macular edema resolved in both cases.

Cystoid macular edema has been reported in four other patients shortly after they started to use latanoprost (19) and other reports have appeared (20–24). A possible explanation is enhanced disruption of the blood–aqueous barrier induced by latanoprost (23).

A review of the published literature (28 eyes in 25 patients) has shown that in all cases there were other associated risk factors, so that a definitive conclusion about a causal relation cannot be reached (25). Nevertheless, latanoprost should be used with caution in patients with risk factors for cystoid macular edema and special surveillance is necessary.

Skin

Hyperpigmentation of the eyelids can occur during latanoprost therapy.

- A 62-year old Korean woman treated with latanoprost for 4 months developed eyelid pigmentation in both upper and lower eyelids of both eyes (26). There was no increase in iris pigmentation. The eyelid pigmentation gradually diminished after withdrawal, but minimal brownish coloration remained along the lower eyelid folds in both eyes at 4 months.
- A 75-year-old woman with open-angle glaucoma who had used latanoprost for 15 months reported that the skin around her eyes was much darker than on the rest of her face (27). The darkening had occurred gradually. Latanoprost was withdrawn; 1 month later there was a discernible lightening of the periocular skin and 2 months after withdrawal the skin was significantly lighter.

Hair

Eyelashes

Latanoprost causes growth of lashes and ancillary hairs around the eyelids, with greater thickness and length of lashes, additional rows of lashes, and conversion of vellus to terminal hairs in canthal areas and regions adjacent to lashes. As well as increased growth, there is also increased pigmentation. Vellus hairs on the lower eyelids also undergo increased growth and pigmentation. Latanoprost caused changes in eyelashes in 26% of 194 patients over 12 months; the changes included increased length, thickness, density, and color (14).

Latanoprost therapy for 2–17 days can cause changes comparable to chronic therapy. The increased number and length of visible lashes are consistent with the ability of latanoprost to induce and prolong anagen growth in telogen (resting) follicles while producing hypertrophic changes in the involved follicles. Laboratory studies suggest that the initiation and completion of the effects of latanoprost on hair growth occur very early in the anagen phase and that the likely target is the dermal papilla.

Latanoprost can even reverse alopecia of the eyelashes (28).

- A 53-year-old woman, with glaucoma and loss of the eyelashes secondary to alopecia following an allergic response to ibuprofen was given latanoprost (29). After 3 weeks her eyelashes were noticeable and 2 months later full growth had occurred.
- Quantitative analysis of eyelash lengthening in 17 patients treated with latanoprost showed a significant increase in eyelash length in the treated eyes (30).

Increased pigmentation of the eyelashes has been reported in a patient treated with latanoprost (31).

Sweat glands

Heavy sweating occurred in a 6-year-old boy with aniridia and glaucoma during treatment with latanoprost eye-drops (32). Other combinations of drugs for glaucoma had been ineffective in reducing the intraocular pressure. He was given latanoprost eye-drops (dose not stated) at night in combination with a beta-blocker during the day. However, at night he had very heavy sweating. His pyjamas had to be changed regularly about 1–2 hours after he went to sleep. When latanoprost was withdrawn, the heavy sweating resolved. When it was restarted, the heavy sweating recurred.

The author commented that systemic absorption occurred for the most part through the mucous membranes of the nose and throat, since the sweating was less severe when the boy's lacrymal points were compressed for 10 minutes after the administration of latanoprost.

Infection risk

Two cases of *H. simplex* virus dermatitis of the periocular skin have been reported in patients using latanoprost (33). Cases of *H. simplex* keratitis are mentioned above, under sensory systems.

References

1. Eisenberg DL, Camras CB. A preliminary risk-benefit assessment of latanoprost and unoprostone in open-angle glaucoma and ocular hypertension. Drug Saf 1999;20(6):505–14.
2. Enyedi LB, Freedman SF. Latanoprost for the treatment of pediatric glaucoma. Surv Ophthalmol 2002;47(Suppl 1):S129–32.
3. Peak AS, Sutton BM. Systemic adverse effects associated with topically applied latanoprost. Ann Pharmacother 1998;32(4):504–5.
4. Veyrac G, Chiffoleau A, Cellerin L, Larousse C, Bourin M. Latanoprost (Xalatan) et effect systémique respiratoire? A propos d'un cas. [Latanoprost (Xalatan) and a systemic respiratory effect? Apropos of a case.] Therapie 1999;54(4):494–6.
5. Weston BC. Migraine headache associated with latanoprost. Arch Ophthalmol 2001;119(2):300–1.
6. Sudesh S, Cohen EJ, Rapuano CJ, Wilson RP. Corneal toxicity associated with latanoprost. Arch Ophthalmol 1999;117(4):539–40.
7. Wand M, Gilbert CM, Liesegang TJ. Latanoprost and *Herpes simplex* keratitis. Am J Ophthalmol 1999;127(5):602–4.
8. Alm A. Prostaglandin derivates as ocular hypotensive agents. Prog Retin Eye Res 1998;17(3):291–312.
9. Teus MA, Arranz-Marquez E, Lucea-Suescun P. Incidence of iris colour change in latanoprost treated eyes. Br J Ophthalmol 2002;86(10):1085–8.
10. Pappas RM, Pusin S, Higginbotham EJ. Evidence of early change in iris color with latanoprost use. Arch Ophthalmol 1998;116(8):1115–16.
11. Camras CB, Neely DG, Weiss EL. Latanoprost-induced iris color darkening: a case report with long-term follow-up. J Glaucoma 2000;9(1):95–8.
12. Grierson I, Lee WR, Albert DM. The fine structure of an iridectomy specimen from a patient with latanoprost-induced eye color change. Arch Ophthalmol 1999;117(3):394–6.
13. Drago F, Marino A, La Manna C. Alpha-methyl-p-tyrosine inhibits latanoprost-induced melanogenesis in vitro. Exp Eye Res 1999;68(1):85–90.
14. Netland PA, Landry T, Sullivan EK, Andrew R, Silver L, Weiner A, Mallick S, Dickerson J, Bergamini MV, Robertson SM, Davis AA; Travoprost Study Group. Travoprost compared with latanoprost and timolol in patients with open-angle glaucoma or ocular hypertension. Am J Ophthalmol 2001;132(4):472–84.
15. Krohn J, Hove VK. Iris cyst associated with topical administration of latanoprost. Am J Ophthalmol 1999;127(1):91–3.
16. Fechtner RD, Khouri AS, Zimmerman TJ, Bullock J, Feldman R, Kulkarni P, Michael AJ, Realini T,

Warwar R. Anterior uveitis associated with latanoprost. Am J Ophthalmol 1998;126(1):37–41.
17. Stewart O, Walsh L, Pande M. Bilateral optic disc oedema associated with latanoprost. Br J Ophthalmol 1999;83(9):1092–3.
18. Callanan D, Fellman RL, Savage JA. Latanoprost-associated cystoid macular edema. Am J Ophthalmol 1998;126(1):134–5.
19. Ayyala RS, Cruz DA, Margo CE, Harman LE, Pautler SE, Misch DM, Mines JA, Richards DW. Cystoid macular edema associated with latanoprost in aphakic and pseudophakic eyes. Am J Ophthalmol 1998;126(4):602–4.
20. Avakian A, Renier SA, Butler PJ. Adverse effects of latanoprost on patients with medically resistant glaucoma. Arch Ophthalmol 1998;116(5):679–80.
21. Gaddie IB, Bennett DW. Cystoid macular edema associated with the use of latanoprost. J Am Optom Assoc 1998;69(2):122–8.
22. Heier JS, Steinert RF, Frederick AR Jr. Cystoid macular edema associated with latanoprost use. Arch Ophthalmol 1998;116(5):680–2.
23. Miyake K, Ota I, Maekubo K, Ichihashi S, Miyake S. Latanoprost accelerates disruption of the blood–aqueous barrier and the incidence of angiographic cystoid macular edema in early postoperative pseudophakias. Arch Ophthalmol 1999;117(1):34–40.
24. Moroi SE, Gottfredsdottir MS, Schteingart MT, Elner SG, Lee CM, Schertzer RM, Abrams GW, Johnson MW. Cystoid macular edema associated with latanoprost therapy in a case series of patients with glaucoma and ocular hypertension. Ophthalmology 1999;106(5):1024–9.
25. Schumer RA, Camras CB, Mandahl AK. Latanoprost and cystoid macular edema: is there a causal relation? Curr Opin Ophthalmol 2000;11(2):94–100.
26. Kook MS, Lee K. Increased eyelid pigmentation associated with use of latanoprost. Am J Ophthalmol 2000;129(6):804–6.
27. Wand M, Ritch R, Isbey EK Jr, Zimmerman TJ. Latanoprost and periocular skin color changes. Arch Ophthalmol 2001;119(4):614–5.
28. Johnstone MA, Albert DM. Prostaglandin-induced hair growth. Surv Ophthalmol 2002;47(Suppl 1):S185–202.
29. Mansberger SL, Cioffi GA. Eyelash formation secondary to latanoprost treatment in a patient with alopecia. Arch Ophthalmol 2000;118(5):718–19.
30. Sugimoto M, Sugimoto M, Uji Y. Quantitative analysis of eyelash lengthening following topical latanoprost therapy. Can J Ophthalmol 2002;37(6):342–5.
31. Reynolds A, Murray PI, Colloby PS. Darkening of eyelashes in a patient treated with latanoprost. Eye 1998;12(Pt 4):741–3.
32. Schmidtborn F. Systemische Nebenwirkung von Latanoprost bei einem Kind mit Aniridie und Glaukom. [Systemic side-effects of latanoprost in a child with aniridia and glaucoma.] Ophthalmologe 1998;95(9):633–4.
33. Morales J, Shihab ZM, Brown SM, Hodges MR. *Herpes simplex* virus dermatitis in patients using latanoprost. Am J Ophthalmol 2001;132(1):114–6.

Latex

General Information

Latex is present in many medical devices, including surgical and examination gloves, catheters, intubation tubes, anesthesia masks, and dental fillers. Reported allergic reactions range from contact urticaria to anaphylaxis (1).

There has been a marked worldwide increase during recent years in the rate of reactions to latex. These reactions are due to either or both:

1. The formulation chemicals (vulcanizers, stabilizers, preservatives). These cause mainly local delayed hypersensitivity reactions. However, some of these chemicals are also carcinogenic, and may have more serious and not immediately apparent consequences.
2. Proteins in the latex. These can cause generalized systemic allergic reactions, including anaphylaxis, which can be severe and life-threatening.

Latex condoms degrade over time. Such degradation has a significant effect on the product's ability to provide a barrier to sexually transmitted agents, including human immunodeficiency virus (HIV). The FDA has issued a final regulation requiring that the labelling of latex condoms shall contain an expiry date based on physical and mechanical testing performed after exposing the product to varying conditions that age latex, both on the outside packaging and on the individual packaging (2). The agency has also stipulated that if a latex condom contains spermicide and if the expiry date based upon spermicidal stability testing is different from the expiry date based on latex integrity testing, the product shall bear only the earlier expiry date.

Organs and Systems

Urinary tract

Urethritis has been described in patients with urinary catheters containing latex (3). In 100 men, the incidence of urethritis with latex catheters was 22% compared with 2% in patients managed with silicone catheters. In all cases, symptoms developed within 12 hours of use and urine specimens were sterile.

Immunologic

Severe anaphylactic reactions have been reported in response to dental work (latex dental dams), barium enemas (latex enema devices), and numerous surgical procedures involving mainly latex gloves and catheters. The two major contributing factors appear to be a hereditary disposition and occupational exposure. The latter has increased rapidly owing to progress in medical technology, the associated increase in the use of medical devices, and increased awareness among health-care professionals of the need to wear protective gloves during various procedures. This increased exposure has meant that a growing number of people have become sensitized to latex proteins; in one study, 6–7% of surgical personnel and 18–40% of patients with spina bifida were sensitive to latex (4). Particularly high-risk circumstances appear to be direct contact of a latex device or air-borne particles from a latex device (for example corn starch carrying latex proteins) with mucous membranes or with tissues exposed as a result of surgical procedures.

FDA investigations, which eventually identified natural latex/natural rubber (NLNR) allergy as an emerging public health concern, were started in response to voluntary reports submitted by physicians, nurses, and technologists (5). The first reports described deaths that occurred during barium enema procedures, before the administration of barium. Over the past decade, the FDA has received more than 1700 reports of severe allergic reactions, including 16 deaths, related to medical devices containing latex. The deaths all occurred in 1989 among children with spina bifida and were caused by a reaction to the latex cuffs used on the tip of barium enema catheters.

In Australia, regulatory changes have been proposed for the labeling and safety requirements of latex-containing devices that directly or indirectly come into contact with body tissues (6). Most latex-containing devices are in this category, and include tubes, catheters, empty containers, syringes, medical gloves, and devices such as condoms and diaphragms. The FDA is requiring all medical devices containing latex to be labeled as such and to carry a caution that latex can cause allergic reactions (7). The FDA has also urged manufacturers of latex containing medical devices to set the protein levels in their products as low as possible. The FDA also requires that "hypoallergenic" claims should not be attached to medical devices, because they incorrectly imply that the devices may be safely used by people who are sensitive to latex.

References

1. Gaignon I, Veyckemans F, Gribomont BF. Latex allergy in a child: report of a case. Acta Anaesthesiol Belg 1991;42(4):219–23.
2. Anonymous. Latex condoms—expiry date. WHO Pharm Newslett 1998;1&2:14.
3. Nacey JN, Tulloch AG, Ferguson AF. Catheter-induced urethritis: a comparison between latex and silicone catheters in a prospective clinical trial. Br J Urol 1985;57(3):325–8.
4. Anonymous. Allergic reactions to Latex-containing medical devices. FDA Med Bull 1991;91(July):2–3.
5. Dillard SF. Natural rubber latex allergy. FDA Med Bull 1997;27(2):4.
6. Anonymous. Latex in devices—regulations concerning health and safety. WHO Pharm Newslett 1995;5/6:19.
7. Anonymous. Latex containing devices—labelling required. WHO Pharm Newslett 1997;1&2:16–17.

Lauraceae

See also Herbal medicines

General Information

The genera in the family of Lauraceae (Table 1) include cinnamon and sassafras.

Cinnamonum camphora

Camphor is a white crystalline substance, obtained from the tree *Cinnamonum camphora* (camphor tree), but the name has also been given to various volatile substances found in different aromatic plants.

Camphor has been used as a substance of abuse for many centuries, both by ingestion and by inhalation. Today it is found in many non-prescription vaporized or topical "cold cures," topical musculoskeletal anesthetic rubs, "cold sore" formulations, sunscreens, and mothballs. It has also been used to procure an abortion (1).

Adverse effects

The acute effects of ingesting camphor were described by Louis Lewin in "Phantastica" (1924):

> After ingestion of 1.2 grains [72 g] the following symptoms occur: an agreeable warmth of the skin, general nervous excitation, a desire to move, tickling of the skin, and a peculiar feeling of ecstasy similar to drunkenness. One addict said that "he saw his destiny full of great possibilities clearly and distinctly before his eyes." This state continued for one and a half hours. After ingestion of 2.4 grains there was an urgent desire to move. All movements were generally facilitated, and when walking the limbs were lifted far more than necessary. Intellectual thought was impossible. There was a flood of ideas, chasing each other with great rapidity, without any one being analysed. The individual lost perception of his identity. After vomiting, awareness returned, although distraction, forgetfulness and vacancy of mind persisted. On awaking the state of intoxication seemed to have been extraordinarily long and full of events of which the subject did not remember any. After 3 hours he was able to pull himself together and return to full consciousness, but the effect on the brain was so potent that unconsciousness and convulsions again occurred within an hour and lasted for half an hour, after which the subject gradually regained his full mental faculties and normal muscle function.

Lewin also described the effects of chronic abuse:

> Loss of the sense of location and brief gaps in memory usually succeed gastric irritation and convulsions when camphor is taken habitually. The lost memories finally reappear, but in a very strange fashion, so that, according to the statement of an addict, all affairs, events, and things that he had forgotten seemed new, as if he had had no previous knowledge of them. Even after he recognized all the members

Table 1 The genera of Lauraceae

Aniba (aniba)
Beilschmiedia (beilschmiedia)
Cassytha (cassytha)
Cinnamomum (cinnamon)
Cryptocarya (cryptocarya)
Endiandra
Eusideroxylon (ironwood)
Laurus (laurel)
Licaria (licaria)
Lindera (spicebush)
Litsea (litsea)
Nectandra (sweetwood)
Ocotea (sweetwood)
Persea (bay)
Sassafras (sassafras)
Umbellularia (California laurel)

of his family, the objects in his room seemed unfamiliar, as if they had just been given to him. In Slovakia convulsive states similar to epilepsy are so common in consumers of camphor that all cases of similar fits are directly attributed to it.

Nervous system
Convulsions can occur after transdermal absorption of camphor (2).

- A 20-month-old girl developed status epilepticus after ingesting camphor and required ventilation. She was treated with intravenous diazepam and phenobarbital and nasogastric-activated charcoal and made a complete neurological recovery (3).

Liver
Hepatotoxicity occurred in a 2-month-old baby after a camphor-containing cold remedy was applied to the skin; liver function tests returned to normal after the remedy was withdrawn (4).

Chronic ingestion of camphor can mimic Reye's syndrome (5).

Skin
Contact dermatitis has been reported from the use of camphor in ear-drops (6). Photo-distributed skin eruptions have been reported after use of a sunscreen containing camphor (7).

Drug overdose
In children exposure to as little as 500 mg of camphor can be fatal (8). More commonly, a dose of 750–1000 mg is associated with seizures and death. Products that contain 10% camphor contain 500 mg in 5 ml.

After taking an unknown amount of a 10% camphor spirit (maximum dose 200 ml), a 54-year-old woman became comatose, having developed tonic-clonic seizures and respiratory failure (9). After gastric lavage, hemoperfusion was performed with amberlite XAD4 but did not alter either the pharmacokinetics of camphor or the course of the intoxication.

Laurus nobilis

Laurus nobilis (laurel) has well-known analgesic, diaphoretic, antipyretic, and diuretic effects (10), and is widely used in rheumatic, pyrexial, and infective disorders (11), as well as in the perfume and soap industries (10).

Adverse effects
Laurel oil obtained from the berries of *L. nobilis* is a potent skin sensitizer, owing to the presence of allergenic sesquiterpene lactones, and is usually seen in aromatherapists or their clients (12–14).

- A 55-year-old woman developed erythema and edema over her knees (12). She had applied laurel oil, obtained from a herbalist, to her knees to relieve joint pain 15 days earlier. After 3 days, the erythema and edema had begun to appear. She had erythema, edema, and papules over her patellae, and eczema around the eye. She was treated with an oral antihistamine and a topical glucocorticoid. Two days later, the lesions worsened and systemic glucocorticoid therapy was needed. The lesions started to heal, leaving slight postinflammatory hyperpigmentation. Patch-testing was performed with a European standard series and commercial laurel oil 1 month later. There was a +++ reaction to the oil only, and no reaction to either fragrance mix or *Myroxylon pereirae* resin in the standard series. The same formulation of laurel oil was negative on patch-testing in 15 control subjects.

Sassafras albidum

Sassafras albidum (sassafras) root contains 1–2% of volatile oil, which in turn consists largely of safrole, a weakly hepatocarcinogenic agent in laboratory animals. Some metabolites of safrole have mutagenic activity in bacteria and weak hepatocarcinogenic effects in rodents. The carcinogenic effect is primarily mediated by the formation of 1′-hydroxysafrole, followed by sulfonation to an unstable sulfate that reacts to form DNA adducts; these metabolites are formed by CYP2C9 and CYP2E1, the latter contributing three-fold more to the metabolic clearance than the former (15).

In one case sassafras tea caused sweating (16).

In Germany, the health authorities have proposed the withdrawal of sassafras-containing medicines, including homeopathic products up to D3, from the market (17). Of particular concern is the uncontrolled availability of sassafras oil because of its use in aromatherapy. Internal use of sassafras oil in recommended doses up to 12 drops/day can lead to a daily intake up to 0.2 g of safrole (18).

References

1. Rabl W, Katzgraber F, Steinlechner M. Camphor ingestion for abortion (case report). Forensic Sci Int 1997;89(1–2):137–40.
2. Piyaraly S, Boumahni B, Raudrant-Sigogne N, Edmar A, Renouil M, Mallet EC. Camphre percutane et convulsion chez un nouveau-né. [Percutaneous camphor and convulsions in a neonate.] Arch Pediatr 1998;5(2):205–6.
3. Emery DP, Corban JG. Camphor toxicity. J Paediatr Child Health 1999;35(1):105–6.
4. Uc A, Bishop WP, Sanders KD. Camphor hepatotoxicity. South Med J 2000;93(6):596–8.
5. Jimenez JF, Brown AL, Arnold WC, Byrne WJ. Chronic camphor ingestion mimicking Reye's syndrome. Gastroenterology 1983;84(2):394–8.
6. Stevenson OE, Finch TM. Allergic contact dermatitis from rectified camphor oil in Earex ear drops. Contact Dermatitis 2003;49(1):51.
7. Marguery MC, Rakotondrazafy J, el Sayed F, Bayle-Lebey P, Journe F, Bazex J. Contact allergy to 3-(4′ methylbenzylidene) camphor and contact and photocontact allergy to 4-isopropyl dibenzoylmethane. Photodermatol Photoimmunol Photomed 1996;11(5–6):209–12.
8. Love JN, Sammon M, Smereck J. Are one or two dangerous? Camphor exposure in toddlers. J Emerg Med 2004;27(1):49–54.
9. Koppel C, Martens F, Schirop T, Ibe K. Hemoperfusion in acute camphor poisoning. Intensive Care Med 1988;14(4):431–3.

10. Ilisulu K. Ilaç ve Baharat Bitkileri. 1st ed. Ankara, 1992:63–75.
11. Yesilada E, Ustun O, Sezik E, Takaishi Y, Ono Y, Honda G. Inhibitory effects of Turkish folk remedies on inflammatory cytokines: interleukin-1alpha, interleukin-1beta and tumor necrosis factor alpha. J Ethnopharmacol 1997;58(1):59–73.
12. Ozden MG, Oztas P, Oztas MO, Onder M. Allergic contact dermatitis from *Laurus nobilis* (laurel) oil. Contact Dermatitis 2001;45(3):178.
13. Schaller M, Korting HC. Allergic airborne contact dermatitis from essential oils used in aromatherapy. Clin Exp Dermatol 1995;20(2):143–5.
14. Keane FM, Smith HR, White IR, Rycroft RJ. Occupational allergic contact dermatitis in two aromatherapists. Contact Dermatitis 2000;43(1):49–51.
15. Ueng YF, Hsieh CH, Don MJ, Chi CW, Ho LK. Identification of the main human cytochrome P450 enzymes involved in safrole 1′-hydroxylation. Chem Res Toxicol 2004;17(8):1151–6.
16. Haines JD Jr. Sassafras tea and diaphoresis. Postgrad Med 1991;90(4):75–6.
17. Arzneimittelkommission der Deutschen Apotheker. Vorinformation Sassafras-haltige Arzneimittel. Dtsch Apoth Ztg 1995;135:366–8.
18. De Smet PAGM. Een alternatieve olie met een luchtje. Pharm Weekbl 1994;129:258.

Lauromacrogols

General Information

Lauromacrogols are mixtures of monolauryl esters of macrogols. They have the following general formula: $C_{12}H_{25}(OCH_2CH_2)_nOH$. Each is named after the number n in its formula. For example, in lauromacrogol 400 (polidocanol), $n = 400$. They have been used as surfactants, spermicides, solvents, and non-ionic emulsifiers.

Lauromacrogol 9 has been used as a sclerosant and local anesthetic.

Lauromacrogol 400 (polidocanol) has been used as a solvent and non-ionic emulsifier that contains 95% hydroxypolyethoxydodecane and 5% ethyl alcohol. In medicaments it has been used as a topical anesthetic, an antipruritic, and a sclerosant.

Organs and Systems

Immunologic

Contact allergic reactions to lauromacrogol 400 have been reported (1). Patch-testing can yield irritant reactions. In a retrospective study of 8739 patients tested with a topical drug patch test series, 3186 patients were tested with 0.5% lauromacrogol 400 in water (2). There was slight irritation in 0.88%, weakly positive reactions in 0.97%, and strongly positive reactions in 0.25%. In 6202 patients tested with a 3% solution of lauromacrogol 400 in petrolatum, there was slight skin irritation in 0.48%, weakly positive reactions in 1.77%, and strongly positive reactions in 0.34%. Among the 649 patients tested with both formulations, concurrence was moderate.

References

1. Frosch PJ, Schulze-Dirks A. Kontaktallergie durch Polidocanol (Thesis). [Contact allergy caused by polidocanol (thesis).] Hautarzt 1989;40(3):146–9.
2. Uter W, Geier J, Fuchs T; IVDK Study Group. Contact allergy to polidocanol, 1992 to 1999. J Allergy Clin Immunol 2000;106(6):1203–4.

Laxatives

General Information

Laxatives can be classified according to their several mechanisms of action:

- bulk-forming laxatives, such as bran, methylcellulose, *Plantago* extracts (ispaghula and psyllium), and sterculia;
- stimulant laxatives, such as the anthraquinones (senna and dantron), bisacodyl, docusate sodium (also a fecal softener), and sodium picosulfate; cascara, castor oil, oxyphenisatin, and phenolphthalein are obsolete stimulant laxatives;
- fecal softeners, such as arachis oil and the obsolete liquid paraffin;
- osmotic laxatives, such as lactulose, lactitol, the polyethylene glycols, magnesium salts, sodium citrate, and phosphates.

General adverse effects of laxatives

If laxatives of any type are heavily used, not necessarily to the point of abuse, diarrhea will be common, as well as a tendency to nausea and fluid and electrolyte imbalance. The possibility of laxative-induced colonic injury, with damage to the autonomic nervous innervation of the large intestine, has been much discussed and was probably a problem with the violent cathartics formerly used (podophyllin, aloes, and cascara), but is not on record with the laxatives normally used today. Chronic abuse of laxatives, such as senna, can cause changes in colonic structure and function.

Habitual, usually secretive, abuse of laxatives is much more common in women than in men and there is overlap with the anorectic/bulimic syndrome. Abuse of irritant agents such as senna and cascara have been the commonest varieties (SED-10, 704), but many proprietary laxatives have been abused. Abuse can lead to a condition characterized by chronic diarrhea, hypokalemia, and fluid depletion. The features also include hypomagnesemia, hypocalcemia, and hypoalbuminemia, with thirst, lassitude, weight loss, edema, and occasionally osteomalacic bone pain and clubbing. In one small series of cases of laxative abusers, pseudo-Bartter's syndrome was induced; the complications included confusion, convulsions, muscle weakness (with or without paralysis or rhabdomyolysis), and bone changes; hypokalemia and hypophosphatemia were common, and when the laxatives were withdrawn some patients suffered prolonged edema (1).

Bulk-forming laxatives

The bulking agents include vegetable fiber products (such as bran), paraffin and methylcellulose (which absorbs water into the intestinal tract), agar (which expands to form a gel), and psyllium seeds or other mucilaginous plant products. Bulking agents are largely free of adverse effects, but any non-absorbable agent can aggravate symptoms associated with pre-existent intestinal stricture. Abdominal bloating due to bacterial fermentation of unabsorbed carbohydrate is a common sequel to excessive intake. The sugar content of some bulk laxatives can be sufficient to impair diabetic control; the vegetable matter in other preparations can cause bezoars and is potentially allergenic.

Plantago species (psyllium and ispaghula)

Plantago seeds are widely used as bulk laxatives under the names of "psyllium" (from *Plantago psyllium* or *Plantago indica*) and "ispaghula" (from *Plantago ovata*).

Psyllium husk combined with microencapsulated paraffin has been compared with standard psyllium for the treatment of constipation in a randomized, double-blind study (2). There was a significant increase in the weekly number of defecations with the combined formulation, which was well tolerated; no adverse effects were reported.

The efficacy, speed of action, and acceptability of ispaghula husk, lactulose, and other laxatives in the treatment of simple constipation in 394 patients have been studied by 65 general practitioners (3). Ispaghula was used by 224 patients and other laxatives by 170. After 4 weeks of treatment ispaghula husk was assessed by the GPs to be superior to the other laxatives. In patients' assessment, ispaghula users had a higher proportion of normal stools and less soiling than patients using other laxatives. Diarrhea and abdominal pain and gripes and were less common with ispaghula. Distension, flatulence, indigestion, and nausea were equally frequent in the two groups.

Esophageal obstruction by a bezoar after ingestion of psyllium has been reported (4).

- A 69-year-old man with Parkinson's disease developed severe dysphagia after taking granules of the bulk laxative Perdiem (82% psyllium and 18% senna formulated as granules). Disimpaction of the bezoar was performed via a rigid endoscope under general anaesthesia.

Occupational exposure to *Plantago* species has resulted in sensitization, with symptoms ranging from rhinitis and lacrimation to more severe respiratory compromise. This problem arises in a more serious form among the personnel of pharmaceutical factories processing psyllium (SEDA-16, 426), and eosinophilia has also been recorded. The allergen appears to reside in the endosperm or embryonic seed components and not in the husk, which is the laxative component; in principle, therefore, it should be feasible to supply a non-antigenic form of purified psyllium husk (SEDA-17, 423).

Ingestion of psyllium has been associated with rare cases of generalized urticarial rash and anaphylactic shock (5,6). The possibility that the intestinal absorption of lithium and other drugs may be inhibited by psyllium should also be considered (7).

Sterculia

The family of *Sterculia* plants yield a fiber that has bulk laxative effects.

Esophageal obstruction after ingestion of sterculia has been reported (8).

- A 91-year-old man presented with complete esophageal obstruction after taking a tablespoonful of sterculia granules (Normacol) without water. There was no predisposing esophageal disease. The severity of obstruction was such that endoscopic clearance was not possible, and the patient required gastrotomy and manual disimpaction of the lower esophagus.

Stimulant laxatives

All of the anthraquinones can cause cramping and abdominal discomfort. Chronic use can be associated with melanosis coli. The urine can be colored red. The possibility of colonic injury has been discussed (see General adverse effects of laxatives in this monograph). Hepatitis, confirmed by rechallenge, has been reported, possibly due to re-absorption of rhein anthron produced in the intestine (SEDA-16, 425).

The Food and Drug Administration (FDA) has ruled that the stimulant laxatives aloe (including aloe extract and aloe flower extract) and cascara sagrada (including casanthranol, cascara fluidextract aromatic, cascara sagrada bark, cascara sagrada extract, and cascara sagrada fluid extract) in over-the-counter formulations are not safe and effective or are misbranded (9).

Anthranoid derivatives occur in various laxative herbs (such as aloe, *Cascara sagrada*, medicinal rhubarb, and senna) in the form of free anthraquinones, anthrones, dianthrones, and/or O- and C-glycosides derived from these substances. They produce harmless discoloration of the urine. Depending on intrinsic activity and dose, they can also produce abdominal discomfort and cramps, nausea, violent purgation, and dehydration. However, they are all mutagenic and carcinogenic and should not be used in the long term.

In an epidemiological study, chronic abusers of anthranoid laxatives (identified by the detection of pseudomelanosis coli) had an increased relative risk of 3.04 (95% CI = 1.18, 4.90) for colorectal cancer (10).

Anatomical changes in the colon have been reported in patients taking chronic stimulant laxatives, defined as laxative ingestion more than three times a week for a year or more (11). Loss of haustra, which suggests neuronal injury, or damage to colonic longitudinal musculature, was seen in eight of 29 patients who used a variety of diphenylmethane and anthranoid laxatives but in none of the 26 patients who were not using these drugs. In 18 consecutive patients who were chronic users of stimulant laxatives, there was loss of haustra in 15 who took bisacodyl, phenolphthalein, senna, or casanthranol.

Aloe species

Aloe species contain laxative anthranoid derivatives, the main active ingredient being isobarbaloin. Large doses are claimed to cause nephritis and use during pregnancy is discouraged, since intestinal irritation might lead to pelvic congestion. Aloe is thought to aggravate hemorrhoids.

- Melanosis coli occurred in a 39-year-old liver transplant patient who took an over-the-counter product containing aloe, rheum, and frangula (12). The typical brownish pigmentation of the colonic mucosa developed over 10 months. The medication was withdrawn and follow-up colonoscopy 1 year later showed normal-looking mucosa. However, a sessile polypoid lesion was found in the transverse colon. Histology showed tubulovillous adenoma with extensive low-grade dysplasia.

Bisacodyl (rINN)

Bisacodyl increases peristalsis by a direct effect on the small intestine. Its only specific adverse effect is abdominal cramping, which a minority of patients find troublesome. As with other laxatives, however, heavy or chronic use can derange the system in various ways, for example hypokalemia with rhabdomyolysis (SEDA-16, 425).

Bisacodyl tablets plus an unrestricted diet and a phosphate enema has been compared with Picolax (sodium picosulfate + magnesium citrate) plus clear fluids in a randomized, single-blind trial in bowel preparation for colonoscopy in 66 children aged 18 months to 16 years (13). Bowel cleansing was significantly better with Picolax. Compliance with both regimens was excellent. Bisacodyl produced significantly more abdominal pain. Some children given Picolax reported vomiting ($n = 3$) and were distressed because of lack of solid food ($n = 6$). The other adverse effects included abdominal discomfort and fecal incontinence.

Bisacodyl suppositories can make the rectal mucosa appear inflamed (14), and this can be mistaken for idiopathic proctitis. However, the effect is transient.

Cascara sagrada

Cascara sagrada has been reported to cause liver damage (15).

- A 48-year-old man developed cholestatic hepatitis and hypertension shortly after he started to use the herbal laxative *Cascara sagrada*, which contains an anthracene glycoside. He took 1 capsule (425 mg of aged *C. sagrada* bark) tds for 3 days and subsequently developed right upper quadrant pain, nausea, abdominal bloating, anorexia, and jaundice. The *Cascara* was withdrawn, but his symptoms persisted and his liver function tests were abnormal. One week later, he developed ascites and jaundice and underwent liver biopsy, which showed moderately severe portal inflammation, intracanalicular bile stasis, portal bridging fibrosis, and mild steatosis. He gradually improved without specific treatment, and 3 months later his ascites and jaundice had resolved.

Dantron (rINN)

Dantron is a synthetic analogue of the anthraquinones. All are bacterial mutagens, and dantron, in addition to being genotoxic as assessed by DNA repair testing, induces intestinal tumors in animals (SED-11, 788) (16). Emodin, aloe-emodin, and dantron probably act by inhibiting the catalytic activity of topoisomerase (17).

Therefore, the anthraquinones should no longer be used, except to treat constipation in patients with terminal cancer (18). For this purpose, dantron is available as co-danthramer (BAN; dantron + poloxamer 188) and co-danthrusate (BAN; dantron + docusate sodium).

Oxyphenisatine (rINN)

Oxyphenisatine, once a very widely used laxative, was withdrawn before 1980 in most countries because of chronic persistent/active hepatitis; a full account will be found in volumes in this series from 1971.

Phenolphthalein (rINN)

Phenolphthalein was once widely used as a laxative for self-treatment, often camouflaged in chocolate and thus liable to abuse or accidental use; it is now obsolete. Skin rashes of various types are repeatedly reported, sometimes with pruritus. Pigmentation defects have been described. The most serious albeit rare adverse effect on the skin to have been reliably documented is toxic epidermal necrolysis. A fixed drug eruption with bullous erythema multiforme is associated with auto-sensitization, and direct intracellular immunofluorescence is found (19). A hypothesis that phenolphthalein might increase the risk of development of adenomatous colorectal polyps has not been confirmed (20).

The Federal Institute for Drugs and Medical Devices in Germany has recommended that marketing authorizations for phenolphthalein products be revoked, in view of its potential toxic effects (21), including genotoxicity and carcinogenicity (22). Further to the actions taken in the USA and France to withdraw laxative products containing phenolphthalein, the following measures have been taken (23).

Canada After reviewing the benefits and risks associated with the use of phenolphthalein-containing laxatives, Health Canada concluded that there is a risk that phenolphthalein may cause cancer in humans; therefore authority to sell and distribute these products has been revoked.
European Union At a Pharmacovigilance Working Party meeting in September 1997, it was indicated that national competent authorities were either considering immediate suspension of phenolphthalein or were discussing with the relevant marketing authorization holders voluntary withdrawal down to the wholesale level. If voluntary action was not agreed by marketing authorization holders, the national competent authorities concerned would consider suspension of the products.
Japan Manufacturers voluntarily withdrew products containing phenolphthalein.

Rheum palmatum (medicinal rhubarb)

Rhubarb contains the anthranoids, sennosides and rhein. In a study of patients taking regular doses of rhubarb-containing Kampo medicines (extracts or decoctions) and patients taking excess doses, there was tolerance to initial stimulant pain in the abdomen during excess use (24). The authors proposed that the absence of tenderness on pressure over the umbilical region could predict increasing or excess use of rhubarb.

In 14 616 patients who used various Kampo medicines, some of which contained rhubarb, there was no association between the use of rhubarb and the development of gastric carcinoma (25).

Senna

The leaves and fruits of *Cassia angustifolia* and *Cassia senna* contain sennosides, which are laxative anthranoid derivatives. Mutagenicity testing of sennosides has produced negative results in several bacterial and mammalian systems, except for a weak effect in *Salmonella typhimurium* strain TA102 (26,27). There was no evidence of reproductive toxicity of sennosides in rats and rabbits (28). When a standardized formulation containing senna pods (providing 15 mg of sennosides per day) was given to breastfeeding mothers, the suckling infants were only exposed to a non-laxative amount of rhein, which remained a factor of 1000 below the maternal intake of this active metabolite (29). A well-defined purified senna extract was not carcinogenic when given orally to rats in daily doses up to 25 mg/kg for 2 years (30).

Senna is widely used in fairly low doses without serious problems; it is also used in a very high dosage form (X-Prep) to clear the colon before radiological examination. In this form it is generally well tolerated, but it should not be used if there is any predisposition to colonic rupture.

The safety and efficacy of senna have been reviewed (31). Its rhein-anthrone-induced laxative effects occur through two distinct mechanisms, an increase in intestinal fluid transport, which causes accumulation of fluid intraluminally, and an increase in intestinal motility. Senna can cause mild abdominal complaints, such as cramps or pain. Other adverse effects are discoloration of the urine and hemorrhoidal congestion. Prolonged use and overdose can result in diarrhea, extreme loss of electrolytes, especially potassium, damage to the surface epithelium, and impairment of bowel function by damage to autonomic nerves. Abuse of senna has also been associated with melanosis coli, but resolution occurs 8–11 months after withdrawal. Tolerance and genotoxicity do not seem to be problems associated with senna, especially when used periodically in therapeutic doses.

Exceptional complications of senna abuse include hepatitis as well as finger clubbing and hypertrophic osteopathy.

An unusual disulfiram-type reaction reported on one occasion seems to have been due to an interaction of metronidazole with the alcohol present in X-Prep (SEDA-15, 398).

Sodium picosulfate (rINN)

Oral sodium picosulfate and oral sodium phosphate have been compared for bowel preparation before elective colorectal surgery and colonoscopy in randomized studies in 256 patients (32). Oral sodium phosphate was superior to sodium picosulfate on surgical assessment of bowel preparation, fecal residue in the resected specimen, and endoscopic score. However, there was no significant difference with regard to abdominal pain, nausea, vomiting, embarrassment, fear, and fatigue between the two groups.

Oral sodium picosulfate plus magnesium citrate (Picolax) has been compared with a self-administered phosphate enema for bowel preparation before flexible sigmoidoscopy in a randomized, single-blind trial in 1142 subjects (33). A single self-administered phosphate enema about 1 hour before leaving home was a more acceptable and effective method of preparing the distal bowel than oral Picolax. Although more patients felt unwell after taking the enema (15%) than after taking Picolax (7%), over 80% in both groups felt normal. More of the itemized adverse effects were rated as moderate or severe in the Picolax group, including wind, incontinence, and sleep disturbance. Anal soreness was reported more frequently in the enema group. The other reported adverse effects were abdominal pain/cramps, nausea/vomiting, and faintness/dizziness.

Two cases of generalized urticarial skin reactions occurred after a first dose of sodium picosulfate (34). This may have represented an interaction with aminosalicylate derivatives, which were being administered at the same time, or a simple adverse effect to one of the agents.

A dubious case of status epilepticus attributed to picosulfate has been published (SEDA-16, 425).

Fecal softeners

Liquid paraffin

It has been recommended for many years that the use of liquid paraffin should be discontinued because of its propensity to cause malabsorption of fat-soluble vitamins, to leak and soil the perineal skin, and to cause lipid pneumonia if aspirated; at the very least it should be avoided in young children (35).

Osmotic laxatives

The osmotic laxatives include inorganic salts and the synthetic disaccharide, lactulose, as well as magnesium salts and sodium phosphate. Osmotic agents are largely free of adverse effects, apart from flatulence, cramps, and abdominal discomfort.

Lactulose (rINN) and lactitol (rINN)

Lactulose is a non-absorbable disaccharide that is hydrolysed in the large bowel by intestinal bacteria, yielding monosaccharides that act as osmotic agents; it is also metabolized to hydrogen and carbon dioxide.

In a double-blind, placebo-controlled study in 10 healthy volunteers, lactulose powder 10 g/day for 26–33 days was an effective food-grade prebiotic (36). Fecal bifidobacteria increased significantly during lactulose intake, with a concomitant decrease in *Clostridia*.

The most common adverse effects of lactulose are flatulence, cramps, and abdominal discomfort. Non-toxic megacolon has been seen in some elderly patients and, as with other laxatives, there is always a possibility of dependence (SEDA-11, 374).

- Two women aged 88 and 82 taking lactulose for constipation, developed life-threatening dilatation of the bowel (16). Both underwent surgery. One had cancer of the bowel and an uneventful postoperative recovery. No mechanical abnormalities were found in the second patient but she died in respiratory insufficiency after aspiration.

Low-dose polyethylene glycol electrolyte solution and lactulose have been compared in chronic constipation in a randomized multicenter study in 115 patients with chronic constipation (37). After 4 weeks the patients who took polyethylene glycol had a higher number of stools, a lower median daily score for straining at stool, and greater overall improvement than patients who took lactulose. Except that significantly fewer patients who took polyethylene glycol reported flatus, other adverse effects were similar in the two groups and included liquid stools, abdominal pain, bloating, and rumbling.

- Pneumatosis intestinalis and pneumoperitoneum have been reported in a 57-year-old cirrhotic man with colonic inertia who had been taking oral lactulose 30 ml tds (38). Because of constipation the dose of lactulose had been gradually increased to 60 ml qds together with lactulose enemas. Both conditions resolved 3 days after oral lactulose was withdrawn.

Lactitol is another disaccharide, similar to lactulose. It has been claimed to be more palatable and to have fewer adverse effects (SEDA-18, 374), but it has not been used as widely as lactulose.

The effects of lactulose and lactitol in daily doses of 18–36 g for 6 months have been evaluated in a prospective, open study in 31 cirrhotic patients with chronic encephalopathy (38). Mean daily stool frequency (2.5 versus 1.7) and the frequency of reported adverse effects (59 versus 14%) were significantly higher with lactulose. Common adverse effects were nausea, intestinal discomfort, flatulence, and diarrhea.

There has been a systematic review of 30 randomized comparisons in hepatic encephalopathy of lactulose or lactitol with no intervention, placebo, or antibiotics and comparisons of lactulose with lactitol (39). Compared with placebo or no intervention, non-absorbable disaccharides had no statistically significant effect on mortality, but appeared to reduce the risk of no improvement of hepatic encephalopathy. However, this result might have reflected bias, owing to the poor quality of the majority of the studies.

Phosphates

Oral sodium phosphate 90 ml mixed with 300 ml of clear liquid has been compared with 2 liters of polyethylene glycol solution in a colonoscopist-blinded, randomized trial in 100 patients undergoing colonoscopy as a day-care procedure (40). Sodium phosphate was well tolerated and safe and provided bowel cleansing similar to polyethylene glycol. Five patients who received polyethylene glycol and four who received sodium phosphate reported nausea, and eight patients who received polyethylene glycol and one who received sodium phosphate complained of abdominal fullness.

The standard regimen of sodium phosphate used for bowel cleansing before colonoscopy is 40 tablets (60 g). In a randomized, multicenter, endoscopist-blinded trial in 98 patients undergoing colonoscopy, two smaller doses of sodium phosphate, 28 tablets (42 g) and 32 tablets (48 g), were effective (quality of colon cleansing excellent or good in over 80%) and well tolerated (41). The incidences of adverse effects were similar in the two groups. The reported adverse effects were nausea, vomiting, dizziness, and headache.

Tonic-clonic seizures have been reported in four adults who took oral sodium phosphate as Visicol (InKline Pharmaceutical; total 40 tablets) for bowel cleansing before colonoscopy (42). None of the patients had a history of seizures or electrolyte abnormalities. In all cases the seizures were associated with electrolyte abnormalities, mainly hyponatremia, after administration of Visicol.

Aphthous ulcers in the rectal mucosa have been reported in association with the use of Fleet-phospho-soda enema in preparation for colonoscopy in a 54-year-old woman (43).

Bowel cleansing solutions

Colonic ulceration has been attributed to the use of hydrogen peroxide in an enema (44).

- A 13-year-old girl was given 10% hydrogen peroxide as an enema for constipation. She developed severe rectal bleeding, and colonoscopy showed mucosal ulceration up to the splenic flexure. Histology confirmed ulceration due to traumatic burns. She improved gradually on conservative treatment, and 2 months later a repeat colonoscopy was normal.

References

1. Meyers AM, Feldman C, Sonnekus MI, Ninin DT, Margolius LP, Whalley NA. Chronic laxative abusers with pseudo-idiopathic oedema and autonomous pseudo-Bartter's syndrome. A spectrum of metabolic madness, or new lights on an old disease? S Afr Med J 1990;78(11):631–6.
2. Chicouri MJ. Estudo clinico do psyllium husk associado a parafina microencapsulada no tratamento da constipacao intestinal essencial. Rev Bras Med 2001;58:672–6.
3. Dettmar PW, Sykes J. A multi-centre, general practice comparison of ispaghula husk with lactulose and other laxatives in the treatment of simple constipation. Curr Med Res Opin 1998;14(4):227–33.
4. Shulman LM, Minagar A, Weiner WJ. Perdiem causing esophageal obstruction in Parkinson's disease. Neurology 1999;52(3):670–1.
5. Lantner RR, Espiritu BR, Zumerchik P, Tobin MC. Anaphylaxis following ingestion of a psyllium-containing cereal. JAMA 1990;264(19):2534–6.
6. Spence JD, Huff MW, Heidenheim P, Viswanatha A, Munoz C, Lindsay R, Wolfe B, Mills D. Combination therapy with colestipol and psyllium mucilloid in patients with hyperlipidemia. Ann Intern Med 1995;123(7):493–9.
7. Perlman BB. Interaction between lithium salts and ispaghula husk. Lancet 1990;335(8686):416.
8. Brown DC, Doughty JC, George WD. Surgical treatment of oesophageal obstruction after ingestion of a granular laxative. Postgrad Med J 1999;75(880):106.
9. Food and Drug Administration, HHS. Status of certain additional over-the-counter drug category II and III active ingredients. Final rule. Fed Regist 2002;67(90):31125–7.
10. Siegers CP, von Hertzberg-Lottin E, Otte M, Schneider B. Anthranoid laxative abuse—a risk for colorectal cancer? Gut 1993 Aug;34(8):1099–101.
11. Joo JS, Ehrenpreis ED, Gonzalez L, Kaye M, Breno S, Wexner SD, Zaitman D, Secrest K. Alterations in colonic anatomy induced by chronic stimulant laxatives: the cathartic colon revisited. J Clin Gastroenterol 1998;26(4):283–6.

12. Willems M, van Buuren HR, de Krijger R. Anthranoid self-medication causing rapid development of melanosis coli. Neth J Med 2003;61(1):22–4.
13. Pinfield A, Stringer MD. Randomised trial of two pharmacological methods of bowel preparation for day case colonoscopy. Arch Dis Child 1999;80(2):181–3.
14. Sand P. Tgn pa inflammation og blodning i rektalslimhinden ved behandling af rektal obstipation med fosfatklysma og bisakodyl-rektaltube. [Signs of inflammation and hemorrhage in the rectal mucosa during therapy of rectal constipation with phosphate enemata and bisacodyl rectal tube.] Ugeskr Laeger 1978;140(34):2041–4.
15. Nadir A, Reddy D, Van Thiel DH. *Cascara sagrada*-induced intrahepatic cholestasis causing portal hypertension: case report and review of herbal hepatotoxicity. Am J Gastroenterol 2000;95(12):3634–7.
16. van der Vliet HJ, van Bodegraven AA. Megacolon tijdens lactulosetherapie. [Megacolon during treatment with lactulose.] Ned Tijdschr Geneeskd 2004;148(20):998–1001.
17. Mueller SO, Stopper H. Characterization of the genotoxicity of anthraquinones in mammalian cells. Biochim Biophys Acta 1999;1428(2–3):406–14.
18. Anonymous. Laxatives containing dantron—voluntary withdrawal. WHO Pharm Newslett 1998;112:4.
19. Shelley WB, Schlappner OL, Heiss HB. Demonstration of intercellular immunofluorescence and epidermal hysteresis in bullous fixed drug eruption due to phenolphthalein. Br J Dermatol 1972;86(2):118–25.
20. Longnecker MP, Sandler DP, Haile RW, Sandler RS. Phenolphthalein-containing laxative use in relation to adenomatous colorectal polyps in three studies. Environ Health Perspect 1997;105(11):1210–2.
21. Anonymous. Laxatives containing phenolphthalein—recommendation to revoke marketing authorization. WHO Pharm Newslett 1997,112:3.
22. Anonymous. Laxatives containing dantron and phenolphthalein-unacceptable ingredients in OTC drug products. WHO Pharm Newslett. 1999;3,4:3.
23. Anonymous. Laxatives containing phenolphthalein—voluntary withdrawal. WHO Pharm Newslett 1998;112: 4–5.
24. Mantani N, Kogure T, Sakai S, Kainuma M, Kasahara Y, Niizawa A, Shimada Y, Terasawa K. A comparative study between excess-dose users and regular-dose users of rhubarb contained in Kampo medicines. Phytomedicine 2002;9(5):373–6.
25. Mantani N, Sekiya N, Sakai S, Kogure T, Shimada Y, Terasawa K. Rhubarb use in patients treated with Kampo medicines—a risk for gastric cancer? Yakugaku Zasshi 2002;122(6):403–5.
26. Mengs U. Toxic effects of sennosides in laboratory animals and in vitro. Pharmacology 1988;36(Suppl 1):180–7.
27. Sandnes D, Johansen T, Teien G, Ulsaker G. Mutagenicity of crude senna and senna glycosides in *Salmonella typhimurium*. Pharmacol Toxicol 1992;71(3 Pt 1):165–72.
28. Mengs U. Reproductive toxicological investigations with sennosides. Arzneimittelforschung 1986;36(9):1355–8.
29. Faber P, Strenge-Hesse A. Relevance of rhein excretion into breast milk. Pharmacology 1988;36(Suppl 1):212–20.
30. Lydén-Sokolowski A, Nilsson A, Sjöberg P. Two-year carcinogenicity study with sennosides in the rat: emphasis on gastro-intestinal alterations. Pharmacology 1993;47(Suppl 1): 209–15.
31. Mascolo N, Capasso R, Capasso F. Senna. A safe and effective drug. Phytother Res 1998;12(Suppl 1):S143–5.
32. Yoshioka K, Connolly AB, Ogunbiyi OA, Hasegawa H, Morton DG, Keighley MR. Randomized trial of oral sodium phosphate compared with oral sodium picosulphate (Picolax) for elective colorectal surgery and colonoscopy. Dig Surg 2000;17(1):66–70.
33. Atkin WS, Hart A, Edwards R, Cook CF, Wardle J, McIntyre P, Aubrey R, Baron C, Sutton S, Cuzick J, Senapati A, Northover JM. Single blind, randomised trial of efficacy and acceptability of oral picolax versus self administered phosphate enema in bowel preparation for flexible sigmoidoscopy screening. BMJ 2000;320(7248): 1504–9.
34. McBride K. Sodium picosulphate: reaction or drug interaction? Clin Radiol 1992;45(4):290.
35. Anonymous. Liquid paraffin—restricted indications and availability. Int Pharm J 1990;4:205.
36. Tuohy KM, Ziemer CJ, Klinder A, Knobel Y, Pool-Zobel BL, Gibson GR. A human volunteer study to determine the prebiotic effects of lactulose powder on human colonic microbiota. Microb Ecol Health Dis 2002;14:165–73.
37. Attar A, Lemann M, Ferguson A, Halphen M, Boutron MC, Flourie B, Alix E, Salmeron M, Guillemot F, Chaussade S, Menard AM, Moreau J, Naudin G, Barthet M. Comparison of a low dose polyethylene glycol electrolyte solution with lactulose for treatment of chronic constipation. Gut 1999;44(2):226–30.
38. Shibasaki K, Tsuboi Y, Hasegawa K, Toshima M, Soga K. Effects of long-term administration of lactitol or lactulose in cirrhotic patients with chronic hepatic encephalopathy. Ther Res 2001;22:899–907.
39. Als-Nielsen B, Gluud LL, Gluud C. Non-absorbable disaccharides for hepatic encephalopathy: systematic review of randomised trials. BMJ 2004;328(7447):1046.
40. Reddy DN, Rao GV, Sriram PV. Efficacy and safety of oral sodium phosphate versus polyethylene glycol solution for bowel preparation for colonoscopy. Indian J Gastroenterol 2002;21(6):219–21.
41. Rex DK, Chasen R, Pochapin MB. Safety and efficacy of two reduced dosing regimens of sodium phosphate tablets for preparation prior to colonoscopy. Aliment Pharmacol Ther 2002;16(5):937–44.
42. Mackey AC, Shaffer D, Prizont R. Seizure associated with the use of Visicol for colonoscopy. N Engl J Med 2002;346(26):2095.
43. Berthelet O, Rolachon A, Papillon E, Fournet J. Lésions rectales induites par la préparation colique Fleet-Phospho-soda®. [Rectal mucosal lesions associated with Fleet-Phospho-soda.] Gastroenterol Clin Biol 2001;25(4): 437–9.
44. Bollen P, Goossens A, Hauser B, Vandenplas Y. Colonic ulcerations caused by an enema containing hydrogen peroxide. J Pediatr Gastroenterol Nutr 1998;26(2):232–3.

Lead

General Information

Lead is a heavy soft bluish-gray metal (symbol Pb; atomic no. 82) that is widespread as different salts in minerals such as chromite (oxide), crocoisite (chromate), Jamesonite and zinkenite (sulfides), mimetite (arsenate and chloride), pyromorphite (phosphate and chloride), and vanadinite (vanadate and chloride).

Lead has no place in internal medical treatment, although lead acetate has retained a very small place as an astringent. Its toxic effects are known primarily from environmental and occupational exposure and occasionally from the use of alternative remedies or cosmetics. For example, lead sulfide in eye-drops originating in India has caused lead poisoning, and lead has been found in some supposed aphrodisiacs from India. Children with circulating lead concentrations in excess of 600 ng/ml have impaired intellectual performance and electrocardiographic changes, and at any age excessive intake can cause encephalopathy, neuropathies, anemia, anorexia, colic, and renal damage. Lead poisoning from occupational and environmental sources continues to be reported. The biological chemistry of lead has been reviewed (1).

No significant effects have been attributed to lead as a contaminant in infant formulas or total parenteral nutrition. In an investigation of the protective effect of calcium supplements against lead absorption, 103 infants aged 3.5–6.0 months were randomly assigned to receive an infant formula (iron-fortified, containing 465 micrograms/ml of calcium and 317 micrograms/ml of phosphate) or the same formula with added calcium glycerophosphate (1800 micrograms/ml of calcium and 1390 micrograms/ml of phosphate) for 9 months (2). There was no significant difference between the groups in the mean ratio of urinary calcium to creatinine, serum calcium, or serum phosphorus, nor any change in iron status. At month 4, the median increase was 0.07 μmol/l in the control group and 0.04 μmol/l in the supplemented group. This significant effect was attenuated during the latter half of the trial, with overall increases in blood lead of 0.12 μmol/l in controls and 0.10 μmol/l in the supplemented group. Supplementation did not have a measurable effect on urinary calcium excretion, calcium homeostasis, or iron status. The significant effect on blood lead concentration was expected, although it was not sustained during the whole study, and so no prevention could be concluded.

Herbal remedies

Raised blood lead concentrations in an adult have been attributed to an Asian remedy for menstrual cramps ("Koo Sar Pills") (3).

- A Cambodian woman, her husband, and their two children were screened at a free lead-screening event sponsored by a nursing school community health promotion. The husband and children had normal blood lead concentrations, but the woman had a concentration of 440 ng/ml. She reported no symptoms associated with lead poisoning (for example, muscle pains or weakness, headaches, or loss of appetite). Samples of any medicines, teas, or cosmetics that she had used that might have been the source of the lead were analysed. Lead was found only in bottles of red tablets, at concentrations of 3.5 ppm from one bottle and 1.2 ppm in a second bottle. For 3–4 years she had taken six of these tablets a day on 7 days of each month to treat menstrual cramps. She stopped taking them, and her blood lead concentrations fell from 280 to 12 ng/ml over 6 months. Further laboratory analysis of other bottles showed lead in amounts of 12.5 ppm in tablets from a third bottle and 4.5 ppm in tablets from a fourth bottle. The tablets were traced to a San Francisco-based Hong Kong company who sold them in packages with the brand name listed on the outside of the package as "Koo So Pills" and on the package insert as "Koo Sar Pills." The package literature was written in Chinese. Lead was not among the 11 listed ingredients. The insert stated "These medical pills are good for general debility." The directions for dosage were one pill taken with warm water twice a day (not six per day). The lead content in samples purchased at different shops in San Francisco was 2.7 ppm (0.9 micrograms/tablet) and 4.3 ppm (1.4 micrograms/tablet).

No other cases of lead poisoning have been reported in association with Koo Sar tablets, and it is thought that the varying lead concentrations in the different tablets resulted from varying amounts of lead present during the manufacture of the red dye.

- A 23-year-old Asian butcher developed diffuse abdominal pain, vomiting, and diarrhea, followed by constipation (4). He had a sinus tachycardia and generalized abdominal tenderness without peritonism. His serum bilirubin concentration and alanine transaminase activity were raised, but alkaline phosphatase activity, albumin concentration, and prothrombin time were normal. He had a blood lead concentration of 767 ng/ml and a raised zinc protoporphyrin concentration, diagnostic of lead poisoning. He had taken an herbal medicine, purchased in India, for vague ailments. He stopped taking it, and 3 months later was asymptomatic, with normal liver function tests and marked falls in blood lead (387 ng/ml) and zinc protoporphyrin.

Lead toxicity has been reported in a child who was exposed to lead in a Tibetan herbal remedy (5).

- A 5-year-old Indian boy had static encephalopathy, seizures, and developmental delay from neonatal asphyxia and was referred to a hematologist for persistent anemia (hemoglobin 9.2 g/dl) without basophilic stippling, refractory to iron therapy. He was alert and active but nonverbal, able to stand with support but not able to walk, and had no focal neurological defects. Skeletal and abdominal X-rays showed no lead lines and no gastric lead particles. He had normal iron stores and normal hemoglobin electrophoresis. The blood lead concentration was 860 ng/ml. He was given EDTA and dimercaprol (BAL), and his lead concentration fell to 256 ng/ml. His mother had been giving him a Tibetan herbal vitamin, in the form of tablets, three times a day for the previous 5 years. A traditional medicine healer had told her that the tablets were pure medicinal herbs and plants prepared according to ancient Tibetan pharmacological traditions. They were said to be free from harmful or toxic substances and would actually promote brain growth and improve his mental capabilities. The tablets were produced in India and each was individually wrapped. They were analysed for lead, arsenic, cadmium, and mercury, and it was estimated that he had ingested about 63 g of lead over 4 years. Seven months later his blood lead concentration was 760 ng/ml and he was given EDTA and BAL. On day 2 he had a tonic-clonic seizure lasting 1 minute and his urinary lead concentration was 2310 ng/ml. On discharge his blood lead concentration was 413 ng/ml. During the next 4 years he had a further six chelation treatments with succimer when his lead concentration was over 450 ng/ml. After 4 years his lead concentration was 245 ng/ml.

Topical lead

A 64-year-old woman had treated extensive ulcers of both legs with daily dressings of diachylon ointment, containing 15% lead oxide, for more than a year. She then developed general weakness, loss of weight, anemia, hypotension, and neuropathy. Lead concentrations in the blood were increased three-fold and urinary lead concentrations ten-fold, and a diagnosis of percutaneous lead intoxication was made. Treatment with dimercaptopropane sulfonic acid resulted in considerable reduction of the lead deposits, and the symptoms of poisoning subsided (6).

Second-Generation Effects

Fetotoxicity

Intrauterine lead intoxication has been reported.

- A 24-year-old pregnant woman, who had recently emigrated from India, had periodically over the course of 9 years taken tablets prescribed by an Ayurvedic doctor for a gastrointestinal complaint. The tablets had a high lead content. She presented at 30 weeks gestation with abdominal pain and progressive confusion, culminating in seizures (7). Her erythrocytes showed typical basophilic stippling and her blood lead concentration was 5.2 (reference range 0.06–0.6) μmol/l. She was given intramuscular dimercaprol and intravenous calcium disodium edetate and 36 hours later had an antepartum hemorrhage; labor was induced and she gave birth by vaginal delivery to a 1.6 kg girl, who was flaccid and areflexic and did not move in response to noxious stimuli, but had spontaneous ocular movements. She had bilateral diaphragmatic palsy. The cord blood lead concentration was 7.6 μmol/l, the erythrocyte porphyrin concentration was 20 (reference range 0.4–1.7) μmol/l, and radiography of the long bones showed increased bone density adjacent to the metaphyses. The infant was given chelation dimercaprol (4 mg/kg every 4 hours) and intravenous calcium disodium edetate 50 mg/kg. The blood lead concentration initially rose to 12 μmol/l and then fell rapidly over the next few days. A high urinary lead concentration on day 4 (52 μmol/l) showed that lead was being excreted. Facial, bulbar, proximal limb, and diaphragmatic muscle activity improved.

References

1. Godwin HA. The biological chemistry of lead. Curr Opin Chem Biol 2001;5(2):223–7.
2. Sargent JD, Dalton MA, O'Connor GT, Olmstead EM, Klein RZ. Randomized trial of calcium glycerophosphate-supplemented infant formula to prevent lead absorption. Am J Clin Nutr 1999;69(6):1224–30.
3. Anonymous. Asian remedy for menstrual cramps ("Koo Sar Pills")—lead poisoning in an adult reported. WHO Pharm Newslett 1999;5/6:6.
4. Anderson NR, Gama R, Kapadia S. Herbal remedy poisoning presenting with acute abdomen and raised urine porphyrins. Ann Clin Biochem 2001;38(Pt 4):408–10.
5. Moore C, Adler R. Herbal vitamins: lead toxicity and developmental delay. Pediatrics 2000;106(3):600–2.
6. Bialonczyk C, Partsch H, Donner A. Bleivergiftung durch langzeitanwendung von Diachylonsalbe. [Lead poisoning caused by long-term use of Diachylon ointment.] Z Hautkr 1989;64(12):1118–20.
7. Tait PA, Vora A, James S, Fitzgerald DJ, Pester BA. Severe congenital lead poisoning in a preterm infant due to a herbal remedy. Med J Aust 2002;177(4):193–5.

Lefetamine

General Information

Lefetamine is an opioid receptor partial agonist, which combines the actions of amphetamines with opioid-like effects. It was a drug of abuse in Japan in the 1950s and later also in Italy (1). In 10 opiate addicts, lefetamine relieved acute opiate withdrawal symptoms and did not precipitate withdrawal symptoms in stable addicts (2).

During ordinary use sedation, tiredness, gastrointestinal disturbances, headache, sweating, and flushing have been observed with lefetamine (3).

References

1. Janiri L, Mannelli P, Pirrongelli C, Lo Monaco M, Tempesta E. Lephetamine abuse and dependence: clinical effects and withdrawal syndrome. Br J Addict 1989;84(1):89–95.
2. Mannelli P, Janiri L, De Marinis M, Tempesta E. Lefetamine: new abuse of an old drug—clinical evaluation of opioid activity. Drug Alcohol Depend 1989;24(2):95–101.
3. De Angelis L. Lefetamine hydrochloride. Drugs Today 1983;19:82.

Leflunomide

General Information

The prodrug leflunomide (*N*-(4′-trifluoromethylphenyl)-5-methylisoxazole-4-carboxamide) is an isoxazole derivative. Its main metabolite is the active compound, A77 1726 (1).

Mechanism of action

A77 1726 inhibits dihydro-rate dehydrogenase, the rate-limiting enzyme in pyrimidine synthesis. It inhibits the proliferation of T and B cells, and probably acts via the production and action of interleukin-2. Besides its immunomodulatory action, A77 1726 also has an anti-inflammatory action by inhibition of nuclear factor kappa B (NFκB), tumor necrosis factor alfa (TNF-α), and interleukin 1 beta (IL-1β), and increased production of transforming growth factor beta-1 (TGF-β1) (2–5).

Pharmacokinetics

After oral administration, leflunomide undergoes rapid metabolism in the gut wall, plasma, and liver to A77 1726 (M1), peak plasma concentrations of which are reached after 6–12 hours. A77 1726 is highly (99%) bound to plasma proteins. Its pharmacokinetics are not affected by food, and dosage requirements are not influenced by age or sex. Enterohepatic recirculation and biliary recycling contribute to the long half-life of 2 weeks. About 90% of a single dose of leflunomide is eliminated, 43% in the urine, primarily as leflunomide glucuronides and an oxalinic acid derivative of A77 1726, and 48% in the feces, primarily as A77 1726. Impaired renal function can result in increased plasma concentrations of A77 1726. Elimination of A77 1726 can be dramatically increased by using colestyramine or activated charcoal (6,7).

Indications and clinical efficacy

Leflunomide has anti-inflammatory, immunosuppressive, and virustatic effects. Its efficacy has been demonstrated in patients with rheumatoid arthritis and psoriatic arthritis and other conditions in randomized, double-blind, placebo-controlled trials and other studies (8–32), and it was approved for treatment of adult rheumatoid arthritis in August 1998 (Table 1) (33). In three large phase III trials (US301, $n = 482$; MN301, $n = 358$; MN302, $n = 999$), leflunomide was as effective and well tolerated as methotrexate and sulfasalazine and superior to placebo (34). These data were confirmed by a meta-analysis (35,36). Leflunomide is therefore indicated for patients with rheumatoid arthritis who have failed first-line disease modifying anti-rheumatic drug therapy on the basis of efficacy, safety, and costs (36). It is effective as monotherapy and in combination with methotrexate or infliximab (6).

Clinical experience with leflunomide in patients with other autoimmune diseases is limited. Extended indications for the use of leflunomide include treatment of Crohn's disease in patients who are intolerant of standard immunomodulator therapy (31), chronic sarcoidosis (32), maintenance therapy of complete or partial remission in Wegener's granulomatosis (30), and mild to moderate systemic lupus erythematosus (29) (Table 1).

Leflunomide has been used as an immunosuppressive agent in kidney and liver transplant recipients to spare calcineurin inhibitors and glucocorticoids and to slow progression of chronic kidney graft dysfunction (28,37) (Table 1).

In animals, leflunomide had excellent antiviral activity against cytomegalovirus (CMV). It is currently indicated as second-line therapy for CMV disease after solid organ transplantation and in recipients intolerant of ganciclovir (38). Leflunomide also reduces HIV replication by about 75% at concentrations that can be obtained with conventional dosing (39).

General adverse drug reactions

The safety profile of leflunomide has been said to be excellent, with no myelosuppressive or nephrotoxic adverse effects (40,41). Its major adverse effects are gastrointestinal symptoms (diarrhea and nausea), abnormal liver function tests, skin rashes and pruritus, allergic reactions, alopecia, infections, weight loss, and hypertension (35,42–45). Minor adverse effects are musculoskeletal disorders. Rare adverse effects include sepsis, pancytopenia, interstitial lung disease, hypertriglyceridemia, vasculitis, aseptic meningitis, reversible neuropathy, and serious skin reactions (35,46–49).

In 3325 patients who took leflunomide, the rate of drug withdrawal was 42% within 33 months after approval by the US Food and Drugs Administration, and was more likely in patients who received a loading dose. The most common causes of discontinuation were inefficacy (30%), gastrointestinal symptoms (29%), non-adherence to therapy or loss to follow-up (14%), and raised liver enzymes (5%) (50).

However, the rate of adverse effects associated with leflunomide was significantly lower than with methotrexate and other disease-modifying antirheumatic drugs (DMARDs) in an analysis of 40 594 patients with rheumatoid arthritis (8,51). The incidences of adverse events per 1000 patient-years were as follows:

- no DMARDs: 383
- methotrexate: 145
- leflunomide monotherapy: 94
- methotrexate + other DMARDs: 70
- leflunomide + other DMARDs: 59
- leflunomide + methotrexate: 43
- other DMARDs: 143.

Leflunomide monotherapy also had the lowest rate of hepatic events in the DMARD monotherapy groups.

Further developments

Synthetic malononitrilamides (MNA) have been derived from A77 1726. FK778 is the most promising derivative, because of its much shorter half-life. It also blocks replication of herpesvirus in vitro and in vivo. It has therefore been used as part of an immunosuppressive regimen and as an antiviral agent after solid organ transplantation (52). FK778 is under investigation in a phase II trial after kidney transplantation (53).

Organs and Systems

Cardiovascular

The incidence of hypertension in patients with rheumatoid arthritis taking leflunomide 25 mg/day was 11% in a phase II trial (54). During phase III trials, there was new-onset hypertension in 2.1–3.7% (9,10). Increased sympathetic drive has been implicated in its pathogenesis, because leflunomide-induced hypertension is accompanied by an increased heart rate (55). However, this hypothesis remains to be tested.

Pulmonary hypertension has been described in association with leflunomide (56).

Respiratory

Respiratory symptoms in the MN301, US301, and MN302 trials in patients with rheumatoid arthritis included respiratory infections (21–27%), bronchitis (5–8%), increased cough (4–5%), rhinitis (2–5%), pharyngitis (2–3%), pneumonia (2–3%), and sinusitis (1–5%) (9,10,12).

Table 1 Summary of the efficacy of leflunomide in controlled trials

Disease	Type of study; duration	Intervention	Outcome	References
Rheumatoid arthritis	Double-blind, randomized, controlled trial; 24 weeks	Leflunomide 50–100 mg/day for 1 day, then 5–25 mg/day ($n = 300$) versus placebo ($n = 102$)	Leflunomide 10 and 25 mg/day was significantly more effective than placebo	(8)
Rheumatoid arthritis	Double-blind, randomized, controlled trial; 12 months	Leflunomide 100 mg/day for 3 days, thereafter 20 mg/day ($n = 182$) versus methotrexate 7.5–15 mg/week ($n = 180$) versus placebo ($n = 118$)	American College of Rheumatology response and success rates were: leflunomide 52% and 41%, methotrexate 46% and 35%, and placebo 26% and 19%	(9)
Rheumatoid arthritis	Double-blind, randomized, controlled trial; 24 weeks	Leflunomide 100 mg/day for 3 days, then 20 mg/day ($n = 133$) versus sulfasalazine 2 g/day ($n = 133$) versus placebo ($n = 92$)	American College of Rheumatology 20 response rates were: leflunomide 55%, sulfasalazine 56%, and placebo 29%	(10,11)
Rheumatoid arthritis	Double-blind, randomized, controlled trial; 52 weeks	Leflunomide 100 mg/day for 3 days, then 20 mg/day ($n = 501$) versus methotrexate 7.5–15 mg/day ($n = 498$)	Both drugs effective, although methotrexate resulted in significantly greater improvement in tender and swollen joint counts compared with leflunomide	(12)
Rheumatoid arthritis	Double–blind, randomized, controlled trial; 6 months	Leflunomide 100 mg/day for 3 days, then 20 mg/day ($n = 133$) versus sulfasalazine 0.5–2 g/day ($n = 133$), versus placebo ($n = 92$)	Leflunomide slowed disease progression as early as 6 months, and there was continued retardation of radiographic progression at 2 years	(13)
Rheumatoid arthritis	Follow-up study; 2 years	Leflunomide ($n = 98$) versus methotrexate ($n = 101$)	American College of Rheumatology 20, 50, and 70 response rates for leflunomide versus methotrexate were 79 versus 67%, 56 versus 43%, and 26 versus 20%	(14)
Rheumatoid arthritis	Follow-up study; 2 years	Leflunomide 20 mg/day versus sulfasalazine 2 g/day	American College of Rheumatology 20 response rates were 82% leflunomide versus 60% sulfasalazine after 24 months	(15)
Rheumatoid arthritis	Follow-up study; 5 years	Leflunomide 10–20 mg/day (phase III) continued ($n = 214$)	American College of Rheumatology 20, 50, and 70 response rates after 1 year were maintained for up to 5 years	(16)
Rheumatoid arthritis	Single-center experience; 32 weeks	Leflunomide 100 mg/day for 3 days, then 20 mg/day plus infliximab 3 mg/kg at 2, 4, 8, 16, and 24 weeks ($n = 20$)	11/20 withdrawn (four infliximab infusion reactions, one Stevens–Johnson syndrome); the other patients achieved American College of Rheumatology 20 and 70 response rates in >80% and 46%	(17)
Rheumatoid arthritis	Double-blind randomized controlled trial; 24 weeks	Leflunomide 100 mg/day for 2 days, then 10 mg/day ($n = 130$) versus placebo ($n = 133$), both with methotrexate 10–25 mg/day	American College of Rheumatology 20 rates at 24 weeks: leflunomide + methotrexate 46% versus placebo + methotrexate 20%; similar drug withdrawal and adverse events rates	(18)
Rheumatoid arthritis	Multicenter experience; 24 weeks	Leflunomide 100 mg/day for 3 days, then 20 mg/day ($n = 969$)	191 withdrawn (107 adverse events, 26 lack of efficacy, 58 other reasons); 24% good and 45% moderate responses on the disease activity score, and 61%, 34%, and 9.6% achieved American College of Rheumatology 20, 50, and 70 response rates	(19)
Rheumatoid arthritis	Single-center experience; 3 months	Leflunomide 100 mg/day for 3 days, then 20 mg/day plus infliximab 3 mg/kg at 0, 6, and every 8 weeks ($n = 17$)	20 adverse effects in 13 patients; 8 discontinued	(20)
Rheumatoid arthritis	Single-center experience; 24 weeks,	Leflunomide 100 mg/day for 3 days, then 100 mg/week ($n = 50$)	American College of Rheumatology 20, 50, and 70 response rates at 24 weeks were 74%, 64%, and 28% (five withdrawn, six lost to follow-up)	(21)

Continued

Table 1 Continued

Disease	Type of study; duration	Intervention	Outcome	References
Rheumatoid arthritis	Single-center experience; 6 months	Leflunomide 100 mg/day for 3 days, then 20 mg/day ($n = 378$)	American College of Rheumatology 20, 50, and 70 response rates at 6 months were 48%, 25%, and 12%	(22)
Rheumatoid arthritis	Extension of double-blind, randomized, controlled trial; 48 weeks	Leflunomide + methotrexate continued ($n = 96$) and placebo + methotrexate switched to leflunomide 10 mg/day + methotrexate ($n = 96$)	American College of Rheumatology 20 response rate was 59% at 24 weeks and 55% at 48 weeks in patients maintained on leflunomide + methotrexate, and patients switched from placebo to leflunomide + methotrexate increased their American College of Rheumatology 20 response rates from 25% at 24 weeks to 57% at 48 weeks	(23)
Rheumatoid arthritis	Double-blind, randomized, controlled trial; 24 weeks	Leflunomide 10 mg/day and 100 mg on day 3 ($n = 202$) versus 20 mg/day and 100 mg on days 1–3 ($n = 200$)	American College of Rheumatology (20 response rates: leflunomide 10 mg 50% and 20 mg 57%; adverse events: leflunomide 10 mg 15% and 20 mg 12%	(24)
Rheumatoid arthritis	Multicenter experience; 11–911 days	Leflunomide 100 mg/day for 3 days, then 20 mg/day ($n = 136$)	76% clinical response after 12 months, but 76/136 (56%) leflunomide withdrawn (29% adverse drug reactions and 13% lack of efficacy)	(25)
Psoriatic arthropathy, psoriasis	Double-blind, randomized, controlled trial; 24 weeks	Leflunomide 100 mg/day for 3 days, then 20 mg/day ($n = 95$) versus placebo ($n = 91$)	Leflunomide 59% and placebo 30% were responders at 24 weeks according to the psoriatic arthritis response criteria	(26)
Psoriasis	Phase II study; 12 weeks	Leflunomide 20 mg/day ($n = 8$)	6/8 clinical effectiveness (psoriasis area and severity index score 20 at baseline versus 13 at 12 weeks)	(27)
Liver and kidney transplant recipients	Single-center experience	Leflunomide dosage adjusted to a trough concentration of 100 μg/ml ($n = 53$)	Immunosuppressive potency in liver and kidney transplant recipients, allowing dosage reduction of calcineurin inhibitors and glucocorticoids, but anemia might be dose-limiting after kidney transplantation	(28)
Systemic lupus erythematosus	Single-center experience, double-blind, randomized, controlled trial; 24 weeks	Leflunomide 100 mg/day for 3 days, then 100 mg/day ($n = 6$) versus placebo ($n = 6$)	Disease activity fell significantly in both groups after 6 months, and the reduction in SLE disease activity index from baseline to 24 weeks was significantly greater with leflunomide than with placebo	(29)
Wegener's granulomatosis	Phase II study; 52 weeks	Leflunomide 20–40 mg/day ($n = 20$)	Maintenance of complete or partial remission after cyclophosphamide + glucocorticoid therapy resulted in one major and eight minor relapses	(30)
Crohn's disease	Single-center experience; 3 years	Leflunomide 20 mg/day ($n = 12$)	8/12 clinical responses; seven continued maintenance therapy and one relapsed after follow-up of 6–78 weeks	(31)
Chronic sarcoidosis	Single-center experience; 1 year	Leflunomide 100 mg/day for 3 days, then 10–20 mg/day ($n = 32$; 17 leflunomide and 15 leflunomide + methotrexate)	Complete or partial responses in 13/17 leflunomide and in 12/15 leflunomide + methotrexate	(32)

In Japan, acute interstitial pneumonia due to leflunomide has been mentioned as a serious and severe adverse effect, with an incidence of 1.1% and a fatal outcome in 0.36% (57–59).

- A 49-year-old man with rheumatoid arthritis taking methotrexate developed a skin eruption and a severe non-productive cough after taking leflunomide for 17 days (58). He died of respiratory failure 128 days after the diagnosis of acute interstitial pneumonia.
- A 54-year-old woman with rheumatoid arthritis developed an interstitial pneumonia 2 weeks after the end of a 6-week course of treatment with leflunomide (60).

The onset of the pneumonia was preceded by raised serum liver enzymes and hypertension. The acute respiratory failure improved with prednisolone and colestyramine.

However, clinical trials and subsequent observational studies outside Japan have not suggested that leflunomide causes an excess of pulmonary adverse effects (61).

Nervous system

Leflunomide can cause a peripheral reversible neuropathy (49,62–65). This neuropathy is usually axonal in nature, affecting multiple sensory or motor nerves of distal extremities. The mean time of onset of peripheral neuropathy was 6 months after the start of leflunomide therapy, with a range of 3 days to 3 years. Neurological improvement was more likely after drug withdrawal within 30 days after the onset of the symptoms of neuropathy compared with continuous administration (63).

Peripheral neuropathy attributed to leflunomide was observed in two patients (49).

- A 76-year-old man, with an 18-month history of seropositive rheumatoid arthritis, chronic emphysema, and pulmonary fibrosis, developed polymyalgia and was treated with glucocorticoids and azathioprine. Azathioprine was withdrawn after a rise in aspartate transaminase. He was then given leflunomide 100 mg over 3 days followed by 10 mg/day as a maintenance dosage. After 2 weeks, he developed a sensory neuropathy with a stocking distribution up to the malleoli and leflunomide was withdrawn 4 weeks later. During this time he had also been taking prednisolone, tramadol, disodium etidronate, indoramin, and celecoxib, none of which is known to cause neuropathy. Glucose, vitamin B12, serum folate, thyroid function, serum proteins, Bence–Jones protein electrophoresis, cryoglobulins, anti-neutrophil cytoplasmic antibodies, antinuclear antibodies, the Venereal Disease Research Laboratory test, and hepatitis B and C serology were all normal or negative. Nerve conduction was consistent with motor sensory axonal peripheral neuropathy of the lower limbs. On review 3 months after withdrawal of leflunomide, there was clear subjective and objective improvement of the neuropathy, confirmed by repeat nerve conduction studies.
- A 69-year-old woman with a 10-year history of seropositive erosive rheumatoid arthritis, previously treated with gold salts followed by methotrexate, started to take leflunomide and 3 months later reported numbness in the fingertips and feet bilaterally, with a glove-and-stocking sensory neuropathy involving all fingertips and extending to the mid-shins. Leflunomide was withdrawn. Other medications included prednisolone, lansoprazole, simvastatin, losartan, and amiodarone, which she had been taking for a long time without adverse effects. Screening tests for neuropathy, as in the previous case, were normal or negative. There was no cord or nerve root compression on magnetic resonance imaging of the cervical spine. Nerve conduction studies confirmed a sensory motor peripheral neuropathy. She reported marked improvement in her symptoms 3 months after withdrawal of treatment, and this was confirmed on clinical examination and repeat nerve conduction studies.

One case of leflunomide-induced aseptic meningitis has been reported (48).

Metabolism

Life-threatening hypertriglyceridemia has been described during treatment with leflunomide (46).

Hematologic

Pancytopenia, thrombocytopenia, and anemia can occur during leflunomide treatment (21,66–68). The risk of pancytopenia is increased when it is used in combination with methotrexate and in elderly patients. Its course can be fatal and the time of onset ranges from 11 days to 4 years (66). Anemia has been reported in renal transplant recipients (28).

Leflunomide-associated thrombocytosis and leukocytosis resolved after colestyramine washout and withdrawal of leflunomide (69).

Mouth and teeth

In the MN301, US301, and MN302 trials, mouth ulceration occurred in 3–5% (9,10,12).

Gastrointestinal

In the MN301, US301, and MN302 trials, gastrointestinal symptoms consisted of diarrhea (22–27%), nausea (13%), dyspepsia (6–10%), abdominal pain (6–8%), mouth ulceration (3–5%), vomiting (3–5%), anorexia (3%), and gastroenteritis (1–3%) (9,10,12). Diarrhea and nausea are more common in patients who receive a loading dose, but the onset of action can be delayed without the loading dose (36). Gastrointestinal symptoms occur mainly during the first 6 months after initiation of leflunomide. The severity of symptoms was mild. If there is severe diarrhea and/or weight loss, withdrawal of leflunomide and endoscopic examination is advised, since ulcerative and microscopic colitis have been detected under such circumstances (70). The pathophysiology of leflunomide-associated diarrhea and weight loss is unclear. Weight loss of 9–24 kg was observed in five of 70 patients who took leflunomide, despite normal concentrations of thyroid-stimulating hormone and no other gastrointestinal complaints (44).

Liver

Leflunomide can cause abnormal liver function tests, but the risk of serious and non-serious hepatic adverse events is not higher than with methotrexate (71). In the MN301, US301, and MN302 trials, there were abnormal liver enzymes in 6–10% (9,10,12). The co-administration of methotrexate is a risk factor (18,72–74). According to the National Cancer Institute Common Toxicity Criteria, 8.9% of patients developed grade 2 or 3 hepatotoxicity within the first year, mainly within 6 months and in combination with methotrexate, after the start of leflunomide therapy based on liver enzyme determinations (72). The use of folate was also associated with less frequent changes in liver function tests (9,10,12). Nevertheless, leflunomide can cause severe liver injury (75–78), estimated at a rate of one in 200 users (79). Leflunomide is therefore not recommended in patients with significant liver impairment or evidence of infection with hepatitis B or C virus (80).

A CYP2C9 polymorphism has been implicated in the pathogenesis of leflunomide hepatotoxicity (77).

- A 67-year-old woman with rheumatoid arthritis developed diarrhea and raised liver enzymes after taking leflunomide for 15 days. Histologically, the liver showed acute hepatitis. She was homozygous for the CYP2C9*3 allele. The liver damage subsided within a few weeks.

Urinary tract

Interstitial nephritis occurred in one case of chronic overdose of leflunomide (81).

Skin

Adverse effects of leflunomide on the skin in patients with rheumatoid arthritis include alopecia (9–17%), rash (11–12%), pruritus (5–6%), dry skin (3%), and eczema (1–3%) (9,10,12). Single cases of an erythema multiforme-like drug eruption (82), exfoliative dermatitis (83), a lichenoid drug reaction (84), and skin ulceration (85) have been reported.

Immunologic

In the treatment of rheumatoid arthritis leflunomide can cause a vasculitis, and acute necrotizing vasculitis is rare but serious (47,86).

Long-Term Effects

Mutagenicity

A minor metabolite of leflunomide, 4-Trifluoromethylaniline, was mutagenic in vitro (87).

Tumorigenicity

Male mice had an increased incidence of lymphoma at an oral leflunomide dose of 15 mg/kg, and female mice had a dose-related increased incidence of bronchoalveolar adenomas and carcinomas beginning at 1.5 mg/kg (87).

Second-Generation Effects

Fertility

Leflunomide did not affect fertility in rats (87).

Teratogenicity

In oral embryocytotoxicity and teratogenicity studies in rats and rabbits, leflunomide was embryocytotoxic (growth retardation, embryolethality) and teratogenic (malformations of the head, rump, vertebral column, ribs, and limbs) (87). Not only is leflunomide teratogenic and fetotoxic in animals, but its active metabolite is detectable in plasma up to 2 years after withdrawal. Therefore, the fetus could have in utero exposure to leflunomide up to 2 years after the end of treatment. Leflunomide has been classified as pregnancy category X by the Food and Drug Administration (87,88). However, experience in a very small group of pregnant women who took leflunomide and continued their pregnancy to term gave no indication of an increase in teratogenesis (89). Nevertheless, the majority of 30 pregnant women were elected to interrupt their pregnancies, except three patients (87). At present, withdrawal of leflunomide is mandatory before pregnancy, and colestyramine treatment is advised to wash out leflunomide (80,87,90,91). Both men and women who want to have a child should discontinue leflunomide and take colestyramine to wash it out. Leflunomide has not been studied in children, possibly because of its cytotoxic nature. In particular, its teratogenic potential may be a concern when treating adolescent girls (92).

Lactation

Breastfeeding by nursing mothers is not recommended, because it is unknown if leflunomide is excreted in human milk (80,87).

Drug Administration

Drug dosage regimens

Leflunomide is taken orally. In most regimens it is begun with a loading dose of 100 mg/day over 3 days followed by a maintenance dosage of 10–20 mg/day. Leflunomide 100 mg/week had similar effectiveness and less toxicity in open trials compared with daily dosing (21,93).

Drug–Drug Interactions

Infliximab

The administration of infliximab after or simultaneously with leflunomide seems to be safe and effective in patients with rheumatoid arthritis (20,94,95).

Rifampicin

Multiple doses of rifampicin increase leflunomide concentrations (96).

Warfarin

A case of probable interaction of leflunomide with warfarin has been reported (97).

- A 49-year-old man with resistant rheumatoid arthritis took leflunomide 100 mg/day for 3 days. His international normalized ratio (INR) had been stable for 1 year while he was taking warfarin, and 2 days before starting treatment with leflunomide it was 3.4. After he took the second dose of leflunomide, he developed gross hematuria. His INR had risen to 11, and warfarin was withdrawn. The hematuria resolved spontaneously several hours later, but his INR remained raised for the next 2 days, even though he had stopped taking warfarin. He was given intravenous vitamin K 1 mg on the third day, and 12 hours later the INR fell to 1.9.

Subsequently he began taking warfarin again, but at a lower dose of 1 mg/day, which was sufficient to maintain his INR within the target range.

A77 1726 inhibits CYP2C9 and might increase the systemic availability of CYP2C9 substrates, such as warfarin and phenytoin (97,98).

Management of Adverse Drug Reactions

Usually, overdosage and adverse events can be managed by dosage reduction, the addition of colestyramine, and symptomatic therapy (36). However, in one study in patients with rheumatoid arthritis, leflunomide 10 mg/day compared with 20 mg/day was associated with less efficacy and more adverse events leading to treatment withdrawal (24). Colestyramine 3 × 8 g/day for 11 days is recommended to wash out leflunomide, if A77 1726 plasma concentrations do not fall to 0.02 mg/l or less, additional colestyramine is advised. Without this washout procedure, it can take up to 2 years to reach A77 1726 plasma concentrations of 0.02 mg/l. Oral activated charcoal 50 g every 6 hours for 24 hours also reduced plasma A77 1726 concentrations (80).

Plasma A77 1726 concentrations can be measured by high-performance liquid chromatography (99,100). Monitoring of platelets, white blood cells, hemoglobin, and alanine transaminase activity is advised at baseline, monthly for 6 months, and every 6–8 weeks thereafter. Leflunomide should be withdrawn if pulmonary symptoms such as cough and dyspnea start or worsen (80).

References

1. Bartlett RR, Schleyerbach R. Immunopharmacological profile of a novel isoxazol derivative, HWA 486, with potential antirheumatic activity—I. Disease modifying action on adjuvant arthritis of the rat. Int J Immunopharmacol 1985;7(1):7–18.
2. Imose M, Nagaki M, Kimura K, Takai S, Imao M, Naiki T, Osawa Y, Asano T, Hayashi H, Moriwaki H. Leflunomide protects from T-cell-mediated liver injury in mice through inhibition of nuclear factor kappaB. Hepatology 2004;40(5):1160–9.
3. Manna SK, Mukhopadhyay A, Aggarwal BB. Leflunomide suppresses TNF-induced cellular responses: effects on NF-kappa B, activator protein-1, c-Jun N-terminal protein kinase, and apoptosis. J Immunol 2000;165(10):5962–9.
4. Breedveld FC, Dayer JM. Leflunomide: mode of action in the treatment of rheumatoid arthritis. Ann Rheum Dis 2000;59(11):841–9.
5. Manna SK, Aggarwal BB. Immunosuppressive leflunomide metabolite (A77 1726) blocks TNF-dependent nuclear factor-kappa B activation and gene expression. J Immunol 1999;162(4):2095–102.
6. Kremer JM. What I would like to know about leflunomide. J Rheumatol 2004;31(6):1029–31.
7. Rozman B. Clinical pharmacokinetics of leflunomide. Clin Pharmacokinet 2002;41(6):421–30.
8. Mladenovic V, Domljan Z, Rozman B, Jajic I, Mihajlovic D, Dordevic J, Popovic M, Dimitrijevic M, Zivkovic M, Campion G, et al. Safety and effectiveness of leflunomide in the treatment of patients with active rheumatoid arthritis. Results of a randomized, placebo-controlled, phase II study. Arthritis Rheum 1995;38(11):1595–603.
9. Strand V, Cohen S, Schiff M, Weaver A, Fleischmann R, Cannon G, Fox R, Moreland L, Olsen N, Furst D, Caldwell J, Kaine J, Sharp J, Hurley F, Loew-Friedrich I. Treatment of active rheumatoid arthritis with leflunomide compared with placebo and methotrexate. Leflunomide Rheumatoid Arthritis Investigators Group. Arch Intern Med 1999;159(21):2542–50.
10. Smolen JS, Kalden JR, Scott DL, Rozman B, Kvien TK, Larsen A, Loew-Friedrich I, Oed C, Rosenburg R. Efficacy and safety of leflunomide compared with placebo and sulphasalazine in active rheumatoid arthritis: a double-blind, randomised, multicentre trial. European Leflunomide Study Group. Lancet 1999;353(9149):259–66.
11. Smolen JS. Efficacy and safety of the new DMARD leflunomide: comparison to placebo and sulfasalazine in active rheumatoid arthritis. Scand J Rheumatol Suppl 1999;112:15–21.
12. Emery P, Breedveld FC, Lemmel EM, Kaltwasser JP, Dawes PT, Gomor B, Van Den Bosch F, Nordstrom D, Bjorneboe O, Dahl R, Horslev-Petersen K, Rodriguez De La Serna A, Molloy M, Tikly M, Oed C, Rosenburg R, Loew-Friedrich I. A comparison of the efficacy and safety of leflunomide and methotrexate for the treatment of rheumatoid arthritis. Rheumatology (Oxford) 2000;39(6):655–65.
13. Larsen A, Kvien TK, Schattenkirchner M, Rau R, Scott DL, Smolen JS, Rozman B, Westhovens R, Tikly M, Oed C, Rosenburg R; European Leflunomide Study Group. Slowing of disease progression in rheumatoid arthritis patients during long-term treatment with leflunomide or sulfasalazine. Scand J Rheumatol 2001;30(3):135–42.
14. Cohen S, Cannon GW, Schiff M, Weaver A, Fox R, Olsen N, Furst D, Sharp J, Moreland L, Caldwell J, Kaine J, Strand V. Two-year, blinded, randomized, controlled trial of treatment of active rheumatoid arthritis with leflunomide compared with methotrexate. Utilization of Leflunomide in the Treatment of Rheumatoid Arthritis Trial Investigator Group. Arthritis Rheum 2001;44(9):1984–92.
15. Scott DL, Smolen JS, Kalden JR, van de Putte LB, Larsen A, Kvien TK, Schattenkirchner M, Nash P, Oed C, Loew-Friedrich I; European Leflunomide Study Group. Treatment of active rheumatoid arthritis with leflunomide: two year follow up of a double blind, placebo controlled trial versus sulfasalazine. Ann Rheum Dis 2001;60(10):913–23.
16. Kalden JR, Schattenkirchner M, Sorensen H, Emery P, Deighton C, Rozman B, Breedveld F. The efficacy and safety of leflunomide in patients with active rheumatoid arthritis: a five-year followup study. Arthritis Rheum 2003;48(6):1513–20.
17. Kiely PD, Johnson DM. Infliximab and leflunomide combination therapy in rheumatoid arthritis: an open-label study. Rheumatology (Oxford) 2002;41(6):631–7.
18. Kremer JM, Genovese MC, Cannon GW, Caldwell JR, Cush JJ, Furst DE, Luggen ME, Keystone E, Weisman MH, Bensen WM, Kaine JL, Ruderman EM, Coleman P, Curtis DL, Kopp EJ, Kantor SM, Waltuck J, Lindsley HB, Markenson JA, Strand V, Crawford B, Fernando I, Simpson K, Bathon JM. Concomitant leflunomide therapy in patients with active rheumatoid arthritis despite stable doses of methotrexate. A randomized, double-blind, placebo-controlled trial. Ann Intern Med 2002;137(9):726–33.
19. Dougados M, Emery P, Lemmel EM, de la Serna R, Zerbini CA, Brin S, van Riel P. Efficacy and safety of leflunomide and predisposing factors for treatment

response in patients with active rheumatoid arthritis: RELIEF 6-month data. J Rheumatol 2003;30(12):2572–9.

20. Godinho F, Godfrin B, El Mahou S, Navaux F, Zabraniecki L, Cantagrel A. Safety of leflunomide plus infliximab combination therapy in rheumatoid arthritis. Clin Exp Rheumatol 2004;22(3):328–30.
21. Jaimes-Hernandez J, Robles-San Roman M, Suarez-Otero R, Davalos-Zugasti ME, Arroyo-Borrego S. Rheumatoid arthritis treatment with weekly leflunomide: an open-label study. J Rheumatol 2004;31(2):235–7.
22. Nyugen M, Kabir M, Ravaud P. Short-term efficacy and safety of leflunomide in the treatment of active rheumatoid arthritis in everyday clinical use. Clin Drug Invest 2004;24(2):103–12.
23. Kremer J, Genovese M, Cannon GW, Caldwell J, Cush J, Furst DE, Luggen M, Keystone E, Bathon J, Kavanaugh A, Ruderman E, Coleman P, Curtis D, Kopp E, Kantor S, Weisman M, Waltuck J, Lindsley HB, Markenson J, Crawford B, Fernando I, Simpson K, Strand V. Combination leflunomide and methotrexate (MTX) therapy for patients with active rheumatoid arthritis failing MTX monotherapy: open-label extension of a randomized, double-blind, placebo controlled trial. J Rheumatol 2004;31(8):1521–31.
24. Poor G, Strand V; Leflunomide Multinational Study Group. Efficacy and safety of leflunomide 10 mg versus 20 mg once daily in patients with active rheumatoid arthritis: multinational double-blind, randomized trial. Rheumatology (Oxford) 2004;43(6):744–9.
25. Van Roon EN, Jansen TL, Mourad L, Houtman PM, Bruyn GA, Griep EN, Wilffert B, Tobi H, Brouwers JR. Leflunomide in active rheumatoid arthritis: a prospective study in daily practice. Br J Clin Pharmacol 2004;58(2):201–8.
26. Kaltwasser JP, Nash P, Gladman D, Rosen CF, Behrens F, Jones P, Wollenhaupt J, Falk FG, Mease P; Treatment of Psoriatic Arthritis Study Group. Efficacy and safety of leflunomide in the treatment of psoriatic arthritis and psoriasis: a multinational, double-blind, randomized, placebo-controlled clinical trial. Arthritis Rheum 2004;50(6):1939–50.
27. Tlacuilo-Parra JA, Guevara-Gutierrez E, Rodriguez-Castellanos MA, Ornelas-Aguirre JM, Barba-Gomez JF, Salazar-Paramo M. Leflunomide in the treatment of psoriasis: results of a phase II open trial. Br J Dermatol 2004;150(5):970–6.
28. Williams JW, Mital D, Chong A, Kottayil A, Millis M, Longstreth J, Huang W, Brady L, Jensik S. Experiences with leflunomide in solid organ transplantation. Transplantation 2002;73(3):358–66.
29. Tam LS, Li EK, Wong CK, Lam CW, Szeto CC. Double-blind, randomized, placebo-controlled pilot study of leflunomide in systemic lupus erythematosus. Lupus 2004;13(8):601–4.
30. Metzler C, Fink C, Lamprecht P, Gross WL, Reinhold-Keller E. Maintenance of remission with leflunomide in Wegener's granulomatosis. Rheumatology (Oxford) 2004;43(3):315–20.
31. Prajapati DN, Knox JF, Emmons J, Saeian K, Csuka ME, Binion DG. Leflunomide treatment of Crohn's disease patients intolerant to standard immunomodulator therapy. J Clin Gastroenterol 2003;37(2):125–8.
32. Baughman RP, Lower EE. Leflunomide for chronic sarcoidosis. Sarcoidosis Vasc Diffuse Lung Dis 2004;21(1): 43–8.
33. Kaltwasser JP, Behrens F. Leflunomide: long-term clinical experience and new uses. Expert Opin Pharmacother 2005;6(5):787–801.
34. Li EK, Tam LS, Tomlinson B. Leflunomide in the treatment of rheumatoid arthritis. Clin Ther 2004;26(4):447–59.
35. Osiri M, Shea B, Robinson V, Suarez-Almazor M, Strand V, Tugwell P, Wells G. Leflunomide for the treatment of rheumatoid arthritis: a systematic review and metaanalysis. J Rheumatol 2003;30(6):1182–90.
36. Maddison P, Kiely P, Kirkham B, Lawson T, Moots R, Proudfoot D, Reece R, Scott D, Sword R, Taggart A, Thwaites C, Williams E. Leflunomide in rheumatoid arthritis: recommendations through a process of consensus. Rheumatology (Oxford) 2005;44(3):280–6.
37. Hardinger KL, Wang CD, Schnitzler MA, Miller BW, Jendrisak MD, Shenoy S, Lowell JA, Brennan DC. Prospective, pilot, open-label, short-term study of conversion to leflunomide reverses chronic renal allograft dysfunction. Am J Transplant 2002;2(9):867–71.
38. John GT, Manivannan J, Chandy S, Peter S, Jacob CK. Leflunomide therapy for cytomegalovirus disease in renal allograft recepients. Transplantation 2004;77(9): 1460–1.
39. Schlapfer E, Fischer M, Ott P, Speck RF. Anti-HIV-1 activity of leflunomide: a comparison with mycophenolic acid and hydroxyurea. AIDS 2003;17(11):1613–20.
40. First MR. An update on new immunosuppressive drugs undergoing preclinical and clinical trials: potential applications in organ transplantation. Am J Kidney Dis 1997;29(2):303–17.
41. Shoker AS. Immunopharmacologic therapy in renal transplantation. Pharmacotherapy 1996;16(4):562–75.
42. van Riel PL, Smolen JS, Emery P, Kalden JR, Dougados M, Strand CV, Breedveld FC. Leflunomide: a manageable safety profile. J Rheumatol Suppl 2004;71:21–4.
43. Hoi A, Littlejohn GO. Aminotransferase levels during treatment of rheumatoid arthritis with leflunomide in clinical practice. Ann Rheum Dis 2003;62(4):379.
44. Coblyn JS, Shadick N, Helfgott S. Leflunomide-associated weight loss in rheumatoid arthritis. Arthritis Rheum 2001;44(5):1048–51.
45. Hewitson PJ, Debroe S, McBride A, Milne R. Leflunomide and rheumatoid arthritis: a systematic review of effectiveness, safety and cost implications. J Clin Pharm Ther 2000;25(4):295–302.
46. Laborde F, Loeuille D, Chary-Valckenaere I. Life-threatening hypertriglyceridemia during leflunomide therapy in a patient with rheumatoid arthritis. Arthritis Rheum 2004;50(10):3398.
47. Macdonald J, Zhong T, Lazarescu A, Gan BS, Harth M. Vasculitis associated with the use of leflunomide. J Rheumatol 2004;31(10):2076–8.
48. Cohen JD, Jorgensen C, Sany J. Leflunomide-induced aseptic meningitis. Joint Bone Spine 2004;71(3):243–5.
49. Carulli MT, Davies UM. Peripheral neuropathy: an unwanted effect of leflunomide? Rheumatology (Oxford) 2002;41(8):952–3.
50. Siva C, Eisen SA, Shepherd R, Cunningham F, Fang MA, Finch W, Salisbury D, Singh JA, Stern R, Zarabadi SA. Leflunomide use during the first 33 months after food and drug administration approval: experience with a national cohort of 3,325 patients. Arthritis Rheum 2003;49(6):745–51.
51. Cannon GW, Holden WL, Juhaeri J, Dai W, Scarazzini L, Stang P. Adverse events with disease modifying antirheumatic drugs (DMARD): a cohort study of leflunomide compared with other DMARD. J Rheumatol 2004;31(10):1906–11.
52. Fitzsimmons WE, First MR. FK778, a synthetic malononitrilamide. Yonsei Med J 2004;45(6):1132–5.
53. Vanrenterghem Y, van Hooff JP, Klinger M, Wlodarczyk Z, Squifflet JP, Mourad G, Neuhaus P, Jurewicz A, Rostaing L, Charpentier B, Paczek L, Kreis H, Chang R, Paul LC, Grinyo JM, Short C. The effects of FK778 in combination with tacrolimus and

steroids: a phase II multicenter study in renal transplant patients. Transplantation 2004;78(1):9–14.

54. Rozman B. Clinical experience with leflunomide in rheumatoid arthritis. Leflunomide Investigators' Group. J Rheumatol Suppl 1998;53:27–32.
55. Rozman B, Praprotnik S, Logar D, Tomsic M, Hojnik M, Kos-Golja M, Accetto R, Dolenc P. Leflunomide and hypertension. Ann Rheum Dis 2002;61(6):567–9.
56. Martinez-Taboada VM, Rodriguez-Valverde V, Gonzalez-Vilchez F, Armijo JA. Pulmonary hypertension in a patient with rheumatoid arthritis treated with leflunomide. Rheumatology (Oxford) 2004;43(11):1451–3.
57. McCurry J. Japan deaths spark concerns over arthritis drug. Lancet 2004;363(9407):461.
58. Kamata Y, Nara H, Kamimura T, Haneda K, Iwamoto M, Masuyama J, Okazaki H, Minota S. Rheumatoid arthritis complicated with acute interstitial pneumonia induced by leflunomide as an adverse reaction. Intern Med 2004;43(12):1201–4.
59. Ito S, Sumida T. Interstitial lung disease associated with leflunomide. Intern Med 2004;43(12):1103–4.
60. Takeishi M, Akiyama Y, Akiba H, Adachi D, Hirano M, Mimura T. Leflunomide induced acute interstitial pneumonia. J Rheumatol 2005;32(6):1160–3.
61. Scott DL. Interstitial lung disease and disease modifying anti-rheumatic drugs. Lancet 2004;363(9416):1239–40.
62. Bharadwaj A, Haroon N. Peripheral neuropathy in patients on leflunomide. Rheumatology (Oxford) 2004;43(7):934.
63. Bonnel RA, Graham DJ. Peripheral neuropathy in patients treated with leflunomide. Clin Pharmacol Ther 2004;75(6):580–5.
64. Kopp HG, Moerike K, Kanz L, Hartmann JT. Leflunomide and peripheral neuropathy: a potential interaction between uracil/tegafur and leflunomide. Clin Pharmacol Ther 2005;78(1):89–90.
65. Martin K, Bentaberry F, Dumoulin C, Longy-Boursier M, Lifermann F, Haramburu F, Dehais J, Schaeverbeke T, Begaud B, Moore N. Neuropathy associated with leflunomide: a case series. Ann Rheum Dis 2005;64(4):649–50.
66. Chan J, Sanders DC, Du L, Pillans PI. Leflunomide-associated pancytopenia with or without methotrexate. Ann Pharmacother 2004;38(7–8):1206–11.
67. Hill RL, Topliss DJ, Purcell PM. Pancytopenia associated with leflunomide and methotrexate. Ann Pharmacother 2003;37(1):149.
68. Auer J, Hinterreiter M, Allinger S, Kirchgatterer A, Knoflach P. Severe pancytopenia after leflunomide in rheumatoid arthritis. Acta Med Austriaca 2000;27(4):131–2.
69. Koenig AS, Abruzzo JL. Leflunomide induced fevers, thrombocytosis, and leukocytosis in a patient with relapsing polychondritis. J Rheumatol 2002;29(1):192–4.
70. Verschueren P, Vandooren AK, Westhovens R. Debilitating diarrhoea and weight loss due to colitis in two RA patients treated with leflunomide. Clin Rheumatol 2005;24(1):87–90.
71. Suissa S, Ernst P, Hudson M, Bitton A, Kezouh A. Newer disease-modifying antirheumatic drugs and the risk of serious hepatic adverse events in patients with rheumatoid arthritis. Am J Med 2004;117(2):87–92.
72. van Roon EN, Jansen TL, Houtman NM, Spoelstra P, Brouwers JR. Leflunomide for the treatment of rheumatoid arthritis in clinical practice: incidence and severity of hepatotoxicity. Drug Saf 2004;27(5):345–52.
73. Cannon GW, Kremer JM. Leflunomide. Rheum Dis Clin North Am 2004;30(2):295–309.
74. Gao JS, Wu H, Tian J. [Treatment of patients with juvenile rheumatoid arthritis with combination of leflunomide and methotrexate.] Zhonghua Er Ke Za Zhi 2003;41(6): 435–8.
75. Schiemann U, Kellner H. Gastrointestinale Nebenwirkungen der Therapie rheumatischer Erkrankungen. [Gastrointestinal side effects in the therapy of rheumatologic diseases.] Z Gastroenterol 2002;40(11):937–43.
76. Anonymous. Severe liver damage with leflunomide. Prescrire Int 2001;10(55):149.
77. Sevilla-Mantilla C, Ortega L, Agundez JA, Fernandez-Gutierrez B, Ladero JM, Diaz-Rubio M. Leflunomide-induced acute hepatitis. Dig Liver Dis 2004;36(1):82–4.
78. Thomasset SC, Ong SL, Large SR. Post-coronary artery bypass graft liver failure: a possible association with leflunomide. Ann Thorac Surg 2005;79(2):698–9.
79. Moynihan R. FDA officials argue over safety of new arthritis drug. BMJ 2003;326(7389):565.
80. Aventis Pharmaceuticals Inc. Arava Tablets (leflunomide) 10 mg, 20 mg, 100 mg. Product information, 2005.
81. Haydar AA, Hujairi N, Kirkham B, Hangartner R, Goldsmith DJ. Chronic overdose of leflunomide inducing interstitial nephritis. Nephrol Dial Transplant 2004;19(5):1334–5.
82. Fischer TW, Bauer HI, Graefe T, Barta U, Elsner P. Erythema multiforme-like drug eruption with oral involvement after intake of leflunomide. Dermatology 2003;207(4):386–9.
83. Bandyopadhyay D. Exfoliative dermatitis induced by leflunomide therapy. J Dermatol 2003;30(11):845–6.
84. Canonne-Courivaud D, Carpentier O, Dejobert Y, Hachulla E, Delaporte E. Toxidermie lichenoïde au léflunomide (Arava). [Lichenoid drug reaction to leflunomide.] Ann Dermatol Venereol 2003;130(4):435–7.
85. McCoy CM. Leflunomide-associated skin ulceration. Ann Pharmacother 2002;36(6):1009–11.
86. Holm EA, Balslev E, Jemec GB. Vasculitis occurring during leflunomide therapy. Dermatology 2001;203(3):258–9.
87. Brent RL. Teratogen update: reproductive risks of leflunomide (Arava); a pyrimidine synthesis inhibitor: counseling women taking leflunomide before or during pregnancy and men taking leflunomide who are contemplating fathering a child. Teratology 2001;63(2):106–12.
88. De Santis M, Straface G, Cavaliere A, Carducci B, Caruso A. Paternal and maternal exposure to leflunomide: pregnancy and neonatal outcome. Ann Rheum Dis 2005;64(7):1096–7.
89. Brent RL. Utilization of animal studies to determine the effects and human risks of environmental toxicants (drugs, chemicals, and physical agents). Pediatrics 2004;113(Suppl 4):984–95.
90. Kaplan MJ. Leflunomide Aventis Pharma. Curr Opin Investig Drugs 2001;2(2):222–30.
91. Ostensen M. Disease specific problems related to drug therapy in pregnancy. Lupus 2004;13(9):746–50.
92. Ilowite NT. Current treatment of juvenile rheumatoid arthritis. Pediatrics 2002;109(1):109–15.
93. Jakez-Ocampo J, Richaud-Patin Y, Granados J, Sanchez-Guerrero J, Llorente L. Weekly leflunomide as monotherapy for recent-onset rheumatoid arthritis. Arthritis Rheum 2004;51(1):147–8.
94. Flendrie M, Creemers MC, Welsing PM, van Riel PL. The influence of previous and concomitant leflunomide on the efficacy and safety of infliximab therapy in patients with rheumatoid arthritis; a longitudinal observational study. Rheumatology (Oxford) 2005;44(4):472–8.
95. Hansen KE, Cush J, Singhal A, Cooley DA, Cohen S, Patel SR, Genovese M, Sundaramurthy S, Schiff M. The safety and efficacy of leflunomide in combination with infliximab in rheumatoid arthritis. Arthritis Rheum 2004;51(2):228–32.
96. Kale VP, Bichile LS. Leflunomide: a novel disease modifying anti-rheumatic drug. J Postgrad Med 2004;50(2): 154–7.

97. Lim V, Pande I. Leflunomide can potentiate the anticoagulant effect of warfarin. BMJ 2002;325(7376):1333.
98. Rettie AE, Jones JP. Clinical and toxicological relevance of CYP2C9: drug-drug interactions and pharmacogenetics. Annu Rev Pharmacol Toxicol 2005;45:477–94.
99. Chan V, Charles BG, Tett SE. Rapid determination of the active leflunomide metabolite A77 1726 in human plasma by high-performance liquid chromatography. J Chromatogr B Analyt Technol Biomed Life Sci 2004;803(2):331–5.
100. Schmidt A, Schwind B, Gillich M, Brune K, Hinz B. Simultaneous determination of leflunomide and its active metabolite, A77 1726, in human plasma by high-performance liquid chromatography. Biomed Chromatogr 2003;17(4):276–81.

Lentinan

General Information

Lentinan is an immunomodulating glucan that is extracted from the mushroom *Lentinus edodes*. It has been used in small numbers of patients with gastric cancers (1–3) and malignant effusions (4). It has also been used in HIV-positive patients (5) and to ameliorate impairment of natural killer cell activity after cardiopulmonary bypass (6).

General adverse effects

The incidence of adverse effects due to lentinan, particularly those requiring withdrawal, is low (5). Of 98 patients with HIV infection, treatment had to be withdrawn in four because of adverse effects; other adverse effects included one case each of an anaphylactoid reaction, back pain, leg pain, depression, rigors, fever, chills, granulocytopenia, and raised liver enzymes (5).

Organs and Systems

Hematologic

Leukopenia occurred in one of 19 patients with unresectable or recurrent gastric cancers when they were given lentinan 2 mg/kg intravenously together with TS-1 (tegafur + gimestat + otastat potassium in a molar ratio of 10:4:10) 80 mg/m^2/day (7).

Skin

Skin rashes have been noted in 4% of patients treated with lentinan (8).

References

1. Taguchi T. Clinical efficacy of lentinan on patients with stomach cancer: end point results of a four-year follow-up survey. Cancer Detect Prev Suppl 1987;1:333–49.
2. Qing ZJ, Ming QX, Zhong TF. Clinical evaluation of antitumor effects of lentinan combined with chemotherapy in the treatment of various malignancies. Gan To Kagaku Ryoho 1997;24(Suppl 1):1–8.
3. Nakano H, Namatame K, Nemoto H, Motohashi H, Nishiyama K, Kumada K. A multi-institutional prospective study of lentinan in advanced gastric cancer patients with unresectable and recurrent diseases: effect on prolongation of survival and improvement of quality of life. Kanagawa Lentinan Research Group. Hepatogastroenterology 1999;46(28):2662–8.
4. Kawaoka T, Yoshino S, Hazama S, Tangoku A, Oka M. [Clinical evaluation of intrapleural or peritoneal administration of lentinan and OK-432 for malignant effusion.] Gan To Kagaku Ryoho 2003;30(11):1562–5.
5. Gordon M, Guralnik M, Kaneko Y, Mimura T, Goodgame J, DeMarzo C, Pierce D, Baker M, Lang W. A phase II controlled study of a combination of the immune modulator, lentinan, with didanosine (ddI) in HIV patients with CD4 cells of 200–500/mm^3. J Med 1995;26(5–6):193–207.
6. Hamano K, Gohra H, Katoh T, Fujimura Y, Zempo N, Esato K. The preoperative administration of lentinan ameliorated the impairment of natural killer activity after cardiopulmonary bypass. Int J Immunopharmacol 1999;21(8):531–40.
7. Nimura H, Mitsumori N, Tsukagoshi S, Nakajima M, Atomi Y, Suzuki S, Kusano M, Yoshiyuki T, Tokunaga A. [Pilot study of TS-1 combined with lentinan in patients with unresectable or recurrent advanced gastric cancer.] Gan To Kagaku Ryoho 2003;30(9):1289–96.
8. Chihara G, Tagushi T. Lentinan: biological activities and possible clinical use. EOS Riv Immunol Immunofarmacol 1982;2:93.

Lercanidipine

See also Calcium channel blockers

General Information

Lercanidipine is a third-generation dihydropyridine for once-daily dosing in hypertension. It has similar antihypertensive efficacy and tolerability to other calcium channel blockers (1).

Reference

1. McClellan KJ, Jarvis B. Lercanidipine: a review of its use in hypertension. Drugs 2000;60(5):1123–40.

Lesopitron

General Information

Lesopitron is a non-benzodiazepine anxiolytic drug. Its structure is similar to that of buspirone, and it is an agonist at central serotonin (5-HT$_{1A}$) receptors.

A 6-week, double-blind, randomized, parallel, phase II, single-center, outpatient study has been performed to study the efficacy and safety of lesopitron 40–80 mg/day compared with lorazepam 2–4 mg/day and placebo in 161 patients with generalized anxiety disorder (1). The most common adverse events associated with lesopitron were somnolence, headache, and dyspepsia, compared with headache, somnolence, and insomnia with lorazepam. Patients treated with placebo mainly experienced headache, somnolence, and pharyngitis.

Reference

1. Fresquet A, Sust M, Lloret A, Murphy MF, Carter FJ, Campbell GM, Marion-Landais G. Efficacy and safety of lesopitron in outpatients with generalized anxiety disorder. Ann Pharmacother 2000;34(2):147–53.

Letosteine

General Information

Letosteine is taken orally to loosen bronchial secretions and facilitate expectoration (SEDA-5, 170) (SEDA-7, 191) (1).

Organs and Systems

Gastrointestinal

Two of 37 patients experienced gastralgia and vomiting, severe enough to stop therapy (SEDA-7, 191). In another series of 40 patients, five had gastralgia and nausea, requiring withdrawal of therapy in three.

Reference

1. Arroll B. Non-antibiotic treatments for upper-respiratory tract infections (common cold). Respir Med 2005;99(12):1477–84.

Leukotriene receptor antagonists

General Information

The leukotriene receptor antagonists are antagonists of cysteinyl leukotrienes at $CysLT_1$ receptors and include zafirlukast, montelukast, and pranlukast.

Therapeutic studies

Placebo-controlled studies

The efficacy and tolerability of montelukast, in combination with a selective histamine H_1 receptor antagonist (loratadine), has been investigated in a randomized, double-blind, crossover study for 2 weeks in 125 asthmatic subjects (mean FEV_1 67% predicted), who took montelukast 10 mg plus loratadine 20 mg or placebo od for 2 weeks (1). The subjects were symptomatic, in that their mean baseline daily use of $beta_2$-adrenoceptor agonists was 5.1 inhaled metered doses. During the study, the percentage increase in FEV_1 from baseline was significantly greater with montelukast plus loratadine than with montelukast alone (14 versus 9.7%). The most common adverse events during the trial were headache and upper respiratory tract infection (each in about 10% of subjects). There were no significant differences in the frequencies of adverse experiences between montelukast plus loratadine and montelukast alone. Ten patients withdrew because of an adverse event; six had exacerbation of asthma requiring steroid administration (three in each of the two arms of the study). One patient taking montelukast plus loratadine and four taking montelukast alone had transient self-limiting laboratory abnormalities.

The acute effects of intravenous and oral montelukast on airway function have been compared in a randomized, double-blind, crossover study in 51 asthmatic patients (mean FEV_1 63.8% predicted) (2). The intravenous dose (7 mg) was known to produce a comparable AUC to that obtained with an oral dose of 10 mg. FEV_1 was measured at 0.25, 0.5, 1, and 2 hours and then at regular intervals up to 24 hours after dosing. After intravenous and oral montelukast, the FEV_1 AUC_{0-24} was significantly greater than after placebo (mean increases 21, 16, and 7.8% for intravenous, oral, and placebo respectively). The mean percentage change in FEV_1 for intravenous montelukast was greater than for oral montelukast in the first hour (18 versus 13%). The most frequently reported adverse events included headaches, which occurred in three patients taking placebo, four taking oral montelukast, and one taking intravenous montelukast. Influenza was reported in two patients taking placebo. It was noteworthy that there were no local adverse events at the intravenous site of the montelukast administration. This study has raised the possibility that a bolus dose of intravenous montelukast may have a role in the management of acute exacerbations of asthma.

Organs and Systems

Respiratory

Leukotriene receptor antagonists and Churg–Strauss syndrome

Churg–Strauss syndrome is a rare form of allergic granulomatous vasculitis, first described in 1951, characterized by the histological findings of eosinophilic tissue infiltration, extravascular eosinophil granulomas, and necrotizing vasculitis. It develops in patients with a history of upper airway disease (especially allergic rhinitis and sinusitis) and asthma. There are different definitions of the syndrome, and it is important to know which definition is being used when the results of different incidence studies are being compared. Clinically the syndrome has been defined (3) as a combination of asthma, peripheral eosinophilia (over 1.5×10^9/l), and a systemic vasculitis involving two or more extrapulmonary organs. Recognized clinical risk factors include moderate to severe asthma, chronic sinusitis, and a recent reduction in systemic corticosteroid therapy (4). An important feature is the phasic developmental pattern of the disease, and corticosteroid therapy suppresses some manifestations of the syndrome, leading to incomplete disease. Churg and colleagues labeled these cases "formes frustes" of Churg–Strauss syndrome (5). Careful monitoring must be ensured when tapering corticosteroids in steroid-dependent patients to avoid development of incomplete disease.

Presentation

Of 22 asthmatic patients taking leukotriene receptor antagonists who developed Churg–Strauss syndrome, 13 had used zafirlukast, eight montelukast, and one pranlukast (6). All had used inhaled or oral glucocorticoids. The onset of the syndrome was at 2 days to 10 months after starting treatment with the leukotriene receptor antagonist; the interval between the last dose of oral steroids and the recognized onset of Churg–Strauss syndrome ranged from 3 days to 8 months. In several patients the signs and symptoms of Churg–Strauss syndrome became manifest after the start of leukotriene receptor antagonist treatment and tapering of inhaled/oral steroids (13 of 23 patients).

Eight patients with steroid-dependent asthma, who had been able to either discontinue or reduce their oral glucocorticoid requirement subsequent to starting treatment with zafirlukast, developed Churg–Strauss syndrome (7).

- Two 50-year-old men, both using inhaled glucocorticoids, presented with Churg–Strauss syndrome after taking montelukast for 4–5 months, not related to steroid tapering (8). One had a history of asthma and recurrent sinusitis for 5 years with intermittent short-course oral glucocorticoids and continued inhaled steroids, whereas the other had had asthma for 1 year treated with only inhaled glucocorticoids.
- Two women (aged 60 and 62 years) with allergic rhinitis and asthma, one using inhaled glucocorticoids and the other oral glucocorticoids, developed Churg–Strauss syndrome after taking montelukast (9). In the woman using oral steroids, dosage reduction preceded the onset of the syndrome; in the woman using inhaled steroids there was no dosage reduction. The authors also presented the case of a 54-year-old man with a history of Churg–Strauss syndrome who relapsed after taking montelukast.
- A 50-year-old man with a history of severe asthma and tapering of prednisone took montelukast and developed an erythematous rash and mononeuritis multiplex; skin biopsy confirmed the diagnosis of Churg–Strauss syndrome (10).
- A 54-year-old man with no history of glucocorticoid therapy presented with systemic symptoms and a purpuric rash after taking zafirlukast; the diagnosis was Churg–Strauss syndrome (11).
- An 18-year-old woman with childhood asthma, using inhaled glucocorticoids and zafirlukast, developed Churg–Strauss syndrome 10 days after starting to use rokitamycin (12).

Other case reports of interest include pulmonary eosinophilia in association with montelukast (13) and the clinical exacerbation of ulcerative colitis in a patient with steroid-dependent asthma after the introduction of zafirlukast (14). Drug-induced lupus syndrome has been reported in a child with an onset 10 days after beginning treatment with zafirlukast. The child had not been taking oral glucocorticoids (15).

Mechanism

It was originally postulated that the patients had a primary eosinophilic disorder, which was unmasked by the reduction (or withdrawal) of glucocorticoids, which was possible because the addition of zafirlukast had controlled their asthma. A subsequent report of two patients, who were not taking systemic glucocorticoids and developed Churg–Strauss syndrome in association with zafirlukast, raised some doubts about the hypothesis (16). However, there must be uncertainty about implicating zafirlukast in one of these cases, as there appeared to be a delay of 2 months from the withdrawal of zafirlukast to the onset of symptoms, which were subsequently attributed to Churg–Strauss syndrome.

- A 52-year-old woman developed Churg–Strauss syndrome some 12 weeks after beginning treatment with pranlukast and 8 weeks after discontinuing low-dose oral prednisolone (5 mg on alternate days) (17).
- Churg–Strauss syndrome has been reported with montelukast in a patient who had not taken oral glucocorticoids. Symptoms developed within 2 days of beginning treatment with montelukast (18).

The hypothesis of unmasking of Churg–Strauss syndrome (meaning either unmasking of a previously contained pathological condition or the clinical declaration of a "forme fruste") after reduction of glucocorticoid dosage (4,19) is supported by the fact that Churg–Strauss syndrome has also been reported in asthmatic patients who taper their doses of glucocorticoid after the introduction of other antiasthmatic drugs (4). It seems unlikely that leukotriene receptor antagonists themselves provoke Churg–Strauss syndrome, since none of the established mechanisms of adverse drug reactions provides a plausible explanation for the association (4).

There remains the unlikely possibility that in some cases there is direct allergy to the drugs, manifesting as a granulomatous angiitis. In any event, clinicians should be aware of this possibility, although it is rare, and discontinue the drugs in cases of suspicion and undertake appropriate investigations.

Incidence

There are sufficient cases of Churg–Strauss syndrome to estimate its incidence as probably less than one per 20 000 patients. Whilst this may be more than the estimated incidence of this syndrome in the general population, this apparent increase in incidence does not of itself implicate the drugs as being causal. For example, there may be increased detection related to the increased vigilance associated with the introduction of this new class of drugs. If the antileukotriene drugs are implicated in some way in the development of Churg–Strauss syndrome, the precise mechanism is uncertain. Unmasking pre-existing Churg–Strauss syndrome by permitting glucocorticoid withdrawal is one possibility. Another possibility is that the drugs elicit an allergic response that manifests itself as a granulomatous angiitis, a phenomenon that has been reported rarely with other drugs.

The incidence of Churg–Strauss syndrome among asthmatic patients has been calculated in a cohort study of 36 230 patients with asthma (20). The incidence rates of definite Churg–Strauss syndrome were 0–67 cases per million per year, depending on the definition used. The small number of cases did not allow subgroup analysis. The occurrence of Churg–Strauss syndrome during leukotriene receptor antagonist therapy could therefore be coincidental, because the rate of 64 cases per million patients per year in association with leukotriene receptor antagonists is comparable to the estimated rate of 18–74 cases per million patients per year in the asthma population observed before the introduction of these drugs (4,6,19). Large epidemiological studies, including data on glucocorticoid-naive patients using leukotriene receptor antagonists, are needed to address this question further.

Liver

Asymptomatic increases in serum liver enzymes, to two or three times the upper limit of the reference ranges, were reported in 1.5% of over 4000 patients in the premarketing clinical trials of zafirlukast, but no severe hepatotoxicity was reported. With more extensive use of zafirlukast, some case reports of severe liver injury appeared. Three patients developed severe liver injury after taking zafirlukast 20 mg bd for several months (21). The evidence that zafirlukast was the probable cause of the hepatic injury was based on the rigorous exclusion of other causes of acute hepatitis, liver biopsies with histological characteristics consistent with toxic injury, the presence of hypersensitivity suggestive of a drug reaction in one patient, and inadvertent rechallenge in one patient. In one case a liver transplant was required. The authors stated that the mechanism of the drug-induced hepatotoxicity was not known but they speculated that it may be of immunological origin or, alternatively, that metabolism by CYP2C9 may create toxic metabolites. Whatever the mechanism, hepatotoxicity with zafirlukast is rare. The Acute Liver Failure Study Group, a consortium of 20 academic medical institutions in the USA cooperating in the prospective collection of data on acute liver failure, has not identified any other cases of acute liver injury associated with zafirlukast.

Urinary tract

Glomerulonephritis has been attributed to montelukast (22).

- A 46-year-old woman developed a severe systemic inflammatory reaction characterized by eosinophilia and necrotizing glomerulonephritis. About 4 months after montelukast was added to her existing treatment with budesonide, formoterol, and terbutaline for asthma. At the time of her initial presentation she was treated with azithromycin and amoxicillin, but these drugs were discounted as possible causes as her illness had already begun before she was treated with them. Once the diagnosis was made, montelukast was withdrawn and she improved with glucocorticoids over the next 4 months.

From the limited detail of this brief case report, it is by no means certain that montelukast was the cause of the systemic illness.

References

1. Reicin A, White R, Weinstein SF, Finn AF Jr, Nguyen H, Peszek I, Geissler L, Seidenberg BC. Montelukast, a leukotriene receptor antagonist, in combination with loratadine, a histamine receptor antagonist, in the treatment of chronic asthma. Arch Intern Med 2000;160(16):2481–8.
2. Dockhorn RJ, Baumgartner RA, Leff JA, Noonan M, Vandormael K, Stricker W, Weinland DE, Reiss TF. Comparison of the effects of intravenous and oral montelukast on airway function: a double blind, placebo controlled, three period, crossover study in asthmatic patients. Thorax 2000;55(4):260–5.
3. Lanham JG, Elkon KB, Pusey CD, Hughes GR. Systemic vasculitis with asthma and eosinophilia: a clinical approach to the Churg–Strauss syndrome. Medicine (Baltimore) 1984;63(2):65–81.
4. Lilly CM, Churg A, Lazarovich M, Pauwels R, Hendeles L, Rosenwasser LJ, Ledford D, Wechsler ME. Asthma therapies and Churg–Strauss syndrome. J Allergy Clin Immunol 2002;109(1):S1–19.
5. Churg A, Brallas M, Cronin SR, Churg J. Formes frustes of Churg–Strauss syndrome. Chest 1995;108(2):320–3.
6. Jamaleddine G, Diab K, Tabbarah Z, Tawil A, Arayssi T. Leukotriene antagonists and the Churg–Strauss syndrome. Semin Arthritis Rheum 2002;31(4):218–27.
7. Wechsler ME, Garpestad E, Flier SR, Kocher O, Weiland DA, Polito AJ, Klinek MM, Bigby TD, Wong GA, Helmers RA, Drazen JM. Pulmonary infiltrates, eosinophilia, and cardiomyopathy following corticosteroid withdrawal in patients with asthma receiving zafirlukast. JAMA 1998;279(6):455–7.
8. Guilpain P, Viallard JF, Lagarde P, Cohen P, Kambouchner M, Pellegrin JL, Guillevin L. Churg–Strauss syndrome in two patients receiving montelukast. Rheumatology (Oxford) 2002;41(5):535–9.
9. Solans R, Bosch JA, Selva A, Orriols R, Vilardell M. Montelukast and Churg–Strauss syndrome. Thorax 2002;57(2):183–5.
10. Gal AA, Morris RJ, Pine JR, Spraker MK. Cutaneous lesions of Churg–Strauss syndrome associated with montelukast therapy. Br J Dermatol 2002;147(3):618–19.
11. Soy M, Ozer H, Canataroglu A, Gumurdulu D, Erken E. Vasculitis induced by zafirlukast therapy. Clin Rheumatol 2002;21(4):328–9.
12. Richeldi L, Rossi G, Ruggieri MP, Corbetta L, Fabbri LM. Churg–Strauss syndrome in a case of asthma. Allergy 2002;57(7):647–8.
13. Franco J, Artes MJ. Pulmonary eosinophilia associated with montelukast. Thorax 1999;54(6):558–60.
14. Kroegel C, Reissig A, Hengst U, Petrovic A, Hafner D, Grahmann RP. Ulcerative colitis following introduction of zafirlukast and corticosteroid withdrawal in severe atopic asthma. Eur Respir J 1999;14(1):243.
15. Finkel TH, Hunter DJ, Paisley JE, Finkel RS, Larsen GL. Drug-induced lupus in a child after treatment with zafirlukast (Accolate). J Allergy Clin Immunol 1999;103(3 Pt 1):533–4.
16. Green RL, Vayonis AG. Churg–Strauss syndrome after zafirlukast in two patients not receiving systemic steroid treatment. Lancet 1999;353(9154):725–6.
17. Kinoshita M, Shiraishi T, Koga T, Ayabe M, Rikimaru T, Oizumi K. Churg–Strauss syndrome after corticosteroid withdrawal in an asthmatic patient treated with pranlukast. J Allergy Clin Immunol 1999;103(3 Pt 1):534–5.
18. Tuggey JM, Hosker HS. Churg–Strauss syndrome associated with montelukast therapy. Thorax 2000;55(9):805–6.
19. Masi AT, Hamilos DL. Leukotriene antagonists: bystanders or causes of Churg–Strauss syndrome? Semin Arthritis Rheum 2002;31(4):211–17.
20. Loughlin JE, Cole JA, Rothman KJ, Johnson ES. Prevalence of serious eosinophilia and incidence of Churg–Strauss syndrome in a cohort of asthma patients. Ann Allergy Asthma Immunol 2002;88(3):319–25.
21. Reinus JF, Persky S, Burkiewicz JS, Quan D, Bass NM, Davern TJ. Severe liver injury after treatment with the

leukotriene receptor antagonist zafirlukast. Ann Intern Med 2000;133(12):964–8.

22. Goransson LG, Omdal R. A severe systemic inflammatory reaction following therapy with montelukast (Singulair). Nephrol Dial Transplant 2000;15(7):1054–5.

Levamisole

General Information

Levamisole is the levorotatory isomer of tetramisole. Originally used only as an antihelminthic drug, it acts by paralysing the musculature of susceptible nematodes so that they are expelled by peristalsis. It is rapidly metabolized and excreted, with a half-life of about 4 hours.

Use in infective conditions

Treatment of ascariasis with a single oral dose of levamisole 2.5 mg/kg is effective, with evidence of toxicity in under 1% of patients.

Levamisole has been used experimentally in leprosy, particularly in combination with dapsone. This combination was used in a documented series of Indian patients, some currently lepromatous and others in the course of a leprosy reaction (1). When using doses sufficient to provide as good an effect as that obtained with clofazimine + dapsone in a comparison group, adverse effects were limited to gastrointestinal intolerance (which was usually mild), affecting only five of the 30 patients treated; an incidental case developed pyrexia.

Use in non-infective conditions

Levamisole has immunostimulatory activity by modulating the cell-mediated immune response and restoring T cell functions. It has therefore been used extensively and for extended periods of time in various rheumatic and other chronic diseases, in aphthous ulceration, nephrotic syndrome, warts, and malignancies, such as cancers of the head and neck and, in combination with 5-fluorouracil, colorectal cancer (SEDA-20, 348). Under these conditions, its adverse effects are more frequent and rather different because of the differing dosage scheme and presumably also the greater sensitivity of the individual, quite apart from the fact that it is often used in combination, for example with 5-fluorouracil; some 5% of patients fail to complete the course of treatment because of adverse effects. Most of the material in this record is necessarily derived from experience with long-term treatment; where possible a distinction will be drawn between adverse effects occurring under these conditions and those experienced during the acute treatment of tropical disorders.

Observational studies

Aphthous stomatitis

Levamisole has been used in the treatment of recurrent aphthous stomatitis (2) and its value reviewed (3). In four of seven placebo-controlled studies there was a reduction in the frequency and duration of aphthous ulcers during levamisole treatment. Efficacy did not differ whether levamisole was given routinely or started at the first sign of ulcers. In most patients levamisole was well tolerated. Of 128 patients who took levamisole, two withdrew as result of adverse effects (nausea and flu-like symptoms). The most frequent adverse effects were dysgeusia (21%) and nausea (16%). The other adverse effects occurred in less than 10% of the patients and included dysosmia, headaches, diarrhea, flu-like symptoms, and rash, but not all may have been due to levamisole. Levamisole rarely results in objective clinical improvement, and the associated adverse effects discourage its use.

Cancers

In 63 patients with stage III and stage IV squamous cell carcinomas of the oral cavity, oropharynx, hypopharynx, and larynx, with no distant metastases, randomized to either adjuvant oral chemotherapy with futraful, uracil, and levamisole ($n = 29$) or no treatment ($n = 34$), oral chemotherapy showed a trend of better control of distant tumor recurrence (4). However, there was no statistically significant improvement in overall long-term survival. Of the 29 patients who received adjuvant oral chemotherapy, 17 finished the 1-year course without withdrawing. In nine patients futraful, uracil, and levamisole was withdrawn because of local, regional, or distant metastases. Three patients withdrew after 4 months because of vomiting and mucositis. One developed a mild gastric upset and completed the course. There were no major hematological or nephrotoxic adverse effects.

Candidiasis

In two patients with thymoma associated with myasthenia gravis, who both had recurrent oral candidiasis after thymectomy, radiotherapy, and chemotherapy levamisole was added as adjunctive therapy in combination with oral nystatin (5). Oral candidiasis responded favorably and substantial relief was obtained, with a concurrent increase in T cells and CD4/CD8 ratio, suggesting restoration of T cell immunity. Adverse effects were not mentioned.

Glomerulonephritis

In an extensive review of the treatment of minimal lesion glomerulonephritis the use of levamisole was briefly mentioned (6). The author concluded that levamisole has a beneficial effect in this disorder, although no new studies have appeared in recent years and well-controlled studies are scarce. Levamisole appears to be well tolerated in this condition. The adverse effects were neutropenia, rash, and raised liver transaminases.

Nephrotic syndrome

In 11 children with nephrotic syndrome, of whom five were glucocorticoid-sensitive, six glucocorticoid-resistant, and all resistant to other immunosuppressive drugs, levamisole 2.5 mg/kg was given every 48 hours for up to 18 months (7). Two patients were also given ciclosporin. All the patients in the steroid-sensitive group but none in the steroid-resistant group reacted favorably to levamisole, with disappearance of protein from the urine. There were serious adverse effects in two patients: one developed a transient leukopenia 2 months after the start of treatment and another developed a severe exacerbation of pre-existing psoriasis, although that may have been due to the withdrawal of cyclophosphamide.

Levamisole 2 mg/kg on alternate days was given to 25 glucocorticoid-dependent children with frequent relapses of idiopathic nephrotic syndrome (8). The steroid was tapered, and continued for 3–14 months. During treatment with levamisole the relapse frequency was reduced by 40%. Two patients developed mild transient leukopenia, which disappeared 2 weeks after withdrawal. One had a slight rash that disappeared while treatment was continued and one complained of epigastric pain, which led to drug withdrawal.

In a detailed review of the management of nephrotic syndrome in childhood, levamisole was advocated as a weak but effective glucocorticoid-sparing agent (9). In a prospective study in 20 children (aged 3–15 years; 16 boys, 4 girls) with steroid-dependent minimal-change nephrotic syndrome, there were no significant adverse effects during adjunctive therapy with levamisole, which led to successful withdrawal of glucocorticoids after 2 months in 11 children (10).

Pediculosis capitis

In 28 patients with pediculosis capitis (aged 7–12 years) levamisole was given in a dose of 3.5 mg/kg for 10 days; there were no adverse reactions (11).

Rheumatoid arthritis

The possible benefits of levamisole in rheumatoid arthritis are generally outweighed by its adverse effects (SEDA-11, 277) (12).

Comparative studies

Colorectal cancer

The efficacy of levamisole has been studied in several studies of patients with colorectal carcinoma (13–15). In a phase III trial 5-fluorouracil alone, 5-fluorouracil with levamisole, and 5-fluorouracil with hepatic irradiation have been compared in patients with residual, non-measurable, intra-abdominal metastases after resection of colorectal carcinoma (13). The adverse effects were as expected, and there were no differences between any of the treatments. The main adverse effects were hematological and gastrointestinal. However, analysis of life-threatening adverse effects showed some slight differences: there were fewer than expected in the 5-fluorouracil alone group, and more than expected in the 5-fluorouracil plus hepatic irradiation group. There was no treatment advantage for any of the combinations over 5-fluorouracil alone.

Levamisole combined with 5-fluorouracil in the adjuvant treatment of resected colon cancer has been studied in a prospective, randomized trial in which 891 patients were randomized to receive either intensive fluorouracil and leucovorin combined with levamisole, or a standard regimen of fluorouracil plus levamisole (16). The patients were then again randomized to receive either 6 or 12 months of treatment. Standard fluorouracil plus levamisole was not as effective as fluorouracil, levamisole, and leucovorin, and treatment for 12 months was not superior to treatment for 6 months. Unfortunately, there was no treatment arm with fluorouracil and leucovorin only, which is now widely considered to be the treatment of choice. Serious grade 3–4 adverse effects were more frequent in the three-drug treatment groups, and consisted of diarrhea (13 versus 3 patients in the 6-month groups, 17 versus 7 in the 12-month groups) and stomatitis (10 versus 3 in the 6-month groups, 11 versus 6 in the 12-month groups). Leukopenia occurred more frequently in the standard treatment groups (10 versus 18, one of whom died, in the 6-month groups, and 13 patients, one of whom died, versus 14, one of whom died). There were four treatment-associated deaths.

In another study combined intravenous and intraperitoneal fluorouracil plus leucovorin was compared with standard treatment with fluorouracil and levamisole in 241 patients with resected stage 3 or high-risk stage 2 colon cancers (17). In the combined treatment group there was an increased disease-free interval, an estimated 43% reduction in death rate, and a reduction in local tumor recurrence. Adverse effects were relatively uncommon and were generally judged to be mild to moderate; they were slightly more common in those treated with fluorouracil and levamisole, and consisted of nausea and vomiting (18 versus 14%), diarrhea (16 versus 10%), mucositis (17 versus 12%), granulocytopenia (29 versus 23%), and thrombocytopenia (5 versus 3%). Four cases of unspecified nervous system toxicity were noted in those given fluorouracil plus levamisole. There was abdominal pain during or shortly after intraperitoneal drug administration in 19% of patients. Overall 53% of the patients given fluorouracil plus levamisole and 56% of those given fluorouracil plus leucovorin had mild to moderate adverse effects. Severe reactions, requiring a 20% dosage reduction of fluorouracil, were more common in the fluorouracil plus levamisole arm (13 versus 3%). There were no deaths. Unfortunately, in this study no patients were treated with fluorouracil and leucovorin intravenously only.

It is likely that most of these reported adverse effects, although perhaps enhanced by levamisole, except for the nervous system toxicity noted in a few individuals, were caused by fluorouracil. This has been further emphasized by a dose-finding study to determine the maximum tolerated dose of levamisole in the treatment of colon cancer in 38 patients with advanced non-resectable colon cancer, treated with fluorouracil 450 mg/m^2 by rapid intravenous infusion for 5 days (18). Levamisole was given orally three times daily for 5 days every 5 weeks until disease progression. The main dose-limiting toxic effects were nausea and vomiting and an unpleasant metallic taste. The dose used was about five times the total amount of levamisole given in the standard fluorouracil plus levamisole regimen. Levamisole enhanced the gastrointestinal toxicity of fluorouracil, with anorexia, nausea, vomiting, and occasional diarrhea, but did not enhance the bone-marrow suppression associated with fluorouracil. Increasing the dose of levamisole to 150 mg/m^2 tds for 5 days resulted in significant nervous system toxicity, with confusion, vertigo, and severe vomiting. None of the patients treated with this dosage were able to complete the course.

Fluorouracil plus leucovorin has been compared with fluorouracil plus levamisole and combined fluorouracil plus leucovorin and levamisole in 2151 patients with Dukes B and C colon cancers (19). The regimens were as follows:

- fluorouracil plus leucovorin: six 8-week cycles of leucovorin 500 mg/m^2 as a 2-hour infusion repeated weekly for six doses and fluorouracil 500 mg/m^2, given as an intravenous bolus 1 hour after the start of the leucovorin infusion, also weekly for six doses; the cycle was repeated after a rest period of 2 weeks;
- fluorouracil plus levamisole: fluorouracil 350 mg/m^2 as an intravenous bolus daily for five consecutive days, then once weekly starting on day 29 and levamisole orally tds for 3 days and repeated every 14 days;
- fluorouracil plus leucovorin plus levamisole: the same fluorouracil plus leucovorin treatment as described above, with the addition of levamisole in the dose used in the fluorouracil plus levamisole group.

There was a small prolongation of the disease-free interval and overall survival in favor of fluorouracil plus leucovorin, although of borderline statistical significance. Information on toxicity was obtained in 98% of the patients. Eighteen died while on chemotherapy, four in the fluorouracil plus leucovorin group, three in the fluorouracil plus levamisole group, and 11 in the fluorouracil plus leucovorin and levamisole group. Grade 3–4 toxicity was reported equally in the three groups: fluorouracil plus leucovorin 35%, fluorouracil plus leucovorin and levamisole 36%, and fluorouracil plus levamisole 28%. They consisted mainly of adverse effects attributed to fluorouracil, such as diarrhea, vomiting, and stomatitis. Hematological toxicity was minimal (less than 2% in grades 3–4) and not significantly different across the groups. Neurotoxicity was rare. Ataxia was the most frequent neurological disorder, in 2% of the patients who received fluorouracil plus levamisole and in 1% of the patients in the other two groups combined.

QUASAR was a study of the effects of a higher dose of leucovorin or the addition of levamisole to 5-fluorouracil and leucovorin on survival in 4927 patients with colorectal cancer with no evidence of residual disease after resection (14). High-dose leucovorin was not associated with a survival or recurrence benefit compared with low-dose leucovorin. The addition of levamisole had no apparent survival benefit compared with placebo, with slightly more deaths in patients assigned to levamisole than placebo. Tumor recurrences were also higher in those who took levamisole. Dermatological adverse effects were significantly more frequent in those who took levamisole compared with placebo.

In 680 patients with curatively resected stage III colon cancer, adjuvant treatment with 5-fluorouracil plus leucovorin was significantly more effective than 5-fluorouracil plus levamisole in reducing tumor relapse and improving survival (15). There were fewer adverse effects in those given 5-fluorouracil plus levamisole compared with 5-fluorouracil plus leucovorin (820 versus 1190); the difference was mainly due to gastrointestinal toxicity. Only a few patients developed grade 3 or grade 4 adverse effects. There were no treatment-related deaths in either group.

The Gastrointestinal Intergroup has studied postoperative adjuvant chemotherapy and radiation therapy in 1659 patients with T3/4 and lymph-node-positive rectal cancer after potentially curative surgery to try to improve chemotherapy and to determine the risk of systemic and local failure (20). There was no advantage to regimens containing leucovorin or levamisole over bolus 5-fluorouracil alone in the adjuvant treatment of rectal cancer when combined with irradiation. Local and distant recurrence rates were still high, especially in T3 and T4 lymph node positive patients, even with full adjuvant chemoradiation therapy.

Nephrotic syndrome

In a retrospective analysis in 51 children with glucocorticoid-dependent nephrotic syndrome, the ability of levamisole to reduce the relapse rate and to spare prednisone therapy was compared with that of cyclophosphamide (21). Apart from one patient who had a spontaneously resolving skin rash with levamisole and three patients who had transient neutropenia with cyclophosphamide, there were no other clinically significant adverse effects.

Warts

In 44 patients with multiple recalcitrant warts randomized to either oral cimetidine 30 mg/kg/day in three doses for 12 weeks, or 30 mg/kg/day for 12 weeks plus levamisole 2.5 mg/kg for 2 days per week, cimetidine plus levamisole produced significant improvement (22). Adverse effects of levamisole were infrequent, except for a metallic taste in one patient and nausea in two. In one patient the nausea was severe enough to necessitate withdrawal. There were no significant changes in leukocyte count or differential counts.

Placebo-controlled studies

Colorectal cancer

Fluorouracil (370 mg/m^2) plus high-dose (175 mg) or low-dose (25 mg) folinic acid and either active or placebo levamisole has been evaluated in 4927 patients with colorectal cancer (23). Levamisole produced a significant excess of adverse dermatological events. Serious unexpected adverse events were rare. The authors concluded that the inclusion of levamisole in chemotherapy regimens for colorectal cancer does not delay recurrence or improve survival.

Organs and Systems

Cardiovascular

Hypotension has been attributed to levamisole (24).

Nervous system

Several reports point to a condition that can best be described as multifocal inflammatory leukoencephalopathy, occurring in about four cases in every thousand, during treatment with levamisole either alone (25) or in combination with 5-fluorouracil (SEDA-21, 321) (26,27). It presents with confusion, ataxia, dysarthria, diplopia, focal neurological signs, and seizures, and has been extensively discussed and reviewed (28).

One large literature survey (29) concluded that 6% of patients taking long-term levamisole, mostly for malignancies, experienced "sensory stimulation," for example in the form of "hyperalert states" or insomnia, although depression is less commonly on record. Diplopia and tremor have been observed, whilst a number of children treated for juvenile rheumatoid arthritis or nephrotic syndrome have developed generalized convulsions and coma, with EEG abnormalities suggestive of encephalitis (SED-12, 771) (30); the condition recovers spontaneously, but for a time anticonvulsants may be needed.

- A 65-year-old man developed impaired cognition and a disturbed gait 6 months after the removal of a Dukes C colon cancer with adjuvant chemotherapy with fluorouracil and levamisole. Three months later he developed arthralgias in the hands, elbows, and knees, followed 1 month later by intermittent monocular diplopia, an ataxic gait, and deteriorating cognitive function. An MRI scan of the brain showed multiple small round and oval hyperintense lesions in the periventricular white matter, without surrounding edema or mass effect. Most of the lesions showed ring enhancement after intravenous gadolinium. The cerebrospinal fluid protein content was raised, but cytology was normal. A stereotactic biopsy of one of the lesions showed marked cellularity of the white matter, with mononuclear cells in both the parenchyma and perivascular areas, and severe demyelination of the white matter with relative preservation of the axons. Most of the parenchymal cells were macrophages, containing myelin debris. All the findings were consistent with a diagnosis of multifocal inflammatory leukoencephalopathy after treatment with levamisole. The adjuvant therapy was discontinued and he was treated with methylprednisolone 1 g/day intravenously for 3 days, followed by dexamethasone 4 mg qds orally. Within weeks he started to improve, with resolution of the ataxia and improved cognitive function. However, there was residual mild left hemiparesis and he remained moderately unsteady on his feet. The glucocorticoids were slowly tapered and an MRI scan several weeks later still showed multiple patchy areas of bright signal, corresponding to the previous demyelination, but without enhancement. A further MRI scan after 1 year showed complete resolution. His neurological condition and performance had further improved, but there was residual impairment of short-term memory.

The authors suggested that this syndrome may be more common than supposed, and that it is likely that levamisole is the main causal factor, since the same symptoms have been described after treatment with high-dose levamisole alone, but that the effect may be enhanced by the co-administration of fluorouracil, which potentiates the immunostimulatory action of levamisole. Although there is no conclusive evidence of the value of glucocorticoids in this syndrome, an adequate course of glucocorticoids is advised, comparable to the treatment of multiple sclerosis.

- A 57-year-old man had a Dukes C colon cancer removed and was given adjuvant chemotherapy with fluorouracil and levamisole at 4-week intervals (31). Four months later he developed insomnia, diplopia, and a reduced level of consciousness. He was disoriented in time and place, but there were no focal neurological defects. The cerebrospinal fluid protein concentration was slightly raised. A provisional diagnosis of fluorouracil/levamisole-induced neural toxicity was made and he was treated with dexamethasone 4 mg qds. There was an improvement in orientation after 3 days of treatment, but he remained mentally dull. After 28 days of therapy the corticosteroids were tapered. An MRI scan showed multiple focal hyperintensities, with involvement of both deep and subcortical white matter. The lesions were not associated with a mass effect and were mildly enhanced by gadolinium. At 30 months follow-up the patient was well without evidence of relapse. An MRI scan at 24 months showed small, residual, hyperintense lesions, which were not further enhanced by gadolinium, consistent with gliotic scars.
- A 3-year-old girl who took levamisole 100 mg bd for 3 days for anorexia suddenly developed hyperkinesia, paresthesia, fidgetiness, an unstable gait, and frequent falling (32). An MRI scan of the brain did not show any demyelinating changes. She recovered fully within 48 hours without any specific intervention.

The authors suggested that levamisole overdose had contributed to the profound encephalitis-like effects.

Fatal viral encephalitis due to enterovirus type 71 has been reported during use of levamisole (33).

Psychological, psychiatric

Anxiety and depression have been associated with levamisole (34).

Psychosis has also been reported (35).

- A 28-year-old man, without a psychiatric history, developed a paranoid psychosis. He had been taking levamisole twice a week in an unspecified dose for 2 years for a stage 4 melanoma and metastatic lymph nodes in the axilla. Physical examination, a CT scan, an electroencephalogram, and standard laboratory tests were all normal. He was treated with perphenazine, with partial success, but after tapering of the dose his symptoms reappeared. It was thought likely that the psychosis had been caused by levamisole, which was discontinued. Three weeks later he had recovered completely. Levamisole was not reintroduced.

Hematologic

Agranulocytosis has often been reported during long-term treatment with levamisole. Most cases are reversible and transient, but deaths have occurred. In 3900 patients on whom data were available to the manufacturers, there were 88 cases of agranulocytosis and 43 of leukopenia; such dyscrasias occurred in 4% of patients with rheumatoid arthritis and 2% of oncological cases (29). In other published material the incidence has sometimes been higher; such differences do not appear to be related to the dose or duration of therapy. Agranulocytosis is more prevalent in rheumatoid patients with an HLA-B27 genotype (SEDA-7, 317). Children are also susceptible, and fatal outcomes because of hematological disorders have been described in cases of juvenile rheumatoid arthritis treated intermittently with levamisole. Other deaths have occurred in adults concurrently taking glucocorticoids for several years.

Agranulocytosis can be asymptomatic and, since it occurs unpredictably, regular monitoring of the leukocyte count is advisable, especially in patients concurrently receiving combination chemotherapy. Whilst the mechanism is not clear, granulocyte-agglutinating antibodies have been found, suggesting that levamisole acts as a hapten on the leukocyte membrane.

Thrombocytopenia has been reported in a woman with rheumatoid arthritis; it recurred after rechallenge (36).

Gastrointestinal

Nausea, vomiting, and diarrhea are very common in patients taking levamisole, and are sometimes accompanied by abdominal pain or constipation, although when such symptoms occur it is not always clear that they are due to the drug rather than to its interaction with the disease.

Exacerbation of peptic ulceration has been described, and mouth ulcers and abnormalities of taste sensation can be troublesome in patients taking long-term therapy.

Liver

Neither animal nor most human studies point to hepatotoxicity, but in a series of 11 patients with pyoderma treated with levamisole two had increases in aspartate transaminase activity. Liver toxicity has also been reported in a child with nephrosis (37).

Urinary tract

There has been one published case of uremia (38) and one of a reversible nephropathy in a patient with rheumatoid arthritis (39).

Skin

Type I allergic reactions have caused pruritic rashes and urticaria.

Ischemic necrosis of the skin, reversible on withdrawal, has been documented (40).

Single cases of erythema multiforme and erythema nodosum have been observed (SEDA-7, 317).

Two patients developed lichenoid skin eruptions, which subsided when the drug was stopped, although one of these was left with severe scarring, alopecia of the scalp, and widespread atrophic and hyperpigmented skin lesions.

A healed varicose ulcer has been observed to break down after treatment (41).

Necrotizing vasculitis

Cutaneous necrotizing vasculitis with histological changes resembling a type III hypersensitivity reaction has been described in patients taking levamisole (42,43). In a well-documented case, a widespread vasculitic rash, chiefly affecting the limbs, appeared in a woman with rheumatoid arthritis treated for 2 months. In these cases, serum complement was normal and there were no circulating immune complexes, although a histamine skin wheal test produced a vasculitis at a clinically non-affected site. Both cases were reversible.

- Leukocytoclastic vasculitis has been attributed to levamisole in a 7-year-old boy with glucocorticoid-dependent nephrotic syndrome (44).

The authors estimated that about 0.5% of patients treated with levamisole develop cutaneous vasculitis with circulating autoantibodies.

Five of 160 children with nephrotic syndrome developed distinctive vascular purpura (45). They had taken levamisole for a mean of 24 months when they developed purpuric erythematous macules, which evolved to ecchymotic and necrotic purpura. The lesions were mostly on the external ear. Biopsies obtained from the ear lesions in four patients showed vasculopathic reaction patterns, ranging from leukocytoclastic and thrombotic vasculitis to vascular occlusive disease without true vasculitis. There were anticardiolipin, antinuclear, and/or antineutrophil cytoplasmic antibodies in four patients. The lesions resolved within 2–3 weeks after levamisole withdrawal, whereas anticardiolipin and antineutrophil cytoplasmic antibodies disappeared after 2–14 months only. A direct effect of levamisole on the endothelial cells or levamisole-induced or unmasked latent immunological abnormalities was suspected.

Musculoskeletal

Arthritis has occurred in patients with Crohn's disease or Behçet's disease treated with levamisole (46,47), although it is well known that this can occur with either disease irrespective of drug treatment.

Muscle pain can be severe when levamisole is given with 5-fluorouracil for colonic cancer (48), or there can be a painless rise in creatine kinase activity (49).

Immunologic

Allergic reactions often reflect the effects of the drug or of parasitic breakdown products. They include pruritic skin eruptions, arthritic pain and swelling, muscular pain and swelling, especially in patients already suffering from rheumatoid arthritis, Sjögren's syndrome (50), or psoriatic arthropathy. Skin reactions of various types can occur and type III reactions have been noted. Influenza-like symptoms might be an unusual form of type I allergy or a consequence of restoration of cellular immunity.

Disseminated autoimmune disease has been described during treatment with levamisole for nephrotic syndrome (51).

- An 8-year-old boy had a 5-year history of steroid-dependent nephrotic syndrome. After half a year of glucocorticoid treatment he was given levamisole 2.5 mg/kg on alternate days for 1 year, with complete suppression of the proteinuria. The proteinuria reappeared after withdrawal of levamisole, and glucocorticoids and levamisole were reintroduced as before. Two years later, while still taking levamisole, he developed hepatosplenomegaly, a low-grade fever, and a Coombs' negative hemolytic anemia. The anticardiolipin IgM titer was high, p-ANCA antibodies were positive, C3 was moderately low and antinuclear anti-DNA antibodies were negative. Levamisole was withdrawn. Two weeks later the clinical parameters had normalized and 4 weeks later the liver enlargement had disappeared. Although p-ANCA antibodies persisted at 1 month the anticardiolipin IgM titer had returned to normal. After 6 months there still was splenomegaly but no other symptoms, and proteinuria was absent.

The same group of authors have also described a distinctive vasculitis with circulating antibodies in children with nephrotic syndrome associated with long-term levamisole, presenting with purpura of the ears (45).

- Four boys and one girl (mean age 10 years) had had nephrotic syndrome for 2–8 years and had taken levamisole orally in doses of 1.7–2.5 mg/kg/day for 16–44 months (mean 24 months). All had a sudden onset of rapidly enlarging purpuric and erythematous macules progressing to the formation of necrotic areas, purpuric plaques, and hemorrhagic bullae. The pinnae were involved in all five. In three there were also lesions on the cheek or lower limbs. One had fever and another complained of arthralgia. Routine laboratory tests were all normal. Antibodies to extractable nuclear antigen, cryoglobulin, rheumatoid factor, Coombs' test, circulating immune complexes, and complement and components were all negative or normal. However, antiphospholipid antibodies and/or anticardiolipin IgG and IgM were positive in three patients, p-ANCA was positive in three, and c-ANCA in one. Antinuclear antibodies were positive in two patients and anti-double stranded DNA antibodies were positive in one. Biopsies of the skin lesions in four patients showed vasculitis, ranging from a leukocytoclastic and thrombotic vasculitis to vascular occlusive disease without true vasculitis. Two patients had a hypersensitivity vasculitis in the superficial and deep dermis, with neutrophilic infiltration of the vessel walls and fibrinoid necrosis. Features of panniculitis with occlusion of deep and superficial blood vessels by fibrin-platelet thrombi were found in one patient. The lesions completely resolved in all patients within 2–3 weeks after the withdrawal of levamisole. The serum autoantibodies had disappeared in all cases after 2–14 months.

Although leucocytoclastic immune-complex vasculitis induced by levamisole is well known, this specific presentation with involvement of the ears has not been described before.

Second-Generation Effects

Teratogenicity

Animal studies do not point to a teratogenic effect, but there are insufficient human data to assess the safety of levamisole in pregnancy, and the WHO recommends delaying treatment until after pregnancy when possible.

Susceptibility Factors

Age

The adverse effects that occur after monotherapy with levamisole in children with nephrotic syndrome include taste disturbance (dysgeusia), arthralgia, myalgia, anxiety, sleep disturbances, depression, neutropenia, diarrhea, nausea, and vomiting.

Hepatic disease

Levamisole is mostly metabolized to *para*-hydroxylevamisole (52). It should not be used in severe hepatic disease, nor should it be combined with hepatotoxic antihelminthic drugs or other drugs presenting risks to the liver.

Other features of the patient

Both Sjögren's syndrome (50) and psoriatic arthropathy (53) are conditions in which levamisole is probably better avoided because of the risk of hypersensitivity reactions.

In the treatment of the hyperimmunoglobulin E recurrent infection syndrome (Job's syndrome), infectious complications are more serious when levamisole is given, even where there is normal chemotactic responsiveness (54).

The risk of severe adverse reactions is greater in lymphatic filariasis (55).

Drug Administration

Drug overdose

Acute overdose of levamisole has been described (56).

- A 43-year-old man treated himself with a levamisole enema of 10 g (33 times the therapeutic dose) for a gastrointestinal worm infestation. Soon after he developed malaise, tachycardia, nausea, vertigo, and profuse diarrhea. He lost consciousness and developed generalized seizures and a respiratory arrest. He was intubated, ventilated, and treated with clonazepam. His condition improved after 4 hours. He remained somnolent for 6 hours, and was nauseated and vomited for 24 hours. There was hypokalemia after the diarrhea, raised creatine kinase activity, and a leukocytosis. An electrocardiogram showed ST depression. By the fourth day all his symptoms had subsided.

The symptoms in this case were attributed to the cholinergic effect that levamisole has at this high dose.

Drug–Drug Interactions

Salicylates

Levamisole increases serum concentrations of salicylates, but the effect does not appear to have any clinical consequences (57).

Warfarin

Levamisole and 5-fluorouracil interact with warfarin to produce bleeding (58). The mechanism of this effect is unclear, but the reports are sufficiently clear to point to the need for careful monitoring when this drug combination is used.

References

1. Sharma L, Thalliath GH, Girgia HS, Sen PC. A comparative evaluation of levamisole in leprosy. Indian J Lepr 1985;57(1):11–16.
2. Porter SR, Hegarty A, Kaliakatsou F, Hodgson TA, Scully C. Recurrent aphthous stomatitis. Clin Dermatol 2000;18(5):569–78.
3. Barrons RW. Treatment strategies for recurrent oral aphthous ulcers. Am J Health Syst Pharm 2001;58(1):41–53.
4. Lam P, Yuen AP, Ho CM, Ho WK, Wei WI. Prospective randomized study of post-operative chemotherapy with levamisole and UFT for head and neck carcinoma. Eur J Surg Oncol 2001;27(8):750–3.
5. Lai WH, Lu SY, Eng HL. Levamisole aids in treatment of refractory oral candidiasis in two patients with thymoma associated with myasthenia gravis: report of two cases. Chang Gung Med J 2002;25(9):606–11.
6. Bargman JM. Management of minimal lesion glomerulonephritis: evidence-based recommendations. Kidney Int Suppl 1999;70:S3–16.
7. Tenbrock K, Muller-Berghaus J, Fuchshuber A, Michalk D, Querfeld U. Levamisole treatment in steroid-sensitive and steroid-resistant nephrotic syndrome. Pediatr Nephrol 1998;12(6):459–62.
8. Kemper MJ, Amon O, Timmermann K, Altrogge H, Muller-Wiefel DE. Die Behandlung des häufig Rezidivierenden steroidsensiblen idiopathischen nephrotischen Syndroms im Kindersalter mit Levamisol. [The treatment with levamisole of frequently recurring steroid-sensitive idiopathic nephrotic syndrome in children.] Dtsch Med Wochenschr 1998;123(9):239–43.
9. Holt RCL, Webb NJA. Management of nephrotic syndrome in childhood. Curr Paediatr 2002;12:551–60.
10. Donia AF, Amer GM, Ahmed HA, Gazareen SH, Moustafa FE, Shoeib AA, Ismail AM, Khamis S, Sobh MA. Levamisole: adjunctive therapy in steroid dependent minimal change nephrotic children. Pediatr Nephrol 2002;17(5):355–8.
11. Namazi MR. Levamisole: a safe and economical weapon against pediculosis. Int J Dermatol 2001;40(4):292–4.
12. Pinals RS, Robertson F, Blechman WJ. A double-blind comparison of high and low doses of levamisole in rheumatoid arthritis. J Rheumatol 1981;8(6):949–51.
13. Witte RS, Cnaan A, Mansour EG, Barylak E, Harris JE, Schutt AJ. Comparison of 5-fluorouracil alone, 5-fluorouracil with levamisole, and 5-fluorouracil with hepatic irradiation in the treatment of patients with residual, nonmeasurable, intra-abdominal metastasis after undergoing resection for colorectal carcinoma. Cancer 2001;91(5):1020–8.
14. Kerr DJ. A United Kingdom Coordinating Committee on Cancer Research study of adjuvant chemotherapy for colorectal cancer: preliminary results Semin Oncol 2001;28 (1 Suppl 1):31–4.
15. Porschen R, Bermann A, Loffler T, Haack G, Rettig K, Anger Y, Strohmeyer G; Arbeitsgemeinschaft Gastrointestinale Onkologie. Fluorouracil plus leucovorin as effective adjuvant chemotherapy in curatively resected stage III colon cancer: results of the trial adjCCA-01. J Clin Oncol 2001;19(6):1787–94.
16. O'Connell MJ, Laurie JA, Kahn M, Fitzgibbons RJ Jr, Erlichman C, Shepherd L, Moertel CG, Kocha WI, Pazdur R, Wieand HS, Rubin J, Vukov AM, Donohue JH, Krook JE, Figueredo A. Prospectively randomized trial of postoperative adjuvant chemotherapy in patients with high-risk colon cancer. J Clin Oncol 1998;16(1):295–300.
17. Scheithauer W, Kornek GV, Marczell A, Karner J, Salem G, Greiner R, Burger D, Stoger F, Ritschel J, Kovats E, Vischer HM, Schneeweiss B, Depisch D. Combined intravenous and intraperitoneal chemotherapy with fluorouracil + leucovorin vs fluorouracil + levamisole for adjuvant therapy of resected colon carcinoma. Br J Cancer 1998;77(8):1349–54.
18. Reid JM, Kovach JS, O'Connell MJ, Bagniewski PG, Moertel CG. Clinical and pharmacokinetic studies of high-dose levamisole in combination with 5-fluorouracil in patients with advanced cancer. Cancer Chemother Pharmacol 1998;41(6):477–84.
19. Wolmark N, Rockette H, Mamounas E, Jones J, Wieand S, Wickerham DL, Bear HD, Atkins JN, Dimitrov NV, Glass AG, Fisher ER, Fisher B. Clinical trial to assess the relative efficacy of fluorouracil and leucovorin, fluorouracil and levamisole, and fluorouracil, leucovorin, and levamisole in patients with Dukes' B and C carcinoma of the colon: results from National Surgical Adjuvant Breast and Bowel Project C-04. J Clin Oncol 1999;17(11):3553–9.
20. Tepper JE, O'Connell M, Niedzwiecki D, Hollis DR, Benson AB 3rd, Cummings B, Gunderson LL, Macdonald JS, Martenson JA, Mayer RJ. Adjuvant therapy in rectal cancer: analysis of stage, sex, and local control—final report of intergroup 0114. J Clin Oncol 2002;20(7):1744–50.
21. Alsaran K, Grisaru S, Stephens D, Arbus G. Levamisole vs. cyclophosphamide for frequently-relapsing steroid-dependent nephrotic syndrome. Clin Nephrol 2001;56(4): 289–94.
22. Parsad D, Pandhi R, Juneja A, Negi KS. Cimetidine and levamisole versus cimetidine alone for recalcitrant warts in children. Pediatr Dermatol 2001;18(4):349–52.
23. Pak CY. Correction of thiazide-induced hypomagnesemia by potassium-magnesium citrate from review of prior trials. Clin Nephrol 2000;54(4):271–5.
24. Holcombe RF, Li A, Stewart RM. Levamisole and interleukin-2 for advanced malignancy. Biotherapy 1998;11(4):255–8.
25. Lucia P, Pocek M, Passacantando A, Sebastiani ML, De Martinis C. Multifocal leucoencephalopathy induced by levamisole. Lancet 1996;348(9039):1450.
26. Savarese DM, Gordon J, Smith TW, Litofsky NS, Licho R, Ragland R, Recht L. Cerebral demyelination syndrome in a patient treated with 5-fluorouracil and levamisole. The use of thallium SPECT imaging to assist in noninvasive diagnosis—a case report. Cancer 1996;77(2):387–94.
27. Vaughn DJ, Haller DG. The role of adjuvant chemotherapy in the treatment of colorectal cancer. Hematol Oncol Clin North Am 1997;11(4):699–719.
28. Recht LD, Primavera JM. Case records of the Massachusetts General Hospital. Weekly clinicopathological exercises. Case 24–1999. Neurologic disorder in a 65-year-old man after treatment of colon cancer. N Engl J Med 1999;341(7):512–19.
29. Symoens J, Veys E, Mielants M, Pinals R. Adverse reactions to levamisole. Cancer Treat Rep 1978;62(11): 1721–30.
30. Palcoux JB, Niaudet P, Goumy P. Side effects of levamisole in children with nephrosis. Pediatr Nephrol 1994;8(2):263–4.
31. Yeo W, Tong MM, Chan YL. Multifocal cerebral demyelination secondary to fluorouracil and levamisole therapy. J Clin Oncol 1999;17(1):431–3.
32. Dubey AK, Gupta RK, Sharma RK. Levamisole induced ataxia. Indian Pediatr 2001;38(4):417–19.
33. Mabin D, Castel Y, Le Fur JM, Alix D, Chastel C, Le Roy JP. Encéphalite aiguë virale mortelle au cours d'un traitement par le lévamisole. [Acute viral encephalitis with fatal issue during treatment by levamisole.] Nouv Presse Med 1978;7(45):4143.

34. Hsu WH. Toxicity and drug interactions of levamisole. J Am Vet Med Assoc 1980;176(10 Spec No):1166–9.
35. Jeffries JJ, Cammisuli S. Psychosis secondary to long-term levamisole therapy. Ann Pharmacother 1998;32(1):134–5.
36. Parkinson DR, Cano PO, Jerry LM, Capek A, Shibata HR, Mansell PW, Lewis MG, Marquis G. Complications of cancer immunotherapy with levamisole. Lancet 1977;1(8022):1129–32.
37. Bulugahapitiya DT. Liver toxicity in a nephrotic patient treated with levamisole. Arch Dis Child 1997;76(3):289.
38. Lesquesne M, Floquet J. Les effets secondaires au cours des traitements prolongés par le lévamisole notamment dans le polyarthrites. [Side effects during prolonged treatment with levamisole, especially in polyarthritis.] Nouv Presse Med 1976;5(6):358–9.
39. Hansen TM, Petersen J, Halberg P, Permin H, Ullman S, Brun C, Larsen S. Levamisole-induced nephropathy. Lancet 1978;2(8092 Pt 1):737.
40. Menni S, Pistritto G, Gianotti R, Ghio L, Edefonti A. Ear lobe bilateral necrosis by levamisole-induced occlusive vasculitis in a pediatric patient. Pediatr Dermatol 1997;14(6):477–9.
41. El-Ghobarey AF, Mavrikakis M, Morgan I, Mathieu JP. Delayed healing of varicose ulcer with levamisole. BMJ 1977;1(6061):616.
42. Scheinberg MA, Bezerra JB, Almeida FA, Silveira LA. Cutaneous necrotising vasculitis induced by levamisole. BMJ 1978;1(6110):408.
43. Laux-End R, Inaebnit D, Gerber HA, Bianchetti MG. Vasculitis associated with levamisole and circulating auto-antibodies. Arch Dis Child 1996;75(4):355–6.
44. Bagga A, Hari P. Levamisole-induced vasculitis. Pediatr Nephrol 2000;14(10–11):1057–8.
45. Rongioletti F, Ghio L, Ginevri F, Bleidl D, Rinaldi S, Edefonti A, Gambini C, Rizzoni G, Rebora A. Purpura of the ears: a distinctive vasculopathy with circulating auto-antibodies complicating long-term treatment with levamisole in children. Br J Dermatol 1999;140(5):948–51.
46. Segal AW, Pugh SF, Levi AJ, Loewi G. Levamisole-induced arthritis in Crohn's disease. BMJ 1977;2(6086):555.
47. Siklos P. Levamisole-induced arthritis. BMJ 1977;2(6089):773.
48. Buecher B, Blanc JF, Magnien F, Bechade D, Lapprand M, Oddes B. Des myalgies sevères: un effet indésirable inhabituel du lévamisole associé au 5-fluorouracile. [Severe myalgias: an unusual undesirable effect of levamisole combined with 5-fluorouracil.] Gastroenterol Clin Biol 1996;20(4):407–8.
49. Cersosimo RJ, Lee JM. Creatine kinase elevation associated with 5-fluorouracil and levamisole therapy for carcinoma of the colon. A case report. Cancer 1996;77(7):1250–3.
50. Balint G, el-Ghobary A, Capell H, Madkour M, Dick WC, Ferguson MM, Anwar-ul-haq M. Sjögren's syndrome: a contraindication to levamisole treatment? BMJ 1977;2(6099):1386–7.
51. Barbano G, Ginevri F, Ghiggeri GM, Gusmano R. Disseminated autoimmune disease during levamisole treatment of nephrotic syndrome. Pediatr Nephrol 1999;13(7):602–3.
52. Kouassi E, Caille G, Lery L, Lariviere L, Vezina M. Novel assay and pharmacokinetics of levamisole and p-hydroxy-levamisole in human plasma and urine. Biopharm Drug Dispos 1986;7(1):71–89.
53. Trabert U, Rosenthal M, Muller W. Therapie entzundlich-rheumatischer Krankheiten mit Levamisol, einer immunmodulierenden Substanz. [Therapy of inflammatory-rheumatic diseases with levamisol, an immunity modulating substance.] Schweiz Med Wochenschr 1976;106(39):1293–301.
54. Swim AT, Bradac C, Craddock PR. Levamisole in Job's syndrome. N Engl J Med 1982;307(24):1528–9.
55. Merlin M, Carme B, Kaeuffer H, Laigret J. Activité du lévamisole (Solaskil) dans la filariose lymphatique a *Wuchereria bancrofti* (varieté *pacifica*). [Activity of levamisole (Solaskil) in lymphatic filariasis caused by *Wuchereria bancrofti* (variety *pacifica*).] Bull Soc Pathol Exot Filiales 1976;69(3):257–65.
56. Joly C, Palisse M, Ribbe D, De Calmes O, Genevey P. Intoxication aiguë au lévamisole. [Acute levamisole poisoning.] Presse Med 1998;27(15):717.
57. Rumble RH, Brooks PM, Roberts MS. Interaction between levamisole and aspirin in man. Br J Clin Pharmacol 1979;7(6):631–3.
58. Wehbe TW, Warth JA. A case of bleeding requiring hospitalization that was likely caused by an interaction between warfarin and levamisole. Clin Pharmacol Ther 1996;59(3):360–2.

Levetiracetam

See also Antiepileptic drugs

General Information

Levetiracetam is a piracetam derivative used in the treatment of refractory partial seizures. In trials it has shown an excellent tolerability profile. The main dose-related adverse effects are sedation, fatigue, and headache. Other possible adverse effects include dizziness, unsteadiness, diplopia, nausea, infection, memory impairment, and disturbances of mood and behavior, although in controlled trials the incidence of most of these was no greater than with placebo (1).

The pharmacology, clinical pharmacology, uses, and adverse reactions and interactions of levetiracetam have been reviewed (2–6).

The safety profile of levetiracetam has been reviewed (7). The authors assessed the integrated summary of safety reports submitted for regulatory review in order to obtain information about abnormal laboratory test values and adverse events collected during the overall levetiracetam development program. The analysis included 3347 patients exposed to levetiracetam in clinical trials for epilepsy, cognition, and anxiety disorders. Safety data from all the studies showed a similar pattern of adverse effects, predominantly somnolence, weakness, and dizziness, which occurred most often during the first month of treatment. Laboratory tests that changed significantly in placebo-controlled trials nevertheless stayed in the reference ranges. The incidences of any types of allergic reactions were similar between levetiracetam and placebo (0.3% and 0.2%). Cases of common cold and upper respiratory infection were significantly more frequent with levetiracetam than placebo (13 versus 7.5%), but were not preceded by low neutrophil counts that might have suggested impaired immunological status. There was worsening of seizures (an increase of over 25%) in 14% of patients taking levetiracetam and 26% of patients taking placebo. There were nine sudden, unexplained deaths; the overall mortality rates and standardized mortality rates were higher in the placebo group (1.8% levetiracetam versus 2.5% placebo). Behavioral problems occurred in 5.2–14% of those taking co-careldopa; it is doubtful whether the difference is significant. On the other hand, some patients become hypertensive; they may be individuals who absorb or metabolize the drug at an abnormal rate. Levodopa can cause ventricular dysrhythmias in patients with pre-existing cardiac disorders. Transient flushing of the skin is common; palpitation is unusual.

Respiratory

An isolated case of respiratory dysrhythmia has been reported (5); it was dose-related and impeded adequate treatment, but was ultimately suppressed with tiapride.

Two men with Parkinson's disease, aged 66 and 78 years, developed abnormal respiration (tachypnea and irregularity in the depth of breathing) when levodopa was either introduced at a dose of 300 mg/day in the first case or increased from 300 to 600 mg/day in the other (6). The authors cited a number of earlier similar reports.

Nervous system

Ever since the introduction of levodopa as the mainstay of antiparkinsonian therapy, there has been concern that it may be toxic, causing long-term damage to dopamine neurons. Three reviews have addressed this question in the light of experimental and clinical evidence over the last 30 years. One reviewer concluded that there is no evidence for irreversible levodopa-induced damage in man, only for reversible adverse effects associated with neuronal dysfunction but not neuronal death (7). Others reached broadly the same conclusion, although they noted that there is in vitro evidence of damage associated with oxidative metabolism of levodopa (8). They also described potential toxicity from levodopa in animals in which the nigrostriatal pathway is already damaged by other means. A third reviewer has pointed out that levodopa therapy is an entirely non-physiological means of dopamine replacement, arguing that the intermittent nature of the dopaminergic stimulus provided by most therapies, particularly levodopa, predisposes to motor complications (9). He suggested that more continuous activation of dopamine receptors could minimize or eliminate these problems.

Asterixis, a jerky relaxation of tonically contracted postural muscles, was observed in some patients with structural lesions of the brain or metabolic encephalopathy who were taking levodopa, but not in patients with Parkinson's disease (10).

For most patients fluctuations are variations in the severity of motor manifestations of Parkinson's disease. However, other types of fluctuations can also occur, many of which are of non-motor in nature: these include sensory fluctuations (pain and paresthesia), akathisia or restless legs, autonomic fluctuations (dyspnea, tachycardia, pallor, blood pressure changes, dysphagia, penile erection, urinary frequency) or cognitive effects, such as hallucinations, depression, hypomania, or hypersexuality.

An unusual symptom of Parkinson's disease is apraxia of eyelid opening, a particular aspect of the difficulty in initiating movements (11).

- A 76-year-old woman with atypical Parkinsonism had a poor motor response to levodopa and developed apraxia. An increase in dosage (to levodopa 300 mg/day with benserazide 75 mg/day and selegiline 200 mg/day) caused worsening of the apraxia. Drug withdrawal caused no motor deterioration, but the apraxia disappeared. Challenge with subcutaneous apomorphine reinitiated the symptom, strongly supporting its dopaminergic origin in this patient.

The authors cited the therapeutic use of botulinum toxin in a similar case, but this was ineffective in their patient.

A less well defined adverse effect of levodopa is sedation. This has been studied in 22 volunteers given levodopa 200 mg with benserazide 50 mg or triazolam 0.125 mg or placebo in a randomized crossover design (12). Both active drugs caused drowsiness, more particularly triazolam. During a further 11 days of treatment with levodopa 600 mg/day sedation persisted. Two points are worth noting. First, triazolam was presumably chosen because of its short half-life, but it is a somewhat risky choice, given its known psychiatric adverse effects. Secondly, the very rapid increase in levodopa dosage, from 200 to 600 mg/day, would be unrealistic in a clinical context, when dosage titration would be much more gradual. It is therefore hard to assess the practical relevance of this study.

The advantages and disadvantages of levodopa have been summarized, with particular focus on adverse effects and their management (13). The author concluded that there is no convincing evidence for neurotoxicity of levodopa in humans.

Neurologists from New York and Yugoslavia have noted the variable time to the development of motor complications after starting levodopa (14). Of 40 patients (21 men, mean age 67 years), 17 were at Hoehn and Yahr stage I at the start of levodopa therapy, 13 at stage II, and 10 at stage III. The median times to the development of motor fluctuations were respectively 64, 55, and 14 months in the three groups and the times to onset of dyskinesias were similar. This reinforces the clinical experience of neurologists in general.

Dyskinesias

Dyskinesias occurring during long-term use of levodopa have been classified in various ways. One system presents them as falling broadly into three groups:

- "On" dyskinesias—These coincide with periods of clinical response to the drug; they include chorea, myoclonus, and dystonic movements. They are enhanced by dopamine receptor agonists and reduced by dopamine receptor antagonists.
- "Off" dyskinesias—These coincide with periods of poor response and comprise mainly dystonic postures, affecting in particular the feet; they are inhibited by both dopamine receptor agonists and antagonists.
- "Dysphasic dyskinesias"—These occur at the beginning and end of "on" periods. They involve repetitive stereotyped movements of the lower limbs, and they too react well to both dopamine receptor agonists and antagonists.

There is reason to believe that dyskinesias during prolonged levodopa treatment result from an interaction between the levodopa and the underlying condition rather than from one or the other. In many cases of severe Parkinson's disease one can speak of a "peak dose dyskinesia," which is only problematic when the patient is taking a relatively high dose, which tends to be most marked on the most severely diseased side, and which responds to dosage reduction (15).

The long-term consequences of levodopa therapy have been considered in a review by predominantly Canadian authors, but whose senior author was Oleh Hornykiewicz, the doyen of the dopamine concept of Parkinson's disease (16). Their conclusions were not at all unexpected. Levodopa was given to 42 patients (30 men, mean disease duration of 16 years, mean follow-up about 9 years). There were adverse effects in over 70%: dyskinesias in 62%, on–off effects in about 17%, and end-of-dose wearing-off in about 7% (the last perhaps surprisingly low). Dyskinesia was not only the most common but also the earliest adverse effect. It should be noted that the mean levodopa dosage in this population was rather low, only 500 mg/day.

An interesting case report has drawn attention to the fact that severe response fluctuations can occur soon after the start of treatment in patients with severe disease (17).

- Two men aged 76 and 72 years presented with advanced symptoms of Parkinson's disease and were treated with levodopa. Disabling dyskinesia occurred within days of reaching maintenance dosages of levodopa (1–1.5 g/day with benserazide).

Clearly, the disease status of the patients was the determinant for this adverse reaction, not the duration of levodopa therapy.

In 17 parkinsonian patients three tests of proprioception were carried out 1 hour after the administration of levodopa or a dopamine receptor agonist (18). Although data were not provided for individual patients, there was an overall 11–31% deterioration in the mean scores in all three of the tests. There was no difference between patients with and without dyskinesias, but the authors suggested that abnormal proprioception may be a factor in drug-induced dyskinesia.

There is some evidence that the atypical neuroleptic drug clozapine can alleviate levodopa-induced dyskinesia while itself providing additional relief in Parkinson's disease (SEDA-18, 159); clozapine may also relieve levodopa-induced psychosis (SEDA-17, 166).

"Start hesitation" (paradoxical akinesia) is the name given to sudden episodes during which the patient feels a sensation of extreme heaviness of the feet and finds himself unable to start walking; the legs tremble and the patient falls forward; the condition can improve if the levodopa dosage is reduced.

The "on–off effect" seen after prolonged therapy in some patients is characterized by sudden swings between severe parkinsonian symptoms (with freedom from adverse effects) and normal mobility (but with marked adverse drug effects). It is likely that unexplained variations in dopamine concentrations in the central nervous system are responsible; the condition has been seen less often since combinations with decarboxylase inhibitors came into general use.

Hiccups, an unusual form of dyskinesia, have been attributed to levodopa (19).

- An 80-year-old man with Parkinson's disease and dementia developed worsening bradykinesia, and the dose of co-careldopa was increased from 12.5/50 mg bd to 25/100 mg bd. Two days later, he developed hiccups, which lasted for 1 week and which ceased when the dosage was reduced to the previous level. Ocular dyskinesias have been described in a 60-year-old Spanish man who showed intermittent upward and leftward deviations of gaze associated with peak concentrations of levodopa, in doses of up to 800 mg/day plus benserazide (20).

It should be noted that the patient was and apparently still is taking pramipexole and amantadine in addition to levodopa.

Sleep disorders

Daytime sleepiness and nocturnal wakefulness can both occur in relation to dopaminergic drug therapy, but sleep attacks are rare (21). Many factors beside drug treatment can lead to sleep disorders in parkinsonian patients, including the disease process itself and episodes of sleep apnea; some are skeptical about the existence of sleep attacks as a phenomenon distinct from increased general drowsiness (22), although others disagree. Neurologists from King's College London have concluded that all dopaminergic drugs are capable of causing sleepiness and that in a minority of patients it may take the form of a narcolepsy-like phenotype, possibly amenable to improvement by selegiline or modafinil; they have recommended that affected individuals should not drive (23). Although it was their view that this is a class effect of dopamine agonists, they nevertheless suggested that switching from one agonist to another may sometimes be helpful.

Some remarkable case reports have previously been published (SEDA-25, 169) and reports continue to appear, supplemented by prospective studies and other analyses. For instance, 11 studies involving ropinirole or pramipexole in a total of 2066 patients have been reviewed (24). Four of these (two each with ropinirole and pramipexole) were placebo-controlled. The pooled relative risk of somnolence was 4.98 compared with placebo: there was a non-significant trend for greater somnolence with ropinirole, but the confidence intervals were much wider than with pramipexole. In the other studies levodopa alone was compared with levodopa plus the newer drugs; the relative risk was 2.06 compared with levodopa alone. It must be borne in mind that somnolence and sleep attacks may be separate phenomena, although this is controversial.

The whole field of sleep disorders in Parkinson's disease has been reviewed in a consecutive series of 320 patients from Houston, with analysable data from 303 (sex distribution unknown) (25). The mean age was 67 years and the mean duration of the disease was 9.1 years. All the patients completed the Epworth Sleepiness Scale and answered specific questions about falling asleep while driving and about the restless legs syndrome. The mean sleepiness score was 11.1, values greater than 10 being regarded as abnormal. As one would expect, just over half the patients had scores at that level. Higher scores correlated with longer duration and greater severity of the disease, with male sex, and with the use of dopamine receptor agonists. There was no apparent difference in

The efficacy of clozapine has been described in 60 patients with levodopa-induced neuropsychiatric syndromes (32 assigned to the active drug and 28 to placebo) (72). The mean age was 72 years, the mean duration of disease was 12 years (Hoehn and Yahr stage 3.2), and the mean levodopa dosage was 774 mg/day. At a dose of up to 50 mg/day, clozapine significantly improved psychotic features, with minimal effects on parkinsonian symptoms. Clozapine caused somnolence but was otherwise well tolerated.

References

1. Barbeau A, Roy M. Six-year results of treatment with levodopa plus benzerazide in Parkinson's disease. Neurology 1976;26(5):399–404.
2. Goetz CG, Tanner CM, Nausieda PA. Weekly drug holiday in Parkinson disease. Neurology 1981;31(11):1460–2.
3. Vlay SC. Isoproterenol-induced bradyarrhythmias. Am Heart J 1991;122(4 Pt 1):1169.
4. Rosin MA, Braun M 3rd. Malignant melanoma and levodopa. Cutis 1984;33(6):572–4.
5. De Keyser J, Vincken W. L-dopa-induced respiratory disturbance in Parkinson's disease suppressed by tiapride. Neurology 1985;35(2):235–7.
6. Rice JE, Antic R, Thompson PD. Disordered respiration as a levodopa-induced dyskinesia in Parkinson's disease. Mov Disord 2002;17(3):524–7.
7. Agid Y. Levodopa: is toxicity a myth? Neurology 1998;50(4):858–63.
8. Jenner PG, Brin MF. Levodopa neurotoxicity: experimental studies versus clinical relevance. Neurology 1998;50(6 Suppl 6):S39–43.
9. Chase TN. Levodopa therapy: consequences of the nonphysiologic replacement of dopamine. Neurology 1998;50(5 Suppl 5):S17–25.
10. Glantz R, Weiner WJ, Goetz CG, Nausieda PA, Klawans HL. Drug-induced asterixis in Parkinson disease. Neurology 1982;32(5):553–5.
11. Defazio G, De Mari M, De Salvia R, Lamberti P, Giorelli M, Livrea P. "Apraxia of eyelid opening" induced by levodopa therapy and apomorphine in atypical parkinsonism (possible progressive supranuclear palsy): a case report. Clin Neuropharmacol 1999;22(5):292–4.
12. Andreu N, Chale JJ, Senard JM, Thalamas C, Montastruc JL, Rascol O. L-Dopa-induced sedation: a double-blind cross-over controlled study versus triazolam and placebo in healthy volunteers. Clin Neuropharmacol 1999;22(1):15–23.
13. Jankovic J. Levodopa strengths and weaknesses. Neurology 2002;58(4 Suppl 1):S19–32.
14. Kostic VS, Marinkovic J, Svetel M, Stefanova E, Przedborski S. The effect of stage of Parkinson's disease at the onset of levodopa therapy on development of motor complications. Eur J Neurol 2002;9(1):9–14.
15. Horstink MW, Zijlmans JC, Pasman JW, Berger HJ, van't Hof MA. Severity of Parkinson's disease is a risk factor for peak-dose dyskinesia. J Neurol Neurosurg Psychiatry 1990;53(3):224–6.
16. Rajput AH, Fenton ME, Birdi S, Macaulay R, George D, Rozdilsky B, Ang LC, Senthilselvan A, Hornykiewicz O. Clinical-pathological study of levodopa complications. Mov Disord 2002;17(2):289–96.
17. Onofrj M, Paci C, Thomas A. Sudden appearance of invalidating dyskinesia–dystonia and off fluctuations after the introduction of levodopa in two dopaminomimetic drug naive patients with stage IV Parkinson's disease. J Neurol Neurosurg Psychiatry 1998;65(4):605–6.
18. O'Suilleabhain P, Bullard J, Dewey RB. Proprioception in Parkinson's disease is acutely depressed by dopaminergic medications. J Neurol Neurosurg Psychiatry 2001;71(5):607–10.
19. Collins DR, Wanklyn P. Hiccoughs—an unusual dyskinetic side-effect of L-dopa. Age Ageing 2002;31(5):405–6.
20. Linazasoro G, Van Blercom N, Lasa A, Indakoetxea B, Ruiz J. Levodopa-induced ocular dyskinesias in Parkinson's disease. Mov Disord 2002;17(1):186–7.
21. Stacy M. Sleep disorders in Parkinson's disease: epidemiology and management. Drugs Aging 2002;19(10):733–9.
22. Cantor CR, Stern MB. Dopamine agonists and sleep in Parkinson's disease. Neurology 2002;58(4 Suppl 1):S71–8.
23. Chaudhuri KR, Pal S, Brefel-Courbon C. "Sleep attacks" or "unintended sleep episodes" occur with dopamine agonists: is this a class effect? Drug Saf 2002;25(7):473–83.
24. Etminan M, Samii A, Takkouche B, Rochon PA. Increased risk of somnolence with the new dopamine agonists in patients with Parkinson's disease: a meta-analysis of randomised controlled trials. Drug Saf 2001;24(11):863–8.
25. Ondo WG, Dat Vuong K, Khan H, Atassi F, Kwak C, Jankovic J. Daytime sleepiness and other sleep disorders in Parkinson's disease. Neurology 2001;57(8):1392–6.
26. Pal S, Bhattacharya KF, Agapito C, Chaudhuri KR. A study of excessive daytime sleepiness and its clinical significance in three groups of Parkinson's disease patients taking pramipexole, cabergoline and levodopa mono and combination therapy. J Neural Transm 2001;108(1):71–7.
27. Sanjiv CC, Schulzer M, Mak E, Fleming J, Martin WR, Brown T, Calne SM, Tsui J, Stoessl AJ, Lee CS, Calne DB. Daytime somnolence in patients with Parkinson's disease. Parkinsonism Relat Disord 2001;7(4):283–6.
28. Montastruc JL, Brefel-Courbon C, Senard JM, Bagheri H, Ferreira J, Rascol O, Lapeyre-Mestre M. Sleep attacks and antiparkinsonian drugs: a pilot prospective pharmacoepidemiologic study. Clin Neuropharmacol 2001;24(3):181–3.
29. Ferreira JJ, Thalamas C, Montastruc JL, Castro-Caldas A, Rascol O. Levodopa monotherapy can induce "sleep attacks" in Parkinson's disease patients. J Neurol 2001;248(5):426–7.
30. Micallef-Roll J, Rihet P, Hasbroucq T, Possamai C, Blin O. Levodopa-induced drowsiness in healthy volunteers: results of a choice reaction time test combined with a subjective evaluation of sedation. Clin Neuropharmacol 2001;24(2):91–4.
31. Hobson DE, Lang AE, Martin WR, Razmy A, Rivest J, Fleming J. Excessive daytime sleepiness and sudden-onset sleep in Parkinson disease: a survey by the Canadian Movement Disorders Group. JAMA 2002;287(4):455–63.
32. O'Suilleabhain PE, Dewey RB Jr. Contributions of dopaminergic drugs and disease severity to daytime sleepiness in Parkinson disease. Arch Neurol 2002;59(6):986–9.
33. Ulivelli M, Rossi S, Lombardi C, Bartalini S, Rocchi R, Giannini F, Passero S, Battistini N, Lugaresi E. Polysomnographic characterization of pergolide-induced sleep attacks in idiopathic PD. Neurology 2002;58(3):462–5.
34. Moller JC, Stiasny K, Hargutt V, Cassel W, Tietze H, Peter JH, Kruger HP, Oertel WH. Evaluation of sleep and driving performance in six patients with Parkinson's disease reporting sudden onset of sleep under dopaminergic medication: a pilot study. Mov Disord 2002;17(3):474–81.
35. Ferreira JJ, Galitzky M, Thalamas C, Tiberge M, Montastruc JL, Sampaio C, Rascol O. Effect of ropinirole on sleep onset: a randomized, placebo-controlled study in healthy volunteers. Neurology 2002;58(3):460–2.
36. Winkelman AC, DiPalma JR. Drug treatment of parkinsonism. Semin Drug Treatm 1972;1:10.
37. Soliman IE, Park TS, Berkelhamer MC. Transient paralysis after intrathecal bolus of baclofen for the treatment of

post-selective dorsal rhizotomy pain in children. Anesth Analg 1999;89(5):1233–5.
38. Vazquez A, Jimenez-Jimenez FJ, Garcia-Ruiz P, Garcia-Urra D. "Panic attacks" in Parkinson's disease. A long-term complication of levodopa therapy. Acta Neurol Scand 1993;87(1):14–18.
39. Presthus J, Holmsen R. Appraisal of long-term levodopa treatment of parkinsonism with special reference to therapy limiting factors. Acta Neurol Scand 1974;50(6):774–90.
40. Giovannoni G, O'Sullivan JD, Turner K, Manson AJ, Lees AJ. Hedonistic homeostatic dysregulation in patients with Parkinson's disease on dopamine replacement therapies. J Neurol Neurosurg Psychiatry 2000;68(4):423–8.
41. Goetz CG, Leurgans S, Pappert EJ, Raman R, Stemer AB. Prospective longitudinal assessment of hallucinations in Parkinson's disease. Neurology 2001;57(11):2078–82.
42. Sommer BR, Wise LC, Kraemer HC. Is dopamine administration possibly a risk factor for delirium? Crit Care Med 2002;30(7):1508–11.
43. Anonymous. Levodopa (Larodopa). For the relief of symptoms associated with Parkinson's disease and syndrome. Clin Pharmacol Ther 1970;11(6):921–4.
44. Galea-Debono A, Jenner P, Marsden CD, Parkes JD, Tarsy D, Walters J. Plasma DOPA levels and growth hormone response to levodopa in parkinsonism. J Neurol Neurosurg Psychiatry 1977;40(2):162–7.
45. Rayfield EJ, George DT, Eichner HL, Hsu TH. L-dopa stimulation of glucagon secretion in man. N Engl J Med 1975;293(12):589–91.
46. Granerus AK, Jagenburg R, Svanborg A. Kaliuretic effect of L-dopa treatment in parkinsonian patients. Acta Med Scand 1977;201(4):291–7.
47. Markham CH, Treciokas LJ, Diamond SG. Parkinson's disease and levodopa. A five-year follow-up and review. West J Med 1974;121(3):188–206.
48. Jotkowitz S. Urinary retention as complication of levodopa therapy. JAMA 1976;235(24):2586.
49. Goldberg LI. L-dopa effect on renal function. N Engl J Med 1977;297(2):112–13.
50. Lisi P. Pemfigo eritemosa indotto dall'associazione levodopa-carbidopa. Ann Ital Dermatol Clin Sper 1983;37.
51. Marshall A, Williams MJ. Alopecia and levodopa. BMJ 1971;2(752):47.
52. Honda H, Gindin RA. Gout while receiving levodopa for Parkinsonism. JAMA 1972;219(1):55–7.
53. Toru M, Matsuda O, Makiguchi K, Sugano K. Neuroleptic malignant syndrome-like state following a withdrawal of antiparkinsonian drugs. J Nerv Ment Dis 1981;169(5):324–7.
54. Mizuno Y, Takubo H, Mizuta E, Kuno S. Malignant syndrome in Parkinson's disease: concept and review of the literature. Parkinsonism Relat Disord 2003;9(Suppl 1):S3–9.
55. De Mari M, Zenzola A, Lamberti P. Antiparkinsonian treatment in pregnancy. Mov Disord 2002;17(2):428–9.
56. Makoff AJ, Graham JM, Arranz MJ, Forsyth J, Li T, Aitchison KJ, Shaikh S, Grunewald RA. Association study of dopamine receptor gene polymorphisms with drug-induced hallucinations in patients with idiopathic Parkinson's disease. Pharmacogenetics 2000;10(1):43–8.
57. Grandas F, Galiano ML, Tabernero C. Risk factors for levodopa-induced dyskinesias in Parkinson's disease. J Neurol 1999;246(12):1127–33.
58. Cosentino C, Torres L, Scorticati MC, Micheli F. Movement disorders secondary to adulterated medication. Neurology 2000;55(4):598–9.
59. Hunter KR, Boakes AJ, Laurence DR, Stern GM. Monoamine oxidase inhibitors and L-dopa. BMJ 1970;3(719):388.
60. Goldberg LI, Whitsett TL. Cardiovascular effects of levodopa. Clin Pharmacol Ther 1971;12(2):376–82.
61. Duvoisin RC. Antagonism of levodopa by papaverine. JAMA 1975;231(8):845–6.
62. Posner DM. Antagonism of levodopa by papaverine. JAMA 1975;233(7):768.
63. Kissel P, Tridon P, Andre JM. Levodopa–propranolol therapy in parkinsonian tremor. Lancet 1974;1(7854):403–4.
64. Carter AB. Pyridoxine and Parkinsonism. BMJ 1973;4(5886):236.
65. Leon AS, Spiegel HE, Thomas G, Abrams WB. Pyridoxine antagonism of levodopa in parkinsonism. JAMA 1971;218(13):1924–7.
66. Feldman JM, Lebovitz HE. Levodopa and tests for urinary glucose. N Engl J Med 1970;283(19):1053–4.
67. Wolcott GJ, Hackett TN Jr. Levodopa and tests for ketonuria. N Engl J Med 1970;283(27):1522.
68. Colzi A, Turner K, Lees AJ. Continuous subcutaneous waking day apomorphine in the long term treatment of levodopa induced interdose dyskinesias in Parkinson's disease. J Neurol Neurosurg Psychiatry 1998;64(5):573–6.
69. Verhagen Metman L, Del Dotto P, van den Munckhof P, Fang J, Mouradian MM, Chase TN. Amantadine as treatment for dyskinesias and motor fluctuations in Parkinson's disease. Neurology 1998;50(5):1323–6.
70. Jankovic J, Lai E, Ben-Arie L, Krauss JK, Grossman R. Levodopa-induced dyskinesias treated by pallidotomy. J Neurol Sci 1999;167(1):62–7.
71. Merims D, Ziv I, Djaldetti R, Melamed E. Riluzole for levodopa-induced dyskinesias in advanced Parkinson's disease. Lancet 1999;353(9166):1764–5.
72. The French Clozapine Parkinson Study Group. Clozapine in drug-induced psychosis in Parkinson's disease. Lancet 1999;353(9169):2041–2.

Levofloxacin

See also Fluoroquinolones

General Information

Levofloxacin, the levorotatory (*S*)-enantiomer of the racemate ofloxacin, is an oral and parenteral fluoroquinolone that has bactericidal activity against a wide spectrum of Gram-negative and Gram-positive bacilli (including *Streptococcus pneumoniae*), as well as atypical respiratory pathogens.

In patients with meningitis, levofloxacin penetration in cerebrospinal fluid and the liquor-to-plasma ratio was assessed at 2 hours after dosing in five patients with spontaneous acute bacterial meningitis. Cerebrospinal fluid levofloxacin concentration at 2 hours after dosing was 2.0 μg/ml, and the liquor-to-plasma ratio at 2 hours after dosing was 0.35 (1).

Observational studies

In 10 patients who took levofloxacin 500 mg/day and rifampicin 600 mg/day for 2–6 months, there were no adverse reactions in 46% of patients, occasional digestive symptoms in 40%, and mild diarrhea in 13%; these patients also took unspecified anti-inflammatory drugs (2). There was sleeplessness in 6% but neither tendinitis nor changes in liver function.

In a prospective, multicenter open trial, 313 patients with clinical signs and symptoms of bacterial infections of the respiratory tract, skin, or urinary tract were treated with levofloxacin (3). Of these, 134 patients had a pathogen recovered from the primary infection site and had an MIC of the pathogen to levofloxacin determined. Levofloxacin generated clinical and microbiological response rates of about 95%. These response rates included pathogens such as *Streptococcus pneumoniae* and *Staphylococcus aureus*. In a logistic regression analysis, the clinical outcome was predicted by the ratio of peak plasma concentration to MIC and site of infection. Microbiological eradication was predicted by the peak concentration/MIC ratio. Both clinical and microbiological outcomes were most likely to be favorable if the peak concentration/MIC ratio was at least 12.

Of 17 individuals with suspected latent multidrug-resistant tuberculosis treated with pyrazinamide and levofloxacin, 11 developed musculoskeletal adverse effects related to therapy, 5 had nervous system effects, and 15 had raised liver enzymes, uric acid, or creatinine kinase (4).

Comparative studies

In comparative trials involving commonly used regimens, levofloxacin had equivalent if not greater activity in the treatment of community-acquired pneumonia, acute bacterial exacerbations of chronic bronchitis, acute bacterial sinusitis, acute pyelonephritis, and complicated urinary tract infection (5).

General adverse effects

The adverse effects rates of levofloxacin are 1.3% for nausea, 0.1% for anxiety, 0.3% for insomnia, and 0.1% for headache. No levofloxacin-related adverse events were reported at a rate higher than 1.3%, and most were less common. High-dose levofloxacin (750 mg) was also well tolerated. Surveillance data reported low adverse event rates: nausea 0.8%, rash 0.5%, abdominal pain 0.4%, and diarrhea, dizziness, and vomiting 0.3%. The adverse drug reactions rate for levofloxacin is still one of the lowest of any fluoroquinolone, at 2% compared with 2–10% for other fluoroquinolones (6–9).

Organs and Systems

Cardiovascular

Preclinical and clinical trial data and data from phase IV studies have suggested that levofloxacin causes prolongation of the QT interval (10). There were cardiovascular problems in 1 in 15 million prescriptions compared with 1–3% of patients taking sparfloxacin, who had QT_c prolongation to over 500 ms. Polymorphous ventricular tachycardia with a normal QT interval has been associated with oral levofloxacin in the absence of other causes (6,9,11,12).

Among 23 patients who took levofloxacin 500 mg/day there was prolongation of the QT_c interval by more than 30 ms in four patients and 60 ms in two patients (13). There was absolute QT interval prolongation to over 500 ms in four patients, one of whom developed torsade de pointes.

Phlebitis can occur during parenteral administration of levofloxacin. High concentrations of levofloxacin (5 mg/ml) significantly reduced intracellular ATP content in cultured endothelial cells and reduced ADP, GTP, and GDP concentrations (14). These in vitro data suggest that high doses of levofloxacin are not compatible with maintenance of endothelial cell function and may explain the occurrence of phlebitis. Commercial formulations should be diluted and given into large veins.

Respiratory

Eosinophilic pneumonia complicated by bronchial asthma has been attributed to levofloxacin (15).

- A 76-year-old woman took levofloxacin for a productive cough with non-segmental infiltration in both lung fields. She developed eosinophilia in both the peripheral blood (24%) and the sputum (10%), airflow limitation, hypoxemia, and increased airway responsiveness to methacholine. Bronchoalveolar lavage fluid showed increased total cells and a 55% increase in eosinophils, and the CD4/CD8 ratio was reduced to 0.8. Histological features included increased infiltration of eosinophils in the alveolar and interstitial compartments and goblet cell metaplasia. Levofloxacin was withdrawn, and her symptoms improved without steroid therapy. A leukocyte migration test for levofloxacin was weakly positive.

Nervous system

Levofloxacin can cause seizures (16). In one study convulsions occurred in two per million prescriptions (9,17).

- A 75-year-old white woman was given oral levofloxacin (500 mg on day 1 followed by 250 mg/day) for ischemic toes (16). After three doses she had a seizure. One month later, she was challenged with ciprofloxacin 400 mg intravenously every 12 hours and again had a seizure.
- A 74-year-old white woman was given oral levofloxacin 500 mg/day for bacterial pneumonia and had a seizure after five doses (16).

Sensory systems

Taste disturbance occurred in less than three per million prescriptions of levofloxacin (9).

Gastrointestinal

Of 48 patients taking pyrazinamide 30 mg/kg/day plus levofloxacin 500 mg/day for 1 year, 27 discontinued therapy within 4 months owing to adverse events. Gastrointestinal intolerance was the major adverse event that resulted in early withdrawal (18).

Levofloxacin can cause pseudomembranous colitis due to *Clostridium difficile* (19).

Liver

In a study based on European and international data from about 130 million prescriptions, the adverse effects profile of levofloxacin was compared with that of other fluoroquinolones; there was a low rate of hepatic abnormalities (1/650 000) (6). However, two cases of severe acute liver toxicity were reported in patients who had received intravenous levofloxacin (20,21).

Pancreas

Two case reports have suggested that levofloxacin can cause pancreatitis (22).

Urinary tract

Two reports have suggested that levofloxacin can cause tubulointerstitial nephritis (23). A case of nephrotoxicity and purpura associated with levofloxacin has also been reported; allergic interstitial nephritis or vasculitis was believed to be the underlying pathologic process (24).

- A 73-year-old white man took levofloxacin for a lower urinary tract infection for 3 days and developed palpable purpura and erythematous skin lesions over the lower limbs and trunk, with a markedly reduced urine output. Serum creatinine was 560 μmol/l (6.4 mg/dl). Levofloxacin was withdrawn, and prednisone, furosemide, and intravenous fluids were given. The patient recovered fully over the next 4 weeks.

Skin

In a double-blind, randomized study in 30 healthy adults oral levofloxacin (500 mg/day for 5 days) had a low photosensitizing potential (25), as it did in preclinical animal studies and postmarketing surveillance (26). In preclinical studies levofloxacin was 20 times less phototoxic than sparfloxacin. Phototoxicity occurs in only 1 in 1.8 million cases.

Levofloxacin can cause a rash similar to the ampicillin rash in patients with infectious mononucleosis (27).

- A 78-year-old woman developed a rash with blistering 2 days after completing a course of levofloxacin (28). The rash progressed to toxic epidermal necrolysis in 7 days. She was treated with intravenous fluids and wound dressings. Her condition improved and she was discharged after 22 days.

Musculoskeletal

Tendinopathy has been reported with levofloxacin. Four cases of Achilles tendinitis have been reported in patients taking levofloxacin (29). Two were on chronic dialysis, one was a kidney transplant recipient, and one had chronic vasculitis. In all four cases, tendinitis had an acute onset with bilateral involvement and was incapacitating. In three cases the onset was early during levofloxacin treatment and in one case it began 10 days after the end of treatment. All the patients recovered completely after 3–8 weeks.

Old age, renal dysfunction, and concomitant corticosteroid therapy are predisposing risk factors (30,31). Tendon rupture occurred in less than four per million prescriptions (9).

Immunologic

Anaphylactic and anaphylactoid reactions are rare adverse events after the administration of fluoroquinolones (about 0.46–1.2 per 100 000 patients).

- On two occasions a 49-year-old asthmatic woman who took levofloxacin for a chest infection developed worse respiratory distress, requiring intubation (32). The second reaction was accompanied by a marked skin reaction.

An in vitro study in rat peritoneal mast cells showed that levofloxacin-mediated release of histamine may be closely linked to activation of pertussis toxin-sensitive G proteins (33).

Susceptibility Factors

The pharmacokinetics of intravenous levofloxacin have been studied in intensive care unit patients during continuous venovenous hemofiltration or hemodiafiltration (34,35). Levofloxacin clearance was substantially increased during both types of continuous renal replacement therapy. Levofloxacin 250 mg/day maintained effective plasma drug concentrations in these patients.

Drug–Drug Interactions

Chinese medicines

Chinese medicines did not influence the systemic availability or renal excretion of levofloxacin (36).

Efavirenz

Levofloxacin pharmacokinetics in HIV-positive patients were not altered by steady-state treatment with efavirenz (37).

HIV protease inhibitors

Levofloxacin pharmacokinetics in HIV-positive patients were not altered by steady-state treatment with nelfinavir (37).

Lithium

Co-administration with levofloxacin can cause severe lithium toxicity; the authors did not discuss the mechanism (38).

Theophylline

Theophylline clearance was reduced by levofloxacin plus clarithromycin in a 59-year-old Japanese man, who had stimulation, insomnia, and tachycardia due to theophylline toxicity (39).

The mechanism was probably inhibition of theophylline metabolism by CYP1A2 and CYP3A4.

Warfarin

Enhanced hypoprothrombinemia has been reported when levofloxacin was given with warfarin (40–42).

References

1. Villani P, Viale P, Signorini L, Cadeo B, Marchetti F, Villani A, Fiocchi C, Regazzi MB, Carosi G. Pharmacokinetic evaluation of oral levofloxacin in human immunodeficiency virus-infected subjects receiving concomitant antiretroviral therapy. Antimicrob Agents Chemother 2001;45(7):2160–2.
2. Ortega M, Soriano A, Garcia S, Almela M, Alvarez JL, Tomas X, Mensa J, Soriano E. Perfil de tolerabilidad y seguridad de levofloxacinoen tratamientos prolongados. [Tolerability and safety of levofloxacinin long-term treatment.] Rev Esp Quimioter 2000;13(3):263–6.
3. Preston SL, Drusano GL, Berman AL, Fowler CL, Chow AT, Dornseif B, Reichl V, Natarajan J, Corrado M. Pharmacodynamics of levofloxacin: a new paradigm for early clinical trials. JAMA 1998;279(2):125–9.
4. Papastavros T, Dolovich LR, Holbrook A, Whitehead L, Loeb M. Adverse events associated with pyrazinamide and levofloxacin in the treatment of latent multidrug-resistant tuberculosis. CMAJ 2002;167(2):131–6.
5. Wimer SM, Schoonover L, Garrison MW. Levofloxacin: a therapeutic review. Clin Ther 1998;20(6):1049–70.
6. Carbon C. Comparison of side effects of levofloxacin versus other fluoroquinolones. Chemotherapy 2001;47(Suppl 3): 9–14; discussion 44–8.
7. Rossi C, Sternon J. Les fluoroquinolones de troisième et quatrième generations. [Third and fourth generation fluoroquinolones.] Rev Med Brux 2001;22(5):443–56.
8. Chow AT, Fowler C, Williams RR, Morgan N, Kaminski S, Natarajan J. Safety and pharmacokinetics of multiple 750-milligram doses of intravenous levofloxacin in healthy volunteers. Antimicrob Agents Chemother 2001;45(7):2122–5.
9. Kahn JB. Latest industry information on the safety profile of levofloxacin in the US. Chemotherapy 2001;47(Suppl 3):32–7; discussion 44–8.
10. Owens RC Jr, Ambrose PG. Torsades de pointes associated with fluoroquinolones. Pharmacotherapy 2002;22(5):663–8; discussion 668–72.
11. Scotton PG, Pea F, Giobbia M, Baraldo M, Vaglia A, Furlanut M. Cerebrospinal fluid penetration of levofloxacin in patients with spontaneous acute bacterial meningitis. Clin Infect Dis 2001;33(9):e109–11.
12. Paltoo B, O'Donoghue S, Mousavi MS. Levofloxacin induced polymorphic ventricular tachycardia with normal QT interval. Pacing Clin Electrophysiol 2001;24(5):895–7.
13. Carbon C. Tolérance de la lévofloxacine, dossier clinique et données de pharmacovigilance. [Levofloxacin adverse effects, data from clinical trials and pharmacovigilance.] Therapie 2001;56(1):35–40.
14. Armbruster C, Robibaro B, Griesmacher A, Vorbach H. Endothelial cell compatibility of trovafloxacin and levofloxacin for intravenous use. J Antimicrob Chemother 2000;45(4):533–5.
15. Fujimori K, Shimatsu Y, Suzuki E, Arakawa M, Gejyo F. [Levofloxacin-induced eosinophilic pneumonia complicated by bronchial asthma.] Nihon Kokyuki Gakkai Zasshi 2000;38(5):385–90.
16. Kushner JM, Peckman HJ, Snyder CR. Seizures associated with fluoroquinolones. Ann Pharmacother 2001;35(10):1194–8.
17. Pedros A, Emilio Gomez J, Angel Navarro L, Tomas A. Levofloxacino y sindrome confusional agudo. [Levofloxacin and acute confusional syndrome.] Med Clin (Barc) 2002;119(1):38–9.
18. Fleisch F, Hartmann K, Kuhn M. Fluoroquinolone-induced tendinopathy: also occurring with levofloxacin. Infection 2000;28(4):256–7.
19. Casado Burgos E, Vinas Ponce G, Lauzurica Valdemoros R, Olive Marques A. Tendinitis por levofloxacino. [Levofloxacin-induced tendinitis.] Med Clin (Barc) 2000;114(8):319.
20. Gates GA. Safety of ofloxacin otic and other ototopical treatments in animal models and in humans. Pediatr Infect Dis J 2001;20(1):104–7; discussion 120–2.
21. Karim A, Ahmed S, Rossoff LJ, Siddiqui RK, Steinberg HN. Possible levofloxacin-induced acute hepatocellular injury in a patient with chronic obstructive lung disease. Clin Infect Dis 2001;33(12):2088–90.
22. Spahr L, Rubbia-Brandt L, Marinescu O, Armenian B, Hadengue A. Acute fatal hepatitis related to levofloxacin. J Hepatol 2001;35(2):308–9.
23. Wood ML, Schlessinger S. Levaquin induced acute tubulointerstitial nephritis—two case reports. J Miss State Med Assoc 2002;43(4):116–17.
24. Famularo G, De Simone C. Nephrotoxicity and purpura associated with levofloxacin. Ann Pharmacother 2002;36(9):1380–2.
25. Boccumini LE, Fowler CL, Campbell TA, Puertolas LF, Kaidbey KH. Photoreaction potential of orally administered levofloxacin in healthy subjects. Ann Pharmacother 2000;34(4):453–8.
26. Mennecier D, Thiolet C, Bredin C, Potier V, Vergeau B, Farret O. Pancreatite aiguë survenant après la prise de lévofloxacine et de methylprédnisolone. [Acute pancreatitis after treatment by levofloxacin and methylprednisolone.] Gastroenterol Clin Biol 2001;25(10):921–2.
27. Paily R. Quinolone drug rash in a patient with infectious mononucleosis. J Dermatol 2000;27(6):405–6.
28. Digwood-Lettieri S, Reilly KJ, Haith LR Jr, Patton ML, Guilday RJ, Cawley MJ, Ackerman BH. Levofloxacin-induced toxic epidermal necrolysis in an elderly patient. Pharmacotherapy 2002;22(6):789–93.
29. Lou HX, Shullo MA, McKaveney TP. Limited tolerability of levofloxacin and pyrazinamide for multidrug-resistant tuberculosis prophylaxis in a solid organ transplant population. Pharmacotherapy 2002;22(6):701–4.
30. Ozawa TT, Valadez T. *Clostridium difficile* infection associated with levofloxacin treatment. Tenn Med 2002;95(3):113–15.
31. Aros C, Flores C, Mezzano S. Tendinitis aquiliana asociada al uso de levofloxacino: comunicacion de cuatro casos. [Achilles tendinitis associated with levofloxacin: report of 4 cases.] Rev Med Chil 2002;130(11):1277–81.
32. Smythe MA, Cappelletty DM. Anaphylactoid reaction to levofloxacin. Pharmacotherapy 2000;20(12):1520–3.
33. Mori K, Maru C, Takasuna K, Furuhama K. Mechanism of histamine release induced by levofloxacin, a fluoroquinolone antibacterial agent. Eur J Pharmacol 2000;394(1):51–5.
34. Malone RS, Fish DN, Abraham E, Teitelbaum I. Pharmacokinetics of levofloxacin and ciprofloxacin during continuous renal replacement therapy in critically ill patients. Antimicrob Agents Chemother 2001;45(10):2949–54.
35. Yagawa K. Latest industry information on the safety profile of levofloxacin in Japan. Chemotherapy 2001;47(Suppl 3):38–43. discussion 44–8.
36. Iunda IF, Kushniruk IuI. [Functional state of the testis after the use of certain antibiotics and nitrofuran preparations.] Antibiotiki 1975;(9):843–6.
37. Nakamura H, Ohtsuka T, Enomoto H, Hasegawa A, Kawana H, Kuriyama T, Ohmori S, Kitada M. Effect of levofloxacin on theophylline clearance during theophylline and clarithromycin combination therapy. Ann Pharmacother 2001;35(6):691–3.
38. Takahashi H, Higuchi H, Shimizu T. Severe lithium toxicity induced by combined levofloxacin administration. J Clin Psychiatry 2000;61(12):949–50.

39. Gheno G, Cinetto L. Levofloxacin–warfarin interaction. Eur J Clin Pharmacol 2001;57(5):427.
40. Jones CB, Fugate SE. Levofloxacin and warfarin interaction. Ann Pharmacother 2002;36(10):1554–7.
41. Hansen E, Bucher M, Jakob W, Lemberger P, Kees F. Pharmacokinetics of levofloxacin during continuous venovenous hemofiltration. Intensive Care Med 2001;27(2):371–5.
42. Ravnan SL, Locke C. Levofloxacin and warfarin interaction. Pharmacotherapy 2001;21(7):884–5.

Levosalbutamol

See also Beta$_2$-adrenoceptor agonists and salbutamol

General Information

Levosalbutamol is the (*R*)-enantiomer of the beta$_2$-adrenoceptor agonist salbutamol. It has been suggested to have a better therapeutic index than racemic salbutamol. As levosalbutamol has a much higher receptor affinity than the (*S*)-enantiomer, the therapeutic effects of racemic salbutamol are assumed to be mediated by levosalbutamol. However, toxicity of levosalbutamol is unrelated to beta$_2$-receptor binding, and so the (*S*)-enantiomer may significantly contribute to the toxicity of racemic salbutamol.

The issue of enantioselective efficacy and safety of salbutamol has been reviewed (1). Interest in "chiral switch," that is the replacement of the racemic formulation by the pharmacologically active (*R*)-enantiomer levosalbutamol, may be hampered by enantiomeric interconversion in vivo and marked interindividual variation in salbutamol pharmacokinetics and pharmacodynamics, owing to complex interactions between genetic and environmental effects. The authors concluded that the advantage of levosalbutamol over the racemic formulation appears to be small with respect to efficacy and controversial with respect to safety. Two large crossover studies with multiple inhaled doses of (*S*)-salbutamol in asthmatic patients showed no evidence of adverse effects on FEV$_1$ (2,3).

The effects of two doses of inhaled levosalbutamol (0.63 and 1.25 mg) and racemic salbutamol (1.25 and 2.50 mg) on FEV$_1$ have been studied in a randomized, double-blind trial in 362 asthmatic patients over 4 weeks (4). The average peak FEV$_1$ for levosalbutamol was significantly greater than that for racemic salbutamol after the first dose but not at week 4. The possible superior bronchodilatation achieved with lower doses of levosalbutamol may be more cost-effective (5).

References

1. Ramsay CM, Cowan J, Flannery E, McLachlan C, Taylor DR. Bronchoprotective and bronchodilator effects of single doses of (S)-salbutamol, (R)-salbutamol and racemic salbutamol in patients with bronchial asthma. Eur J Clin Pharmacol 1999;55(5):353–9.
2. Anastasiadis PG, Anninos P, Assimakopoulos E, Koutlaki N, Kotini A, Galazios G. Fetal heart rate patterns in normal and ritodrine-treated pregnancies, detected by magnetocardiography. J Matern Fetal Med 2001;10(5):350–4.
3. Gokay Z, Ozcan T, Copel JA. Changes in fetal hemodynamics with ritodrine tocolysis. Ultrasound Obstet Gynecol 2001;18(1):44–6.
4. Boulton DW, Fawcett JP. The pharmacokinetics of levosalbutamol: what are the clinical implications? Clin Pharmacokinet 2001;40(1):23–40.
5. Cockcroft DW, Swystun VA. Effect of single doses of S-salbutamol, R-salbutamol, racemic salbutamol, and placebo on the airway response to methacholine. Thorax 1997;52(10):845–8.

Lidocaine

See also Local anesthetics

General Information

Lidocaine is the most widely used aminoamide local anesthetic agent, with a low toxic potential; its effects are mostly typical for this class of drug. It can be given by injection or topically and is also combined with prilocaine in Emla for topical administration. It is also used as an antidysrhythmic drug and has occasionally been used in other conditions, such as multiple sclerosis, chronic daily headache, migraine and cluster headaches, and neuropathic pain, such as postherpetic neuralgia.

Local anesthetic gels and creams used liberally on traumatized epithelium can be rapidly absorbed, resulting in systemic effects, such as convulsions, particularly if excessive quantities are used. This has been highlighted in the case of a 40-year-old woman who developed seizures after lidocaine gel 40 ml was injected into the ureter during an attempt to remove a stone (1). Site of administration is also important, as local conditions, particularly vascularity, affect the rate of absorption. Adverse effects of lidocaine when it is used as a local anesthetic can also occur after inadvertent intravascular injection.

The incidence of adverse effects to lidocaine in antidysrhythmic dosages is low. In one series of 750 patients given lidocaine intravenously for cardiac dysrhythmias, adverse reactions occurred in only 47 (6.3%) and were thought to have been life-threatening in 12 (1.6%) (2). However, the risk of adverse effects is dose-related and increases at intravenous infusion rates of around 3 mg/minute (3). Most of the adverse effects are on the cardiovascular and central nervous systems. Nervous system toxicity is directly related to blood concentrations, with symptoms that include light-headedness, headache, dizziness, tremor, confusion, tinnitus, dysarthria, paresthesia, alterations in the level of consciousness from drowsiness to coma, respiratory depression, and convulsions. Cardiovascular effects, including dysrhythmias and very rarely worsening of cardiac function, only occur at very high blood concentrations. The intravenous dose of lidocaine required to produce cardiovascular collapse is seven times that which causes seizures. Risks of serious systemic effects do not increase with age. Deaths have occurred with voluntary intoxication, primarily because of the cardiac effects.

The active metabolites of lidocaine, glycinexylidide and monoethylglycinexylidide, are toxic and intravenous infusion should not continue for more than 24–48 hours.

Hypersensitivity reactions are rare, and not all reports are clear, but cases do occur and are usually mild (SED-12, 255) (4). Some patients are highly sensitive to lidocaine, yet insensitive to other aminoamide local anesthetics (5), and the reverse has also been found (SEDA-14, 109). True anaphylaxis with rechallenge has been documented (6). A few cases of contact dermatitis have been reported.

Even topical administration of lidocaine continues to generate reports with tragic outcomes, as absorption from mucosal surfaces is underestimated.

- A patient due to have a bronchoscopy was given an overdose of lidocaine to anesthetize the airway by an inexperienced health worker. He was then left unobserved and subsequently developed convulsions and cardiopulmonary arrest (7). He survived with severe cerebral damage.

His lidocaine concentration was 24 μg/ml about 1 hour after initial administration (a blood concentration over 6 μg/ml is considered to be toxic).

Drug studies

Lidocaine has been used to treat some of the symptoms of multiple sclerosis in 30 patients with painful tonic seizures, attacks of neuralgia, paroxysmal itching, and Lhermitte's sign (8). Lidocaine was given by intravenous infusion for 5.5 hours in a maintenance dose of 2.0–2.8 mg/kg/hour after a loading dose, and the mean steady-state concentration was 2.4 μg/ml. Lidocaine almost completely abolished the paroxysmal symptoms and markedly alleviated the persistent symptoms of multiple sclerosis. Adverse effects were not specifically mentioned, but in one case, when the plasma concentration of lidocaine rose above 3.5 μg/ml, weakness of the left leg became marked and was associated with an extensor plantar response; this disappeared when the lidocaine was replaced by saline single-blind, but subsequently the positive symptoms recurred.

Intravenous lidocaine has been used to treat severe chronic daily headache in 19 patients (three men, median age 37 years) (9). There were adverse effects during four infusions of lidocaine: hyperkalemia (6.4 mmol/l), which did not resolve after withdrawal of lidocaine; transient hypotension (75/50 mmHg), which was attributed to concomitant droperidol; an unspecified abnormality of cardiac rhythm and on another occasion a transient bradycardia; and chest pain with a normal electrocardiogram, fever, and intractable nausea. The study was neither randomized nor placebo-controlled, and in no case was the adverse event strongly associated with the administration of lidocaine.

In a double-blind, placebo-controlled study of the use of intravenous lidocaine for neuropathic pain, 16 patients were given 5 ml/kg intravenously over 30 minutes (10). Lidocaine was better than placebo in relieving pain. The major adverse effect was light-headedness, which occurred in seven patients given lidocaine and none given saline. Other adverse effects included somnolence, nausea and vomiting, dysarthria or garbled speech, blurred vision, and malaise. In two patients the rate of infusion had to be reduced because of adverse effects.

Organs and Systems

Cardiovascular

Lidocaine can cause dysrhythmias and hypotension. The dysrhythmias that have been reported include sinus bradycardia, supraventricular tachycardia (11), and rarely torsade de pointes (12). There have also been rare reports of cardiac arrest (2) and worsening heart failure (13). Lidocaine can also cause an increased risk of asystole after repeated attempts at defibrillation (14). Lidocaine may increase mortality after acute myocardial infarction, and it should be used only in patients with specific so-called warning dysrhythmias (that is frequent or multifocal ventricular extra beats, or salvos) (15).

Sinus bradycardia has been seen after a bolus injection of 50 mg, atrioventricular block after a dose of 800 mg given over 12 hours, and left bundle branch block after a mere subconjunctival injection of 2% lidocaine.

- High-grade atrioventricular block has been reported in a 14-day-old infant who was given lidocaine 2 mg/kg intravenously (SED-12, 255) (16).

A death due to ventricular fibrillation after 50 mg and another due to sinus arrest after 100 mg have been reported (SED-12, 255) (17). Two cases of ventricular fibrillation and cardiopulmonary arrest occurred after local infiltration of lidocaine for cardiac catheterization (SEDA-21, 136).

Lidocaine does not usually cause conduction disturbances, but two cases have been reported in the presence of hyperkalemia (18).

- A 57-year-old man with a wide-complex tachycardia was given lidocaine 100 mg intravenously and immediately became asystolic. Resuscitation was unsuccessful.
- A 31-year-old woman had a cardiac arrest and was resuscitated to a wide-complex tachycardia, which was treated with intravenous lidocaine 100 mg. She immediately became asystolic but responded to calcium chloride.

In both cases there was severe hyperkalemia, and the authors suggested that hyperkalemia-induced resting membrane depolarization had increased the number of inactivated sodium channels, thus increasing the binding of lidocaine and potentiating its effects.

The degree of hypotension occurring after epidural anesthesia with alkalinized lidocaine (with adrenaline) was greater than with a standard commercial solution (SED-12, 255) (19).

In 23 patients there was a significant dose-dependent reduction in blood pressure following submucosal infiltration of lidocaine plus adrenaline compared with saline plus adrenaline for orthognathic surgery (20). The study was randomized but small; larger studies are needed to confirm effects that could easily have been due to multifactorial causes in patients undergoing general anesthesia.

Respiratory

Topical anesthesia of the airways is commonly used to facilitate endoscopy and sometimes manipulation of the airways. This can result in an increase in airway flow resistance, possibly due to laryngeal dysfunction (21). Lidocaine spray 10%, used for upper airways anesthesia for fiberoptic intubation in a grossly obese patient, caused acute airway obstruction. The patient went on to have a percutaneous tracheotomy, and it was postulated that the local anesthetic had abolished laryngeal receptors responsible for airway maintenance, or that laryngospasm and reduced muscle tone due to the lidocaine might have been the cause (SEDA-22, 140).

Life-threatening bronchospasm can occur after either spinal or topical use of lidocaine. In one series of patients being treated with lidocaine spray 40 mg for persistent cough, there was an increase of airway resistance (SED-12, 255) (22).

Ear, nose, throat

Local anesthesia to the larynx, for example with 4% lidocaine, is generally safe. Laryngeal edema has been reported in a few cases and could be due to the propellant rather than to lidocaine itself (23).

Intranasal 4% lidocaine has been used for migraine and cluster headaches with success and few serious adverse effects: a bitter taste was common and some patients complained of nasal burning and oropharyngeal numbness (SEDA-20, 127).

Lidocaine gel is not recommended for lubrication of laryngeal masks. It confers no benefits and increases the incidence of adverse effects such as intraoperative hiccups, postoperative hoarseness, nausea, vomiting, and tongue paresthesia (24).

Nervous system

Nervous system toxicity is most often seen with rapid intravenous infusion (3,25,26). The effects include headache, dizziness, tremor, confusion, tinnitus, dysarthria, paresthesia, respiratory depression, altered level of consciousness (from drowsiness to coma), and convulsions.

Two cases have illustrated the effects of lidocaine in precipitating partial seizures in patients with a previous history of epilepsy (27).

- A 36-year-old woman developed chest pain and ventricular tachycardia. She had a 14-year history of right-sided focal motor seizures controlled with phenytoin. After receiving intravenous lidocaine 100 mg to treat the dysrhythmias, she developed a typical seizure involving the right side of her face and arm. She was given a loading dose of phenytoin and the seizure abated. However, the ventricular tachycardia persisted and was treated with additional lidocaine 50 mg followed by an infusion of 3.3 mg/minute; 6 hours later she had a generalized seizure with a venous blood lidocaine concentration of 21 μg/ml. The infusion was stopped and the seizure was treated with intravenous diazepam 10 mg.
- A 41-year-old woman with a long-standing history of focal and secondarily generalized seizures controlled with carbamazepine underwent cerebral arteriography, during which she was inadvertently given lidocaine 20 mg via an intra-arterial catheter in the right internal carotid artery; within 20 seconds she had a focal seizure.

These two patients had their typical partial seizures triggered by high doses of lidocaine. In both cases the serum concentrations of their usual anticonvulsants were initially low. The first patient received a loading dose of phenytoin after the partial seizure, was then given a second bolus of lidocaine and an infusion, and then had a second seizure, which was generalized. There was no evidence that this second seizure evolved from the left seizure focus. The authors concluded that lidocaine can activate seizure foci in patients with a history of partial seizures and that this may be more likely if the serum concentrations of anticonvulsants are low. However, therapeutic concentrations of antiepileptic drugs may not prevent generalized seizures that result from the widespread lowering of seizure threshold caused by high concentrations of lidocaine.

A tonic-clonic seizure occurred after the application of 400 mg of lidocaine jelly to traumatized ureteric mucosa (SEDA-22, 142).

- A 54-year-old woman who was given lidocaine, 200 mg intravenously, for ventricular fibrillation during cardiopulmonary bypass, had a tonic-clonic seizure (28). The seizure occurred immediately after the administration of lidocaine and was relieved by the intravenous administration of thiopental and midazolam. Her ventricular fibrillation responded to procainamide 1 g intravenously over 10 minutes.

The pharmacokinetics of lidocaine are altered by cardiopulmonary bypass, because of hemodilution, changed protein binding, the exclusion of the lungs as an organ for first-pass elimination, altered acid-base balance, and sometimes drug interactions. In particular, reduced protein binding may have contributed in this case to the risk of seizure, but plasma lidocaine concentrations were not measured.

- A 30-year-old woman received two 5 g applications of 40% lidocaine cream with occlusion by plastic wrap during and after laser therapy to areas of her skin (29). She developed dizziness and headache postoperatively, followed 45 minutes later by light-headedness, increasing dizziness, and confusion. The dressings were removed. The lidocaine concentration was 2.7 μg/ml 7 hours later.

It is recommended that repeat applications of lidocaine, especially in high-concentration formulations, be avoided and the area of application limited.

- A 16-year-old woman had had an adverse reaction after administration of an unknown local anesthetic agent for a dental procedure. Patch testing had elicited similar symptoms with lidocaine only, and 20 minutes after subcutaneous lidocaine 0.05 mg she developed perioral paresthesia, nausea, vomiting, vertigo, dizziness, mild agitation, drowsiness, and euphoria. Hemodynamic parameters remained stable but her symptoms were thought to be part of a genuine non-allergic, neuropsychiatric reaction, as the patch testing was double-blind and placebo-controlled (30).

Transient and permanent nerve damage can occur after regional anesthesia, particularly neuraxial anesthesia. The mechanism of this nerve damage is unclear. Some studies have shown an indirect effect. However, in crayfish giant axon, lidocaine had a dose- and time-dependent effect on isolated nerve function in vitro (31). At high concentrations lidocaine caused irreversible conduction block and total loss of resting membrane potential. These results in an isolated nerve suggest a direct neurotoxic effect of lidocaine.

Sensory systems

Tinnitus and visual disturbances are early components of a systemic toxic reaction to lidocaine.

Eyes

A potentially beneficial effect of lidocaine has been studied in a randomized, double-blind, placebo-controlled study of the effects of preinstillation of lidocaine on tropicamide-induced mydriasis (32). Pupillary diameter was significantly increased by the instillation of lidocaine before tropicamide. It was thought that lidocaine can enhance intraocular penetration and hence potentiate the effect of tropicamide.

Double vision and difficulty in focusing have been attributed to lidocaine applied to the tongue (33).

- A 22-year-old man developed double vision and difficulty in focusing after using 2% viscous lidocaine for a painful tongue ulcer. He used viscous 2% lidocaine 10 ml hourly and developed symptoms when the daily dose exceeded 240 ml (4800 mg of lidocaine hydrochloride) after 10 days of use. At that time his serum lidocaine concentration was 6.7 μg/ml. His symptoms persisted when the serum concentration of lidocaine fell to below toxic concentrations, implying that metabolites of lidocaine had contributed.

Temporary blindness, an unusual feature of lidocaine toxicity, has been reported in an otherwise healthy young woman (34).

- A 21-year-old 50 kg woman, previously fit, was to have an open reduction and fixation of a fractured proximal phalanx with intravenous regional anesthesia. As a result of misreading the vial label, 30 ml (600 mg) of 2% lidocaine was injected, and this inadvertent error was immediately recognized. The decision was made to continue with the procedure, which was uneventful, with a tourniquet time of 45 minutes. At this point the patient complained of severe tourniquet pain, and without the anesthesiologist's knowledge the cuff was deflated. Immediately she developed a tachycardia, complained of visual disturbances, and became unconscious. She had a seizure, which lasted 30 seconds and resolved with midazolam. She became more alert, but complained of reduced vision. Neurological examination was normal, apart from temporary blindness; this fully resolved within 10 minutes. There were no long-term neurological or visual sequelae.

The authors suggested that the visual symptoms could have occurred as a result of occipital lobe seizure activity or subcortical stimulation, due to the acute high cerebral concentration of lidocaine. The speed of spontaneous resolution was consistent with the pharmacokinetics of lidocaine.

Pupillary mydriasis occurred in a neonate who was given intravenous lidocaine 3 mg/kg/hour as an anticonvulsant (35).

Taste

Taste disturbance has been reported with lidocaine (36).

- A 73-year-old woman was given a Nadbath Rehman block behind the left pinna to provide motor blockade of cranial nerve VII, before retrobulbar block for cataract surgery. Several minutes later she complained of a metallic taste in her mouth. After surgery she had altered taste sensation on the anterior left side of the tongue, with recovery a day later.

The author postulated this to be due to block of the chorda tympani, which runs with cranial nerve VII close to the site of the Nadbath Rehman block.

Metabolism

High systemic doses of lidocaine can cause transient hypoglycemia (SED-12, 255) (37).

Electrolyte balance

There has been one report of hypokalemia (2.2 mmol/l), probably due to potassium channel blockade, after administration of high-dose intravenous lidocaine (8 mg/l) for raised intracranial pressure (SEDA-21, 136).

Hematologic

Severe thrombocytopenic purpura with a lidocaine-mediated antiplatelet IgM antibody has been reported (SED-12, 255) (38).

Three cases of lidocaine-induced methemoglobinemia have been reported in patients undergoing topical anesthesia of the airway and oropharynx (39).

- A 26-year-old woman undergoing bronchoscopy received lidocaine jelly 2% to each nostril, lidocaine solution 2% sprayed on the throat, and 10 ml of lidocaine solution 2% into the trachea. She was also given intravenous diazepam 5 mg and pethidine 75 mg and intramuscular atropine 0.6 mg. She developed dyspnea and cyanosis after the procedure and despite 100% oxygen, her SpO_2 was 85%. Her methemoglobin concentration was 14%.
- A 61-year-old woman was given 15 ml of lidocaine solution 2% and lidocaine spray 4% for topical anesthesia of the throat and oropharynx before upper gastrointestinal endoscopy. She was also sedated with intravenous midazolam 2 mg and pethidine 75 mg. She became cyanosed and desaturated (SpO_2 78%) immediately after the procedure. Her SpO_2 did not recover, despite 100% oxygen. Her methemoglobin concentration was 37%.
- In preparation for transesophageal echocardiogram, a 73-year-old woman was given 15 ml of lidocaine solution 2% and lidocaine spray 4% to anesthetize the oropharynx, plus intravenous midazolam 1 mg and pethidine 12.5 mg. She very rapidly became cyanosed, but remained

asymptomatic. Her SpO_2 was 85% on oxygen 2 l/minute and her methemoglobin concentration was 25%.

Liver

Liver damage due to lidocaine has rarely been reported. However, severe liver damage has been reported shortly after the withdrawal of mexiletine 300 mg/day and the introduction of lidocaine 1000 mg/day, although lidocaine in the same dose had been used during the previous week (40). The lidocaine was withdrawn and the liver enzymes normalized after treatment with prednisolone.

Skin

Topical 5% lidocaine to 33 patients with postherpetic neuralgia in a crossover trial provided significantly more pain relief than a vehicle patch placebo (41). There was no difference in reported adverse effects: skin redness or rash was reported by 9 in the lidocaine patch phase and 11 in the placebo phase. One patient stopped using the placebo patch owing to red irritated skin, which resolved after the application of lidocaine patches.

Treatment of 27 HIV-infected patients with distal sensory polyneuropathy (the most common neurological disorder associated with HIV) with 5% lidocaine gel resulted in effective analgesia in 75% of patients; three had dry skin and one had blisters (42).

In a phase IV trial, 66% patients with postherpetic neuralgia gained relief from a 5% lidocaine patch applied to the most painful area of the body (43). The lidocaine patch was well tolerated, a rash being the most common adverse effect, in 14% of patients.

Several cases of contact dermatitis have been reported with lidocaine. Generalized exfoliative dermatitis has also been noted once. Local inflammation and necrosis, possibly due to mechanical pressure, are both complications at the injection site.

- A 60-year-old woman was given infiltration anesthesia with lidocaine hydrochloride for removal of a melanoma (44). She developed an itchy dermatitis over the area 36 hours later. Conventional patch testing was negative at 48 and 72 hours to lidocaine and mepivacaine (both amides), as was intracutaneous testing with lidocaine 2%, mepivacaine 2%, and bupivacaine 0.5%. However, intradermal testing at 1/100 dilutions was positive, with itching and erythema at 48 hours with lidocaine and mepivacaine, suggesting delayed hypersensitivity to these drugs, but not with bupivacaine.

It has previously been reported that lidocaine and mepivacaine have a high degree of cross-reactivity not seen with bupivacaine.

Sexual function

Two cases of impotence after anesthesia for elective circumcision in adults have been described (SED-12, 256) (45), but it is very doubtful whether this was a pharmacological and not merely a psychological effect.

Immunologic

There have been 62 reports of allergic contact dermatitis to lidocaine worldwide between 1972 and 1996; 49 were in Australia and several showed cross-reactivity with other amide local anesthetics, such as bupivacaine, mepivacaine, and prilocaine (46).

Body temperature

There is no reliable evidence to support reports of malignant hyperthermia due to local anesthetic agents. In 307 dental patients susceptible to malignant hyperthermia who received local anesthesia, only one had ever developed symptoms suggestive of malignant hyperthermia, after mepivacaine and on another occasion lidocaine (47). Both reactions resolved without specific therapy. There has been one case report of cyanosis, muscle rigidity, tachycardia, tachypnea, a temperature of 41.5°C, and loss of consciousness in a patient who received epidural lidocaine and bupivacaine (48). However, perioperative stress may itself be a potential trigger of malignant hyperthermia.

Death

In New York City, five of 50 000 deaths over a 5-year period were associated with tumescent liposuction; all had received lidocaine in doses of 10–40 mg/kg in association with general anesthesia and/or intravenous sedation and analgesia (49). Three patients died as a result of severe acute intraoperative hypotension and bradycardia with no identified cause, one died of fluid overload, and another died of pulmonary embolism. The authors speculated that lidocaine toxicity or lidocaine-related drug interactions could have contributed to some of the deaths, but other causes could not be ruled out.

In California, six cases of cardiac arrest or severe hypoxemia associated with outpatient liposuction resulted in four deaths over a 3.5-year period, all in women aged 38–62 years; one had a cardiac arrest after sedation and the administration of local anesthetic but before liposuction was started, four had respiratory difficulties and cardiac arrest after liposuction, and one had respiratory difficulties during liposuction (50). Whether the cause of morbidity and mortality in any of these cases was related to local anesthetic toxicity was not mentioned.

A weak solution of lidocaine has sometimes been injected into excess fat before liposuction, so that the procedure can be carried out without general anesthesia. The technique is generally regarded as safe (51). However, deaths are increasingly reported, associated with local anesthetic toxicity or drug interactions (49).

A 19-year-old healthy volunteer undergoing bronchoscopy was given about 1200 mg of lidocaine to anesthetize the airway and was sent home after the procedure, despite complaining of chest pain. Shortly afterwards she had a tonic-clonic seizure and cardiopulmonary arrest and died 2 days later. The research protocol had failed to specify an upper dose limit for lidocaine (52).

Second-Generation Effects

Fetotoxicity

Because of rapid transfer across the placenta and the prolonged half-life of lidocaine in neonates, lidocaine can cause fetal acidosis (SEDA-8, 127). Fetal bradycardia is usually observed only in those fetuses with pre-existing heart rate deceleration. Despite massive intoxication at birth, one child had normal behavioral development at 7 months of age (SED-12, 256) (53).

Lactation

Low concentrations of lidocaine and its metabolite monoethylglycinexylidide (MEGX) have been found in breast milk after a dental procedure, but no risk seems to be involved (54).

Susceptibility Factors

Age

Children

Two reports have illustrated the need for particular care when using local anesthetics in neonates and small children. A 2-year-old child died from the combined effects of chloral hydrate, lidocaine, and nitrous oxide for a dental procedure (55). The doses used were not clarified, but in postmortem blood the plasma concentration of lidocaine was 12 μg/ml. The level and adequacy of perioperative monitoring was also not clear.

A neonate who needed a tracheostomy 10 days after a tracheoesophageal fistula repair was given intravenous lidocaine, 1 mg/kg followed 15–20 minutes later by 0.7 mg/kg. Immediately after, tonic-clonic seizures developed. The child recovered, with no observable ill effects at 6 months.

The authors pointed out that the dose of lidocaine used was well within recommended dosage limits. However, they stressed that a more appropriate dosing schedule should be worked out for neonates.

Lidocaine pharmacokinetics tend to follow a single compartment model in neonates, with an increased half-life, and substantially reduced protein binding, leading to a much larger volume of distribution than in adults, but an increased proportion of unbound drug (56).

Elderly people

In the elderly, some local anesthetics (including lidocaine and bupivacaine) have longer durations of action (57).

Sex

That sex differences can affect lidocaine pharmacokinetics is suggested by a report of higher blood concentrations in men than in women after administration of the same dose (SED-12, 256) (58).

Hepatic disease

In patients with heart and liver disease, the dosage requirement of lidocaine is reduced; the half-life of lidocaine is substantially longer in patients with liver disease (59).

Other features of the patient

The adverse effects of lidocaine are dose-related, and are more common in people of light weight and in patients with acute myocardial infarction or congestive cardiac failure. There is also an increased risk of central nervous system effects during cardiopulmonary bypass (60). In cardiac failure, shock, and postoperatively, there are reductions in both the metabolism and the apparent volume of distribution of lidocaine; dosages should be altered accordingly (61).

Drug Administration

Drug additives

The addition of dextran to a lidocaine + adrenaline solution used for infiltration reduced the absorption of both (62).

Alkalinization of local anesthetic solutions should theoretically lead to a faster onset of effect and prolonged anesthesia. However, raising the pH of the solution can cause the local anesthetic to precipitate out of solution, and one study with 2% lidocaine has shown no difference in quality or onset of anesthesia (SEDA-20, 129).

Adrenaline 1:100 000, added to lidocaine 2%, has caused full-thickness skin necrosis when used for ambulatory phlebectomy for varicose veins (SEDA-21, 136).

Drug administration route

Creams and gels

Cutaneous absorption of lidocaine is negligible through normal skin after short-term application. However, when applied to erosive lesions over large body areas, significant absorption may occur. When the drug is applied to mucous membranes, blood levels simulate those resulting from intravenous injection. Local anesthetic creams and gels used liberally on traumatized epithelium can be rapidly absorbed, resulting in systemic effects, such as convulsions, particularly if excessive quantities are used. This has been highlighted in the case of a 40-year-old woman who developed seizures after lidocaine gel 40 ml was injected into the ureter during an attempt to remove a stone (1).

Topical administration of lidocaine to the nasal mucosa occasionally causes severe methemoglobinemia in patients who have the heterozygous form of NADH methemoglobin reductase deficiency (63).

Subcutaneously in liposuction

Some have suggested that lidocaine is unnecessary and potentially toxic in liposuction, and that it provides no postoperative pain relief (64). Others think that lidocaine toxicity is not a major cause of death during liposuction, stating that all reported deaths after liposuction have been associated with general anesthesia or sedation, including the five in New York, and that doses of lidocaine higher than those used in these cases (10–40 mg/kg) are routinely used in tumescent liposuction, no deaths having been reported (50,65). It is possible that adrenaline, high pressure injection, removal of lidocaine by liposuction, and the development of tolerance all contribute to delay in absorption and lack of toxic symptoms at higher than expected plasma concentrations (66).

Patches

Lidocaine is available as a topical analgesic in an adhesive patch formulation for the pain of postherpetic neuralgia.

The pharmacokinetics and safety of the 5% lidocaine patches have been studied in 20 healthy volunteers, who applied four patches to the skin either every 24 hours or every 12 hours for 3 days (67). Mean steady-state plasma concentrations were 186 and 225 ng/ml respectively, well below those required for an antidysrhythmic effect (1500 ng/ml) or a risk of toxicity (5000 ng/ml). The patches were well tolerated, with no major cutaneous adverse effects. This is in line with data from postmarketing surveillance studies, which have shown that since the availability of lidocaine patches in 1999, no adverse cardiac or other serious adverse events have been reported (68).

The pharmacokinetics of lidocaine in patches have been investigated in two studies. In 20 healthy volunteers, 5% lidocaine patches were applied for 18 hours/day on 3 consecutive days (69). The mean peak concentrations on days 1, 2, and 3 were 145, 153, and 154 ng/ml respectively; the median values of t_{max} were 18.0, 16.5, and 16.5 hours; and the mean trough concentrations were 83, 86, and 77 ng/ml. The patches were well tolerated; local skin reactions were generally minimal and self-limiting. In 20 healthy volunteers, 4 lidocaine patches were applied every 12 or 24 hours on 3 consecutive days (67). The mean maximum-plasma lidocaine concentrations at steady state were 225 and 186 ng/ml respectively. There was no loss of sensation at the site of application. No patient had edema and most cases of erythema were very slight. No systemic adverse events were judged to be related to the patches.

Drug overdose

Inadvertent intravenous injection of lidocaine 1 g resulted in asystole, apnea, and tonic-clonic seizures, with full recovery after 6 hours of intensive resuscitation (SED-12, 256) (70).

Fatal accidental overdose has been reported in a child (71).

- An 18-month-old infant died after swallowing an unknown amount of 2% viscous lidocaine. He rapidly became unwell at home, with convulsions, followed by an asystolic cardiorespiratory arrest. He was intubated and resuscitated by paramedics, but continued to have seizures. He was given anticonvulsants and cardiorespiratory resuscitation was unsuccessful. Toxicological tests identified high concentrations of lidocaine and its metabolites.

Owing to the rare but serious poisonings reported to date, 2% viscous lidocaine should not be prescribed for children under 6 years of age.

An unusual case of homicide using an overdose of intravenous lidocaine has been described (72).

- A 32-year-old man, who had been in hospital for several months because of acute intermittent porphyria and chronic pancreatitis, had a seizure and an asystolic cardiac arrest. Resuscitation was unsuccessful. There was a suspicion of patient mistreatment by one of the attending nurses, and toxicological analyses showed high blood concentrations of lidocaine, diazepam, phenytoin, and promethazine. Diazepam and phenytoin had been administered during resuscitation but lidocaine had not.

The cause of death was given as a ventricular dysrhythmia caused by a lidocaine overdose (total dose about 1500 mg); a nurse was later arrested and tried for murder.

Drug–Drug Interactions

Argatroban

The thrombin inhibitor argatroban had no effect on the pharmacokinetics of intravenous lidocaine 1.5 mg/kg for 10 minutes followed by 2 mg/kg/hour for 16 hours in 12 healthy volunteers; the argatroban was given as an intravenous infusion of 2 μg/kg/minute for 16 hours (73).

Beta-adrenoceptor antagonists

The combination of lidocaine with beta-adrenoceptor antagonists is associated with a slightly increased risk of some minor non-cardiac adverse events (dizziness, numbness, somnolence, confusion, slurred speech, and nausea and vomiting) (74). The combination is not associated with an increased risk of dysrhythmias.

Some beta-blockers reduce hepatic blood flow and inhibit microsomal enzymes, reducing the clearance of lidocaine; there is a clinically significant increase in the plasma concentration of lidocaine during concomitant propranolol therapy (75).

Cimetidine

Cimetidine inhibits the metabolism of lidocaine (76,77) and reduces protein binding, increasing toxicity.

Erythromycin

The effects of erythromycin, an inhibitor of CYP3A4, on the pharmacokinetics of lidocaine have been studied in nine healthy volunteers. Steady-state oral erythromycin had no effect on the plasma concentration versus time curve of lidocaine after intravenous administration, but erythromycin increased the plasma concentrations of the major metabolite of lidocaine, MEGX (78). It is not clear what the interpretation of these results is, particularly since the authors did not study enough subjects to detect what might have been small but significant changes in various disposition parameters of lidocaine and did not report unbound concentrations of lidocaine or its metabolites. However, whatever the pharmacokinetic explanation, the clinical relevance is that one would expect that erythromycin would potentiate the toxic effects of lidocaine that are mediated by MEGX.

Itraconazole

The effects of itraconazole, an inhibitor of CYP3A4, on the pharmacokinetics of lidocaine have been studied in nine healthy volunteers. Steady-state oral itraconazole had no effect on the plasma concentration versus time curve of lidocaine after intravenous administration nor on the plasma concentrations of the major metabolite of lidocaine, MEGX (78).

Mexiletine

An interaction of lidocaine with mexiletine, which resulted in toxic concentrations of lidocaine, has been reported (79).

- An 80-year-old man with a dilated cardiomyopathy was given a lidocaine infusion started at 90 mg/hour for a ventricular tachycardia. He was already taking mexiletine 400 mg/day, and the plasma concentration was within the usual target range; however, the dose was reduced to 200 mg/day to avoid possible adverse effects. Intermittent ventricular tachycardia persisted, and so the lidocaine infusion was increased to 120 mg/day, but adverse effects (involuntary movements, muscle rigidity) were observed. The lidocaine infusion was stopped and within 20 minutes the adverse effects abated; the lidocaine concentration was 6.84 μg/ml. The ventricular tachycardia persisted, lidocaine was restarted at a lower rate, and the oral dose of mexiletine was increased to 450 mg/day. This resulted in an unexpectedly high concentration of lidocaine and the lidocaine concentration was significantly higher while the mexiletine dose was high.

Further studies suggested that mexiletine had displaced lidocaine from tissue binding sites. The authors suggested that this finding has implications for loading doses and acute effects of lidocaine in the concurrent therapy of lidocaine and mexiletine and highlighted the importance of close monitoring of lidocaine concentrations in this setting.

Opioid analgesics

A synergistic interaction of intrathecal fentanyl 100 μg and morphine 0.5 mg, given before induction, with systemically administered lidocaine 200 mg 4 hours later for ventricular tachycardia, resulted in potentiation of opioid effects in a 74-year-old man with major heart disease after coronary artery bypass grafting; during the 5 minutes after lidocaine he had a respiratory arrest with loss of consciousness and miotic pupils, all reversed by naloxone (80). The proposed mechanism was thought to be a reduction in calcium ion concentrations in opioid-sensitive CNS sites.

Propafenone

The CNS toxicity of lidocaine was increased in 11 healthy volunteers who simultaneously received propafenone, which reduced the metabolism of lidocaine (81).

Propofol

Propofol dose-dependently reduced the threshold for lidocaine-induced convulsions in rats (82). Higher doses of propofol completely abolished convulsions. However, there was no difference in the dose of lidocaine that caused cardiac arrest and death, when it was given with three different propofol infusions and placebo.

Ranitidine

Ranitidine inhibits the clearance of lidocaine (77).

Suxamethonium

Procaine and cocaine are esters that are hydrolysed by plasma cholinesterase and may therefore competitively enhance the action of suxamethonium (83). Chloroprocaine may have a similar action. Lidocaine also interacts, although the mechanism is not clear unless very high doses are used (84).

References

1. Pantuck AJ, Goldsmith JW, Kuriyan JB, Weiss RE. Seizures after ureteral stone manipulation with lidocaine. J Urol 1997;157(6):2248.
2. Pfeifer HJ, Greenblatt DJ, Koch-Weser J. Clinical use and toxicity of intravenous lidocaine. A report from the Boston Collaborative Drug Surveillance Program. Am Heart J 1976;92(2):168–73.
3. Greenspon AJ, Mohiuddin S, Saksena S, Lengerich R, Snapinn S, Holmes G, Irvin J, Sappington E, et al. Comparison of intravenous tocainide with intravenous lidocaine for treating ventricular arrhythmias. Cardiovasc Rev Rep 1989;10:55–9.
4. Adriani J, Coffman VD, Naraghi M. The allergenicity of lidocaine and other amide and related local anesthetics. Anesthesiol Rev 1986;13:30–6.
5. Bonnet MC, du Cailar G, Deschodt J. Anaphylaxie à la lidocaine. [Anaphylaxis caused by lidocaine.] Ann Fr Anesth Reanim 1989;8(2):127–9.
6. Kennedy KS, Cave RH. Anaphylactic reaction to lidocaine. Arch Otolaryngol Head Neck Surg 1986;112(6):671–3.
7. Avery JK. Routine procedure—bad outcome. Tenn Med 1998;91(7):280–1.
8. Sakurai M, Kanazawa I. Positive symptoms in multiple sclerosis: their treatment with sodium channel blockers, lidocaine and mexiletine. J Neurol Sci 1999;162(2):162–8.
9. Hand PJ, Stark RJ. Intravenous lignocaine infusions for severe chronic daily headache. Med J Aust 2000;172(4):157–9.
10. Attal N, Gaude V, Brasseur L, Dupuy M, Guirimand F, Parker F, Bouhassira D. Intravenous lidocaine in central pain: a double-blind, placebo-controlled, psychophysical study. Neurology 2000;54(3):564–74.
11. Ziegelbaum M, Lever H. Acute urinary retention associated with flecainide. Cleve Clin J Med 1990;57(1):86–7.
12. Krikler DM, Curry PV. Torsade de pointes, an atypical ventricular tachycardia. Br Heart J 1976;38(2):117–20.
13. Gottlieb SS, Packer M. Deleterious hemodynamic effects of lidocaine in severe congestive heart failure. Am Heart J 1989;118(3):611–12.
14. Weaver WD, Fahrenbruch CE, Johnson DD, Hallstrom AP, Cobb LA, Copass MK. Effect of epinephrine and lidocaine therapy on outcome after cardiac arrest due to ventricular fibrillation. Circulation 1990;82(6):2027–34.
15. Tisdale JE. Lidocaine prophylaxis in acute myocardial infarction. Henry Ford Hosp Med J 1991;39(3–4):217–25.
16. Garner L, Stirt JA, Finholt DA. Heart block after intravenous lidocaine in an infant. Can Anaesth Soc J 1985;32(4):425–8.
17. Hansoti RC, Ashar PN. Atrioventicular block and ventricular fibrillation due to lidocaine therapy. Bombay Hosp J 1975;17:26.
18. McLean SA, Paul ID, Spector PS. Lidocaine-induced conduction disturbance in patients with systemic hyperkalemia. Ann Emerg Med 2000;36(6):615–18.
19. Parnass SM, Curran MJ, Becker GL. Incidence of hypotension associated with epidural anesthesia using alkalinized

and nonalkalinized lidocaine for cesarean section. Anesth Analg 1987;66(11):1148–50.
20. Enlund M, Mentell O, Krekmanov L. Unintentional hypotension from lidocaine infiltration during orthognathic surgery and general anaesthesia. Acta Anaesthesiol Scand 2001;45(3):294–7.
21. Beydon L, Lorino AM, Verra F, Labroue M, Catoire P, Lofaso F, Bonnet F. Topical upper airway anaesthesia with lidocaine increases airway resistance by impairing glottic function. Intensive Care Med 1995;21(11):920–6.
22. Howard P, Cayton RM, Brennan SR, Anderson PB. Lignocaine aerosol and persistent cough. Br J Dis Chest 1977;71(1):19–24.
23. Ryder W. "Two cautionary tales". Anaesthesia 1994;49(2):180–1.
24. Keller C, Sparr HJ, Brimacombe JR. Laryngeal mask lubrication. A comparative study of saline versus 2% lignocaine gel with cuff pressure control. Anaesthesia 1997;52(6):592–7.
25. Stargel WW, Shand DG, Routledge PA, Barchowsky A, Wagner GS. Clinical comparison of rapid infusion and multiple injection methods for lidocaine loading. Am Heart J 1981;102(5):872–6.
26. Olthoff D, Vetter B, Deutrich C, Burkhardt U. Pharmakokinetische Untersuchungen zu den Ursachen der erhohten Neurotoxizität des Lidokains während kardiochirurgischer Operationen. [Pharmacokinetic studies on the causes of increased neurotoxicity of lidocaine during heart surgery.] Anaesthesiol Reanim 1989;14(4):207–14.
27. DeToledo JC, Minagar A, Lowe MR. Lidocaine-induced seizures in patients with history of epilepsy: effect of antiepileptic drugs. Anesthesiology 2002;97(3):737–9.
28. Lee DL, Ayoub C, Shaw RK, Fontes ML. Grand mal seizure during cardiopulmonary bypass: probable lidocaine toxicity. J Cardiothorac Vasc Anesth 1999,13(2):200 2.
29. Goodwin DP, McMeekin TO. A case of lidocaine absorption from topical administration of 40% lidocaine cream. J Am Acad Dermatol 1999;41(2 Pt 1):280–1.
30. Anibarro B, Seoane FJ. Adverse reaction to lidocaine. Allergy 1998;53(7):717–18.
31. Kanai Y, Katsuki H, Takasaki M. Graded, irreversible changes in crayfish giant axon as manifestations of lidocaine neurotoxicity in vitro. Anesth Analg 1998;86(3):569–73.
32. Ghose S, Garodia VK, Sachdev MS, Kumar H, Biswas NR, Pandey RM. Evaluation of potentiating effect of a drop of lignocaine on tropicamide-induced mydriasis. Invest Ophthalmol Vis Sci 2001;42(7):1581–5.
33. Yamashita S, Sato S, Kakiuchi Y, Miyabe M, Yamaguchi H. Lidocaine toxicity during frequent viscous lidocaine use for painful tongue ulcer. J Pain Symptom Manage 2002;24(5):543–5.
34. Sawyer RJ, von Schroeder H. Temporary bilateral blindness after acute lidocaine toxicity. Anesth Analg 2002;95(1):224–6.
34. Berger I, Steinberg A, Schlesinger Y, Seelenfreund M, Schimmel MS. Neonatal mydriasis: intravenous lidocaine adverse reaction. J Child Neurol 2002;17(5):400–1.
36. Bigeleisen PE. An unusual presentation of metallic taste after lidocaine injections. Anesth Analg 1999;89(5): 1239–40.
37. Janda A, Salem C. Hypoglykämie durch Lidocain-Überdosierung. [Hypoglycemia caused by lidocaine overdosage.] Reg Anaesth 1986;9(3):88–90.
38. Stefanini M, Hoffman MN. Studies on platelets: XXVIII: acute thrombocytopenic purpura due to lidocaine (Xylocaine)-mediated antibody. Report of a case. Am J Med Sci 1978;275(3):365–71.
39. Karim A, Ahmed S, Siddiqui R, Mattana J. Methemoglobinemia complicating topical lidocaine used during endoscopic procedures. Am J Med 2001;111(2):150–3.
40. Kakinoki K, Tachibana Y, Yonejima H, Ogino H, Satomura Y, Unoura M. A case of mexiletine and lidocaine induced severe liver injury. Acta Hepatol Jpn 2000;41:812–16.
41. Galer BS, Rowbotham MC, Perander J, Friedman E. Topical lidocaine patch relieves postherpetic neuralgia more effectively than a vehicle topical patch: results of an enriched enrollment study. Pain 1999;80(3):533–8.
42. Dorfman D, Dalton A, Khan A, Markarian Y, Scarano A, Cansino M, Wulff E, Simpson D. Treatment of painful distal sensory polyneuropathy in HIV-infected patients with a topical agent: results of an open-label trial of 5% lidocaine gel. AIDS 1999;13(12):1589–90.
43. Anonymous. Lidocaine patch shown to relieve postherpetic neuralgia. J Pharm Technol 2001;17:154.
44. Scala E, Giani M, Pirrotta L, Guerra EC, Girardelli CR, De Pita O, Puddu P. Simultaneous allergy to ampicillin and local anesthetics. Allergy 2001;56(5):454–5.
45. Palmer JM, Link D. Impotence following anesthesia for elective circumcision. JAMA 1979;241(24):2635–6.
46. Weightman W, Turner T. Allergic contact dermatitis from lignocaine: report of 29 cases and review of the literature. Contact Dermatitis 1998;39(5):265–6.
47. Minasian A, Yagiela JA. The use of amide local anesthetics in patients susceptible to malignant hyperthermia. Oral Surg Oral Med Oral Pathol 1988;66(4):405–15.
48. Klimanek J, Majewski W, Walencik K. A case of malignant hyperthermia during epidural analgesia. Anaesth Resusc Intensive Ther 1976;4(2):143–5.
49. Rao RB, Ely SF, Hoffman RS. Deaths related to liposuction. N Engl J Med 1999;340(19):1471–5.
50. Ginsberg MM, Gresham L; Vermeulen C, Serra M, Roujeau JC; Talmor M, Barie PS; Klein JA; Rigel DS, Wheeland RG; Schnur P, Penn J, Fodor PB. Deaths related to liposuction. N Engl J Med 1999;341(13):1000–3.
51. Klein JA. Tumescent technique for local anesthesia improves safety in large-volume liposuction. Plast Reconstr Surg 1993;92(6):1085–100.
52. Day RO, Chalmers DR, Williams KM, Campbell TJ. The death of a healthy volunteer in a human research project: implications for Australian clinical research. Med J Aust 1998;168(9):449–51.
53. Kim WY, Pomerance JJ, Miller AA. Lidocaine intoxication in a newborn following local anesthesia for episiotomy. Pediatrics 1979;64(5):643–5.
54. Lebedevs TH, Wojnar-Horton RE, Yapp P, Roberts MJ, Dusci LJ, Hackett LP, Ilett K. Excretion of lignocaine and its metabolite monoethylglycinexylidide in breast milk following its use in a dental procedure. A case report. J Clin Periodontol 1993;20(8):606–8.
55. Engelhart DA, Lavins ES, Hazenstab CB, Sutheimer CA. Unusual death attributed to the combined effects of chloral hydrate, lidocaine, and nitrous oxide. J Anal Toxicol 1998;22(3):246–7.
56. Resar LM, Helfaer MA. Recurrent seizures in a neonate after lidocaine administration. J Perinatol 1998;18(3): 193–5.
57. Chauvin M. Toxicité aiguë des anesthésiques locaux en fonction du terrain. [Acute toxicity of local anesthetics as a function of the patient's condition.] Ann Fr Anesth Reanim 1988;7(3):216–23.
58. Bruguerolle B, Isnardon R, Valli M, Vadot G. Influence du sexe sur les taux plasmatiques de lidocaine en anesthésie dentaire. Thérapie (Paris) 1982;37:593.
59. Thomson PD, Rowland M, Melmon KL. The influence of heart failure, liver disease, and renal failure on the disposition of lidocaine in man. Am Heart J 1971;82(3):417–21.
60. Bauer LA, Brown T, Gibaldi M, Hudson L, Nelson S, Raisys V, Shea JP. Influence of long-term infusions on lidocaine kinetics. Clin Pharmacol Ther 1982;31(4): 433–7.
61. Kumana CR. Therapeutic drug monitoring—antidysrhythmic drugs. In: Richens A, Marks V, editors. Therapeutic

Drug Monitoring. Ch 16A. London, Edinburgh: Churchill-Livingstone, 1981:370.
62. Adams HA, Biscoping J, Kafurke H, Muller H, Hoffmann B, Boerner U, Hempelmann G. Influence of dextran on the absorption of adrenaline-containing lignocaine solutions: a protective mechanism in local anaesthesia. Br J Anaesth 1988;60(6):645–50.
63. Kotler RL, Hansen-Flaschen J, Casey MP. Severe methaemoglobinaemia after flexible fibreoptic bronchoscopy. Thorax 1989;44(3):234–5.
64. Perry AW, Petti C, Rankin M. Lidocaine is not necessary in liposuction. Plast Reconstr Surg 1999;104(6):1900–2.
65. Klein JA. Lidocaine is not necessary in liposuction: discussion. Plast Reconstr Surg 1999;104:1903–6.
66. Rubin JP, Bierman C, Rosow CE, Arthur GR, Chang Y, Courtiss EH, May JW Jr. The tumescent technique: the effect of high tissue pressure and dilute epinephrine on absorption of lidocaine. Plast Reconstr Surg 1999;103(3):990–1002.
67. Gammaitoni AR, Alvarez NA, Galer BS. Pharmacokinetics and safety of continuously applied lidocaine patches 5%. Am J Health Syst Pharm 2002;59(22):2215–20.
68. Galer BS. Effectiveness and safety of lidocaine patch 5%. J Fam Pract 2002;51(10):867–8.
69. Gammaitoni AR, Davis MW. Pharmacokinetics and tolerability of lidocaine patch 5% with extended dosing. Ann Pharmacother 2002;36(2):236–40.
70. Finkelstein F, Kreeft J. Massive lidocaine poisoning. N Engl J Med 1979;301(1):50.
71. Nisse P, Lhermitte M, Dherbecourt V, Fourier C, Leclerc F, Houdret N, Mathieu-Nolf M. Intoxication mortelle après ingestion accidentelle de Xylocaine visqueuse a 2% chez une jeune enfant. [Fatal intoxication after accidental ingestion of viscous 2% lidocaine in a young child.] Acta Clin Belg Suppl 2002;(1):51–3.
72. Kalin JR, Brissie RM. A case of homicide by lethal injection with lidocaine. J Forensic Sci 2002;47(5):1135–8.
73. Inglis AM, Sheth SB, Hursting MJ, Tenero DM, Graham AM, DiCicco RA. Investigation of the interaction between argatroban and acetaminophen, lidocaine, or digoxin. Am J Health Syst Pharm 2002;59(13):1258–66.
74. Wyse DG, Kellen J, Tam Y, Rademaker AW. Increased efficacy and toxicity of lidocaine in patients on beta-blockers. Int J Cardiol 1988;21(1):59–70.
75. Naguib M, Magboul MM, Samarkandi AH, Attia M. Adverse effects and drug interactions associated with local and regional anaesthesia. Drug Saf 1998;18(4):221–50.
76. Jackson JE, Bentley JB, Glass SJ, Fukui T, Gandolfi AJ, Plachetka JR. Effects of histamine-2 receptor blockade on lidocaine kinetics. Clin Pharmacol Ther 1985;37(5): 544–8.
77. Kowalsky SF. Lidocaine interaction with cimetidine and ranitidine: a critical analysis of the literature. Adv Ther 1988;5:229–44.
78. Isohanni MH, Neuvonen PJ, Palkama VJ, Olkkola KT. Effect of erythromycin and itraconazole on the pharmacokinetics of intravenous lignocaine. Eur J Clin Pharmacol 1998;54(7):561–5.
79. Maeda Y, Funakoshi S, Nakamura M, Fukuzawa M, Kugaya Y, Yamasaki M, Tsukiai S, Murakami T, Takano M. Possible mechanism for pharmacokinetic interaction between lidocaine and mexiletine. Clin Pharmacol Ther 2002;71(5):389–97.
80. Jensen E, Nader ND. Potentiation of narcosis after intravenous lidocaine in a patient given spinal opioids. Anesth Analg 1999;89(3):758–9.
81. Ujhelyi MR, O'Rangers EA, Fan C, Kluger J, Pharand C, Chow MS. The pharmacokinetic and pharmacodynamic interaction between propafenone and lidocaine. Clin Pharmacol Ther 1993;53(1):38–48.
82. Lee VC, Moscicki JC, DiFazio CA. Propofol sedation produces dose-dependent suppression of lidocaine-induced seizures in rats. Anesth Analg 1998;86(3):652–7.
83. Matsuo S, Rao DB, Chaudry I, Foldes FF. Interaction of muscle relaxants and local anesthetics at the neuromuscular junction. Anesth Analg 1978;57(5):580–7.
84. Usubiaga JE, Wikinski JA, Morales RL, Usubiaga LE. Interaction of intravenously administered procaine, lidocaine and succinylcholine in anesthetized subjects. Anesth Analg 1967;46(1):39–45.

Lidoflazine

See also Calcium channel blockers

General Information

Lidoflazine is a calcium channel blocker (1). The use of lidoflazine in patients with microvascular angina has been associated with malignant ventricular dysrhythmias (SEDA-16, 199).

Reference

1. Janssen PA. Pharmacologie et effets cliniques de la lidoflazine. [Pharmacology and clinical effects of lidoflazine.] Actual Pharmacol (Paris) 1970;23:135–61.

Liliaceae

See also Herbal medicines

General Information

The genera in the family of Liliaceae (Table 1) include various types of lily, amarylis, asphodel, crocus, daffodil, fritillary, hyacinth, onions (including garlic), snowdrop, and tulip.

Food allergy to spices accounts for 2% of all cases of food allergies but 6.4% of cases in adults. Prick tests to native spices in 589 patients with food allergies showed frequent sensitization to the Liliaceae garlic, onion, and chive (4.6% of prick tests in children, 7.7% of prick tests in adults) (1).

Allium sativum

Allium sativum (garlic, camphor of the poor, da suan, poor man's treacle, rustic treacle, stinking rose) contains a variety of amino acids and steroids, including ajoene, alliin, allicin, glutamyl-*S*-allylcysteine, and glutamyl-*S*-(2-carboxy-1-propyl)-cysteinglycine. Traditionally it has been used as an antiseptic, diaphoretic, diuretic, expectorant, and stimulant and in the treatment of asthma, hoarseness, cough, difficulty in breathing, chronic bronchitis, leprosy, tubercular consumption, whooping-cough, worms, epilepsy, rheumatism, dropsy, and hysteria. In modern times it has been used as a hypolipidemic (2), although its effect is small (3).

Table 1 The genera of Liliaceae

Aletris (colicroot)
Allium (onion)
Alstroemeria (lily of the Incas)
Amaryllis (amaryllis)
Amianthium (amianthium)
Androstephium (funnel lily)
Asparagus (asparagus)
Asphodelus (asphodel)
Astelia (pineapple grass)
Bloomeria (golden star)
Brodiaea (brodiaea)
Calochortus (mariposa lily)
Camassia (camas)
Chamaelirium (chamaelirium)
Chionodoxa (chionodoxa)
Chlorogalum (soap plant)
Chlorophytum (chlorophytum)
Clintonia (blue bead)
Colchicum (crocus)
Convallaria (lily of the valley)
Cooperia (rain lily)
Cordyline (cordyline)
Crinum (swamp lily)
Curculigo (curculigo)
Dasylirion (sotol)
Dianella (dianella)
Dichelostemma (snake lily)
Disporum (fairy bells)
Echeandia (echeandia)
Eremocrinum (eremocrinum)
Erythronium (fawn lily)
Eucharis (Amazon lily)
Fritillaria (fritillary)
Gagea (gagea)
Galanthus (snowdrop)
Gloriosa (flame lily)
Habranthus (copper lily)
Harperocallis (harperocallis)
Hastingsia (rush lily)
Helonias (helonias)
Hemerocallis (day lily)
Hesperocallis (desert lily)
Hippeastrum (hippeastrum)
Hosta (plantain lily)
Hyacinthoides (hyacinthoides)
Hyacinthus (hyacinth)
Hymenocallis (spider lily)
Hypoxis (star grass)
Kniphofia (red hot poker)
Leucocrinum (star lily)
Loucojum (snowflake)
Lilium (lily)
Liriope (lily turf)
Lloydia (alp lily)
Lophiola (lophiola)
Lycoris (lycoris)
Maianthemum (may flower)
Medeola (Indian cucumber)
Melanthium (bunch flower)
Merendera
Milla (milla)
Muilla (muilla)
Muscari (grape hyacinth)
Narcissus (daffodil)
Narthecium (asphodel)
Nolina (bear grass)
Nothoscordum (false garlic)
Odontostomum (Hartweg's doll's-lily)
Ophiopogon (ophiopogon)
Ornithogalum (star of Bethlehem)
Ornithoglossum
Pleea (pleea)
Pleomele (hala pepe)
Polygonatum (Solomon's seal)
Ruscus (broom)
Schoenocaulon (feathershank)
Schoenolirion (sunnybell)
Scilla (scilla)
Scoliopus (fetid adder's tongue)
Stenanthium (featherbells)
Sternbergia (winter daffodil)
Streptopus (twisted stalk)
Tofieldia (tofieldia)
Tricyrtis (tricyrtis)
Trillium (trillium)
Tristagma (springstar)
Triteleia (triteleia)
Triteleiopsis (Baja lily)
Tulipa (tulip)
Uvularia (bellwort)
Veratrum (false hellebore)
Xerophyllum (bear grass)
Zephyranthes (zephyr lily)
Zigadenus (death camas)

Adverse effects

Respiratory

Occupational inhalation of garlic powder can lead to asthma (4).

Nervous system

A spontaneous spinal epidural hematoma resulting in paraplegia in an 87-year-old patient was attributed to chronic excessive use of garlic cloves (5).

Hematologic

Bleeding due to impaired platelet function has been attributed to garlic (6).

- A 54-year-old woman underwent strabismus surgery and had bilateral retrobulbar hemorrhages intraoperatively. In the absence of other possible causes, the authors thought that the bleeding had been due to garlic pills prescribed by a naturopath. On the day of surgery, she had taken five pills, equivalent to about 5 g of fresh garlic bulb. Platelet function, measured 2 weeks later, was normal.

Garlic has well-documented effects on platelet aggregation (7).

Skin

Topical administration of garlic can lead to allergic contact dermatitis or burn-like skin lesions (8).

- A 50-year-old Romanian man was advised by his herbalist to treat his asthma with a compress of freshly crushed garlic (9). He wore the compress on his forehead overnight and subsequently developed second-degree burns in this area. Specific IgE RAST tests for garlic were negative. He was treated conservatively and made an uneventful recovery.

- Two Korean patients used topical garlic for pruritus and subsequently developed irritant contact dermatitis of the treated skin areas (10). Withdrawal resulted in full recovery.

Of about 1000 patients with occupational skin diseases, five had occupational allergic contact dermatitis from spices (11). They were chefs or workers in kitchens, coffee rooms, and restaurants. In all cases the dermatitis affected the hands. The causative spices were garlic, cinnamon, ginger, allspice, and clove. The same patients had positive patch-test reactions to carrot, lettuce, and tomato.

Drug interactions

The antiplatelet activity of garlic might lead to over-anticoagulation when garlic and warfarin are administered concomitantly (12). However, evidence of such an effect is scanty (13).

Colchicum autumnale

Colchicum autumnale (autumn crocus) and other *Colchicum* species belong to the family known as the Colchicaceae, a proposed subdivision of the Liliaceae. They contain colchicine and related alkaloids. Other members of the Colchicaceae include *Gloriosa* species and *Merendera* species. *C. autumnale* (autumn crocus) is the traditional source of colchicine, which is covered in a separate monograph.

Another plant subdivision, the Wurmbaeoideae, includes *Androcymbium* species, *Iphigenia* species, and *Wurmbea* species, which also contain colchicine. *Iphigenia indica* (shan cigu) is a traditional Chinese herbal medicine (14).

Ruscus aculeatus

Ruscus aculeatus (butcher's broom, knee holy, knee holly, knee holm, Jew's myrtle, sweet broom, pettigree) has been used topically for vasoconstrictor treatment of varicose veins and hemorrhoids (15), and for chronic venous insufficiency, both alone (16,17) and in the combination known as Cyclo 3 fort, marketed in France, which contains an extract of *R. aculeatus* 150 mg, hesperidin methyl chalcone 150 mg, ascorbic acid 100 mg, and metesculetol.

In a meta-analysis of the efficacy of Cyclo 3 fort in patients with chronic venous insufficiency 20 double-blind, randomized, placebo-controlled studies and 5 randomized comparison studies in 10 246 subjects were included (18). Cyclo 3 fort significantly reduced the severity of pain, cramps, heaviness, and paresthesia compared with placebo. There were also significant reductions in venous capacity and severity of edema.

Adverse effects

Gastrointestinal

Chronic diarrhea has been described with Cyclo 3 fort and attributed to a disturbance of gastrointestinal motility (SEDA-16, 205) (SEDA-17, 244). However, the mechanism may be immunological, since lymphocytic colitis has occasionally been reported (19).

Skin

R. aculeatus can cause allergic contact dermatitis (20).

Veratrum species

The rhizome and root of *Veratrum album* (white hellebore) and the rhizome of *Veratrum viride* (green hellebore) contain many alkaloids, including hypotensive ester alkaloids and jervine. *Veratrum californicum* contains the alkaloids cyclopamine, cycloposine, and jervine.

Adverse effects

Among the major toxic symptoms of the veratrum alkaloids are vomiting, hypotension, and bradycardia.

V. californicum is teratogenic activity in livestock (21).

Drug overdose

Veratrum poisoning can cause heartburn and vomiting, bradydysrhythmias, atrioventricular dissociation, and vasodilatation with hypotension (22,23). It can be fatal (24).

Of 12 patients, aged 20–80 years, with acute hellebore (*V. album*) intoxication, 10 had a sinus bradycardia at about 40/minute, shortening of the PR interval down to 0.08–0.12 seconds and of the QT_c interval down to 0.32–0.36 seconds, transient right and incomplete left bundle-branch block, atrial and ventricular extra beats, nodal rhythm ($n = 1$), and altered ventricular repolarization (25). The authors suggested that the bradycardia due to *V. album* is caused by a reflex increase in vagal tone and responds to atropine.

Five patients with acute accidental poisoning with *V. album* rapidly developed nausea, vomiting, abdominal pain, hypotension, and bradycardia (26). In four cases the electrocardiogram showed sinus bradycardia and in one there was complete atrioventricular block with an ectopic atrial bradycardia and an intermittent idioventricular rhythm. Symptomatic treatment and/or atropine led to recovery within a few hours.

References

1. Moneret-Vautrin DA, Morisset M, Lemerdy P, Croizier A, Kanny G. Food allergy and IgE sensitization caused by spices: CICBAA data (based on 589 cases of food allergy). Allerg Immunol (Paris) 2002;34(4):135–40.
2. Neil A, Silagy C. Garlic: its cardio-protective properties. Curr Opin Lipidol 1994;5(1):6–10.
3. Stevinson C, Pittler MH, Ernst E. Garlic for treating hypercholesterolemia. A meta-analysis of randomized clinical trials. Ann Intern Med 2000;133(6):420–9.
4. Canduela V, Mongil I, Carrascosa M, Docio S, Cagigas P. Garlic: always good for the health? Br J Dermatol 1995;132(1):161–2.
5. Rose KD, Croissant PD, Parliament CF, Levin MB. Spontaneous spinal epidural hematoma with associated platelet dysfunction from excessive garlic ingestion: a case report. Neurosurgery 1990;26(5):880–2.

6. Carden SM, Good WV, Carden PA, Good RM. Garlic and the strabismus surgeon. Clin Experiment Ophthalmol 2002;30(4):303–4.
7. Briggs WH, Xiao H, Parkin KL, Shen C, Goldman IL. Differential inhibition of human platelet aggregation by selected *Allium* thiosulfinates. J Agric Food Chem 2000;48(11):5731–5.
8. Lee TY, Lam TH. Contact dermatitis due to topical treatment with garlic in Hong Kong. Contact Dermatitis 1991;24(3):193–6.
9. Baruchin AM, Sagi A, Yoffe B, Ronen M. Garlic burns. Burns 2001;27(7):781–2.
10. Yim YS, Park CW, Lee CH. Two cases of irritant contact dermatitis due to garlic. Korean J Dermatol 2001;39:86–9.
11. Kanerva L, Estlander T, Jolanki R. Occupational allergic contact dermatitis from spices. Contact Dermatitis 1996;35(3):157–62.
12. Sunter WH. Warfarin and garlic. Pharm J 1991;246:722.
13. Vaes LP, Chyka PA. Interactions of warfarin with garlic, ginger, gingko, or ginseng: nature of the evidence. Ann Pharmacother 2000;34(12):1478–82.
14. De Smet PA. Health risks of herbal remedies. Drug Saf 1995;13(2):81–93.
15. MacKay D. Hemorrhoids and varicose veins: a review of treatment options. Altern Med Rev 2001;6(2):126–40.
16. Vanscheidt W, Jost V, Wolna P, Lucker PW, Muller A, Theurer C, Patz B, Grutzner KI. Efficacy and safety of a Butcher's broom preparation (*Ruscus aculeatus* L. extract) compared to placebo in patients suffering from chronic venous insufficiency. Arzneimittelforschung 2002;52(4):243–50.
17. Beltramino R, Penenory A, Buceta AM. An open-label, randomized multicenter study comparing the efficacy and safety of Cyclo 3 Fort versus hydroxyethyl rutoside in chronic venous lymphatic insufficiency. Angiology 2000;51(7):535–44.
18. Boyle P, Diehm C, Robertson C. Meta-analysis of clinical trials of Cyclo 3 Fort in the treatment of chronic venous insufficiency. Int Angiol 2003;22(3):250–62.
19. Tysk C. Lakemedelsutlost enterokolit. Viktig differentialdiagnos vid utredning av diarre och tarmblodning. [Drug-induced enterocolitis. Important differential diagnosis in the investigation of diarrhea and intestinal hemorrhage.] Lakartidningen 2000;97(21):2606–10.
20. Landa N, Aguirre A, Goday J, Raton JA, Diaz-Perez JL. Allergic contact dermatitis from a vasoconstrictor cream. Contact Dermatitis 1990;22(5):290–1.
21. James LF. Teratological research at the USDA-ARS poisonous plant research laboratory. J Nat Toxins 1999;8(1):63–80.
22. Festa M, Andreetto B, Ballaris MA, Panio A, Piervittori R. Un caso di avvelenamento da veratro. [A case of veratrum poisoning.] Minerva Anestesiol 1996;62(5):195–6.
23. Quatrehomme G, Bertrand F, Chauvet C, Ollier A. Intoxication from *Veratrum album*. Hum Exp Toxicol 1993;12(2):111–15.
24. Gaillard Y, Pepin G. LC-EI-MS determination of veratridine and cevadine in two fatal cases of *Veratrum album* poisoning. J Anal Toxicol 2001;25(6):481–5.
25. Marinov A, Koev P, Mirchev N. [Electrocardiographic studies of patients with acute hellebore (*Veratrum album*) poisoning.] Vutr Boles 1987;26(6):36–9.
26. Garnier R, Carlier P, Hoffelt J, Savidan A. Intoxication aiguë alimentaire par l'ellebore blanc (*Veratum album* L.). Données cliniques et analytiques. A propos de 5 cas. [Acute dietary poisoning by white hellebore (*Veratrum album* L.). Clinical and analytical data. A propos of 5 cases.] Ann Med Interne (Paris) 1985;136(2):125–8.

Lincosamides

General Information

The two established members of the group of antibiotics known as the lincosamides, lincomycin and its semisynthetic derivative clindamycin, have a narrow antibacterial spectrum involving mostly Gram-positive species and some obligate anerobes, such as *Bacteroides*. Like chloramphenicol and erythromycin, they combine with a subunit of bacterial ribosomes and interfere with protein synthesis.

Whereas oral lincomycin has a systemic availability of about 40%, which may be further compromised by food, clindamycin is absorbed from the gastrointestinal tract about 90–100%. Both are eliminated mainly by hepatic metabolism and biliary excretion.

Observational studies

Long-term oral clindamycin therapy has been successfully used in a 36-year-old woman with late-stage AIDS who presented with disseminated, nodular cutaneous lesions and underlying osteomyelitis due to a microsporidial infection with an Encephalitozoon-like species (1).

Comparative studies

In a multicenter, double-blind, randomized trial in 87 patients, clindamycin + primaquine was compared with co-trimoxazole as therapy for AIDS-related *Pneumocystis jiroveci* pneumonia; efficacy was similar. In patients with a PaO_2 under 70 mmHg, clindamycin + primaquine was associated with fewer adverse events and less glucocorticoid use, but more rashes (2).

In a prospective, open, randomized trial clindamycin (600 mg tds) and quinine (650 mg tds) were compared with atovaquone (750 mg bd) plus azithromycin (500 mg on day 1 followed by 250 mg/day) in 58 patients with non-life-threatening babesiosis (3). Bacterial response was complete 3 months after the end of treatment. Adverse effects were reported by 72% of those who received clindamycin and quinine compared with 15% of those who received atovaquone and azithromycin. The most common adverse effects with clindamycin and quinine were tinnitus (39%), diarrhea (33%), and impaired hearing (28%); the symptoms had resolved in 73% of the patients assigned to clindamycin/quinine 3 months after the start of therapy and in 100% after 6 months.

In 233 women with bacterial vaginosis, a 3-day regimen of clindamycin (intravaginal ovules, 100 mg/day) was as effective as a 7-day regimen of oral metronidazole (500 mg bd) and better tolerated (4). Treatment-related adverse events were reported more often with metronidazole, and systemic symptoms, such as nausea and taste disturbance, accounted for most of the difference between the groups.

Placebo-controlled studies

In a 10-week, multicenter, double-blind study 480 patients with moderate to moderately severe acne were randomized to receive twice-daily 5% benzoyl peroxide, 1% clindamycin, 5% benzoyl peroxide plus 1% clindamycin, or vehicle, all topically (5). There were significantly greater reductions in the numbers of inflammatory and total lesions in patients who used combination therapy compared with those who used any of its three individual components. The most frequent adverse effect, dry skin, occurred to a similar extent with the combination and with benzoyl peroxide alone.

General adverse effects

The direct toxicity of the lincosamides is relatively low (SED-7, 389) (6). The adverse effects of clindamycin may be well below 1%. In a tertiary care center, adverse reactions to clindamycin were reported in 0.47% of 3896 courses, and in half of these events an effect of other medications could not be excluded (7). However, clindamycin has not been given in as high doses as lincomycin.

The most common adverse effect is diarrhea, which occurs in as many as 10–20% of patients. The most serious gastrointestinal complication is colitis due to *Clostridium difficile*, which occurs with about equal frequency after oral and parenteral treatment (8,9). Skin rashes, urticaria, and angioedema have been reported with lincomycin, but are rare. In contrast, maculopapular and pruritic eruptions occur after 1–2 weeks of treatment in up to 10% of patients taking clindamycin. Clindamycin has also been incriminated in one case of Stevens–Johnson syndrome and in one of anaphylaxis; in the latter, hemagglutinating antibodies were found against clindamycin and lincomycin (10). Leukocytoclastic angiitis associated with clindamycin is rare. If a similar angiitis can also occur in the colon, the question arises whether some cases of antibiotic-associated colitis might be caused by the drug itself rather than by bacterial toxins. Tumor-inducing effects have not been reported.

Organs and Systems

Cardiovascular

Rapid intravenous infusion of large doses of lincomycin (600 mg in 5–10 minutes) can cause flushing and a sensation of warmth for about 10 minutes.

- A patient who received 200 mg/kg of lincomycin experienced nausea, vomiting, hypotension, dyspnea, and electrocardiographic changes for 20 minutes (SED-7, 389) (11).

Rapid intravenous infusion of lincomycin 1–2 g can cause phlebitis.

Clindamycin can prolong the QT interval and cause ventricular fibrillation (12). Cardiac arrest associated with rapid intravenous administration of clindamycin has been reported (SEDA-8, 258) (13).

Nervous system

Clindamycin, either alone or in combination with neuromuscular blocking drugs or aminoglycosides, has been associated with neuromuscular blockade.

- A 58-year-old woman who was accidentally overdosed with 2400 mg (40 mg/kg) of clindamycin during anesthesia (with tubocurarine and suxamethonium induction) developed prolonged neuromuscular blockade, unresponsive to intravenous calcium or cholinesterase inhibitors (edrophonium and neostigmine), and required assisted ventilation for 11 hours (14). It seems likely that the large dose of clindamycin used in this case produced sustained neuromuscular blockade in the absence of non-depolarizing relaxants and after full recovery from suxamethonium.

Neuromuscular function

Lincosamide antibiotics can produce neuromuscular block postjunctionally by interacting with the open state of the acetylcholine receptor-channel complex. Lipophilicity, rather than stereochemistry of the molecule, is important for open-channel blockade affecting primarily the "off" rate of channel blocking (15). Neuromuscular blockade after clindamycin has been reported (16).

- A 44-year-old woman with mild asthma and mitral valve prolapse was given intravenous clindamycin 300 mg, methylprednisolone 125 mg, and midazolam 2 mg 30 minutes before surgery. Suxamethonium 120 mg was given and general anesthesia was induced with fentanyl 0.1 mg and propofol 120 mg, and maintained with 60% nitrous oxide in oxygen, desflurane, and a single dose of propofol 80 mg. Five hours after uneventful surgery and about 20 minutes after another intravenous dose of clindamycin 600 mg, she complained of profound weakness and had bilateral ptosis, difficulty in speaking, and rapid shallow respiration. Her weakness rapidly became more profound, and she was given neostigmine 4 mg and glycopyrrolate 0.8 mg, after which her muscle strength returned to normal. Electromyography showed no evidence of neuromuscular disease, and acetylcholine receptor antibodies were negative.

An in vitro study has shown a direct effect of clindamycin on nicotinic but not muscarinic acetylcholine receptors (17). This may explain improvement of tremor on treatment with clindamycin in a patient with Parkinson's disease. On each of three occasions, the tremor almost completely disappeared shortly after the start of therapy with clindamycin but reappeared within 1–3 days after withdrawal.

Sensory systems

In a prospective study subconjunctival injections of clindamycin did not produce any general adverse effects (18). However, conjunctival inflammation and keratitis were observed in one of 13 cases, caused by an error in the administered concentration of clindamycin, which was too high.

Hematologic

Granulocytopenia and thrombocytopenia have been described in a few patients taking lincosamides.

However, a cause-and-effect relation has not been unequivocally established.

Lymphadenitis has been attributed to clindamycin (19).

- A 54-year-old woman with paraplegia due to spina bifida was treated with clindamycin, ciprofloxacin, and gentamicin for osteomyelitis of the ischium and acetabulum, but developed painful swelling of lymph nodes in the neck, which she said occurred with each dose of clindamycin. Withdrawal of gentamicin had no effect, but withdrawal of clindamycin resolved the adenitis over 7 days; the ciprofloxacin was continued.

Gastrointestinal

Drug-induced esophagitis is rare, accounting for about 1% of all cases of esophagitis. An incidence of 3.9 in 100 000 has been reported. After the first description, there have been more than 250 observations, with more than 50 different drugs. Among those, the principal antibiotics included tetracyclines (doxycycline, metacycline, minocycline, oxytetracycline, and tetracycline), penicillins (amoxicillin, cloxacillin, penicillin V, and pivmecillinam), clindamycin (20), co-trimoxazole, erythromycin, lincomycin, spiramycin, and tinidazole. Doxycycline alone was involved in one-third of all cases. Risk factors included prolonged esophageal passage, due to motility disorders, stenosis, cardiomegaly, the formulation, supine position during drug ingestion, and failure to use liquid to wash down the tablet. Direct toxic effects of the drug (pH, accumulation in epithelial cells, non-uniform dispersion) also seem to contribute to the development of drug-induced esophagitis (21). Clindamycin should be taken with a meal or followed by a glass of water (22).

The most prominent adverse reaction of the lincosamides is diarrhea, which varies from mildly loose bowel movements to life-threatening pseudomembranous colitis (see monograph on Beta-lactam antibiotics). Almost all antimicrobial drugs have been associated with severe diarrhea and colitis; however, lincomycin and clindamycin have been particularly incriminated. The incidence of clindamycin-induced diarrhea in hospital is 23%. Diarrhea resolves promptly after withdrawal in most cases. It seems to be dose-related and may result from a direct action on the intestinal mucosa. Severe colitis due to *C. difficile* is not dose-related and occurs in 0.01–10% of recipients. Clustering of cases in time and place suggests the possibility of cross-infection. Even low doses of clindamycin, in some cases after topical administration, can cause marked alterations in several intestinal functions related to bowel flora (23). There was reduced susceptibility of *C. difficile* to clindamycin in 80% of French isolates in 1997 (24). Lincomycin was among the antibiotics that were most often associated with the development of antibiotic-associated diarrhea in a Turkish study of 154 patients; other associated antibiotics were azithromycin and ampicillin (25).

In a one-year retrospective study at a tertiary hospital in Spain, 17% of 148 episodes of diarrhea associated with *C. difficile* developed after therapy with clindamycin (26). The possible association of toxin-positive *C. difficile*-induced colitis and the use of clindamycin phosphate vaginal cream for bacterial vaginosis has been reported in a 25-year-old white woman postpartum (27).

In a prospective study patients treated with antibiotics, including clindamycin, for 3 days had a significantly lower frequency of antibiotic-associated diarrhea than those treated for longer periods (28).

Restricting the use of clindamycin has been successful in terminating outbreaks of *C. difficile* diarrhea associated with its use (29). Between 1989 and 1992, outbreaks of diarrhea due to a clindamycin-resistant strain of *C. difficile* occurred in different parts of the USA. Resistance was mediated by the ermB gene. The use of clindamycin was a specific risk factor for diarrhea due to this strain (30).

- A young otherwise healthy nurse developed severe diarrhea and vomiting, profuse ascites, pleural effusion, abdominal tenderness, peritoneal irritation, and systemic toxicity 10 days after taking oral clindamycin for a dental infection (31). Although the assay for *C. difficile* was repeatedly negative, features compatible with pseudomembranous colitis were seen at sigmoidoscopy, and the diagnosis was confirmed histologically.

Topical application of clindamycin to the skin has been used in acne vulgaris. However, percutaneous absorption can occur (SEDA-8, 160) and several cases of diarrhea have been reported, including cases of pseudomembranous colitis (32).

Clindamycin can rarely cause antibiotic-associated diarrhea after short-term use as vaginal cream (33).

Liver

Since the lincosamides are eliminated by biliary excretion, toxicity would be expected in patients with liver disease. High doses of clindamycin may be hepatotoxic (34). Abnormal liver function tests during treatment with lincomycin are rare, and only in patients who had taken large doses (over 4 g/day) for more than 3 weeks (6). In another series, intravenous lincomycin 4–18 g/day was not associated with renal or hepatic toxicity (SED-7, 388).

Skin

The most common adverse events in patients using clindamycin/benzoyl peroxide were dry skin, peeling, erythema, and rash (35,36). However, withdrawal rates due to adverse events were low (0–0.8%).

- A 57-year-old Caucasian woman with a history of ocular toxoplasmosis, treated with intravitreal clindamycin (1 mg/0.1 ml) and dexamethasone (0.4 mg/0.1 ml), developed a generalized erythematous macular rash over the scalp, face, arms, thighs, and trunk 2 days after the start of treatment (37).

Precautions are necessary to avoid ultraviolet radiation after taking photoreactive drugs (38). Metabolism of lincomycin can lead to the formation of reactive oxygen species and cause tissue injury and damage to various cellular macromolecules, which can result in phototoxicity. Typical photosensitivity with a maculopapular eruption has been observed with lincomycin in two patients treated intramuscularly (6).

- Toxic epidermal necrolysis has been described in a 50-year-old insulin-dependent diabetic who received clindamycin (300 mg 8-hourly) (39). On the seventh day, he developed flu-like symptoms, fever, and an erythematous rash, associated with sloughing of 30% of the body surface after a further 4 days (when Nikolsky's sign became positive). He was given oral methylprednisolone 32 mg and eventually made a full recovery.

Lincomycin can cause acne rosacea (40).

A fixed drug eruption has been reported in a patient taking clindamycin (12).

- In a 38-year-old non-atopic man, a generalized pruriginous maculopapular eruption with lip edema and facial erythema developed after 10 days of treatment with oral clindamycin phosphate (300 mg qds) and amoxicillin (500 mg qds) for bronchopneumonia (24). A patch test was positive 2 months later for clindamycin phosphate but negative for penicillin, amoxicillin, ampicillin, and erythromycin. Prick tests and intradermal tests were all negative. Oral rechallenge with clindamycin phosphate 300 mg was positive.

Acute, generalized, exanthematous pustulosis has been associated with clindamycin (41).

Immunologic

Although the risk of drug hypersensitivity is increased in patients with AIDS, clindamycin hypersensitivity has been considered to be relatively uncommon, despite its widespread use, with rash developing in about 9% of patients. However, in a retrospective survey of 50 patients with AIDS recruited in a European multicenter study of treatment for *Toxoplasma* encephalitis, the incidence of rash in 26 patients given pyrimethamine plus clindamycin was 58%, compared with 75% in those given pyrimethamine plus sulfadiazine, a non-significant difference (42). Treatment was initially continued throughout the duration of hypersensitivity, and was tolerated in all patients taking pyrimethamine plus clindamycin, but had to be withdrawn in half of those taking pyrimethamine plus sulfadiazine. Stevens–Johnson syndrome developed in two patients and fatal toxic epidermal necrolysis in one. Thus, the continuation of treatment despite a rash was more likely to succeed with pyrimethamine plus clindamycin but was potentially hazardous with pyrimethamine plus sulfadiazine.

In a prospective study, true-positive patch tests were seen in four of six patients with known clindamycin hypersensitivity, while 22 healthy controls were negative; there was one false positive and one false negative reaction (43).

Successful desensitization has been described in a 35-year-old woman who developed a generalized rash after taking clindamycin (600 mg 6-hourly) and pyrimethamine for 12 days for AIDS-associated cerebral toxoplasmosis; the rash resolved after withdrawal of clindamycin (44). Subsequent oral rechallenge was performed (without pretreatment with glucocorticoids or antihistamines), starting with three doses of 20 mg on day 1, 40 mg on day 2, 80 mg on day 3, and so on, until a dose of 600 mg qds was reached on day 7. A transient rash lasting 5 hours developed after the second dose of 600 mg. She remained free from adverse reactions for the duration of follow-up (13 months).

Infection risk

Superinfection with resistant strains of *Pseudomonas*, *Proteus*, or staphylococci has been observed with lincosamides. Suppression of *Bacteroides* in the intestinal flora may be related to the proliferation of *C. difficile*, which is important in causing pseudomembranous colitis. Excessive growth of *Candida* on the skin occurred when lincomycin was applied topically (6).

Long-Term Effects

Drug resistance

Staphylococcus aureus, pneumococci, Group A streptococci, and viridans streptococci acquire resistance in vitro to the lincosamides regularly, easily, and quickly (SED-8, 638). In endometrial cultures taken after clindamycin therapy, the occurrence of clindamycin-resistant anerobic bacteria was significantly higher than before therapy (45). Their similar mechanism of action has been used to explain cross-resistance between the macrolide antibiotics and the lincosamides. Among erythromycin-resistant staphylococci, 50% of the isolated strains were also resistant to lincomycin (SED-6, 304). In patients who need long-term suppressive therapy, but who are allergic to penicillin, the development of such combined resistance of the oropharyngeal flora can be a serious clinical problem.

The erythromycin ribosomal methylase (erm) genes encode 23S ribosomal RNA methylases. This modification results in reduced binding of all known macrolides, lincosamides, and streptogramin B to the ribosome (MLS resistance). Novel triazine-containing methyltransferase inhibitors that may reverse erm-mediated resistance are under development (46).

The MLS resistance was found in four of 137 consecutive clinical isolates of *Streptococcus pyogenes* (47). In two, both ermB and ermTR genes were present. In the other two, these genes were not identified, suggesting a new mechanism of high-level resistance to these antibiotics. Erm genes were detected in 45% of 173 strains of *Streptococcus pneumoniae* isolated from surveillance studies in day-care centers in Central Italy (48). From 387 clinical strains of erythromycin-resistant strains of *S. pyogenes* isolated in Italian laboratories from 1995 to 1998, 31% were assigned to the inducible and 17% to the constitutive MLS resistance phenotype (49). Resistance to erythromycin increased to 33% in 1997 among community-acquired isolates of *S. pneumoniae* from central Italy (50). Most carried an erm gene and were also resistant to clindamycin. Regulatory regions located upstream of the erm genes were amplified and sequenced in clinical isolates of enterococci and streptococci with either inducible or constitutive resistance. Expression of constitutive resistance in two strains of *S. pneumoniae* and *Enterococcus faecalis* could be accounted for by a large deletion or a DNA duplication within the regulatory regions respectively (51). In 294 macrolide-, lincosamide-, and/or streptogramin-resistant clinical isolates of *S. aureus* and coagulase-negative staphylococci isolated in 1995 from 32 French hospitals, ermA or ermC genes were found in 88% (52). Genes related to linA/linA′ and conferring resistance to lincomycin were detected in one strain of *S. aureus* and 7 strains of coagulase-negative staphylococci.

A resistance gene, named linB, which encodes a lincosamide nucleotidyltransferase catalysing the adenylation of the hydroxyl group in position 3 of the molecules of lincomycin and clindamycin has been characterized in a clinical isolate of *Enterococcus faecium* (53). Expression of linB was also observed in *Escherichia coli* and *S. aureus*, and the spread of this gene in other clinical isolates of *E. faecium* has been suggested.

In *Brachyspira hyodysenteriae* (formerly *Serpulina hyodysenteriae*) isolates, resistance to clindamycin was associated with a transversion mutation in the nucleotide position homologous with position 2058 of the *E. coli* 23S rRNA gene (54).

There was a significant increase in the rate of resistance in clinical strains of *Bacteroides fragilis* from Canada (20% in 1997) (55). This trend was also observed in a prospective multicenter survey from the USA (56).

Among *P. acnes* isolated from acne lesions, a resistance level of 4% (of 50 strains) and 6.8% (of 70 strains) were found in Japanese and German studies respectively (57,58).

Of 302 clinical isolates of *S. pyogenes* from Portugal, 108 were resistant to erythromycin, and 86 also had a constitutive resistance to clindamycin (MLSB phenotype) (59). Four isolates had a phenotype characterized by low-level erythromycin resistance and high-level clindamycin resistance. In another European study of 286 *S. pneumoniae* strains, 7% were resistant to penicillin, and 35% were also resistant to clindamycin (60). Of 3205 group A streptococcal strains from Canada, only 18 and 2 strains respectively showed inducible and constitutive resistance to clindamycin (61). Among 180 strains of the *Streptococcus milleri* group isolated in Spain, 17% were resistant to clindamycin (62).

An increase in resistance to clindamycin has been found in group B streptococcal strains causing neonatal infection (63).

Second-Generation Effects

Pregnancy

In pregnant women with bacterial vaginosis, a 7-day regimen of 2% vaginal clindamycin cream was effective and did not alter the rates of preterm deliveries or peripartum infections (64,65).

Fetotoxicity

Although lincomycin penetrates the fetal circulation, no fetal abnormalities were related to lincomycin administration in 302 women who had completed a course of lincomycin therapy (500 mg every 6 hours) for 1 week; all three trimesters of pregnancy were included (66).

Drug Administration

Drug formulations

Whereas only about 4% of clindamycin from a vaginal cream was systemically absorbed, systemic absorption was in the range of 30% when clindamycin was intravaginally administered as a phosphate ovule (67).

Drug–Drug Interactions

Ciclosporin

In two patients who had lung transplants and were taking an immunosuppressive regimen that included ciclosporin, the addition of clindamycin (600 mg tds) resulted in a significant reduction in ciclosporin concentrations (68).

Ganglion blocking agents

Clindamycin may potentiate the effects of some ganglion blocking agents (69).

Macrolides

Antagonism between the lincosamides and the macrolide antibiotics has been observed in vitro and was explained by binding to the same subunit of bacterial ribosomes (70). This mechanism of bacteriostatic action also suggests that the lincosamides might prevent the bactericidal action of the penicillins and the cephalosporins.

Non-depolarizing neuromuscular blocking drugs

Clindamycin and lincomycin potentiate the action of non-depolarizing neuromuscular blocking drugs, such as pancuronium and D-tubocurarine. The lincosamide-induced block cannot be reliably reversed pharmacologically (71).

References

1. Kester KE, Turiansky GW, McEvoy PL. Nodular cutaneous microsporidiosis in a patient with AIDS and successful treatment with long-term oral clindamycin therapy. Ann Intern Med 1998;128(11):911–14.
2. Toma E, Thorne A, Singer J, Raboud J, Lemieux C, Trottier S, Bergeron MG, Tsoukas C, Falutz J, Lalonde R, Gaudreau C, Therrien R. Clindamycin with primaquine vs. trimethoprim–sulfamethoxazole therapy for mild and moderately severe *Pneumocystis carinii* pneumonia in patients with AIDS: a multicenter, double-blind, randomized trial (CTN 004). CTN-PCP Study Group. Clin Infect Dis 1998;27(3):524–30.
3. Krause PJ, Lepore T, Sikand VK, Gadbaw J Jr, Burke G, Telford SR 3rd, Brassard P, Pearl D, Azlanzadeh J, Christianson D, McGrath D, Spielman A. Atovaquone and azithromycin for the treatment of babesiosis. N Engl J Med 2000;343(20):1454–8.
4. Paavonen J, Mangioni C, Martin MA, Wajszczuk CP. Vaginal clindamycin and oral metronidazole for bacterial vaginosis: a randomized trial. Obstet Gynecol 2000;96(2):256–60.
5. Leyden JJ, Berger RS, Dunlap FE, Ellis CN, Connolly MA, Levy SF. Comparison of the efficacy and safety of a combination topical gel formulation of benzoyl peroxide and clindamycin with benzoyl peroxide, clindamycin and vehicle gel

Some feel that 1% lindane is safe when used properly (1,5), but precautionary recommendations have been made (3):

(a) a hot soapy bath before treatment is not necessary;
(b) application for 24 hours may be too long, 6 hours having a cure rate of 96%;
(c) a concentration weaker than 1% may be adequate;
(d) lindane should not be repeated within 8 days, and then only if active parasites can still be demonstrated;
(e) lindane 1% should be used with extreme caution, if at all, in pregnant women, very small infants, and people with massively excoriated skin.

There has been concern from animal experiments that lindane may be mutagenic, carcinogenic, and teratogenic; in therapeutic use, however, such hazards are highly unlikely (1,2).

Organs and Systems

Nervous system

In 1976, the US Food and Drug Administration (FDA) published a "Gamma Benzene Hexachloride (Kwell) Alert," based in part on several poorly documented cases of convulsions after topical treatment with lindane (6). Indeed, several authors have reported convulsions (7–9), but in most cases lindane had been inappropriately used (4,7), while another case took place in unusual therapeutic circumstances (prematurity, marasmus, pneumonia, congestive heart failure, ventricular septal defect) (8). A child with convulsions after the application of lindane had tuberous sclerosis and may therefore have had a reduced threshold for convulsions (9).

Hematologic

Anemia, possibly caused by topical lindane, has been described (10).

Urinary tract

Urinary retention has been ascribed to lindane (SEDA-10, 131).

Skin

Acute generalized exanthematous pustulosis has been attributed to topical lindane (11).

Immunologic

Henoch-Schönlein purpura, possibly caused by topical lindane, has been described (12).

References

1. Rasmussen JE. The problem of lindane. J Am Acad Dermatol 1981;5(5):507–16.
2. Shacter B. Treatment of scabies and pediculosis with lindane preparations: an evaluation. J Am Acad Dermatol 1981;5(5):517–27.
3. Solomon LM, Fahrner L, West DP. Gamma benzene hexachloride toxicity: a review Arch Dermatol 1977;113(3):353–7.
4. Telch J, Jarvis DA. Acute intoxication with lindane (gamma benzene hexachloride). Can Med Assoc J 1982;126(6):662–3.
5. Kramer MS, Hutchinson TA, Rudnick SA, Leventhal JM, Feinstein AR. Operational criteria for adverse drug reactions in evaluating suspected toxicity of a popular scabicide. Clin Pharmacol Ther 1980;27(2):149–55.
6. Food and Drug Administration. Gamma benzene hexachloride (Kwell) alert. FDA Drug Bull 1976;6:28.
7. Lee B, Groth P. Scabies: transcutaneous poisoning during treatment. Pediatrics 1977;59(4):643.
8. Pramanik AK, Hansen RC. Transcutaneous gamma benzene hexachloride absorption and toxicity in infants and children. Arch Dermatol 1979;115(10):1224–5.
9. Matsuoka LY. Convulsions following application of gamma benzene hexachloride. J Am Acad Dermatol 1981;5(1):98–9.
10. Morgan DP, Roberts RJ, Walter AW, Stockdale EM. Anemia associated with exposure to lindane. Arch Environ Health 1980;35(5):307–10.
11. Juan WH, Yang LC, Hong HS. Acute generalized exanthematous pustulosis induced by topical lindane. Dermatology 2004;209(3):239–40.
12. Fagan JE. Henoch-Schonlein purpura and gamma-benzene hexachloride. Pediatrics 1981;67(2):310–11.

Lipsticks, substances used in

General Information

Branched-chain fatty acid esters, such as glyceryl di-isostearate and di-isostearyl malate, have replaced castor oil and lanolin as major components of lipsticks.

Palmitate-related substances are viscous oils used in cosmetics and topical medicaments. In lipsticks they replace castor oil (1). Allergic reactions to lipsticks have been reported to be caused by a variety of allergens, for example azo dyes, colophony, lanolin, castor oil, sunscreens, and para-tertiary butylphenol.

Organs and Systems

Immunologic

The fatty acid esters have low allergenic potential but cases of contact allergy has been reported, in one case to di-isostearyl malate (patch-tested in 7.7% in petrolatum) (2), and in another case to glyceryl monoisostearate monomyristate in a 23-year-old woman, who had cheilitis from her lipstick (3).

- A 17-year-old woman developed pruritic edematous erythema on her lips after using a lipstick containing isopalmitate (4). A patch test with 10% isopalmitate in petrolatum was positive on day 3, with six negative controls.
- A 27-year-old woman developed papules, scales, and slight swelling of her lips (5). A patch test with isopalmityl diglyceryl sebacate, 10% in petrolatum, was positive.

References

1. Sai S. Lipstick dermatitis caused by castor oil. Contact Dermatitis 1983;9(1):75.
2. Guin JD. Allergic contact cheilitis from di-isostearyl malate in lipstick. Contact Dermatitis 2001;44(6):375.
3. Asai M, Kawada A, Aragane Y, Tezuka T. Allergic contact cheilitis due to glyceryl monoisostearate monomyristate in a lipstick. Contact Dermatitis 2001;45(3):173.
4. Kimura M, Kawada A. Contact dermatitis due to 2-hexyldecanoic acid (isopalmitate) in a lipstick. Contact Dermatitis 1999;41(2):99–100.
5. Suzuki K, Matsunaga K, Suzuki M. Allergic contact dermatitis due to isopalmityl diglyceryl sebacate in a lipstick. Contact Dermatitis 1999;41(2):110.

Lisinopril

See also Angiotensin converting enzyme inhibitors

General Information

Lisinopril is a non-sulfhydryl ACE inhibitor. It has been used in patients with hypertension, heart failure, myocardial infarction, and diabetic nephropathy.

Organs and Systems

Cardiovascular

An updated and comprehensive review of the use of lisinopril in congestive heart failure has been published (1), including a section on tolerability and details of the ATLAS (Assessment with Treatment with Lisinopril and Survival) trial. The tolerance of high doses of lisinopril (32.5–35 mg od) in heart failure, one of the issues addressed by this trial, was not significantly different from that of low doses (2.5–5 mg od). Since high doses were more effective than low doses, the authors recommended that more aggressive use of ACE inhibitors is warranted (2). However, this conclusion is valid only in the conditions of the trial, with careful and slow dose escalation. With such a strategy, most patients with heart failure can be titrated successfully to high maintenance doses.

Shock after myocardial infarction has been attributed to an ACE inhibitor (3).

- A 42-year-old woman suffered an acute anterior myocardial infarction, initially associated with pulmonary edema. After hemodynamic stabilization she was given lisinopril 10 mg orally. Two hours later she developed circulatory failure in conjunction with acute renal insufficiency. Right heart catheterization showed markedly reduced systemic vascular resistance but a normal cardiac index. After the usual causes of cardiogenic shock had been ruled out, repeated fluid challenges and intravenous noradrenaline failed to improve her hemodynamic status. She was therefore given angiotensin II intravenously (5–7.5 μg/minute), which immediately and markedly raised the systematic vascular resistance and resulted in subsequent regression of shock. She was discharged after an otherwise uneventful course.

Endocrine

The syndrome of inappropriate antidiuretic hormone secretion (SIADH) has been attributed to lisinopril (4).

- A 76-year-old woman taking lisinopril 20 mg/day and metoprolol for hypertension developed headaches, nausea, and a tingling sensation in her arms. Her serum sodium was 109 mmol/l, with a serum osmolality of 225 mosm/kg, urine osmolality of 414 mosm/kg, and urine sodium of 122 mmol/l. She had taken diclofenac 75 mg/day for arthritic pain for 6 years and naproxen for about 1 month. Propoxyphene napsylate and paracetamol had then been substituted and zolpidem had been started. A diagnosis of SIADH was postulated and thyroid and adrenal causes were excluded. Lisinopril was withdrawn and fluid was restricted to 100 ml/day. The serum sodium gradually corrected to 143 mmol/l.

The authors referred to three other similar cases, in two of which the diagnosis may have been confused by the concomitant use of diuretics in patients with heart failure. However, the present and one other case had occurred without co-existing risk factors for hyponatremia. They discussed a synergistic effect of zolpidem and/or diclofenac, and suggested a potential mechanism involving noninhibition of brain ACE, which leaves brain angiotensin II receptors exposed to high circulating concentrations of angiotensin which would strongly stimulate thirst and the release of antidiuretic hormone.

Pancreas

Several cases of pancreatitis have been reported with ACE inhibitors, including lisinopril.

- A 67-year-old man without other risk factors developed acute pancreatitis only 3 hours after taking lisinopril. The originality of this case resides in the fact that the patient had experienced a similar but less severe reaction to the medication 3 months before. Thus, this case probably represents the first time a patient was rechallenged with lisinopril and had a more severe adverse reaction (5).
- A 42-year-old woman, who was taking lisinopril, nicardipine, metoprolol, simvastatin, omeprazole, an estrogen, and sublingual glyceryl trinitrate, presented with epigastric pain and vomiting (6). Pancreatitis was diagnosed on the grounds of raised activities of lipase (200 IU/l) and amylase (117 IU/l) and diffuse homogeneous enlargement of the head and body of the pancreas on CT scan. The pancreatic enzyme activities normalized 5 days after lisinopril and simvastatin withdrawal. Two months later she was taking estrogen and simvastatin, but not lisinopril. Her amylase and lipase were normal.

The temporal relation in the second case suggests that lisinopril was causative. The authors raised the possibility that the concomitant use of an estrogen and simvastatin, as well as a history of familial hypertriglyceridemia, may have predisposed her to pancreatitis.

Skin

Worsening of pre-existing cold urticaria has been associated with lisinopril (7).

- A 43-year-old Caucasian man had a history of mild cold urticaria during the preceding 10 years. Shortly after starting to take lisinopril 20 mg/day and hydrochlorothiazide 25 mg/day for hypertension his condition worsened considerably and he had several bouts of severe cold urticaria. On one occasion, after swimming in water at 24°C, he developed severe urticaria and angioedema, and required emergency hospital admission. Standard ice-cube and cold-water immersion tests were strongly positive within 1 minute. Tests for a variety of causative factors were negative, and a diagnosis of acquired cold urticaria was made. Lisinopril was withdrawn, he was given valsartan 80 mg/day, and the dose of hydrochlorothiazide was reduced to 12.5 mg/day. During the next 24 weeks he had only mild symptoms of cold urticaria. Repeat ice-cube and cold-water immersion tests were negative at 1 and 3 minutes, but positive at 5 minutes.

The authors cited evidence that the kallikrein/kinin system is involved in cold urticaria, that ACE inhibitors increase wheal-and-flare reactions to cutaneously applied bradykinin, and that ACE inhibitor therapy is associated with raised plasma kinin concentrations. They therefore recommended avoidance of ACE inhibitors in patients with cold urticaria.

Erythema multiforme has been attributed to lisinopril (8).

- A 68-year-old man who had taken lisinopril 10 mg/day for several years stopped taking it temporarily because of a cough. It was then restarted in a dosage of 5 mg/day and a few days later he developed several bean-sized non-pruritic erythematous plaques with scales over the whole body, particularly on the chest. The appearance was of seborrheic dermatitis, but histology showed the features of erythema multiforme. The eruptions cleared completely a few days after lisinopril withdrawal. Two months later, a rechallenge test was positive.

Sexual function

Lisinopril 20 mg/day has been compared with atenolol 100 mg/day in a 16-week, double-blind, randomized, controlled trial in 90 hypertensive men aged 40–49 and without a history of sexual dysfunction. The number of occasions on which they had sexual intercourse fell during the first month in both groups (9). Subsequently, sexual activity tended to recover with lisinopril but not atenolol. The authors suggested that lisinopril may cause only a temporary reduction in sexual function.

Drug–Drug Interactions

Clozapine

Raised clozapine blood concentrations have been reported after the introduction of lisinopril (10).

- A 39-year-old man with schizophrenia and diabetes, who had taken clozapine 300 mg/day and glipizide 10 mg/day for a year, took lisinopril 5 mg/day for newly diagnosed hypertension. On several occasions afterwards he had roughly a doubling of his blood concentrations of clozapine and norclozapine. He had typical effects of clozapine toxicity. After replacement of lisinopril by diltiazem, the blood concentrations of clozapine and norclozapine returned to the values that were present before lisinopril was introduced.

The information given here was sketchy and there was no information on the timing of blood samples relative to the dose of clozapine. Clozapine is metabolized by CYP1A2 and CYP3A4, but there is no evidence that lisinopril affects these pathways.

Tizanidine

Hypotension followed the addition of tizanidine to lisinopril (11).

- A 10-year-old boy developed hypotension and reduced alertness. His blood pressure was 56/24 mmHg and his heart rate 88/minute. He had a history of a hypoxic ischemic insult to the central nervous system, subsequent hypertension, and spastic quadriplegia. His blood pressure had been controlled for the last 10 months with lisinopril (dose not stated). Tizanidine had been added 1 week before admission for spasticity. Lisinopril and tizanidine were withdrawn and his blood pressure rose to 149/89 mmHg over the next day. He was discharged and lisinopril was restarted but not tizanidine. He had no further problems with hypotension.

The authors interpreted the finding as a consequence of limited ability of the patient to respond to hypotension because of simultaneous blockade of the sympathetic system with the centrally acting alpha$_2$-adrenoceptor agonist tizanidine.

References

1. Simpson K, Jarvis B. Lisinopril: a review of its use in congestive heart failure. Drugs 2000;59(5):1149–67.
2. Massie BM, Armstrong PW, Cleland JG, Horowitz JD, Packer M, Poole-Wilson PA, Ryden L. Toleration of high doses of angiotensin-converting enzyme inhibitors in patients with chronic heart failure: results from the ATLAS trial. The Assessment of Treatment with Lisinopril and Survival. Arch Intern Med 2001;161(2):165–71.
3. Desachy A, Normand S, Francois B, Cassat C, Gastinne H, Vignon P. Choc refractaire après administration d'un inhibiteur de l'enzyme de conversion. Interêt d'un traitement par angiotensine II. [Refractory shock after converting enzyme inhibitor administration. Usefulness of angiotensin II.] Presse Méd 2000;29(13):696–8.
4. Shaikh ZH, Taylor HC, Maroo PV, Llerena LA. Syndrome of inappropriate antidiuretic hormone secretion associated with lisinopril. Ann Pharmacother 2000;34(2):176–9.
5. Gershon T, Olshaker JS. Acute pancreatitis following lisinopril rechallenge. Am J Emerg Med 1998;16(5):523–4.
6. Miller LG, Tan G. Drug-induced pancreatitis (lisinopril). J Am Board Fam Pract 1999;12(2):150–3.
7. Kranke B, Mayr-Kanhauser S. Cold urticaria and angiotensin converting enzyme inhibitor. Acta Derm Venereol 2002;82(2):149–50.
8. Horiuchi Y, Matsuda M. Eruptions induced by the ACE inhibitor, lisinopril. J Dermatol 1999;26(2):128–30.
9. Fogari R, Zoppi A, Corradi L, Mugellini A, Poletti L, Lusardi P. Sexual function in hypertensive males treated

with lisinopril or atenolol: a cross-over study. Am J Hypertens 1998;11(10):1244–7.
10. Abraham G, Grunberg B, Gratz S. Possible interaction of clozapine and lisinopril. Am J Psychiatry 2001;158(6):969.
11. Johnson TR, Tobias JD. Hypotension following the initiation of tizanidine in a patient treated with an angiotensin converting enzyme inhibitor for chronic hypertension. J Child Neurol 2000;15(12):818–19.

Lisuride

General Information

Lisuride is a dopamine receptor agonist that is used as an alternative drug in the treatment of Parkinson's disease. The pattern of adverse effects is similar to that seen with most of the ergot alkaloids (SEDA-10, 118). The adverse effects that occurred after subcutaneous administration were so troublesome that the subcutaneous formulation was eventually unmarketable.

Organs and Systems

Respiratory

In one instance to date, pleuropulmonary disease has been observed. Effusions were present but apparently there was no significant fibrosis, and the condition was almost completely reversible.

Nervous system

Vasoconstriction due to ergot-related dopamine receptor agonists can affect the cerebral circulation (1).

- A 33-year-old woman was discharged from hospital after a normal delivery, taking lisuride 0.2 mg/day for suppression of lactation. Within a day, she complained of throbbing headache, which was followed by right hemiparesis and then a generalized tonic-clonic seizure starting from the right arm. She had widespread segmental vasoconstriction in the cerebral arteries and two intracerebral hemorrhages. She recovered fully within 1 month.

The authors commented that there have been at least seven reported cases of postpartum ergot-related angiopathy with bromocriptine and ergonovine.

Because of its serotoninergic properties, lisuride can cause more psychiatric complications than expected (2).

References

1. Roh JK, Park KS. Postpartum cerebral angiopathy with intracerebral hemorrhage in a patient receiving lisuride. Neurology 1998;50(4):1152–4.
2. Kapfhammer HP, Ruther E. Dopaminagonisten in der Therapie des Parkinsonsyndroms. [Dopamine agonists in the therapy of Parkinson syndrome.] Nervenarzt 1985;56(2):69–81.

Lithium

General Information

Lithium is an alkaline earth element that is used medicinally in the form of salts such as lithium chloride and lithium carbonate. Its main use is in the prevention or attenuation of recurrent episodes of mania and depression in individuals with bipolar mood disorder (manic depression). Lithium also has clearly established antimanic activity, although its relatively slow onset of action often necessitates the use of ancillary drugs, such as antipsychotic drugs and/or benzodiazepines, at the start of therapy. If lithium alone is ineffective for recurrent bipolar mood disorder, combining it or replacing it with carbamazepine or valproate may be of value; reports with lamotrigine and olanzapine are also encouraging.

Lithium also has antidepressant activity in bipolar disorder, has prophylactic value in recurrent major depression, and is a useful augmenting agent for antidepressant-resistant depression. Other uses in psychiatry include schizoaffective disorder, emotional instability, and pathological aggression. The point prevalence of lithium use has been estimated to be as high as 1 in 1000 people in populations in industrial countries. The complex relation between sub-syndromal manifestations of bipolar disorder, particularly cognitive dysfunction, and the role that lithium might play in alleviating or aggravating this problem have been discussed in a thoughtful review (1).

The well-established effectiveness of long-term lithium in reducing manic-depressive morbidity includes a reduced risk of suicide and suicidal behavior. For example, in one study, suicidal acts per 1000 patient-years were 23 before lithium, 3.6 during lithium, 71 in the first year after withdrawal, and 23 in subsequent years (2). In another study, suicide rates during treatment with lithium were 31 per 1000 person-years (emergency department suicide attempts), 11 per 1000 person-years (suicide attempts resulting in hospitalization), and 1.7 per 1000 person-years (suicide deaths); the risk of suicide death was 2.7 times higher during treatment with divalproex than during treatment with lithium (3). A retrospective study divided high-risk patients into excellent, moderate, and poor responders to lithium and showed that no further suicide attempts occurred in 93%, 83%, and 49% respectively (4). The substantial reduction in suicidal tendency in the poor responder group suggested an anti-suicidal effect of lithium beyond its mood-stabilizing properties, although the psychosocial benefits of lithium clinic treatment could have been contributing factors.

Since bipolar disorder is a condition for which long-term treatment is usually necessary, both acute and long-term adverse effects are important, especially since patients in remission are often less likely to tolerate them (5). With this in mind, one might consider some speculatively positive findings involving the neurotropic and neuroprotective effects of lithium (6). The concentration of bcl-2, a cytoprotective protein, was upregulated by lithium in both rodent brains and human neuronal cells, as was the concentration of *N*-acetylaspartate, a marker of neuronal viability and function, in human gray matter

(7). In addition, a 3-dimensional magnetic resonance imaging study with quantitative brain-tissue segmentation showed that treatment with lithium for 4 weeks increased the total volume of gray matter by about 3% in eight of 10 patients in the depressed phase of bipolar I disorder.

Beneficial nonpsychiatric uses of lithium

Some collateral drug effects that are not related to the intended therapeutic effect are potentially beneficial. Several beneficial effects of lithium, besides its action in bipolar disorder, have been described.

Nervous system

There has been a spate of publications describing the neuroprotective effects of lithium. By inhibiting glycogen synthase kinase-3, lithium inhibits tau hyperphosphorylation and protects against β-amyloid-induced cell death, suggesting a possible role in the treatment of Alzheimer's disease (8,9). Studies in mice and cell lines show that lithium reduces gp120-associated neurotoxicity, suggesting that it may be useful in preventing progression of HIV-associated cognitive deterioration (10). Low-dose lithium reduced infarct volume and neurological deficits in a rat model of transient focal cerebral ischemia (11).

Overall, the evidence that lithium has neuroprotective and neurotropic effects through a variety of mechanisms is striking (12), although whether those findings will evolve into therapies of practical clinical value remains to be seen.

Chronic cluster headache has responded to lithium (13).

Sensory systems

In cultured mouse retinal ganglion cells, lithium supported the survival and regeneration of axons (14). This led the authors to the very speculative suggestion that lithium might be useful in treating conditions such as glaucoma, optic neuritis, and other neuron loss disorders.

Endocrine

Lithium blocks the release of iodine and thyroid hormones from the thyroid and has been used to treat hyperthyroidism, as an adjunct to radioiodine therapy (15–18) and in metastatic thyroid carcinoma (19). However, it can also cause hyperthyroidism. Lithium enhanced the efficacy of radioiodine in 23 patients (20), but was ineffective in a larger comparison of lithium ($n = 175$) or radioiodine alone ($n = 175$) (21). In 24 patients with Graves' disease, lithium attenuated or prevented increases in thyroid hormone concentration after methimazole withdrawal and radioiodine treatment (15,22).

Lithium has been used, with several other drugs, to treat four patients with amiodarone-associated thyrotoxicosis, but the drugs were ineffective in two patients, who required thyroidectomy (23). One hopes that the authors actually used milligram amounts of lithium carbonate rather than the microgram amounts listed in the article.

Metabolism

Lithium therapy in a 17-year-old man with Kleine–Levin syndrome led to remission of the characteristic manifestations, including hyperphagia (24).

Hematologic

Lithium has beneficial granulocytopoietic effects (25–27). For example, lithium carbonate (800–900 mg/day) effectively corrected neutropenia due to chemotherapy or radiotherapy in over 85% of 100 cancer patients (28). The potential benefit and possible risks of using lithium to treat clozapine-induced neutropenia/agranulocytosis have been reviewed (29).

- A 29-year-old man with agranulocytosis, who could not tolerate granulocyte-colony stimulating factor, had normalization of peripheral granulocyte counts when he took lithium carbonate 800 mg/day (30).
- A 16-year-old with severe aplastic anemia failed to respond to treatment with corticosteroids plus an androgen and to antilymphocyte globulin, but had a strikingly positive response to the combination of lithium and an androgen derivative (31). Leukopenia and thrombocytopenia recurred 2 months after lithium was withdrawn and responded to reintroduction of the drug.

The potential of lithium to prevent or treat clozapine-induced granulocytopenia has been reviewed (29). In a study of 38 patients on clozapine for schizophrenia or schizoaffective disorder, the addition of lithium increased the leukocyte count (32). A 20-year-old man with olanzapine-induced neutropenia 5 mg/day was able to tolerate 20 mg/day while taking lithium (33).

Skin

Lithium succinate is used topically to treat seborrheic dermatitis (34). A topical 8% lithium gluconate ointment was more effective than a placebo ointment in treating 129 patients with facial seborrheic dermatitis (complete remission in 29 versus 3.8%) (35).

Immunologic and infections

Comments on the generally favorable effects of lithium on immune function have been summarized (36). The antiviral and neuroprotective properties of lithium were mentioned in a review of the immune system and bipolar disorder (37). The potential benefit of lithium in treating AIDS and AIDS-related dementia, owing in part to its cytokine-regulating and neuroprotective effects, has been reviewed (38). Genital *Herpes simplex* infection has responded to lithium (39).

- Lithium had an antiviral effect in a 44-year-old woman whose psychiatric symptoms did not improve but who had complete suppression of *Herpes labialis* for 2 years (after a 30-year history of at least twice-yearly episodes) followed by a recurrence, only 5 days after stopping the drug (40).

Cancers

In one study, there was a lower risk of cancer in both 609 lithium patients and 2396 psychiatric controls compared with the general population, and in the lithium group, there was a nonsignificant trend toward an even lower risk of nonepithelial tumors (41).

Lithium gamolenate, a compound with in vitro antitumor activity, given intravenously or orally, was ineffective in treating advanced pancreatic adenocarcinoma ($n = 278$) (42). Adverse effects attributed to lithium (type unspecified) were reported in two of 93 in the oral group (mean serum lithium 0.15 mmol/l), five of 90 with low-dose intravenous administration (mean serum lithium 0.4 mmol/l), and seven of 95 with the high-dose intravenous administration (mean serum lithium 0.8 mmol/l).

Pharmacokinetics

Ionized lithium is readily absorbed from the gastrointestinal tract and is excreted almost entirely by the kidney, which ordinarily clears it at a rate of about one-quarter to that of creatinine clearance (43).

A reduction in glomerular filtration rate (GFR) will reduce lithium clearance, as will a negative sodium balance. Lithium is not metabolized and is not bound to plasma proteins.

Lithium is easily, inexpensively, and accurately measurable in the serum, and serum concentration determination is a useful adjunct to monitoring its therapeutic efficacy and avoiding toxicity (44).

Both immediate-release and modified-release formulations of lithium carbonate are available. Peak blood concentrations are lower and occur more slowly with modified-release formulations than with immediate-release formulations, but all formulations are supposed to deliver equivalent amounts of lithium per millimole. The effectiveness of lithium should not be altered by the formulation used or the number of daily doses (assuming full adherence to therapy), but if it is given once a day the 12-hours serum lithium concentration will be somewhat higher than if the same amount is given in divided doses.

Standardizing the timing of blood sampling to about 12 hours after the last dose (which is preferably taken in the morning) will do much to avoid the vagaries of absorption and should provide a consistency that will allow accurate comparisons across samples (44). Blood concentrations are most useful if a steady state has been reached before sampling (4–5 days after starting treatment or after a dosage change).

Recommended serum lithium concentrations for the treatment of mania and for maintenance treatment are not uniformly agreed on, although differences of opinion are not large. For example, a concentration of 0.5–0.8 mmol/l has been advised for patients starting treatment, with the recognition that both lower and higher concentrations may be necessary. In US product monographs, concentration ranges for acute mania (1.0–1.5 mmol/l) and long-term treatment (0.6–1.2 mmol/l) tend to be higher than currently practiced (mania 0.8–1.2 mmol/l; long-term 0.6–1.0 mmol/l) and considerably higher than concentrations recommended in Europe. While there is uniform agreement that the serum concentration should be kept as low as is compatible with therapeutic efficacy, there is as yet no accurate way to predict this concentration in an individual. Within the target range, one can generally expect efficacy to increase with blood concentration, but at a price—adverse effects are likely to increase. Elderly people will require a lower dosage of lithium to achieve a given serum concentration, and they tend to be more sensitive to adverse effects than younger individuals, but whether they respond better to lower concentrations is unclear.

The frequency with which blood concentrations should be measured varies with the stage of the illness and with a number of patient factors (including age, associated illnesses, concomitant medications, and diet). Generally, concentrations are measured every 5–7 days during the start of therapy, and then less and less often as stability occurs and persists. In reliable patients taking long-term treatment, concentrations may be measured every 3–4 or even 6 months.

Instruction and information

The safe and effective use of lithium is best ensured by close collaboration among patients, physicians, and significant others, all of whom must remain well-informed and up to date about treatment guidelines, benefits, adverse effects, risks, and precautions. While verbal communication and education is invaluable, it should be constructively supplemented with written information (45,46).

Comparative studies

The availability of anticonvulsant mood stabilizers has led to comparative studies with lithium. A review of the comparative efficacy and tolerability of drug treatments for bipolar disorder included tolerability comparisons of lithium versus carbamazepine, lithium versus valproate semisodium, and lithium versus other medications (47).

In 29 patients, the burden of taking lithium ($n = 17$) was compared with that of valproate ($n = 12$) using a visual analogue scale. Adverse effects were common but not significantly different between drugs (48), a finding that contrasts with the common impression that valproate is better tolerated. Indeed, a telephone interview of 11 adolescents taking lithium and 32 taking valproate found more adverse effects, poorer compliance, and greater perceived burden in the lithium group. There was a non-significant trend toward more weight gain with valproate (mean 12 kg) than with lithium (mean 9 kg) (49).

In a 4-week, placebo-controlled study of lithium in 40 hospitalized children and adolescents (mean age 12.5 years) with aggression related to conduct disorder, lithium was "statistically and clinically superior to placebo" (50). Although there were no dropouts related to adverse events, nausea, vomiting, and increased urinary frequency occurred significantly more often in the lithium group. The 55% incidence of vomiting with lithium (versus 20% with placebo) may have been related to the relatively high mean serum lithium concentration of 1.07 mmol/l (range 0.78–1.55 mmol/l).

Lithium versus carbamazepine

In a 2-year, double-blind study, lithium was superior to carbamazepine in prophylactic efficacy, although it caused more adverse effects (Table 1) (51).

Lithium versus divalproex

In a randomized, placebo-controlled, 12-month maintenance comparison of lithium and divalproex in 372 bipolar I outpatients, neither active drug was more effective than placebo on the primary outcome measure—the time to recurrence of any mood episode (52). While a history of intolerance to either lithium or divalproex was an

Table 1 Adverse effects of lithium and carbamazepine in a double-blind trial (in %)

Adverse effect	Lithium ($n = 42$)	Carbamazepine ($n = 46$)
Difficulty concentrating	45	33
Thirst	41	22
Hand tremor	31	4
Blurred vision	26	11
Reduced appetite	21	9
Increased appetite	17	33
Weakness	14	4

exclusion criterion, it was not stated whether or not prior nonresponders were entered and, if so, how many. The following adverse effects were significantly more frequent:

(a) with lithium than with placebo: nausea, diarrhea, and tremor;
(b) with divalproex than with placebo: tremor, weight gain, and alopecia;
(c) with lithium than with divalproex: polyuria, thirst, tachycardia, akathisia, and dry eyes;
(d) with divalproex than with lithium: sedation, infection, and tinnitus.

Unfortunately, all dropouts were pooled, whether due to adverse events or noncompliance, making overall tolerability comparisons impossible.

General adverse effects

The adverse effects of lithium have been reviewed (5,53–55). The adverse effects of lithium range widely in intensity and can be a major cause of nonadherence to therapy. However, with proper attention to the prevention and management of adverse effects, most patients can be treated effectively and safely. Withdrawal of lithium is almost always followed by resolution of adverse effects, although certain problems can sometimes persist (for example renal).

Adverse effects that can occur at concentrations in the target range, especially in the upper part of the range, include mild cognitive complaints, postural tremor, hypothyroidism, weight gain, leukocytosis, hypercalcemia, loss of appetite, nausea, loose stools, acne, and psoriasis. Renal adverse effects include impaired concentrating ability and polyuria with secondary polydipsia. Cardiac adverse effects are rarely symptomatic and are usually reversible. Lithium does not cause physiological dependence, although there may be an increased risk of early recurrence if it is withdrawn rapidly.

When 60 patients (22 men, 38 women) who had taken lithium for 1 year or more (mean 6.9 years; mean serum concentration 0.74 mmol/l) were interviewed about adverse effects, 60% complained of polyuria–polydipsia syndrome (serum creatinine concentrations were normal) and 27% had hypothyroidism requiring treatment (56). Weight gain was more common in women (47 versus 18%) as were hypothyroidism (37 versus 9%) and skin problems (16 versus 9%), while tremor was more common in men (54 versus 26%). Weight gain of over 5 kg in the first year of treatment was the only independent variable predictive of hypothyroidism.

The severity of lithium toxicity depends on the magnitude and duration of exposure and idiosyncratic factors. Manifestations of acute toxicity range in intensity from mild (tremor, unsteadiness, ataxia, dysarthria) to severe (impaired consciousness, neuromuscular irritability, seizures, heart block, and renal insufficiency), and the sequels of toxicity range from none at all to permanent neurological damage (often cerebellar) to death. Causes of raised serum lithium concentrations include increased intake and reduced excretion (due to kidney disease, low sodium intake, drug interactions). Whether long-term lithium use carries a risk of progressive renal insufficiency in a few patients continues to be debated. Reviews have addressed lithium toxicity in the elderly (57) and lithium intoxication with an emphasis on the kidney (58).

Dose- and time-related adverse effects

During initiation and stabilization of treatment, adverse effects, such as gastrointestinal upset, tremor, dysphoria, fatigue, muscle weakness, unsteadiness, thirst, and excessive urination, are not uncommon, but they usually abate with time. Such adverse effects are more likely to occur at higher dosages or higher serum concentrations and can usually be avoided or attenuated by proper attention to dosage, clinical and laboratory monitoring, and, if necessary, the use of adjunctive medication.

Long-term use of lithium is sometimes associated with weight gain, polyuria and polydipsia, and thyroid dysfunction (see below), but many patients have been treated successfully for several decades without developing treatment-limiting adverse effects. However, long-term success should not breed complacency, since there is an ever-present risk of recurrence (if concentrations are too low) and toxicity (if concentrations are too high).

Treatment of toxicity

Two patients with lithium toxicity (serum concentrations 3.5 and 4.2 mmol/l) had the well-recognized rebound increase in serum concentrations after the end of hemodialysis. Both died during hospitalization from what was cryptically described as "unrelated events" (59).

- A 49-year-old with severe lithium toxicity was treated successfully with continuous veno-venous hemodiafiltration; the serum lithium concentration fell from 3.0 to 0.93 mmol/l after 7 hours and there was no rebound increase after the end of the procedure (60). The maximum lithium clearance was 28 ml/minute which is considerably lower than usually attained with hemodialysis.

An all too common treatment error in the face of severe toxicity is "watchful waiting," during which the patient's condition is more likely to worsen than improve.

Organs and Systems

Cardiovascular

Cardiovascular disease is not a contraindication to lithium, but the risks may be greater, in view of factors such as fluid and electrolyte imbalance and the use of concomitant medications. Close clinical and laboratory monitoring is necessary, and an alternative mood stabilizer may be preferred. While long-term tricyclic antidepressant therapy may be more cardiotoxic than lithium, the newer antidepressants (SSRIs and others) seem to be safe.

In two studies of 277 and 133 patients taking long-term lithium, there was no evidence of increased cardiovascular mortality compared with the general population (61,62). While the latter study reported on 16-year mortality, it did not provide information about which patients continued to take lithium after the first 2 years.

Blood pressure

Lithium does not affect blood pressure adversely, nor does it benefit blood pressure, although lithium hippurate was used to treat arterial hypertension in the 1920s.

Cardiac dysrhythmias

Nonspecific, benign ST-T wave electrocardiographic changes are the most common cardiovascular effects of lithium.

- A 13-year-old boy taking lithium developed a "pseudo-myocardial infarct pattern" on the electrocardiogram; this may have been an overinterpretation of nonspecific T-wave changes (63).

A very uncommon adverse effect involves sinus node dysfunction (extreme bradycardia, sinus arrest, sinoatrial block), which can be associated with syncopal episodes, perhaps due to hypothyroidism (64,65). In such cases, lithium must either be withdrawn or continued in the presence of a pacemaker. At therapeutic concentrations, other cardiac conduction disturbances have been reported, sometimes in conjunction with hypercalcemia (66), but are uncommon.

Two reviews of the cardiac effects of psychotropic drugs briefly mentioned lithium and dysrhythmias, with a focus on sinus node dysfunction (67,68), reports of which, as manifested by bradycardia, sinoatrial block, and sinus arrest, continue to accumulate in association with both toxic (69) and therapeutic (70,71) serum lithium concentrations. The rhythm disturbance normalized in some cases when lithium was stopped (69,71), persisted despite discontinuation (70), or was treated with a permanent cardiac pacemaker (71). Of historical interest is the observation that the first patient treated with lithium by Cade developed manifestations of toxicity in 1950, including bradycardia (72).

There have been several reports of bradycardia and sinus node dysfunction.

- During an episode of lithium toxicity (serum concentration 3.86 mmol/l), a 42-year-old woman developed sinus bradycardia that required a temporary pacemaker (69). There was marked prolongation of sinus node recovery time. Lithium was withdrawn and the patient underwent hemodialysis once daily for 3 days; sinus node recovery time normalized. The presence of non-toxic concentrations of carbamazepine may have contributed to the condition.
- A 65-year-old man taking lithium for 2 years, with therapeutic concentrations, developed sinus bradycardia (30 beats/minute), which remitted when the drug was stopped and recurred when it was restarted (73). Implantation of a permanent pacemaker allowed lithium to be continued.
- Asymptomatic bradycardia occurred in three of 15 patients treated for mania with a 20 mg/kg oral loading dose of slow-release lithium carbonate (74).
- A 9-year-old boy whose serum lithium concentration was 1.29 mmol/l had a sinus bradycardia with a junctional escape rhythm (40 beats/minute), which normalized at a lower lithium concentration (75).
- A 58-year-old woman with lithium toxicity developed an irregular bradycardia (as low as 20 beats/minute), which resolved during hemodialysis; persistent sinoatrial conduction delay suggested that she was predisposed to the bradydysrhythmia (76).
- A 52-year-old man took an overdose of lithium (serum concentration 4.58 mmol/l) and developed asymptomatic sinus bradycardia with sinus node dysfunction and multiple atrial extra beats, which resolved after hemodialysis (77).
- A 66-year-old woman with pre-existing first-degree AV block, developed sinus bradycardia, a junctional rhythm, a prolonged QT interval, and syncopal episodes (serum lithium concentration 1.4 mmol/l in a 40-hours sample) about 2 weeks after beginning lithium therapy. She was treated successfully with a pacemaker and a lower dose of lithium (78).
- A 36-year-old man became hypomanic after lithium was withdrawn because of symptomatic first-degree atrioventricular block (although, how first-degree block could have caused symptoms is unclear) (79).
- A 44-year-old woman developed atropine-resistant but isoprenaline-sensitive bradycardia (36 beats/minute), thought to be due to sinus node dysfunction related to lithium, fentanyl, and propofol (65).
- A 52-year-old man with a serum lithium concentration of 4.58 mmol/l had sinus node dysfunction with multiple atrial extra beats and an intraventricular conduction delay, which normalized following hemodialysis (77). Two patients, a 58-year-old woman and a 74-year-old woman, developed sick sinus syndrome while taking lithium but were able to continue taking it after pacemaker implantation (80,81).
- A 59-year-old woman with syncope and sick sinus syndrome, which remitted when lithium was withdrawn, recurred when lithium was restarted, and then persisted despite lithium withdrawal; after a pacemaker was implanted she was treated successfully with lithium for 7 years (80).

Lithium can also occasionally cause tachycardia.

- A 59-year-old man was noted to have tachycardia, a shortened QT interval, and nonspecific ST-T changes, while hospitalized with lithium-associated hypercalcemia (82).

An extension of a previously published study (66) added a third comparator group of 18 hypercalcemic non-lithium treated patients and compared them with 12 hypercalcemic lithium patients, 40 normocalcemic lithium patients, and 20 normocalcemic bipolar patients taking anticonvulsant mood stabilizers (83). Both hypercalcemic groups had more conduction abnormalities than the other

Both goiter and hypothyroidism continue to be reported as complications of lithium therapy (81,176,177).

In a cross-sectional study of 121 patients taking lithium, there was no difference in thyroid function tests among those taking treatment for 0.7–6 months, 7–10 months, or 61–240 months. However, when compared with healthy volunteers ($n = 24$) and prelithium controls ($n = 11$), there was a significant increase in radioiodine uptake in all lithium groups. Serum TSH concentrations were higher in prelithium patients than controls and highest in those taking lithium. Being from an iodine-deficient area appeared to predispose lithium patients to abnormally high TSH values and clinical hypothyroidism (178).

In 1989, in 150 patients at different stages of lithium therapy, thyroid function was assessed and subsequently 118 were reassessed at least once and 54 completed a 10-year follow-up (179). The annual rates of new cases of thyroid dysfunction were subclinical hypothyroidism 1.7%, goiter 2.1%, and autoimmunity 1.4%. While these figures were little different from those found in the general population, the authors acknowledged that lithium was a potential cause of thyroid dysfunction.

Of 42 bipolar patients who had taken lithium for 4–156 months, three had subclinical hypothyroidism, three had subclinical hyperthyroidism, and one was overtly hyperthyroid (177). Ultrasonography showed that goiter was present in 38% and mild thyroid dysfunction was suggested in 48% because of an apparent increased conversion of free T4 to free T3. There was no correlation between the duration of lithium therapy and thyroid abnormalities.

Hypothyroidism

Lithium-induced hypothyroidism has been briefly reviewed (180). Some patients develop more persistent subclinical hypothyroidism (TSH over 5 mU/l, free thyroxine normal) and others overt hypothyroidism (higher risk in women, in those with pre-existing thyroid dysfunction, and those with a family history of hypothyroidism). Since subclinical hypothyroidism is not necessarily asymptomatic, treatment with thyroxine may be necessary in this group (181), as well as in those with more obvious hypothyroidism (182).

The prevalence of thyroperoxidase antibodies was higher in 226 bipolar patients (28%) than in population- and psychiatric-control groups (3–18%). While there was no association with lithium exposure, the presence of antibodies increased the risk of lithium-induced hypothyroidism (183).

Thyroid function tests in 101 lithium maintenance patients were compared with their baseline values and with results in 82 controls without psychiatric or endocrine diagnoses. With hypothyroidism defined as a serum TSH above the reference range, 8 patients were hypothyroid at baseline, and another 40 became so during treatment. Women over 60 years of age were at slightly higher risk and had higher TSH values. Patients with a positive family history of hypothyroidism had raised TSH concentrations sooner after starting lithium (3.7 versus 8.7 years). Whether any patients became clinically hypothyroid was not noted (it was stated that those with grade II hypothyroidism were almost free of symptoms) (184).

Serum TSH concentrations were raised (10 mU/l or more) in 13 of 61 children aged 5–17 years taking lithium and valproate for up to 20 weeks (185).

In a review of lithium-induced subclinical hypothyroidism (TSH over 5 mU/l, free thyroxine normal), a prevalence of up to 23% in lithium patients was contrasted with up to 10% in the general population. It was stressed that subclinical hypothyroidism from any cause can be associated with subtle neuropsychiatric symptoms, such as depression, impaired memory and concentration, and mental slowing and lethargy, as well as with other somatic symptoms. Management guidelines were discussed (181).

An abstract reported that 23% of 61 children and adolescents taking lithium and divalproex sodium for up to 20 weeks had a TSH concentration over 10 mU/l (reference range 0.2–6.0); however, no clinical information was provided (186). Another abstract reported that the prevalence of thyroperoxidase antibodies was higher in bipolar outpatients (28% of 226) than in psychiatric inpatients with any diagnosis (10% of 2782) or healthy controls (14% of 225), but this was not related to lithium exposure; on the other hand, hypothyroidism was associated with lithium exposure, especially in the presence of antithyroid antibodies (187).

When 22 men and 38 women who had taken lithium for at least a year (mean 6.9 years) for bipolar disorder were evaluated for adverse effects, hypothyroidism requiring thyroid supplementation was found in 16 (14 women and 2 men); 9 had a goiter (56). The area from which some of the patients came was known to have a high background incidence of thyroid dysfunction.

The observation that Canada, with ample nutritional iodine, has a relatively high rate of lithium-related hypothyroidism compared with relatively low rates in iodine-deficient countries such as Italy, Spain, and Germany led to the suggestion that ambient iodine may play a role in the genesis of this condition (188). This is reminiscent of the association of amiodarone with hypothyroidism or hyperthyroidism in iodine-replete and iodine-deficient areas respectively (SEDA-10, 148).

Case reports of adverse thyroid effects of lithium have included the following:

- A 56-year-old man taking lithium whose TSH concentration was abnormally high (50 mU/l) (189).
- A 44-year-old woman who had taken lithium for 10 years and who developed swelling of the right lobe of the thyroid and hypothyroidism (65).
- A 63-year-old woman taking long-term lithium who developed subclinical hypothyroidism and primary hyperparathyroidism (190).

Hyperthyroidism

Despite the predominantly antithyroid effects of lithium, thyrotoxicosis continues to be described during treatment and after withdrawal (191–193). In a retrospective review of 201 patients taking lithium (mean duration 6.4 years), hypothyroidism requiring supplemental thyroxine developed in 10% (3.4% of men, 15% of women) after a mean duration of 56 months. Women over 50 years of age tended to have an earlier onset. Two patients developed goiter requiring surgery and two others developed thyrotoxicosis (182).

Reports of hyperthyroidism associated with lithium include one in a woman who was also hypercalcemic with a normal parathyroid hormone (PTH) concentration (194) and two discovered while treating lithium toxicity (195).

- A 27-year-old man developed thyrotoxicosis while taking lithium (193).
- A 52-year-old woman became thyrotoxic 2 months after stopping long-term lithium therapy; the authors briefly reviewed 10 previous reports (196).
- A woman with lithium-associated hyperthyroidism lost 2 kg over 3 months, suggesting that lithium may have indirectly caused the weight loss (197).

Thyroiditis

A retrospective record review of 300 patients with Graves' disease and 100 with silent thyroiditis who had undergone thyroid scans showed that the likelihood of lithium exposure was 4.7 times higher in the latter, suggesting a link between lithium and thyrotoxicosis caused by silent thyroiditis (198).

- A 30-year-old man, who had taken lithium for 16 years for bipolar disorder and long-term ciclosporin and prednisolone after a bone-marrow transplant, developed subacute thyroiditis associated with a diffusely enlarged gland that showed heterogeneous echogenicity, but without a clear relation to lithium (199).

Goiter

Euthyroid or hypothyroid goiter can also complicate lithium therapy, although the goiter is seldom of clinical importance and tends to resolve on withdrawal or with thyroxine treatment. In one ultrasound study, there was a 44% incidence of goiter in patients who had taken lithium for 1–5 years compared with 16% in a control group; cigarette smoking was associated with a greater size and frequency of goiter in both groups (200).

Hyperthyroidism has also been associated with lithium use and withdrawal, although a cause-and-effect relation has been more difficult to establish. In fact, lithium has been used with some success to treat hyperthyroidism, particularly in conjunction with propylthiouracil (201) and ^{131}I (16).

Parathyroid and calcium

Mild rises in serum calcium and PTH concentrations have been associated with long-term use of lithium, and, in a review, 27 reports of parathyroid adenoma and 11 of hyperplasia were mentioned (202). The hypercalcemia and raised PTH concentrations are often reversible on withdrawal, but surgical intervention may be necessary. So far, long-term lithium therapy has not emerged as a risk factor for reduced bone mineral density or osteoporosis (203). In one study, there was a greater frequency of electrocardiographic conduction defects in hypercalcemic patients taking lithium than in normocalcemic patients taking lithium (66).

Of 537 patients who had parathyroid glands excised for hyperparathyroidism, 12 (2.2%) had been taking lithium and 11 (2.0%) had been taking it long-term (mean 15.3 years, range 2–30). Manifestations included fatigue, bone pain and fracture, and abdominal pain and constipation. Six had a single adenoma and five had multigland hyperplasia. All resumed lithium, but one had a recurrence after 3 years and one had increased PTH concentrations, but a normal serum calcium. A literature review detected 27 prior reports of parathyroid adenoma and 11 of hyperplasia associated with lithium (202).

When 15 euthymic bipolar patients who had taken lithium for a mean of 49 months were compared with 10 nonlithium euthymic bipolar controls, the former had significantly higher total serum calcium concentrations and intact PTH (iPTH) concentrations (204). The authors advised baseline and periodic serum calcium and iPTH concentrations and bone density measurements in all lithium patients, although whether the benefit outweighs cost is open to question.

Ten patients who had taken lithium for less than 1 year and 13 who had taken it for more than 3 years were assessed for alterations in bone metabolism and parathyroid function (203). There were no differences in bone mineral density, serum calcium concentration, or PTH concentration, but both groups had increased bone turnover and the long-term group had nonsignificantly higher calcium and PTH concentrations (including one hyperparathyroid patient who had an adenoma excised). The authors' conclusion that lithium therapy is not a risk factor for osteoporosis needs to be tempered by the small sample size, the case of adenoma, and the blood concentration trends.

Total serum calcium and iPTH concentrations were measured in 15 patients taking long-term lithium and 10 lithium-naïve patients; both were significantly higher in the lithium group (205). While the number of lithium patients with abnormally high concentrations was not stated, mean iPTH concentrations were almost twice the upper limit of the reference range (102 versus 55 pg/ml).

Parathyroid tumors from nine patients with lithium-associated hyperparathyroidism (six multiglandular, three uniglandular) were compared with 13 nonlithium-associated sporadic parathyroid tumors with regard to gross genomic alterations (206). Gross chromosomal alterations were absent in most of the lithium group and were more common in the sporadic group.

In 53 patients studied prospectively at 1, 6, 12, and 24 months, lithium increased serum PTH concentrations (apparent by 6 months) and increased renal reabsorption of calcium in the absence of a significant change in serum calcium (207). A prospective study of 101 lithium maintenance patients and 82 healthy controls showed higher serum calcium concentrations during lithium treatment than at baseline or in the controls, and higher calcium serum concentrations in those lithium patients over 60 years of age (184).

When compared with 12 healthy matched controls, 13 women who had taken lithium for a mean of 8 (range 3–16) years had higher mean ionized and total calcium concentrations, but mean plasma parathormone concentrations did not differ. In eight of the women taking lithium, the calcium concentration was above the upper end of the reference range, and in one the parathormone concentration was abnormally high (208).

Of 15 patients taking long-term lithium who had surgery for primary hyperparathyroidism, 14 had adenomas

(11 single, 3 double) and one had four-gland hyperplasia. All restarted lithium successfully after surgery, except one who again developed hyperparathyroidism, resulting in removal of another adenoma (209).

Hyperparathyroidism was considered a possible cause of treatment-resistant manic psychosis in a patient taking lithium (210).

- Hypercalcemia and raised PTH concentrations improved in a woman who had taken lithium for over 20 years after she was switched to divalproex (211).
- A 64-year-old woman who had taken lithium for over 10 years was admitted with altered consciousness, agitation, and disorientation. The serum calcium was 3.35 mmol/l (reference range 2.1–2.6 mmol/l) and the PTH concentration was raised. With hydration and conversion from lithium to valproate, the serum calcium concentration normalized, but 2 years later disorientation and hypercalcemia recurred and a 150 mg parathyroid adenoma was removed surgically (212).
- A 53-year-old woman who had taken lithium for 9 years and carbamazepine for 3 years and had a 3-month history of lethargy was found to be hypercalcemic with a raised concentration of iPTH. She was saved from parathyroid surgery when withdrawal of lithium resolved the hypercalcemia (213).
- A 51-year-old man who had taken lithium for over 10 years presented with nausea, vomiting, anorexia, hypercalcemia (3.1 mmol/l), and increased PTH concentration (iPTH 110 ng/l). Abnormalities resolved after an oxyphilic parathyroid adenoma was excised (214).

Other reports of hyperparathyroidism in patients taking lithium have included the following:

- Three cases among 26 cases of chronic lithium poisoning (215).
- A 78-year-old man who had taken lithium for 30 years who presented with dehydration, azotemia, hypernatremia, hypercalcemia, and increased PTH concentrations (216).
- A 63-year-old woman taking long-term lithium therapy (190).
- A woman who had taken lithium for 15 years who became hypercalcemic and stopped taking lithium, but 2 years later had two parathyroid adenomas removed surgically (217).
- A 42-year-old man who had taken lithium for 17 years and who had raised serum calcium and PTH concentrations which normalized after removal of a parathyroid adenoma (218).
- A 59-year-old man with hypercalcemia and increased PTH concentrations 3 months after starting lithium, which normalized after lithium was withdrawn (82).
- Three cases from Denmark (219) and one from Spain (220);
- A 78-year-old woman who had taken lithium for 25 years (221).
- A 74-year-old man who had an adenoma resected (81).
- Two 77-year-old women who developed hyperparathyroidism which was managed medically (81).
- A 39-year-old (sex unspecified) whose adenoma was resected after taking lithium for 10 years (209).
- A 59-year-old woman with hyperparathyroidism (222).

A lithium chloride solution caused changes in gravicurvature, statocyte ultrastructure, and calcium balance in pea root, believed to be due to effects of lithium on the phosphoinositide second messenger system (223). The implications with regard to human parathyroid function are obscure.

Metabolism

Diabetes mellitus

It has been reported that diabetes mellitus is three times more common in bipolar patients than in the general population (224). However, lithium does not appear to increase the risk of diabetes mellitus, and its use in patients with pre-existing diabetes is generally safe, assuming that the diabetes is well controlled.

When lithium toxicity has been reported in patients with diabetes mellitus, it has been attributed to impaired glucose intolerance (225).

- An increased lithium dosage requirement in a hyperglycemic 40-year-old woman was attributed to the osmotic diuretic effect of glycosuria, increasing lithium excretion (226).
- Two patients with diabetes mellitus developed lithium toxicity (serum concentrations 3.3 and 3.0 mmol/l) in association with impaired consciousness, and hyperglycemia that resolved after intravenous insulin and fluids (227).

While the authors of the second report concluded that impaired glucose tolerance had predisposed to lithium intoxication, the opposite is also possible.

When a 45-year-old man with severe lithium-induced diabetes insipidus developed hyperosmolar, nonketotic hyperglycemia, it was suggested that poorly controlled diabetes mellitus may have contributed to the polyuria (228). Prior contact with a female patient who had developed hyperosmolar coma secondary to lithium-induced diabetes insipidus (229) allowed physicians 4 years later to treat her safely after a drug overdose and a surgical procedure, by avoiding intravenous replacement fluids with a high dextrose content (despite stopping lithium several years earlier, the patient continued to put out 10 liters of urine daily) (230).

Difficulty in attaining a therapeutic serum concentration of lithium despite increased doses was attributed to increased renal clearance due to the osmotic effect of glycosuria in a 44-year-old man with poorly controlled diabetes mellitus (226).

Weight gain

Weight gain, a well-recognized adverse effect of lithium, occurs in one-third to two-thirds of patients (231). It is more common in those with prior weight problems and at higher dosages of lithium. Possible mechanisms include complex effects on carbohydrate and lipid metabolism, mood stabilization itself, lithium-induced hypothyroidism, the use of high-calorie beverages to treat lithium-induced polydipsia, and the concomitant use of other weight-gaining drugs (for example valproate, olanzapine, mirtazapine). Recognizing and managing weight gain early in the course of treatment can do much to ensure continued adherence to lithium regimens. Two reviews of weight gain with psychotropic drugs mentioned lithium (232,233).

Risk and magnitude

In a review of psychotropic drug-induced weight gain, the prevalence and magnitude of the problem with lithium was discussed together with risk factors, mechanisms, and management (231). Adolescent inpatients treated with risperidone ($n = 18$) or conventional antipsychotic drugs ($n = 19$) over 6 months gained more weight than a control group but concomitant treatment with lithium was not a contributing factor (234).

A review of psychotropic drugs and weight gain included a brief summary of lithium-related weight gain (235). A retrospective evaluation of 176 patients taking long-term lithium showed that weight gain was an adverse effect in 18%. While 34% of the total did not adhere to treatment because of somatic adverse effects, no specific adverse effect (including weight gain) was associated with nonadherence (236).

The prevalence of overweight (BMI 25–29) and obesity (BMI 30 or more) was determined in 89 euthyroid bipolar patients and 445 reference subjects. The rate of obesity in patients taking only lithium was 1.5 times greater than in the reference population (a nonsignificant difference), compared with a statistically significant 2.5 times greater rate associated with antipsychotic drugs (237).

The prevalence of overweight (BMI 20 or more) and obesity (BMI 30 or more) has been evaluated in 89 euthymic bipolar patients and 445 age- and sex-matched controls (237). The bipolar women were more overweight and more obese than the controls and the bipolar men were more obese but not more overweight. Obesity was clearly related to antipsychotic drug use and less so to lithium and anticonvulsants (but patients taking lithium alone had an obesity rate 1.5 times that of the general population).

A review of the effects of mood stabilizers on weight included a section on lithium in which the authors concluded that lithium-related weight gain occurs in one-third to two-thirds of patients, with a mean increase of 4–7 kg; possible mechanisms were discussed (238).

An open chart review of 74 hospitalized patients showed a mean weight gain of 6.3 kg and an increase in BMI of 2.1 kg/m^2 after they had taken lithium for a mean of 89 days (239). Of 47 lithium-treated patients, 14 gained at least 5% of their baseline BMI, 6 gained over 10%, and 2 gained over 15% during an acute treatment phase of unspecified duration, while during the 1-year maintenance phase 11 gained over 5% and 2 gained over 10% (240).

Comparative studies

In a 1-year, placebo-controlled study of bipolar I prophylaxis ($n = 372$), weight gain with divalproex, but not with lithium, was significantly more common than with placebo (52). A patient who gained 18 kg over 18 months while taking lithium and perphenazine lost 16 kg when the latter was changed to loxapine (she also participated in a weight loss program) (241). Whether lithium played a role in the weight gain was unclear.

In a 12-month maintenance study, weight gain was an adverse event in 21% of patients taking divalproex, 13% of those taking lithium, and 7% of those taking placebo (52). The divalproex/placebo difference was statistically significant, but the lithium/placebo difference was not.

Mechanism

In 15 consecutive patients, serum leptin concentrations were measured at baseline and after 8 weeks of lithium treatment. There was a significant mean increase of 3.5 ng/ml and serum leptin correlated positively with weight gain (5.9 kg), increased BMI (24–27), and clinical efficacy (242). The authors suggested that leptin might play a role in lithium-induced weight gain.

Management

The Expert Consensus Guideline Series, Medication Treatment of Bipolar Disorder 2000, has recommended to "continue present medication, focus on diet and exercise" as the preferred first-line treatment for managing weight gain in patients taking lithium or divalproex. The next approach was to continue medication and add topiramate. Second-line treatments included switching from divalproex to lithium or vice versa, reducing the dosage, and switching to another drug. The addition of an appetite suppressant was a lower second-line recommendation (243).

Nutrition

In a review of naturally occurring dietary lithium (food and water sources), the author acknowledged that human lithium deficiency states have not been identified, but concluded that lithium should be considered an essential element, a conclusion reached on rather shaky grounds (244).

Electrolyte balance

Potassium

Episodes of acute hypokalemic paralysis have been associated with long-term lithium therapy (245).

- A 25-year-old man, who had taken lithium for 5 years, awakened from sleep unable to move his limbs and had a generalized flaccid paralysis with a serum potassium concentration of 2.1 mmol/l (245). Lithium was withdrawn and he responded to treatment with intravenous potassium chloride.

The diagnosis of acute hypokalemic paralysis was attributed to lithium but without confirmation by rechallenge it was unclear whether this was causal or coincidental.

Sodium

Hypernatremia can occur secondary to dehydration in patients taking lithium and is not uncommon in association with lithium poisoning. Lithium-induced diabetes insipidus is often a contributing factor.

Mineral balance

Fluid and sodium balance are important to the safe use of lithium. Both dehydration and a negative sodium balance (for example a low salt intake, diuretic-induced sodium loss) will reduce renal lithium clearance and predispose to toxicity (246). Hyponatremia (for example, secondary to polydipsia or SIADH) may also increase the risk of lithium toxicity (247).

When nine trace elements were measured in whole blood (oven dried, moisture-free) from controls, pre-lithium, and lithium patients, there were many changes related to lithium, but none appeared to be clinically important (248).

Fluid balance

Edema associated with lithium is uncommon (249,250). It is usually restricted to the legs, and is usually transient or intermittent. If treatment is necessary, the intermittent and cautious use of a loop diuretic may be helpful (but see drug–drug interactions).

Dehydration, secondary to lithium-induced nephrogenic diabetes insipidus, was thought to be the cause of a superior sagittal sinus thrombosis in a 30-year-old woman who presented with confusion, papilledema, and a left hemiparesis (251).

Hematologic

The most common hematological effect of lithium is a benign leukocytosis (252), consisting primarily of mature granulocytes, which is reversible on withdrawal. An increase in platelet count is a much less consistent finding (253), and there are no clinically important effects on erythrocytes. Despite anecdotal reports to the contrary, epidemiological studies have shown no increased risk of leukemia with lithium (254). The leukocyte-inducing effects of lithium have been used with some success to treat granulocytopenia (25,26).

The effects of lithium on hemopoiesis have been studied in 100 patients who had developed chronic granulocytopenia after cancer chemotherapy or radiotherapy (255). The mean leukocyte count rose by 46%, but there were no changes in platelet or erythrocyte counts. However, there was a significant increase in platelet count in those whose baseline values were below 150×10^9/l. Lithium was well tolerated (mean serum concentration 0.59 mmol/l).

Granulocyte counts and granulocyte colony-stimulating factor (G-CSF) concentrations were measured in 18 patients before and after 1 and 4 weeks of lithium treatment, and compared with values in 20 patients taking long-term lithium (256). At week 4, the granulocyte count was significantly higher than at baseline or at week 1, or in the long-term group. There was only a nonsignificant increase in G-CSF concentration at weeks 1 and 4. The granulocyte count in those taking long-term lithium did not differ significantly from the baseline values in the other group.

A retrospective review of inpatients showed higher leukocyte and granulocyte counts in those taking lithium alone ($n = 38$) compared with those taking antipsychotic drugs alone ($n = 207$); lymphocyte counts were not affected. Rises in leukocyte counts above normal occurred in 18% of those taking lithium and 6% of those taking antipsychotic drugs (252). The neutrophil-stimulating effect of lithium was used to advantage to successfully re-treat a patient with clozapine several years after stopping it because of neutropenia (257). Likewise, lithium was used to successfully stimulate neutrophil production in a patient with clozapine-induced neutropenia and in another with clozapine-induced agranulocytosis (recovery was as fast as seen with colony-stimulating factor and twice as rapid as expected spontaneously) (25).

In eight patients with bipolar disorder, lithium for 3–4 weeks increased neutrophil count by 88% and also caused a significant increase in CD34+ cells (although three patients had no increase in either) (258).

- A lithium-treated bipolar patient with acute myeloid leukemia had an unusually great increase in CD34+ cells following administration of G-CSF, suggesting a boosting effect from lithium (259).
- After he had failed to respond to combined treatment with corticosteroids and androgens and to antilymphocyte globulin, a 16-year-old with aplastic anemia responded to lithium combined with an androgen derivative, relapsed when lithium was stopped, and responded again when it was restarted (31).

Of 39 patients taking lithium, 18% had neutrophilia and 15% had raised activity of polymorphonuclear elastase (a marker of granulocyte activation) (260). In keeping with these observations, a chart review of 38 patients taking clozapine showed an increase in leukocyte count when lithium was added (32). A man with olanzapine-induced neutropenia (with a prior history of risperidone-induced neutropenia), which normalized with drug withdrawal, had no difficulty when the drug was reintroduced after the patient had been treated with lithium (33).

When 50 bipolar lithium patients were compared with 30 healthy controls, platelet counts were similar, but the lithium group had higher concentrations of plasma beta-thromboglobulin and platelet factor 4, suggesting lithium-induced platelet activation (253).

A cross-sectional study showed a 20% lower serum vitamin B12 concentration in patients taking lithium ($n = 81$) than in controls ($n = 14$) (serum and erythrocyte folate concentrations were normal) (261).

Mouth and teeth

A comprehensive review of psychoactive drug-induced hyposalivation and hypersalivation included a discussion of lithium-induced dry mouth (common) and sialorrhea (262). A review of dental findings and their management in patients with bipolar disorder briefly mentioned that xerostomia, sialadenitis, dysgeusia, and stomatitis have been attributed to lithium (263). Dry mouth is common and can be due to lithium-induced polyuria, a direct effect on thirst, salivary gland hypofunction, or other drugs (262). Hypersalivation attributable to lithium is rare (264).

A review of drug-induced oral ulceration mentioned lithium as a possible cause, based on two older references (265,266).

- An 8-year-old taking lithium citrate for 6 months developed waxing and waning areas of denuded papillae on her tongue, diagnosed as benign migratory glossitis (geographic tongue) and attributed to lithium (267).

The issue has been raised of whether oral lithium therapy was responsible for failure of titanium dental implants in a 62-year-old man (268).

Gastrointestinal

Lithium can cause loss of appetite, nausea, and at times vomiting and loose stools, especially early in therapy, but these can be minimized by the passage of time and by making dosage increases gradually (52). Gastrointestinal symptoms can also be an early warning sign of lithium intoxication.

In a 12-month maintenance study, lithium (n = 94) was not unexpectedly associated with more nausea (45 versus 31%) and diarrhea (46 versus 30%) than placebo (n = 94) (52).

- A 72-year-old man who had recently started to take lithium developed severe nausea, vomiting, and oliguric renal insufficiency which was initially attributed to lithium toxicity, until a serum lithium concentration of only 0.35 mmol/l directed evaluation to the correct diagnosis of acute gastric volvulus (269).
- An 80-year-old woman taking lithium developed constipation, nausea, vomiting, and abdominal pain after starting to take amfebutamone. A diagnosis of acute paralytic ileus was made and attributed to amfebutamone, although an amfebutamone–lithium interaction could not be excluded (270).
- In an 80-year-old woman a 2-month history of diarrhea, nausea, and abdominal distress attributed to irritable bowel syndrome was ultimately determined to be due to early lithium intoxication (271). Her lithium concentration when she was hospitalized was 1.2 mmol/l, although she had taken no lithium for the previous 10 days. Treatment with a thiazide diuretic contributed to the toxicity.

Pancreas

Of 47 cases of drug-induced pancreatitis reported to the Danish Committee on Adverse Drug Reactions between 1968 and 1999, one involved lithium (plus a neuroleptic drug) (272). Whether lithium was causally involved is not known.

- A 78-year-old woman taking lithium had hyperamylasemia and hyperlipasemia in the absence of gastrointestinal symptoms. Ultrasound examination showed the pancreas and liver to be normal. She also had hyperparathyroidism and renal dysfunction (221).

Urinary tract

There have been several reviews of the effects of lithium on the kidney (273–276).

In a retrospective study, 114 patients who had taken lithium for 4–30 years were compared with 94 unmedicated age- and sex-matched controls with regard to changes in creatinine concentrations (277). Of the patients taking lithium, 21% had blood creatinine concentrations that had increased gradually and were now over the top of the reference range. This finding was associated with episodes of lithium intoxication and with diseases and other medications that could also affect glomerular function. Sex, psychiatric diagnosis, duration of treatment, cumulative dose, and serum lithium concentrations did not predict an abnormal creatinine concentration.

Renal function was assessed in 10 patients taking long-term lithium (over 3 years, mean 80 months), 10 taking short-term lithium (3 years or less, mean 16 months), and 10 lithium-naïve patients (171). Blood urea nitrogen and serum creatinine concentrations were within the reference ranges and did not differ among the groups, but 24-hour creatinine clearance was significantly lower in those taking long-term lithium (73 versus 125 and 150 ml/minute). There were no significant differences among the groups in urine osmolality after 8-hour water deprivation and desmopressin, but partial nephrogenic diabetes insipidus was diagnosed in four long-term and two short-term patients and hypothalamic diabetes insipidus in two long-term patients. The authors concluded that long-term lithium therapy is a risk factor for renal impairment.

In a retrospective review of lithium concentrations in 2210 psychiatric hospital patients, 151 (6.8%) had serum lithium concentrations of 1.5 mmol/l or more. Of those with high serum concentrations, 10 (6.6%) had a raised blood urea nitrogen or serum creatinine concentration (278). In a retrospective study of 114 patients who had taken lithium for 4–30 years and 94 matched unmedicated subjects, 21% of those taking lithium had blood creatinine concentrations greater than 1.5 mg/ml [sic]; comparative figures were not given for the controls (277). Raised creatinine concentrations tended to be associated with episodes of lithium toxicity and drugs or diseases that could alter glomerular function.

Renal disease is not a contraindication to lithium, but it does complicate its use, and alternative mood stabilizers should be considered. Despite the diverse effects of lithium on the kidney, most patients find it to be generally well tolerated; nevertheless, monitoring should include periodic testing of renal function. In one case, a psychiatrist and family physician were sued for failing to monitor renal function in a patient who developed renal insufficiency (279). The distribution of monitoring guidelines in the area of Aberdeen, Scotland, led to an increase in the number of lithium patients who had at least once-yearly serum creatinine concentration measurements from 71% to 78%, still leaving 22% without adequate renal function monitoring (280).

To what extent long-term treatment with lithium impairs GFR is a matter of continued study (275). Lithium does not appear to impair GFR consistently, especially if correction is made for age-related changes in kidney function, although in one study there was an age-related reduction in 21% of 142 patients who had taken lithium for at least 15 years (281). There have been a few case reports of progressive renal insufficiency attributed to lithium, but it has not been possible to establish a cause-and-effect relation with absolute certainty.

In a review of the renal and metabolic complications of lithium, the example of a 78-year-old woman taking long-term lithium who had urinary incontinence, moderate renal insufficiency, a 5–7 litres 24-hour urine volume, and thyroid and parathyroid abnormalities was used to set the scene (221).

In a historical cohort study, changes in renal function in 86 patients taking lithium were evaluated first after a median treatment duration of 5.8 years and again after 16 years (282). Maximum plasma osmolality was reduced in nine of 63 patients in the initial study and in 24 of 63 at follow-up. Other findings included increased serum creatinine (in one of 76 patients initially and eight of 76 at follow-up) and reduced GFR (in three of 29 patients initially and six of 29 at follow-up); only the latter of these changes was not significant. The authors noted that this progressive impairment in renal dysfunction was greater than expected for age and advised strict surveillance of renal function in patients taking long-term lithium.

In a retrospective review of 6514 renal biopsies, there were 24 patients with renal insufficiency who had taken lithium for a mean duration of 13.6 years (range 2–25 years); the histological changes included chronic tubulointerstitial nephropathy (100%), cortical and medullary tubular cysts (63%) or tubular dilatation (33%), global glomerulosclerosis (100%), and focal segmental glomerulosclerosis (50%) (283). Only two had a history of acute lithium toxicity. Clinical findings included proteinuria (42%), nephrotic syndrome (25%), nephrogenic diabetes insipidus (87%), and hypertension (33%). Despite lithium withdrawal, either seven (abstract) or eight (text) of nine patients with an initial serum creatinine of over 221 μmol/l (2.5 mg/dl) progressed to end-stage renal insufficiency, whereas this occurred in only one of ten with lower creatinine concentrations. The study design was such that the risk of renal insufficiency with long-term lithium therapy could not be established and the possibility of alternative causes could not be excluded.

Two studies in rats have potential implications for humans. In rats with mild to severe lithium-induced nephropathy, urine *N*-acetyl-β-D-glucosaminidase was an early indicator of renal insufficiency (284). Both ^{6}Li and ^{7}Li caused reduced urine concentrating ability and increased urine volume and renal tubular lesions, but ^{6}Li was more nephrotoxic (285). The authors suggested that eliminating ^{6}Li from pharmaceutical products might reduce nephrotoxicity (although ^{6}Li accounts for only about 7% of the lithium in such products).

Concentrating ability

Lithium often impairs renal concentrating ability, an effect that is related in part to both dosage and duration of treatment (273,275). While it is initially reversible on withdrawal, it may eventually become irreversible and indicative of structural tubular damage. Impaired concentration is of no clinical consequence in itself, but it may go hand in hand with polyuria (lithium-induced nephrogenic diabetes insipidus), which can sometimes be a social and occupational nuisance and can increase the risk of toxicity secondary to dehydration. These problems can be minimized if the maintenance serum concentration is low, but whether single daily dosing is kinder to the kidney has yet to be resolved. Since the defect is at the level of the kidney (both before and after the site of cyclic AMP generation and probably involving the water channel protein aquaporin-2, a vasopressin-regulated water channel protein (286)), vasopressin (ADH) is unlikely to be effective. A thiazide and/or potassium-sparing diuretic (especially amiloride) can reduce the urine volume, although serum lithium concentrations can rise at the same time. Avoiding hypokalemia is essential, but whether dietary potassium supplementation can also be helpful is not known. Inositol is no longer considered promising.

In a comparison of patients taking long-term lithium ($n = 10$) or short-term lithium ($n = 9$) and bipolar patients not taking lithium ($n = 10$), there was significantly lower creatinine clearance and renal concentrating ability in the long-term group (287).

Acute and chronic renal insufficiency

Renal insufficiency was attributed to lithium in a 40-year-old who had had nontoxic concentrations for 15 years (interstitial nephropathy on biopsy) (288) and in a 55-year-old woman who had taken lithium for 6 years (serum creatinine 141 μmol/l (289). A few patients develop progressive renal insufficiency that can best be attributed to lithium (275).

Chronic renal insufficiency (creatinine clearance under 80 ml/minute), for which there was no apparent alternative explanation, developed in 53 patients taking long-term lithium (mean 17.7 years); 7 required periodic dialysis (290).

After taking lithium for 6 years, a 55-year-old woman developed mild renal insufficiency (serum creatinine 1.6 mg/dl) and lithium was withdrawn (289).

Interstitial nephritis

Lithium-associated changes in kidney morphology include an acute, reversible, and possibly lithium-specific distal tubular lesion and a chronic, nonspecific, and tubulointerstitial nephritis (291). The differential diagnosis of the latter is extensive, and it is not clear if lithium is causative. Lithium received a brief mention in a review of tubulointerstitial nephritis (291).

- A 48-year-old man taking lithium and chlorprothixene had a creatinine clearance of 60 ml/minute and a renal biopsy showing chronic interstitial nephritis (292).
- Lithium-induced interstitial nephritis (serum creatinine 2.3 mg/dl) occurred in an 89-year-old woman who had taken lithium for 29 years (81).

Nephrogenic diabetes insipidus

There have been several case reports of lithium-related nephrogenic diabetes insipidus, sometimes associated with dehydration and lithium intoxication (216,293–296).

Nephrogenic diabetes insipidus has been specifically reviewed in the context of a case in which resolution did not occur despite withdrawal of lithium (297).

Nephrogenic diabetes insipidus secondary to lithium led to severe dehydration in two patients who required intravenous rehydration followed by a thiazide diuretic to reduce urine volume (294). One patient had persistent polyuria (6.7 l/day) 57 months after stopping lithium (211).

- A 77-year-old woman who had taken lithium for 10 years developed delirium, hypernatremia, prerenal azotemia, and a serum lithium concentration of 1.4 mmol/l; her condition was attributed to dehydration related to partial nephrogenic diabetes insipidus (293).
- Eight years after stopping lithium because of polydipsia and polyuria, a 55-year-old woman was hospitalized with lethargy, coma, and hypernatremia (sodium concentration 156 mmol/l) after her fluid intake had been restricted (297).

- A 30-year-old woman who became dehydrated secondary to lithium-induced nephrogenic diabetes insipidus developed a superior sagittal sinus thrombosis (251).
- A 78-year-old woman who had taken lithium for 25 years had hypotonic polyuria (4.7 l/day), mild renal insufficiency, and hyperparathyroidism attributed to lithium (221).
- Nephrogenic diabetes insipidus resulted in dehydration and hypernatremia in a 78-year-old man who had taken lithium for 30 years (216).
- Nephrogenic diabetes insipidus in a 63-year-old woman was treated successfully with lithium withdrawal and amiloride (298).

Nephrotic syndrome

Nephrotic syndrome (proteinuria, edema, hypoalbuminemia, hyperlipidemia) is a rare and idiosyncratic complication of lithium therapy; it usually resolves on withdrawal, and can recur on rechallenge (299,300). Lithium-associated nephrotic syndrome occurred in a 59-year-old woman with lithium toxicity (serum concentration 1.9 mmol/l) whose renal biopsy showed focal segmental glomerulosclerosis. Lithium withdrawal led to resolution of edema and marked improvement in proteinuria and albuminemia (300).

- An 83-year-old man developed nephrotic syndrome while taking lithium (301).
- An 11-year-old boy who had taken lithium for an unstated duration developed nephrotic syndrome with focal glomerulosclerosis which remitted fully after lithium was withdrawn (299).
- A 59-year-old woman with lithium-associated nephrotic syndrome (focal segmental glomerulosclerosis on biopsy) had resolution of edema and pleural effusions and marked improvement in albuminemia and proteinuria after withdrawal of lithium (300).

Renal tubular acidosis

Incomplete distal renal tubular acidosis has been attributed to lithium, but appears to be of no clinical significance (302).

Skin

In a review of skin reactions to mood stabilizers, a wide variety of reactions attributed to lithium were mentioned, but the authors did not critically evaluate the data on which the reports had been based (303).

In a review of acute skin reactions to psychotropic drugs, alopecia, psoriasiform, acneiform, and lichenoid eruptions, and drug-induced lupus were attributed to lithium, but critical comment was not provided (304).

There have been anecdotal reports of papular and nonpapular rashes, pityriasis versicolor, hidradenitis suppurativa, and nail dystrophy (305,306), although causal relations are difficult to establish.

In a review of lichenoid drug eruptions, lithium was implicated in one patient with ulcerative oral lesions and in another with ulcerative genital lesions (307).

- A 60-year-old man developed systemic swelling, redness, and pruritus 1 month after starting to take lithium; it was attributed to the drug based on positive patch and challenge tests (308).
- A 55-year-old man who had taken lithium and haloperidol for 11 years developed hyperkeratotic follicular papules on his scalp, extremities, and trunk, which on biopsy were suggestive of follicular mycoses fungoides (309). He also had a 1-year history of scalp, axillary, and pubic hair loss. Following replacement of lithium with valproate, his hair regrew and the papules cleared almost completely in 3 months.

A man and a woman developed vegetating plaques with peripheral pustules (halogenoderma) after taking lithium for 6 and 8 years respectively (310). No follow-up information was provided and it could not be established whether the lesions were caused by, worsened by, or unrelated to lithium.

Acne

Acne can occur or worsen during lithium treatment (311). In a comparison of 51 patients taking lithium with 57 patients taking other psychotropic drugs, there were secondary skin reactions in 45% of the former and 25 of the latter; while acne (33 versus 9%) and psoriasis (6 versus 0%) were more common in the lithium group, the only statistically significant association was acne in males (312).

- Six months after beginning lithium, a man in his late twenties developed severe truncal acne which worsened over 5 years, at which time lithium was withdrawn (313). Nevertheless, the lesions were still present 4 years later, leading to the conclusion that lithium had caused irreversible acne.

In this case, the association could have been coincidental.

Alopecia

Hair loss in psychopharmacology has been reviewed (314). It appears to be an uncommon and unpredictable adverse effect of lithium. Hypothyroidism is occasionally involved. Hair texture can also be altered (315).

- A 36-year-old woman had taken lithium for 4 months when her scalp hair became thinner and stopped growing. She continued to take lithium, and 2 months later was diagnosed and treated for hypothyroidism, after which her hair became curlier but did not grow longer or fuller.

Darier's disease

Darier's disease (follicular keratosis) can be exacerbated by lithium (316,317).

- In a woman who had had keratosis follicularis (Darier's disease) since she was 16, the condition worsened when she was given lithium at age 50 (and improved when she switched to valproate) (317).

However, despite reports that Darier's disease is worsened by lithium, a 52-year-old man noted no exacerbation despite taking lithium for many years (318).

Psoriasis

Psoriasis can occur or worsen during lithium treatment (311). Before psoriasis can be treated effectively, lithium may have to be withdrawn. In a comparison of 51 patients taking lithium with 57 patients taking other psychotropic drugs, there were secondary skin reactions in 45% of the former and 25% of the latter; while acne (33 versus 9%) and psoriasis (6 versus 0%) were more common in the lithium group, the only statistically significant association was acne in males (312).

- A 42-year-old woman taking lithium developed psoriasis which resolved when the drug was withdrawn (319). Brief mention was made of two patients (age and sex unstated) taking lithium whose psoriasis improved with oral omega-3 fatty acids (320).
- Lithium worsened psoriasis in a 54-year-old woman; improvement followed withdrawal (321).

Hair, nails, sweat glands

Hair loss in psychopharmacology has been reviewed (314). It appears to be an uncommon and unpredictable adverse effect of lithium. Hypothyroidism is occasionally involved. Hair texture can also be altered (315).

- A 36-year-old woman had taken lithium for 4 months when her scalp hair became thinner and stopped growing. She continued to take lithium, and 2 months later was diagnosed and treated for hypothyroidism, after which her hair became curlier but did not grow longer or fuller.

Musculoskeletal

Despite lithium-induced increases in serum calcium and PTH concentrations, most recent studies have not shown a reduction in bone mineral density or increased risks of osteoporosis or bone fractures (322). In 26 patients who had taken lithium for at least 10 years, bone mineral density did not differ from controls (323).

A patient with a diffuse sensorimotor peripheral neuropathy also developed rhabdomyolysis during the acute episode in association with a serum lithium concentration of 3.1 mmol/l and a serum sodium of 163 mmol/l (114).

Sexual function

Despite occasional reports of reduced libido and erectile dysfunction, lithium causes little in the way of sexual dysfunction in men or women (324). In a brief review of the sexual adverse effects of psychotropic drugs, reduced libido and arousal with lithium were mentioned in passing, particularly when it was combined with other drugs (which, of course, makes it difficult to implicate lithium) (325).

Reproductive system

In a cross-sectional pilot study of 22 bipolar women taking lithium ($n = 10$), divalproex ($n = 10$), or both ($n = 10$), there was an increased number of ovarian follicles in one woman taking lithium, but no evidence of hormonal changes suggestive of polycystic ovary syndrome in any patient (326). The small sample size was a limiting factor.

When 22 women with bipolar disorder (10 taking lithium alone, 10 taking divalproex alone, and 2 taking both) were evaluated for polycystic ovary syndrome, none had typical hormonal screening abnormalities (326). Some type of menstrual dysfunction was present in all ten women taking lithium alone, but it predated use of the drug in all but one.

Compared with 13 women taking placebo, 10 women taking lithium carbonate 900 mg/day for one menstrual cycle had no significant alterations in reproductive hormone concentrations (327).

In an in vitro study, LY294002, a phosphatidylinositol-3-kinase inhibitor, overcame impaired human sperm motility induced by lithium chloride (328).

At blood concentrations within the human target range, oral lithium caused degenerative changes in testicular morphology in spotted munia (*Lonchura punctulata*), a seasonally breeding subtropical finch (329). Lithium at a serum concentration of about 0.6 mmol/l reduced sperm motility, number, and viability, and markedly altered testicular histopathology in *Viscacha*, a nocturnal rodent from the pampas of Argentina (330). How these findings might relate to effects in men is open to question.

Immunologic

Lithium is not an allergen. Allergic reactions that have been reported in patients taking lithium have been attributed to excipients in the formulation (331), as in a case of leukocytoclastic vasculitis (332).

In a brief report, evidence has been presented that short-term exposure to lithium (less than 2 months) caused alterations in the expression of histocompatibility antigens (333).

In 10 healthy volunteers, lithium caused increases in interleukin-4 and interleukin-10 concentrations and falls in interleukin-2 and interferon concentrations (334). In in vitro studies of monocytes from women with breast cancer, lithium chloride suppressed production of interleukin-8 and induced production of interleukin-15 (335,336). The clinical implications of these findings are unclear.

The immunomodulatory effects of lithium have been reviewed (337,338). Lithium

(a) stimulated the production of pro-inflammatory cytokines and negative immunoregulatory cytokines or proteins in nine healthy subjects (339);
(b) altered the expression of human leukocyte antigens (HLA) in 11 of 15 subjects (333);
(c) normalized manifestations of mild immune activation in 17 rapid cycling bipolar patients (340).

The clinical implications of these findings are unclear.

The very complex antiviral and immunomodulatory effects of lithium have been reviewed (341). In 15 inpatients, lithium produced changes in a number of histocompatibility antigens, but whether these have any clinical implications is unknown (342).

Death

The 1997 Annual Report of the American Association of Poison Control Centers Toxic Exposure Surveillance System listed nine lithium-associated deaths and provided some clinical details in seven cases, including serum concentrations of 2.4–7.8 mmol/l (343).

Long-Term Effects

Drug abuse

Lithium is not a drug of abuse or dependence, although when one bipolar alcohol abuser was prevented from drinking, he tried to get a "buzz" by increasing his lithium dose to the point of toxicity (serum concentration 3.0 mmol/l) (344). The only other suggestion of abuse appeared in 1977 when passing mention to the "fairly recent (over the past 2 years or so) abuse of lithium" by poly-drug abusers (345).

Drug tolerance

In a review of whether the prophylactic efficacy of lithium was transient or persistent, the authors concluded that "the balance of evidence does not indicate a general loss of lithium efficacy" (346). A similar conclusion was reached in a study of 22 patients who had taken lithium for at least 20 years (347). There was no change in affective morbidity over the second 10 years compared with the first 10 years. However, individual exceptions could not be excluded.

Drug withdrawal

Three issues have been addressed:

(a) does rapid withdrawal increase recurrence risk?
(b) how common is post-withdrawal refractoriness to the reinstitution of lithium?
(c) does withdrawal increase the risk of thyrotoxicosis?

Recurrence risk

Abrupt or rapid withdrawal of lithium is not associated with a physical withdrawal reaction, but there does appear to be an increased risk of early recurrence of mania and depression compared with more gradual withdrawal (348,349), although this conclusion has been questioned (350). Data from Italy have suggested that gradual withdrawal of lithium (over 15–30 days) was associated with a markedly reduced risk of early recurrence of mania and depression and a much greater likelihood of prolonged stability compared with rapid discontinuation (over 1–14 days) (348). There was a marked increase in suicidal acts during the first year after lithium withdrawal; after that the risk returned to what it had been before the start of lithium treatment. The increased risk in the first year exceeded that expected from increased affective morbidity alone. There was a 1.95-fold greater risk, during this first year in those who discontinued lithium rapidly, although this was not statistically significant (351).

Of 30 patients with major depressive disorder who had responded to lithium augmentation for antidepressant-resistant depression, 15 were switched to placebo over 1–7 days (352). Two became manic, and it was suggested that lithium withdrawal may have uncovered latent bipolar disorder (353).

When 21 elderly patients with a major depressive episode who had responded to lithium augmentation had lithium withdrawn gradually (over 2–12 weeks), 9 relapsed but none became manic (354). Whether gradual withdrawal protected against withdrawal mania or whether there were no latent bipolar patients in the study is unknown.

A retrospective study of lithium withdrawal in pregnant and nonpregnant women showed similar rates and times of recurrence, including a higher risk of early occurrence with rapid withdrawal (1–14 days) versus gradual withdrawal (15–30 days) (355). How to balance the first trimester fetal risk of greater lithium exposure during gradual withdrawal with the greater maternal risk of potentially devastating relapse after rapid withdrawal remains a challenge.

There is a higher risk of postpartum recurrence of bipolar disorder in women who have discontinued lithium; the protective effect of restarting lithium late in pregnancy or soon after delivery has been emphasized (355).

The observation that rapid or abrupt lithium withdrawal might be associated with a more immediate or higher likelihood of recurrence has gathered further support from a reanalysis of data from a double-blind lithium maintenance study, in which the benefits of low serum concentrations (0.4–0.6 mmol/l) and standard serum concentrations (0.8–1.0 mmol/l) were compared (356). Recurrence rates were greater only in those whose concentrations were abruptly reduced from standard to low at the start of the study. The authors suggested that rapid dosage reduction, rather than a low maintenance concentration itself, accounted for their initial conclusion that standard concentrations were more effective than low concentrations.

Others have concluded that withdrawal mania is "a major and sinister complication of the everyday use of lithium" (357). Withdrawal of effective lithium therapy was associated with an increased risk of suicide and suicidal acts, especially during the first 12 months. Gradual withdrawal (over 15–30 days) was associated with half the rate of suicidal acts compared with more rapid withdrawal (strong trend toward statistical significance) (358).

Refractoriness to retreatment

In 28 patients who had responded to lithium treatment of mania or schizoaffective mania and who had recurrences after withdrawal, there were equally good responses to retreatment with lithium (359). These findings add to the evidence that lithium discontinuation-induced refractoriness is the exception rather than the rule. However, the issue of whether post-withdrawal refractoriness to reintroduction of lithium is a real phenomenon and, if so, how often it occurs continues to be debated (360). Three patients failed to respond to the reintroduction of lithium, despite having had sustained beneficial responses before withdrawal (361).

Risk of thyrotoxicosis

Lithium withdrawal may be associated with an outpouring of thyroid hormone in predisposed individuals; there have been reports of thyrotoxicosis (192) and a thyrotoxic crisis (192) after lithium withdrawal.

- A 37-year-old man who had taken lithium and sulpiride for 14 years and who was a long-time smoker without respiratory symptoms or a history of asthma had lithium withdrawn because of an asymptomatic bradycardia (44 beats/minute) (70). Six weeks later, he developed symptoms of asthma, including nocturnal cough, exertional wheezing, increased airway resistance, and a low FEV1, attributed to lithium withdrawal.

Mutagenicity

In 18 patients taking benzodiazepines and/or neuroleptic drugs, there were increased chromosomal aberrations and increased sister chromatid exchange, but there were no significant differences between this group and another group of 18 patients taking lithium in addition to benzodiazepines and/or antipsychotic drugs (362).

Tumorigenicity

There is no evidence that lithium causes or promotes the growth of tumors. Since tumors are not rare events over a lifetime, and since lithium is taken for long periods of time, any apparent association is likely to be coincidental.

Second-Generation Effects

Fertility

Intramuscular lithium chloride produced subtherapeutic blood concentrations (by human standards) in male rose-ringed parakeets, but significantly reduced testicular weight and caused widespread degenerative changes in the testes (363). Fertility was not assessed directly.

Pregnancy

The treatment of bipolar disorder during pregnancy and lactation has been reviewed, with reference to lithium-related maternal, fetal, and neonatal toxicity, morphological and behavioral teratogenicity, carcinogenicity and mutagenicity, and miscellaneous effects (364–376). Elsewhere, the effects of lithium, valproic acid, and carbamazepine during pregnancy (377) and drug-induced congenital defects (with only a brief mention of lithium) (378) have been reviewed. A more specific review dealing with the use of drugs during pregnancy in women with renal disease mentioned the need for lithium-dosage reduction in such cases (379).

Pregnancy in bipolar women was found to be a "risk-neutral" condition, in that it neither protected against nor increased episode risk in a comparison of 42 pregnant with 42 nonpregnant women who stopped lithium either rapidly (over 1–14 days) or gradually (over 15–30 days). Stopping lithium was not "risk-neutral," and the risk was especially high in those who stopped rapidly (380) (see also Withdrawal effects). These observations must be balanced against the low but real risk of teratogenesis from first trimester lithium exposure (381).

- A 37-year-old woman with severe bipolar disorder, who continued to take lithium throughout pregnancy, had a normal delivery (382).

Teratogenicity

While there is an increased risk of teratogenesis (particularly cardiovascular) from exposure to lithium in the first trimester, this risk has been overstated initially because of selection bias (380,381,383,384). Subsequently, case-control and cohort studies have substantially reduced, but not eliminated, such concerns (385). The risk of major malformations from exposure to lithium in the first trimester appears to be lower than from exposure to carbamazepine or valproate.

The teratogenic effects of lithium have been reviewed in several articles (364,365,386); two reviews of drug-related congenital malformation briefly mentioned lithium and cardiovascular teratogenesis (378,387). The authors concluded that while the risk of cardiovascular malformation is lower than once believed, it is nevertheless increased.

The cardiovascular teratogenicity of lithium has been summarized in a review of managing bipolar disorder during pregnancy and postpartum (371). While the risk of Ebstein's anomaly is increased, likely 10–20 times more than in the general population, the absolute risk (0.05–0.10%) is small. Fetal ultrasonography was advised at 18–20 weeks of gestation in cases of first trimester lithium exposure (386).

In a review of all pregnancies in Leiden in The Netherlands between 1994 and 2002, none of the 20 children of mothers who had taken lithium had major problems or congenital anomalies (388).

There is no evidence that children exposed to lithium during pregnancy who are born without malformations develop other than normally.

Fetotoxicity

Hypoglycemia, requiring temporary glucagon and glucose supplementation, was noted in a neonate whose mother had taken lithium throughout pregnancy (cord lithium concentration 1.73 mmol/l) (370).

Reports of fetal goiter and a variety of other lithium-related adverse events in newborns have been reviewed (386).

In 20 infants exposed to lithium during labor and delivery, there were higher rates of perinatal complications (65%) and special care nursery admissions (45%) than in nonexposed infants, although most complications were transient (389). An infant who died shortly after birth had oromandibular-limb hypogenesis spectrum which was speculatively attributed to lithium that the mother had taken during most of her pregnancy (390).

A neonate whose mother had taken lithium throughout pregnancy developed a supraventricular tachycardia (240/minute) which was treated successfully with adenosine (391). Another newborn girl exposed to lithium in utero had asymptomatic cardiomegaly that resolved by 1 month of age (226).

Transient polyuria in two newborns was attributed to the lithium their mothers had taken throughout pregnancy (370,391).

Neonates born to mothers taking lithium included a boy with a goiter and chemical hypothyroidism who required temporary treatment with oral thyroxine for 11 weeks (392), a girl with respiratory distress, cardiomegaly, hyperbilirubinemia, nephrogenic diabetes insipidus, and hypoglycemia who responded to various treatments and eventually remitted fully (370), and a preterm infant with a supraventricular tachycardia and temporary polyuria associated with 20% weight loss (391). The mother of the preterm infant developed polyhydramnios during pregnancy, which was attributed to lithium-induced fetal polyuria.

Lactation

Lithium concentrations in breast milk are about 40% of maternal serum concentrations, although the range is wide (369,393,394). Because of this, breastfeeding is often discouraged (394), although the authors of a comprehensive review of the use of mood stabilizers during breastfeeding have pointed out that there is a paucity of information to support adverse effects of lithium in breastfeeding infants—one case of toxicity in a 2-month-old with an intercurrent infection (serum lithium 1.4 mmol/l) and one report of lethargy and cyanosis at days 5 and 6 (infant serum concentration 0.6 mmol/l on day 5) secondary to fetal and breast milk exposure. However, there have been only two reports of lithium toxicity attributed to breastfeeding (395,396). Others, however, have stated that "lithium should only be used with great caution ..." (397); "[breastfeeding by women taking lithium] has been repeatedly discouraged in the literature" (398); "... it also seems unwise to expose infants unnecessarily to lithium" (394). Lithium has also been stated to be "an excellent example of a drug that requires monitoring and case-by-case assessment so that nursing mothers can be successfully treated" (393).

In a review of the use of psychotropic drugs during breastfeeding, it was briefly mentioned that lithium was not advisable, but was justified under certain circumstances (399). Lithium was also briefly discussed in a review of xenobiotics and breastfeeding (400).

Breast-milk lithium concentrations were measured in 11 women taking lithium carbonate 600–1,500 mg/day (401). Maternal serum concentrations were available in only three and infant concentrations in two. No infants had adverse effects that could be attributed to lithium, and the authors calculated that infant lithium exposure was low, leading them to challenge the general contraindication to breastfeeding under such circumstances.

In its 2001 Policy Statement, the American Academy of Pediatrics Committee on Drugs modified its earlier contraindication to lithium during breastfeeding by listing it with "drugs that have been associated with significant effects on some nursing infants, and should be given to nursing mothers with caution" (402).

The Motherisk Team in Toronto has recommended use of the Exposure Index (the maternal milk/plasma ratio times 100 divided by the infants' clearance in ml/kg/minute) to determine the advisability of breastfeeding when a mother is taking lithium (396). However, this approach does not seem very practical.

Given the extremely high risk of postpartum recurrence in bipolar patients, the issue is not whether the mother should take a mood stabilizer (she should), but whether the baby should be breastfed. A review of mood stabilizers during breastfeeding reaffirmed that there are only two reported cases of infant lithium toxicity associated with breastfeeding (one of which involved both fetal and breast milk exposure) (395). The following recommendations were made in the case of a mother taking lithium who chooses to breastfeed:

(a) educate her about the manifestations of toxicity;
(b) explain the risks of dehydration;
(c) consider partial or total formula supplements during episodes of illness or dehydration;
(d) suspend breastfeeding if toxicity is suspected;
(e) check infant and maternal serum lithium concentrations.

Susceptibility Factors

Age

Whether elderly patients taking lithium received proper monitoring was questioned in a case note audit of 91 patients, over 40% of whom had deviations from practice standards. These included absence of pretreatment laboratory tests, infrequent monitoring of serum lithium concentrations, lack of adequate adverse effects documentation, and the use of risky concomitant drugs (403). In a placebo-controlled study, there was poor tolerance of lithium augmentation of antidepressants in 76% (13/17) of elderly (mean age 70 years) patients at a mean serum concentration of 0.63 mmol/l, due to tremor and muscle twitches, cognitive disturbance, tiredness and sedation, and gastrointestinal upsets (404).

In a cross-sectional study of 12 octogenarians (average age 84 years) who had taken lithium for an average of 54 months (mean serum concentration 0.42 mmol/l), none became toxic and none had to stop treatment because of adverse effects. Transient renal function abnormalities were noted: one patient developed nephrogenic diabetes insipidus and one became hypothyroidic (405). For lithium therapy in very old people, the authors advised close monitoring in a specialized setting.

Renal disease

While there are no absolute contraindications to lithium, patients with advanced kidney disease or unstable fluid/electrolyte balance may be more safely treated with an alternative mood stabilizer, such as carbamazepine, valproate, lamotrigine, or olanzapine.

Other features of the patient

Factors that put patients at risk of lithium intoxication are those that increase intake (deliberately or accidentally), reduce excretion (kidney disease, dehydration, low sodium intake, drug interactions), or reduce body water (dehydration secondary to fluid restriction, vomiting, diarrhea, or polyuria) (45). Patients with lithium-induced polyuria are at a particular risk of toxicity if their ability to replace fluids is compromised (for example by anesthesia, over-sedation, CNS trauma).

Thyrotoxicosis was considered a possible contributor to lithium toxicity in two patients, possibly by increasing tubular lithium reabsorption through induction of the sodium-hydrogen antiporter (195).

Two patients developed lithium intoxication (serum concentrations 3.3 and 3.0 mmol/l) in association with poorly controlled diabetes mellitus, suggesting that the latter is a risk factor (227).

A review of the effects of obesity on drug pharmacokinetics briefly mentioned that the steady-state volume of distribution of lithium correlated with ideal body weight and fat-free mass but not with total body weight (406). Lithium clearance was greater in those with obesity than in lean controls, suggesting that obese patients may require larger maintenance doses to maintain target serum concentrations.

Drug Administration

Drug formulations

Despite the availability of modified-release lithium formulations for several decades, there continues to be a paucity of information about their efficacy and tolerability compared with less expensive immediate-release formulations (407).

Brain lithium concentrations (measured by magnetic resonance spectroscopy) after the use of a modified-release formulation (Lithobid SR) or an immediate-release formulation have been compared in a crossover design in 12 patients with bipolar disorder (408). There were higher brain concentrations with the modified-release formulation, but whether this has clinical implications requires further study.

Formulations of lithium carbonate tablets with various binding substances have been discussed (409).

A modified-release formulation (Carbolithium Once-A-Day) produced a reduction in peak/trough lithium ratio compared with a standard formulation (410), and an interim analysis of an open switch to the modified-release formulation suggested better tolerability and efficacy at 4 weeks ($n = 27$) and 6 weeks ($n = 15$) (411). A paucity of detail, however, prevents firm conclusions.

A modified-release multi-particulate lithium capsule has been described consisting of five copolymer-coated prolonged-release tablets and one standard tablet, each 6 mm in size (412).

Following an overdose with a sustained-release formulation (8,000 mg of Teralithe 400 LP), the appearance of clinical symptoms (vomiting and dizziness) was delayed for 35 hours, despite a serum lithium concentration of 2.38 mmol/l at 15 hours and 3.12 mmol/l at 25 hours (413).

A woman taking conventional lithium developed lithium toxicity after two doses of a homeopathic formulation, "Lithium carb. 30"; a paucity of detail allows no conclusions to be drawn from this observation (414).

Drug additives

Gelatin is derived from natural pork and beef products and is present in some lithium formulations. Since certain religions forbid the consumption of gelatin, knowing that it is present in Eskalith capsules and Eskalith CR and absent in Eskalith tablets (not available in the USA) and Lithobid SR might influence prescribing practices under certain circumstances (415). The same would apply to other lithium products.

Drug dosage regimens

In an open-label pilot study of rapid administration of slow-release lithium (20 mg/kg/day in two divided doses) for acute mania, five of 15 patients completed 10 days of treatment, seven improved sooner and were discharged, two withdrew because of adverse effects (bradycardia in one and tremor, fatigue, and diarrhea in the other; and one patient appears not to have been accounted for) two other patients also had asymptomatic bradycardia (74).

A review of loading strategies in acute mania included a section on lithium (416).

A small study of brain lithium concentrations measured by magnetic resonance spectroscopy showed higher brain:serum lithium concentration ratios in subjects taking a single daily dose ($n = 5$) than in those taking a twice-daily regimen ($n = 3$) (417). Even to speculate about the possible clinical implications of this finding would be premature.

Drug administration route

Intravenous

To determine the safety of using lithium chloride dilution to measure cardiac output, the pharmacokinetic and toxic effects of intravenous lithium chloride have been studied in six conscious healthy Standardbred horses (418). The mean peak serum concentration was 0.56 mmol/l. There were neither toxic effects nor significant changes in laboratory studies, electrocardiograms, or gastrointestinal motility. Three horses had increased urine output.

A similar study was performed in patients undergoing cardiac surgery and healthy volunteers; the highest dose of lithium chloride was 0.6 mmol given intravenously five times at 2-minute intervals (419). Unfortunately, no mention was made of tolerability or adverse effects.

When 10 volunteers were given 500 ml of a 0.1% lithium carbonate solution (13.5 mmol of lithium) intravenously over 1 hour, the peak serum concentration was 0.93 mmol/l, the elimination half-life was 7.8 hours, and there were no adverse effects (420).

Drug overdose

There are three forms of lithium overdose:

(a) acute (abrupt overdose in a drug-naïve person);
(b) chronic (gradual accumulation, reaching toxic concentrations);
(c) acute-on-chronic (abrupt overdose by a person already taking lithium), which can also be due to a drug interaction.

Thus, the term overdose (57,421,422) can be misleading, because poisoning can develop not only as a result of overdosage but also by a fall in lithium clearance. Of 205 cases of lithium poisoning reported to the Ontario Canada Regional Poison Information Centre in 1996, 12 were acute overdoses (someone else's tablets), 19 were chronic poisonings, and 174 were acute-on-chronic poisonings. Over 80% had no or minimal symptoms, two patients died, and one had persistent renal sequelae (423). A retrospective study of 97 cases of lithium poisoning treated at a regional center in Australia over 13 years found severe neurotoxicity in 28 cases (26 were cases of chronic and two of acute-on-chronic poisonings) (215). Risk factors were nephrogenic diabetes insipidus, older age, abnormal thyroid function, and impaired renal function.

Early signs of intoxication include ataxia, dysarthria, coarse tremor, weakness, and drowsiness. More advanced toxicity can involve progressively impaired consciousness, neuromuscular irritability (myoclonic jerks), seizures, cardiac dysrhythmias, and renal insufficiency. A reversible Creutzfeldt–Jakob-like syndrome has been described (103). The severity of intoxication depends on both the extent and duration of exposure to raised lithium concentrations, as well as idiosyncratic factors.

When the Marseilles Poisons Centre analysed information on lithium overdose between 1991 and 2000, in addition to an unspecified number of suicide attempts and accidental poisonings in children, the next most frequent reports were prescription misinterpretation ($n = 43$), dehydration in the elderly ($n = 35$), renal insufficiency ($n = 15$), and diuretic interactions ($n = 8$) (424).

The 2000 Annual Report of the American Association of Poison Control Centers Toxic Exposure Surveillance System listed six lithium-related deaths (four cases of intentional suicide and two of therapeutic error) and two other deaths in which lithium was not listed as the primary cause (425). A total of 4663 lithium-related exposures were reported, in which death was the outcome in 13 and a major life-threatening event or cause of significant disability in 267.

A chart review of psychiatric hospital admissions between 1990 and 1996 showed that 6.8% of 2210 patients who were given lithium had at least one serum concentration of 1.5 mmol/l or over (43% of these were increased at admission) and of those only 28% had signs and symptoms of toxicity (278).

In another case, following an overdose with a modified-release formulation, the appearance of clinical symptoms (vomiting and dizziness) was delayed for 35 hours, despite a serum lithium concentration of 2.38 mmol/l at 15 hours and 3.12 mmol/l at 25 hours (413).

The distribution of clinical practice guidelines in Northeast Scotland had no impact on whether appropriate action was taken for high serum lithium concentrations (80% before the guidelines, 82% after). There was no significant difference in proper attention to high concentrations between those in primary care alone (77%) and those in shared care (85%) (280).

In a retrospective study of 114 patients admitted to a toxicological ICU with suspected lithium intoxication, 81 had definite intoxication; 78% were deliberate overdoses, and 22% were accidental (due, for example, to renal insufficiency, dehydration, drug interactions, poor compliance, drunkenness). Most were treated conservatively with gastric lavage and forced diuresis; hemodialysis was used only in 3–6%. Two of those who took a deliberate overdose and one of those who took an accidental overdose died (426).

Cases of lithium toxicity in a municipal hospital over a 10-year period involved eight women (mean age 66 years); neurological symptoms were the most common presentations (92). Two were acute overdoses and the rest were chronic intoxications. There was one death (group not specified).

Convincing manifestations of toxicity have occasionally been reported in patients with concentrations within the preferred target range (sometimes called "therapeutic" concentrations) (427). While full recovery is often the case, improvement may lag many days behind the fall in serum lithium concentration. Unfortunately, both persistent neurological damage (characteristically cerebellar) and deaths have occurred. The risk of an adverse outcome from toxicity can be minimized by prompt and comprehensive treatment (428–430), which should include gastric lavage and ion exchange resins for acute overdose, volume expansion to restore fluid and electrolyte balance and improve kidney function, and in severe cases, hemodialysis. Hemodiafiltration has also been used, and while this technique eliminates rebound increases in lithium concentration after dialysis, it is also less efficient than hemodialysis.

The 1998 Annual Report of the American Association of Poison Control Centers Toxic Exposure Surveillance System listed three lithium-related fatal exposures (two intentional and one a therapeutic error) and three other fatalities in which lithium was not the primary cause of death. A total of 4486 lithium-related poison exposure cases were reported, in which the outcome was death in five and a major life-threatening event or cause-significant residual disability in 212 (431).

A study of drug intoxication in the south of Brazil reported 2938 cases of drug ingestion, 25 of which involved lithium (including 14 suicide attempts) (432).

Of 133 patients 40 who had begun treatment with lithium died over an observation period of 16 years. Suicide (in 11 cases) was twice as common as in the general population, but it was more likely to occur in lithium noncompliant patients (433). It is important to be aware that suicidal behavior is actually reduced in patients who are compliant with long-term lithium therapy (although still somewhat higher than in the general population).

The 2001 Annual Report of the American Association of Poison Control Centers Toxic Exposure Surveillance System included six fatal exposures to lithium, three of which were intentional suicides. A total of 4607 exposures to lithium were reported, and death was the outcome in eight (434). A retrospective review of eight cases of lithium poisoning included one death (92).

Other reports include the following:

- A 71-year-old woman developed lithium toxicity (serum concentration 2.1 mmol/l) because of increased absorption of urinary lithium from the bowel following urinary diversion with ileal conduits for stress incontinence (435).
- A 29-year-old man who overdosed on 8,000 mg of a sustained-release lithium formulation had a serum concentration of 3.12 mmol/l 25 hours later, but only became symptomatic (with vomiting and dizziness) 35 hours later; his symptoms resolved with hemodialysis (413).
- A 72-year-old woman developed an acute confusional state, gait instability, and blepharospasm and apraxia of eyelid opening (24 hours serum concentration 1.8 mmol/l), which resolved after withdrawal (436).
- In the presence of high lithium concentrations (2.6 and 1.6 mmol/l), two patients had high amplitude of the primary complex in median nerve somatosensory evoked potentials, which normalized as concentrations fell (437).
- Two women with lithium toxicity and stormy clinical courses were found to be hyperthyroid (195).
- A 32-month-old boy developed lithium toxicity after ingesting a relative's tablets (438).
- A 46-year-old man became toxic after an initially unrecognized pontine hemorrhage (439).
- A 39-year-old woman took an overdose of lithium tablets, was given a single dose of haloperidol, and developed neuroleptic malignant syndrome (131).
- A 62-year-old woman developed persistent cerebellar and extrapyramidal sequelae at a serum concentration of 3.61 mmol/l (107).

Management

An all too common treatment error in the face of severe toxicity is "watchful waiting," during which the patient's condition is more likely to worsen than improve.

Hemodialysis (295,440,441), sometimes with additional continuous venovenous hemofiltration dialysis (442,443), continues to be described as a successful intervention for lithium poisoning. Peritoneal dialysis is a far less efficient way to clear lithium from the body. One patient treated in this way had permanent neurological abnormalities and another died; a third toxic patient who also had diabetic ketoacidosis died after treatment with hydration and insulin (444). On the other hand, a 51-year-old woman who took 50 slow-release lithium carbonate tablets (450 mg) had a serum lithium concentration of 10.6 mmol/l 13 hours later, but no evidence of neurotoxicity or nephrotoxicity. She was treated conservatively with intravenous fluids and recovered fully (445). Acute lithium overdose is often better tolerated than chronic intoxication.

Several reports have described severe poisoning responding to treatment that included hemodialysis or hemodiafiltration:

- A 57-year-old man, serum lithium concentration 3.1 mmol/l (446).
- A 52-year-old woman, serum lithium concentration 3.2 mmol/l (446).
- A 58-year-old woman, serum lithium concentration 4.0 mmol/l (76).
- A 52-year-old man, serum lithium concentration 4.6 mmol/l (77).
- A 40-year-old man, serum lithium concentration 5.4 mmol/l (447).
- A 39-year-old man, serum lithium concentration 5.9 mmol/l, with renal insufficiency associated with a polydrug overdose (448).

Some patients recovered from severe intoxication without dialysis:

- A 24-year-old woman, who survived a lithium carbonate overdose (5600 mg; serum concentration 4.0 mmol/l) with conservative treatment (449).
- A 55-year-old woman, serum lithium concentration 4.5 mmol/l, who was left with residual slurred speech (450).
- A 52-year-old woman, serum lithium concentration 10.6 mmol/l after an acute overdose (445).

In a small number of patients for whom hemodialysis was recommended, the outcomes were similar in those who were actually dialysed and those who were not, leading the authors to conclude that dialysis should be reserved for the more severe cases (451).

- Two teenagers with neurological toxicity (serum concentrations 5.4 mmol/l and 4.81 mmol/l) were treated successfully with hemodialysis followed by continuous venovenous hemofiltration, which prevented a post-dialysis rebound in serum lithium concentrations (442).
- An agitated, confused, disoriented 52-year-old woman who took an overdose of lithium recovered fully after high-volume continuous venovenous hemofiltration (452).

In an in vitro study, bentonite was an effective adsorbent of lithium; the authors suggested that it be explored as an overdose treatment (450).

Product monographs written by pharmaceutical companies and published by the Canadian Pharmacists Association in the Compendium of Pharmaceutical Specialties have been reviewed with regard to the adequacy of lithium overdose management advice (453). All five were rated "fair" for listing essential interventions for managing overdose but "poor" for warning against contraindicated interventions, and all contained misleading or dangerous information. All in all, a dismal showing.

Drug–Drug Interactions

General

Drug interactions with lithium have been reviewed (454–458); another review focused on interactions in the elderly (458). A review of drug interactions with lithium considered both pharmacokinetic interactions [for example diuretics, nonsteroidal anti-inflammatory drugs (NSAIDs)] and pharmacodynamic interactions (for example antipsychotic drugs, SSRIs) and summarized the most important ones in tabular form (454).

Alcohol

Excessive use of alcohol can interfere with adherence to lithium therapy. Alcohol does not itself appear to alter lithium pharmacokinetics (459).

Anesthetics

Sinus bradycardia (36/minute) developed in a 44-year-old woman taking lithium who received fentanyl and propofol (65).

Angiotensin converting enzyme (ACE) inhibitors

There have been scattered reports of lithium toxicity associated with the use of ACE inhibitors and attributed to reduced lithium excretion (458,460). This is not a predictable interaction.

- A 57-year-old man developed confusion, lethargy, ataxia, and myoclonus in conjunction with a serum lithium concentration of 2.6 mmol/l 4 days after starting to take captopril 50 mg tds (460).

In rats, ramipril reduced renal lithium clearance and increased fractional lithium reabsorption in association with decreased systolic blood pressure and decreased sodium excretion. These effects were attenuated by icatibant, a specific bradykinin B2 receptor antagonist (461).

Angiotensin-2 receptor antagonists

There have been occasional reports of lithium toxicity in patients taking angiotensin receptor blockers.

- A 58-year-old bipolar woman with previously stable therapeutic lithium concentrations was hospitalized with a 10-day history of confusion, disorientation, and agitation 8 weeks after starting to take candesartan 16 mg/day. Both drugs were withdrawn, the serum

lithium concentration fell from a high of 3.25 mmol/l, and she was again maintained on her usual therapeutic concentration of lithium (462).
- Lithium toxicity occurred in an elderly patient after the addition of losartan (463).
- A 51-year-old woman developed symptoms of lithium toxicity (serum concentration 1.4 mmol/l) while taking valsartan, which resolved when the valsartan was replaced by diltiazem (serum lithium concentration 0.8 mmol/l) (464).

Anticonvulsants

The combination of lithium with an anticonvulsant mood stabilizer can be beneficial. There have been reports of lithium/carbamazepine neurotoxicity, but on the other hand, lithium can benefit carbamazepine-induced leukopenia. There do not appear to be clinically important pharmacokinetic interactions of lithium with gabapentin (465), lamotrigine, valproate, or topiramate (although one subject did have a 70% fall in lithium concentration) (466). In a review of pharmacokinetic interactions between antiepileptic drugs and psychotropic drugs, there were no clinically significant interactions of lithium with gabapentin, lamotrigine, valproate, or topiramate, although serum lithium concentrations were reduced slightly by topiramate (466).

Although reviews have generally been favorable regarding the combination of lithium with anticonvulsants (466–468), there have been occasional anecdotal reports of possible interactions.

Carbamazepine

Lithium intoxication in a 33-year-old man was attributed to carbamazepine-induced renal insufficiency (469).

A case report suggested an association between lithium and carbamazepine in causing sinus node dysfunction (69).

Lamotrigine

In an open crossover study in 20 healthy men, the serum lithium concentration was slightly lower (0.65 versus 0.71 mmol/l) when lamotrigine 100 mg/day was added for 6 days, but the difference was not statistically significant (470).

Topiramate

In a 42-year-old woman, the serum lithium concentration rose from 0.5 to 1.4 mmol/l after she increased her topiramate dose from 500 to 800 mg/day (471). The authors speculated that topiramate had interfered with lithium excretion. On the other hand, in a crossover study in healthy volunteers, 6 days of treatment with topiramate did not significantly alter serum lithium concentrations; however, the maximum topiramate dose was only 200 mg/day and one subject did have about a 70% fall in lithium C_{max} and AUC (472).

Valproate

In rats, lithium pretreatment reduced the plasma half-life of valproate by 25% and increased urinary excretion of valproate glucuronide (473).

Antidepressants

Adverse interactions of lithium with tricyclic antidepressants, SSRIs, and monoamine oxidase inhibitors have been reviewed (474). In reviews of antidepressants and the serotonin syndrome, a possible contributory role has been suggested for lithium, based on case reports with tricyclic antidepressants, SSRIs, trazodone, and venlafaxine (139,475).

Lithium augmentation of antidepressants is a well-established treatment for resistant depression and is usually well tolerated with all classes of antidepressants, although there have been a few reports of the serotonin syndrome with SSRIs (474). It is possible that shared adverse effects could be magnified by combining lithium with various antidepressants (for example tremor, weight gain, gastrointestinal upset). Hyponatremia secondary to the SIADH has been linked to SSRIs and tricyclic antidepressants, especially in elderly patients, and could predispose to lithium toxicity.

In 28 of 75 patients taking lithium, 24-hour urine volumes were over 3 l/day, and this group had a greater duration of lithium exposure (6.0 versus 3.9 years) (476). There was no relation between polyuria and serum lithium concentrations or dosing regimens, but there was an association with the concurrent use of serotonergic antidepressants (odds ratio 4.25).

Amfebutamone

Although data have suggested that amfebutamone has approximately the same seizure potential as the tricyclic compounds (SEDA-8, 30) (477), the manufacturers reported an increased risk of seizures in patients taking over 600 mg/day in combination with lithium or antipsychotic drugs (SEDA-10, 20) (478).

- A 45-year-old man taking lithium, amfebutamone, and venlafaxine developed a prolonged seizure after ECT, thought to have been caused by a lowering of the seizure threshold due to amfebutamone (although a role of the other two drugs could not be excluded) (123).

Mirtazapine

In a placebo-controlled, crossover study in 12 healthy men, lithium and mirtazapine had no effect on the pharmacokinetics of each other and there was no difference in psychometric testing between the addition of lithium and placebo (479).

Nefazodone

In 12 healthy volunteers, there were no clinically significant alterations in blood concentrations of lithium or nefazodone and its metabolites when the drugs were co-administered (480). The addition of lithium for 6 weeks to nefazodone in 14 treatment-resistant patients produced no serious adverse effects and no dropouts (481). Lithium augmentation of nefazodone in 13 treatment-resistant depressed patients was associated with a variety of annoying adverse effects, but none led to treatment withdrawal (482).

SSRIs

The authors of a thorough literature review of 503 patients treated with lithium and SSRIs (483) acknowledged that conclusions would be hedged with qualifications and equivocations but suggested the following:

(a) "when lithium is added to SSRIs new, nonserious, events occur frequently";
(b) "serotonin syndrome is associated with combined lithium/SSRI therapy, but is rare";
(c) "the evidence for the efficacy of lithium add-on to SSRIs is at best provisional".

There was no systematic evidence that SSRIs alter serum lithium concentrations.

Fluoxetine
Lithium toxicity has also been reported during co-administration with fluoxetine (484).

- After 4 hours of mild, intermittent, hot-weather work, a 45-year-old man taking fluoxetine and lithium (serum concentration not mentioned) collapsed, became comatose, convulsed, and was febrile (42°C); consciousness returned after 6 days but cerebellar symptoms and atrophy persisted (485). It was suggested that disruption of temperature regulation had been caused by a synergistic effect of the two drugs (although he had taken neither drug for 36 hours before the episode).

Fluvoxamine
Six patients taking a stable dose of fluvoxamine had a minor increase in plasma fluvoxamine concentration (from 67 to 76 ng/ml) 2 weeks after starting to take unspecified doses of lithium; this is unlikely to be of clinical significance (486).

Paroxetine
Serum lithium concentrations were unchanged when breakthrough depression was treated double blind by the addition of paroxetine (20–40 mg/day, $n = 19$) and the combination was generally well tolerated (487).

- A 20-year-old woman taking lithium and risperidone became catatonic 5–7 days after the addition of paroxetine, leading to speculation that this was due to an interaction between the three drugs (488). Of 17 patients 4 who had paroxetine added to lithium as an adjunctive antidepressant developed symptoms suggestive of emerging serotonin syndrome (for example nausea, vomiting, diarrhea, sweating, anxiety, oversleeping) (489).

Tricyclic antidepressants
Amitriptyline
Serum lithium concentrations were unchanged when breakthrough depression was treated double blind by the addition of amitriptyline (75–150 mg/day, $n = 23$) and the combination was generally well tolerated (487).

- A 34-year-old woman took amitriptyline 300 mg each night for several years (490). Six days after starting to take lithium 300 mg tds, she had several generalized tonic-clonic seizures. A second episode occurred on re-exposure to lithium.

Doxepin
An interaction of lithium with doxepin has been described.

- A 65-year-old man who took lithium and doxepin for 13 years presented with a 6-month history of myoclonic jerking of both arms, which resolved when both drugs were stopped (491).

Whether this represented a drug interaction or a single drug effect is unclear.

Six patients taking a stable dose of fluvoxamine had a minor increase in plasma fluvoxamine concentration (from 67 to 76 ng/ml) 2 weeks after starting to take unspecified doses of lithium; this is unlikely to be of clinical significance (486).

Antimicrobial drugs

Two reviews of drug interactions with antibiotics briefly and incompletely discussed lithium (492,493).

Quinolones

- A 56-year-old man with normal renal function and therapeutic lithium concentrations became toxic (serum concentration 2.53 mmol/l 24 hours after the last dose) with renal impairment (serum creatinine 141 μmol/l; 1.6 mg/dl) within days of starting levofloxacin. Both symptoms and laboratory abnormalities resolved with withdrawal of both lithium and levofloxacin (494).

Trimethoprim

- A 40-year-old woman developed nausea, malaise, impaired concentration, trembling, unsteadiness, diarrhea, and muscle spasm in association with a serum lithium concentration of 2.1 mmol/l while taking trimethoprim 300 mg/day (495).
- A 42-year-old woman developed symptoms of lithium toxicity and a raised serum concentration (2.1 mmol/l) while taking trimethoprim (495).

This interaction may be due to an amiloride-like diuretic effect of trimethoprim, causing lithium retention.

Antipsychotic drugs

In a discussion of drug interactions with antipsychotic drugs, the literature on lithium was reviewed (496). Caution was advised when lithium is combined with antipsychotic drugs, especially with high dosages of high-potency drugs. In a review of acute, life-threatening, drug-induced neurological syndromes, the controversy of whether lithium increases the risk of neuroleptic malignant syndrome was mentioned briefly (497) (see also Nervous system).

While it is still not clear whether there is a unique encephalopathic interaction of lithium with haloperidol, there is a consensus that the judicious use of these two drugs in combination should be safe. In general, caution is advised if lithium is combined with antipsychotic drugs, especially with high dosages of high-potency drugs (496). There have been reports of neuroleptic malignant syndrome in patients taking lithium plus antipsychotic drugs, but a causal relation has not been established (498).

The risk of extrapyramidal adverse effects may be increased when lithium is combined with antipsychotic drugs.

Erythrocyte/plasma lithium concentration ratios were lower in patients taking phenothiazines or haloperidol than in those taking lithium alone (499,500), and the former group had a higher incidence of neurological and renal adverse effects (500).

- A 59-year-old man taking lithium, haloperidol, and carbamazepine had impaired memory, impaired attention, and an encephalopathy-like pattern on the electroencephalogram that normalized when haloperidol was withdrawn (501). Olanzapine 5 mg/day was added, and 3 weeks later he became disoriented. Surprisingly, the olanzapine was continued and he remained disoriented.

Amisulpride
In a placebo-controlled, parallel-design, double-blind study in 24 male volunteers, amisulpride 100 mg bd for 7 days did not alter lithium pharmacokinetics (502).

Amoxapine
The neuroleptic malignant syndrome occurred in a 63-year-old man when lithium was added to amoxapine (129).

Aripiprazole
A review of aripiprazole included a brief mention of no apparent pharmacokinetic interaction with lithium (503).

Chlorpromazine
The neuroleptic malignant syndrome in a 49-year-old man was attributed to a combination of lithium and chlorpromazine (504).

Clozapine
Seizures and other neurological effects have been described in a few cases when lithium was added to clozapine (505). Five treatment-resistant patients were treated successfully with a combination of clozapine and lithium with no clinically significant adverse events (506). However, a 59-year-old woman developed neurotoxic symptoms 3 days after lithium was added to clozapine; the symptoms resolved when both drugs were stopped and recurred with rechallenge (507).

- Multisystem organ failure occurred shortly after clozapine was added to a therapeutic dose of lithium in a 23-year-old woman (508). Improvement occurred when clozapine was stopped and the toxicity was attributed to clozapine.

Haloperidol
The neuroleptic malignant syndrome has been described when lithium was added to haloperidol (131).

- A pharmacodynamic drug interaction could not be excluded when a 60-year-old man developed delirium at a serum lithium concentration of 0.97 mmol/l when taking lithium and haloperidol (99).

Olanzapine
The neuroleptic malignant syndrome occurred when lithium was added to olanzapine (130).

- A 13-year-old boy with rhabdomyolysis ascribed to olanzapine was also taking lithium, so that a drug interaction could not be excluded (63).
- A 16-year-old boy developed the neuroleptic malignant syndrome when his olanzapine dose was increased (509).

In a double-blind study of 344 patients inadequately responsive to lithium or valproate who were randomized to olanzapine or lithium for 6 weeks, 21% gained weight on lithium plus olanzapine compared with 4.9% taking lithium and placebo (510). Whether lithium contributed to weight gain in the olanzapine group is unclear.

Quetiapine
In an open study in 10 patients, the addition of quetiapine 250 mg tds did not significantly alter serum lithium concentrations (511).

Risperidone
There were no changes in lithium pharmacokinetics when risperidone was substituted open-label for another neuroleptic drug in 13 patients (512). On the other hand, an 81-year-old man had an acute dystonic reaction 4 days after lithium was added to a regimen of risperidone, valproic acid, and benzatropine (513).

- A 17-year-old man had taken risperidone for 2 years without adverse effects, but 12 weeks after lithium was added, he reported prolonged erections (lasting 1–3 hours) 2–5 times daily; risperidone was tapered and withdrawn and the problem resolved (514).

In an in vitro study, there was no visible precipitate formation when lithium citrate syrup was mixed with risperidone solution (515).

Ziprasidone
In 34 healthy men, ziprasidone did not alter serum lithium concentrations or renal lithium clearance (516).

In a placebo-controlled, open-label study in 25 healthy subjects there were no changes in serum lithium concentration or renal lithium clearance when ziprasidone (40–80 mg/day) was added for 7 days (516).

Anxiolytics

There has been a well-documented case of profound hypothermia in a patient taking lithium and diazepam; it did not occur with either drug alone (517). Otherwise, benzodiazepines and lithium have proven to be compatible.

Calcitonin

Serum lithium concentration should be monitored at the start of calcitonin therapy.

Serum lithium concentrations fell significantly within 3 days of starting calcitonin in four women (518), due to increased renal clearance of lithium (518,519).

After they had received 100 units of salmon calcitonin subcutaneously for 3 days, four patients had a 30% mean reduction in serum lithium concentration, which was attributed to reduced absorption and/or increased renal excretion (518).

Calcium channel blockers

Lithium clearance is reduced by about 30% by nifedipine (520).

389. Viguera AC, Howlett SA, Cohen LS, Nonacs RM, Stoller J. In: Neonatal outcome associated with lithium use during pregnancy. Presented at the NCDEU 40th Annual Meeting, May 30–June 2, Boca Raton, FL; 2000. New Clinical Drug Evaluation Unit Program: Poster number: 49.
390. Tekin M, Ellison J. Oromandibular-limb hypogenesis spectrum and maternal lithium use. Clin Dysmorphol 2000;9(2):139–41.
391. Zegers B, Andriessen P. Maternal lithium therapy and neonatal morbidity. Eur J Pediatr 2003;162(5):348–9.
392. Frassetto F, Tourneur Martel F, Barjhoux CE, Villier C, Bot BL, Vincent F. Goiter in a newborn exposed to lithium in utero. Ann Pharmacother 2002;36(11):1745–8.
393. Moretti ME, Lee A, Ito S. Which drugs are contraindicated during breastfeeding? Practice guidelines. Can Fam Physician 2000;46:1753–7.
394. Yoshida K, Smith B, Kumar R. Psychotropic drugs in mothers' milk: a comprehensive review of assay methods, pharmacokinetics and of safety of breast-feeding. J Psychopharmacol 1999;13(1):64–80.
395. Chaudron LH, Jefferson JW. Mood stabilizers during breastfeeding: a review. J Clin Psychiatry 2000;61(2):79–90.
396. Koren G, Moretti M, Ito S. Continuing drug therapy while breastfeeding. Part 2. Common misconceptions of physicians. Can Fam Physician 1999;45:1173–5.
397. Austin MP, Mitchell PB. Use of psychotropic medications in breast-feeding women: acute and prophylactic treatment. Aust NZ J Psychiatry 1998;32(6):778–84.
398. Llewellyn A, Stowe ZN. Psychotropic medications in lactation. J Clin Psychiatry 1998;59(Suppl 2):41–52.
399. Burt VK, Suri R, Altshuler L, Stowe Z, Hendrick VC, Muntean E. The use of psychotropic medications during breast-feeding. Am J Psychiatry 2001;158(7):1001–9.
400. Howard CR, Lawrence RA. Xenobiotics and breastfeeding. Pediatr Clin North Am 2001;48(2):485–504.
401. Moretti ME, Koren G, Verjee Z, Ito S. Monitoring lithium in breast milk: an individualized approach for breast-feeding mothers. Ther Drug Monit 2003;25(3):364–6.
402. Ward RM, Bates BA, Benitz WE, Burchfield DJ, Ring JC, Walls RP, Walson PD. Transfer of drugs and other chemicals into human milk. Pediatrics 2001;108(3):776–89.
403. Olugbemi E, Katona C. Case note audit of lithium use in the elderly. Aging Ment Health 1998;2:151–4.
404. Stoudemire A, Hill CD, Lewison BJ, Marquardt M, Dalton S. Lithium intolerance in a medical-psychiatric population. Gen Hosp Psychiatry 1998;20(2):85–90.
405. Fahy S, Lawlor BA. Lithium use in octogenarians. Int J Geriatr Psychiatry 2001;16(10):1000–3.
406. Cheymol G. Effects of obesity on pharmacokinetics implications for drug therapy. Clin Pharmacokinet 2000;39(3):215–31.
407. Kilts CD. The ups and downs of oral lithium dosing. J Clin Psychiatry 1998;59(Suppl 6):21–6.
408. Henry ME, Moore CM, Demopolas C, Cote J, Renshaw PF. A comparison of brain lithium levels attained with immediate and sustained release lithium. Biol Psychiatry 2001;49(Suppl 8):119S.
409. Gazikolovic E, Obrenovic D, Nicovic Z. Formulaciji tableta litijom-karbonata razlicitim sredstvima za vezivanje. [Formulation of lithium carbonate tablets with various binding substances.] Vojnosanit Pregl 2001;58(6):641–4.
410. Castrogiovanni P. A novel slow-release formulation of lithium carbonate (Carbolithium Once-A-Day) vs standard Carbolithium: a comparative pharmacokinetic study. Clin Ter 2002;153(2):107–15.
411. Durbano F, Mencacci C, Dorigo D, Riva M, Buffa G. The long-term efficacy and tolerability of carbolithium once a day: an interim analysis at 6 months. Clin Ter 2002;153(3):161–6.
412. Pietkiewicz P, Sznitowska M, Dorosz A, Lukasiak J. Lithium carbonate 24-hours extended-release capsule filled with 6 mm tablets. Boll Chim Farm 2003;142(2):69–71.
413. Astruc B, Petit P, Abbar M. Overdose with sustained-release lithium preparations. Eur Psychiatry 1999;14(3):172–4.
414. Owen D. Interactions between homeopathy and drug treatment. Br Homeopath J 2000;89(1):60.
415. Sattar SP. Pinals DA. When taking medications is a sin. Psychiatr Serv 2002;53(2):213–4.
416. Carroll BT, Thalassinos A, Fawver JD. Loading strategies in acute mania. CNS Spectr 2001;6(11):919–22, 930.
417. Soares JC, Boada F, Spencer S, Mallinger AG, Dippold CS, Wells KF, Frank E, Keshavan MS, Gershon S, Kupfer DJ. Brain lithium concentrations in bipolar disorder patients: preliminary (7)Li magnetic resonance studies at 3 T. Biol Psychiatry 2001;49(5):437–43.
418. Hatfield CL, McDonell WN, Lemke KA, Black WD. Pharmacokinetics and toxic effects of lithium chloride after intravenous administration in conscious horses. Am J Vet Res 2001;62(9):1387–92.
419. Jonas MM, Linton RAF, O'Brien TK, Band DM, Linton NWF, Kelly F, Burden TJ, Chevalier SFA, Thompson RPH, Birch NJ, Powell JJ. The pharmacokinetics of intravenous lithium chloride in patients and normal volunteers. J Trace Microprobe Techn 2001;19:313–20.
420. Waring WS, Webb DJ, Maxwell SR. Lithium carbonate as a potential pharmacological vehicle. Intravenous kinetics of single-dose administration in healthy subjects. Eur J Clin Pharmacol 2002;58(6):431–4.
421. Scharman EJ. Methods used to decrease lithium absorption or enhance elimination. J Toxicol Clin Toxicol 1997;35(6):601–8.
422. Kores B, Lader MH. Irreversible lithium neurotoxicity: an overview. Clin Neuropharmacol 1997;20(4):283–99.
423. Bailey B, McGuigan M. Lithium poisoning from a poison control center perspective. Ther Drug Monit 2000;22(6):650–5.
424. Anonymous. Lithium overdose. Prescrire Int 2003;12(63):19.
425. Litovitz TL, Klein-Schwartz W, White S, Cobaugh DJ, Youniss J, Omslaer JC, Drab A, Benson BE. 2000 Annual report of the American Association of Poison Control Centers Toxic Exposure Surveillance System. Am J Emerg Med 2001;19(5):337–95.
426. Montagnon F, Said S, Lepine JP. Lithium: poisonings and suicide prevention. Eur Psychiatry 2002;17(2):92–5.
427. Bell AJ, Ferrier IN. Lithium induced neurotoxicity at therapeutic levels: an aetiological review. Lithium 1994;5:181.
428. Groleau G. Lithium toxicity. Emerg Med Clin North Am 1994;12(2):511–31.
429. Kasahara H, Shinozaki T, Nukariya K, Nishimura H, Nakano H, Nakagawa T, Ushijima S. Hemodialysis for lithium intoxication: preliminary guidelines for emergency. Jpn J Psychiatry Neurol 1994;48(1):1–12.
430. Okusa MD, Crystal LJ. Clinical manifestations and management of acute lithium intoxication. Am J Med 1994;97(4):383–9.
431. Litovitz TL, Klein-Schwartz W, Caravati EM, Youniss J, Crouch B, Lee S. 1998 Annual Report of the American Association of Poison Control Centers Toxic Exposure Surveillance System. Am J Emerg Med 1999;17(5):435–87.
432. De Almeida Teixeira A, Machado MF, Ferreira WM, Torres JB, Brunstein MG, Barros HMT, Barros E. Lithium acute intoxication: epidemiologic study of the causes. J Bras Psiquiatr 1999;48:399–403.
433. Brodersen A, Licht RW, Vestergaard P, Olesen AV, Mortensen PB. Dodeligheden blandt patienter med affektiv sygdom der pategynder lithium behandling. En 16-ar s

opfolgning. [Mortality in patients with affective disorder who commenced treatment with lithium. A 16-year follow-up.] Ugeskr Laeger 2001;163(46):6428–32.
434. Litovitz TL, Klein-Schwartz W, Rodgers GC Jr, Cobaugh DJ, Youniss J, Omslaer JC, May ME, Woolf AD, Benson BE. 2001 Annual Report of the American Association of Poison Control Centers Toxic Exposure Surveillance System. Am J Emerg Med 2002;20(5):391–452.
435. Alhasso A, Bryden AA, Neilson D. Lithium toxicity after urinary diversion with ileal conduit. BMJ 2000;320(7241):1037.
436. Micheli F, Cersosimo G, Scorticati MC, Ledesma D, Molinos J. Blepharospasm and apraxia of eyelid opening in lithium intoxication. Clin Neuropharmacol 1999;22(3):176–9.
437. Vollhardt M, Ferbert A. [Influence of hypocalcemia and high serum levels of lithium on the amplitude of N20/P25 components of median nerve SEP.] EEG-Labor 1999;21:65–70.
438. Ochoa ER, Farrar HC, Shirm SW. Lithium poisoning in a toddler with fever and altered consciousness. Case presentation and discussion. J Invest Med 2000;48:612.
439. Novak-Grubic V, Tavcar R. Lithium intoxication secondary to unrecognized pontine haemorrhage. Acta Psychiatr Scand 2001;103(5):400–1.
440. Peces R, Pobes A. Effectiveness of haemodialysis with high-flux membranes in the extracorporeal therapy of life-threatening acute lithium intoxication. Nephrol Dial Transplant 2001;16(6):1301–3.
441. Danel V, Rhodes AS, Saviuc P, Hanna J. Intoxication grave par le lithium: à propos de deux cas. JEUR 2001;14:134–6.
442. Meyer RJ, Flynn JT, Brophy PD, Smoyer WE, Kershaw DB, Custer JR, Bunchman TE. Hemodialysis followed by continuous hemofiltration for treatment of lithium intoxication in children. Am J Kidney Dis 2001;37(5):1044–7.
443. Beckmann U, Oakley PW, Dawson AH, Byth PL. Efficacy of continuous venovenous hemodialysis in the treatment of severe lithium toxicity. J Toxicol Clin Toxicol 2001;39(4):393–7.
444. Suraya Y, Yoong KY. Lithium neurotoxicity. Med J Malaysia 2001;56(3):378–81.
445. Nagappan R, Parkin WG, Holdsworth SR. Acute lithium intoxication. Anaesth Intensive Care 2002;30(1): 90–2.
446. Ilagan MC, Carlson D, Madden JF. Lithium toxicity: two case reports. Del Med J 2002;74(6):263–70.
447. De Ridder K, De Meester J, Demeyer I, Verbeke J, Nollet G. [Management of a case of lithium intoxication.] Tijdschr Geneeskd 2002;58:769–72.
448. Kerbusch T, Mathot RA, Otten HM, Meesters EW, van Kan HJ, Schellens JH, Beijnen JH. Bayesian pharmacokinetics of lithium after an acute self-intoxication and subsequent haemodialysis: a case report. Pharmacol Toxicol 2002;90(5):243–5.
449. Yoshimura R, Yamada Y, Ueda N, Nakamura J. Changes in plasma monoamine metabolites during acute lithium intoxication. Hum Psychopharmacol 2000;15(5): 357–60.
450. Ponampalam R, Otten EJ. In vitro adsorption of lithium by bentonite. Singapore Med J 2002;43(2):86–9.
451. Bailey B, McGuigan M. Comparison of patients hemodialyzed for lithium poisoning and those for whom dialysis was recommended by PCC but not done: what lesson can we learn? Clin Nephrol 2000;54(5):388–92.
452. van Bommel EF, Kalmeijer MD, Ponssen HH. Treatment of life-threatening lithium toxicity with high-volume continuous venovenous hemofiltration. Am J Nephrol 2000;20(5):408–11.
453. Brubacher JR, Purssell R, Kent DA. Salty broth for salicylate poisoning? Adequacy of overdose management advice in the 2001 Compendium Pharmaceuticals Specialties. CMAJ 2002;167(9):992–6.
454. Muller-Oerlinghausen B. Drug interactions with lithium. A guide for clinicians. CNS Drugs 1999;11:41–8.
455. Jefferson JW, Greist JH, Ackerman DL, Carroll JA. Lithium Encyclopedia for Clinical Practice. 2nd edn. Washington DC: American Psychiatric Press, 1987.
456. Janicak PG, Davis JM. Pharmacokinetics and drug interactions. In: Sadock BJ, Sadock VA, editors. Kaplan & Sadock's Comprehensive Textbook of Psychiatry. 7th ed. Philadelphia: Lippincott, Williams & Wilkins, 2000;2:2250–9.
457. DeVane CL, Nemeroff CB. 2000 Guide to psychotropic drug interactions. Primary Psychiatry 2000;7:40–68.
458. Sproule BA, Hardy BG, Shulman KI. Differential pharmacokinetics of lithium in elderly patients. Drugs Aging 2000;16(3):165–77.
459. Schou M. Treatment of Manic-Depressive Illness: A Practical Guide. 3rd edn. Basel: Karger; 1989.
460. Ventura JM, Igual MJ, Borrell C, Lozano MD, Maiques FJ, Alos M. Toxicidad de litio inducida por captoprilo. A propósito de un caso. [Lithium toxicity induced by captopril. A case study.] Farm Hosp 2000;24:166–9.
461. Bagate K, Grima M, De Jong W, Imbs JL, Barthelmebs M. Effects of icatibant on the ramipril-induced decreased in renal lithium clearance in the rat. Naunyn Schmiedebergs Arch Pharmacol 2001;363(3):281–7.
462. Zwanzger P, Marcuse A, Boerner RJ, Walther A, Rupprecht R. Lithium intoxication after administration of AT1 blockers. J Clin Psychiatry 2001;62(3):208–9.
463. Blanche P, Raynaud E, Kerob D, Galezowski N. Lithium intoxication in an elderly patient after combined treatment with losartan. Eur J Clin Pharmacol 1997;52(6):501.
464. Leung M, Remick RA. Potential drug interaction between lithium and valsartan. J Clin Psychopharmacol 2000;20(3):392–3.
465. Frye MA, Kimbrell TA, Dunn RT, Piscitelli S, Grothe D, Vanderham E, Cora-Locatelli G, Post RM, Ketter TA. Gabapentin does not alter single-dose lithium pharmacokinetics. J Clin Psychopharmacol 1998;18(6):461–4.
466. Spina E, Perucca E. Clinical significance of pharmacokinetic interactions between antiepileptic and psychotropic drugs. Epilepsia 2002;43(Suppl 2):37–44.
467. Wang PW, Ketter TA. Pharmacokinetics of mood stabilizers and new anticonvulsants. Psychopharmacol Bull 2002;36(1):44–66.
468. Pies R. Combining lithium and anticonvulsants in bipolar disorder: a review. Ann Clin Psychiatry 2002;14(4): 223–32.
469. Mayan H, Golubev N, Dinour D, Farfel Z. Lithium intoxication due to carbamazepine-induced renal failure. Ann Pharmacother 2001;35(5):560–2.
470. Chen C, Veronese L, Yin Y. The effects of lamotrigine on the pharmacokinetics of lithium. Br J Clin Pharmacol 2000;50(3):193–5.
471. Pinninti NR, Zelinski G. Does topiramate elevate serum lithium levels? J Clin Psychopharmacol 2002;22(3):340.
472. Doose DR, Kohl KA, Desai-Krieger D, Natarajan J, Van Kammen DP. The effect of topiramate of lithium serum concentration. Presented at the 37th Annual Meeting of the American College of Neuropsychopharmacology, 14–18 December, Las Croabas, Puerto Rico; 1998.
473. Yoshioka H, Ida S, Yokota M, Nishimoto A, Shibata S, Sugawara A, Takiguchi Y. Effects of lithium on the pharmacokinetics of valproate in rats. J Pharm Pharmacol 2000;52(3):297–301.

474. Schweitzer I, Tuckwell V. Risk of adverse events with the use of augmentation therapy for the treatment of resistant depression. Drug Saf 1998;19(6):455–64.
475. Sternbach H. Serotonin syndrome: how to avoid, identify & treat dangerous drug interactions. Current Psychiatry 2003;2:15,16,19,24.
476. Movig KL, Baumgarten R, Leufkens HG, van Laarhoven JH, Egberts AC. Risk factors for the development of lithium-induced polyuria. Br J Psychiatry 2003;182:319–23.
477. Peck AW, Stern WC, Watkinson C. Incidence of seizures during treatment with tricyclic antidepressant drugs and bupropion. J Clin Psychiatry 1983;44(5 Part 2):197–201.
478. Dufresne RL, Weber SS, Becker RE. Bupropion hydrochloride. Drug Intell Clin Pharm 1984;18(12):957–64.
479. Sitsen JM, Voortman G, Timmer CJ. Pharmacokinetics of mirtazapine and lithium in healthy male subjects. J Psychopharmacol 2000;14(2):172–6.
480. Laroudie C, Salazar DE, Cosson JP, Cheuvart B, Istin B, Girault J, Ingrand I, Decourt JP. Pharmacokinetic evaluation of co-administration of nefazodone and lithium in healthy subjects. Eur J Clin Pharmacol 1999;54(12):923–8.
481. Hawley C, Sivakumaran T, Huber TJ, Ige AK. Combination therapy with nefazodone and lithium: safety and tolerability in fourteen patients. Int J Psychiatry Clin Pract 1998;2:251–4.
482. Hawley C, Sivakumaran T, Ochocki M, Ratnam S, Huber T. A preliminary safety study of combined therapy with nefazodone and lithium. Int J Neuropsychopharmacol 1999;2(Suppl 1):S30–1.
483. Hawley CJ, Loughlin PJ, Quick SJ, Gale TM, Sivakumaran T, Hayes J, McPhee S. Efficacy, safety and tolerability of combined administration of lithium and selective serotonin reuptake inhibitors: a review of the current evidence. Hertfordshire Neuroscience Research Group. Int Clin Psychopharmacol 2000;15(4):197–206.
484. Salama AA, Shafey M. A case of severe lithium toxicity induced by combined fluoxetine and lithium carbonate. Am J Psychiatry 1989;146(2):278.
485. Epstein Y, Albukrek D, Kalmovitc B, Moran DS, Shapiro Y. Heat intolerance induced by antidepressants. Ann N Y Acad Sci 1997;813:553–8.
486. Takano A, Suhara T, Yasuno F, Ichimiya T, Inoue M, Sudo Y, Suzuki K. Characteristics of clomipramine and fluvoxamine on serotonin transporter evaluated by PET. Int Clin Psychopharmacol 2002;17(Suppl 2):S84–5.
487. Bauer M, Zaninelli R, Muller-Oerlinghausen B, Meister W. Paroxetine and amitriptyline augmentation of lithium in the treatment of major depression: a double-blind study. J Clin Psychopharmacol 1999;19(2):164–71.
488. Shad U, Preskorn SH, Izgur Z. Failure to consider drug–drug interactions as a likely cause of behavioral deterioration in a patient with bipolar disorder. J Clin Psychopharmacol 2000;20(3):390–2.
489. Fagiolini A, Buysse DJ, Frank E, Houck PR, Luther JF, Kupfer DJ. Tolerability of combined treatment with lithium and paroxetine in patients with bipolar disorder and depression. J Clin Psychopharmacol 2001;21(5):474–8.
490. Solomon JG. Seizures during lithium-amitriptyline therapy. Postgrad Med 1979;66(3):145–6,148.
491. Evidente VG, Caviness JN. Focal cortical transient preceding myoclonus during lithium and tricyclic antidepressant therapy. Neurology 1999;52(1):211–3.
492. Joos AA. Pharmakologische Interaktionen von Antibiotika und psychopharmaka. [Pharmacologic interactions of antibiotics and Psychotropic drugs.] Psychiatr Prax 1998;25(2):57–60.
493. Hersh EV. Adverse drug interactions in dental practice: interactions involving antibiotics. Part II of a series. J Am Dent Assoc 1999;130(2):236–51.
494. Takahashi H, Higuchi H, Shimizu T. Severe lithium toxicity induced by combined levofloxacin administration. J Clin Psychiatry 2000;61(12):949–50.
495. de Vries PL. Lithiumintoxicatie bij gelijktijdig gebruik van trimethoprim. [Lithium intoxication due to simultaneous use of trimethoprim.] Ned Tijdschr Geneeskd 2001;145(11):539–40.
496. ZumBrunnen TL, Jann MW. Drug interactions with antipsychotic agents. Incidence and therapeutic implications. CNS Drugs 1998;9:381–401.
497. Richard IH. Acute, drug-induced, life-threatening neurological syndromes. Neurologist 1998;4:196–210.
498. Schou M. Adverse lithium–neuroleptic interactions: are there permanent effects? Hum Psychopharmacol 1990;5:263.
499. Ahmadi-Abhari SA, Dehpour AR, Emamian ES, Azizabadi-Farahani M, Farsam H, Samini M, Shokri J. The effect of concurrent administration of psychotropic drugs and lithium on lithium ratio in bipolar patients. Hum Psychopharmacol 1998;13:29–34.
500. Dehpour AR, Emamian ES, Ahmadi-Abhari SA, Azizabadi-Farahani M. The lithium ratio and the incidence of side effects. Prog Neuropsychopharmacol Biol Psychiatry 1998;22(6):959–70.
501. Swartz CM. Olanzapine-lithium encephalopathy. Psychosomatics 2001;42(4):370.
502. Chaufour S, Borgstein NG, Van Den Eynde W, Bernard F, Canal M, Zieleniuk I, Pinquier JL. Repeated administrations of amisulpride (A) do not modify lithium carbonate (L) pharmacokinetics in healthy volunteers. Clin Pharmacol Ther 1999;65:143.
503. Taylor DM. Aripiprazole: a review of its pharmacology and clinical use. Int J Clin Pract 2003;57(1):49–54.
504. Leber K, Malek A, D'Agostino A, Adelman HM. A veteran with acute mental changes years after combat. Hosp Pract (Off Ed) 1999;34(6):21–2.
505. Edge SC, Markowitz JS, DeVane CL. Clozapine drug–drug interactions: a review of the literature. Hum Psychopharmacol 1997;12:5–20.
506. Moldavsky M, Stein D, Benatov R, Sirota P, Elizur A, Matzner Y, Weizman A. Combined clozapine-lithium treatment for schizophrenia and schizoaffective disorder. Eur Psychiatry 1998;13:104–6.
507. Lee SH, Yang YY. Reversible neurotoxicity induced by a combination of clozapine and lithium: a case report. Zhonghua Yi Xue Za Zhi (Taipei) 1999;62(3):184–7.
508. Patton S, Remick RA, Isomura T. Clozapine—an atypical reaction. Can J Psychiatry 2000;45(4):393–4.
509. Berry N, Pradhan S, Sagar R, Gupta SK. Neuroleptic malignant syndrome in an adolescent receiving olanzapine–lithium combination therapy. Pharmacotherapy 2003;23(2):255–9.
510. Tohen M, Chengappa KN, Suppes T, Zarate CA Jr, Calabrese JR, Bowden CL, Sachs GS, Kupfer DJ, Baker RW, Risser RC, Keeter EL, Feldman PD, Tollefson GD, Breier A. Efficacy of olanzapine in combination with valproate or lithium in the treatment of mania in patients partially nonresponsive to valproate or lithium monotherapy. Arch Gen Psychiatry 2002;59(1):62–9.
511. Munera PA, Perel JM, Asato M. Medication interaction causing seizures in a patient with bipolar disorder and cystic fibrosis. J Child Adolesc Psychopharmacol 2002;12(3):275–6.
512. Demling J, Huang ML, De Smedt G. Pharmacokinetics and safety of combination therapy with lithium and risperidone in adult patients with psychosis. Int J Neuropsychopharmacol 1999;2:S63.

513. Durrenberger S, de Leon J. Acute dystonic reaction to lithium and risperidone. J Neuropsychiatry Clin Neurosci 1999;11(4):518–9.
514. Owley T, Leventhal B, Cook EH Jr. Risperidone-induced prolonged erections following the addition of lithium. J Child Adolesc Psychopharmacol 2001;11(4):441–2.
515. Park SH, Gill MA, Dopheide JA. Visual compatibility of risperidone solution and lithium citrate syrup. Am J Health Syst Pharm 2003;60(6):612–3.
516. Apseloff G, Mullet D, Wilner KD, Anziano RJ, Tensfeldt TG, Pelletier SM, Gerber N. The effects of ziprasidone on steady-state lithium levels and renal clearance of lithium. Br J Clin Pharmacol 2000;49(Suppl 1):61S–4S.
517. Naylor GJ, McHarg A. Profound hypothermia on combined lithium carbonate and diazepam treatment. BMJ 1977;2(6078):22.
518. Passiu G, Bocchetta A, Martinelli V, Garau P, Del Zompo M, Mathieu A. Calcitonin decreases lithium plasma levels in man. Preliminary report. Int J Clin Pharmacol Res 1998;18(4):179–81.
519. Bachofen M, Bock H, Beglinger C, Fischer JA, Thiel G. [Calcitonin, a proximal-tubular-acting diuretic: lithium clearance measurements in humans.] Schweiz Med Wochenschr 1997;127(18):717 52.
520. Bruun NE, Ibsen H, Skott P, Toftdahl D, Giese J, Holstein-Rathlou NH. Lithium clearance and renal tubular sodium handling during acute and long-term nifedipine treatment in essential hypertension. Clin Sci (Lond) 1988;75(6):609–13.
521. Pinkofsky HB, Sabu R, Reeves RR. A nifedipine-induced inhibition of lithium clearance. Psychosomatics 1997;38(4):400–1.
522. Price WA, Giannini AJ. Neurotoxicity caused by lithium-verapamil synergism. J Clin Pharmacol 1986;26(8): 717–9.
523. Price WA, Shalley JE. Lithium–verapamil toxicity in the elderly. J Am Geriatr Soc 1987;35(2):177–8.
524. Dubovsky SL, Franks RD, Allen S. Verapamil: a new antimanic drug with potential interactions with lithium. J Clin Psychiatry 1987;48(9):371–2.
525. Tariq M, Morais C, Sobki S, Al Sulaiman M, Al Khader A. Effect of lithium on cyclosporin induced nephrotoxicity in rats. Ren Fail 2000;22(5):545–60.
526. Colussi G, Rombola G, Surian M, De Ferrari ME, Airaghi C, Benazzi E, Malberti F, Minetti L. Lithium clearance in humans: effects of acute administration of acetazolamide and furosemide. Kidney Int Suppl 1990;28:S63–6.
527. Hurtig HI, Dyson WL. Lithium toxicity enhanced by diuresis. N Engl J Med 1974;290(13):748–9.
528. Finley PR, Warner MD, Peabody CA. Clinical relevance of drug interactions with lithium. Clin Pharmacokinet 1995;29(3):172–91.
529. Pyevich D, Bogenschutz MP. Herbal diuretics and lithium toxicity. Am J Psychiatry 2001;158(8):1329.
530. Perlman BB. Interaction between lithium salts and ispaghula husk. Lancet 1990;335(8686):416.
531. Hendy MS, Dove AF, Arblaster PG. Mazindol-induced lithium toxicity. BMJ 1980;280(6215):684–5.
532. Verduijn M. Lithiumtoxiciteit door mazindol: Patiënt sprak niet te volgen taal. [Lithium toxicity caused by mazindol: the patient spoke incomprehensible language.] Pharm Weekbl 1998;133:1901.
533. O'Regan JB. Letter: Adverse interaction of lithium carbonate and methyldopa. Can Med Assoc J 1976;115(5):385–6.
534. Teicher MH, Altesman RI, Cole JO, Schatzberg AF. Possible nephrotoxic interaction of lithium and metronidazole. JAMA 1987;257(24):3365–6.
535. Hill GE, Wong KC, Hodges MR. Potentiation of succinylcholine neuromuscular blockade by lithium carbonate. Anesthesiology 1976;44(5):439–42.
536. Hill GE, Wong KC, Hodges MR. Lithium carbonate and neuromuscular blocking agents. Anesthesiology 1977;46(2):122–6.
537. Naguib M, Koorn R. Interactions between psychotropics, anaesthetics and electroconvulsive therapy: implications for drug choice and patient management. CNS Drugs 2002;16(4):229–47.
538. Haas DA. Adverse drug interactions in dental practice: interactions associated with analgesics. Part III in a series. J Am Dent Assoc 1999;130(3):397–407.
539. Ragheb M. The clinical significance of lithium–nonsteroidal anti-inflammatory drug interactions. J Clin Psychopharmacol 1990;10(5):350–4.
540. Sussman N, Magid S. Psychiatric manifestations of nonsteroidal anti-inflammatory drugs. Prim Psychiatry 2000;7:26–30.
541 Montvale NJ, Physicians' Desk Reference. Medical Economics Company, Inc; 2001:2484.
542. Davies NM, McLachlan AJ, Day RO, Williams KM. Clinical pharmacokinetics and pharmacodynamics of celecoxib: a selective cyclo-oxygenase-2 inhibitor. Clin Pharmacokinet 2000;38(3):225–42.
543. Davies NM, Gudde TW, de Leeuw MA. Celecoxib: a new option in the treatment of arthropathies and familial adenomatous polyposis. Expert Opin Pharmacother 2001;2(1):139–52.
544. Rossat J, Maillard M, Nussberger J, Brunner HR, Burnier M. Renal effects of selective cyclooxygenase-2 inhibition in normotensive salt-depleted subjects. Clin Pharmacol Ther 1999;66(1):76–84.
545. Gunja N, Graudins A, Dowsett R. Lithium toxicity: a potential interaction with celecoxib. Intern Med J 2002;32(9–10):494.
546. Lundmark J, Gunnarsson T, Bengtsson F. A possible interaction between lithium and rofecoxib. Br J Clin Pharmacol 2002;53(4):403–4.
547. Sajbel TA, Carter GW, Wiley RB. Pharmacokinetics/pharmacodynamics/pharmacometrics/drug metabolism. Pharmacotherapy 2001;21:380.
548. Bocchia M, Bertola G, Morganti D, Toscano M, Colombo E. Intossicazione da litio e uso di nimesulide. [Lithium poisoning and the use of nimesulide.] Recenti Prog Med 2001;92(7–8):462.
549. Reimann IW, Frolich JC. Effects of diclofenac on lithium kinetics. Clin Pharmacol Ther 1981;30(3):348–52.
550. Monji A, Maekawa T, Miura T, Nishi D, Horikawa H, Nakagawa Y, Tashiro N. Interactions between lithium and non-steroidal antiinflammatory drugs. Clin Neuropharmacol 2002;25(5):241–2.
551. Ragheb M. Ibuprofen can increase serum lithium level in lithium-treated patients. J Clin Psychiatry 1987;48(4):161–3.
552. Bailey CE, Stewart JT, McElroy RA. Ibuprofen-induced lithium toxicity. South Med J 1989;82(9):1197.
553. Joseph DiGiacomo. Interview with F Flach. Risk management issues associated with psychopharmacological treatment. Essent Psychopharmacol 2001;4:137–50.
554. Iyer V. Ketorolac (Toradol) induced lithium toxicity. Headache 1994;34(7):442–4.
555. Cold JA, ZumBrunnen TL, Simpson MA, Augustin BG, Awad E, Jann MW. Increased lithium serum and red blood cell concentrations during ketorolac coadministration. J Clin Psychopharmacol 1998;18(1):33–7.
556. Danion JM, Schmidt M, Welsch M, Imbs JL, Singer L. Interaction entre les anti-inflammatoires non steroidiens et les sels de lithium. [Interaction between non-steroidal anti-inflammatory agents and lithium salts.] Encephale 1987;13(4):255–60.

557. Turck D, Heinzel G, Luik G. Steady-state pharmacokinetics of lithium in healthy volunteers receiving concomitant meloxicam. Br J Clin Pharmacol 2000;50(3):197–204.
558. Levin GM, Grum C, Eisele G. Effect of over-the-counter dosages of naproxen sodium and acetaminophen on plasma lithium concentrations in normal volunteers. J Clin Psychopharmacol 1998;18(3):237–40.
559. Kerry RJ, Owen G, Michaelson S. Possible toxic interaction between lithium and piroxicam. Lancet 1983;1(8321):418–9.
560. Nadarajah J, Stein GS. Piroxicam induced lithium toxicity. Ann Rheum Dis 1985;44(7):502.
561. Walbridge DG, Bazire SR. An interaction between lithium carbonate and piroxicam presenting as lithium toxicity. Br J Psychiatry 1985;147:206–7.
562. Jones MT, Stoner SC. Increased lithium concentrations reported in patients treated with sulindac. J Clin Psychiatry 2000;61(7):527–8.
563. Apseloff G, Wilner KD, von Deutsch DA, Gerber N. Tenidap sodium decreases renal clearance and increases steady-state concentrations of lithium in healthy volunteers. Br J Clin Pharmacol 1995;39(Suppl 1):25S–8S.
564. Gardner DM, Lynd LD. Sumatriptan contraindications and the serotonin syndrome. Ann Pharmacother 1998;32(1):33–8.
565. Donovan JL, DeVane CL. A primer on caffeine pharmacology and its drug interactions in clinical psychopharmacology. Psychopharmacol Bull 2001;35(3):30–48.
566. Gai MN, Thielemann AM, Arancibia A. Effect of three different diets on the bioavailability of a sustained release lithium carbonate matrix tablet. Int J Clin Pharmacol Ther 2000;38(6):320–6.
567. Gupta S, Austin R, Devanand DP. Lithium and maintenance electroconvulsive therapy. J ECT 1998;14(4):241–4.
568. Jha AK, Stein GS, Fenwick P. Negative interaction between lithium and electroconvulsive therapy—a case-control study. Br J Psychiatry 1996;168(2):241–3.
569. Schou M. Lithium and electroconvulsive therapy: adversaries, competitors, allies? Acta Psychiatr Scand 1991;84(5):435–8.
570. Lippmann SB, El-Mallakh R. Can electroconvulsive therapy be given during lithium treatment? Lithium 1994;5:205–9.
571. Nordt SP, Cantrell FL. Elevated lithium level: a case and brief overview of lithium poisoning. Psychosom Med 1999;61(4):564–5.
572. Van Osch-Gevers M, Draaisma JMTh, Verzijl JM. Een 20 maanden oude peuter met onbegrepen convulsies. [A 20-month-old toddler suffering from unexplained convulsions.] Pharm Weekbl 1999;134:1163–4.
573. Lovell RW, Bunker WW. Lithium assay errors. Am J Psychiatry 1997;154(10):1477.
574. Linder MW, Keck PE Jr. Standards of laboratory practice: antidepressant drug monitoring. National Academy of Clinical Biochemistry. Clin Chem 1998;44(5):1073–84.
575. Namnyak S, Hussain S, Davalle J, Roker K, Strickland M. Contaminated lithium heparin bottles as a source of pseudobacteraemia due to *Pseudomonas fluorescens*. J Hosp Infect 1999;41(1):23–8.
576. He GR, Cheng W, Huang YY. [Effect of heparin lithium as anticoagulant in assay of FT3, FT4 and TSH.] Di Yi Jun Yi Da Xue Xue Bao 2002;22(8):721–3.
577. Geller B, Cooper TB, Sun K, Zimerman B, Frazier J, Williams M, Heath J. Double-blind and placebo-controlled study of lithium for adolescent bipolar disorders with secondary substance dependency. J Am Acad Child Adolesc Psychiatry 1998;37(2):171–8.
578. Rohde LA, Szobot C. Lithium in bipolar adolescents with secondary substance dependency. J Am Acad Child Adolesc Psychiatry 1999;38(1):4.
579. Geller B. Lithium in bipolar adolescents with secondary substance dependency. J Am Acad Child Adolesc Psychiatry 1999;38:4.
580. Seidel S, Kreutzer R, Smith D, McNeel S, Gilliss D. Assessment of commercial laboratories performing hair mineral analysis. JAMA 2001;285(1):67–72.

Lobeline

General Information

Lobeline is derived from the plant *Lobelia inflata* (Indian tobacco). It is both an agonist and an antagonist at nicotinic receptors, although it is not structurally related to nicotine (1). It inhibits nicotine- and amphetamine-induced dopamine release by interacting with the tetrabenazine-binding site on the monoamine transporter. It also inhibits dopamine re-uptake. It has been used in smoking cessation, but is ineffective (2).

Nausea, vomiting, coughing, tremor, and dizziness have been noted with an average dose of lobeline. It can also cause nausea, sweating, and palpitation when inhaled from a cigarette.

Drug Administration

Drug overdose

Profuse sweating, paresis, tachycardia, hypotension, hypothermia, convulsions, coma, and death can occur in overdosage.

References

1. Dwoskin LP, Crooks PA. A novel mechanism of action and potential use for lobeline as a treatment for psychostimulant abuse. Biochem Pharmacol 2002;63(2):89–98.
2. Stead LF, Hughes JR. Lobeline for smoking cessation. Cochrane Database Syst Rev 2000;(2):CD000124.

Local anesthetics

General Information

Local anesthetics typically contain a hydrophilic tertiary amine group linked to a lipophilic ester or amide. The most commonly used local anesthetics are either amides or esters, as shown in Table 1. The aminoester anesthetics cause adverse reactions more commonly than local anesthetics in the amide group. The esters are typically metabolized by de-esterification by esterases, such as pseudocholinesterase in the plasma or esterases in the liver. Metabolism occurs rapidly, and so these agents have short durations of action after they reach the systemic circulation. The amides are mainly metabolized in the liver, by *N*-dealkylation followed by oxidation by CYP isozymes. Metabolism of these drugs occurs more slowly.

The potency of a local anesthetic depends on its lipophilicity (Table 2) (1); the more lipophilic, the more potent.

Local anesthetics can be classified as follows (2):

(a) low potency, short duration of action (for example procaine);
(b) intermediate potency, intermediate duration of action (for example lidocaine, prilocaine);
(c) high potency, long duration of action (for example ropivacaine).

Local anesthetics have a wide range of effects. They inhibit sodium, potassium, and calcium ion channels, alpha-adrenoceptors, and phosphatidylinositol signalling. They also cause dysrhythmias when injected directly into the brain. Local anesthetics are also mitochondrial poisons and impair oxidative phosphorylation.

The adverse effects of local anesthetics are well established (3,4). The safety advantages claimed for newer agents have to be treated with much reserve. With increasing experience, discovery of optimal doses, and understanding of potency differences, the tolerability of newer agents is often found to be similar to that of substances that have been used for much longer.

The adverse effects of local anesthetics fall broadly into four groups (5):

(a) Effects attributable to the technique itself rather than to the agent used, for example needle damage to a vessel or nerve.
(b) Local and regional effects of the drug, which may be related to its anesthetic activity or a consequence of irritation or allergy.
(c) Systemic effects, most usually seen if the agent is inadvertently injected into a blood vessel in sufficient quantities.
(d) Effects of additives, notably vasoconstrictors to prolong the local effect, hyaluronidase to promote penetration, and preservatives to prevent bacterial contamination or degradation (6).

The possibility must always be anticipated that when a local anesthetic is administered, some of it will reach organs or tissues for which it was not originally destined, either because it has been incorrectly administered or because some anatomical or other idiosyncrasy of the patient has resulted in unexpected diffusion or leakage of the agent beyond its intended location. The main problems that result relate either to effects on the nervous system or adverse effects resulting from unintended entry into the general circulation. Very occasionally, infections are transmitted (SEDA-16, 129).

Systemic toxicity is most likely to occur if a local anesthetic is accidentally injected into a vessel in sufficient quantity (7). Even with appropriate local administration, there is inevitably some diffusion of the local anesthetic into the body from the site at which it is applied, varying with local blood flow and the technique; intercostal block, for example, rapidly produces high plasma concentrations, while subcutaneous infiltration leads to much lower concentrations more slowly. The amount of local anesthetic used is another contributory factor.

Although the effects are usually mild, systemic toxicity related to local anesthesia can be fatal: in one study of 53 deaths after the use of local anesthetics there was no evidence of allergy (SED-11, 217) (8). In preventing systemic complications from local anesthesia, such measures as close monitoring of patients, the administration of intravenous fluids before major regional block, the immediate availability of drugs and equipment to treat systemic toxicity, preoxygenation, injection of a test dose, and incremental dosing are important measures.

Some distinction must be made between the main groups of local anesthetics as to the frequency of complications. Hypersensitivity reactions, for example, are relatively less common with the aminoamides, such as bupivacaine, cinchocaine, etidocaine, lidocaine, mepivacaine, prilocaine, and ropivacaine, than with the aminoesters. However, the systemic toxic effects of individual local anesthetics differ: bupivacaine, cinchocaine, and tetracaine are the most toxic. Furthermore, the individual characteristics of the patient (for example age, sex, body weight, and cardiac, renal, and hepatic function) are important (SEDA-17, 134).

The early recognition of complications can be very difficult if a local anesthetic is administered during

Table 1 Structural groups of some commonly used local anesthetics (durations of action in parentheses)

Amides
- Articaine
- Bupivacaine (2–8 hours)
- Cinchocaine (2–3 hours)
- Etidocaine (2–6 hours)
- Levobupivacaine
- Lidocaine (1–2 hours)
- Mepivacaine (1.5–3 hours)
- Prilocaine (1–2 hours)
- Ropivacaine (4–6 hours)

Esters of benzoic acid
- Cocaine

Esters of meta-aminobenzoic acid
- Proxymetacaine

Esters of para-aminobenzoic acid
- Benzocaine
- Chloroprocaine
- Oxybuprocaine
- Procaine (30–45 minutes)
- Propoxycaine
- Tetracaine

Table 2 Partition coefficients (*n*-octanol/water) of some local anesthetics

Local anesthetic	Partition coefficient
Benzocaine	1.44
Procaine	2.51
Mepivacaine	2.69
Prilocaine	2.73
Lidocaine	3.40
Bupivacaine	4.05
Etidocaine	4.19
Tetracaine	4.32
Oxybuprocaine	4.38

general anesthesia, to prevent postoperative pain, since unconscious or sedated patients will not recognize the early signs of problems, such as traumatic paresthesia (9).

In a general review of the systemic toxicity of local anesthetics interesting trends were identified (10). The incidence of systemic toxicity has been falling during the last 20 years, most probably due to increased awareness of the potential cardiotoxicity of long-acting aminoamide local anesthetics. Steps to guard against unintentional intravascular injection have been increasingly used. These include aspiration, incremental injection, dose limitation, and the use of test doses. The most studied test dose is adrenaline 15 micrograms, which reliably produces a tachycardia in healthy subjects within 20 seconds of intravascular injection. Specifically, the incidence of cardiotoxicity has also fallen; several case series of systemic toxicity have been published in recent years, reporting only nervous system toxicity but no cases of cardiotoxicity. This contradicts previous estimates of the risk of cardiotoxicity, which suggested an incidence of 10% of all systemic toxicity reactions, reconfirming the impression of increased carefulness of healthcare professionals.

Organs and Systems

Cardiovascular

Cardiovascular complications are not uncommon in the course of local anesthesia; however, most changes are moderate, involving mild peripheral vasodilatation and reduced cardiac output with a change in heart rate.

Local anesthetics reduce myocardial contractility and rate of conduction (11). They also cause direct vasoconstriction or vasodilatation of vascular smooth muscle (12) and central stimulation of the autonomic nervous system (13).

Cardiac arrest and marked myocardial depression, in which hypoxia plays a critical role, have been reported.

Cardiovascular collapse can be severe and refractory to treatment; most fatal cases involve bupivacaine.

The cardiovascular system is more resistant to the toxic effects of local anesthetics than the nervous system. Mild circulatory depression can precede nervous system toxicity, but seizures are more likely to occur before circulatory collapse. The intravenous dose of lidocaine required to produce cardiovascular collapse is seven times that which causes seizures. The safety margin for racemic bupivacaine is much lower. The stereospecific levorotatory isomers levobupivacaine and ropivacaine are less cardiotoxic, and have a higher safety margin than bupivacaine, but not lidocaine; in the case of ropivacaine this may be at the expense of reduced anesthetic potency (14,15). Toxicity from anesthetic combinations is additive.

A comparison of the cardiotoxicity of the two stereoisomers of ropivacaine and bupivacaine on the isolated heart showed that both compounds had negative inotropic and negative chronotropic effects irrespective of the stereoisomer used, but bupivacaine had greater effects compared with ropivacaine at equal concentrations (16). Atrioventricular conduction time showed stereoselectivity for bupivacaine at clinical concentrations; the R(+) isomer had a greater effect in lengthening atrioventricular conduction time, but the less fat-soluble ropivacaine only showed stereoselectivity at concentrations far greater than those used clinically. Similar to the negative inotropic and chronotropic effects, bupivacaine produced greater effects on atrioventricular conduction time than ropivacaine at equal concentrations. This important study has confirmed speculations that not only the stereospecificity of ropivacaine but also its physicochemical properties contribute to its cardiac safety.

Current concepts of resuscitation after local anesthetic cardiotoxicity have been reviewed (17). Vasopressin may be a logical vasopressor in the setting of hypotension, rather than adrenaline, in view of the dysrhythmogenic potential of the latter. Amiodarone is probably of use in the treatment of dysrhythmias. Calcium channel blockers, phenytoin, and bretyllium should be avoided. In terms of new modes of therapy targeted at the specific action of local anesthetics, lipid infusions, propofol, and insulin/glucose/potassium infusions may all have a role, but further research is necessary.

Nervous system

Central nervous system effects of low concentrations of local anesthetics are mainly sedation and confusion; high concentrations are more likely to cause seizures (18).

The first sign of systemic toxicity can be mild sedation or diminished alertness. Dizziness, tinnitus, metallic tastes, muscle twitching, perioral numbness, visual disturbances, disorientation, and light-headedness are the most frequently reported adverse nervous system effects (19).

However, as the blood concentrations achieved are sometimes higher than one would anticipate, toxicity can occasionally prove much more severe than expected, for example frank convulsions, sometimes progressing to respiratory arrest and loss of consciousness. The management of local anesthetic-induced convulsions has been reviewed (20).

Local anesthetic-induced seizures have been reported more often with bupivacaine, particularly in combination with chloroprocaine (SEDA-20, 123). Ropivacaine-induced seizures have also been reported (21,22).

Severe seizures have been reported after topical use of TAC, a combination of tetracaine, adrenaline, and cocaine, in children (23,24).

Endocrine

Local anesthetics generally have only slight endocrine and metabolic adverse effects, without clinical repercussions.

Hematologic

Methemoglobinemia has been reported with benzocaine, Cetacaine (a mixture of benzocaine, butyl aminobenzoate, and tetracaine), cocaine, lidocaine, novocaine, and prilocaine. Acquired methemoglobinemia can result from exposure to chemicals that contain an aniline group, such as benzocaine and procaine, or to those that are transformed to metabolites that contain an aniline group, such as lidocaine and prilocaine. Toxic blood concentrations of local anesthetics, aberrant hemoglobin, and NADH-methemoglobin reductase deficiency are critical factors that favor the onset of methemoglobinemia. However, methemoglobinemia can occur even in the absence of such risk factors. Young children are most likely to experience clinical effects, but topical use (for example of Cetacaine) has very occasionally caused severe problems even in adults (25). Intravenous methylthioninium chloride (methylene blue) 1–2 mg/kg and oxygen are usually recommended when methemoglobinemia exceeds 30%.

There have again been several reports of methemoglobinemia following topical anesthesia (26,27). Most have been associated with topical benzocaine, and the patients recovered fully after the administration of methylthioninium chloride.

- A neonate born at 24 weeks had a rectal biopsy under general anesthesia and was intubated with an endotracheal tube that had been lubricated with lidocaine jelly 1 g and after the biopsy a rectal pack soaked in about 1 g of benzocaine lubricant; 30 minutes after surgery she developed cyanosis, with a methemoglobin concentration of 45% (28).

The authors postulated that either local anesthetic could have been responsible, but that the oxidant effects of the two agents may have been additive. They highlighted the need for awareness of seemingly minor uses of medications in neonates.

Liver

Reduced hepatic clearance, as well as relative overdosage, of local anesthetics can lead to systemic toxicity, as illustrated by three patients who underwent topicalization of the oropharynx for transesophageal echocardiography with lidocaine 10% spray or 2% viscous and subsequently became confused and drowsy (SEDA-21, 135).

Immunologic

Systemic hypersensitivity reactions are not a frequent problem in local anesthesia. Systemic toxicity or allergy to additives (hyaluronidase, bisulfate, parabens) has sometimes been mistakenly classified as hypersensitivity to local anesthetics (SEDA-17, 135) (29). Well-documented case reports are very few, relating particularly to the older aminoesters; this appears to be because these agents have the highly antigenic para-aminobenzoic acid as a metabolite (SEDA-13, 98). The incidence of true allergy is actually very low, probably less than 1% of all the adverse effects attributable to these substances (SEDA-20, 123).

Allergic reactions to aminoamide local anesthetics are unusual, but type I hypersensitivity reactions are described, and life-threatening anaphylaxis can rarely occur (SEDA-21, 136) (SEDA-22, 134). Cross-reaction between amides also occurs, for example articaine, bupivacaine, lidocaine, and prilocaine (SEDA-22, 134).

Type IV delayed hypersensitivity reactions are uncommon, but allergic contact dermatitis and localized erythema and blistering have been reported (SEDA-21, 136).

- A 58-year-old man with a urological stoma used a catheter lubricated with Braum Monodose ointment (30). After almost 2 years, he developed severe pruritus and squamous erythematous plaques in the peristomal skin. Patch tests were positive with the lubricant ointment and one of its constituents, tetracaine.

Both anaphylactoid reactions and bronchospasm have occasionally been reported, although the latter may have been due to sympathetic nervous blockade leading to unopposed parasympathetic effects (SEDA-18, 143) (31).

Contact hypersensitivity also occurs. Benzocaine is a potent skin sensitizer, and several cases of contact dermatitis to lidocaine have been reported. In many cases there is no cross-reactivity between different local anesthetics.

- A 79-year-old man developed a weeping dermatitis of the perianal skin, buttocks, and proximal thighs (32). In the previous 3 weeks, he had used Proctosedyl cream which contains cinchocaine (dibucaine). Patch tests were positive with Proctosedyl cream and 5% cinchocaine in petrolatum, while benzocaine, lidocaine, and clioquinol were negative.
- A 62-year-old woman had a systemic contact dermatitis several days after topical administration of DoloPosterine ointment for hemorrhoids (33). She had erythematous vesicular lesions on her perianal area and an edematous erythematous rash on her upper thighs, elbow flexures, axillae, and face. Patch tests with the ointment and its constituents were positive with DoloPosterine and dibucaine 5% in petrolatum; patch tests with benzocaine and other local anesthetics were negative.
- A 71-year-old Japanese man developed an itchy erythematous papular eruption after using an over-the-counter medicament for skin wounds (Makiron) for 1 month (34). Patch tests with the constituents showed positive reactions to dl-chlorphenamine maleate and cinchocaine hydrochloride (both 1% in petrolatum). Patch tests with lidocaine hydrochloride and mepivacaine hydrochloride showed no cross-sensitization.

However, some sensitized patients do cross-react with various related local anesthetic agents or chemically similar compounds, including some muscle relaxants (SEDA-15, 117). On the other hand, cross-reactivity between aminoesters and aminoamides seems unlikely and does not appear to be on record. Although cross-reactivity between amide local anesthetics is uncommon, it has been reported.

- A 26-year-old woman, 6 months pregnant, developed local redness and itching after exposure to topical agents containing lidocaine, and a further similar reaction to bupivacaine, also with swelling, 8 hours after injection (35). She had a history of anaphylaxis to an unidentified agent, and a patch test was performed using mepivacaine, lidocaine, and ropivacaine; all resulted in strong reactions after 48 hours, while patch testing was negative with chloroprocaine. She subsequently had a cesarean section under spinal anesthesia with chloroprocaine with no adverse reaction.
- A 39-year-old man was investigated for three episodes of facial swelling following dental procedures over 2 years. The swelling always occurred on the same side as the dental procedure and about 12 hours after it, took a couple of days to resolve, did not respond to

antihistamines, and was not associated with a rash, laryngeal edema, or bronchospasm. He was admitted twice and treated with intravenous antibiotics for cellulitis. He also reported a history of a rash after penicillin but no previous reactions to local anesthetics. All blood tests, including full blood count, C3 and C4 concentrations, and C1 esterase inhibitor activity and function were normal; an antinuclear antibody test was negative, IgE concentrations were not raised, and latex-specific IgE was not detected. Skin prick, intradermal, and subcutaneous tests were carried out with isotonic saline, lidocaine, prilocaine, and procaine; these did not show immediate reactions, but 2 days later a wheal appeared at the lidocaine site. There was a less intense reaction with prilocaine and none with saline or procaine.

The authors concluded that sensitization to lidocaine must have taken place during previous procedures and that cross-reactivity with another amide type local anesthetic, prilocaine, had also occurred.

Contact dermatitis was reported in three hemodialysis patients who used Emla cream repeatedly as analgesia for AV fistula cannulation (SEDA-21, 136).

Twenty patients with a prior history of generalized and/or local skin reactions after local anesthetics were examined with intradermal testing and patch testing; in 10 of them a lymphocyte transformation test was performed to investigate whether they had T cell sensitization to local anesthetics, which might have been responsible for their symptoms (36). Only two had a positive intradermal test, whereas six had a positive patch test and six had a positive lymphocyte transformation test, suggesting that allergic skin symptoms could be mediated by T cells in some patients who do not have evidence of an IgE-mediated reaction.

- A 20-year-old woman, who had had eight previous uneventful exposures to local anesthetics for dental procedures, received an injection of 1% lidocaine for treatment of an in-growing toenail; 12 hours later she developed widespread urticaria lasting a week accompanied by bronchospasm and abdominal discomfort (37). A skin prick test gave a slight positive reaction, and later a positive intradermal injection provided evidence of a true type I hypersensitivity reaction. Following negative skin and intradermal tests with prilocaine, subsequent dental treatment 12 months later was performed using prilocaine with no untoward effects.
- A 70-year-old woman received a peribulbar block using 10 ml of 2% lidocaine, 0.75% bupivacaine (50/50), and hyaluronidase 500 units for cataract extraction; 12 hours later she awoke with a painful, swollen eye (38). There was marked swelling, erythema, tenderness of the eyelids, and a tense orbit, with reduced visual acuity, marked restriction of eye movements, and conjunctival chemosis. There was no hematoma or evidence of infection, but allergy could not be ruled out. Four days later, she received tetracaine eye drops and local infiltration with lidocaine for further suturing and again developed similar symptoms and signs in that eye, with swelling extending to the cheek; follow-up showed persistent ocular dysfunction.

The second patient had had previous exposure to prilocaine, lidocaine, and bupivacaine without problems. The author proposed a diagnosis of lidocaine allergy, although hyaluronidase as the antigen could not be excluded.

- A 23-year-old woman developed an allergic contact dermatitis after applying an over-the-counter proprietary antipruritic jelly containing 0.1% cinchocaine chloride, and a "caine" mixture (5% benzocaine, 1% cinchocaine hydrochloride, 1% procaine hydrochloride) (39). She had positive patch testing to both components.

Allergic reactions attributed to local anesthetics can be due to excipients in the formulation (40).

- A 69-year-old woman developed hypesthesia of all four limbs lasting several hours after three gastroscopies using lidocaine jelly; although the symptom was not typical of an allergic reaction, intradermal tests and nasal provocation tests were performed. The intradermal tests were negative, but the nasal provocation tests were positive for carboxymethylcellulose, a suspending agent used in lidocaine jelly; this caused ipsilateral nasal congestion and dysesthesia of the tongue and the ipsilateral temporal region within 30 minutes. A drug-induced lymphocyte stimulation test was also positive for carboxymethylcellulose.

Hypersensitivity to carboxymethylcellulose may have contributed to this patient's unusual symptoms.

The use of skin testing to identify a causative drug allergen has been repeatedly advocated by several groups, but their advice has not always been followed. Intradermal testing can be helpful in distinguishing between safe and unsafe agents in patients with a history of allergy to local anesthesia.

Various types of immunodepressant effects of local anesthetics can be detected by laboratory testing, although they may have no clinical significance. Lidocaine dose-dependently inhibits EA rosetting by human lymphocytes. In vitro depression of human leukocyte random motility and phagocytosis has also been reported (SED-11, 220) (41).

When injected into the skin, local anesthetics often cause pseudo-allergic reactions, with similar symptoms to immediate type allergy (42). However, true immediate hypersensitivity to local anesthetics is extremely rare.

- A 50-year-old man had local infiltrations a few days after an injection of lidocaine and dexamethasone (43). Prick and intradermal tests were negative after 20 minutes. However, lidocaine produced a positive patch test after 2 days, with erythema and papules.

Second-Generation Effects

Fertility

The use of in vitro fertilization has raised the question of whether the use of local anesthetics during oocyte removal is innocuous or not. Pharmacological concentrations of anesthetic agents are found in follicular fluid (44). No clinical effects have been noted, but knowledge of the behavioral effects of lidocaine on offspring in rats must cause some concern (SEDA-15, 117).

Pregnancy

It seems most unlikely that local anesthetics have any adverse effect on the fetus when used during pregnancy (45). However, the risks of local anesthetic toxicity may be greater in pregnancy because an increase in the unbound fraction of local anesthetic and physiological changes increase the transfer of local anesthetic into the central nervous system. The authors of a report of systemic symptoms in a pregnant patient suggested the precautionary use of a lower dose of local anesthetic than usual and a longer tourniquet time, to increase the safety of this technique during pregnancy (46).

Susceptibility Factors

Age

Children

Neonates and infants absorb local anesthetics more rapidly after topical application to the airways, and peak plasma concentrations can be reached within 1 minute of application. In the first few months of life they have a larger volume of distribution, reduced hepatic clearance, and lower concentrations of albumin and alpha$_1$-acid glycoprotein (47).

Drug Administration

Drug administration route

Local anesthetics can be given by many different routes, each of which has its own particular adverse effects. In this section the following routes of administration are covered:

- Brachial plexus anesthesia
- Buccal anesthesia
- Caudal anesthesia
- Cervical plexus anesthesia
- Dental anesthesia
- Digital anesthesia
- Epidural anesthesia
- Intercostal nerve anesthesia
- Interpleural anesthesia
- Intra-articular anesthesia
- Intradermal anesthesia
- Intrathecal (spinal) anesthesia
- Intravenous regional anesthesia
- Laryngeal anesthesia
- Lumbar plexus anesthesia
- Nasal anesthesia
- Neck anesthesia
- Obstetric anesthesia
- Ocular anesthesia
- Oropharyngeal anesthesia
- Otic anesthesia
- Paravertebral anesthesia
- Perianal anesthesia
- Peritonsillar anesthesia
- Respiratory anesthesia
- Sciatic nerve anesthesia
- Stellate ganglion anesthesia
- Subcutaneous anesthesia
- Submucosal anesthesia
- Urinary tract anesthesia

Brachial plexus anesthesia

The systemic complications of brachial plexus anesthesia are similar to those seen with others if sufficient drug enters the circulation. Injections outside the axillary sheath result in higher plasma concentrations of local anesthetic than intrasheath injection (SEDA-22, 135). However, several other complications are specific to this route. Local complications include hematoma and infection. Horner's syndrome, temporary phrenic nerve blockade, and peripheral neuropathies have been reported (SEDA-18, 142).

The adverse effects of ropivacaine and bupivacaine have been compared in 104 patients who received 30 ml of either 0.75% ropivacaine or 0.5% bupivacaine for subclavian perivascular brachial plexus block (48). There were similar incidences of nausea (33 and 28%), vomiting (8 and 14%), and Horner's syndrome (8 and 6%), and one patient who received bupivacaine developed a tonic-clonic generalized seizure 8 minutes after injection, suggestive of systemic toxicity.

Patient-controlled interscalene analgesia (PCIA) with ropivacaine 0.2% has been compared with patient-controlled intravenous analgesia (PCIVA) with an opioid in 35 patients after elective major shoulder surgery (49). Although hemidiaphragmatic excursion on the non-operated side was increased in the PCIA group 24 and 48 hours after the initial block, pulmonary function was similar in both groups. Pain was significantly better controlled in the PCIA group at 12 and 24 and the PCIA group had a lower incidence of nausea and vomiting (5.5 versus 60%).

Cardiovascular

Cardiovascular complications can arise from unintended stellate ganglion block (SEDA-21, 131).

- A 67-year-old man had an axillary plexus block for a right palmar fasciectomy with mepivacaine 850 mg and adrenaline 225 micrograms. Twenty minutes later he became agitated and confused and an electrocardiogram showed fast atrial fibrillation. Rapid systemic absorption of the combination of high-dose mepivacaine and adrenaline in a patient who was also taking amiodarone, sotalol, captopril, and amiloride for pre-existing cardiac disease was felt to be responsible (50).

Pulmonary embolism has been attributed to brachial plexus block.

- A 43-year-old man with end-stage renal disease became acutely hypoxic after an interscalene brachial plexus block with 35 ml of 1.5% mepivacaine for primary placement of an arteriovenous fistula in the left arm (51). He had been undergoing hemodialysis for 1 month using subclavian and internal jugular vascular catheters for temporary access. Immediately after an apparently straightforward block, his oxygen saturation fell from 99 to 85%, he complained of chest pain and shortness of breath, and he developed hemoptysis. A CT scan suggested acute pulmonary embolism.

The authors proposed that manipulations and vasodilatation related to the interscalene block may have facilitated the dislodgement of a pre-existing thrombus in the arm.

Respiratory

Large volumes (30–40 ml) of local anesthetics for interscalene block cause hemidiaphragmatic paresis in nearly all patients. An interscalene brachial plexus block in 11 volunteers using 10 ml of either 0.25% bupivacaine or 0.5% bupivacaine, both with adrenaline 1:200 000, resulted in significant impairment of lung function (forced vital capacity fell by 75% and FEV_1 by 78%) and in hemidiaphragmatic excursion in those given 0.5% bupivacaine, but not 0.25% bupivacaine (52). The authors suggested that 10 ml of 0.25% bupivacaine provides adequate anesthesia, with only occasional interference with respiratory function.

However, reducing the volume of local anesthetic (1.5% mepivacaine) from 40 to 20 ml, and applying proximal digital pressure, did not reduce the incidence or intensity of diaphragmatic paralysis during interscalene block in 20 patients, in whom arterial oxygen saturation fell significantly (53).

- A 55-year-old man with newly diagnosed non-small-cell lung cancer developed difficulty in breathing, cyanosis, agitation, and confusion, 10 minutes after interscalene supplementation of an axillary nerve block with only 3 ml of 2% mepivacaine with adrenaline (54). He was anesthetized, intubated, and ventilated. Surgery proceeded and postoperative radiographic examination of the lungs showed ipsilateral elevation of the diaphragm with reduced respiratory excursion. Phrenic nerve block after the interscalene injection was the postulated cause of the deterioration in respiratory function. He was successfully extubated at the end of the procedure.

Pneumothorax has occasionally been observed (55). The axillary technique is recommended to prevent this complication (56).

Phrenic nerve palsy, resulting in paralysis of the ipsilateral hemidiaphragm, can rarely cause severe respiratory compromise, depending on pre-existing lung dysfunction. In unpremedicated patients who underwent supraclavicular brachial plexus block for upper limb surgery, blocks were performed using a peripheral nerve stimulator and 0.5 ml/kg of bupivacaine 0.375% (57). Spirometric and ultrasonographic assessments of diaphragmatic function were made at intervals. Of 30 patients, 15 had complete paralysis of the hemidiaphragm, 5 had reduced diaphragmatic movement, and 10 had no change. Those with complete paralysis all had significant reductions in pulmonary function and those with reduced or normal movement had minimal changes. Only one of the patients had respiratory symptoms and the oxygen saturation remained unchanged. This may not be the case, however, in patients with significant pre-existing respiratory disease or in obese people; the authors therefore suggested caution in choosing this approach as a safer alternative to general anesthesia in such individuals.

Two cases of respiratory compromise after infraclavicular brachial plexus blockade have been described (58).

- An 84-year-old woman weighing 74 kg had a past history of hypertension, emphysema, and ischemic heart disease. She had an infraclavicular brachial plexus block with 40 ml (400 mg) of prilocaine 1% and 10 ml (75 mg) of ropivacaine 0.75%, and 20 minutes later developed difficulty in breathing and became desaturated. She had received midazolam 2 mg before the block.
- A 47-year-old woman with a history of hypertension, gastric reflux, and obesity was premedicated with oxazepam 10 mg and had an infraclavicular brachial plexus block with the same doses of ropivacaine and prilocaine as in the first case; 10 minutes later she developed dyspnea and became desaturated.

Each patient's symptoms settled with supplementary oxygen, and surgery proceeded uneventfully. In both instances a chest X-ray showed a raised hemidiaphragm on the side of the block, but pneumothorax was excluded. The respiratory compromise was probably caused by paresis of the ipsilateral diaphragm due to blockade of the phrenic nerve, which is likely to occur after an infraclavicular plexus block but is well tolerated in most patients. Dyspnea in these two patients may have resulted from several factors. Both had been lightly sedated with benzodiazepines (although both were alert and cooperative, so this probably had a minimal contribution). The first had emphysema, which may have been an important factor; in such patients diaphragmatic function is important for sufficient gas exchange and a 50% loss of function can result in significant impairment. The second woman was obese, and obesity is associated with a reduction in functional residual capacity and respiratory function, so she may have had reduced respiratory reserve. The authors suggested that in patients with reduced pulmonary reserve, infraclavicular brachial plexus blockade should be avoided and an axillary approach considered. In addition they speculated that a smaller volume of local anesthetic may reduce the risk of phrenic nerve blockade.

Nervous system

Neurological injury after peripheral blockade has an incidence of less than 1%. However, it has been suggested that for axillary nerve blocks, neurological damage is more likely if paresthesia is the endpoint for location of the nerve sheath, in contrast to the transarterial method. This is probably due to the increased likelihood of direct damage from a needle, intraneural injection of local anesthetic, or toxicity of the local anesthetic to the nerve (59). However, published results on this issue remain contradictory (60).

Ropivacaine is less toxic than bupivacaine. However, there have been reports of brachial plexus blockade after ropivacaine, associated with unusual symptoms of nervous system toxicity; none of the patients recalled the events and there were no subsequent sequelae (61).

- A 46-year-old man received an axillary nerve block using 40 ml of 0.5% ropivacaine with 1:200 000 adrenaline and 45 seconds later developed a sinus tachycardia and started screaming, appearing terrified. He struck out violently with all limbs and sat upright, attempting to leave the bed. The pulse oximeter reading (SpO_2) fell to 90% and his symptoms were interpreted as a seizure and treated successfully with 100% oxygen, sodium thiopental, and intubation.

- A 60-year-old woman received an interscalene block using 30 ml of 0.5% ropivacaine with 1:200 000 adrenaline. Immediately after the injection, she sat up and began screaming in a loud high-pitched voice, appearing terrified and enraged. She then attempted to get off the stretcher in an uncoordinated manner and became unresponsive to verbal commands. She had a sinus tachycardia and hypotension. Treatment with 100% oxygen and propofol was effective.
- A 76-year-old woman received an interscalene block using 20 ml of 0.75% ropivacaine with 1:400 000 adrenaline. At the end of the injection, she sat up and appeared extremely terrified; she screamed twice, fell back on the stretcher, and began moving the unblocked arm and both legs in clonic movements, remaining unresponsive to verbal command. She had a sinus tachycardia and hypertension (205/70 mmHg). The seizure abated with thiopental.

The authors suggested that these signs of anxiety, vocalization, and agitation may have been due to the administration of ropivacaine formulated exclusively as the *S*(–) enantiomer, which has a spectrum of nervous system and cardiovascular toxicity different from the racemic mixture.

Reverse arterial flow can cause nervous system toxicity, even during peripheral regional blocks with only small volumes of local anesthetic (62).

- A 47-year-old woman received an axillary brachial plexus block with 3 ml of 1% lidocaine after negative aspiration. She became dysphoric 30 seconds later, with muscle twitching in the face and distal arms, became unresponsive, and required ventilation.

During a study of 104 adults to compare the efficacy and safety of 40 ml of 0.75% ropivacaine (300 mg) and 40 ml of 0.5% bupivacaine (200 mg) for axillary plexus block, significantly more patients reported postoperative dizziness in the ropivacaine group (5 versus 0) (63). However, this occurred 4–5 hours after the injection in two patients and the day after in the other three, and was therefore unlikely to have been due to high serum concentrations. One patient developed dizziness, dysarthria, and unconsciousness, with convulsions shortly after an injection of ropivacaine, indicating an intravenous injection.

In some cases adjuvants should be considered as well as the local anesthetic after a toxic reaction (64).

- A 52-year-old woman received an axillary plexus block with 20 ml of 1% ropivacaine, clonidine 70 micrograms, and 15 ml of 1% mepivacaine with 1:400 000 adrenaline. Generalized tonic-clonic seizure activity developed, even though careful incremental aspiration was performed. She was still comatose 90 minutes later, but this was reversed by intravenous naloxone.

The authors suggested that clonidine could have been responsible for the maintenance of her unconscious state.

Axillary blockade using high-dose mepivacaine with adrenaline was performed in 50 patients, each of whom received 850 mg of mepivacaine; two patients had symptoms of toxicity associated with this combination (euphoria, dizziness, and tinnitus) 13 and 15 minutes after the procedure with doses of 14.1 and 16.4 mg/kg of mepivacaine respectively (65). One patient who received 10.9 mg/kg developed hypertension and atrial fibrillation, became agitated, and lost consciousness 12 minutes after the block was performed, and required beta-blockade and midazolam before waking up 15 minutes later. Another received 6.5 mg/kg, became light-headed, agitated, and hypertensive, and reported whole body numbness 18 minutes later, with resolution of symptoms after 10 minutes with beta-blockade. The author thought that adrenaline had probably been responsible for the reaction in the first patient. As high-dose mepivacaine did not greatly improve the quality of the block and can obviously produce serious systemic reactions, it would be prudent to limit the dose to under 10 mg/kg.

Horner's syndrome is a well-recognized complication of interscalene brachial plexus block, stellate ganglion block, and occasionally epidural blockade. It occurs when the local anesthetic reaches the cervical sympathetic trunk and is usually transient. However, persistent Horner's syndrome is a rare complication, and may represent traumatic interruption of the cervical sympathetic chain. Cases of prolonged Horner's syndrome related to prevertebral hematoma formation at the site of continuous interscalene blockade have been described (66).

- A 48-year-old obese woman had a 22G interscalene catheter inserted under local anesthesia via a short-bevel stimulating needle. Anesthesia was achieved using 0.6% ropivacaine 40 ml followed by an infusion of ropivacaine 0.2% for effective analgesia. On day 3, she reported blurred vision and a painful neck swelling. She had developed a hematoma around the catheter insertion site (confirmed by ultrasound) and had an ipsilateral Horner's syndrome including myosis, ptosis, enophthalmos, ipsilateral anhidrosis, and conjunctival hyperemia.
- An interscalene catheter was inserted in an awake 20-year-old woman for analgesia after shoulder surgery. Analgesia was achieved with ropivacaine 0.2% as a 30 ml bolus followed by an infusion of the same solution. One day later she had visual disturbance and neck swelling due to a hematoma between the prevertebral and scalene muscles.

Neither patient was taking NSAIDs, aspirin, or anticoagulants. Catheters were removed immediately on diagnosis of hematoma formation. There was no neurological or sympathetic fiber damage to the upper limb in either patient, as tested by electroneuromyography and sympathetic skin response. Remission in both cases occurred within 1 year. There has been one previous report of prolonged Horner's syndrome in the absence of any obvious technical complication (67). Further studies into the use of interscalene catheters are needed to assess their propensity to cause this rare complication.

In 60 patients receiving patient-controlled interscalene analgesia with either ropivacaine 0.2% or bupivacaine 0.15%, there was a significant reduction in hand motor function and an increased incidence of paresthesia in the bupivacaine group, with no difference in pain scores (68).

This finding contrasts with that in a comparison of epidural bupivacaine or ropivacaine, in which there was no difference in motor function between the two groups (69).

Inadvertent injection into the subarachnoid space, occasionally causing cerebral or neurological problems, is a life-threatening complication of brachial plexus anesthesia. It can also cause postdural puncture headache (SEDA-21, 131).

Interscalene block can cause paralysis of the arm.

- A 33-year-old woman received combined regional and general anesthesia for a shoulder repair (70). Preoperatively an interscalene catheter was placed uneventfully. The next day, she had almost complete paralysis of the arm with hypesthesia of dermatomes C5–7. The symptoms persisted and 4.5 months later, during surgical exploration of the brachial plexus, electrical stimulation of the three trunks was possible and there were electrophysiological signs of recovery. Despite extensive neurophysiological tests a clear cause could not be established and there was no improvement at 2 years.

Sensory systems

- An intolerable metallic taste appeared and disappeared in a 48-year-old woman within hours of infusion of bupivacaine via an axillary catheter, and its severity changed with the rate of infusion (71). The mechanism was postulated to be through sodium channels or taste bud disturbances.

Psychological, psychiatric

- A 59-year-old woman, grade ASA I, had psychiatric effects associated with local anesthetic toxicity after receiving bupivacaine 50 mg and mepivacaine 75 mg for an axillary plexus block. She complained of dizziness and a "near death experience" (72).

Hematologic

Methemoglobinemia has been reported in a woman who received a combination of local anesthetics (73).

- A 60-year-old woman with medical problems including severe coronary vascular disease and anemia, taking multiple medications, including isosorbide dinitrate, received axillary plexus blockade with bupivacaine 150 mg + 10 ml of 1% lidocaine injected into the operative field; 90 minutes later her SpO_2 fell to 85–89% on oxygen 10 l/minute. She became drowsy, disoriented, and tachypneic, and an arterial blood gas showed a metabolic acidosis and a methemoglobin concentration of 6.4%. Her mental status improved 10 minutes after methylthioninium chloride and sodium bicarbonate; her SpO2 rose to 96% on air, her methemoglobin concentration fell to 1.6%, and her acidosis partly resolved.

The authors assumed that displacement of lidocaine from protein binding by bupivacaine, in combination with metabolic acidosis and treatment with nitrates, had caused methemoglobinemia.

Susceptibility factors

Mepivacaine toxicity has been studied in 10 patients with end-stage chronic renal insufficiency undergoing vascular access surgery (74). These patients represent a high-risk group for general anesthesia, as they often have concomitant coronary artery disease, hypertension, and diabetes. Brachial plexus block is often used: as well as avoiding systemic effects, it enhances regional blood flow. However, high doses of local anesthetic are required, and this block carries one of the highest rates of seizures. In this study, following axillary block with mepivacaine 650 mg, plasma concentrations were greater than the threshold of 6 micrograms/ml, above which signs of nervous system toxicity reportedly occur. The authors suggested that the absence of nervous system signs may have been due to slow systemic absorption of the local anesthetic. Peak concentrations occurred after 60–90 minutes, but were still high at 150 minutes, raising the question of more prolonged monitoring after these blocks.

Buccal anesthesia

Persistent hiccup, paralysis of cranial nerves, and systemic toxicity are the main complications of local anesthesia in the mouth (75–77). Trismus has been seldom reported (78–80).

Caudal anesthesia

In a study in 60 anesthetized children undergoing minor subumbilical surgery caudal blocks, 0.2% ropivacaine, 0.25% racemic bupivacaine, and 0.25% levobupivacaine (all 1 ml/kg) were compared (81). All the blocks were successful in terms of intraoperative and early postoperative analgesia. Ropivacaine, but not levobupivacaine, was associated with less motor block during the first postoperative hour compared with racemic bupivacaine. However, the lower concentration of ropivacaine will have biased this result.

Caudal block with bupivacaine in children provides adequate analgesia in the early postoperative period, but additional analgesia is often required as the block wears off. Two studies have looked at adjuvants to prolong the analgesic effect.

The first was a randomized, controlled trial in 60 boys undergoing unilateral herniorrhaphy (82). They received 0.25% bupivacaine 1 ml/kg or the same dose of bupivacaine plus 1.5 mg/kg tramadol, or tramadol 1.5 mg/kg alone made up to the same volume. Caudal administration of bupivacaine plus tramadol resulted in more effective analgesia, with a longer period without demand for additional analgesia postoperatively without increases in any adverse effects. The second was a study of the addition of midazolam to caudal bupivacaine in 30 children undergoing genitourinary surgery (83). They randomly received 0.25% bupivacaine 0.5 ml/kg or the same dose of bupivacaine plus midazolam 50 micrograms/kg. There were no untoward events in either group. Fewer required additional analgesia in the first 6 hours postoperatively in the bupivacaine plus midazolam group than with bupivacaine alone: 27% compared with 60%. Midazolam prolonged analgesia with no increase in adverse effects.

In 165 children receiving caudal anesthesia with fentanyl 1 mg/kg and bupivacaine 4 mg/kg, there were adverse effects in only six, two of whom required postoperative ventilation. This was felt to be due to their pathology and not the anesthetic. However, there was no comment on the presence or absence of specific local anesthetic adverse effects, and an unusually high dose of bupivacaine was used, 4 mg/kg, twice that recommended by the manufacturers and greater than that used by most pediatric anesthetists (2.5–3 mg/kg) (SEDA-20, 124).

Caudal bupivacaine has been successfully combined with clonidine, ketamine, diamorphine, and buprenorphine, with increased duration of anesthesia and a low incidence of adverse effects (SEDA-20, 124) (SEDA-21, 131).

Awake regional anesthesia for inguinal hernia repair in former preterm infants has been suggested, in order to avoid life-threatening respiratory complications that can occur after general anesthesia. Caudal anesthesia is becoming a more popular technique for this purpose. To prolong the duration of anesthesia and to reduce the postoperative need for analgesics in these infants, caudal clonidine has been considered useful.

- A former preterm infant had two awake caudal anesthetics for herniotomy within 3 weeks (84). The first was uneventful with bupivacaine 0.25% at 35 weeks of age. At 38 weeks, the baby had intraoperative and postoperative bouts of apnea after inadvertent administration of bupivacaine 0.125% plus clonidine.

There has been a report of T wave changes on the electrocardiogram during caudal administration of local anesthetics (85).

- A 4.2 kg 2-month-old baby was given a caudal injection under general anesthesia for an inguinal hernia repair. A mixture of 1% lidocaine 2 ml and 0.25% bupivacaine 2 ml was injected. Every 1 ml was preceded by an aspiration test and followed by observation for electrocardiographic changes for 20 seconds. On administration of the third 1 ml dose, there was a significant increase in T wave amplitude. The aspiration test was repeated and was positive for blood. The caudal injection was stopped and the electrocardiogram returned to normal after 35 seconds. The baby remained cardiovascularly stable with no postoperative sequelae.

Previous reports have suggested that an increase in T wave amplitude could result from inadvertent intravascular administration of adrenaline-containing local anesthetics. This is the first case report of local anesthetics alone causing significant T wave changes.

Inadvertent dural puncture is a recognized complication in up to 1% of caudal anesthetics. It can be due to excessive needle insertion or sacral abnormalities. Potentially serious consequences, such as total spinal anesthesia, can result (SEDA-21, 131).

In eight episodes of toxic methemoglobinemia in seven premature infants after the combination of caudal anesthesia (prilocaine 5.4–6.7 mg/kg) and Emla cream (prilocaine 12.5 mg) for herniotomy, the highest methemoglobin concentration 5.5 hours after anesthesia was 31% (86). All the infants were symptomatic, with mottled skin, pallor, cyanosis, and poor peripheral perfusion. The most severe symptoms occurred at 3–8 hours and disappeared within 10–20 hours. The authors stressed the importance of recognizing the poor tolerance of premature infants to methemoglobinemia and that whereas topical prilocaine is relatively safe, caudal administration is not.

Cervical plexus anesthesia

Nervous system

Deep cervical plexus block can cause ipsilateral phrenic nerve palsy. A patient with pre-existing respiratory disease and a contralateral raised hemidiaphragm developed hypoxia and respiratory distress when given 20 ml of plain bupivacaine 0.375% by this route for carotid endarterectomy (87). Local anesthetic spread resulted in presumed stellate ganglion block, which caused nasal congestion and aggravated the respiratory distress. The symptoms resolved without intubation, but the authors advised against deep cervical plexus block in patients with diaphragmatic motion abnormalities or chronic respiratory disease.

Nerve palsies can occur during deep cervical plexus anesthesia.

- A woman complained of being unable to clear secretions effectively from her throat, had a paroxysm of coughing, and developed a large neck hematoma requiring surgical re-exploration (88).
- A 71-year-old man complained of difficulty in breathing and was desaturated on pulse oximetry for 5 minutes after cervical plexus blockade (89). He required tracheal intubation, was ventilated for 110 minutes, and was then successfully extubated. It was thought that the most likely diagnosis was cardiorespiratory failure exacerbated by phrenic nerve blockade.
- A 67-year-old man developed transient hemiparesis and facial nerve palsy before becoming unconscious and apneic 10 minutes after a right cervical plexus block (89). His trachea was intubated without the need for anesthetic drugs and he was ventilated. Hypotension was treated with intravenous ephedrine. He woke up, started breathing, and was extubated 75 minutes later. The authors postulated brainstem anesthesia following accidental injection of local anesthetic into a dural cuff as a cause of loss of consciousness.

Hemidiaphragmatic paralysis can occur with cervical plexus anesthesia and can be particularly risky in cases of pre-existing airways obstruction (90).

Infiltration of even small doses of a local anesthetic in the region of the carotid artery is likely to cause nervous system toxicity if injected intra-arterially (91).

- A 76-year-old man had already received a deep and superficial cervical plexus block for an awake carotid endarterectomy. One hour later, during manipulation of the carotid artery discomfort was treated with infiltration of 1 ml of 0.5% lidocaine in that region. Immediately he became unresponsive, with generalized tonic-clonic seizure activity of the face and arms. He was given 100% oxygen and within 30 seconds the seizure terminated spontaneously with no sequelae.

This demonstrates the requirement for constant vigilance in a patient undergoing awake carotid endarterectomy.

Dental anesthesia

Dental anesthesia is generally safe and effective. However, it can cause adverse effects, ranging from mild to severe, perhaps a reflection of the number of dental anesthesias performed.

Systemic effects, such as dizziness, tachycardia, agitation, nausea, tremor, syncope, seizures, and bronchospasm, are a definite risk with local anesthesia in a vascular area. A wide range of patients present for dental surgery, and it is important that an adequate medical history be taken and accurate doses calculated on an individual basis. Low concentrations of adrenaline should be used.

Complication rates increase with premedication at home, and pre-existing disease or risk factors, such as pregnancy, cardiovascular disease, and allergies. Articaine and lidocaine with epinephrine 1:200 000 were associated with a low incidence of complications (3.1 and 0%), whilst mepivacaine and articaine with adrenaline 1:100 000 caused the most frequent complications (7.2 and 6.1%) (SEDA-22, 135).

Cardiovascular

Acute hypertension leading to myocardial infarction and pulmonary edema has been described after the use of mepivacaine with levonordefrin (92).

Nervous system

An unexplained case of permanent neurological deficit, consisting of left facial palsy, right sensorineural hearing loss, gait ataxia, and hemisensory loss in the body and face, has been described after inferior alveolar nerve block (93).

Facial paralysis is occasionally reported and is not necessarily due to poor technique; in one case vascular spasm seemed to provide an explanation (SED-12, 252).

- An 8-year-old girl received prilocaine for a dental procedure performed under 70% oxygen/30% nitrous oxide (94). The dose of 288 mg was 2.7 times higher than the recommended safe dose of 6 mg/kg. Toward the end of the procedure, she became unconscious and had a convulsion.

Two reviews have highlighted the fact that the degree and incidence of neurological damage after dental anesthesia is probably underestimated. Some drugs, such as articaine and prilocaine, seem to cause a higher incidence of paresthesia than others (SEDA-20, 124).

In seven subjects articaine with adrenaline caused distortion of lingual nerve function with effects on vowel pronunciation and therefore the potential to impair speech (95).

- A 49-year-old man developed uvular deviation as a result of palatal muscle paralysis following intraoral mandibular block of the inferior alveolar nerve with 1.8 ml of 2% lidocaine with adrenaline 1 in 100 000 (96). A few minutes after injection he had swallowing difficulties and a foreign body sensation in his throat. There was paralysis of the velum palatinum, with deviation of the uvula towards the non-paralysed side opposite the point of anesthetic infiltration. This resolved after the anesthetic had worn off.

The authors suggest that a high inferior alveolar nerve block can easily affect the mandibular nerve if the anesthetic solution diffuses to the internal trunk of the third trigeminal branch and the supply to the tensor veli palatini.

Sensory systems

Adverse ocular effects, such as ptosis, are on record (SEDA-15, 118). Transient dizziness, diplopia, and partial blindness have been reported after the entry of lidocaine with adrenaline into the ophthalmic artery following mandibular block (97). A similar case after posterior alveolar block resulted in dizziness and diplopia for 3 hours when the patient stood up, possibly due to the entry of local anesthetic into the ophthalmic artery (SEDA-22, 135).

Ophthalmological complications after intraoral anesthesia occurred in 14 cases over 15 years (98). The most common symptom was diplopia. Three patients developed Horner's syndrome, with ptosis, enophthalmos, and miosis on the same side as the anesthesia. Three patients developed mydriasis and ptosis. There was complete resolution in all patients. The authors postulated that direct diffusion of anesthetic solution from the pterygomaxillary fossa through the sphenomaxillary cavity to the orbit had caused the ophthalmological effects.

- A 45-year-old man developed temporary monocular blindness, ophthalmoplegia, ptosis, and mydriasis immediately after a mandibular block injection (99). Unidentified intra-arterial injection into the maxillary artery, with backflow of the local anesthetic solution to the middle meningeal artery was the postulated cause.

Additives

Additives in local anesthetic solutions can cause allergic reactions (100).

- A 34-year-old man developed swelling and redness of the face after receiving lidocaine as Lignospan® for dental treatment. Patch testing showed allergic contact dermatitis due to the preservative disodium ethylenediamine tetra-acetic acid (EDTA).

Digital anesthesia

Digital anesthesia with 1% lidocaine plus adrenaline was performed on 23 patients for surgery to finger injuries; 11 patients received adrenaline 1:200 000, and 12 received 1:100 000 (101). A digital tourniquet was also used, but no patient developed ischemic symptoms. The authors discussed the usefulness of adrenaline as an additive to local anesthetic solutions in prolonging regional block, reducing the dose of local anesthetic required. They stated that an extensive search of the literature had revealed no sound clinical evidence to support the widely held opinion that adrenaline contributes to the risk of gangrene when it is used in digital blocks.

Epidural anesthesia

The accidental transformation of epidural to subarachnoid block can be dramatic, and tracheal intubation and ventilatory support may be necessary (102). Severe hypotension can result after inadvertent intrathecal local anesthesia (SEDA-21, 131). In women in labor, fetal bradycardia can occur. Postdural puncture headache can also be a sign of catheter migration.

Long-term epidural catheters can be highly effective in the management of chronic pain of malignant and non-malignant origin, but they can also cause complications. Infection and extravasation of fluid to the paraspinal tissue resulting in inadequate analgesia have been described in a patient with non-Hodgkin's lymphoma (103). Another patient with non-Hodgkin's lymphoma had a tunnelled thoracic epidural for analgesia and presented with spinal cord compression. Laminectomy showed a mass consisting of white chalk-like drug-related precipitate around the catheter tip. As the solvent for bupivacaine contains sodium hydroxide and sodium chloride, the authors assumed that the mass was a precipitate of sodium hydroxide (104).

- A 1-year-old boy inadvertently received ropivacaine 6 mg intravenously over 2 hours when his epidural infusion was incorrectly connected to his intravenous cannula (40). He had already received ropivacaine 28 mg via his epidural catheter. He suffered no overt adverse effects.

In a dose-finding study for the combination of 0.2% ropivacaine with fentanyl for thoracic epidural analgesia in 224 patients undergoing major abdominal surgery, each received fentanyl in concentrations of 0, 1, 2, or 4 micrograms/ml; effective pain relief was provided by all the combinations and the degree of motor block was low overall and did not differ significantly among the groups (105). Hypotension was most common during the first postoperative 24 hours and was most frequent in those given fentanyl 4 micrograms/ml. Although the combination with fentanyl 4 micrograms/ml improved the quality of analgesia, there was a higher incidence of adverse effects, such as hypotension, nausea, and pruritus.

Patient-controlled epidural analgesia is increasingly being used, as it reduces the need for adjustment of epidural infusion rates by anesthetic personnel. In a retrospective survey of 1057 patients who received postoperative patient-controlled epidural analgesia using bupivacaine 0.1% plus fentanyl 5 micrograms/ml, on the first postoperative day 93% of the patients had adequate analgesia and 96% reported no nausea; two patients had an episode of respiratory depression and one patient was unrousable (106). Hypotension occurred in 4.3%, but there were no cases of epidural hematoma or abscess. Despite these adverse events, the authors concluded that patient-controlled epidural analgesia was effective and safe on surgical wards. The large amount of fentanyl in the solution they used is most probably the reason for the rare, potentially life-threatening adverse effects.

The amount of bupivacaine with fentanyl used in patient-controlled epidural analgesia was significantly less than with a continuous infusion of the same mixture in a group of 54 patients (mean age 71 years) after total knee arthroplasty (107). However, 10% of the patients were too confused to use the PCEA device. Despite the advantages of analgesic dosage reductions, a constant infusion may prove more appropriate in this age group.

Patient-controlled epidural analgesia (0.05% bupivacaine and fentanyl 4 micrograms/ml) has been studied prospectively in 1030 patients requiring postoperative analgesia (108). Pruritus was the most common adverse effect, with an incidence of 17%, with two susceptibility factors: age (under 58 years) and increased consumption of analgesia (over 9 ml/hour). The incidence of nausea was 15% and of sedation 13%; female sex was a slight risk factor for both. Hypotension had an incidence of 6.8% and motor block of 2%; lumbar placement of the epidural catheter was the strongest risk factor. Respiratory depression occurred in 0.3%.

The effects of single-dose epidural analgesia with lidocaine and morphine have been studied in 60 women undergoing elective cesarean section (109). The patients received morphine sulfate 4 mg and 2% lidocaine 18–20 ml. Four patients proceeded to general anesthesia owing to failure of the epidural block to reach T6, 48% of patients complained of discomfort during surgery, and 23% needed supplementary analgesia. Perioperative adverse effects were hypotension 29%, bradycardia 3.6%, and shivering 5.4%. Postoperative adverse effects were pruritus 45% and nausea and vomiting 35%. Apgar scores at 1 and 5 minutes were 8 or over. At 2 hours and 24 hours, two babies had transient tachypnea and one had mild respiratory distress. Maternal and neonatal venous concentrations of morphine, measured at delivery, were low. The authors recommended this technique for elective cesarean section in uncomplicated obstetric patients. This study had no control group and reported a high incidence of unwanted effects and a high perioperative failure rate. Mean analgesic duration of morphine was reported as 24 hours. However, 75% of patients required additional analgesia after 12 hours. There was no record of the incidence of postoperative maternal respiratory depression.

Comparative studies

After thoracotomy, 106 patients received a thoracic epidural infusion of either 0.1% or 0.2% bupivacaine, both with fentanyl 10 micrograms/ml, compared with epidural fentanyl alone; there was no difference in the number of episodes of postoperative hypotension (systolic pressure below 90 mmHg) or in the number of interventions for postoperative hypotension, but intraoperative vasopressors were used significantly more in the bupivacaine groups (110). In addition, two patients given 0.2% bupivacaine reported slight weakness of both hands and another a right-sided Horner's syndrome and weakness of the right hand. There was a similar incidence of nausea and pruritus in all the groups; however, the incidence of respiratory depression with fentanyl was high (4.2%).

Random allocation of 150 women in labor to either an intermittent epidural bolus, a continuous epidural infusion, or patient-controlled epidural analgesia with 0.125% bupivacaine and sufentanil 0.5 micrograms/ml resulted in significantly more frequent motor blockade with continuous infusion compared with intermittent boluses (22 versus 4%), with similar frequencies of pruritus, hypotension, and high sensory level in each group (111).

In 52 patients who received either epidural bupivacaine (0.10–0.28 mg/kg/hour) or lidocaine (0.44–0.98 mg/kg/hour), both with epidural morphine, there were no significant differences in the times to mobilize, motor function (as measured by the Bromage grade), and the incidence of hypotension (112). Most of the patients had no motor blockade, and the Bromage grade did not help predict which of them could be mobilized.

In 90 parturients who received epidural analgesia during labor with bolus administration of either 10 ml of 0.125% bupivacaine or 0.125% ropivacaine, each with sufentanil 7.5 micrograms, there were comparable onset times and duration of analgesia in the two groups, but patients given ropivacaine had significantly less motor blockade after the third and subsequent epidural injections compared with those given bupivacaine: 93% of those given ropivacaine had no motor impairment compared with 66% of those given bupivacaine (113). There were no differences in hemodynamic effects and pruritus.

An epidural infusion of 0.2% ropivacaine plus sufentanil has been compared with 0.175% bupivacaine plus sufentanil in 86 patients postoperatively after major gastrointestinal surgery; there was no statistically significant difference in the incidence of adverse effects (respiratory depression, sedation, nausea, vomiting, pruritus, and motor blockade), but those given ropivacaine mobilized more quickly (114).

In 60 women who underwent elective cesarean section under epidural anesthesia, 0.5% levobupivacaine or 0.5% bupivacaine (30 ml) were equally efficacious in terms of anesthesia (115). The incidence and severity of motor blockade, hypotension, changes in QT interval, nausea, and vomiting were not significantly different, and neither were the neonatal Apgar scores.

Drug combinations are often used in epidural anesthesia to enhance the analgesic effect and minimize adverse effects. Continuous epidural analgesia (0.125% bupivacaine 12.5 mg/hour and morphine 0.25 mg/hour) has been compared with patient-controlled analgesia (morphine) in 60 patients after major abdominal surgery. Analgesia was superior in the epidural group, satisfaction and sedation scores were similar in both groups, whilst episodes of moderate nocturnal postoperative hypoxemia (SaO_2 85–90%) were more frequent in the epidural group (116).

The addition of opioids to local anesthetic to improve the efficacy of epidural analgesia for cesarean section has been advocated (109,117). A test dose of lidocaine 60 mg was given to 24 patients undergoing elective cesarean section, followed by either bupivacaine 45 mg or bupivacaine 45 mg plus fentanyl 50 micrograms (117). Sensory blockade to T6 was achieved in both groups, but pain scores were significantly lower in the fentanyl group. Rescue fentanyl on uterine exteriorization was required in 40% of the control group, but in none in the fentanyl group. There were no significant differences in adverse effects, specifically pruritus, hypotension, nausea and vomiting, maternal respiratory depression, and Apgar scores.

Cardiovascular

Hypotension is a frequent adverse effect of epidural anesthesia. In a comparison of the effects of bupivacaine and ropivacaine in 60 women undergoing cesarean section, 90% had a fall in blood pressure to below 90 mmHg, or by more than 30% of baseline (118).

Abrupt onset of arterial hypotension is also a complication of cervical epidural anesthesia, particularly in elderly patients (119). However, supplementation with adrenaline in this high-risk group is no longer defensible; it is better to be cautious with dosage and to monitor the patient closely.

- Severe hypotension during a lumbar epidural anesthetic in a 61-year-old woman taking amitriptyline was refractory to high doses of ephedrine and other indirect alpha-adrenergic agents (120). It eventually responded to one dose of noradrenaline 200 micrograms, illustrating the importance of the choice of vasopressor for treating hypotension in the presence of chronic tricyclic antidepressant use.
- A 27-year-old woman developed significant myocardial depression and pulmonary edema after administration of 5 ml of bupivacaine 0.5% via an epidural catheter (121). The bupivacaine followed a test dose of 3 ml lidocaine 2%.

Although initial aspiration on the epidural catheter was negative, the most likely explanation must be inadvertent intravascular administration of lidocaine and bupivacaine.

Unusually, a mother and her child died after repeated administration of a local anesthetic for cesarean section; pulmonary edema was believed to have been the cause (122).

Intracardiac conduction disturbances should not be considered as absolute contraindications to epidural anesthesia: there were only nine cases of sinus bradycardia, easily reversed with atropine sulfate, in 66 patients (123). However, rare cases of complete heart block and complete left bundle branch block have occurred (SEDA-21, 132) (124).

Unexpected cardiopulmonary arrest can result from accidental dural puncture during epidural blockade (SEDA-22, 136).

- Asystolic cardiac arrest has been described in a 55-year-old man who underwent partial hepatectomy under combined general and epidural anesthesia (125). During postoperative recovery he developed asystole followed by ventricular fibrillation. Resuscitation was unsuccessful.

The authors concluded that in the absence of any other abnormality the arrest had been the result of an autonomic imbalance due to spreading sympathetic block, although other postoperative causes of death should not be discarded.

Respiratory

Respiratory depression was noted in 0.24% of patients in a Chinese series of 10 978 epidural blocks (SED-12, 254) (126). Direct paralysis of respiration probably plays an important role. Respiratory depression with adverse cardiovascular effects after miscalculated dose requirements or a misplaced catheter has also been described (SEDA-22, 136).

In 15 patients receiving lidocaine 300 mg plus adrenaline by cervical epidural injection, the upper cervical nerve roots C3, 4, and 5 were anesthetized. None of the patients had pre-existing pulmonary disease. Only one had symptoms of impaired pulmonary function at 20 minutes after epidural, and complained of dyspnea, with a reduction in maximum inspiratory pressure, FEV_1, FVC, and SpO_2. Four patients had a bradycardia requiring atropine, eight complained of nausea, and one developed hypotension requiring ephedrine. At 20 minutes after the epidural, all the patients had a maximum reduction in FEV_1 and FVC, ranging from 12 to 16% of preanesthetic measurements. The authors felt that as the maximum inspiratory pressure was virtually unchanged, this suggested that the motor function of the phrenic nerve was mostly intact, despite analgesia of the C3, 4, and 5 dermatomes (127).

Nervous system

Peripheral paresthesia, in 1.13% of patients in a Chinese series (SED-12, 254) (126) and 0.16% of patients in a Japanese study of 15 884 epidurals (128), is the most frequent neurological deficit attributed to spinal and epidural analgesia.

High spinal block has previously been reported as a rare complication of epidural anesthesia.

- A 31-year-old woman in labor had an epidural catheter sited at L3/4 (129). A test dose of 0.25% bupivacaine 10 ml was followed 90 minutes later by another 10 ml. After a further 90 minutes she required cesarean section, had a block to T7, and was topped up with 0.75% ropivacaine 10 ml. Within minutes she developed arm weakness, and over the next 15 minutes developed further ascending block requiring intubation. Three hours later the block had regressed to T8 and she had no further complications.

The cause was thought to be subdural injection, although other mechanisms could not be excluded; for example the catheter could have been partly intrathecal and the ultimate distribution of the dose could have been related to the speed of injection or catheter migration before the final dose was given.

Lumbar extradural analgesia with bupivacaine increases intracranial pressure in some patients, apparently those who already have some reduced intracranial compliance, and who may be at risk (130). A sudden increase in intracranial pressure, due to an increased volume in the caudal space, can precipitate respiratory arrest because of direct midbrain stimulation.

- A watershed cerebral infarct with subsequent full recovery occurred in a 70-year-old man 8 hours after a hypotensive event following an incremental bolus of 1% lidocaine 10 ml via an established epidural catheter (131).

A cause-and-effect relation cannot be established in such cases.

Epidural anesthesia can mask a neurological deficit, such as nerve compression of the femoral nerve and lateral femoral cutaneous nerve of the thigh from the lithotomy position (SEDA-22, 137).

- Neurological effects after accidental intravenous injection of a large dose of levobupivacaine (142 mg) have been described during epidural anesthesia (132).
- A 77-year-old woman had epidural anesthesia, following negative aspiration, with a 3 ml test dose of 0.75% levobupivacaine with 1:200 000 adrenaline and then incremental doses up to a total of 17 ml of 0.75% levobupivacaine. During the final 5 ml of injection, she became disoriented and drowsy, with slurred speech, immediately followed by excitation with shouting and writhing about. She was given thiopental for seizure prophylaxis with high-flow oxygen, and the excitatory signs abated. The catheter was withdrawn 1 cm and blood was freely aspirated. The serum levobupivacaine concentration 14 minutes later was 2.7 micrograms/ml.

Transient radicular irritation

Transient radicular irritation has been reported (SEDA-21, 130) (SEDA-22, 137).

- A 38-year-old woman underwent cystoscopy and urethral dilatation in the lithotomy position under continuous epidural anesthesia at the L3–4 interspace with 3 ml of 1.5% lidocaine with adrenaline 1:200 000 as a test dose, followed by a total of 15 ml of 2% lidocaine with adrenaline 1:200 000 in incremental doses (133). The operation was uneventful, but 4 hours later she developed severe bilateral buttock and posterior leg pain, described as "deep, aching, and excruciating," worse when immobile, and better when standing; there were no other symptoms and ibuprofen gave immediate relief.

The authors stressed that transient radicular irritation can occur after epidural administration, despite the lower concentrations of lidocaine in the cerebrospinal fluid.

- Transient neurological symptoms have been reported in two parturients who received lidocaine 45 mg with adrenaline 5 micrograms/ml as a test dose followed by bupivacaine (134). One patient received a single dose of bupivacaine 12.5 mg and the other received a total of 62 mg bupivacaine administered as two 5 ml and one 3 ml bolus of 0.25% bupivacaine followed by an infusion of 0.125% bupivacaine at 5 ml/hour for 4 hours 40 minutes. Both patients later developed reversible burning lower back, buttock pain, and leg pain; there was nothing to suggest intrathecal administration of local anesthetic in either case. Both patients gave birth in the lithotomy position, which may have been contributory.
- Severe burning pain in the buttocks, thighs, and calves has been described in a 5-year-old boy who was given 0.25% bupivacaine and morphine epidurally for perioperative and postoperative analgesia (135).

Two unexplained cases of back and leg pain have been separately described (SEDA-20, 125).

Motor block

Prolonged profound motor block occurred in two patients using patient-controlled epidural analgesia with 0.1% ropivacaine subsequent to spinal bupivacaine for cesarean section (136). One of them developed pressure sores on both heels. The authors hypothesized that epidural ropivacaine may interact with intrathecal bupivacaine to prolong its effects and advised caution when this combination is used, as unexpected motor block can ensue.

The optimal concentration of lumbar epidural ropivacaine in terms of adverse effects and quality of analgesia has been studied in 30 patients using patient-controlled epidural analgesia after lower abdominal surgery (137). Each solution provided comparable analgesia, but motor block was significantly more common and more intense with 0.2% ropivacaine + 4 micrograms/ml fentanyl than with 0.1% ropivacaine + 2 micrograms/ml fentanyl or 0.05% ropivacaine + 1 microgram/ml fentanyl. The amount of ropivacaine used by the 0.1% ropivacaine group was significantly higher than in the other two groups, implying that the concentration rather than the amount of ropivacaine is a primary determinant of motor block with patient-controlled epidural analgesia. The authors recommended the use of ropivacaine in concentrations under 0.2% to reduce motor blockade while still providing effective analgesia.

Epidural solutions containing 0.125% levobupivacaine with and without fentanyl 4 micrograms/ml produced a greater degree of motor blockade only in the first 6 hours of patient-controlled epidural analgesia compared with fentanyl alone in groups of 22 patients after total hip or knee arthroplasty (138).

- An 85-year-old woman undergoing elective right total knee replacement had prolonged motor blockade of her left leg when her epidural ropivacaine (0.2% at 8–10 ml/hour) infusion was discontinued on the third postoperative day; normal motor function had returned by the sixth postoperative day (139).

Paraplegia can result, and can be prevented by early recognition, appropriate investigation, and immediate surgical intervention.

- Delayed onset, prolonged coma, and flaccid quadriplegia occurred in a 22-year-old woman 2 hours after an injection of fentanyl 100 micrograms and 10 ml bupivacaine 0.25%, given in divided doses (4, 3, and 3 ml) via an epidural catheter (140). At the time of the initial attempt at insertion she had complained of severe cervico-occipital pain with loss of resistance to air injection. Despite negative aspiration of CSF, the physician suspected intrathecal injection of air and abandoned the attempt at epidural catheter placement at that level. An epidural catheter was successfully inserted one level higher. Within 1 hour of the original epidural injection, she developed hypotension requiring ephedrine, and a surprisingly high sensory block to T6 with profound lower limb motor blockade. This progressed 2 hours later to upper limb weakness, with respiratory failure requiring intubation and ventilation. She remained unconscious for 9 hours after the initial intubating dose of thiopental. She was able to move all of her limbs 26 hours later and was successfully extubated 43 hours later.

In this case the authors felt that although the initial picture looked like the effects of subdural injection of bupivacaine and fentanyl, the prolonged coma with high motor blockade was more reminiscent of total spinal injection. They postulated that delayed total spinal anesthesia had occurred in this patient as a result of the epidural administration of a large quantity of bupivacaine and fentanyl via a hole made in the dura during the first attempt at epidural insertion.

Accidental subdural block can also lead to rapidly developing high block, patchy block, and symptoms such as myoclonus and anxiety (SEDA-20, 125) (SEDA-22, 136).

Total spinal anesthesia

Permanent or temporary deficits of spinal cord function are caused either by cord ischemia after arterial hypotension, or by cord compression due to an epidural or subdural hematoma or infection, or injury to the spinal cord and nerve roots as a consequence of needle puncture, introduction of a catheter, or chemical irritation.

Total spinal anesthesia is a potentially life-threatening complication of epidural anesthesia.

- A 68-year-old man developed total spinal anesthesia after the administration of 20 ml of ropivacaine 1% without a prior test dose via an epidural catheter, which was inadvertently placed intrathecally (83). Initial aspiration of both the Touhy needle and the catheter failed to identify the intrathecal position of the catheter. The patient noted weakness in his right leg immediately after the end of the injection. This was followed by weakness in his right arm, asystole, apnea, and loss of consciousness. Ventricular escape beats were noted and sinus rhythm returned after mask ventilation with 100% oxygen and the administration of atropine 1 mg and ephedrine 50 mg. He was able to open his eyes, but remained apneic and was therefore intubated and ventilated. Cardiovascular stability was maintained with incremental boluses of ephedrine to a total of 60 mg. He regained consciousness and was successfully extubated 145 minutes later. All sensory and motor deficits had resolved within 8 hours and no neurological deficit or transient neurological symptoms were detected 5 days later.

This complication emphasizes the fact that aspiration is not sufficient to identify an intrathecal catheter position and that a large dose of a local anesthetic should never be administered without a prior test dose.

- Total spinal anesthesia was suspected in a 46-year-old man who was found unconscious and apneic with no palpable cardiac output 20 minutes after a high thoracic (T2/3) epidural injection of 3 ml lidocaine 1% and 3 ml bupivacaine 0.125% (141). Following initial cardiopulmonary resuscitation he was admitted to the intensive care unit, where treatment included mechanical lung ventilation, thiamylal infusion, and cooling to a core temperature of 33–34°C. The thiamylal was withdrawn after 17 days and he was warmed and successfully extubated the next day. He was discharged after a further 4 months of rehabilitation with no relevant neurological consequences.

Horner's syndrome

Horner's syndrome (miosis, ptosis, anhidrosis, and vasodilatation, with increased temperature of the affected side) can result from epidural anesthesia. A report of Horner's syndrome due to a thoracic epidural catheter has highlighted the fact that small doses of local anesthetic can block the sympathetic fibers to the face, particularly when the catheter tip is close to T2 (142). The same symptoms have been reported after obstetric epidural anesthesia (143).

Horner's syndrome has been reported after lumbar epidural block in two other patients who were having lumbar epidural anesthesia for chronic pain treatment (144). The authors suggested that this complication had probably occurred through anatomical changes in the epidural space, leading to a high degree of sympathetic blockade.

A left-sided Horner's syndrome has been reported following a lumbar epidural with ropivacaine for cesarean section (145). The symptoms resolved after 5 hours. The most likely cause was high sympathetic block, possibly facilitated by left lateral positioning, leading to cephalad spread of the local anesthetic. The authors also wondered whether the physicochemical properties of ropivacaine favor its effect on sympathetic fibers over bupivacaine.

Metabolism
A small reduction in glucose concentrations, rarely leading to hypoglycemic coma, can occur (SEDA-16, 130). This effect is in keeping with the finding that the catabolic stress response to surgery may be suppressed by epidural analgesia (SED-12, 254) (146). However, in one study, thoracic epidural administration produced a degree of hyperglycemia (SED-12, 252) (147).

- Symptomatic hypoglycemia occurred in a healthy 30-year-old primigravida after a second 5 ml bolus of 0.25% bupivacaine administered epidurally during labor (148). She developed an altered mental state, which responded rapidly to 50 ml of 50% dextrose administered intravenously.

Urinary tract
Epidural anesthesia increases the risk of urinary retention (149).

Musculoskeletal
Occasionally orthopedic patients have developed compartment syndrome postoperatively during epidural infusions of bupivacaine/fentanyl mixtures. However, although "aggressive analgesia" was blamed for the resulting disasters, there seems to have been a remarkable lack of adequate pressure area care, correct positioning, and regular review of both patients and splints (SEDA-22, 136).

Infection risk
Contamination of catheters, with subsequent clinical infection, is a potential hazard of epidural analgesia. But not every suspected infection is what it seems; aseptic meningitis has been described after an intradural injection of bupivacaine with methylprednisolone acetate (150).

Death
Inadvertent intravenous administration, due to the accidental placement of an epidural catheter in a vein, is a high-risk complication; deaths have been reported (151).

Pregnancy
Patient-controlled epidural analgesia using either 0.125% ropivacaine with fentanyl 2 micrograms/ml or 0.125% bupivacaine with fentanyl 2 micrograms/ml was studied in 50 patients during labor. Significantly more patients receiving bupivacaine developed motor blockade; 68% of patients in the bupivacaine group developed minimal motor block (Bromage score = 1), while the majority (68%) of patients in the ropivacaine group had no motor blockade. The incidences of adverse effects were similar in both groups. Hypotension occurred in 24% of the ropivacaine group and 16% of the bupivacaine group. Pruritus occurred in 56% of the ropivacaine group and 52% of the bupivacaine group (152).

In 122 women who received 20 ml of either ropivacaine 7.5 mg/ml or bupivacaine 5 mg/ml for epidural anesthesia during elective cesarean section, there were no significant differences in adverse effects, such as the incidence of hypotensive episodes, bradycardia, or nausea and vomiting; however, there was a greater median fall in systolic blood pressure in those given ropivacaine (24 versus 16%) (153). Efficacy and neonatal tolerability were similar in the two groups. This, together with its lesser cardiotoxicity, favors ropivacaine as an alternative to bupivacaine in this setting.

The possibility of increased maternal mortality is a topic of debate. In 1979 there were 150 maternal deaths (0.27 per 1000 births) in Germany, of which 15–25% were apparently related to regional anesthesia, with such complications as hypotension, systemic toxicity, total spinal block, hematoma, catheter rupture, and uterine injury (SED-12, 253) (154). However, obstetric regional anesthesia is regarded as being safer than general anesthesia, whatever the choice of drug, if competently and carefully performed.

Fetotoxicity
Maternal hypotension and excessive placental transfer of local anesthetics and other drugs, for example narcotics or sedatives, given to the mother before or during delivery are the main causes of neonatal death related to the use of these agents in obstetrics. However, deaths are very infrequent (155).

In about 10% of cases, obstetric use of epidural anesthesia will cause some bradycardia in the fetus, but this is not always a clinical problem (SEDA-15, 119). However, accidental intravenous injection of bupivacaine can lead to both maternal convulsions and severe fetal bradycardia (156).

The question of possible neurobehavioral effects in the child as a consequence of obstetric analgesia is still debated; although impairment of visual and neurological performance, reduced alertness, and alterations in walking and muscle tone have all been reported, most authors have found normal Apgar scores and psychomotor development after obstetric anesthesia (SED-12, 253) (157,158), and any functional defects noted at birth are likely to be transient (159).

The effects of low concentrations of epidural bupivacaine on the developing neonatal brain has been studied in infant rhesus monkeys, to decide if there was a detrimental relation between perinatal analgesia with epidural bupivacaine and later infant development (160). The monkeys, whose mothers had been given epidurals at term (but not during labor) were subjected to a battery of neurobehavioral tests for 1 year. The authors concluded that epidural bupivacaine did not cause neonatal abnormalities or specific cognitive defects, but that it may delay the normal course of behavioral development. It is difficult to extrapolate the results of this small study to human obstetrics.

Susceptibility factors
Epidural infusions of bupivacaine are often used in children. However, there are concerns about the increased incidence of adverse effects in infants, owing to reduced hepatic clearance and serum protein binding. In 22 infants

aged 1–7 months who received a continuous infusion of bupivacaine 0.375 mg/kg/hour for 2 days during and after surgery, the unbound and total serum concentrations of bupivacaine were measured, along with presurgical and postsurgical concentrations of $alpha_1$ acid glycoprotein (161). The concentrations of $alpha_1$ acid glycoprotein increased markedly after surgery. However, because of reduced clearance unbound concentrations of bupivacaine increased to over 0.2 micrograms/ml in two infants younger than 2 months. The authors proposed a maximum dosage rate of 0.25 mg/kg/hour in infants younger than 4 months and 0.3 mg/kg/hour in older infants.

Intercostal nerve anesthesia

High spinal anesthesia after inadvertent injection is a possible complication of intercostal nerve block (SED-12, 252). Pneumothorax is another reported complication (55).

Interpleural anesthesia

Interpleural administration of local anesthetics has been followed by Horner's syndrome and increased skin temperature, apparently pointing to an effect on the sympathetic nervous system (162). Pneumothorax or infection can also result. Interpleural administration of local anesthetics can produce high serum drug concentrations and a risk of systemic toxicity (SEDA-21, 13), possibly increased by the addition of adrenaline (SEDA-20, 126).

Intra-articular anesthesia

Intra-articular anesthesia has been used successfully in many patients, with few adverse effects (SEDA-20, 126). However, it is not always safe; at least one death has occurred from bupivacaine used in this way (163). Intra-articular anesthesia in the knee joint was followed in one case by necrosis of the knee ligament and the skin, apparently due to localized drug-induced embolism (164).

Intradermal anesthesia

Intradermal local anesthetic solutions can cause considerable pain on injection. Additives, such as hyaluronidase, which are used to enhance the analgesic effect of local anesthetics, can often exacerbate this (165). Infiltration from the inside of a wound can be less painful than through intact skin (166).

The order of injection can affect the pain of local anesthetic infiltration with buffered lidocaine; in a sequence of two injections the second injection was consistently reported to be more painful than the first. This finding has important consequences with regard to trial design in this area of research (167). Buffered lidocaine warmed to 37°C was less painful than warmed plain lidocaine, plain lidocaine, and buffered lidocaine in a randomized controlled trial in 26 volunteers (168).

Intrathecal (spinal) anesthesia

Intrathecal anesthesia has been compared with general anesthesia in 33 patients with pre-eclamptic toxemia undergoing cesarean section (169). The complications after general anesthesia were more serious, with a 4.3% mortality, whereas complications after spinal anesthesia were less serious and easily manageable, notably intraoperative hypotension (47%), difficulty in locating the subarachnoid space (29%), and intraoperative vomiting (6%).

Hyperbaric ropivacaine 0.25% has been compared with hyperbaric bupivacaine 0.25% in a crossover study in 18 volunteers who received an intrathecal anesthetic; the doses were 4, 8, or 12 mg (170). More patients had lumbosacral back pain after intrathecal ropivacaine compared with bupivacaine (5 versus 1), although this difference was not significant; the back pain lasted 3–5 days and was mild to moderate in intensity.

Intrathecal isobaric ropivacaine (15 mg) has been compared with intrathecal isobaric bupivacaine (10 mg) in 100 patients having transurethral resection of the bladder or prostate (171). Median cephalad spread of blocks was two segments higher for both pinprick and cold with bupivacaine compared with ropivacaine. Onset time to anesthesia was the same in both groups. Significantly more patients in the ropivacaine group complained of painful sensations at the surgical site (16 versus 0%). There was no difference in anesthetic duration, the incidence, intensity, onset, and duration of motor blockade, or the incidence of hypotension in the two groups. There were no cases of transient neurological symptoms. The authors concluded that ropivacaine 15 mg is less potent than bupivacaine 10 mg for intrathecal analgesia.

Continuous intrathecal anesthesia with 10 ml of 0.25% bupivacaine over 24 hours has been compared with continuous epidural anesthesia with 48 ml of 0.25% bupivacaine over 24 hours during the first 2 days after hip replacement in 102 patients (172). Continuous spinal anesthesia provided better analgesia and more patient satisfaction, but significantly more patients had motor blockade during the day of surgery and the first postoperative day. There was a significantly higher incidence of nausea and vomiting with continuous epidural anesthesia (39 versus 21).

When a pneumatic tourniquet was used in intrathecal anesthesia, pain was twice as frequent with tetracaine (60%) as with bupivacaine (25%) (173). However, using bupivacaine and tetracaine together seems to produce a more prolonged analgesic effect without inducing more hypotension than either agent alone (SEDA-18, 143).

In 80 patients undergoing lower extremity or lower abdominal surgery randomized to receive hyperbaric bupivacaine 10 mg alone or in combination with fentanyl 12.5 micrograms intrathecally, those given fentanyl had significantly longer duration of analgesia with no reported sedation or respiratory depression (174). Pruritus occurred in 20% of patients given fentanyl and shivering occurred significantly more often in those given bupivacaine only (30 versus 12.5%).

The addition of low doses of clonidine and neostigmine to intrathecal bupivacaine + fentanyl in 30 patients in labor significantly increased the duration of analgesia but was associated with significantly more emesis (175).

In a comparison of intrathecal bupivacaine 10 mg and bupivacaine 7.5 mg combined with ketamine 25 mg, in 30 healthy women there was no extension of postoperative analgesia or reduction in postoperative analgesic requirements in those given ketamine (176). Those given ketamine had a shorter duration of motor blockade, but had an increased incidence of adverse effects, and the study was abandoned after 30 patients.

Intrathecal blockade with 0.5% isobaric bupivacaine 10 mg has been compared with 0.5% isobaric bupivacaine 5 mg combined with fentanyl 25 micrograms (diluted to 2 ml with isotonic saline) in 32 patients undergoing elective cesarean section (177). The bupivacaine + fentanyl combination was associated with significantly less hypotension than bupivacaine alone (31 versus 94%) and a near 10-fold reduction in the mean ephedrine requirement (2.8 versus 23.8 mg). There were also significant differences in the incidence of nausea (31 versus 69%) and the median time to peak block (8 versus 10 minutes) with bupivacaine plus fentanyl. The authors advised further large-scale studies to quantify the minimum dose of bupivacaine plus fentanyl for single-dose spinal anesthesia.

An isobaric solution of sameridine given intrathecally in doses of 15, 20, and 23 mg has been compared with hyperbaric lidocaine 100 mg in 100 volunteers (178). Sameridine has both local anesthetic and opioid analgesic properties. There was one incident of transient paresthesia with sameridine 20 mg and two cases of bradycardia with lidocaine; the incidence of hypotension was more frequent with lidocaine, but pruritus was more common with sameridine.

Cardiovascular

Hypotension is the most frequent adverse effect of spinal anesthesia; in one very large series it occurred in 22% of the subarachnoid group (179), but the actual figures differ with the anesthetic, its concentration, and the definition of hypotension used. For example single-dose spinal anesthesia causes significantly more hypotension and bradycardia than continuous spinal anesthesia (180). Hypotension may be more of a problem with tetracaine or lidocaine than with bupivacaine in equivalent doses (SEDA-12, 35), and the incidence is less when the patient is in the lateral rather than the sitting position. However, using bupivacaine and tetracaine together seems to produce a more prolonged analgesic effect without inducing more hypotension than either agent alone (SEDA-18, 143). Hypotension is also reported with intrathecal opioids and opioid/local anesthetic combinations; sufentanil appears to predominate in these reports (SEDA-21, 132) (SEDA-22, 137).

Hypotension can be prevented or treated with vasopressors and/or fluids (SED-12, 254) (SEDA-18, 143) (181–183). A comparison of these approaches showed that ephedrine alone is less effective than ephedrine and colloid (184), and metaraminol, with or without colloid, is better than colloid alone (185).

The effect of baricity on the hemodynamic effects of intrathecal 0.5% bupivacaine has been measured by recording invasive systolic blood pressure and central venous pressure in 36 men given plain bupivacaine 0.5%, heavy bupivacaine 0.5% (in dextrose 8%), or a mixture of the two (in dextrose 4%) (186). Heavy bupivacaine caused more rapid falls in central venous pressure and systolic blood pressure than plain bupivacaine. However, it was subsequently remarked that both 4 and 8% dextrose are significantly hyperbaric relative to adult cerebrospinal fluid, implying that the 4% solution should have behaved more like the 8% solution (187).

In 191 women who had had cesarean sections under spinal anesthesia using hyperbaric bupivacaine 12–15 mg and morphine 0.25 mg, who were transferred to the recovery room on a stretcher with the upper body either flexed 30° or supine during transport 10% of each group had a greater than 20% fall in systolic blood pressure unaffected by position (188). The authors recommended routine monitoring of the blood pressure and pulse after transfer to the stretcher, and suggested that raising the head for the comfort of the mother during transport does not increase the risk of hypotension.

Isobaric bupivacaine 4 mg combined with fentanyl 20 micrograms has been compared with isobaric bupivacaine 10 mg alone in 20 patients over the age of 70 undergoing surgery for fractured neck of femur (114). Hypotension was defined as a systolic blood pressure less than 90 mmHg or a fall in mean arterial pressure of more than 25%. Significantly more patients given bupivacaine only had hypotension (90 versus 10%). The mean dosage requirement of ephedrine was higher with bupivacaine only (32 versus 0.5 mg) and two patients in this group required phenylephrine, while no patient given bupivacaine plus fentanyl did. No patient in either group complained of perioperative pain or required supplementary analgesia intraoperatively.

In young infants similar problems with blood pressure occur, and some changes in heart rate may be found, but tend to be transient (SEDA-12, 154) (189).

Intrathecal blockade for cesarean section using 0.5% hyperbaric bupivacaine at three different doses of 7.5 mg, 8.75 mg, and 10 mg has been studied in a double-blind comparison in 60 patients (190). There was no significant difference in maximum block height, but more of the patients who were given the two lower doses had moderate visceral pain requiring rescue ketamine. Bupivacaine 10 mg was associated with significantly more bradycardia, and 7.5 and 8.75 mg with significantly more hypotension. Motor block lasted significantly longer with 10 mg. The outcome was good in all the infants, although one baby whose mother had received bupivacaine 10 mg had an Apgar score below 10 at 5 minutes. The authors concluded that the use of bupivacaine 7.5 mg avoids hypotension, bradycardia, and prolonged block.

Bradycardia occurs in some 3% of spinal anesthetics in adults. Bradycardia can lead to cardiac arrest, either by direct block of the sympathetic innervation of the heart (in unintended high block) or as a consequence of insufficient venous return. In 900 cases of major anesthetic mishaps giving rise to compensation claims, there were 14 cases of cardiac arrest under spinal anesthesia, of which six were fatal (191). Myocardial infarction and cardiac arrest preceded by atrioventricular block have also been described.

- A 68-year-old man was given 0.5% bupivacaine 4 ml or spinal anesthesia, and 5 minutes later complained of nausea and developed hypotension, loss of consciousness, and a tonic-clonic seizure. He had first-degree heart block 4 minutes after subarachnoid injection, followed 1 minute later by third-degree heart block, and then asystole. He was successfully resuscitated. Proposed theories included a reflex bradycardia resulting from reduced venous return and/or unopposed vagal tone due to thoracic sympathectomy induced by spinal anesthesia (192).

Bradycardia has been reported to follow spinal anesthesia in association with urinary retention (193).

- A receding spinal block to level L1–2 gave rise to acute bradycardia (34–40/minute) and transient loss of consciousness in a 31-year-old man 5 hours after spinal anesthesia; on waking he complained of severe low back pain, and although he had no symptoms of urinary retention, urinary catheterization yielded 900 ml of urine with immediate relief of symptoms.

Slow injection of hyperbaric bupivacaine 8 mg has been compared with hyperbaric bupivacaine 15 mg used to achieve bilateral block in 30 patients of ASA grades I–II (194). There was significantly greater cardiovascular stability in the patients who had a unilateral spinal block.

Respiratory

Respiratory arrest is one of the most serious potential adverse effects of spinal anesthesia, either due to brainstem depression in high block or rostral spread of opioids after the use of combined techniques (SEDA-21, 132) (SEDA-22, 137).

Immediate respiratory arrest has been reported after the administration of intrathecal bupivacaine and fentanyl (195).

- A 26-year-old woman in labor was given an epidural for analgesia. After 2 hours and total doses of bupivacaine 77.5 mg and fentanyl 190 micrograms, the epidural was removed owing to failure. A subsequent intrathecal injection of bupivacaine 2.5 mg plus fentanyl 10 micrograms was followed 4 minutes later by apnea and loss of consciousness. She was rapidly intubated and regained consciousness after 15 minutes, at which time her sensory level was T8 to pinprick. She was extubated after 30 minutes.

The authors concluded that the respiratory depression had been due to excessive cephalad spread of fentanyl, possibly facilitated by the volume of bupivacaine that had previously been injected epidurally.

Bronchospasm has been reported in two obstetric patients, possibly due to thoracic sympathetic blockade in one and hypersensitivity in the other (SEDA-21, 132).

There is a potential risk that spinal anesthesia will cause apnea in premature infants. However, spinal anesthesia with a sound technique has been used safely in high-risk infants. Tetracaine was used in 142 such cases; only two infants had serious adverse effects, one with unexplained but treatable apnea and one in whom too high a block resulted in respiratory arrest (196).

Two former preterm infants (postconceptual age 38 weeks) both received spinal anesthetics for inguinal herniorrhaphy (block level T4–6) (197). No other medications were given. Both infants had frequent episodes of perioperative apnea and associated bradycardia. One had a 20-second bout of apnea, with an oxygen saturation of 70% and a heart rate of 80/minute, the other a 30-second bout of apnea, with a saturation of 70% and a heart rate of 60/minute. These episodes persisted for 8 hours into the postoperative period in one of the infants.

- A patient who was receiving modified-release morphine for malignant pain had a respiratory arrest after intrathecal bupivacaine 12.5 mg. She recovered after treatment with naloxone. Another patient who was taking modified-release morphine was given intrathecal morphine 10 mg and bupivacaine 7.5 mg. He had respiratory distress and became comatose. Morphine-induced respiratory depression was not diagnosed and the patient subsequently died. In both cases, respiratory distress and sedation was probably due to opioid action in the absence of the stimulating effect of pain on respiration, due to the intrathecal bupivacaine (198).
- A 20-year-old woman who received a combined spinal epidural for labor had a respiratory arrest 23 minutes after the administration of sufentanil 10 micrograms and bupivacaine 2.5 mg (199).

Nervous system

- A 40-year-old woman developed acute aphasia and a change in mental status 15 minutes after the intrathecal administration of sufentanil 10 micrograms and isobaric bupivacaine 2.5 mg as part of a combined spinal epidural anesthetic for analgesia during labor (200). She appeared to be in a dissociated state, had apparent difficulty swallowing, and was aphasic, but able to follow simple commands. She had sensory block to T6 on the right and T8 on the left, with no motor block. The neurological picture resolved about 100 minutes after the anesthetic; an exact etiology could not be established.
- A similar case has been reported 20 minutes after the intrathecal administration of 0.5% hyperbaric bupivacaine 2 ml for cesarean section (201). She became unresponsive then apneic for a short time. There were no changes in heart rate or blood pressure and no loss of airway protection. She slowly regained consciousness over the next hour without any consequences.

The authors were unclear about the cause and suggested subdural injection, as the slow onset, stable hemodynamics, and rapid recovery were suggestive of this complication. However, other causes, including a psychogenic response, are possibilities.

- New onset, severe lightning pain after repeated subarachnoid blockade occurred in a 48-year-old man with pre-existing neuropathic pain after incomplete spinal cord injury, similar to previous reports in patients with phantom limb pain (202).

Postural headache is a common complication of spinal anesthesia (so-called postdural puncture headache). It is caused by CSF leakage through the puncture site. The incidence has been greatly reduced by the use of smaller-gauge and pencil-point spinal needles. However, headache (or psychosis) can be the presenting sign of subdural hematoma, which has twice been observed in women given spinal anesthesia for childbirth (SEDA-18, 143).

- A 30-year-old patient developed aseptic meningitis 24 hours after spinal anesthesia with bupivacaine plus fentanyl; it resolved without sequelae within 48 hours (203).

Conus medullaris syndrome has been reported after consecutive intrathecal injections of hyperbaric 1%

tetracaine, followed by hyperbaric 5% lidocaine with adrenaline, in a patient with diabetic neuropathy (SEDA-21, 130).

Less frequent neurological complications are bladder dysfunction or sphincter paresis (204), intracranial hypertension, and convulsions, the latter reflecting systemic toxicity.

- A 36-year-old man had two generalized tonic-clonic convulsions after receiving intrathecal tetracaine 8 mg to supplement inadequate block established by intrathecal administration of tetracaine 10 mg (205). His seizures were controlled with intravenous thiamylal sodium. He regained consciousness, but complained of dizziness and blurred vision. He had a sensory block to T4–5.

The authors excluded total spinal anesthesia as a cause of the seizures, on the basis of the sensory level and the lack of hypotension.

Cauda equina syndrome

Cauda equina syndrome is the triad of bilateral paraparesis or paraplegia of the muscles of the legs and buttocks, saddle anesthesia plus sensory deficits below the groin, and incompetence of bladder and rectal sphincters, causing incontinence of urine and feces.

Cauda equina syndrome has been reported after the use of microcatheters for continuous intrathecal anesthesia. The concern was sufficient reason for the FDA to withdraw microcatheters from the US market after 11 cases of cauda equina in 1992 (SEDA-21, 129) (206). It has now become obvious that a confounding factor was the use of hyperbaric solutions pooling around lumbosacral nerve roots, aggravated by the poor mechanics of microcatheters and the use of inappropriate amounts; the authors of one study argued that the problem was not evident with the use of low concentrations of isobaric local anesthetics administered via microcatheters (207).

Six cases of the syndrome have also been reported after "single-shot" spinal anesthesia at the L3–4 interspace with 5% hyperbaric lidocaine (208).

- A 55-year-old man was given 5% hyperbaric lidocaine 100 mg intrathecally in the sitting position for transurethral resection of the prostate in the lithotomy position, with no complications. However, the next day he complained of persistent numbness of the perianal, scrotal, penile, and sacral regions, and both legs. He also had difficulty in defecation and weakness of both quadriceps muscles. Despite normal MRI scanning, electromyography, and electroneurography, he had no neurological improvement, even 1.5 years after the operation.
- A 59-year-old woman received 5% hyperbaric lidocaine 60 mg for an operation on a toe. That evening she complained of urinary and bowel incontinence; 5 months later she had urinary stress incontinence and bowel incontinence, with absent anal reflexes. There was also reduced sensation over the medial side of the foot.
- A 48-year-old woman had spinal anesthesia for hallux valgus surgery and had pain radiating to the left buttock during insertion of the needle. Hyperbaric 5% lidocaine 100 mg was injected, with no associated paresthesia. One month later, she complained of persistent numbness of the perianal and sacral regions and had sensory loss in these regions, which failed to improve over 6 months.
- A 31-year-old man had spinal anesthesia with 5% hyperbaric lidocaine 100 mg for fasciotomy. His systolic blood pressure briefly fell to 90 mmHg and he was given ephedrine. He later complained of persistent numbness of the entire right leg, right scrotum, right side of the penis, and right buttock, and had difficulty in micturition; there was no improvement one month later, and he had reduced pain and temperature sensation in the right leg, intact touch sensation, and weakness of right hip extension. His neurological state did not improve over a year.
- A 37-year-old woman had varicose vein surgery under spinal anesthesia with 5% hyperbaric lidocaine 120 mg in two injections followed by a general anesthesia, because the spinal block was inadequate. Postoperatively she complained of persistent numbness in the right buttock, difficulty in micturition, and bowel incontinence. She had reduced sensation in the perianal region and both labia majora, with a large residual urine volume. An MRI scan was normal, but electromyography, electroneurography, and cystometry 4 months later showed denervation of the pelvic muscles, partial denervation of the detrusor muscle, and signs of re-innervation. After 5 months her condition remained much the same.
- A 59-year-old man had spinal anesthesia for hallux valgus surgery with 5% hyperbaric lidocaine 75 mg. The next day he had persistent perianal numbness, difficulty in micturition, and a large residual urine volume. An MRI scan was normal and he had reduced perianal and scrotal sensation, difficulty in defecation, and erectile impotence. He was no better 5 months later.

The authors stated that at least some of the cases had probably resulted from neurotoxicity of hyperbaric lidocaine, most often in the absence of obvious maldistribution. They recommended that hyperbaric lidocaine should be used in concentrations not exceeding 2% and in a total dose no greater than 60 mg.

- A 75-year-old woman with a history of lumbar laminectomy, but no neurological deficit, received an intrathecal injection of 4 ml of 0.5% bupivacaine with preservatives at the L4–5 level using a 22-gauge spinal needle for a total knee replacement (209). Intraoperatively she complained of severe low back pain, which improved 8 hours later. In parallel, she developed persistent sensory loss to L1 and flaccid paralysis of both legs. An MRI scan was normal, but myelography showed inflammation of the cauda equina; 2 months later she developed hydrocephalus and had adhesive arachnoiditis of the thoracolumbar region. Her neurological condition did not improve over 2 years.

A retrospective review of 603 continuous spinal anesthetics (127 had microcatheters) showed three patients with postoperative paresthesia, one of whom was from the microcatheter group (210). One patient, who had received anesthesia via a macrocatheter with 5% lidocaine, developed sensory cauda equina syndrome.

- A 57-year-old man with pre-existing severe vascular disease was given bupivacaine 12.5 mg with 1:1000 adrenaline 0.2 ml for incision and drainage of a thigh abscess (211). After 2–3 minutes he complained of "severely painful warmth" on the anterior of both thighs. The pain resolved with onset of the block, but the next morning he had symptoms of cauda equina syndrome. Some perineal sensation returned over the next few days.

The authors suggested that the neurological deficit had been due to anterior spinal artery insufficiency secondary to intrathecal bupivacaine and adrenaline. They questioned the use of adrenaline in patients with multi-organ vascular disease.

- A man with severe vascular disease was given general and epidural anesthesia with 2% isobaric lidocaine plus adrenaline for a popliteal distal vein bypass graft (212). The epidural inadvertently became a total spinal, which was discovered at the end of the operation. He developed cauda equina syndrome, confirmed by electromyography. He was unable to turn or sit up by himself for a month and at 12 months was walking with a cane and needed self-catheterization and medication for neuropathic pain.

The cauda has a tenuous blood supply, and in this patient with pre-existing vascular disease, perioperative hypotension and the use of intrathecal adrenaline may have precipitated ischemia in an area with very poor reserve. To follow this with an accidental large dose of lidocaine, which is neurotoxic in animals when directly applied and theorized to cause interruption of nerve blood supply, would add insult to injury. The authors questioned the wisdom of performing continuous epidural anesthesia in such patients, when frequent neurological assessments cannot be performed.

Bupivacaine has recently been implicated in two cases of cauda equina syndrome (213). One patient was given 3.6 ml of a hyperbaric 0.5% solution, and the other, 3.5 ml of plain bupivacaine. Spinal stenosis was felt to have contributed to the first case, while the cause of the second was unclear.

- Cauda equina syndrome occurred in a 55-year-old woman who underwent spinal anesthesia with a 22 G needle in the L4–5 interspace (214). On needle insertion, she felt radiating pain in her right leg. The needle was immediately withdrawn and repositioned. Pain-free intrathecal injection of 2.0 ml of hyperbaric cinchocaine 0.24% with adrenaline 66 micrograms resulted in block to L1. Surgery was carried out in the supine position. Three days postoperatively, she had enuresis and reduced perineal sensation, without bowel dysfunction or lower limb symptoms. There was sensory loss at S2–5. The symptoms persisted, required self-catheterization and systemic steroids, and disappeared on the 19th postoperative day.

The cause of this transient neurological deficit was unclear, but the authors suggested that the following factors may have contributed:

- direct nerve damage;
- local anesthetic toxicity;
- adrenaline effects.

Transient radicular irritation

Neurological sequelae of intrathecal anesthesia are rare and usually minor. However, transient radicular irritation can occur with the use of both isobaric and hyperbaric solutions of local anesthetics. Hyperbaric 5% lidocaine is such a persistent offender that there is little to recommend its use in neuraxial blockade (SEDA-20, 125) (SEDA-21, 129) (SEDA-22, 138). However, others have suggested that lidocaine can be used for intrathecal anesthesia if a short-acting anesthetic is desired (215). There have also been reports with most other local anesthetics, including tetracaine and mepivacaine. High concentrations of hyperbaric 4% mepivacaine are likely to cause transient radicular irritation of the same order of magnitude as 5% lidocaine (216). A randomized study with isobaric mepivacaine 2% administered intrathecally to patients undergoing surgery in the supine position showed an incidence of 7.5% compared with 2.5% with isobaric lidocaine 2% (217). There is a low incidence of transient radicular irritation after intrathecal bupivacaine, but a few cases have been reported (SEDA-20, 125). Bupivacaine and tetracaine have toxic effects on chick neuron cultures in vitro (218).

Since the cause of transient radicular irritation after lidocaine intrathecal anesthesia has not been elucidated, and although non-neurotoxic mechanisms must be considered, it has been recommended that the lowest effective doses and concentrations for intrathecal injection should be used (219).

Presentation Transient radicular irritation causes transient pain in the back, buttocks, and lower extremities, without formal neurological signs or symptoms. It can follow single-dose intrathecal anesthesia. Lidocaine has been reported as the predominant culprit. However, transient radicular irritation has also been reported with bupivacaine, mepivacaine, tetracaine, and prilocaine. Osmolarity, the addition of dextrose, and speed of injection do not contribute, and even reducing the concentration of lidocaine does not alter the incidence (220,221).

Cases involving lidocaine (222–224) and mepivacaine (225,226) have been reported.

- A 50-year-old woman had a right knee arthroscopy under spinal anesthesia with 1% lidocaine 4 ml. The anesthetic and procedure were uncomplicated. At 4 hours she complained of a mild cramp in her buttocks and went home at 6 hours. By the next morning the buttock pain was severe, cramp-like in nature, and radiated down the fronts of both thighs. Walking alleviated it, simple analgesics were ineffective, and lying down made the pain worse. Neurological examination was unremarkable and the pain was gone after 36 hours.
- A 74-year-old man who had a cystoscopy performed in the lithotomy position, reported dull pain in the hips, buttocks, and legs, radiating to the toes after a spinal anesthetic with 5% hyperbaric lidocaine 75 mg. The pain occurred 30 hours after the dural puncture and

disappeared after 18 hours. Three months before he had had a similar anesthetic for a transurethral resection of the prostate and complained of similar but more severe symptoms of transient radicular irritation.

- A 66-year-old woman with unrecognized spinal stenosis had six spinal anesthetics over 3 years. The first five were with lidocaine 2%. After 24–48 hours, she developed pain in the back, hips, buttocks, and thighs, which lasted for 2–3 days. On the sixth occasion she had a spinal anesthetic with 1.5% mepivacaine 4 ml and the next day again had severe back pain radiating bilaterally to the hips and thighs.
- Three patients undergoing minor surgical procedures in the lithotomy position were given a spinal anesthetic with 2% mepivacaine 3 ml. From 6 to 10 hours postoperatively they complained of burning pain in both buttocks radiating to both thighs and calves. Neurological examination in all cases was normal and all symptoms had resolved by 3–5 days postoperatively.
- A 30-year-old man had a left spermatic vein ligature performed in the supine position. He had uncomplicated unilateral spinal anesthesia with 1% hyperbaric bupivacaine 8 mg. Three days later he reported an area of hypesthesia in the L3–4 dermatomes of the left leg. Sensation returned to normal after 2 weeks.

Incidence The incidence of transient radicular irritation varies depending on the local anesthetic used, its baricity, and its concentration. It has been reported to be as high as 37% in patients who receive 5% lidocaine. In a prospective study of 303 parturients undergoing intrathecal anesthesia using 0.75% hyperbaric bupivacaine or 5% lidocaine there were no cases of transient radicular irritation after lidocaine (227). This is remarkable, as significantly more procedures were performed in the lithotomy position in the lidocaine group; the authors wondered if such a low incidence of transient radicular irritation could have been explained by their use of a 1:1 dilution of lidocaine with cerebrospinal fluid.

Transient neurological symptoms have been studied in patients given intrathecal lidocaine 2% or intrathecal prilocaine 2%. In one study of 70 patients transient neurological symptoms occurred in 20% of patients given lidocaine, with no cases in those given prilocaine (228). In another study in 70 patients given intrathecal procaine or lidocaine in a 2:1 dose ratio there were significantly more transient neurological symptoms with lidocaine than with procaine (31 versus 6%) (229). However, in a similar study of 100 patients there was no significant difference in the incidence of transient neurological symptoms, although the trend suggested a lower incidence with prilocaine (4 versus 14.3%) (230).

In 110 patients presenting for knee arthroscopy who were randomized to receive either 1% hypobaric lidocaine 50 mg or 1% hypobaric lidocaine 20 mg + fentanyl 25 micrograms complaints of transient neurological symptoms were nearly ten times more frequent in those given lidocaine 50 mg (33 versus 3.6%) (231). Patients given lidocaine 50 mg also had a greater fall in systolic blood pressure and a greater need for ephedrine.

In a prospective study of 1045 patients receiving spinal anesthesia with 3% hyperbaric lidocaine for anorectal surgery in the prone position, 4 (0.4%) complained of aching, hypesthesia, numbness, and dull pain in both buttocks and legs on the third postoperative day. In three cases the symptoms resolved by day 5 and in one by day 7 (232).

In a retrospective audit of 363 patients receiving spinal anesthesia, of whom 322 received hyperbaric 5% lidocaine 75–100 mg and 41 hyperbaric 0.5% bupivacaine 12.5–15 mg, six patients given lidocaine reported back pain at 24 hours; five of them had undergone arthroscopy. One patient given bupivacaine, who underwent arthroscopy, complained of backache (233).

Over 14 months, 1863 patients received spinal anesthesia, of whom 40% were given bupivacaine, 47% lidocaine, and 13% tetracaine (234). Patients given lidocaine had a significantly higher risk of transient radicular irritation (relative risks 5.1 compared with bupivacaine and 3.2 compared with tetracaine). They were more likely to be men, have outpatient surgery, and have surgery in the lithotomy position. For those who were given lidocaine, the relative risk of transient radicular irritation was 2.6, for those in the lithotomy position 3.6, and for ambulatory surgery 1.6. Most of the patients had resolution of symptoms by 72 hours and all by 6 months.

The incidence of transient radicular irritation with two different local anesthetics used for single-dose spinal anesthesia has been studied in 60 ambulatory patients given spinal anesthesia for knee arthroscopy (235). None of those who were given 1.5% mepivacaine 45 mg developed transient radicular irritation. Six of those given 2% lidocaine 60 mg developed transient radicular irritation, but all symptoms resolved by 1–5 days. The difference between the two groups was significant.

Of 90 patients who received intrathecal hyperbaric lidocaine 5%, mepivacaine 4%, or bupivacaine 0.5%, none in the bupivacaine group developed transient radicular irritation, but 20% in the lidocaine group and 37% in the mepivacaine group complained of a mixture of back and leg pain, classified as transient radicular irritation (216).

When 90 patients received spinal anesthesia for gynecological procedures with 2% lidocaine, 2% prilocaine, or 0.5% bupivacaine (all 2.5 ml in 7.5% glucose), nine of the 30 patients who received lidocaine had transient radicular irritation, defined as pain or dysesthesia in the legs or buttocks, compared with none of the 30 patients who received bupivacaine (236). The symptoms resolved within 48 hours. One of the 30 patients who received prilocaine had transient radicular irritation that lasted for 4 days.

In 200 patients given hyperbaric 5% lidocaine or hyperbaric 5% prilocaine, four developed transient radicular irritation after lidocaine (the patients were supine or prone) compared with one after prilocaine (this patient had a knee arthroscopy) (237). There were no significant differences between the two groups.

When procaine 5% or procaine 5% with fentanyl 20 micrograms was given to 106 patients for spinal anesthesia, the incidence of transient radicular irritation was 0.9% (238). There was nausea and vomiting in 17% of men and 32% of women.

Procaine has been suggested as an alternative to lidocaine for intrathecal use in ambulatory surgery, as it also

bupivacaine, fentanyl 25 micrograms, and morphine 0.2 mg. After 4 minutes she developed hypotension, which was treated with ephedrine. Another 4 minutes later she became agitated and complained of difficulty in swallowing. At this stage she had a block to T4 with no dyspnea, her facial sensation was normal, and phonation was intact; the dysphagia resolved within 30 minutes.

Urinary tract

Urinary retention as a true transient neurological symptom developed after accidental total spinal anesthesia with mepivacaine, which is often considered to be the best agent for intrathecal anesthesia, owing to its low incidence of transient radicular irritation (268).

- A 71-year-old man received an intrathecal anesthetic with 2 ml of 0.3% hyperbaric mepivacaine using a 25-gauge Quincke needle at the L3–4 interspace, before which he had slight hypesthesia in the L5–S1 dermatomes in the right leg, reportedly having originated from the use of local anesthetic in the lumbar spine 16 years before to treat severe lumbago (269). When he was turned supine he started to complain of severe lightning pain in the region of his hypesthetic segments, which completely resolved 4 hours later.

Musculoskeletal

Profound musculoligamental relaxation by high doses of local anesthetics may contribute to the development of postoperative musculoskeletal pain. Of 60 patients who received either spinal anesthesia with hyperbaric 5% lidocaine (85–100 mg) or balanced general anesthesia with neuromuscular blockade, there was transient radicular irritation in eight patients who received spinal anesthesia and in one who received general anesthesia, a significant difference (270). However, there was non-radiating back pain in ten of the patients who received spinal anesthesia and in six of those who received general anesthesia.

Sexual function

For reasons that are not understood, intraoperative penile erection is sometimes observed with neuraxial blockade; it can be followed by prolonged priapism (SEDA-14, 110).

A long-standing belief that intrathecal anesthesia in young men reduces sexual potency was not confirmed in a retrospective study (SEDA-17, 139).

Intravenous regional anesthesia

Systemic toxic reactions are the most common complications of intravenous regional anesthesia, and they occur soon after the tourniquet is released. In cases of early accidental tourniquet release or rupture, deaths have resulted; prilocaine seems to be the safest agent for this technique (271).

- A 74-year-old woman was given prilocaine 400 mg for carpal tunnel surgery. Within 3 minutes, she developed signs of central nervous system toxicity, sweating, and tachycardia. Twenty minutes later, her symptoms had resolved and the cause was found to be a leak in the tourniquet.

The authors used this case to stress the importance of adequately functioning equipment and the relative safety of prilocaine (272).

Methods of reducing the dose of lidocaine used in intravenous regional anesthesia by adding fentanyl 0.05 mg, pancuronium bromide 0.5 mg, or both, have been evaluated in 60 patients undergoing elective forearm, wrist, and hand surgery; the dose of lidocaine used was 100 mg (273). None of the patients had signs of drug toxicity on release of the tourniquet; those who were given all three agents had better anesthesia and muscle relaxation. A separate group of volunteers, in whom the tourniquet was released immediately after injection of the lidocaine/fentanyl/pancuronium mixture, complained of minor adverse effects including mild dizziness and transient visual disturbances and one case of vomiting and moderate hypotension.

A study of lidocaine toxicity in intravenous regional anesthesia showed that two of 24 patients who were given 0.5% lidocaine 40 ml for carpal tunnel decompression had serum lidocaine concentrations above the target range 2 minutes before and 2, 5, and 10 minutes after distal tourniquet deflation (274). However, no patients had signs of central nervous system or cardiovascular toxicity.

Cardiovascular

Chloroprocaine, because of its rapid onset and ester hydrolysis, should be the ideal agent for intravenous regional anesthesia. However, there are reports that it can cause endothelial damage and dysrhythmias after tourniquet deflation (275).

- Phlebitis seems to have been triggered by intravenous regional anesthesia in a 32-year-old smoker who was also taking oral contraceptives (276).

Nervous system

In 15 volunteers, ropivacaine 1.2 and 1.8 mg/kg produced intravenous regional anesthesia as quickly as a conventional dose of lidocaine (3 mg/kg), but with more prolonged anesthesia (55 minutes before loss of pinprick analgesia) and motor block (120 minutes before return of hand grip strength) at the higher dose, suggesting that ropivacaine can provide a greater degree of residual analgesia (277). All the volunteers given lidocaine and only one patient receiving high-dose ropivacaine developed light-headedness and a hearing disturbance when the tourniquet was released after 30 minutes, but with individual peak arterial plasma ropivacaine concentrations lower than the mean values for the group. The authors pointed out the limitations of this study in terms of a small sample size and their inability to determine the safety of ropivacaine for intravenous regional anesthesia.

- A 56-year-old man developed unexplained acute aphasia when the tourniquet was released 20 minutes after the infusion of 0.75% lidocaine 20 ml for wrist surgery (278). He also had light-headedness, but no circumoral numbness or visual or auditory disturbances. He made a spontaneous recovery 20 hours later with no sequelae.

The correlation of nervous system adverse effects with plasma concentrations after the intravenous administration of 40 ml of lidocaine 0.5% plus ropivacaine 0.2% for regional anesthesia has been examined in 10 volunteers (279). The double-cuffed tourniquet was inflated for as long as it could be tolerated. The incidence, duration, and intensity of nervous system adverse effects were recorded at 3, 10, and 30 minutes after tourniquet release and correlated with venous samples. There was a lower incidence and shorter duration of nervous system adverse effects with ropivacaine than with lidocaine; however, the dose of ropivacaine was much lower than that of lidocaine and therefore no clear conclusions can be drawn. In view of the availability of safer and effective alternatives for intravenous regional anesthesia, such as prilocaine and lidocaine, the reasons for using ropivacaine are hard to comprehend.

Sensory systems

Ears

It has been suggested that ropivacaine is a good choice for intravenous regional anesthesia because of its longer duration of action and lower risk of toxicity. In 20 patients scheduled for upper limb surgery who received 40 ml of either ropivacaine 0.2% or lidocaine 0.5% for intravenous regional anesthesia, both agents provided same onset and quality of surgical anesthesia, but ropivacaine gave longer-lasting analgesia in the immediate postoperative period (279). Additionally, one patient in the lidocaine group had tinnitus on release of the tourniquet, while there were no adverse effects in the ropivacaine group.

Taste

When 20 patients each received 40 ml of 0.5% chloroprocaine or 0.5% lidocaine for intravenous regional anesthesia, chloroprocaine caused a significantly higher incidence of a metallic taste (22 versus 0%) than lidocaine; when the study was repeated using alkalinized instead of plain chloroprocaine, there was no significant difference between the groups (280).

Skin

When 20 patients each received 40 ml of 0.5% chloroprocaine or 0.5% lidocaine for intravenous regional anesthesia, chloroprocaine caused a significantly higher incidence of urticaria (28 versus 0%) than lidocaine; when the study was repeated using alkalinized instead of plain chloroprocaine, there was no significant difference between the groups (280).

Laryngeal anesthesia

Local anesthesia to the larynx, for example with 4% lidocaine, is generally safe. Laryngeal edema has been reported in a few cases, perhaps due to the propellant rather than to lidocaine itself (281). An unusual complication is mydriasis if part of the spray is accidentally directed to the eye (SEDA-18, 144).

- A 22-year-old man had a generalized tonic-clonic convulsion and loss of consciousness after an attempted superior laryngeal nerve block using 2% lidocaine 2 ml (282). The seizure was not terminated by intravenous diazepam 10 mg and he was intubated after intravenous thiopental and suxamethonium. He required two boluses of ephedrine 10 mg to maintain his blood pressure. Surgery proceeded uneventfully and he recovered without any sequelae.

The authors postulated vertebral artery injection of local anesthetic as the cause of the seizure and loss of consciousness.

Local anesthesia administered directly into a fracture hematoma can cause systemic absorption and toxicity (SED-12, 252) (283).

Lumbar plexus anesthesia

The combination of lumbar plexus and posterior sciatic nerve block represents an alternative to a neuraxial technique.

- An 80-year-old 41 kg woman was given a combination of a posterior lumbar plexus block and a posterior sciatic nerve block for dynamic hip screw repair of a fractured right neck of femur (284). The lumbar plexus block was technically difficult, requiring three attempts, and 25 ml of ropivacaine 0.75% (187.5 mg), adrenaline (1 in 400 000), and clonidine 50 micrograms was slowly injected, aspirating after every 3 ml. The sciatic nerve block was straightforward, and 20 ml of a solution containing mepivacaine 1.5% (300 mg), adrenaline 1 in 400 000, and clonidine 50 micrograms was injected slowly. She had seizures and dysrhythmias 20 minutes after completion of the block. Cardiopulmonary resuscitation was successful, surgery proceeded under general anesthesia, and she made a full recovery. Blood samples taken 5 minutes after the seizures contained ropivacaine 1.9 micrograms/ml and mepivacaine 3.7 micrograms/ml.

The authors suggested that the timing of events (the neurological signs preceded cardiac toxicity) suggested a toxic reaction to one of the local anesthetics or an overdose from their combination.

Nasal anesthesia

Intranasal 4% lidocaine has been used for migraine and cluster headaches with success and few serious adverse effects: a bitter taste was common and some patients complained of nasal burning and oropharyngeal numbness

Unilateral mydriasis (anisocoria), suggesting serious neurological injury, has been attributed to topical cocaine (285).

- A 51-year-old man developed mydriasis in one eye, with loss of the accommodation reflex, immediately after endoscopic sinus surgery, before which 4% cocaine had been applied to the nasal mucosa on cotton pledglets. There were no surgical or anatomical complications.

The authors suggested a diagnosis of local anesthetic blockade of the nasociliary nerve.

Acute angle closure glaucoma has been attributed to local cocaine (286).

- A 46-year-old woman developed acute angle closure glaucoma 24 hours after the application of topical intranasal 25% cocaine (about 200 mg) for an elective antral washout under general anesthesia. She developed a severe headache around the right eye, with halos and blurring of vision on the same side and associated nausea and vomiting. The next day, when she awoke, she had completely lost the vision in that eye.

Neck anesthesia

With regional anesthesia in the neck there is a risk of inadvertent intra-arterial injection; this could explain one report of convulsions in an elderly woman (287). There is also a risk of subarachnoid injection and pneumothorax.

Obstetric anesthesia

When a local anesthetic is used for episiotomy, there is a risk that the needle will enter the child's scalp; in two cases involving prilocaine, this resulted in cyanosis, methemoglobinemia, and hemolytic anemia (288).

Retroperitoneal hematoma has been reported as a complication of pudendal block, probably due to pudendal artery perforation (SEDA-21, 134).

Prilocaine 3% + felypressin 0.03 IU/ml has been compared with lidocaine 2% + adrenaline 12.5 micrograms/ml in 300 women having large-loop excision of the cervical transformation zone (289). Those who received lidocaine had significantly less blood loss, but were more likely to have adverse effects, including shaking and feeling faint.

Ocular anesthesia

A cluster of 25 cases of transient or permanent diplopia occurred after 13 retrobulbar blocks, 10 peribulbar blocks, and two unknown techniques, possibly related to the non-availability of hyaluronidase, highlighting the likely importance of hyaluronidase in preventing anesthetic-related myopathy in the extraocular muscles (290). Other reports of 21 cases of persistent postoperative diplopia following the peribulbar technique (291) and 4 cases following the retrobulbar technique during the period of non-availability of hyaluronidase support this theory (292). Bupivacaine and lidocaine may be contraindicated for peribulbar or retrobulbar injections without hyaluronidase.

Severe sneezing after ocular local anesthetic injection during intravenous sedation has been linked to photic sneezing. However, in 557 patients there was no relation between the two (293). Severe involuntary sneezing occurred after ocular blockade under thiopental sedation overall in 5.2% and only in 7.6% of those with a history of photic sneezing; peribulbar block had a significantly higher incidence of involuntary sneezing compared with retrobulbar block (24 versus 4.5%). Sneezing can occur with many hypnotics and after injections inside the muscle cone and outside the orbit, without pupillary dilatation or lid elevation (294). Awareness of this phenomenon can facilitate recognition and prompt needle withdrawal to avoid serious problems from sudden head movements during injection.

Ocular explosion occurred in seven cases after periocular anesthetic injections (295). To minimize the incidence of ocular explosion, the authors recommended the following:

(a) use a blunt needle and a 12 ml syringe;
(b) aspirate the plunger and wiggle the syringe before injection;
(c) discontinue the injection if corneal edema or resistance to injection is noted;
(d) inspect the globe for evidence of intraocular injection before ocular massage or placement of a Honan balloon.

Retrobulbar anesthesia

Retrobulbar anesthesia, competently administered, is a safe procedure. In 13 000 patients in whom a curved needle technique was used, the only serious complication was a single case of postoperative ischemic neuropathy (296). However, other centers have experienced recurrent problems with chemosis (up to 30%), sub-conjunctival hemorrhage, and lid hemorrhage before perfecting their technique (SEDA-18, 144).

Inadvertent injection into the subarachnoid space surrounding the optic nerve has on various occasions led to bilateral impairment of vision and ophthalmoplegia, with varying degrees of nervous system and respiratory effects, ranging from pulmonary edema (297) to respiratory arrest (SED-12, 254) (SEDA-21, 133) (298). Similar adverse effects result from diffusion of the local anesthetic toward the cerebrospinal fluid (SEDA-14, 110). Several groups have shown that such complications can occur, especially with higher concentrations, independently of any fault in technique (SED-12, 254) (299). Patients must therefore be closely monitored during ocular anesthesia and surgery. Particular care should be taken in patients with orbital roof defects, as there is potential for local anesthetics to move rapidly into the nervous system, with severe toxic effects (SEDA-20, 126).

On the other hand, headache after bupivacaine-induced block has been traced to the use of a vasoconstrictor additive, and is more likely to occur with noradrenaline than adrenaline (300). Unwanted effects on the eye muscles, occurring in some 1% of retrobulbar blocks, extend to ptosis, horizontal rectus muscle palsy, and lagophthalmos; all recover spontaneously within a matter of weeks (301). It has been postulated that local anesthetics can be myotoxic, causing contracture and subsequent diplopia (302). Tissue pressure, causing ischemia, can also lead to muscle damage and subsequent contracture and strabismus (SEDA-22, 139).

Two cases of vitreous hemorrhage have been observed after retrobulbar block in patients with severe diabetic retinopathy (303).

- A retrobulbar injection in a 45-year-old woman with high myopia was complicated by globe perforation with vitreous and submacular hemorrhage (304).
- In another case, retrobulbar hemorrhage and raised intraocular pressure developed after subtenon block with lidocaine (305).

Retinal vascular occlusion is rare, but it can occur in patients with severe vascular disease, without retrobulbar or optic nerve sheath hemorrhage; the mechanism is unclear (SED-12, 254) (306).

There is a risk of traumatic optic nerve injury with retrobulbar block (SEDA-21, 134).

Complications from retrobulbar block can arise from accidental scleral perforation and intraocular injection of local anesthetic.

- An 86-year-old man scheduled for cataract surgery sustained an inadvertent occult single perforating needle injury with an intraocular injection of 0.5% plain bupivacaine during a retrobulbar block using a long (38 mm) needle (307). He had pain on injection and a raised intraocular pressure, with corneal edema, poor iris detail, and a reduced red reflex. Paracentesis lowered the intraocular pressure and surgery proceeded uneventfully. At 6 weeks, he had a reduction in visual acuity, and a scan identified a vitreous hemorrhage and retinal detachment. Prompt vitreoretinal surgery was performed with reasonable success.

The authors added that retinal toxicity of the local anesthetic agent did not affect the visual outcome in this patient. Scleral perforation is a well-known complication of eye blocks for ophthalmic surgery. The incidence with retrobulbar techniques is 0.075% and with peribulbar blocks 0.0002%. When recognized, ocular perforation usually requires a vitreoretinal procedure and is associated with a poor visual outcome. Risk factors include an anxious or oversedated patient, long sharp needles, superior injection, incorrect angle of needle insertion, and myopic eyes. If the intraocular pressure is increased, paracentesis may acutely reduce it, preventing retinal and optic nerve ischemia and possible permanent visual loss.

Retrobulbar anesthesia can lead to serious systemic toxicity. However, in animal studies accidental intravitreous spread of lidocaine, bupivacaine, or a mixture of the two did not cause long-term retinal damage (308).

Possible techniques to reduce complications include avoiding Atkinson's position, the classical position for retrobulbar block (309), during injection, limiting the volume of solution injected, and the use of shorter needles (310,311).

Retrobulbar anesthesia can be complicated by brainstem anesthesia (312).

- A 79-year-old man received retrobulbar anesthesia using a 1:1 mixture of 2% lidocaine and 0.5% bupivacaine plus hyaluronidase, which was complicated by brainstem anesthesia presenting as dysarthria. Initially there was some resistance to injection and the syringe was withdrawn slightly before injection of 4 ml of solution; 5 minutes later he complained of a strange sensation in his throat, which progressed to difficulty in swallowing and not being able to speak above a whisper. His blood pressure rose to 210/118 and his pulse to 120/minute; he also had signs of involvement of cranial nerves III, VI, and XII. He received glyceryl trinitrate for the hypertension and by 24 hours all the cranial nerve symptoms and signs had resolved.

Two cases of cardiopulmonary arrest after retrobulbar block for corrective squint surgery have been described (313). Both the patients were fit, healthy young men and they received a retrobulbar block with 2% lidocaine 2 ml via a 23G 1.5" needle after negative aspiration. Three minutes later both complained of breathlessness and rapidly became apneic and unresponsive, with unrecordable pulse and blood pressure. Both were resuscitated and became fully alert within 40 minutes. Possible reasons suggested were an allergic reaction, a direct toxic effect, a vasovagal attack, intra-arterial injection, or injection directly into the optic nerve sheath with spread of the local anesthetic into the CSF. The latter seemed to be the most likely in these cases. Since then the authors have altered their technique, including changing the position of gaze and using a short blunt needle. These cases illustrate the need for careful monitoring, knowledge of potential complications, and the ready availability of resuscitation facilities (including appropriately trained personnel familiar with the equipment), even when performing what many regard as minor local anesthetic blocks.

Peribulbar anesthesia

Peribulbar anesthesia is generally considered safer than retrobulbar anesthesia, with a lower incidence of adverse effects. It avoids deep penetration of the orbit and therefore inadvertent subarachnoid injection. It also seems to be safer with regard to the risk of bulb perforation (314).

Cardiovascular

In addition to complications arising from the local anesthetic used during ocular anesthesia, complications can arise as a direct result of the injection. An arteriovenous fistula has been reported (315).

- An arteriovenous fistula of the supraorbital vessels developed in a 75-year-old man after peribulbar anesthesia with a supplementary supranasal injection. He elected to have conservative management and the lesion remained asymptomatic and static in size over 10 months follow-up.

Respiratory

Pulmonary edema has been attributed to lidocaine (316).

- A 74-year-old woman had peribulbar blockade with 4 ml of 2% lidocaine at the inferotemporal approach and then 3 ml at the medial approach. She had a history of mitral stenosis, occasional angina, and possibly myocardial infarction, but denied breathlessness on exertion, nocturnal dyspnea, or orthopnea. She had breathlessness and sweating 10 minutes after the medial injection. She then developed hypoxia and a few minutes later began to cough up pink frothy secretions, required intubation, and developed a sinus tachycardia without acute electrocardiographic or cardiac enzyme changes.

The authors assumed that she had developed neurogenic pulmonary edema, probably worsened by the co-existing myocardial disease.

Sensory systems

Nine patients developed prolonged symptomatic diplopia (predominantly vertical) after peribulbar anesthesia with ropivacaine 1% plus hyalase 750 units (317). The mean time to resolution of the diplopia was 24 hours. The authors stressed the importance of warning patients undergoing peribulbar blockade with ropivacaine of the possibility of prolonged diplopia and queried its future use in routine cataract surgery.

Six cases of global perforation have occurred during routine cataract surgery (SEDA-21, 134). It has incidentally led to contralateral mydriasis, hemiplegic coma, and damage to the infra-orbital nerve (SEDA-18, 144). The contralateral eye may exhibit oculomotor weakness (SEDA-16, 130). Three other reports have highlighted problems.

- A 76-year-old man undergoing trabeculectomy developed bilateral amaurosis after a peribulbar block with 6 ml of a mixture of 2% lidocaine, 0.5% bupivacaine, and hyaluronidase (318). The authors thought it unlikely that the optic nerve sheath had been penetrated and suggested that local spread to the optic nerves via the subarachnoid or subdural space had been responsible.
- A 49-year-old woman had a tonic-clonic seizure about 15 minutes after a peribulbar block for left trabeculectomy (319). She recovered and surgery continued uneventfully. However, she had severe permanent visual loss in that eye, and an MRI scan at 4 weeks showed swelling of the left optic nerve. The authors suggested that some prilocaine had been injected into the nerve sheath, causing the convulsions, local optic nerve swelling, and subsequent optic nerve atrophy.

In 60 patients, peribulbar blockade was performed with either 8 ml of 0.75% ropivacaine or a 1:1 mixture of 2% lidocaine and 0.5% bupivacaine (320). Surgical block was achieved after a similar period of time in each group, but ropivacaine provided a better quality of postoperative analgesia, with no pain reported at 24 hours in 26 (87%) compared with 18 (60%) in the lidocaine + bupivacaine group. One patient given ropivacaine reported unbearable pain due to a high intraocular pressure, and the incidence of postoperative nausea and vomiting was under 7% in both groups.

In 54 patients who received peribulbar anesthesia with either 1% ropivacaine or a mixture of 0.75% bupivacaine + 2% lidocaine there was no significant difference in akinesia scores or adverse effects reported the following day, notably headache, dizziness, nausea, scalp anesthesia, and diplopia, the latter occurring in 26% and 30% respectively (321).

Peribulbar anesthesia with 1% etidocaine, 0.5% bupivacaine, and hyaluronidase has been evaluated in 300 patients (322). The mean volume administered was 17 ml. There was adequate analgesia in 85% of cases, and the other 15% required supplementation with a subtenon block. Akinesia occurred in 82% of cases. Two patients developed generalized seizures, and four developed severe hypotension.

- A rare case of hyphema after peribulbar block with 1% lidocaine 8 ml occurred in a 38-year-old woman with a history of Fuchs' heterochromic iridocyclitis (323).

Postoperative strabismus and diplopia occurred in two of 200 patients undergoing cataract extraction under peribulbar anesthesia; the symptoms resolved spontaneously by 6 months (324).

Hematologic

- A 27-year-old woman with diabetes mellitus, complicated by diabetic retinopathy and chronic renal insufficiency with anemia, developed methemoglobinemia (11%) after peribulbar blockade with prilocaine 80 mg, bupivacaine 30 mg, hyaluronidase, and naphazoline (325). She recovered uneventfully after methylthioninium chloride 1.5 mg/kg.

The authors concluded that she may have been at increased risk of methemoglobinemia as a result of the metabolic acidosis associated with renal insufficiency, since impaired protein binding of prilocaine could have increased the concentrations of ionized prilocaine. Furthermore, the patient was also taking isosorbide dinitrate, which may have predisposed her to methemoglobinemia.

Topical anesthesia

Topical anesthesia in the eye is relatively safe in controlled circumstances, when administered correctly (SEDA-20, 127). There does not seem to be any benefit in warming topical local anesthetic solutions before use (326).

Topical anesthetic abuse, mostly unintentional, remains a persistent cause of keratitis and epithelial defects, leading to continuing ocular pain, visual impairment, and at worst enucleation (SEDA-21, 134) (SEDA-22, 140) (327). Mechanisms include direct toxicity of the local anesthetic or preservative and immunological causes.

In 14 patients, 0.5% proxymetacaine had similar efficacy to 0.4% oxybuprocaine and 0.5% tetracaine but was significantly better tolerated (328).

There have been reports of topical ocular anesthetic abuse.

- A 49-year-old woman developed repeated episodes of severe keratitis after radial keratotomy for myopia (329). After 18 months of repeated hospital admissions, several operations, and considerably reduced visual acuity, it eventually transpired that she had been self-medicating with 1% proparacaine mixed with artificial tears to control pain after her surgery.

Abuse of these medications often results in irreversible corneal damage and visual loss (330). Two patients continued to instil their topical 0.5% tetracaine eye-drops, despite medical advice. The result was bilateral corneal perforation in the first case and a large unilateral descemetocele in the second. Surgery was required to correct the perforations, but the long-term anatomical and functional results were poor. A third patient had obtained 0.5% tetracaine hydrochloride drops over the counter to relieve discomfort in his eye after colleagues at work had attempted to remove a foreign body from his eye. He had developed chronic toxic keratitis and was persuaded to discontinue the eye-drops. With appropriate treatment the cornea returned to normal.

Lidocaine gel 2% has been compared with 0.5% tetracaine drops for topical anesthesia in cataract surgery in 25 patients (331). There were no corneal epithelial or ocular surface complications, demonstrating the safety of the gel, which may provide a more practical and efficient method of anesthesia, because it needs to be applied only once as opposed to three applications of the drops.

Differences in the manufacture of unpreserved lidocaine formulations have been postulated as a cause of transient corneal clouding in patients who were given intraocular unpreserved lidocaine 1% as an adjunct to topical anesthesia (332). Independent analysis of the lidocaine solution associated with corneal clouding found it to be hypotonic and not buffered with bicarbonate compared with the solution that did not cause corneal clouding.

Intracameral anesthesia
Non-preserved intracameral lidocaine 1% is a useful adjunct to topical anesthesia for cataract surgery. In 631 patients, topical anesthesia alone was compared with combined topical and intracameral anesthesia (333) The combination had greater efficacy—only 1% of those given combined anesthesia needing to be converted to general anesthesia compared with 40% of those given topical anesthesia alone. The authors suggest that the key difference between the two methods is reduced sensitivity to the microscope light. Another prospective study in 93 patients showed that intracameral non-preserved lidocaine was both safe and efficacious; four patients reported discomfort and none had measurable endothelial cellular changes (334).

The endothelial toxicity of local anesthetics has been assessed in pigs, as this might be relevant to the safety of agents given by intracameral injection (335). Lidocaine, mepivacaine, and prilocaine were safe, while bupivacaine in clinically effective concentrations resulted in significant cell reduction.

Sub-tenon anesthesia
Sub-tenon infiltration of local anesthesia has recently become increasingly popular for cataract and vitreoretinal surgery; presumed advantages are its safety, speed of onset, and patient compliance. Three cases of persistent diplopia following sub-tenon local anesthesia have been reported (336). Two of the patients were given injections of 4 ml of a mixture of lidocaine 1% or 2% with adrenaline 1 in 100 000 and hyaluronidase 1500 units, and the third was given 4 ml of 0.75% bupivacaine with lidocaine. All had vertical diplopia, consistent with restriction of the inferior rectus muscle, which persisted for 2–9 months. The authors suggested possible mechanisms, including direct trauma to the muscle, inflammation and adhesions, infection, and myotoxicity of local anesthetics. They have since modified their technique, reducing the rate and force of infiltration.

An infectious complication of sub-tenon anesthesia has been reported (337).

- A 63-year-old woman underwent phacoemulsification and lens implantation under sub-tenon block. After the local anesthetic was injected, the eye was prepared with an aqueous solution of povidone iodine and the surgery proceeded uneventfully. At the end, gentamicin and betamethasone were injected subconjunctivally. Over the next few days she developed orbital cellulitis, requiring intravenous antibiotics.

The authors concluded that bacterial contamination of the episcleral space from the ocular surface or skin flora had occurred during or after the sub-tenon injection. They recommended applying topical povidone iodine before the episcleral space is opened, in order to reduce this risk.

Eyelid and conjunctival anesthesia
Local infiltration with prilocaine 2% was significantly more comfortable than lidocaine 2% in a prospective randomized study in 125 patients undergoing minor eyelid procedures (338).

Two cases of transient blindness after subconjunctival injection of 2% mepivacaine 2 ml were reported in patients with advanced refractory glaucoma undergoing diode laser cyclophotocoagulation (339). The authors hypothesized that in patients with advanced optic neuropathy, even subconjunctival anesthesia can result in optic nerve block.

Oropharyngeal anesthesia
Reduced hepatic clearance, as well as relative overdosage, of local anesthetics can lead to systemic toxicity, as illustrated by three patients who underwent topical anesthesia of the oropharynx for transesophageal echocardiography and subsequently became confused and drowsy (SEDA-21, 135).

- Acute bilateral parotid swelling occurred after upper gastrointestinal endoscopy in a 53-year-old woman who had gargled 2% lidocaine solution beforehand; the swelling was associated with difficulty in swallowing and resolved after treatment with intravenous glucocorticoids for 4 days (340).
- A 21-year-old developed seizures, respiratory distress requiring tracheal intubation, severe hypotension, and then bradycardia culminating in asystole and death while gargling with 4% lidocaine 20 ml (800 mg) (341).

The authors strongly advised against exceeding the maximum recommended dose of lidocaine (200 mg), even when using it topically.

Otic anesthesia
Transient vestibular irritation without hearing loss after infiltration of the auditory canal has been incidentally attributed to diffusion of the local anesthetic from the site of injection (342).

Paravertebral anesthesia
Postural headache after thoracic paravertebral nerve anesthesia, and probably reflecting dural entry, has been reported (343). Nerve root damage is another possible complication. Hematuria due to injury to the kidney or ureter is an unusual complication of lumbar paravertebral sympathetic block (344).

An epidural abscess and paraplegia occurred after paravertebral lidocaine infiltration for back pain (SEDA-21, 133).

Among 44 women who received a single paravertebral block with 0.3 ml/kg of 0.5% bupivacaine at the level of T4 for breast surgery, there was one incident of epidural spread of the block with paraparesis for 280 minutes accompanied by unilateral Horner's syndrome for 170 minutes (345).

Post-thoracotomy pain can be treated with thoracic epidural or thoracic paravertebral blockade. In 100 adult patients allocated to receive one of these treatments with preoperative bolus doses of bupivacaine followed by a continuous infusion there was less postoperative respiratory morbidity and significantly better arterial oxygenation in the paravertebral group; nausea (10 versus 2), vomiting (7 versus 2), and hypotension (7 versus 0) were more problematic in the epidural group (346).

Perianal anesthesia

Local anesthetic ointments are widely used to relieve the symptoms of hemorrhoids and anal fissures. Absorption through the mucosa can be considerable; a case of convulsions as a suspected consequence of such treatment has been cited (SED-12, 253) (347).

Peritonsillar anesthesia

A stroke occurred after infiltration of the tonsillar bed with bupivacaine subsequent to tonsillectomy (348).

- A 16-year-old girl undergoing adenotonsillectomy had cardiac asystole for 10 seconds after injection of her adenoid bed with 0.5% bupivacaine 1 ml with adrenaline 5 micrograms/ml. She had already been given an unstated quantity of bupivacaine with adrenaline 5 micrograms/ml injected into her tonsillar fossae. Her cardiac output returned spontaneously, but she had a central medullopontine infarction, confirmed on MRI and CT brain scans. Magnetic resonance angiography showed an abnormal circle of Willis, with absence of both posterior communicating vessels. The authors were unclear as to the exact cause of the cardiac event and stroke, which resulted in a persistent neurological deficit.

Two cases of medullary injury after injections of local anesthetics intraoperatively have been reported (349).

- A 4-year-old child received injections of lidocaine plus adrenaline into the anterior tonsillar pillars and nasopharynx during adenotonsillectomy. After the procedure, he became agitated and dysarthric, vomited, and had abnormal eye movements. He was unable to stand and walk, owing to ataxia. An MRI scan showed a cavity in the right paramedian medulla.
- A 7-year-old boy underwent tonsillectomy, with an injection of lidocaine plus adrenaline into the operative field. After surgery he was lethargic, and during the next 24 hours he developed respiratory distress requiring mechanical ventilation. He was pyrexial (41.8°C) and had cardiomegaly and a left hemiparesis. A cranial MRI scan showed a hemorrhagic lesion in the right paramedian medulla.

Both patients had lesions in the medial medulla supplied by branches of the anterior spinal and vertebral arteries, and although such cases are rare it seems wise, in the light of these reports, to avoid the routine use of adrenaline as an adjunct to local anesthesia for adenotonsillectomy.

Excessive volumes of local anesthetic in a confined space can lead to life-threatening upper airway obstruction. When glossopharyngeal nerve blocks are used for tonsillectomy, children under 15 kg should be given 1 ml or less of 0.25% bupivacaine per tonsil (350).

Respiratory anesthesia

Topical anesthesia of the airways is commonly used to facilitate endoscopy and sometimes manipulation of the airways. This can result in an increase in airway flow resistance, possibly due to laryngeal dysfunction (351). Lidocaine spray 10%, used for upper airways anesthesia for fiber optic intubation in a grossly obese patient, caused acute airway obstruction. The patient went on to have a percutaneous tracheotomy, and it was postulated that the local anesthetic had abolished laryngeal receptors responsible for airway maintenance, or that laryngospasm and reduced muscle tone due to the lidocaine might have been the cause (SEDA-22, 140).

- Unilateral bronchospasm has been described in a 19-year-old woman after the administration of lidocaine 4% 5 ml into the larynx via a Laryngojet injector (352).

Lidocaine gel is not recommended for lubrication of laryngeal masks. It confers no benefits and increases the incidence of adverse effects such as intraoperative hiccups, postoperative hoarseness, nausea, vomiting, and tongue paresthesia (353).

- A patient due to have a bronchoscopy was given an overdose of lidocaine to anesthetize the airway by an inexperienced health worker. He was then left unobserved and subsequently developed convulsions and cardiopulmonary arrest (354). He survived with severe cerebral damage. His lidocaine concentration was 24 micrograms/ml about 1 hour after initial administration (a blood concentration over 6 micrograms/ml is considered to be toxic).
- A 19-year-old healthy volunteer undergoing bronchoscopy was given about 1200 mg of lidocaine to anesthetize the airway and was sent home after the procedure, despite complaining of chest pain. Shortly afterwards she had a tonic-clonic seizure and cardiopulmonary arrest and died 2 days later. The research protocol had failed to specify an upper dose limit for lidocaine (355).

Sciatic nerve anesthesia

Sciatic nerve anesthesia can cause cardiovascular depression (356).

- A 74-year-old man was to receive a combined sciatic nerve and psoas compartment block for a total hip arthroplasty; the classic Labat's approach was used and 30 ml of 0.75% ropivacaine was injected over 1.5 minutes, after which he suddenly became unresponsive and developed tonic–clonic movements. Propofol was administered and the seizure resolved, but he developed sinus bradycardia with progressive lengthening of the QRS interval, which converted to nodal bradycardia. A ventricular escape rhythm at 20/minute with T wave inversion was treated with ephedrine 10 mg and adrenaline 0.1 mg, resulting in supraventricular tachycardia with transient atrial fibrillation.

The authors pointed out that an equipotent dose of bupivacaine would have resulted in worse cardiovascular depression with less chance of successful resuscitation.

Stellate ganglion anesthesia

Inadvertent spinal anesthesia and subsequent nervous system toxicity, for example with transient paralysis or apnea, are the main complications of stellate ganglion block (SEDA-22, 140). It has been suggested that ultrasound guidance when performing the block might improve safety (357). The use of very small test doses and an anterior approach to the stellate ganglion are recommended preventive measures.

Brachial plexus paresis has been reported (358). Accidental block of the recurrent laryngeal nerve can cause hoarseness and occasionally aspiration of saliva (359).

In two women with Raynaud's syndrome, the symptoms were aggravated contralaterally after stellate ganglion block (SEDA-18, 145).

Severe hypertension has been reported after a left-sided block, possibly due to vagal nerve block and unopposed sympathetic output (SEDA-21, 134).

Convulsions are a recognized complication of inadvertent intra-arterial injection during stellate ganglion block; two such cases have been described (360).

- A 28-year-old 75 kg woman underwent stellate ganglion block for symptomatic treatment of Raynaud's syndrome. An anterolateral approach was used, guarding the carotid artery and jugular vein. After an aspiration test was negative in two planes, 5 ml of 1% lidocaine was injected over 2–3 seconds using a 20 G needle. However, a second aspiration test was positive for blood, the needle was pulled back, and on reinjection the patient immediately had a severe generalized tonic-clonic seizure. The patient made a rapid recovery with no further treatment and was fully conscious after 2 minutes.
- A 31-year-old 72 kg man with diabetes, who had had a below-knee amputation in the past, developed Buerger's disease affecting his hands, particularly on the right. He underwent his third stellate ganglion block for symptomatic treatment. An anterior paratracheal approach was used with a 20 G 3.5 cm needle; after an aspiration test was negative in two planes, 1 ml of 1% lidocaine was injected every 2–3 seconds. After one injection, he had an abrupt seizure which was treated with diazepam 10 mg. He made a full recovery and later completed his course of stellate ganglion blocks uneventfully.

It was thought that inadvertent vertebral arterial injection had occurred, with subsequent rapid elimination due to high cerebral blood flow. The authors suggested several precautions to minimize this risk, including using a large-diameter needle and using less than the calculated minimum arterial toxic dose of lidocaine (16.8 mg) as the initial test dose; for subsequent doses they suggested 5 mg.

Subcutaneous anesthesia

When infiltrating local anesthetics into the skin there is always a risk of intravascular injection (SEDA-17, 140), but it can be avoided by back-aspiration of the syringe or continuous advancement of the needle during injection.

Skin infiltration with local anesthetics can cause pain. The pain experienced during skin infiltration of lidocaine, chloroprocaine, and buffered solutions of both has been studied in 22 volunteers in a double-blind, randomized study (361). The pH of the solutions was unrelated to the pain score, but both formulations of chloroprocaine were significantly less painful than lidocaine.

A weak solution of lidocaine has sometimes been injected into excess fat before liposuction, so that the procedure can be carried out without general anesthesia. The technique is generally regarded as safe (362). However, deaths are reported, associated with local anesthetic toxicity or drug interactions (363).

Of 30 volunteers who had subcutaneous slow infusion tumescent anesthesia at 250 ml/hour with three solutions containing lidocaine 2 mg/ml, ropivacaine 0.5 mg/ml mixed with lidocaine 1 mg/ml, and ropivacaine 1 mg/ml alone, all containing adrenaline 1:1 000 000, one had a tingling sensation in the tongue after lidocaine and another went into vasovagal shock (364). In the same paper, 5020 surgical procedures were reported in 3270 patients using different strengths of ropivacaine alone (0.05–0.2%) with a maximum dose of 300 mg, or with a mixture of ropivacaine and prilocaine (0.08–0.3%) with a maximum ropivacaine dose of 160 mg and a maximum prilocaine dose of 300 mg. There was no methemoglobinemia and there were no minor or major adverse effects related to the local anesthetic. The maximum plasma concentrations were low, suggesting that higher maximum doses may be possible, provided adrenaline is added.

- Ventricular tachycardia, severe hypertension, and pulmonary edema developed in a 53-year-old woman soon after she had a skin flap infiltrated with 4 ml of 0.5% lidocaine and 0.0005% adrenaline (20 micrograms) (365).

This has been previously described during general anesthesia but not with a local anesthetic alone, and the author emphasized the risk of severe cardiovascular compromise, even with a small dose of adrenaline.

Five patients with complex regional pain syndrome received a subcutaneous infusion of 10% lidocaine, with successful alleviation of many of their symptoms; initially 200 mg/kg was infused but symptoms of vertigo and slurred speech each occurred in four of them and stuttering in three, so the rate was adjusted to 100–190 mg/hour and serum lidocaine concentrations of 0.1–8.1 micrograms/ml (average 3.7 micrograms/ml); other symptoms, such as aphasia, nausea, fatigue, metallic taste, lightheadedness, and perioral numbness, each occurred in over half of the patients (366).

An iatrogenic tension pneumothorax was the result of breast infiltration with lidocaine and adrenaline before an augmentation procedure (SEDA-20, 127).

Infiltration anesthesia has reportedly caused transient paralysis.

- Transient paraplegia occurred after wound site infiltration with bupivacaine in a 35-year-old woman during removal of a lumboperitoneal shunt that had been inserted 2 years previously for benign intracranial hypertension (367). Under general anesthesia with the patient in the left lateral position, a small incision was made over the right flank and the drain was easily removed. The site was infiltrated with 7.5 ml of 0.5% bupivacaine with adrenaline 1 in 200 000. During recovery, she was anxious and moderately hypotensive and had a flaccid paralysis from T4 down. An MRI scan was normal. She gradually recovered motor function, sensation, and pain at the wound site.

The authors concluded that the local anesthetic may have passed down a fistulous track into the subarachnoid space, producing spinal block.

Submucosal anesthesia

Complications noted at various times with submucosal use include allergic reactions to the parabens present in lidocaine, systemic effects due to general diffusion (which

144. Hogagard JT, Djurhuus H. Two cases of reiterated Horner's syndrome after lumbar epidural block. Acta Anaesthesiol Scand 2000;44(8):1021–3.
145. Zahn PK, Van Aken HK, Marcus AE. Horner's syndrome following epidural anesthesia with ropivacaine for cesarean delivery. Reg Anesth Pain Med 2002;27(4):445–6.
146. Kehlet H, Brandt MR, Hansen AP, Alberti KG. Effect of epidural analgesia on metabolic profiles during and after surgery. Br J Surg 1979;66(8):543–6.
147. Lund J, Stjernstrom H, Jorfeldt L, Wiklund L. Effect of extradural analgesia on glucose metabolism and gluconeogenesis. Studies in association with upper abdominal surgery. Br J Anaesth 1986;58(8):851–7.
148. Jacobs JS, Vallejo R, DeSouza GJ, TerRiet MF. Severe hypoglycemia after labor epidural analgesia. Anesth Analg 2000;90(4):892–3.
149. Olofsson CI, Ekblom AO, Ekman-Ordeberg GE, Irestedt LE. Post-partum urinary retention: a comparison between two methods of epidural analgesia. Eur J Obstet Gynecol Reprod Biol 1997;71(1):31–4.
150. Thomson SJ, Lomax DM, Collett BJ. Chemical meningism after lumbar facet joint block with local anaesthetic and steroids. Anaesthesia 1991;46(7):563–4.
151. Reiz S, Nath S. Cardiotoxicity of local anaesthetic agents. Br J Anaesth 1986;58(7):736–46.
152. Meister GC, D'Angelo R, Owen M, Nelson KE, Gaver R. A comparison of epidural analgesia with 0.125% ropivacaine with fentanyl versus 0.125% bupivacaine with fentanyl during labor. Anesth Analg 2000;90(3):632–7.
153. Bjornestad E, Smedvig JP, Bjerkreim T, Narverud G, Kolleros D, Bergheim R. Epidural ropivacaine 7.5 mg/ml for elective Caesarean section: a double-blind comparison of efficacy and tolerability with bupivacaine 5 mg/ml. Acta Anaesthesiol Scand 1999;43(6):603–8.
154. Dick W. Gefährdung der Mutter durch Allgemeinanaesthesie und Regionalanaesthesie. [Maternal risk from general anaesthesia and regional anaesthesia.] Anaesthesist 1980;29(5):219–25.
155. Douglas MJ. Potential complications of spinal and epidural anesthesia for obstetrics. Semin Perinatol 1991;15(5):368–74.
156. Knitza R, Sirtl C, Wisser J, Rhein R, Fischer B. Zerebraler Krampfanfall nach Periduralanästhesie mit Bupivacain zur Sectio caesarea. [Cerebral convulsion following peridural anesthesia with bupivacaine in cesarean section.] Geburtshilfe Frauenheilkd 1988;48(1):47–9.
157. Muth H, Schliemann F. Zur Periduralanaesthesie in der Geburthilfe. [Peridural anesthesia during labor. Report on 2726 cases.] Med Welt 1981;32(13):420–1.
158. Bratteby LE. Effects on the infant of obstetric regional analgesia. J Perinat Med 1981;9(Suppl 1):54–6.
159. Morikawa S, Ishikawa J, Kamatsuki H, Shinzato Y, Watanabe A, Ishikawa H, Chihara H, Nagata T, Kometani K. [Neurobehavior and mental development of newborn infants delivered under epidural analgesia with bupivacaine..] Nippon Sanka Fujinka Gakkai Zasshi 1990;42(11):1495–502.
160. Golub MS, Germann SL. Perinatal bupivacaine and infant behavior in rhesus monkeys. Neurotoxicol Teratol 1998;20(1):29–41.
161. Meunier JF, Goujard E, Dubousset AM, Samii K, Mazoit JX. Pharmacokinetics of bupivacaine after continuous epidural infusion in infants with and without biliary atresia. Anesthesiology 2001;95(1):87–95.
162. Parkinson SK, Mueller JB, Rich TJ, Little WL. Unilateral Horner's syndrome associated with interpleural catheter injection of local anesthetic. Anesth Analg 1989;68(1):61–2.
163. Abbott PJ Jr, Sullivan G. Cardiovascular toxicity following preincisional intra-articular injection of bupivicaine. Arthroscopy 1997;13(2):282.
164. Wand A, Junger H. Embolia cutis medicamentosa in atypical localisation. Aktuelle Derm 1990;16:128–9.
165. Nevarre DR, Tzarnas CD. The effects of hyaluronidase on the efficacy and on the pain of administration of 1% lidocaine. Plast Reconstr Surg 1998;101(2):365–9.
166. Bartfield JM, Sokaris SJ, Raccio-Robak N. Local anesthesia for lacerations: pain of infiltration inside vs outside the wound. Acad Emerg Med 1998;5(2):100–4.
167. Bartfield JM, Pauze D, Raccio-Robak N. The effect of order on pain of local anesthetic infiltration. Acad Emerg Med 1998;5(2):105–7.
168. Colaric KB, Overton DT, Moore K. Pain reduction in lidocaine administration through buffering and warming. Am J Emerg Med 1998;16(4):353–6.
169. Ahmed SM, Khan RM, Bano S, Ajmani P, Kumar A. Is spinal anaesthesia safe in pre-eclamptic toxaemia patients? J Indian Med Assoc 1999;97(5):165–8.
170. McDonald SB, Liu SS, Kopacz DJ, Stephenson CA. Hyperbaric spinal ropivacaine: a comparison to bupivacaine in volunteers. Anesthesiology 1999;90(4):971–7.
171. Malinovsky JM, Charles F, Kick O, Lepage JY, Malinge M, Cozian A, Bouchot O, Pinaud M. Intrathecal anesthesia: ropivacaine versus bupivacaine. Anesth Analg 2000;91(6):1457–60.
172. Mollmann M, Cord S, Holst D, Auf der Landwehr U. Continuous spinal anaesthesia or continuous epidural anaesthesia for post-operative pain control after hip replacement? Eur J Anaesthesiol 1999;16(7):454–61.
173. Concepcion MA, Lambert DH, Welch KA, Covino BG. Tourniquet pain during spinal anesthesia: a comparison of plain solutions of tetracaine and bupivacaine. Anesth Analg 1988;67(9):828–32.
174. Karakan M, Tahtaci N, Goksu S. The effects of intrathecal bupivacaine and fentanyl in combined spinal epidural anesthesia. Int Med J 2000;7:145–9.
175. Owen MD, Ozsarac O, Sahin S, Uckunkaya N, Kaplan N, Magunaci I. Low-dose clonidine and neostigmine prolong the duration of intrathecal bupivacaine–fentanyl for labor analgesia. Anesthesiology 2000;92(2):361–6.
176. Kathirvel S, Sadhasivam S, Saxena A, Kannan TR, Ganjoo P. Effects of intrathecal ketamine added to bupivacaine for spinal anaesthesia. Anaesthesia 2000;55(9):899–904.
177. Ben-David B, Miller G, Gavriel R, Gurevitch A. Low-dose bupivacaine-fentanyl spinal anesthesia for cesarean delivery. Reg Anesth Pain Med 2000;25(3):235–9.
178. Mulroy MF, Greengrass R, Ganapathy S, Chan V, Heierson A. Sameridine is safe and effective for spinal anesthesia: a comparative dose-ranging study with lidocaine for inguinal hernia repair. Anesth Analg 1999;88(4):815–21.
179. Unzueta Merino MC, Escolan Villen F, Aliaga Font L, Cantallops Pericas B, Sabate Pes A, Aguilar JL, Villar Landeira JM. Revision de las complicaciones de la anestesia espinal en un periodo de 8 anos (1977–1984). [Review of the complications of spinal anesthesia in an 8-year period (1977–1984).] Rev Esp Anestesiol Reanim 1986;33(5):336–41.
180. Holst D, Mollmann M, Karmann S, Wendt M. Kreislaufverhalten unter Spinalanasthesie. Kathetertechnik versus Single-dose-Verfahren. [Circulatory reactions under spinal anesthesia. The catheter technique versus the single dose procedure.] Anaesthesist 1997;46(1):38–42.
181. Critchley LA, Short TG, Gin T. Hypotension during subarachnoid anaesthesia: haemodynamic analysis of three treatments. Br J Anaesth 1994;72(2):151–5.
182. Mark JB, Steele SM. Cardiovascular effects of spinal anesthesia. Int Anesthesiol Clin 1989;27(1):31–9.

183. Hemmingsen C, Poulsen JA, Risbo A. Prophylactic ephedrine during spinal anaesthesia: double-blind study in patients in ASA groups I–III. Br J Anaesth 1989;63(3):340–2.
184. Critchley LA, Stuart JC, Conway F, Short TG. Hypotension during subarachnoid anaesthesia: haemodynamic effects of ephedrine. Br J Anaesth 1995;74(4):373–8.
185. Critchley LA, Conway F. Hypotension during subarachnoid anaesthesia: haemodynamic effects of colloid and metaraminol. Br J Anaesth 1996;76(5):734–6.
186. Critchley LA, Morley AP, Derrick J. The influence of baricity on the haemodynamic effects of intrathecal bupivacaine 0.5%. Anaesthesia 1999;54(5):469–74.
187. Hallworth S, Fernando R. The spread and side-effects of intrathecally administered bupivacaine. Anaesthesia 1999;54(10):1016–17.
188. Bandi E, Weeks S, Carli F. Spinal block levels and cardiovascular changes during post-Cesarean transport. Can J Anaesth 1999;46(8):736–40.
189. Mahe V, Ecoffey C. Spinal anesthesia with isobaric bupivacaine in infants. Anesthesiology 1988;68(4):601–3.
190. Kiran S, Singal NK. A comparative study of three different doses of 0.5% hyperbaric bupivacaine for spinal anaesthesia in elective caesarean section. Int J Obstet Anesth 2002;11(3):185–9.
191. Caplan RA, Ward RJ, Posner K, Cheney FW. Unexpected cardiac arrest during spinal anesthesia: a closed claims analysis of predisposing factors. Anesthesiology 1988;68(1):5–11.
192. Jordi EM, Marsch SC, Strebel S. Third degree heart block and asystole associated with spinal anesthesia. Anesthesiology 1998;89(1):257–60.
193. Coleman MM, Bardwaj A, Chan VV. Back pain and collapse associated with receding subarachnoid blockade. Can J Anaesth 1999;46(5 Pt 1):464–6.
194. Casati A, Fanelli G, Beccaria P, Aldegheri G, Berti M, Senatore R, Torri G. Block distribution and cardiovascular effects of unilateral spinal anaesthesia by 0.5% hyperbaric bupivacaine. A clinical comparison with bilateral spinal block. Minerva Anestesiol 1998;64(7–8):307–12.
195. Kuczkowski KM. Respiratory arrest in a parturient following intrathecal administration of fentanyl and bupivacaine as part of a combined spinal-epidural analgesia for labour. Anaesthesia 2002;57(9):939–40.
196. Sartorelli KH, Abajian JC, Kreutz JM, Vane DW. Improved outcome utilizing spinal anesthesia in high-risk infants. J Pediatr Surg 1992;27(8):1022–5.
197. Tobias JD, Burd RS, Helikson MA. Apnea following spinal anaesthesia in two former pre-term infants. Can J Anaesth 1998;45(10):985–9.
198. Piquet CY, Mallaret MP, Lemoigne AH, Barjhoux CE, Danel VC, Vincent FH. Respiratory depression following administration of intrathecal bupivacaine to an opioid-dependent patient. Ann Pharmacother 1998;32(6):653–5.
199. Katsiris S, Williams S, Leighton BL, Halpern S. Respiratory arrest following intrathecal injection of sufentanil and bupivacaine in a parturient. Can J Anaesth 1998;45(9):880–3.
200. Fragneto RY, Fisher A. Mental status change and aphasia after labor analgesia with intrathecal sufentanil/bupivacaine. Anesth Analg 2000;90(5):1175–6.
201. Chan YK, Gopinathan R, Rajendram R. Loss of consciousness following spinal anaesthesia for caesarean section. Br J Anaesth 2000;85(3):474–6.
202. Wajima Z, Shitara T, Inoue T, Ogawa R. Severe lightning pain after subarachnoid block in a patient with neuropathic pain of central origin: which drug is best to treat the pain? Clin J Pain 2000;16(3):265–9.
203. Robles Romero M, Gonzalez Mesa JM, de las Heras Rosas MA, Rojas Caracuel MA, Garcia Perez A, Hurtado Leiva F. Meningitis aseptica tras anestesia intradura. [Aseptic meningitis after intradural anesthesia.] Rev Esp Anestesiol Reanim 2000;47(5):226.
204. Schou H, Hole P. Neurologic deficit following spinal anesthesia. Acta Anaesthesiol Belg 1987;38(3):241–3.
205. Chen IC, Lin CS, Chou HM, Peng TH, Liu CH, Wang CF, Lin IS. Unexpected recurrent seizures following repeated spinal injections of tetracaine—a case report. Acta Anaesthesiol Sin 2000;38(2):103–6.
206. Benson JS. U.S. Food and Drug Administration safety alert: cauda equina syndrome associated with use of small-bore catheters in continuous spinal anesthesia. AANA J 1992;60(3):223.
207. Standl T, Eckert S, Schulte am Esch J. Microcatheter continuous spinal anaesthesia in the post-operative period: a prospective study of its effectiveness and complications. Eur J Anaesthesiol 1995;12(3):273–9.
208. Loo CC, Irestedt L. Cauda equina syndrome after spinal anaesthesia with hyperbaric 5% lignocaine: a review of six cases of cauda equina syndrome reported to the Swedish Pharmaceutical Insurance 1993–1997. Acta Anaesthesiol Scand 1999;43(4):371–9.
209. Uefuji T. [Persistent neurological deficit and adhesive arachnoiditis following spinal anesthesia with bupivacaine containing preservatives..] Masui 1999;48(2):176–80.
210. Horlocker TT, McGregor DG, Matsushige DK, Chantigian RC, Schroeder DR, Besse JA. Neurologic complications of 603 consecutive continuous spinal anesthetics using macrocatheter and microcatheter techniques. Perioperative Outcomes Group. Anesth Analg 1997;84(5):1063–70.
211. Tetzlaff JE, Dilger J, Yap E, Smith MP, Schoenwald PK. Cauda equina syndrome after spinal anaesthesia in a patient with severe vascular disease. Can J Anaesth 1998;45(7):667–9.
212. Lee DS, Bui T, Ferrarese J, Richardson PK. Cauda equina syndrome after incidental total spinal anesthesia with 2% lidocaine. J Clin Anesth 1998;10(1):66–9.
213. Kubina P, Gupta A, Oscarsson A, Axelsson K, Bengtsson M. Two cases of cauda equina syndrome following spinal-epidural anesthesia. Reg Anesth 1997;22(5):447–50.
214. Akioka K, Torigoe K, Maruta H, Shimizu N, Kobayashi Y, Kaneko Y, Shiratori R. A case of cauda equina syndrome following spinal anesthesia with hyperbaric dibucaine. J Anesth 2001;15(2):106–7.
215. Gisvold SE. Lidocaine may still be an excellent drug for spinal anaesthesia. Acta Anaesthesiol Scand 1999;43(4):369–70.
216. Salmela L, Aromaa U. Transient radicular irritation after spinal anesthesia induced with hyperbaric solutions of cerebrospinal fluid-diluted lidocaine 50 mg/ml or mepivacaine 40 mg/ml or bupivacaine 5 mg/ml. Acta Anaesthesiol Scand 1998;42(7):765–9.
217. Salazar F, Bogdanovich A, Adalia R, Chabas E, Gomar C. Transient neurologic symptoms after spinal anaesthesia using isobaric 2% mepivacaine and isobaric 2% lidocaine. Acta Anaesthesiol Scand 2001;45(2):240–5.
218. Saito S, Radwan I, Obata H, Takahashi K, Goto F. Direct neurotoxicity of tetracaine on growth cones and neurites of growing neurons in vitro. Anesthesiology 2001;95(3):726–33.
219. Hampl K, Schneider M, Corbey MP, Bach AB, Dahlgren N. Transient radicular irritation after spinal anaesthesia with Xylocain. Acta Anaesthesiol Scand 1999;43(3):359–65.
220. Neal JM, Pollock JE. Can scapegoats stand on shifting sands? Reg Anesth Pain Med 1998;23(6):533–7.
221. deJong RH. In my opinion: spinal lidocaine: a continuing enigma. J Clin Monit Comput 1998;14(2):147–8.

traditional tricyclic compounds must be viewed with skepticism (SEDA-11, 14). However, lofepramine is safer than conventional tricyclic antidepressants in overdose.

References

1. d'Elia G, Borg S, Hermann L, Lundin G, Perris C, Raotma H, Roman G, Siwers B. Comparative clinical evaluation of lofepramine and imipramine. Psychiatric aspects. Acta Psychiatr Scand 1977;55(1):10–20.
2. Bernik V, Maia E. Therapeutical and clinical evaluation of a new antidepressant drug, lofepramin (EMD 31.802), in comparison to amitriptyline in the treatment of depression. Rev Bras Clin Ter 1978;7:43.

Loganiaceae

See also Herbal medicines

General Information

The genera in the family of Loganiaceae (Table 1) include strychnos and trumpet flower.

Strychnos nux-vomica

The dried ripe seeds of *Strychnos nux-vomica* (nux vomica) contain the alkaloids strychnine and brucine, together with traces of other alkaloids.

Adverse effects

Strychnine is a powerful convulsant, which can cause serious and even lethal poisoning (1).

Maqianzi, the dried ripe seed of *S. nux-vomica* contains 1.0–1.4% each of strychnine and brucine. It has been used as a herbal remedy for rheumatism, musculoskeletal injuries, and limb paralysis.

- A 42-year-old woman with neck pain took 15 g of maqianzi in two doses 7 hours apart (recommended dose 0.3–0.6 g) (2). One hour after she took the second dose she suddenly developed tonic contractions of all her limbs and carpopedal spasm lasting 5 minutes, difficulty in breathing, chest discomfort, and perioral numbness. She complained of muscle pain and tiredness and had hyperventilation and weakness of all four limbs. All her symptoms gradually subsided over the next few hours.

Table 1 The genera of Loganiaceae

Fagraea
Gelsemium (trumpet flower)
Labordia (labordia)
Mitreola (hornpod)
Spigelia (pinkroot)
Strychnos (strychnos)

References

1. Wang Z, Zhao J, Xing J, He Y, Guo D. Analysis of strychnine and brucine in postmortem specimens by RP-HPLC: a case report of fatal intoxication. J Anal Toxicol 2004;28(2):141–4.
2. Chan TY. Herbal medicine causing likely strychnine poisoning. Hum Exp Toxicol 2002;21(8):467–8.

Lomefloxacin

See also Fluoroquinolones

General Information

Lomefloxacin is a fluoroquinolone antibacterial drug with actions and uses similar to those of ciprofloxacin.

Organs and Systems

Gastrointestinal

In a multicenter, prospective, randomized study of oral lomefloxacin 400 mg/day in 182 patients with chronic bacterial prostatitis, the most frequent adverse events were gastrointestinal disorders (1).

Skin

Photosensitivity was found in 44 (1.03%) of 4276 patients treated with lomefloxacin in Japan. Most cases were not severe and improved after withdrawal. Risk factors for a sensitivity reaction were age over 60 years with concomitant diseases and complications, total amount of lomefloxacin over 20 g, treatment for longer than 30 days, and previous treatment with a quinolone (2).

In eight patients (mean age 69 years) with eczematous or acute sunburn-like lesions in photo-exposed areas, who took lomefloxacin for 1 week to several months, phototoxicity appeared to be the main mechanism of photosensitivity, particularly in older patients with concomitant diseases and long-term use of the drug (3).

References

1. Naber KG; European Lomefloxacin Prostatitis Study Group. Lomefloxacin versus ciprofloxacin in the treatment of chronic bacterial prostatitis. Int J Antimicrob Agents 2002;20(1):18–27.
2. Arata J, Horio T, Soejima R, Ohara K. Photosensitivity reactions caused by lomefloxacin hydrochloride: a multicenter survey. Antimicrob Agents Chemother 1998;42(12):3141–5.
3. Oliveira HS, Goncalo M, Figueiredo AC. Photosensitivity to lomefloxacin. A clinical and photobiological study. Photodermatol Photoimmunol Photomed 2000;16(3):116–20.

Lonazolac

See also Non-steroidal anti-inflammatory drugs

General Information

Lonazolac, an arylacetic acid derivative, causes adverse effects like those of other NSAIDs. Gastrointestinal disturbances are followed in frequency by nervous system and skin reactions. The extent of gastrointestinal blood loss is similar to that with diclofenac (1). Cholestatic hepatitis has also been reported (SEDA-8, 106).

Reference

1. Uthgenannt H, Arent H. Uber den Einfluss von 3-(4-Chlorphenyl-) 1-phenyl-1H-pyrazol-4-Essigsäure (Lonazolac-Ca), Diclofenac-Na und Indometacin auf die gastrointestinale Blutausscheidung. [Effect of 3-(4-chlorphenyl-) 1-phenyl-1H-pyrazole-4-acetic acid (lonazolac-Ca), diclofenac-Na and indomethacin on the gastrointestinal blood loss.] Wien Klin Wochenschr 1982;94(13):345–9.

Loperamide

General Information

Loperamide is an opioid whose action is almost completely restricted to the gut. Recognition of its consequent safety, if it is appropriately used, has led to its being released in many countries for sale without prescription. It nevertheless has some central activity, and nausea, dizziness, dry mouth, abdominal pain, ileus, and lethargy all occur in a minority of users, with occasional reports of more serious central reactions, such as a possible association with delirium in a child (1).

The effectiveness of loperamide 4, 8, and 12 mg in reducing symptoms of lactose intolerance has been investigated in an open study in 19 subjects (2). Loperamide 8 mg significantly improved symptom scores to a similar extent as lactase tablets. Four subjects complained of delayed constipation and abdominal cramps related to loperamide.

Organs and Systems

Gastrointestinal

Some cases of necrotizing enterocolitis have been reported in infants with paralytic ileus after treatment for mild diarrhea (3). This is only one of the good reasons to avoid the drug in young children; the most important is that diarrhea in infants should not be suppressed pharmacologically (4).

Second-Generation Effects

Teratogenicity

To determine whether loperamide in pregnancy is associated with an increased risk of birth malformations, birth outcomes in 105 women who had taken loperamide during pregnancy (89 during the first trimester) were compared with the outcomes in women matched for age, smoking, alcohol, and other exposures (5). There were no differences in the frequencies of birth malformations between the two groups. However, 21 of the women had babies that were 200 g smaller than babies in the control group.

References

1. Schwartz RH, Rodriquez WJ. Toxic delirium possibly caused by loperamide. J Pediatr 1991;118(4 Pt 1):656–7.
2. Szilagyi A, Torchinsky A, Calacone A. Possible therapeutic use of loperamide for symptoms of lactose intolerance. Can J Gastroenterol 2000;14(7):581–7.
3. Chow CB, Li SH, Leung NK. Loperamide associated necrotising enterocolitis. Acta Paediatr Scand 1986;75(6):1034–6.
4. Chetley A. Not for children. In: Chetley A, editor. Problem Drugs. London and Atlantic Highlands: Zed Books, 1995.
5. Einarson A, Mastroiacovo P, Arnon J, Ornoy A, Addis A, Malm H, Koren G. Prospective, controlled, multicentre study of loperamide in pregnancy. Can J Gastroenterol 2000;14(3):185–7.

Lopinavir and ritonavir

See also Protease inhibitors

General Information

Lopinavir and ritonavir are nucleoside analogue reverse transcriptase inhibitors that are used in combination in the treatment of AIDS.

The pharmacology, clinical pharmacology, uses, adverse effects, and interactions of lopinavir + ritonavir have been reviewed (1).

Observational studies

In studies of combining ritonavir with fluconazole (2) and ritonavir with mefloquine (3) there were no significant effects, and dosage adjustment is not warranted.

Placebo-controlled studies

In a randomized, double-blind study in 70 patients taking a regimen containing protease inhibitors, lopinavir + ritonavir 400/100 mg or 400/200 mg bd was substituted (4). On day 15 nevirapine 200 mg bd was added and NRTIs were changed to include at least one NRTI not previously taken. Despite a more than four-fold reduction in phenotypic susceptibility to the pre-entry protease inhibitor in 63% of the patients, mean plasma HIV-1 RNA concentrations fell by 1.14 log copies/ml after 2 weeks. At week 48, 86% had plasma HIV-1 RNA concentrations of under 400 copies/ml, and 76% under 50 HIV-1 RNA copies/ml. Mean CD4 cell counts increased by 125 cells/μl. The most common adverse events were diarrhea ($n = 16$) and weakness ($n = 4$). There were rises in gamma-glutamyltransferase activity ($n = 18$), total cholesterol ($n = 17$), and triglycerides ($n = 17$), and transient rises in transaminase activities ($n = 11$). Three patients discontinued therapy because of drug-related adverse events.

General adverse effects

In early monotherapy studies, including 62 and 87 patients (5,6), in which the potent antiretroviral effect of ritonavir was first demonstrated, the most common adverse events were nausea, diarrhea, headache, circumoral paresthesia, and altered taste sensation. Nausea, vomiting, and diarrhea are common during the start of therapy and usually disappear over the first few weeks of treatment. These adverse effects can be markedly reduced by using a step-up approach, increasing to the full dose over six days. General weakness, circumoral paresthesia, and taste disturbance occur in 5–10% of patients and are seldom dose-limiting.

Ritonavir does not have a broad therapeutic margin, and patients with higher ritonavir concentrations are at a higher risk of neurological or gastrointestinal adverse effects. It is feasible to individualize the dosage regimen with the aid of plasma concentration measurement and close observation of adverse effects, and there is a close relation between the two; this may enable one to increase substantially the percentage of patients who tolerate ritonavir without risking underdosage (7).

An important consideration in the use of all HIV-1 protease inhibitors, but of ritonavir in particular, is their potential for drug interactions through their effects on cytochrome P450 isozymes. The various interactions of ritonavir with other anti-HIV drugs have recently been reviewed (8).

Organs and Systems

Cardiovascular

Two of 16 patients taking lopinavir + ritonavir developed so-called inflammatory edema, which resolved on withdrawal and recurred after rechallenge (9). In three of eight patients inflammatory edema occurred 1–4 weeks after they started to take regimens that contained lopinavir + ritonavir (10). The edema affected the feet, ankles, and calves and was associated in one case with fever and in another with a transient rash; in one case the left shoulder and groin were also affected. All three recovered completely within 1–4 weeks despite continued drug treatment, but 7 months later one had a relapse that required withdrawal of lopinavir + ritonavir.

From a case in which there was positive dechallenge and rechallenge it has been concluded that edema of the lower limbs can be an adverse effect of ritonavir in some HIV-positive patients (11). The authors suspected a relation to the drug's vasodilatory activity. However, it should also be borne in mind that ritonavir has caused reversible renal insufficiency, which should be looked for in any patient who develops edematous changes.

Nervous system

Myasthenia has been attributed to ritonavir (12).

- A 71-year-old man with an 8-year history of HIV infection developed slurred speech, difficulty in climbing stairs, bilateral ptosis, and lateral rectus weakness 3 weeks after having started to take ritonavir (1200 mg/day). All his signs worsened with prolonged testing, and edrophonium produced improvement in ptosis and speech. Specific electromyographic testing confirmed myasthenia gravis. Computed tomography of the chest was normal. After withdrawal of ritonavir the signs and symptoms partly resolved by 3 months.

A definite causal link with ritonavir could not be established, but the authors speculated that ritonavir may have unmasked myasthenia gravis in this patient.

Sensory systems

Ototoxicity has been attributed to lopinavir + ritonavir (13).

- A 46-year-old man took a regimen containing lopinavir + ritonavir, and 4 weeks later complained of reduced auditory acuity accompanied by lancinating pain. Audiology showed mild to moderate bilateral sensorineural hearing loss. On withdrawal and use of efavirenz his hearing recovered.

Based on the time-course and the effect of withdrawal, lopinavir/ritonavir appears to have been the causative agent in this case.

Gastrointestinal

In a prospective, randomized trial in 100 patients, the most common adverse effects of lopinavir + ritonavir included abnormal stools, diarrhea, and nausea (14).

Urinary tract

In a retrospective analysis of 87 HIV-positive patients taking ritonavir in combination with two nucleoside analogues, serum creatinine increased in 12 cases by 66 (5–242)% from 66 (range 46–102) μmol/l, with a median glomerular filtration rate (GFR) of 116 ml/minute (60–202). Ten of the 12 patients had other risk factors for nephrotoxicity, such as dehydration or use of nephrotoxic drugs (15). It is prudent to monitor renal function in patients receiving ritonavir, particularly in the presence of other risk factors for renal dysfunction.

Three patients developed reversible renal insufficiency 10–12 days after starting treatment including ritonavir (16).

Reproductive system

Four women taking ritonavir developed hypermenorrhea, strongly suggesting that this can occur as a complication of ritonavir treatment (17).

Immunologic

Subcutaneous non-tuberculous granulomatous lesions developed in a 48-year-old HIV-positive man when he was given ritonavir (18).

Susceptibility Factors

Age

The adverse effects commonly observed with ritonavir in adults are reportedly similar in children (19). Of 51 children aged 6 months to 18 years who took escalating doses of a liquid formulation of ritonavir (from 250 up to 400 mg/m^2 every 12 hours), seven withdrew because of gastrointestinal toxicity and four because of grade three hepatic transaminase rises. Both serum triglyceride and cholesterol concentrations increased significantly from baseline within 12 weeks of treatment.

Drug–Drug Interactions

Carbamazepine

Ritonavir can interact with carbamazepine (20).

- A 49-year-old woman with a long history of HIV infection developed worsening ataxia leading to two falls. Four days before admission she had had her antiretroviral drugs changed from zidovudine, lamivudine, and indinavir to ritonavir, saquinavir, and efavirenz. She was also taking carbamazepine to control generalized seizures resulting from a previous right thalamic infarction. The change in antiretroviral therapy resulted in an increase in serum carbamazepine concentration from 6.9 to 20 μg/ml. Serum concentrations in the usual target range were eventually achieved by a sixth of the dose of carbamazepine that had been required before starting ritonavir.

As saquinavir is only a mild inhibitor of CYP3A4 and efavirenz is an inducer, this effect was attributed to the potent inhibitor ritonavir.

Coumarin anticoagulants

Ritonavir can dangerously increase warfarin concentrations (21).

In contrast, ritonavir has been reported to reduce the effect of acenocoumarol (22).

- A 46-year-old man with prosthetic cardiac valves took acenocoumarol and later started to take stavudine, lamivudine, and ritonavir 600 mg bd. His INR fell markedly. Although the dose of acenocoumarol was progressively increased to three times the original dose, it was impossible to achieve the previous INR, and ritonavir was withdrawn.

Ecstasy

Ritonavir can interact with methylenedioxymetamfetamine (MDMA, ecstasy) (23).

- A 32-year old HIV-positive man who added ritonavir 600 mg bd to his existing antiretroviral regimen of zidovudine and lamivudine became unwell within hours after having ingested two and a half tablets of ecstasy, estimated to contain 180 mg of methylenedioxymetamfetamine. He was hypertonic, sweating profusely, tachypneic, tachycardic, and cyanosed. Shortly after, he had a tonic-clonic seizure and cardiorespiratory arrest. Attempts at resuscitation were unsuccessful. Blood concentrations obtained postmortem showed an concentration of 4.56 μg/ml, in the range of that reported in a patient with a life-threatening illness and symptoms similar to this patient after an overdose of 18 tablets of MDMA.

Ritonavir inhibits CYP2D6, which is the principal pathway by which MDMA is metabolized.

Ergot alkaloids

Ergot alkaloids are among the many medications that are contraindicated in patients taking ritonavir. One patient developed severe ergotism after taking ritonavir and ergotamine for 13 days (24), and other cases of ischemia of the lower limbs or elsewhere in the periphery have been reported in patients taking both ritonavir and ergotamine (25–27).

Fentanyl

By inhibiting CYP3A4, ritonavir can significantly inhibit the metabolism of fentanyl, and considerable caution is needed (28).

Ketoconazole

In 12 patients taking ritonavir and saquinavir for HIV infection, ketoconazole significantly increased the AUC, the plasma concentration at 12 hours, and the half-life of ritonavir by 29, 62 and 31% respectively (29). Similar increases of 37, 94, and 38% were recorded for saquinavir. CSF concentrations of ritonavir were raised by 178% by ketoconazole, but there was no significant change in CSF concentrations of saquinavir.

Methadone

Withdrawal symptoms, and the need to increase the dose of methadone, in a 51-year-old man previously stable on a maintenance dosage, have been attributed to ritonavir (30).

Rifamycins

In a pilot, non-randomized study, HIV-infected patients with tuberculosis were treated with regimens containing rifampicin and ritonavir (31). Despite the effects on CYP3A4, there was no significant interaction; plasma ritonavir concentrations remained sufficiently high and rifampicin concentrations did not rise to the toxic range.

Statins

An interaction of ritonavir with simvastatin reportedly resulted in rhabdomyolysis (32).

- A 51-year-old woman taking zidovudine, lamivudine, indinavir, and simvastatin started to take ritonavir and after 1 week developed diffuse muscle weakness and body aches. Creatine kinase (total and the MB isozyme), lactate dehydrogenase, and transaminases were all raised. There were crystals and hemoglobin in the urine.

Presumably this interaction occurred through inhibition of CYP3A4 by ritonavir.

References

1. Qazi NA, Morlese JF, Pozniak AL. Lopinavir/ritonavir (ABT-378/r). Expert Opin Pharmacother 2002;3(3):315–27.

2. Koks CH, Crommentuyn KM, Hoetelmans RM, Burger DM, Koopmans PP, Mathot RA, Mulder JW, Meenhorst PL, Beijnen JH. The effect of fluconazole on ritonavir and saquinavir pharmacokinetics in HIV-1-infected individuals. Br J Clin Pharmacol 2001;51(6):631–5.
3. Khaliq Y, Gallicano K, Tisdale C, Carignan G, Cooper C, McCarthy A. Pharmacokinetic interaction between mefloquine and ritonavir in healthy volunteers. Br J Clin Pharmacol 2001;51(6):591–600.
4. Benson CA, Deeks SG, Brun SC, Gulick RM, Eron JJ, Kessler HA, Murphy RL, Hicks C, King M, Wheeler D, Feinberg J, Stryker R, Sax PE, Riddler S, Thompson M, Real K, Hsu A, Kempf D, Japour AJ, Sun E. Safety and antiviral activity at 48 weeks of lopinavir/ritonavir plus nevirapine and 2 nucleoside reverse-transcriptase inhibitors in human immunodeficiency virus type 1-infected protease inhibitor-experienced patients. J Infect Dis 2002; 185(5):599–607.
5. Markowitz M, Saag M, Powderly WG, Hurley AM, Hsu A, Valdes JM, Henry D, Sattler F, La Marca A, Leonard JM, et al. A preliminary study of ritonavir, an inhibitor of HIV-1 protease, to treat HIV-1 infection. N Engl J Med 1995;333(23):1534–9.
6. Danner SA, Carr A, Leonard JM, Lehman LM, Gudiol F, Gonzales J, Raventos A, Rubio R, Bouza E, Pintado V, et al. A short-term study of the safety, pharmacokinetics, and efficacy of ritonavir, an inhibitor of HIV-1 protease. European-Australian Collaborative Ritonavir Study Group. N Engl J Med 1995;333(23):1528–33.
7. Gatti G, Di Biagio A, Casazza R, De Pascalis C, Bassetti M, Cruciani M, Vella S, Bassetti D. The relationship between ritonavir plasma levels and side-effects: implications for therapeutic drug monitoring. AIDS 1999;13(15):2083–9.
8. Hsu A, Granneman GR, Bertz RJ. Ritonavir. Clinical pharmacokinetics and interactions with other anti-HIV agents. Clin Pharmacokinet 1998;35(4):275–91.
9. Lascaux AS, Lesprit P, Bertocchi M, Levy Y. Inflammatory oedema of the legs: a new side-effect of lopinavir. AIDS 2001;15(6):819.
10. Eyer-Silva WA, Neves-Motta R, Pinto JF, Morais-De-Sa CA. Inflammatory oedema associated with lopinavir-including HAART regimens in advanced HIV-1 infection: report of 3 cases. AIDS 2002;16(4):673–4.
11. Dol L, Geffray L, el Khoury S, Cevallos R, Veyssier P. Oedèmes des members inférieurs chez un patient seropositif pour le VIH: effet secondaire du ritonavir? [Edema of the lower extremities in a HIV seropositive patient: secondary effect of ritonavir?] Presse Méd 1999;28(2):75.
12. Saadat K, Kaminski HJ. Ritonavir-associated myasthenia gravis. Muscle Nerve 1998;21(5):680–1.
13. Williams B. Ototoxicity may be associated with protease inhibitor therapy. Clin Infect Dis 2001;33(12):2100–2.
14. Murphy RL, Brun S, Hicks C, Eron JJ, Gulick R, King M, White AC Jr, Benson C, Thompson M, Kessler HA, Hammer S, Bertz R, Hsu A, Japour A, Sun E. ABT-378/ritonavir plus stavudine and lamivudine for the treatment of antiretroviral-naive adults with HIV-1 infection: 48-week results. AIDS 2001;15(1):F1–9.
15. Bochet MV, Jacquiaud C, Valantin MA, Katlama C, Deray G. Renal insufficiency induced by ritonavir in HIV-infected patients. Am J Med 1998;105(5):457.
16. Duong M, Sgro C, Grappin M, Biron F, Boibieux A. Renal failure after treatment with ritonavir. Lancet 1996;348(9028):693.
17. Nielsen H. Hypermenorrhea associated with ritonavir. Lancet 1999;353(9155):811–12.
18. Kawsar M, El-Gadi S. Subcutaneous granulomatous lesions related to ritonavir therapy in a HIV infected patient. Int J STD AIDS 2002;13(4):273–4.
19. Mueller BU, Nelson RP Jr, Sleasman J, Zuckerman J, Heath-Chiozzi M, Steinberg SM, Balis FM, Brouwers P, Hsu A, Saulis R, Sei S, Wood LV, Zeichner S, Katz TT, Higham C, Aker D, Edgerly M, Jarosinski P, Serchuck L, Whitcup SM, Pizzuti D, Pizzo PA. A phase I/II study of the protease inhibitor ritonavir in children with human immunodeficiency virus infection. Pediatrics 1998;101(3 Pt 1):335–43.
20. Burman W, Orr L. Carbamazepine toxicity after starting combination antiretroviral therapy including ritonavir and efavirenz. AIDS 2000;14(17):2793–4.
21. Newshan G, Tsang P. Ritonavir and warfarin interaction. AIDS 1999;13(13):1788–9.
22. Llibre JM, Romeu J, Lopez E, Sirera G. Severe interaction between ritonavir and acenocoumarol. Ann Pharmacother 2002;36(4):621–3.
23. Henry JA, Hill IR. Fatal interaction between ritonavir and MDMA. Lancet 1998;352(9142):1751–2.
24. Vila A, Mykietiuk A, Bonvehi P, Temporiti E, Uruena A, Herrera F. Clinical ergotism induced by ritonavir. Scand J Infect Dis 2001;33(10):788–9.
25. Montero A, Giovannoni AG, Tvrde PL. Leg ischemia in a patient receiving ritonavir and ergotamine. Ann Intern Med 1999;130(4 Pt 1):329–30.
26. Liaudet L, Buclin T, Jaccard C, Eckert P. Drug points: severe ergotism associated with interaction between ritonavir and ergotamine. BMJ 1999;318(7186):771.
27. Rosenthal E, Sala F, Chichmanian RM, Batt M, Cassuto JP. Ergotism related to concurrent administration of ergotamine tartrate and indinavir. JAMA 1999;281(11):987.
28. Olkkola KT, Palkama VJ, Neuvonen PJ. Ritonavir's role in reducing fentanyl clearance and prolonging its half-life. Anesthesiology 1999;91(3):681–5.
29. Khaliq Y, Gallicano K, Venance S, Kravcik S, Cameron DW. Effect of ketoconazole on ritonavir and saquinavir concentrations in plasma and cerebrospinal fluid from patients infected with human immunodeficiency virus. Clin Pharmacol Ther 2000;68(6):637–46.
30. Geletko SM, Erickson AD. Decreased methadone effect after ritonavir initiation. Pharmacotherapy 2000;20(1):93–4.
31. Moreno S, Podzamczer D, Blazquez R, Iribarren JA, Ferrer E, Reparaz J, Pena JM, Cabrero E, Usan L. Treatment of tuberculosis in HIV-infected patients: safety and antiretroviral efficacy of the concomitant use of ritonavir and rifampin. AIDS 2001;15(9):1185–7.
32. Cheng CH, Miller C, Lowe C, Pearson VE. Rhabdomyolysis due to probable interaction between simvastatin and ritonavir. Am J Health Syst Pharm 2002;59(8):728–30.

Loratadine

See also Antihistamines

General Information

Loratadine is a second-generation antihistamine (SEDA-18, 182) (SEDA-19, 174) (SEDA-22, 178).

Organs and Systems

Cardiovascular

In contrast to astemizole and terfenadine, loratadine is generally believed to be free of adverse cardiac effects. However, there is some evidence that it could be associated with atrial dysrhythmias. In human atrial myocytes loratadine rate-dependently inhibited the transient outward potassium current at therapeutic concentrations, possibly providing a basis for supraventricular dysrhythmias (1). However, during prolonged exposure (3 months) of healthy adult men to four times the recommended daily dose (40 mg/day) there was no change in the electrocardiogram that would suggest QT_c prolongation or any evidence of cardiac dysrhythmias (2).

Prolonged QT interval and symptomatic ventricular tachycardia has been described in a patient who took loratadine plus quinidine, but is most likely to have been attributable to the quinidine and the patient's cardiac condition (SEDA-19, 174).

The pharmacokinetics, electrocardiographic effects, and tolerability of loratadine syrup have been studied in 161 children aged 2–5 years (3). A single-dose open study was performed to characterize the pharmacokinetic profiles of loratadine and its metabolite desloratadine, and a randomized, double-blind, placebo-controlled, parallel-group study was performed to assess the tolerability of loratadine syrup 5 mg after multiple doses. Electrocardiographic parameters were not altered by loratadine compared with placebo. There were no clinically important changes in other tolerability assessments.

In healthy adults loratadine 10 mg/day had no effects on the electrocardiogram when co-administered for 10 days with therapeutic doses of ketoconazole or cimetidine (4).

Liver

Two cases of severe hepatotoxicity in patients using loratadine have been reported (5).

Skin

Loratadine caused erythematous, edematous, pruriginous skin eruptions in a 19-year-old woman who complained of at least three episodes of eruptions located at the same sites each time (6). An oral challenge with loratadine was positive, and cetirizine and ebastine caused no cutaneous reaction. Histopathology suggested a fixed drug eruption.

Drug–Drug Interactions

Nefazodone

Nefazodone is a phenylpiperazine antidepressant that is predominantly metabolized by CYP3A. In a randomized, double-blind, double-dummy, parallel-group, multiple-dose study in healthy men and women who were given loratadine 20 mg od or nefazodone 300 mg every 12 hours, the plasma loratadine concentrations were significantly increased by co-administration of nefazodone (7). The mean QT_c interval was unchanged by loratadine alone, but was markedly prolonged with co-administration of nefazodone, and the extent of prolongation correlated with the plasma loratadine concentration.

References

1. Crumb WJ Jr. Rate-dependent blockade of a potassium current in human atrium by the antihistamine loratadine. Br J Pharmacol 1999;126(3):575–80.
2. Affrime MB, Brannan MD, Lorber RR, Danzig MR, Cuss F. A 3-month evaluation of electrocardiographic effects of loratadine in healthy individuals. Adv Ther 1999;16:149–57.
3. Salmun LM, Herron JM, Banfield C, Padhi D, Lorber R, Affrime MB. The pharmacokinetics, electrocardiographic effects, and tolerability of loratadine syrup in children aged 2 to 5 years. Clin Ther 2000;22(5):613–21.
4. Kosoglou T, Salfi M, Lim JM, Batra VK, Cayen MN, Affrime MB. Evaluation of the pharmacokinetics and electrocardiographic pharmacodynamics of loratadine with concomitant administration of ketoconazole or cimetidine. Br J Clin Pharmacol 2000;50(6):581–9.
5. Schiano TD, Bellary SV, Cassidy MJ, Thomas RM, Black M. Subfulminant liver failure and severe hepatotoxicity caused by loratadine use. Ann Intern Med 1996;125(9):738–40.
6. Ruiz-Genao DP, Hernandez-Nunez A, Sanchez-Perez J, Garcia-Diez A. Fixed drug eruption due to loratadine. Br J Dermatol 2002;146(3):528–9.
7. Abernethy DR, Barbey JT, Franc J, Brown KS, Feirrera I, Ford N, Salazar DE. Loratadine and terfenadine interaction with nefazodone: Both antihistamines are associated with QTc prolongation. Clin Pharmacol Ther 2001;69(3):96–103.

Lorazepam

See also Benzodiazepines

General Information

Lorazepam is a benzodiazepine with CNS, depressant, anxiolytic, and sedative properties, used as a hypnotic, sedative, and anxiolytic drug.

Comparative studies

In a multicenter, randomized, double-blind comparison of diazepam (0.15 mg/kg followed by phenytoin 18 mg/kg), lorazepam (0.1 mg/kg), phenobarbital (15 mg/kg), and phenytoin (18 mg/kg) in 518 patients with generalized convulsive status epilepticus, lorazepam was more effective than phenytoin and at least as effective as phenobarbital or diazepam plus phenytoin (1). Drug-related adverse effects did not differ significantly among the treatments and included hypoventilation (up to 17%), hypotension (up to 59%), and cardiac rhythm disturbances (up to 9%).

Intramuscular lorazepam 4 mg has been compared with the combination of intramuscular haloperidol 10 mg + promethazine 50 mg in 200 emergency psychiatric patients with agitation, aggression, or violence (2). The treatments were comparably effective and well tolerated overall, but two patients who took lorazepam had moderate adverse effects: one had worse bronchial asthma and one had nausea and dizziness.

Placebo-controlled studies

The use of intravenous benzodiazepines administered by paramedics for the treatment of out-of-hospital status epilepticus has been evaluated in a double-blind, randomized trial in 205 adults (3). The patients presented either with seizures lasting 5 minutes or more or with repetitive generalized convulsive seizures and were randomized to receive intravenous diazepam 5 mg, lorazepam 2 mg, or placebo. Status epilepticus was controlled on arrival at the hospital in significantly more patients taking benzodiazepines than placebo (lorazepam 59%, diazepam 43%, placebo 21%). The rates of respiratory or circulatory complications related to drug treatment were 11% with lorazepam, 10% with diazepam, and 23% with placebo, but these differences were not significant.

Organs and Systems

Respiratory

Patients receiving intravenous benzodiazepines must be monitored for respiratory depression, which may demand artificial ventilation during intensive treatment. Lorazepam may cause less respiratory depression than diazepam at equieffective dosages (SEDA-20, 59).

Psychological, psychiatric

Lorazepam causes some rare adverse effects, including a manic-like reaction on withdrawal, delirium, and paradoxical precipitation of tonic seizures or myoclonus in children (SEDA-19, 35). It can both relieve and worsen behavioral disturbances in demented elderly patients (SEDA-20, 32).

The effects of lorazepam on three neuropsychiatric measures of attention and psychomotor performance have been investigated in 40 patients, 20 of whom were given placebo, 10 were given lorazepam 1 mg, and 10 were given lorazepam 2.5 mg (4). Performance on digit cancellation, digit-symbol substitution, and the Paced Auditory Serial Addition Task was significantly impaired by lorazepam (2.5 mg) and this was significantly worse in the middle-aged subjects compared with the younger. These results suggest that older people are more susceptible to these adverse effects.

Lorazepam disinhibits aggression more than its chemically and kinetically similar analogue oxazepam (5).

Cognition

The psychomotor and amnesic effects of single oral doses of lorazepam 2 mg were studied in 48 healthy subjects in a double-blind, placebo-controlled, randomized, parallel-group study (6). The effects were assessed by a battery of subjective and objective tests that explored mood and vigilance, attention, psychomotor performance, and memory. Vigilance, psychomotor performance, and free recall were significantly impaired by lorazepam.

Lorazepam shares with other benzodiazepines the ability to impair explicit memory, but has a distinct further effect on implicit memory as well (7). However, it impairs memory more than its chemically and kinetically similar analogue, oxazepam (8). The effects of lorazepam 2.5 mg and diazepam 0.3 mg/kg on explicit and implicit memory tasks have been examined in 24 men and 24 women randomly allocated to lorazepam, diazepam, or placebo (7). An implicit word-stem completion task and explicit memory tasks of immediate and delayed word recall and word recognition were administered 90 minutes after drug administration. Both diazepam and lorazepam significantly impaired performance on explicit memory measures. Only lorazepam significantly impaired performance on the implicit memory task.

In a separate study, pharmacokinetic–pharmacodynamic modeling of the psychomotor and amnesic effects of a single oral dose of lorazepam 2 mg was investigated in 12 healthy volunteers in a randomized, double-blind, placebo-controlled, two-way, crossover study using the following tasks: choice reaction time, immediate and delayed cued recall of paired words, and immediate and delayed free recall and recognition of pictures (9). The delayed recall trials were more impaired than the immediate recall trials; similar observations were made with the recognition versus recall tasks.

The effects of lorazepam and diazepam on false memories and related states of awareness have been investigated in 36 healthy volunteers, randomly assigned to one of three groups (placebo, diazepam 0.3 mg/kg, lorazepam 0.038 mg/kg) (10). The results suggested that diazepam and lorazepam cause impaired conscious recollection, associated with true, but not false, memories.

Metabolism

Metabolic acidosis and hyperlactatemia have been attributed to lorazepam (11).

- A 34-year-old woman with a history of renal insufficiency induced by long-term use of cocaine developed respiratory failure and was intubated and sedated with intravenous lorazepam (65 mg, 313 mg, and 305 mg on 3 consecutive days). After 2 days she had a metabolic acidosis, with hyperlactatemia and hyperosmolality. Propylene glycol, a component of the lorazepam intravenous formulation, was considered as a potential source of the acidosis, as she had received more than 40 times the recommended amount over 72 hours. Withdrawal of lorazepam produced major improvements in lactic acid and serum osmolality.

Long-Term Effects

Drug withdrawal

Lorazepam has considerable abuse potential, and poses particular difficulties in withdrawal (12). On the other hand, a sizeable sample ($n = 97$) of chronic users who wanted to discontinue were generally able to use stable or decreasing doses on an as-needed basis (13).

The Omnibus Budget Reconciliation Act of 1987 (OBRA '87) regulations (www.elderlibrary.org) specify when antipsychotic drugs can and cannot be used to treat behavioral disturbances in nursing home residents in the USA. Accordingly, antipsychotic drugs can be used in patients with delirium or dementia only if there are psychotic or agitated features that present a danger to the patient or others. Preventable causes of agitation must be excluded and the nature and frequency of these behaviors must be documented. Non-dangerous agitation, uncooperativeness, wandering, restlessness, insomnia, and impaired memory are insufficient in isolation to justify the use of antipsychotic drugs. With this in mind, the effects of withdrawing haloperidol, thioridazine, and lorazepam have been examined in a double-blind, crossover study in 58 nursing home residents (43 women and 15 men, mean age 86 years), half of whom continued to take the psychotropic drugs that had been prescribed, while the other half were tapered to placebo (14). After 6 weeks, the drugs were tapered to the reverse schedule for another 6 weeks. There were no differences between drug and placebo in functioning, adverse effects, and clinical global impression. Cognitive functioning improved during placebo. The authors concluded that gradual dosage reductions of psychoactive medications must be attempted, unless clinically contraindicated, in an effort to withdraw these drugs. Similar conclusions have been reached in other studies (SEDA-22, 54).

Drug Administration

Drug administration route

The pharmacokinetics of intranasal lorazepam compared with oral administration have been evaluated in 11 volunteers in a randomized, crossover study (15). Lorazepam had favorable pharmacokinetics for intranasal administration compared with standard methods. Intranasal delivery could provide an alternative non-invasive delivery route for lorazepam.

Drug–Drug Interactions

Caffeine

Caffeine aggravates, rather than attenuates, lorazepam-induced impairment in learning and performance (16). This contradicts popular wisdom that stimulants are useful in perking up patients taking benzodiazepines, and invites research into what may be a very dangerous practice in benzodiazepine users, that of taking caffeine before driving or operating machinery (see also General Introduction in the monograph on Benzodiazepines).

Clozapine

Caution has been recommended when starting clozapine in patients taking benzodiazepines (SEDA-19, 55). Three cases of delirium associated with clozapine and benzodiazepines (17) have been reported. There have been several reports of synergistic reactions, resulting in increased sedation and ataxia, when lorazepam was begun in patients already taking clozapine (18).

Haloperidol

A thorough review of the pharmacokinetics of haloperidol, with special emphasis on interactions, has been published (19). The interactions include one with lorazepam.

Moxonidine

When co-administered with lorazepam 0.4 mg, moxonidine increased impairment of attentional tasks (choice, simple reaction time and digit vigilance performance, memory tasks, immediate word recall, delayed word recall accuracy, and visual tracking). These effects should be considered when moxonidine is coadministered with lorazepam, although they were smaller than would have been produced by a single dose of lorazepam 2 mg alone (20).

References

1. Treiman DM, Meyers PD, Walton NY, Collins JF, Colling C, Rowan AJ, Handforth A, Faught E, Calabrese VP, Uthman BM, Ramsay RE, Mamdani MB. A comparison of four treatments for generalized convulsive status epilepticus. Veterans Affairs Status Epilepticus Cooperative Study Group. N Engl J Med 1998;339(12):792–8.
2. Alexander J, Tharyan P, Adams C, John T, Mol C, Philip J. Rapid tranquillisation of violent or agitated patients in a psychiatric emergency setting. Pragmatic randomised trial of intramuscular lorazepam v. haloperidol plus promethazine. Br J Psychiatry 2004;185:63–9.
3. Alldredge BK, Gelb AM, Isaacs SM, Corry MD, Allen F, Ulrich S, Gottwald MD, O'Neil N, Neuhaus JM, Segal MR, Lowenstein DH. A comparison of lorazepam, diazepam, and placebo for the treatment of out-of-hospital status epilepticus. N Engl J Med 2001;345(9):631–7.
4. Fluck E, Fernandes C, File SE. Are lorazepam-induced deficits in attention similar to those resulting from aging? J Clin Psychopharmacol 2001;21(2):126–30.
5. Bond A, Lader M. Differential effects of oxazepam and lorazepam on aggressive responding. Psychopharmacology (Berl) 1988;95(3):369–73.
6. Micallef J, Soubrouillard C, Guet F, Le Guern ME, Alquier C, Bruguerolle B, Blin O. A double blind parallel group placebo controlled comparison of sedative and mnesic effects of etifoxine and lorazepam in healthy subjects. Fundam Clin Pharmacol 2001;15(3):209–16.
7. Le Roi S, Kirby KC, Montgomery IM, Daniels BA. Differential effects of lorazepam and diazepam on explicit and implicit memory. Aust J Psychopharmacol 1999;9:48–54.
8. Curran HV, Schiwy W, Lader M. Differential amnesic properties of benzodiazepines: a dose-response comparison of two drugs with similar elimination half-lives. Psychopharmacology (Berl) 1987;92(3):358–64.
9. Blin O, Jacquet A, Callamand S, Jouve E, Habib M, Gayraud D, Durand A, Bruguerolle B, Pisano P. Pharmacokinetic–pharmacodynamic analysis of amnesic effects of lorazepam in healthy volunteers. Br J Clin Pharmacol 1999;48(4):510–12.
10. Huron C, Servais C, Danion JM. Lorazepam and diazepam impair true, but not false, recognition in healthy volunteers. Psychopharmacology (Berl) 2001;155(2):204–9.
11. Cawley MJ. Short-term lorazepam infusion and concern for propylene glycol toxicity: case report and review. Pharmacotherapy 2001;21(9):1140–4.
12. Lader M. Clin pharmacology of anxiolytic drugs: Past, present and future. In: Biggio G, Sanna E, Costa E, editors. GABA-A Receptors and Anxiety. From Neurobiology to Treatment. New York: Raven Press, 1995:135.
13. Romach M, Busto U, Somer G, Kaplan HL, Sellers E. Clinical aspects of chronic use of alprazolam and lorazepam. Am J Psychiatry 1995;152(8):1161–7.
14. Cohen-Mansfield J, Lipson S, Werner P, Billig N, Taylor L, Woosley R. Withdrawal of haloperidol, thioridazine, and lorazepam in the nursing home: a controlled, double-blind study. Arch Intern Med 1999;159(15):1733–40.
15. Wermeling DP, Miller JL, Archer SM, Manaligod JM, Rudy AC. Bioavailability and pharmacokinetics of lorazepam after intranasal, intravenous, and intramuscular administration. J Clin Pharmacol 2001;41(11):1225–31.
16. Rush CR, Higgins ST, Bickel WK, Hughes JR. Acute behavioral effects of lorazepam and caffeine, alone and in combination, in humans. Behav Pharmacol 1994;5(3):245–54.
17. Jackson CW, Markowitz JS, Brewerton TD. Delirium associated with clozapine and benzodiazepine combinations. Ann Clin Psychiatry 1995;7(3):139–41.

lumefantrine in Thailand may be due to poorer absorption and more resistant parasites in these areas, and the manufacturers have recommended higher doses than were used in these studies (6).

In an open, randomized trial in 260 Tanzanian children, lumefantrine was superior to chloroquine and did not produce major adverse effects (7).

References

1. Ridley RG, Hudson AT. Chemotherapy of malaria. Curr Opin Infect Dis 1998;11:691–705.
2. Fadat G, Louis FJ, Louis JP, Le Bras J. Efficacy of micronized halofantrine in semi-immune patients with acute uncomplicated falciparum malaria in Cameroon. Antimicrob Agents Chemother 1993;37(9):1955–7.
3. Bouchaud O, Basco LK, Gillotin C, Gimenez F, Ramiliarisoa O, Genissel B, Bouvet E, Farinotti R, Le Bras J, Coulaud JP. Clinical efficacy and pharmacokinetics of micronized halofantrine for the treatment of acute uncomplicated falciparum malaria in nonimmune patients. Am J Trop Med Hyg 1994;51(2):204–13.
4. Wildling E, Jenne L, Graninger W, Bienzle U, Kremsner PG. High dose chloroquine versus micronized halofantrine in chloroquine-resistant *Plasmodium falciparum* malaria. J Antimicrob Chemother 1994;33(4):871–5.
5. Toivonen L, Viitasalo M, Siikamaki H, Raatikka M, Pohjola-Sintonen S. Provocation of ventricular tachycardia by antimalarial drug halofantrine in congenital long QT syndrome. Clin Cardiol 1994;17(7):403–4.
6. Fourcade L, Gachot B, De Pina JJ, Heno P, Laurent G, Touze JE. Choc anaphylactique associé au traitement du paludisme par halofantrine. [Anaphylactic shock related to the treatment of malaria with halofantrine.] Presse Méd 1997;26(12):559.
7. Di Perri G, Di Perri IG, Monteiro GB, Bonora S, Hennig C, Cassatella M, Micciolo R, Vento S, Dusi S, Bassetti D, et al. Pentoxifylline as a supportive agent in the treatment of cerebral malaria in children. J Infect Dis 1995;171(5):1317–22.

Lycopodiaceae

See also Herbal medicines

General Information

The family of Lycopodiaceae contains three genera of clubmoss, *Huperzia*, *Lycopodium*, and *Lycopodiella*.

Lycopodium serratum

Lycopodium serratum (clubmoss, Jin bu huan) has been used in Chinese medicine for more than 1000 years. It contains the alkaloid serratidine and triterpenoids, such as oxolycoclavinol, oxoserratenetriol, tohogeninol, and tohogenol.

Adverse effects

Jin bu huan can cause liver damage (1).

- A 49-year-old man developed signs of hepatitis after taking three tablets of Jin bu huan per day for 2 months for insomnia. No other potential causes for the liver damage could be identified. A liver biopsy showed chronic hepatitis with moderate portal and parenchymal lymphocytic inflammation and focal necrosis. The patient stopped taking the herbal remedy and his liver function normalized.

There have been other reports of hepatotoxic effects of Jin bu huan (2).

Overdosage of Jin bu huan can cause central nervous system and respiratory depression with rapid life-threatening bradycardia (3,4).

References

1. Picciotto A, Campo N, Brizzolara R, Giusto R, Guido G, Sinelli N, Lapertosa G, Celle G. Chronic hepatitis induced by Jin Bu Huan. J Hepatol 1998;28(1):165–7.
2. McRae CA, Agarwal K, Mutimer D, Bassendine MF. Hepatitis associated with Chinese herbs. Eur J Gastroenterol Hepatol 2002;14(5):559–62.
3. Centers for Disease Control and Prevention (CDC). Jin bu huan toxicity in adults—Los Angeles, 1993. MMWR Morb Mortal Wkly Rep 1993;42(47):920–2.
4. Centers for Disease Control and Prevention (CDC). Jin bu huan toxicity in children—Colorado, 1993. MMWR Morb Mortal Wkly Rep 1993;42(33):633–6.

Lyme disease vaccine

See also Vaccines

General Information

Lyme disease is a tick-borne, spirochetal zoonosis, characterized by a distinctive skin lesion, systemic symptoms, and neurological, rheumatological, and cardiac involvement, occurring in varying combinations over a period of months to years. *Borrelia burgdorferi* is the causative agent in North America, whereas in Europe three genomic groups (named *Borrelia burgdorferi sensu stricto*, *Borrelia garinii*, and *Borrelia afzelii*) have been identified. Endemic foci have been found in North America, Europe, the former USSR, Japan, and China. In many of these areas, Lyme disease is now the most common vector-borne disease. Because of this epidemiological problem and the severity of the disease, a vaccine was developed. High titers of antibody to outer surface protein A (OspA) of the spirochete prevented *B. burgdorferi* infection in mice and subsequently in immunized hamsters, dogs, and monkeys.

In December 1998, based on many prelicensure clinical trials, the first Lyme disease vaccine (LYMErix, manufactured by the then SmithKline Beecham) was licensed by the Food and Drug Administration (FDA) for individuals aged 15–70 years old (1) and subsequently became commercially available in the USA. In 1999, the Advisory Committee on Immunization Practices (ACIP) made recommendations for Lyme disease vaccine (2), including data on efficacy and safety (SEDA-23, 338). No convincing evidence was found that the vaccine caused serious problems, but discussion about its safety continued and the demand for the vaccine did not reach a sustainable level. Therefore, in February 2002 the vaccine was withdrawn by the manufacturers.

In two overviews the results of various clinical and efficacy trials were summarized (3,4) and the safety, immunogenicity, and efficacy of the vaccine were underlined. The authors considered that the intravector mode of action of the vaccine was unique and opened the door to a new method of preventing insect-borne illnesses in humans.

Dr Neal Halsey, head of the Institute for Vaccine Safety at John Hopkins University, explained that the poor sales had resulted from "public misperception and the promotion of false concerns" (5). Lyme disease researchers consider the Lyme vaccine story in the USA to have been a setback in Lyme disease prevention. Vaccines meeting the specific epidemiological situation in Europe are under development. Lyme disease prevention and prophylaxis has been reviewed (6).

Observational studies

LYMErix safety data reported to the Vaccine Adverse Event Reporting System (VAERS) from 21 December 1998 to 31 October 2000 mentioned reports of adverse events associated with Lyme vaccine in prelicensure trials, including injection site reactions, transient arthralgia and myalgia within 30 days of vaccination, fever, and a flu-like illness (7). Allergic reactions were reported to the VAERS and some could have plausibly been linked to the vaccine because of the short latency between vaccination and reaction onset. No clear patterns in age, sex, time to onset, or vaccine dose were identified, although the unexpected predominance of reports of arthrosis in men might warrant further consideration.

Placebo-controlled studies

The results of two efficacy and safety trials using Lyme disease vaccine with or without adjuvant have been reported. In a double-blind trial, 10 305 subjects at least 18 years old, recruited at 14 sites in areas of the USA where Lyme disease was endemic, were randomly assigned to receive either placebo ($n = 5149$) or OspA vaccine ($n = 5156$) (8). The first two injections were given 1 month apart and 7515 subjects also received a booster dose at 12 months. The efficacy of the vaccine was 68% in the first year of the study in the entire population and 92% in the second year among the 3745 subjects who received a third injection. The vaccine was well tolerated. There was a higher incidence of mild, self-limiting, local and systemic reactions in the vaccine group, but only during the 7 days after vaccination (Table 1). There was no significant increase in the frequency of arthritis or neurological events in vaccine recipients. The authors concluded that OspA vaccine was safe and effective in the prevention of Lyme disease.

In another randomized, double-blind trial in 10 936 subjects in areas of the USA in which Lyme disease is endemic, either recombinant *B. burgdorferi* OspA with adjuvant or placebo was given initially and at 1 and 12 months (9). After two injections, 22 subjects given vaccine and 43 given placebo contracted definite Lyme disease; vaccine efficacy was 49% (95% CI = 15, 69%). In the second year, after the third injection, 16 vaccine recipients and 66 placebo recipients contracted definite Lyme disease; vaccine efficacy was 76% (CI = 58, 86%). The efficacy of the vaccine in preventing asymptomatic infection was 83% in the first year and 100% in the second year. Injection of the vaccine was associated with mild to moderate local or systemic reactions lasting a median of 3 days (Table 2).

Table 1 Percentage incidences of adverse effects within 7 days after injection

Adverse effect	Vaccine	Placebo
First injection		
Number of subjects	5156	5149
Any adverse effect	9.8	4.1
Musculoskeletal	6.4	1.3
Myalgia	5.5	0.6
General	1.8	0.9
Pain at injection site	0.3	0.04
Second injection		
Number of subjects	5050	5034
Any adverse effect	6.1	3.1
Musculoskeletal	3.3	1.1
Myalgia	2.5	0.4
General	1.7	0.8
Pain at injection site	0.8	0.1
Third injection		
Number of subjects	3745	3770
Any adverse effect	11.2	5.5
General	7.3	2.6
Tenderness	2.3	0.2
Pain at injection site	1.5	0.2
Unspecified pain	1.0	0.1
Reaction at injection site	0.8	0.2
Swelling	0.6	0.1
Pain in limb	0.5	0.02
Edema at injection site	0.5	0
Rigors	0.2	0
Skin or subcutaneous tissue	2.1	0.2
Erythematous rash	1.9	0.1

Organs and Systems

Musculoskeletal

Suspicions were expressed in the Mealey Publication's Drug and Medical Device Report that the Lyme disease vaccine LYMErix could cause an incurable form of autoimmune arthritis. It was hypothesized that blood concentrations of OspA after three doses of vaccine place vaccinees classified by genetic type HLA-DR4+ at risk of developing treatment-resistant Lyme arthritis. The premarket trials for the vaccine were assessed by an independent advisory committee, which found no link between Lyme disease immunization and autoimmune arthritis (10). However, the committee stressed the need for long-term surveillance and further studies in those over 70 years and in children, and the effect of the vaccine in patients with chronic arthritis; the possible development of autoimmunity deserves further study (11). After licensing of the vaccine, more than 1 million Americans received it and no unusual adverse effects were reported to the manufacturer (10).

Table 2 Percentages of subjects with symptoms with an overall incidence of at least 1% that were classified as related or possibly related to vaccination or unrelated to vaccination

Symptom	Vaccine	Placebo	*P*-value
*Related or possibly related to vaccination**			
Local at injection site			
Soreness	24.1	7.6	<0.001
Redness	1.8	0.5	<0.001
Swelling	0.9	0.2	<0.001
Systemic: early (<30 days)			
Total*	19.4	15.1	<0.001
Arthralgia	3.9	3.5	0.34
Headache	3.0	2.5	0.14
Myalgias	3.2	1.8	<0.001
Fatigue	2.3	2.0	0.37
Aching	2.0	1.4	0.01
Influenza-like illness	2.0	1.1	<0.001
Fever	2.0	0.8	<0.001
Chills	1.8	0.5	<0.001
Upper respiratory tract infection	1.0	1.1	0.69
Systemic: late (>30 days)			
Total*	4.1	3.4	0.06
Arthralgia	1.3	1.2	0.54
Unrelated to vaccination			
Early (<30 days)	27.1	27.9	0.37
Late (>30 days)	53.3	52.6	0.48

* Totals include all early or late related or possibly related systemic events, not just those with a frequency of at least 1%.

However, subsequently the FDA received some reports of arthritis and Lyme disease after the use of the vaccine (12). Therefore, on 31 January 2001, the FDA's Vaccines and Related Biological Products Advisory Committee held a meeting to evaluate safety data of LYMErix. Among other information, the experts considered a manufacturer's briefing document as well as safety data reported to the VAERS. The Associated Press Report from 31 January 2001 on the FDA meeting on Lyme vaccine read (in part) as follows: "Vaccine Safety experts found no proof that the LYMErix vaccine is dangerous—the rare cases of arthritis and other symptoms could be coincidence. Many reports are of minor complaints or are not believed to have been caused by the vaccine, but the FDA is studying 133 reports of severe arthritis-like symptoms. That's because of a theory that the vaccine might set off an autoimmune reaction where the body attacks its own tissues, particularly in people who carry a certain gene called HLA-4." The panel said that ultimately "no convincing evidence exists that the vaccine causes serious problems", but the experts urged the FDA and the manufacturer to expedite new safety studies and demanded that the Government should act to ensure that patients are told about the possible risks before inoculation. They also urged that the CDC should aggressively distribute a patient-friendly safety fact sheet about LYMErix (13).

A postmarketing assessment cohort study using automated record linkage was initiated at Harvard Pilgrim Health Care (HPHC) in order to address the theoretical concern that immunization with a vaccine containing OspA might cause an autoimmune arthritis and to evaluate whether exposure to the vaccine is a risk factor for Lyme disease, treatment-resistant Lyme disease, rheumatoid arthritis, certain neurological diseases, allergic events, hospitalization, and death (SEDA-24, 367) [http://www.fda.gov/ohrms/dockets/ac/01/slides/3680s2-05_platt.pdf]. The study involves 25 000 HPHC members who are expected to receive the vaccine and 75 000 non-immunized controls. For the most recent report, matched data were available for 2568 vaccinees and 7497 controls. At this stage, the available results do not suggest that the outcomes of interest were more frequent among vaccinees than among non-vaccinees. Having recognized that enrolment into the database is at a slower rate than anticipated, two additional Health Maintenance Organizations in countries where Lyme disease is endemic have been identified and will contribute.

On 30 November 2000, 1.4 million doses of vaccine had been distributed. From January 1999 to the time of the database query, there was no evidence that the incidence of these arthritic conditions was higher than reported in the general population or that they were associated with an autoimmune process (7).

To address further the question of a possible link between Lyme vaccine and arthritis, the FDA is conducting a telephone survey of individuals who have reported arthritic conditions to the VAERS after receiving the vaccine (7). This survey is a census of available and willing individuals who submitted reports that have been coded as arthritis, arthrosis, rheumatoid arthritis, joint disease, and arthralgia. The goals of the survey are to describe the characteristics of these adverse events, to identify concomitant factors that might influence the characteristics of these events, and to describe the relation of the events to immunization. After this survey phase is complete, the VAERS will identify cases of arthritis and will conduct a case-control study to examine the hypothesis that Lyme vaccine causes arthritis. It is planned to compare people who report arthritis after Lyme disease vaccine with two control groups: people who report arthritis to the VAERS after other vaccines and people who report adverse events to the VAERS other than arthritis after Lyme vaccine. All cases will be age-, sex-, and race-matched with controls. All three groups will be tested for DR HLA haplotypes at the allele level and for peripheral blood lymphocyte responses to OspA and leukocyte function-associated antigen-1 (LFA-1). This is an attempt to determine if people who report arthritis after Lyme vaccine have a higher prevalence of certain HLA alleles that are known to be associated with rheumatoid arthritis and have the same third common hypervariable region, while simultaneously having greater peripheral T cell reactivity to OspA and LFA-1. Given the relatively small number of arthritis cases reported after Lyme vaccine, probably only a very high risk will be detectable.

Four cases of arthritis associated with the administration of Lyme vaccine have been reported (14).

- 15 weeks after a third dose of Lyme vaccine a 9-year-old boy developed arthritis, including both knees, the right elbow, the left hip, the right ankle, and the right thumb; he was probably in an asymptomatic phase of natural Lyme infection.

- About 3 months after a third dose of Lyme vaccine a 16-year-old boy developed arthritis of both knees.
- 24 hours after a second dose of Lyme vaccine a 53-year-old man developed flu-like symptoms and arthralgia; he later developed swelling of the finger joints and toe joints.
- 24 hours after a second dose of Lyme vaccine a 43-year-old man developed multiple synovitis.

In all cases the disease was self-limiting and to the knowledge of the authors inconsequential in the long term. They considered that the findings supported post-infectious and mimicry models, by showing that OspA, an outer surface protein of the causative organism of Lyme disease, *B. burgdorferi*, could cause acute arthritis, the possibility that it was associated with a more protracted form of arthritis, and that it perhaps had a modulating effect in individuals with concurrent Lyme infection.

Susceptibility Factors

Genetic factors

From reports containing information on HLA types, clinical descriptions of adverse events in those given Lyme disease vaccine are similar in people with DR4 and non-DR4 HLA haplotypes and do not suggest more inflammatory arthritis in people of DR4 haplotype (15) [http://www.fda.gov/ohrms/dockets/ac/01/briefing/3680b2-06.pdf]. The characteristics of adverse events in people with a self reported history of Lyme disease do not differ substantially from all adverse events after Lyme vaccine.

Drug Administration

Drug dosage regimens

In a randomized study in 956 volunteers aged 17–72 years a shortened immunization schedule of injections at 0, 1, and 2 months were compared with a schedule of injections at 0, 1, and 12 months (16). Adverse events were transient and mild to moderate. Soreness was the most frequently reported local symptom (82%), whereas fatigue (20–22%) was the most frequently reported general symptom. Two volunteers had more serious adverse events: severe chills and shaking in one and an episode of syncope (lasting a few minutes with complete recovery) on the day of the first dose in another. The authors concluded that doses at 0, 1, and 2 months would provide protection during a typical tick-transmission season.

References

1. Anonymous. Lyme disease vaccine. Med Lett Drugs Ther 1999;41(1049):29–30.
2. Advisory Committee on Immunization Practices (ACIP). Recommendations for the use of Lyme disease vaccine. MMWR Recomm Rep 1999;48(RR-7):1–17, 21–5.
3. Thanassi WT, Schoen RT. The Lyme disease vaccine: conception, development, and implementation. Ann Intern Med 2000;132(8):661–8.
4. Onrust SV, Goa KL. Adjuvanted Lyme disease vaccine: a review of its use in the management of Lyme disease. Drugs 2000;59(2):281–99.
5. Immunization News for April 26, 2002. http://www.immunizationinfo.org (accessed 27 April 2002).
6. Hayney MS, Grunske MM, Boh LE, Da Camada CC, Perreault MM. Lyme disease prevention and vaccine prophylaxis. Ann Pharmacother 1999;33(6):723–9.
7. FDA. Vaccines and Related Biological Products Advisory Committee. LYMErix. Lyme Disease Vaccine Safety Update, 31 January 2001. http://www.fda.gov/ohrms/dockets / ac/01/briefing/368ob2.htm (accessed 10 February 2001).
8. Sigal LH, Zahradnik JM, Lavin P, Patella SJ, Bryant G, Haselby R, Hilton E, Kunkel M, Adler-Klein D, Doherty T, Evans J, Molloy PJ, Seidner AL, Sabetta JR, Simon HJ, Klempner MS, Mays J, Marks D, Malawista SE. A vaccine consisting of recombinant *Borrelia burgdorferi* outer-surface protein A to prevent Lyme disease. Recombinant Outer-Surface Protein A Lyme Disease Vaccine Study Consortium. N Engl J Med 1998;339(4):216–22.
9. Steere AC, Sikand VK, Meurice F, Parenti DL, Fikrig E, Schoen RT, Nowakowski J, Schmid CH, Laukamp S, Buscarino C, Krause DS, Cohen S, Boyer J, Hanrahan K, Dalgin P, Dalgin J, Garrett A, Petelaba M, Feder H, Good S, Green J, Miller K, Spiegel M, Daniel G, Jacob R, Maderazo E, Maiorano M, Seidner A, Bruno L. Vaccination against Lyme disease with recombinant *Borrelia burgdorferi* outer-surface lipoprotein A with adjuvant. Lyme Disease Vaccine Study Group. N Engl J Med 1998;339(4):209–15.
10. SmithKline to vigorously defend itself against class action. Mealey Publications Report. Press Release Newswire Association Baltimore, 23 December 1999.
11. Marwick C. Guarded endorsement for Lyme disease vaccine. JAMA 1998;279(24):1937–8.
12. Noble HB. Concerns over reactions to Lyme shots. NewYork Times, 21 November 2000.
13. Associated Press Report, 31 January 2001. Warnings urged for Lyme vaccine. http://www.fda.gov (accessed 1 February 2001).
14. Rose CD, Fawcett PT, Gibney KM. Arthritis following recombinant outer surface protein A vaccination for Lyme disease. J Rheumatol 2001;28(11):2555–7.
15. FDA. LYMErix Safety Data Reported to the Vaccine Adverse Event Reporting System; (VAERS) from December 21, 1998 through October 31, 2000. http://www.fda.gov/ohrms/dockets/ac/01/briefing/3680b2_06.pdf.
16. Schoen RT, Sikand VK, Caldwell MC, Van Hoecke C, Gillet M, Buscarino C, Parenti DL. Safety and immunogenicity profile of a recombinant outer-surface protein A Lyme disease vaccine: clinical trial of a 3-dose schedule at 0, 1, and 2 months. Clin Ther 2000;22(3):315–25.

Lysergide

General Information

Lysergic acid diethylamide (LSD) is a hallucinogen that is usually taken orally. Its initial effects, anticholinergic and sympathomimetic in type, occur within about half an hour and include tachycardia, hyperthermia, mydriasis, piloerection, hypertension, and occasionally nausea and vomiting. The more important psychoactive effects develop 1–2 hours later and can last 24–48 hours. They are principally changes in perception, mood, and behavior, leading in many cases to acute panic, hallucinations, delusions, and in some cases a classical psychosis. Perception may be strikingly heightened and distorted, and initial perceptions may mask and overshadow later sensory perception. Users often grossly exaggerate their mental and emotional capacities, attributing to themselves extraordinary powers. Visual hallucinations, loss of appreciation of time and space, and instability of mood are common. Meaningfulness and a sense of universal union often predominate. A significant problem in street purchase is the uncertain quality and likely impurity of the material obtained. Doses of 25 mg and more are sufficient to cause its psychophysiological effects, which are generally dose-related up to 500 mg. The half-life is about 3 hours, but the effects last considerably longer (1).

Acute panic attacks and hallucinogen-induced psychotic disorder often occur when people with preexisting personality disorder or pre-psychotic personalities use hallucinogens. Suicide and self-injury have been reported. Prolonged psychotic disorders can occur, but psychiatric opinion is divided as to whether these occur only in people with pre-existing disorders or in healthy individuals as well. "Flashbacks" occur particularly when there has been prolonged heavy use, but eventually disappear (SED-11, 83) (1,2). Self-injury and suicide can result (3).

Hypersensitivity reactions are exceedingly rare and no reports have been validated. Tumor-inducing effects are possible, as a consequence of various reports from animal and human studies that chromosomal abnormalities may be associated with exposure to LSD. However, its mutagenic effects in practice are questionable, and no useful evidence for or against its potential for carcinogenicity has been produced (4).

Organs and Systems

Cardiovascular

Vasoconstriction, affecting both cerebral and peripheral circulations, has been associated with LSD (5), but it is not usually significant at ordinary doses in people with a normal circulatory system.

Nervous system

Hallucinogen-induced mood disorder is associated with changes in affect, varying from euphoria to manic-like symptoms, panic/fear, and depression, often occurring within minutes and often varying in the same individual on different occasions. Changes in sensory perception, with a loss of ability to distinguish temporal or spatial reality and sensory hallucinations, particularly visual and tactile, are frequent, with a tendency to assume godlike attributes. These features often merge in a psychosis, particularly with repeated use. Whether chronic psychosis after LSD is the result of the drug or of a combination of the drug and predisposing factors is currently unanswerable (6–8).

The repeated use of LSD is associated not only with psychoses, but also with more specific neurological signs and symptoms, including ataxia, incoordination, dysphasia, paresthesia, and tremor. Convulsions have been reported. "Flashback," or the return of hallucinogenic effects, occurs in almost a quarter of those who have used LSD, particularly if they have also used other CNS stimulants, such as alcohol or marijuana (2,9). They can experience distortions of perception of objects, space, or time, which intrude without warning into reality, resulting in delusions, panic, and unusual images. A "trailing phenomenon" has also been reported, in which the visual perception of objects is reduced to a series of interrupted pictures rather than a constant view (10). The frequency of these events may slowly abate over several years, but in a significant number their incidence later increases (1,3).

Sensory systems

Apart from visual hallucinations (discussed under the section Nervous system in this monograph), diplopia, blurred vision, mydriasis, and other visual disturbances occur (11). Pupillary dilatation, combined with altered sensory appreciation, has led to a number of instances of retinal damage after continued direct exposure to the sun (12).

Hematologic

The only hematological effect reported has been an increased rate of blood clotting associated with severe hyperthermia (13).

Gastrointestinal

Retroperitoneal fibrosis has been reported, not unexpectedly, in view of the structural similarity between LSD and methysergide (3).

Body temperature

Hyperthermia can occur but does so very seldom with usual doses (14). It has been produced experimentally with high doses.

Second-Generation Effects

Teratogenicity

Animal studies have not shown that LSD is teratogenic. Various publications have referred to a high incidence of abortions and congenital abnormalities associated with LSD. However, none of these has shown any consistent pattern of abnormality, and neither has there been an acceptable control group (4).

Susceptibility Factors

People who are predisposed to psychosis, schizophrenia, or a family history thereof, may be at considerable risk of developing LSD psychosis (3,8). People with epilepsy may be more prone to convulsions, with a reduction in convulsant threshold.

Drug–Drug Interactions

Monoamine oxidase inhibitors

Chronic administration of a monoamine oxidase inhibitor causes a subjective reduction in the effects of LSD, perhaps due to differential changes in central serotonin and dopamine receptor systems (15).

Phenothiazines and butyrophenones

Phenothiazines and butyrophenones can counteract the psychoactive effects of LSD and benzodiazepines can depress their effects (16).

Reserpine

Reserpine can accentuate the effects of LSD (17).

Interference with Diagnostic Tests

Ambroxol

A urine sample from a patient with a severe head injury tested positive for LSD (18). The test was carried out using a homogeneous immunoassay CEDIA DAU LSD (Boehringer, Mannheim). Although LSD has a half-life of 3 hours, the patient's urine tested positive for several days. Analysis of the same urine samples using high-performance liquid chromatography (HPLC) failed to detect LSD. LSD screening was then performed in urine samples obtained from ten other patients in the same ward. All samples tested positive for LSD by the CEDIA DAU LSD assay but negative using HPLC. All of the patients were taking ambroxol. Ambroxol was detected in the urine by HPLC. In a volunteer, LSD was not detected in a fasting urine sample. After a dose of ambroxol 15 mg a urine sample obtained 90 minutes later tested positive for LSD. The addition of 50 μl of Mucosolvan juice (which contains ambroxol) to the negative fasting urine sample resulted in a positive test for LSD. The authors concluded that ambroxol should be excluded when LSD screening is performed using the CEDIA DAU LSD test.

References

1. Watson SJ. Hallucinogens and other psychotomimetics: biological mechanisms. In: Barchas JD, Berger PA, Cioranello RD, Elliot GR, editors. Psychopharmacology from Theory to Practise. New York: Oxford University Press, 1977.
2. Alarcon RD, Dickinson WA, Dohn HH. Flashback phenomena. Clinical and diagnostic dilemmas. J Nerv Ment Dis 1982;170(4):217–23.
3. Strassman RJ. Adverse reactions to psychedelic drugs. A review of the literature. J Nerv Ment Dis 1984;172(10):577–95.
4. Tuchmann-Duplessis H. Drug effects on the fetus. In: Avery GS, editor. Monographs on Drugs, vol. 2. London: ADIS, 1975:158.
5. Lieberman AN, Bloom W, Kishore PS, Lin JP. Carotid artery occlusion following ingestion of LSD. Stroke 1974;5(2):213–15.
6. Sarwer-Foner GJ. Some clinical and social aspects of lysergic acid diethylamidel. II. Psychosomatics 1972;13(5):309–16.
7. McWilliams SA, Tuttle RJ. Long-term psychological effects of LSD. Psychol Bull 1973;79(6):341–51.
8. Bowers MB Jr.. Acute psychosis induced by psychotomimetic drug abuse. I. Clinical findings. Arch Gen Psychiatry 1972;27(4):437–40.
9. Tec L. Phenothiazine and biperiden in LSD reactions. JAMA 1971;215(6):980.
10. Asher H. "Trailing" phenomenon—a long lasting LSD side effect. Am J Psychiatry 1971;127:1233.
11. Abraham HD. Visual phenomenology of the LSD flashback. Arch Gen Psychiatry 1983;40(8):884–9.
12. Schatz H, Mendelblatt F. Solar retinopathy from sun-gazing under the influence of LSD. Br J Ophthalmol 1973;57(4):270–3.
13. Klock JC, Boerner U, Becker CE. Coma, hyperthermia and bleeding associated with massive LSD overdose. A report of eight cases. West J Med 1974;120(3):183–8.
14. Friedman SA, Hirsch SE. Extreme hyperthermia after LSD ingestion. JAMA 1971;217(11):1549–50.
15. Bonson KR, Murphy DL. Alterations in responses to LSD in humans associated with chronic administration of tricyclic antidepressants, monoamine oxidase inhibitors or lithium. Behav Brain Res 1996;73(1–2):229–33.
16. Vardy MM, Kay SR. LSD psychosis or LSD-induced schizophrenia? A multimethod inquiry. Arch Gen Psychiatry 1983;40(8):877–83.
17. Resnick O, Krus DM, Raskin M. Accentuation of the psychological effects of LSD-25 in normal subjects treated with reserpine. Life Sci 1965;4(14):1433–7.
18. Rohrich J, Zorntlein S, Lotz J, Becker J, Kern T, Rittner C. False-positive LSD testing in urine samples from intensive care patients. J Anal Toxicol 1998;22(5):393–5.

Lysine acetylsalicylate

General Information

Lysine acetylsalicylate is a soluble form of salicylate developed for intravenous administration in acute pain. Its mode of action and scope of adverse effects are similar to those of aspirin (1), although it has a faster onset of action (2) and causes less gastrointestinal bleeding (3).

References

1. Majluf-Cruz A, Chavez-Ochoa AR, Majluf-Cruz K, Coria-Ramirez E, Pineda Del Aguila I, Trevino-Perez S, Matias-Aguilar L, Lopez-Armenta JC, Corona de la Pena N. Effect of combined administration of clopidogrel and lysine acetylsalicylate versus clopidogrel and aspirin on platelet aggregation and activated GPIIb/IIIa expression in healthy volunteers. Platelets 2006;17(2):105–7.
2. Gurfinkel EP, Altman R, Scazziota A, Heguilen R, Mautner B. Fast Platelet suppression by lysine acetylsalicylate in chronic stable coronary patients. Potential clinical impact over regular aspirin for coronary syndromes. Clin Cardiol 2000;23(9):697–700.
3. Bretagne JF, Fevillu A, Gosselin M, Gastard J. Aspirine et toxicite gastroduodenale. Etude endoscopique en double insu des effects d'un Placébo, de l'aspirine et de l'acétylsalicylate de lysine chez le sujet sain. [Aspirin and gastroduodenal toxicity. A double-blind endoscopic study of the effects of placebo, aspirin and lysine acetylsalicylate in healthy subjects.] Gastroenterol Clin Biol. 1984;8(1):28–32.

contribute significantly to its overall direct costs (monitoring costs, prolonged hospitalization due to complications or treatment failures) and indirect costs (quality of life, loss of productivity, time spent by families and patients receiving medical care). In one study an adverse event in a hospitalized patient was associated on average with an excess of 1.9 days in the length of stay, extra costs of $US2262 (1990–3 values), and an almost two-fold increase in the risk of death. In the outpatient setting, adverse drug reactions result in 2–6% of hospitalizations, and most of them were thought to be avoidable if appropriate interventions had been taken. In a review, economic aspects of antibacterial therapy with macrolides have been summarized and critically evaluated (23).

Organs and Systems

Cardiovascular

Cardiovascular reactions are rare if macrolide antibiotics are used in the absence of susceptibility factors, which include drug interactions, increasing age, female sex, concomitant diseases, and co-morbidity (24).

Respiratory

In an animal model, acute lung injury was inhibited by pretreatment with clarithromycin or roxithromycin, which significantly ameliorated bleomycin-induced increases in the total cell and neutrophil counts in bronchoalveolar lavage fluids and wet lung weight (25). Pretreatment with clarithromycin or roxithromycin also suppressed inflammatory cell infiltration and interstitial lung edema. Pretreatment with azithromycin was much less effective.

Nervous system

Table 2 lists the rates of adverse events affecting the nervous system attributed to erythromycin and newer macrolides.

Sensory systems

Eyes

Bilateral ischemic optic neuropathy can develop secondary to macrolides (26).

Ears

The cochlear toxicity of systemic macrolides, azithromycin, clarithromycin, and erythromycin, has been investigated in guinea pigs by measuring transiently evoked otoacoustic emissions (27). A single intravenous dose of erythromycin 125 mg/kg caused no change in evoked otoacoustic emissions, whereas oral azithromycin 45 mg/kg and intravenous clarithromycin 75 mg/kg reversibly reduced the emission response. This could have been caused by transient dysfunction of the outer hair cells.

Psychological, psychiatric

Although there is no evidence that neuropsychiatric complications of macrolides develop more readily in uremic patients, several factors may predispose toward these adverse effects, such as reduced drug clearance, altered plasma protein binding, different penetration of drug across the blood–brain barrier, and an increased propensity for drug interactions.

Two women, aged 49 and 50 years, developed altered mental status a few days after starting to take clarithromycin for eradication of *H. pylori* (28). There was incoherent speech with perseveration, inability to sustain attention, impaired ability to comprehend, coprolalia, euphoria, restlessness, visual hallucinations, anxiety, and inappropriate affect. Similarly, in three cases, a 46-year-old man, a 39-year-old woman, and a 4-year-old boy, treatment with clarithromycin was followed by nervous system and psychiatric symptoms that included euphoria, insomnia, aggressive behavior, hyperactivity, and emotional lability (29).

Hematologic

Clarithromycin and roxithromycin slightly inhibited the down-regulation of L-selectin expression on neutrophils induced by interleukin-8 stimulation (30). Furthermore, clarithromycin strongly inhibited the interleukin-8-induced up-regulation of the expression of Mac-1, an adhesion molecule, on neutrophils.

Hematological changes with macrolides are very rare. Isolated instances of neutropenia are occasionally reported (31).

Gastrointestinal

The gastrointestinal adverse effects are the most common untoward effects of the macrolides (Table 2). Nausea and vomiting associated with abdominal pain and occasionally diarrhea can be minor and transitory or, in a small percentage of patients, become severe enough to result in premature withdrawal. The rate of these adverse effects varies among the different antibiotics. In general, newer macrolides, such as azithromycin, clarithromycin, or roxithromycin, are better tolerated and cause fewer adverse effects than erythromycin.

Erythromycin is a motilin receptor agonist (2–4). This mechanism may be at least partly responsible for the gastrointestinal adverse effects of macrolides.

Based on observations in dogs and rabbits, clarithromycin is significantly less potent than azithromycin and erythromycin as an agonist for stimulation of smooth muscle contraction (32). A lower rate of gastrointestinal adverse events would therefore be expected with clarithromycin than with azithromycin (Table 2). Since most of these data were compiled from several studies, and since most have not been obtained by direct comparison of the various macrolides in single studies, the rates should be interpreted with caution. They most probably provide only an approximate indication of the rate of adverse events. Small differences in rates between individual macrolides will in most cases not be clinically useful indicators of the true risk for the occurrence of adverse events.

In contrast to the macrolides mentioned above, macrolides with a 16-membered lactone ring (acetylspiramycin, josamycin, leucomycin, midecamycin, rokitamycin, spiramycin, tylocin) have little if any motor-stimulating effects (33,34).

Drug-induced esophagitis is rare, accounting for about 1% of all cases of esophagitis. An incidence of 3.9 in 100 000 has been reported. After the first description, there have been more than 250 observations, with more than 50 different drugs. Among those, the principal antibiotics included tetracyclines (doxycycline, metacycline, minocycline, oxytetracycline, and tetracycline), penicillins (amoxicillin, cloxacillin, penicillin V, and pivmecillinam), clindamycin, co-trimoxazole, erythromycin, lincomycin, spiramycin, and tinidazole. Doxycycline alone was involved in one-third of all cases. Risk factors included prolonged esophageal passage, due to motility disorders, stenosis, cardiomegaly, the formulation, supine position during drug ingestion, and failure to use liquid to wash down the tablet. Direct toxic effects of the drug (pH, accumulation in epithelial cells, non-uniform dispersion) also seem to contribute to the development of drug-induced esophagitis (35).

Liver

Erythromycin can cause two different types of liver damage (36,37), benign increases in serum transaminases, which may or may not recur on rechallenge, and cholestatic hepatitis. Reports of intrahepatic cholestasis with azithromycin (38), clarithromycin (39,40), and josamycin (41) suggest that the newer macrolides are not free of this adverse effect, although the relative risks compared with erythromycin are unclear. Similar involvement of the liver has been seen with the ester of triacetyloleandomycin, but not with the unesterified antibiotic.

Macrolides such as josamycin, midecamycin, and spiramycin, which do not form stable complexes with cytochrome P450, rarely if ever cause cholestatic hepatitis.

Urinary tract

- A 77-year-old man taking regular captopril, furosemide, salbutamol inhaler, vitamin C, and nasal beclomethasone dipropionate took clarithromycin 250 mg bd for sinusitis and bronchitis and 5 days later developed abdominal pain and intermittent fever (42). Laboratory findings included raised serum creatinine and blood urea nitrogen, aspartate transaminase, amylase, lactate dehydrogenase, and creatine kinase (not of the MB isoenzyme). The cause of the non-oliguric renal insufficiency was diagnosed by renal biopsy as interstitial nephritis with eosinophilic infiltrates. During the course of illness he also developed thrombocytopenia.

Skin

Skin rashes and fixed drug eruptions can occur during treatment with various macrolides but are rare (under 1%) (17).

Immunologic

Immunomodulatory effects of macrolides have been repeatedly reported; for example suppression of the release of chemotactic mediators may be important for the clinical effect of roxithromycin in patients with chronic lower respiratory tract infections (43). Both clarithromycin and azithromycin altered cytokine production in human monocytes in vitro (44).

The suppressive activity of macrolide antibiotics on pro-inflammatory cytokine production has also been shown in human peripheral blood monocytes, in which roxithromycin inhibited the in vitro production of interleukin-1 beta and tumor necrosis factor alpha (45). It also suppressed cytokine production after a prolonged pretreatment period in mice. In another mouse model both roxithromycin and clarithromycin inhibited angiogenesis and enhanced the antitumor activity of some cytotoxic agents, suggesting a beneficial effect when combined with such drugs against solid tumors (46,47). Furthermore, growth suppression of human fibroblasts by roxithromycin has been demonstrated both in vitro and in vivo (48).

Azithromycin has been associated with Churg–Strauss syndrome in a patient with atopy (49).

- A 46-year-old man with asthma was treated with oral roxithromycin 300 mg/day for 5 days for purulent rhinitis and 2 weeks later developed arthritis, mononeuritis multiplex, eosinophilia (64%), eosinophilic infiltrations in the bone marrow, raised IgE concentrations, and transient pulmonary infiltrates. Churg–Strauss syndrome was diagnosed.

A similar course of disease had occurred 1 year before, after the administration of azithromycin (50).

Leukocytoclastic vasculitis associated with clarithromycin has been reported in an 83-year-old woman who was treated for pneumonia. All her symptoms resolved after withdrawal and a short course of glucocorticoids (51).

- Henoch–Schönlein purpura developed in an 84-year-old Indian woman 10 days after she started to take clarithromycin (250 mg bd) for pneumonia (52). She was otherwise healthy and taking no regular medications. Histology confirmed a leukocytoclastic vasculitis of superficial vessels, with extravasation of erythrocytes, and direct immunofluorescence showed immunoglobulin A in superficial dermal vessels. Treatment with prednisone (1 mg/kg/day) was required. Most of the symptoms and signs resolved within a few days, but renal function remained impaired.

The authors identified two previous case reports of clarithromycin-induced leukocytoclastic vasculitis.

- A 39-year-old man developed acute angioedema and urticaria 6 hours after taking erythromycin base 500 mg in enteric-coated pellets for acute sinusitis (53). He remembered having taken erythromycin once before without any problem. He had no known allergies and was taking no regular medications, but he had had chemotherapy for non-Hodgkin's lymphoma several years earlier.

The authors identified five previous reports of erythromycin-associated urticarial reactions. However, it was not possible to exclude a reaction to the ingredients of the coated pellets.

Long-Term Effects

Drug tolerance

An area of increasing concern and clinical importance is the increasing macrolide resistance that has been reported over the last several years with some of the common pathogens, particularly *Streptococcus pneumoniae*, group A streptococci, and *Haemophilus influenzae*, and may result in failure of therapy of pneumonia, pharyngitis, and skin infections (54). High rates of resistance of several groups of streptococci to macrolides have been reported from all parts of the world (55–64).

Resistance to erythromycin can develop rapidly and is usually associated with bacterial cross-resistance to the other macrolide antibiotics, and also to the chemically unrelated lincomycins. Resistance has been detected in strains of staphylococci, Group A hemolytic streptococci, viridans streptococci, *Streptococcus pyogenes*, *Neisseria gonorrhoeae*, *Bacteroides fragilis*, and *Clostridium difficile* (65,66). It has tended to occur in hospitals, where either erythromycin or the lincosamides were used extensively, but can also result from multiple drug resistance when other antibiotics are used. Subinhibitory concentrations of erythromycin can cause resistance in staphylococci.

In combination with proton pump inhibitors and other antibiotics, macrolides are still successfully used for the eradication of *H. pylori* infection (67,68). However, resistance of *H. pylori* to macrolides has emerged in a number of countries. The first case of *H. pylori* resistance to clarithromycin has now also been documented in Denmark and follows increased use of this macrolide in eradication regimens (69).

Clinical isolates of *N. gonorrhoeae* with reduced susceptibility to azithromycin are commonly found in Uruguay, and one of the mechanisms involved included mutations in the mtrR gene (70).

Resistance of *H. pylori* to clarithromycin appears to have increased in proportion to clarithromycin use. Clarithromycin resistance arises through mutations that lead to base changes in 23S ribosomal RNA subunits. A rapid PCR hybridization assay with a sensitivity of 97% for the detection of clarithromycin resistance of strains of *H. pylori* has been described (71). Resistance to clarithromycin has a serious impact on the efficiency of eradicating regimens that include clarithromycin (72–74). The reported incidences of primary resistance of *H. pylori* to clarithromycin are 6.1% in the USA, 8% in Austria, 8.7% in Bulgaria, 9.5% in Japan, 10% in Spain, 11% in France, 13% in Nigeria, and 23% in Italy (75–82).

Among strains of *Enterococcus faecium*, resistance against tylosin was mainly detected in strains from poultry, but also in some strains from pork. Among strains of *E. faecium* and *Enterococcus faecalis* isolated from pigs and poultry in Denmark, resistance to tylosin was often observed among isolates from places in which these antimicrobials had been widely used, but rarely among isolates from places in which their use had been limited (83).

Second-Generation Effects

Teratogenicity

In a large case-control surveillance study from Hungary in 38 151 pregnant women, oral erythromycin during pregnancy did not present a detectable teratogenic risk to the fetus (84).

Susceptibility Factors

Allergic reactions to antimicrobials are frequent in patients with Sjögren's syndrome. They are especially susceptible to reactions to penicillins, cephalosporins, and sulfonamides, but reactions to macrolides and tetracyclines also seem to be over-represented in these patients (85).

Drug–Drug Interactions

Alfentanil

The metabolism of alfentanil, a potent short-acting narcotic, is inhibited by macrolide antibiotics, resulting in significant changes in half-life and clearance (86).

Antihistamines

Toxic effects of terfenadine and astemizole have been reported in patients taking concomitant macrolides, especially clarithromycin (87–89,116), typically resulting in prolongation of the QT interval and cardiac dysrhythmias (torsade de pointes) (111). The potential interaction of azithromycin with terfenadine has been evaluated in a randomized, placebo-controlled study in 24 patients who took terfenadine plus azithromycin or terfenadine plus placebo (90). However, azithromycin did not alter the pharmacokinetics of the active carboxylate metabolite of terfenadine or the effect of terfenadine on the QT_c interval.

Only a modest increase in QT_c interval has been observed with concomitant use of erythromycin and the antihistamine ebastine (91).

Clarithromycin (500 mg bd for 10 days) significantly increased the steady-state maximum plasma concentration and the steady-state AUC of loratadine (10 mg/day for 10 days) (92). In contrast, the addition of loratadine did not affect the steady-state pharmacokinetics of clarithromycin or its active metabolite, 14(R)-hydroxyclarithromycin. No QT_c interval exceeded 439 ms in any subject.

Benzodiazepines

Interactions of macrolides with triazolam and midazolam are clinically important. Increased serum concentration, AUC, and half-life, and reduced clearance have been documented (93,94,118). These changes can result in clinical effects, such as prolonged psychomotor impairment, amnesia, or loss of consciousness (95). No interactions between ciprofloxacin and diazepam have been reported (96).

Carbamazepine

Significant increases in serum carbamazepine concentrations due to reduced clearance (97) and prolonged half-life (98,122,123) can result in confusion, somnolence, ataxia, vertigo, nausea, and vomiting in patients taking macrolides (100,124,125). Toxicity can occur rapidly after addition of the macrolide and abate quickly on withdrawal (126). However, a retrospective analysis of 3995 patients treated with azithromycin did not show any pharmacokinetic interaction in patients who were also taking carbamazepine (127,128).

- Carbamazepine toxicity, with dizziness, lethargy, and nystagmus, developed in a 17-year-old boy two days after he started to take clarithromycin 500 mg/day (129). His serum carbamazepine concentration (previously acceptable) rose, but returned to within the target range after withdrawal of clarithromycin.

Ciclosporin

The pharmacokinetics of ciclosporin can be altered by macrolides. Commonly observed changes include increases in ciclosporin AUC and peak plasma concentration and reductions in the time to peak and clearance (102,104,130,131). Ciclosporin concentrations should therefore be monitored, to minimize the risk of toxicity in patients taking certain macrolides. When azithromycin is used concomitantly with ciclosporin, blood ciclosporin concentrations need to be monitored (132).

Cytochrome P450

The frequency and pattern of drug interactions with macrolides is influenced by the chemical structure of the individual macrolide. The most important mechanism determining many drug interactions is the effect of macrolides on the hepatic cytochrome P450, which oxidizes macrolides after binding of the drug to oxidized (Fe_3) cytochrome P450 (126). Binding of the macrolide to group IIIA cytochrome P450 can have one of several consequences: oxidation can result in the formation of a stable iron-metabolite complex, causing either induction of cytochrome P450 and increased metabolism of the antibiotic, or inactivation of cytochrome P450 and inhibition of drug metabolism (126).

Structural properties of the macrolides determine whether the drug metabolizing enzyme is induced or inactivated. Macrolides with a 14-membered lactone ring have a greater potential to inhibit cytochrome P450 than bulkier macrolides with 15-membered or 16-membered lactone rings. It is therefore useful to group the macrolides according to their molecular structure and their potential for drug interactions via cytochrome P450 (Table 3).

The differences in interactions of different macrolides with cytochrome P450 are marked. Troleandomycin is a more potent inhibitor of microsomal drug metabolism than erythromycin, while josamycin, midecamycin, and spiramycin have not so far been incriminated (133,134). Azithromycin does not induce or inhibit cytochrome P450 in rats (135).

The occurrence of an interaction in a particular patient is difficult to predict. Hepatic concentrations of CYP3A4, the activity of which can be estimated by an erythromycin breath test (133), vary at least ten-fold among patients (136,137).

Table 3 Molecular structures of macrolides and the extent of their interactions with cytochrome P450

Degree of interaction	Number of carbon atoms in macrolide ring		
	14	15	16
High	Troleandomycin Erythromycin		
Low	Flurithromycin Clarithromycin Roxithromycin		Josamycin Midecamycin Miocamycin
Not incriminated	Dirithromycin	Azithromycin	Rokitamycin Spiramycin

The variability is compounded by the fact that, in addition to the liver, mucosal cells of the small intestine commonly express CYP3A4, where it is responsible for significant first-pass metabolism of orally administered substrates (137).

Drugs that participate in major CYP3A4 interactions with macrolides are listed in Table 4. Other drugs that may be affected include alprazolam (138), the water-soluble artemisinin analogue artelinic acid (139), gallopamil (140), lovastatin (141), nefazodone (142), and risperidone (143). Pharmacokinetic interactions with clarithromycin, erythromycin, and troleandomycin have been reviewed (144).

Digoxin

The interaction between macrolides and digoxin is not a consequence of altered cytochrome P450 activity. Digoxin is metabolized in the gastrointestinal tract by *Eubacterium lentum* in the bowel flora of about 10% of patients (106). The direct antibacterial effect of macrolides reduces digoxin metabolism and increases its systemic availability (134). The resultant increased digoxin plasma concentrations are associated with severe nausea, vomiting, and dysrhythmias (105,145,146).

Table 4 Summary of major interactions with macrolides

Interacting drug	Azithromycin	Clarithromycin	Erythromycin	Roxithromycin	Reference
Alfentanil	ND	ND	++	ND	(99)
Carbamazepine	–	++	++	–	(100,101)
Ciclosporin	+	ND	++	(+)	(102,103)
Digoxin	ND	++	++	ND	(104,105)
Disopyramide	ND	ND	++	(+)	(106,107)
Methylprednisolone	–	ND	+	ND	(108)
Oral contraceptives	ND	–	ND	–	(109,110)
Rifamycins	+?	++	ND	ND	(111–115)
Terfenadine, astemizole	ND	++	++	ND	(116)
Theophylline	–	+	++	(+)	(29)(101)(117)
Triazolam, midazolam	–	ND	++	(+)	(118)
Warfarin	–	–	++	–	(119,120)
Zidovudine	–	+	ND	ND	(121)

++ clinically relevant
\+ potentially clinically relevant
(+) probably insignificant interaction
– documented lack of interaction
ND no published data
? insufficient information to judge relevance

In Japan, three further attenuated live measles vaccines are licensed for general use:

1. AIK-Cvaccine
2. Biken-CAM vaccine
3. Schwarz-FFB vaccine.

No significant differences have been reported between the three vaccines regarding either immunogenicity or adverse reactions (5).

Data on adverse effects after measles immunization reported in the framework of the US Monitoring System on Adverse Events Following Immunization to the Centers for Disease Control have been published (SEDA-13, 274). Case reports on suspected encephalitis (including two cases with hearing loss) and convulsions have been reviewed (SEDA-8, 299) (SEDA-9, 284) (SEDA-11, 291) (SEDA-12, 283) (SEDA-16, 388); very rare individual case reports on cerebellar ataxia, diffuse retinopathy, optic neuritis, regional lymphadenitis, thrombocytopenic purpura (70% of cases of thrombocytopenic purpura occur following viral diseases; purpura has been reported also following the receipt of measles vaccine), paroxysmal cold hemoglobinuria, parkinsonism, pityriasis lichenoides et varioliformis acuta, nephrosis, and depression of the tuberculin skin test reaction were cited (SED-11, 679) (SED-12, 811) (SEDA-12, 283) (SEDA-16, 389) (SEDA-17, 376).

A review of the data generated in the last 4 years has amply described the continued efforts of the scientific community to monitor and understand true measles vaccine-associated adverse events (6). The rapidity and clarity of this same community's debunking of the spurious associations with Crohn's disease and autism suggests that those charged with vaccination programs have learned from past mistakes.

The immunogenicity and safety of two live attenuated measles vaccine strains (Schwarz strain and AIK-C strain) have been compared in 9-month-old Taiwanese infants in order to find a candidate for an effective measles immunization in the first year of life (7). Because of persisting maternal measles antibody, the commercially available measles vaccines do not produce a sufficient antibody response when given during the first year of life. However, early protection is particularly required in developing countries with high measles morbidity and mortality in infants. Attempts to find suitable candidates for early immunization, including the use of the high-titer Edmonston–Zagreb measles vaccine strain, failed (SED-14, 1078). The Japanese AIK-C measles vaccine strain (derived from the Edmonston strain) has been given to 67 infants and a measles vaccine based on the Schwarz strain was given to 68 infants. The AIK-C strain vaccine caused seroconversion in 65 infants (97%), whereas only 65 infants (70%) seroconverted with the Schwarz strain vaccine. Adverse effects of the two vaccines were comparable: fever 8.8% (Schwarz strain) versus 19% (AIK-C strain); skin rash 13 versus 13%; rhinorrhea 8.8 versus 12%; cough 7.4 versus 6%; diarrhea 2.9 versus 4.5%; poor appetite 2.9 versus 1.5%; irritability 2.9 versus 6%.

Mumps vaccine

Live mumps virus vaccine is available in monovalent (mumps only) form and in combination with measles (MM vaccine) and with measles and rubella (MMR vaccine). Vaccines based on the following mumps vaccine strains are in use:

- The Jeryl Lynn strain is used mainly in vaccines prepared in the USA. The virus was isolated from a female patient in 1963. Vaccines based on Jeryl Lynn strain are mostly used worldwide.
- The Urabe Am9 strain was attenuated in Japan and has been used for the preparation of MMR and other mumps-containing vaccines in Japan and Europe.
- The Rubini strain was isolated in Switzerland and was attenuated by passage in human diploid cells for use in vaccine production.
- The L-3 (Leningrad) strain was derived by combining five isolates of mumps virus from sick children. The attenuated strain is used for vaccine production, especially in Russia.
- The L-3 strain was further attenuated in Zagreb, Croatia, by adaptation and passage in SPF chick embryo fibroblast cell cultures (mumps vaccine strain L-Zagreb).

The most commonly used vaccines have been based on the Urabe Am9 strain and the Jeryl Lynn strain. However, in September 1992 health authorities worldwide were informed by Smith Kline Beecham Biologicals that the company had decided to suspend the distribution of vaccines containing the Urabe Am9 strain, since alternative vaccines were available to maintain the immunization programs established in the various countries.

General adverse effects

Various authors have investigated the immunogenicity and reactogenicity of different mumps vaccine strains. Among adverse reaction reports, episodes of parotitis and low-grade fever have been most prominent. Rash, pruritus, purpura, and other allergic reactions are uncommon, usually mild, and of brief duration (8). Data on adverse effects after immunization with mumps-containing vaccines collected in the framework of MSAEFI have been published (SEDA-13, 274). There have been reports of febrile convulsions, meningitis, orchitis, parotitis, swollen lymph nodes, and thrombocytopenia (SED-12, 813) (SEDA-16, 389) (SEDA-17, 377).

Rubella vaccine

Rubella vaccine is a live attenuated virus vaccine. Most of the vaccines currently manufactured outside Japan are produced in human diploid cells and are based either on the RA 27/3 strain (the most widely used) or the Cendehill strain. In Japan, five different vaccine strains (for example TO 336 and MEQ 11) are produced in two different non-human substrates. In China, another vaccine strain (BRD-2) has been developed and produced in human diploid cells. Its antigenicity and reactogenicity are comparable to those of the RA 27/3 strain.

General adverse effects

Subcutaneous injection is commonly followed by local soreness and induration. Children sometimes develop low grade fever, rash, and lymphadenopathy after immunization. Acute arthritis/arthralgia sometimes occurs.

Measles–mumps–rubella vaccine

In most industrialized countries, measles–mumps–rubella (MMR) vaccine has replaced the former use of single antigen vaccines against measles, mumps, and rubella in childhood immunization programs. Single antigen rubella vaccines are still used in postchildhood rubella prevention. Comparisons of the efficacy and safety of different MMR vaccines and monovalent versus bivalent or trivalent vaccines have been made in various clinical trials (SEDA-14, 285). Minor symptoms (fever, rash, malaise) occurred usually after 5–14 days and lasting for 2–3 days. Occasionally, febrile convulsions have been recorded within 3 weeks of immunization, and mild parotitis occurred rarely in the third week after immunization. On average, the seroconversion rates were between 95 and 99% for measles and rubella, and less for mumps.

In a crossover study among 581 twin pairs aged between 14 months and 6 years only 0.5–4% had adverse reactions to MMR vaccine. The difference between the reaction rate reported in the immunized members of the twin pairs and those reported in the placebo-injected twin sisters or brothers showed that most of the reactions were temporally and not causally related to immunization. Respiratory symptoms, nausea, and vomiting were more frequent in the placebo-injected group than in the MMR-immunized group (9).

General adverse effects

A Vaccine Safety Datalink project has been used to compare adverse events after MMR immunization either at 4–5 years or at 10–12 years (10). Information on events that are plausibly associated with MMR immunization (seizures, pyrexia, malaise/fatigue, musculoskeletal symptoms, rash, edema, induration, lymphadenopathy, thrombocytopenia, aseptic meningitis, joint pain) has been collected from 8514 children who received the vaccine at preschool age and from 18 036 schoolchildren. The results suggested that the risk of events is greater in those aged 10–12 years.

When the MMR immunization program was launched in Finland in 1982, a countrywide surveillance system, including all hospitals and health centers, was established to monitor serious adverse events after immunization. From 1982 to 1996 almost 3 million doses of MMR vaccine were distributed to 1.8 million individuals, mostly children. Most of the reported adverse events were minor or self-limiting events among 437 vaccinees, for example fever, rash, headache, fatigue, nausea, vomiting, transient arthralgia, and swelling of the parotid glands. In all, 173 potentially serious adverse events were evaluated in detail. The assessment of causality is shown in Table 1.

- One 13-month-old boy died 8 days after immunization. Autopsy showed that the cause of death was aspiration of vomit. The most commonly reported neurological adverse events were febrile seizures. Epilepsy was diagnosed in three children; symptoms manifested for the first time 1, 10, and 21 days after immunization. One child was later diagnosed as having severe Lennox–Gastaut syndrome; medical records subsequent to the acute phase were not available for the other two.

In the four cases of encephalitis, a causal relation with MMR vaccine could not be excluded, because no other specific cause was detected. One child with acute

Table 1 Assessment of causality between MMR vaccination and 173 serious events

Event	Number of reports	Number not causally associated with MMR	Possibly causally associated with MMR		
			Number	%	Incidence per 100 000 doses
Respiratory					
Asthma	10	5	5	50	0.2
Pneumonia	12	7	5	42	0.2
Nervous system (n = 77)					
Febrile seizures	52	24	28	54	0.9
Epilepsy	3	2	1	33	0.03
Undefined seizure	4	2	2	50	0.07
Encephalitis	4	1	3	75	0.1
Meningitis	4	4	0	0	0
Guillain–Barré syndrome	2	0	2	100	0.07
Transient gait disturbance	5	0	5	100	0.2
Confusion during fever	3	1	2	67	0.07
Metabolism					
Diabetes	3	3	0	0	0
Reproductive function					
Orchitis	7	6	1	14	0.03
Immunologic (n = 74)					
Anaphylaxis	30	16	14	47	0.5
Henoch–Schönlein purpura	2	1	1	50	0.03
Urticaria	30	5	25	83	0.8
Stevens–Johnson syndrome	1	0	1	100	0.03
Death (n = 1)	1	1	0	0	0

lymphoblastic leukemia (diagnosed after immunization but with symptoms leading to the diagnosis already present at the time of immunization) developed, during immunosuppressive treatment, measles encephalopathy 54 days after immunization and interstitial pneumonia a few days later; 14 years later the leukemia had not relapsed, but she had developed severe epilepsy. The fourth child had *Herpes simplex* encephalitis, with a temporal association between MMR immunization and encephalitis (11). Idiopathic thrombocytopenic purpura was excluded from the analysis, because it has been analysed before (12).

Organs and Systems

Respiratory

Measles

Measles giant-cell pneumonia after measles immunization has been described in a 21-year-old man with AIDS (13).

- A 21-year-old man developed AIDS followed by *Pneumocystis jiroveci* pneumonia. About a year after a booster immunization with MMR vaccine, he developed measles giant-cell pneumonia, confirmed by transbronchial and thoracoscopic lung biopsies. The entire genome of the isolated strain and that of the currently used vaccine strain Moraten were subsequently sequenced and were almost identical.

Taking into consideration the long interval between measles immunization and pneumonia, the causal relation in this case was doubtful.

Nervous system

Measles

The long debate on the degree of risk to the nervous system presented by measles vaccine, especially encephalitis and encephalopathy, is not completely resolved (14). The problem has been analysed by the CDC, Atlanta, Georgia (4,15,16), the Ministry of Health and Welfare, Japan (5), the National Childhood Encephalopathy Study in the United Kingdom (SEDA-11, 285), and investigators in the Northwest Thames region of England (17). However, most investigators, having critically analysed the studies, have concluded that the incidence of suspected cases of encephalitis/encephalopathy after immunization is still much lower than that of natural infection, suggesting that some or most of the reported neurological disorders may be only temporally and not causally related to measles immunization.

Encephalopathy

Claims that cases of encephalopathy followed by permanent brain injury or death were due to measles immunization, submitted to the US National Vaccine Injury Compensation Program, have been reviewed (SED-13, 920) (18). A total of 403 claims of encephalopathy and/or seizure disorders after measles, measles–rubella, measles–mumps–rubella, mumps, or rubella immunization were identified during the period 1970–93. The medical records of these cases were reviewed by physicians in the compensation program to determine, if possible, the cause of injury and the classification of the findings. The inclusion criteria established by the compensation program were met by 48 claims by patients with acute encephalopathy of undetermined cause 2–15 days after immunization with attenuated measles virus. The clustering and peak onset of encephalopathy occurred in 17 patients on days 8 and 9, and the encephalopathy was followed by permanent brain impairment or death. The patients ranged in age from 10 months to 49 months, with a median age of 15 months. There were no cases of encephalopathy of undetermined cause within 15 days after the administration of mumps or rubella vaccine. Table 2 shows the clinical findings and sequelae among the 48 cases. The authors concluded that manifestations of acute encephalopathy among these 48 children were similar to the clinical features of acute encephalopathy described after natural measles. Vaccine-associated measles encephalopathy may be a rare complication of measles immunization. From 1970 to 1993 in the USA, about 75 million children received measles vaccine by age 4 years. The 48 cases of encephalopathy after measles immunization probably represented under-reporting to this passive compensation system. However, given the generous compensation offered in this program, it is reasonable to conclude that most serious cases temporally related to an immunization have been captured. The incidence of 48 cases of encephalopathy possibly caused by 75 million doses of vaccine can reasonably be described as low.

The clinical features of acute and chronic encephalopathy or death in these 48 patients were classified into three groups based on the initial findings of ataxia in 6, behavioral changes in 8, and seizures in 34. The onset of neurological findings varied in severity from ataxia or behavioral changes to prolonged seizures or coma. Fever preceded the onset of acute encephalopathy by several hours to several days in 43 of 48 children. There was a measles-like rash with a post-vaccination onset from day 6 to day 15 in 13 children.

The 1994 report of the Institute of Medicine concluded that the evidence was inadequate to accept or reject a causal relation between MMR and encephalopathy, and it is known that the incidence of encephalitis after measles immunization of healthy children tends to be lower than the observed incidence of encephalitis of unknown cause. Two large studies have been negative. In a study analogous to the British Childhood Encephalopathy Study there were no increased risks of either encephalopathy or neurological sequelae after measles immunization (19). A retrospective case-control study through the CDC Vaccine Safety Datalink assessing the risk for 300 000 doses of MMR found not a single case of encephalitis/encephalopathy within 30 days of the administration of MMR (20). In contrast, the review mentioned above (18) reported an association between measles vaccine and encephalopathy. However, the conclusion of the report of the Institute of Medicine is still valid, namely that evidence is still inadequate to accept or reject a causal relation between measles vaccine and these diseases.

After the publication of the Institute of Medicine report, a literature search for adverse events after measles immunization, limited to publications published in 1994–98, unearthed a considerable amount of data that strengthened the rare association of measles-containing vaccines with postinfectious encephalomyelitis (6). The report has also been criticized as an attempt to establish an adverse event of a vaccine, without a specific laboratory

Table 2 Clinical effects of acute encephalopathy in 48 patients 2–15 days after the first dose of measles, measles–rubella, or measles–mumps–rubella vaccine, and sequelae, 1970–93

Clinical onset	Number	Acute illness	Number	Neurological sequelae	Number
With initial ataxia ($n = 6$)					
Irritability	6	Ataxia	6	Ataxia (chronic)	4
Fever	5	Changed behavior	4	Mental retardation	3
Measles-like rash	3	Mental regression	3	Seizure disorder	1
		Hospitalization		Hearing loss	1
With initial behavioral changes ($n = 8$)					
Lethargy	3	Mental regression	8	Mental retardation	6
Irritability	2	Coma	5	Spastic paresis	5
Confusion	2	Hospitalization	6	Seizure disorder	1
Coma	1	Death	2	Choreoathetosis	1
Fever	6			Death (later)	1
Measles-like rash	1				
With initial seizures ($n = 34$)					
Fever	32	Hospitalization	33	Mental retardation	31
Status epilepticus	17	Mental regression	31	Seizure disorder	23
Generalized	14	Coma	29	Spastic paresis	10
Focal	3	Behavioral changes	5	Death (later)	3
Measles-like rash	9	Death	2		

finding, without a specific syndrome, without comparable data for non-immunized children, and by ignoring or minimizing years of descriptive epidemiology on reactions (21). In reply, the original authors reminded their critic that the US Congress had set up the Vaccine Injury Table to avoid disagreements over causation by making temporal association an important eligibility element for listed conditions (22). Although biologic plausibility is an important standard for assessing causation in medicine, it is less important in law. In the case of the National Vaccine Injury Compensation Program, the statute provided for a legal presumption of causation, if encephalopathy began 5–15 days after measles immunization.

Seizures

As with the administration of other agents that can produce fever, some children develop febrile seizures after receiving measles vaccine. Most of these convulsions are simple febrile seizures and do not in themselves increase the probability of subsequent epilepsy or other neurological disorders. There may be an increased risk of convulsions among children with a prior history of convulsions or those with a history of convulsions in siblings or parents. After analysing data on the increased risk of such children, both the US Immunization Practices Advisory Committee (ACIP) and the Committee on Infectious Diseases of the American Academy of Pediatrics have recommended that children with a history of convulsions should be vaccinated because the benefits of immunization outweigh the risks. According to the ACIP, children at risk could receive antipyretics, starting before the expected onset of fever and continuing for 5–7 days. The Committee on Infectious Diseases was reluctant to recommend prevention with antipyretics, though after the onset of fever these are likely to be effective (16,23).

Epilepsy has been attributed to measles vaccine (24).

- A 23-month-old boy developed Lennox–Gastaut syndrome (an epileptic syndrome caused by an acquired organic brain insult) 14 days after measles immunization with Japanese FL-vaccine, based on AIK-C live attenuated measles vaccine strain. The child's prenatal and perinatal histories and his development until 23 months of life were uneventful. His monozygotic twin brother had no epileptic seizures, but it is not clear from the original paper whether or not the twin received the same vaccine.

Subacute sclerosing panencephalitis

Subacute sclerosing panencephalitis (SSPE) can occur after immunization with live attenuated measles vaccine, but the possible role of measles virus vaccine in the pathogenesis of SSPE has been neither proved nor disproved. However, the frequency seems to be lower than after natural measles. A fall in the reported incidence of SSPE in the USA accompanied the reduction in the reported incidence of measles and following it by about 7 years (25). Similar experience has been reported from Israel (26), Japan (27,28), and the eastern part of Germany (29). There is no evidence of an increased risk of SSPE on revaccination. A different note is sounded from Romania, where epidemiological investigation of SSPE indicated a yearly incidence of 5–6 cases per million inhabitants without any change due to a measles immunization program implemented about 10 years earlier (30).

Using RNA-templated sequencing, vaccine-strain measles virus has been implicated as the cause of death in three immunocompromised children with inclusion body encephalitis (6). The authors referred to a case of measles vaccine virus-associated giant cell pneumonia in a patient with advanced HIV infection.

Mumps

Meningitis

The risk of aseptic meningitis is increased after the administration of the Urabe mumps vaccine strain in mumps vaccine or MMR vaccine. Since 1992, most vaccine manufacturers have decided to suspend the distribution of vaccines containing the Urabe strain, provided that alternative vaccines were available to maintain the immunization programs established in the various countries. In 1997, a mass immunization campaign with an Urabe vaccine strain-containing MMR vaccine was carried out in the city of Salvador, in North-East Brazil (31). There was an increased risk of aseptic meningitis 3 weeks after mass immunization. The estimated risk of aseptic meningitis was 1 in 14 000 doses of MMR vaccine.

To assess the risk of mumps vaccine-associated meningitis, pediatricians were asked to report to the British Paediatric Surveillance Unit (BPSU) all confirmed and suspected cases during 1990–91. The risk based on confirmed cases was estimated to be 1 per 250 000 doses distributed (32). However, data from one district, based on two confirmed cases and one suspected case identified by the Nottingham Public Health Laboratory, suggested a much higher risk, about 1 in 4000 doses (33). To investigate whether the risk observed in Nottingham was atypical or indicative of substantial under-reporting elsewhere, additional studies were initiated. A laboratory study including four independent laboratories identified 13 cases of vaccine-associated meningitis after immunization with Urabe strain vaccines; in one-third of instances, mumps virus characterized as a vaccine-like virus was isolated. The risk estimate of 1 per 11 000 doses distributed was lower than in the Nottingham study but much higher than in the BPSU surveillance. Furthermore, children with a discharge diagnosis of viral meningitis were identified in the Oxford region and their immunization status ascertained. The estimated risk was 4.7 per 100 000 doses. Because there have been no cases of proven vaccine-associated mumps meningitis with isolation of the Jeryl Lynn vaccine virus in the UK, the decision was taken to change to Jeryl Lynn-containing vaccines (32).

Eight cases of mumps vaccine-associated meningitis have occurred in Canada. Mumps viruses have been isolated and characterized by nucleotide sequencing as Urabe Am9-like strains. Urabe mumps vaccine virus-containing vaccines are no longer licensed for sale in Canada (34).

Forsey and colleagues have examined over 80 mumps viruses from around the world; they included 20 isolates found in the cerebrospinal fluid of children with vaccine-associated meningitis in the UK and Ireland and isolates from parotitis and meningitis following mumps immunization from Australia, Belgium, Canada, France, Germany, and Japan (35). They were characterized by PCR and dideoxynucleotide sequencing for the differentiation of wild from attenuated mumps viruses. The isolates were characterized as Urabe Am9-like vaccine strains. The Jeryl Lynn mumps vaccine strain was found in one vaccinee from Germany, but no virus of this type was isolated from a patient with meningitis. Although one cannot conclude from this that Jeryl Lynn is free of such adverse effects, all the evidence points toward a considerable difference between the mumps vaccine strains in the degree of risk. Virological heterogeneity provides a clue for further investigation (36). Commercial mumps vaccine of the Jeryl Lynn strain contains at least two distinct mumps viruses; it has been suggested that this factor contributes significantly to the safety and efficacy of this vaccine (23).

The Global Advisory Committee on Vaccine Safety has considered a comprehensive review of the world literature on the safety of mumps immunization, with special attention to vaccine-associated meningitis. They found no cases of virologically proven aseptic meningitis after mumps immunization based on the Jeryl Lynn vaccine strain. If mumps vaccines based on vaccine strains such as Urabe Am9, Leningrad-3, or Leningrad–Zagreb are being used in mass immunization campaigns, the committee recommends that the potential for clustering of aseptic meningitis cases after the campaign should be taken into consideration. The available data are insufficient to distinguish between the safety profiles of the Urabe Am9, Leningrad-3, and Leningrad–Zagreb strains with regard to vaccine-associated meningitis (37).

Rubella

Adverse effects on the nervous system that have at least temporally been associated with rubella vaccination include myelitis, myeloradiculitis (SEDA-2, 268) (SEDA-20, 292), meningomyelitis (SEDA-10, 291), encephalitis (SEDA-5, 308), peripheral neuropathy (SEDA-12, 284), facial or peripheral paresthesia (SEDA-11, 295) (SEDA-12, 284), and carpal tunnel syndrome (SEDA-12, 284). In many of these cases the causal relation was doubtful. The authors of the report of the Institute of Medicine, National Academy of Sciences, Washington, DC (1991) entitled "Adverse Effects of Pertussis and Rubella Vaccines" (38) considered that there was insufficient evidence to indicate either the presence or absence of a causal relation between RA 27/3 rubella vaccine and radiculoneuritis and other neuropathies.

- Acute disseminated encephalomyelitis occurred in a 14-year-old boy 22 days after rubella immunization (39). The authors suggested that live rubella vaccine can occasionally trigger immunologically mediated demyelination within the nervous system.

It has been suggested that there is insufficient evidence to indicate either the presence or absence of a causal relation between RA 27/3 rubella vaccine and radiculoneuritis and other neuropathies (38), although cases have been reported.

- A 23-year-old woman developed a mild distal demyelination neuropathy 4 weeks after rubella immunization (40). Immunological studies showed the presence of antibodies to the rubella virus proteins and to the myelin basic protein.

The authors suspected that a virus-induced immune response caused an auto-aggressive reaction responsible for demyelination.

Measles–mumps–rubella

A cranial nerve palsy has been attributed to MMR (41).

- A 13-month-old girl developed a recurrent sixth nerve palsy 1 week after MMR immunization. This resolved completely over 8 weeks and recurred 15 weeks after initial onset. Other causes for the sixth nerve palsy were excluded.

Meningitis

Vaccine-associated meningitis is a well-known adverse effect of mumps (or MMR) immunization. Until 1991 the reported incidence was low, but in that year Japanese researchers published the result of a nationwide survey, started in 1989, in which the incidence of vaccine-associated mumps meningitis varied from less than 1 case per 7000 to 1 per 405 from prefecture to prefecture. Meningitis was generally mild and there were no sequelae from the illness. The vaccine used contained the Urabe Am9 strain (42,43). In April 1993, the Ministry of Health and Welfare in Japan decided to interrupt the use of MMR vaccine (44).

A retrospective study was carried out to determine the incidence of vaccine-associated meningitis in Japan after the administration of different locally produced MMR vaccines (MHW MMR vaccine, Takeda MMR vaccine, Biken MMR vaccine, and Kitasato MMR vaccine) (45). Among the three MMR vaccines (Biken vaccine excepted) the incidence of meningitis was about 1 in 500–900 vaccinees. The criteria for inclusion of a case of meningitis were symptoms of meningitis and pleocytosis in the cerebrospinal fluid. In a complementary nationwide comparison of four MMR vaccines conducted in Japan by 1255 pediatricians the total number of vaccinees was 38 203 (46). All were arbitrarily given one of the MMR vaccines produced by three manufacturers (Biken, Kitasato, and Takeda) or the standard MMR vaccine made of designated strains (Biken's mumps Urabe Am9 strain, Kitasato's measles AIK-C strain, and Takeda's rubella To336 strain). The rates of virologically confirmed aseptic meningitis per 10 000 recipients were 16.6, 11.6, 3.2, and 0 for the standard MMR, Takeda MMR, Kitasato MMR, and Biken MMR vaccines respectively. The incidence of convulsions was the highest with the standard MMR vaccine, and the incidence of fever associated with vomiting at 15–35 days (symptoms relevant to aseptic meningitis) were also the highest with the standard MMR vaccine. The incidence of parotitis was the lowest with Takeda MMR vaccine.

The finding that the incidences of aseptic meningitis differed after administration of the standard MMR vaccine or Biken MMR vaccine has inevitably raised questions about the consistency of manufacture of the Urabe Am9 mumps virus vaccines. The National Institute of Health found that the biological characteristics of the Urabe Am9 mumps virus contained in the standard MMR vaccine and in the Biken MMR vaccine were different. The Biken Company reported that the mumps vaccine in the standard MMR vaccine was a mixture of two Urabe Am9 mumps vaccine bulks, one identical to that contained in the Biken MMR vaccine and the other produced by a different manufacturing process.

In 1995, a somewhat different note was sounded from France, where all mumps vaccines produced and marketed at that time contained the Urabe vaccine strain. The incidence of vaccine-associated meningitis was estimated using two different data sources: the national network of hospital virology laboratories and the manufacturer's pharmacovigilance department (47). The risk of vaccine-associated meningitis was assessed at one case per 28 400 doses distributed when using the laboratory network data or one case per 13 000–67 200 doses distributed when using the pharmacovigilance data. The French vaccination committee recommended that the vaccine continue to be used whilst awaiting vaccine containing the Jeryl Lynn strain.

Cases of aseptic meningitis occurring 14–26 days after MMR immunization have been reviewed (48). All the patients had been immunized with the L-Zagreb mumps strain, Edmonston–Zagreb measles strain, and the RA 27/3 rubella strain. The incidence of vaccine-associated meningitis was 9 per 10 000 doses. This finding was similar to that reported for the same mumps vaccine strain by Cizman (49), 10 per 10 000 (SEDA-12, 815), but higher than that found by Kraigher (48).

Transmission of Urabe mumps vaccine strain between siblings has been reported (44). A girl developed parotitis after immunization with Urabe mumps strain; 19 days later her older sister developed mumps. The strain isolated showed molecular biological characteristics typical for the Urabe strain.

The reason for the high incidence of vaccine-associated mumps meningitis has been investigated by a comparison of the nucleotide sequence of the hemagglutinin-neuraminidase gene from vaccine virus with the genes of viruses isolated from patients with vaccine-associated meningitis (50). The analysis showed that the Urabe AM9 vaccine strain is a mixture of viruses that differ at nucleotide 1081: a wild type-like variant A and a variant G. Vaccinees who developed vaccine-associated meningitis or parotitis had predominantly variant A (98–100%), indicating strong selection of the wild type-like variant of the mumps virus.

The incidence of aseptic meningitis after immunization with MMR containing the Jeryl Lynn mumps vaccine strain has been assessed in a Vaccine Safety Datalink project (20). The overall rate of confirmed cases in the study population (children aged 1–2 years) was 172 cases per million children, very close to the background rate of 162 naturally occurring cases per million children aged 1–4 years in Olmsted County, MN. The authors concluded that there is no increased risk of aseptic meningitis after vaccination with MMR including the Jeryl Lynn mumps vaccine strain.

Gait disturbance

An analysis of 41 reports of gait disturbance in 15-month-old children in temporal relation with the first MMR immunization, collected in the framework of the Danish surveillance system for adverse events after immunization, has been reported (51). About 533 000 doses of MMR vaccine were administered to 15-month-old children in Denmark during the 10 years from 1987 to 1996. The number of reported cases of gait disturbance corresponded to a frequency of eight per 100 000 doses of MMR vaccine. The authors considered that the symptoms were characteristic of cerebellar ataxia. The high frequency and mainly mild course of gait disturbances might indicate a mumps-related reaction. The symptoms mainly occurred at 7–14 days after immunization, and the duration was on average 1–2 weeks (range 1 day to over 4 months). Most cases were mild and short-lasting and a longer duration of symptoms seems to be predictive of late sequelae. In the same period about the same number of doses were used for the second MMR immunization without similar reactions. Disturbance of gait has rarely been reported, and the authors listed in their paper two reports from Sweden and Germany in which symptoms were so mild that no invasive investigations were carried out.

Guillain–Barré syndrome

To test the hypothesis that MMR vaccine can cause Guillain–Barré syndrome, a retrospective study has been carried out in Finland, based on linkage of individual immunization records with nation-wide hospital discharge registers (52). MMR vaccine did not cause any increase in the incidence of Guillain–Barré syndrome over background and there was no clustering of cases at any time after the administration of the vaccine. The authors concluded that there is no causal association between MMR immunization and Guillain–Barré syndrome.

Sensory systems

Rubella

Bilateral optic neuritis (53) and retinal vasculitis (SEDA-20, 292) have been attributed to rubella immunization.

Psychological, psychiatric

Measles–mumps–rubella

The suggestion that measles/MMR immunization can cause autism has not been confirmed. Autism is characterized by absorption in self-centered subjective mental activities (such as day-dreams, fantasies, hallucinations), especially when accompanied by marked withdrawal from reality.

History

The scientific and public response to the 1998 publication of Wakefield and colleagues (54), and Wakefield's subsequent press conference, in which he suggested that immunization with MMR might be associated with Crohn's disease and autism was enormous and controversial. For example, Black and colleagues (55) stated that the publicity generated by this paper was out of proportion to the strength of the evidence it contained; Beale (56) suggested that the Lancet would bear a heavy responsibility for acting against the public health interest that the journal usually aims to promote; O'Brien and colleagues (57) considered that the substantial amount of evidence that contradicts the findings of Wakefield and colleagues did not achieve the same prominence in the popular press.

In replying to these letters, Wakefield (58) defended the clinician's duty to his patients and the researcher's obligation to test hypotheses. For his part, the editor of the Lancet pointed out that the paper had been presented with a commissioned commentary in the same issue; peer review had confirmed that the paper merited publication, with suitable revisions and editing, as an early report; finally, he considered that the press had presented the information in a balanced way (59). However, it was subsequently discovered that the work had been sponsored by a pharmaceutical company which had not been declared at the time (60). Furthermore, the children who were included in the study had been selected other than at random. Subsequently, 10 of Wakefield's colleagues withdrew the findings that they had initially reported and one other could not be traced; only Wakefield did not retract (61).

The Lancet then reviewed the developments in the discussion (62), with emphasis on evidence that contradicts the alleged association and new data presented by Wakefield. The last part of the editorial read as follows:

In a new twist, Wakefield's crusade fuelled further anxiety among parents when he and John O'Leary, director of pathology at Coombe Women's Hospital, Dublin, Ireland, presented unpublished data to the US Senate's congressional oversight committee in Washington on April 6 [2000]. The hearing was called by the chairman, Dan Burton, an Indiana Republican, whose grandson has autism and visited the Royal Free Hospital in November last year. At the hearing, six parents of children with autism gave moving testimonies of their children's illness. ... Scientific evidence was presented by six chosen 'experts'. According to Wakefield's testimony, he has now studied more than 150 children with 'autistic enterocolitis'—an unproven association had become a disease—and a detailed analysis of the first 60 cases is to be published in the American Journal of Gastroenterology later this year.

Wakefield presented uninterpretable fragments of results only and concentrated on refuting studies that had contradicted his findings. His conclusions were surprisingly non-committal: 'the virological data indicate that this may be measles virus in some children'; he added that it would be imprudent to interpret the temporal relationship with MMR as a chance finding, in the absence of thorough investigation. O'Leary explained that gut-biopsy material from 24 of 25 children with autism was positive for measles virus compared with one of 15 controls, and that this material was presented to him by Wakefield using 'blinded protocols'. Since the controls are not further described and the details of these findings remain unpublished, this evidence raises far more questions than it answers.

"Autism is a poorly understood neurodevelopmental-disease spectrum with a heart-breaking personal story behind every case. But parents of such children have not been served well by these latest claims made well beyond the publically [sic] available evidence. A congressional hearing, like a press conference, is no place to make controversial scientific assessments. And if scientists question the safety of vaccines without making their evidence fully transparent, harm will be done to many more children than they purport to protect."

Wakefield and Montgomery subsequently raised doubts about the adequacy of the evidence that secured the license for MMR vaccine (63). Particularly in view of the immunosuppressive properties of the measles virus, they suggested that there is a potential for adverse interactions between the component live viruses. They therefore proposed that spaced monovalent measles, mumps, and rubella immunization should replace the use of the combined MMR vaccine. The continuing publications of Wakefield led to reduced MMR coverage in some parts of the UK and to well-publicized concerns about the potential for measles outbreaks among primary school entrants. In an editorial in the British Medical Journal, Elliman and Bedford replied to Wakefield's paper (64). They considered that the current concerns were idiosyncratic and presented reviews confirming the vaccine's safety. The Medicines Control Agency and the Department of Health in the UK rejected any suggestion by Wakefield and colleagues that combined MMR vaccines were licensed prematurely. A review of the licensing of MMR vaccines led to the assurance that the licensing procedure was normal and was based on robust studies (65). This position was shared by the Committee on Safety of Medicines and the Joint Committee on Vaccination and Immunisation. At the end of November 2001, Wakefield left his post at the Royal Free and University College Medical School in London. The college said: "Dr Wakefield's research was no longer in line with the Department of Medicine's research strategy and he left the university by mutual agreement" (66). The WHO strongly endorsed the use of MMR vaccine. The combination vaccine was recommended rather than monovalent presentations. There was no evidence to suggest impaired safety of MMR (67).

In April 2001, the Institute of Medicine's Immunization Safety Review Committee released its report "MMR vaccine and autism". Although scientists generally agreed that most cases of autism result from events that occur in the prenatal period or shortly after birth, there was concern because the symptoms of autism typically do not emerge until the child's second year, and this is the same time at which MMR vaccine is first administered in most developed countries. The committee took also into consideration the papers published by Wakefield and other groups and scientists suggesting evidence of a link between MMR vaccine and Crohn's disease and autism. Following review of the numerous research efforts on the MMR–autism hypothesis the committee concluded in its report "that the evidence favors rejection of a causal relationship at the population level between MMR vaccine and autistic spectrum disorders". Epidemiological evidence showed no association between MMR vaccine and autism, and the committee did not find a proven biological mechanism that would explain such a relation. Therefore, the committee did not recommend a policy review at this time of the licensure of MMR vaccine or of the current schedules and recommendations for MMR administration (68).

A conference of the American Academy of Pediatrics on "new challenges in childhood immunizations" was convened in Oak Brook, IL, on 12–13 June 2000 and reviewed data on what is known about the pathogenesis, epidemiology, and genetics of autism and the available data on hypothesized associations with Crohn's disease, measles, and MMR vaccine. The participants concluded that the available evidence did not support the hypothesis that MMR vaccine causes either Crohn's disease or autism or associated disorders. They recommended continued scientific efforts directed to the identification of the causes of autism (69).

The response to a newly published adverse event due to immunization must be rapid. If the reported association is correct, urgent re-evaluation of the immunization program is necessary. Otherwise, if the reported association is false, a credible counter-message is necessary to minimize the negative impact on the immunization program (6). The rapidity of response to the 1998 publication of Wakefield and colleagues, including the convening of an independent review panel in the UK, was very useful.

Evidence

Two studies suggested a link between measles/MMR immunization and autism. Fudenberg reported that 15 of 40 patients with infantile autism developed symptoms within a week after MMR immunization (70). Wakefield and colleagues evaluated 12 children with chronic enterocolitis and regressive developmental disorders (54). The onset of behavioral symptoms was associated with MMR immunization in eight cases, as reported by the parents. Both reports were non-comparative and anecdotal. By chance alone some cases of autism will occur shortly after immunization, and most children in developed countries receive their first measles or MMR vaccination in the second year of life, when autism typically manifests. The imprecision of the interval between immunization and the onset of behavioral symptoms in the study by Wakefield and colleagues made these data suspect, even before their retraction.

Inaccuracies in the study of Fudenberg, for example referring to hepatitis B vaccine as a live vaccine, cast some doubts on the carefulness of the entire report. Developmental delay is likely to be detected by a gradual awareness over a period of time, not on a particular day. Epidemiological studies in various countries (UK, Sweden, Finland), comparing the introduction and use of vaccines and the incidence of autism, have not supported a relation between measles/MMR vaccine and autism (71–74). Wing reviewed 16 studies in Europe, North America, and Japan and found no increase in autism with increasing use of measles or MMR vaccines (75). An analysis of two large European datasets produced similar results (76). In early 1998, experts in various medical disciplines reviewed the work of the Inflammatory Disease Study Group of the Royal Free Hospital in detail and concluded that there is no evidence for a link between measles/MMR vaccine and either Crohn's disease or autism (77).

Data from an earlier study have been reanalysed to test the hypothesis that MMR vaccine might cause autism but that the induction interval needs to be short (78). Evidence for an increased incidence was sought using the case-series method. The study used data on all MMR vaccines, including booster doses. The results of this study, combined with results obtained earlier by the same authors, provided powerful evidence against the hypothesis that MMR vaccine causes autism at any time after immunization.

Metabolism

Measles–mumps–rubella

A total of 20 cases of type I diabetes mellitus suspected to be induced by MMR immunization have been reported to Behringwerke, Marburg, Germany, probably due to the mumps component (79). The earliest case occurred 3 days after receiving the vaccine and the latest 7 months after immunization. Twelve cases were diagnosed within 30 days of immunization. The investigators considered the cases of diabetes mellitus to have a temporal relation to the immunization. For every 5 million children immunized against mumps 50 spontaneous cases of diabetes mellitus are to be expected by random coincidence within a period of 30 days after immunization. In fact, only 12 cases were reported within 30 days after immunization. Mainly based on this analysis the Deutsche Vereinigung zur Bekämpfung der Viruskrankheiten (DVV) could not confirm the relation between mumps immunization and diabetes mellitus (80).

Hematologic

Measles

Anemia has been reported after measles immunization (81). The vaccine can cause a significant fall in hemoglobin that can persist for 14–30 days and can be difficult to distinguish from iron deficiency.

Rubella

Thrombocytopenic purpura has been attributed to rubella (82). However, the authors of the report of the Institute of Medicine, National Academy of Sciences, Washington, DC (1991) entitled "Adverse Effects of Pertussis and Rubella Vaccines" (38) considered that there was insufficient evidence to indicate either the presence or absence of a causal relation between RA 27/3 rubella vaccine and thrombocytopenic purpura.

Measles–mumps–rubella

There is a relation between MMR vaccination and thrombocytopenic purpura, but not with the measles component itself (18). Thrombocytopenic purpura after MMR has been reviewed, with discussion of pathogenesis and the vaccines and infections associated with this problem (83). Rubella vaccine is one of the most frequently reported causes of thrombocytopenia in Denmark (84). In France, a retrospective epidemiological survey (1984–92) showed that the rates of thrombocytopenic purpura per 100 000 vaccinees were 0.23 for measles vaccine, 0.17 for rubella vaccine, 0.87 for combination MR vaccine, and 0.95 for MMR vaccine (85). Thrombocytopenia was severe and always associated with purpura. Cases of recurrent thrombocytopenic purpura after repeated MMR immunization have been reported (86,87). The Advisory Committee on Immunization Practices (ACIP) of the Centers for Disease Control and Prevention (CDC) has recommended avoiding subsequent doses of MMR when a previous episode of thrombocytopenia occurred in close temporal proximity to the previous immunization, that is within 6 weeks (88,89).

The causal relation between MMR vaccine and idiopathic thrombocytopenic purpura has been confirmed using linkage of immunization records and hospital admission records; the absolute risk within 6 weeks of immunization was 1 per 22 300 doses (90).

Gastrointestinal

Measles–mumps–rubella

The suggestion that measles/MMR immunization can cause Crohn's disease has not been confirmed.

Inflammatory bowel disease (ulcerative colitis and Crohn's disease) is a general term for a group of chronic inflammatory disorders of unknown cause involving the gastrointestinal tract. Despite many attempts to confirm an infectious agent as the cause of disease, no bacterial, viral, or fungal agents have so far been isolated. There is strong evidence for a genetic predisposition.

In 1993 and 1994, researchers in the UK and Sweden suggested that Crohn's disease might be a late result of measles infection at a critical time during early childhood (91,92). In a study of the outcome of maternal measles infection in 25 Swedish babies, three of four children exposed to measles in utero subsequently developed Crohn's disease (93). Whereas wild measles virus was initially implicated, a controversial debate was initiated in 1995, when Thompson and colleagues suggested that attenuated measles vaccine virus might also cause inflammatory bowel disease, having found an increased risk of inflammatory bowel disease in about 3000 immunized individuals compared with about 11 000 non-immunized controls (94). Furthermore, the Inflammatory Bowel Disease Study Group of the Royal Free Hospital, London (Wakefield and colleagues), suggested that measles virus is present in the bowel of patients with Crohn's disease (with evidence from transmission electron microscopy, immunohistochemistry, in situ hybridization, and immunogold electron microscopy) (92,95,96).

Wakefield and colleagues then made two suggestions in a paper in the Lancet (54): that autism is linked to a form of inflammatory bowel disease and that this new syndrome is associated with MMR immunization. Their hypothesis was that MMR vaccine causes non-specific gut injury, allowing the absorption of normally non-permeable peptides, which in turn cause serious developmental disorders. The authors stated that they had not proved an association between measles, mumps, and rubella vaccines and either autism or inflammatory bowel disease. However, there were enough references in the text to lead the reader to the assumption that there is sufficient evidence provided by the study, and by other scientific publications, that there is a link. This paper of Wakefield and colleagues, publicized by a subsequent press conference, resulted in a heated debate and a huge number of letters to the editor of the Lancet, in turn severely criticizing both the article and its implications for immunization programs, blaming the editor for publishing the article, and defending the obligation of clinical researchers to publish provocative findings. Considerable evidence, mainly microbiological and epidemiological, has been collected by others to suggest that the association with MMR does not exist.

The alleged association of measles vaccination with Crohn's disease and autism has also been criticized as being based on poor science and as having been largely refuted by a large volume of stronger work, three types of evidence against the hypothesis (biological, microbiological, and epidemiological) being considered in detail (6).

Several groups have found no evidence of persistence of measles virus in the tissues of patients with Crohn's disease with a very sensitive test (polymerase chain reaction) (97–100). Furthermore, no viral genomic sequences of measles, mumps, and rubella viruses were found in intestinal specimens (100). The results of Iizuka and colleagues (98,101) were particularly interesting—they used the same monoclonal antibody in their immunohistochemical studies that Wakefield and colleagues had used. The antigen recognized could be a measles virus protein, but they considered it much more likely that the previous immunochemical observations were accounted for by antigen mimicry between measles virus and a host protein found in the intestinal tissue of patients with Crohn's disease. Serological studies have also shown lower measles complement fixation titers in patients with Crohn's disease than in controls, not supporting an association of measles vaccine with Crohn's disease (102,103).

The major weaknesses of the epidemiological studies reported by the Inflammatory Bowel Disease Study Group have been discussed in a number of letters to the editor (104,105) and editorials (105). On behalf of the World Health Organization's Expanded Program on Immunization, Lee and colleagues (71) questioned the conclusion that there was a temporal association between immunization and the onset of symptoms, because the study of Wakefield and colleagues had provided data on the interval between immunization and the onset of symptoms in only five of their 12 cases of so-called autism-bowel syndrome, and the age at which the vaccine was given was mentioned in only three. Furthermore, Lee and colleagues criticized the study on the grounds that no patient selection had been made by Wakefield and colleagues, other than the 12 patients referred to them; there were no controls and no blinding of the investigators (71). Payne and Mason (106) made the same comment, that the cases reported by Wakefield and colleagues were highly selected and that the underlying population was unclear.

Several epidemiological studies have failed to confirm an association between measles/measles vaccine and Crohn's disease. For example:

- *Copenhagen*: In a study of 25 mothers with measles during pregnancy there were no cases of Crohn's disease in their children (107).
- *Finland*: Peltola and colleagues (108) reported on over a decade's effort to detect all severe adverse events associated with MMR vaccine distributed in Finland. There was no evidence to support the hypothesis that the vaccine could cause pervasive developmental disorders or inflammatory bowel disease. Comparing the incidence of Crohn's disease and the Finnish data for measles and measles immunization, Pebody and colleagues (109) came to the same conclusion, namely that there is no association between Crohn's disease and measles vaccine.
- *Japan*: A nationwide survey of inflammatory bowel disease was carried out in 1979–93 in children under 16 years of age. From 1979 to 1992 the number of cases of inflammatory bowel disease was almost the same (ulcerative colitis rates 0.08–0.12 per 100 000, Crohn's disease 0.04–0.06 per 100 000). In 1992, the incidence of Crohn's disease rose to 0.10 and in 1993 to 0.12 per 100 000; the incidence rate of ulcerative colitis increased in 1993 to 0.18 per 100 000. Measles immunization (implemented in 1968) was 68% until 1993, and during the 1980s and early 1990s was relatively constant at about 70% (110).
- *UK*: In close to 7 million children who received MR vaccine in a catch-up campaign there was no increase in the number of new cases or exacerbation of existing cases of Crohn's disease (111).
- In an international case-control study of 499 patients with chronic inflammatory bowel disease and 998 control patients from nine countries, there was no difference in the risk of inflammatory bowel disease in association with either natural measles or measles immunization (112).

Pancreas

Mumps

Acute pancreatitis after mumps immunization is very rare and has been reported only sporadically in adolescents.

- A 13-month-old boy presented with an acute abdomen and surgery was performed for a suspected perforated appendicitis (113). The appendix was normal but the pancreas was enlarged, edematous, and covered with fibrin, with areas of superficial necrosis. The serum amylase activity was 528 IU (normal under 200 IU).

Unfortunately the authors reported no data on the vaccine used or the interval between immunization and disease onset.

Measles–mumps–rubella

- A 19-year-old woman who received MMR vaccine developed pancreatitis 11 days later (114). Other causes of pancreatitis could not be implicated.

Skin

Measles

- An 11-month-old boy developed hypertrichosis at the injection site (2.5 × 3 cm) 1 month after measles immunization (115). The hypertrichosis and induration persisted during the follow-up period of 3 months.

Measles–mumps–rubella

Gianotti–Crosti syndrome has been reported in a child immunized with MMR (116).

- Three days after MMR immunization a 15-month-old boy developed a rash, initially on the arms but later involving the legs. Six weeks later he had an extensive, symmetrical, non-follicular, papular eruption on his face, arms, and legs, with striking sparing of his trunk. This was labeled Gianotti–Crosti syndrome, a self-healing non-recurrent erythematous or skin-colored papular eruption with symmetrical distribution on the face, buttocks, and extremities in children.

A wide spectrum of infectious diseases has been associated with this syndrome, and preceding immunization against influenza, diphtheria, pertussis, and poliomyelitis has been reported.

- A 13-year-old girl developed toxic epidermal necrolysis 7 days after being immunized with live attenuated MMR vaccine (117).

Musculoskeletal

Rubella

Acute arthritis/arthralgia due to rubella vaccine occurs more often and tends to be more severe in susceptible women than in children, usually involving the small peripheral joints. Joint symptoms generally begin 3–25 days

500 mg/day) had no effects on body weight, lean body mass, blood pressure, plasma sodium concentration, urinary sodium excretion, or the exchangeable sodium pool (8).

Hematologic

Medroxyprogesterone acetate, administered either orally or by injection, has little or no effect on blood coagulation (23).

The suitability of medroxyprogesterone for women with sickle cell disease has been evaluated in a controlled crossover trial, which showed that both hematological and clinical parameters were improved (24).

Liver

No consistent effects of medroxyprogesterone acetate on liver function have been found, and primary biliary cirrhosis and chronic active hepatitis have appeared to improve during treatment (25).

Musculoskeletal

Subgroups of users of depot medroxyprogesterone acetate may have reduced spinal bone density, but this seems to be reversible after withdrawal, even after several years of drug exposure (26). Bone mineral density in one cross-sectional study was lower among users of depot medroxyprogesterone acetate, but withdrawal was followed by complete recovery of normal bone density (26). A current study in the USA is expected to provide further data on this matter in women who have used medroxyprogesterone acetate for as long as 10 years.

Reproductive system

Poor cycle control is a problem with medroxyprogesterone acetate. Most women using the product have at first either irregular or excessive bleeding and spotting or amenorrhea linked to endometrial atrophy (27); however, only one woman in a thousand bleeds sufficiently to warrant aggressive therapy, such as curettage. As the duration of use increases, amenorrhea becomes more common. Depot medroxyprogesterone acetate is associated with greater variability in menstrual patterns than other hormonal contraceptives (28,29). Bleeding/spotting episodes are infrequent but are prolonged when they occur, and the prevalence of amenorrhea increases over time to more than half of users after the first year. Under 10% of users have bleeding patterns defined as fully satisfactory and acceptable, compared with 85–90% of women not using contraception and the majority of women taking appropriate doses of oral contraceptives. However, with appropriate patient selection and counselling, many users view amenorrhea positively and are content to continue with the medroxyprogesterone. Indeed, because they are often amenorrheic, they may experience improvements in such menstrual cycle conditions as menorrhagia and dysmenorrhea and in iron deficiency anemia. Other potential benefits include reduction in the risk of pelvic inflammatory disease, improvement in sickle cell disease parameters, and lessened seizure frequency in women with epilepsy.

Other effects are generally less prevalent with progestogen-only contraceptives than with combined oral contraceptives because of the absence of an estrogen and a lower dose of the progestogen. Headache, breast tenderness, and less commonly nausea and dizziness have been reported by users of progestogen-only contraceptives, but it is not clear whether progestogen-only contraceptives actually play a causal role. Androgenic adverse effects, such as acne, hirsutism, and weight gain, occur, but rarely.

The reduced penetrability of cervical mucus, which contributes to the contraceptive effect, may well provide some small degree of protection against pelvic inflammatory disease. However, this effect is likely to be less than that exerted by combined oral contraceptives, since the expanded cervical ectropion found among combined oral contraceptive users is not present in users of progestogen-only contraceptives.

Immunologic

Anaphylactic reactions to medroxyprogesterone are very rare.

- A 40-year-old woman developed anaphylactic shock after receiving depot medroxyprogesterone acetate 150 mg intramuscularly (30). She was not taking any other medications, and there was no history of allergy to food or cosmetics. She responded fully to immediate resuscitation. She had another episode when she received another dose 12 weeks later.

Long-Term Effects

Tumorigenicity

The effects of depot medroxyprogesterone acetate on reproductive cancers appear to be similar to those of combined oral contraceptives. Most notably, despite initial concerns about breast cancer in beagle dogs that were given large doses of medroxyprogesterone, a pooled analysis of epidemiological studies concluded that women using medroxyprogesterone are not at increased risk of breast cancer (31). Furthermore, the risk did not increase with increasing duration of use. However, women who had begun use within the past 5 years had significantly increased risk, perhaps because of accelerated growth of pre-existing tumors or increased surveillance.

Another review, dating from 1994, concluded that depot medroxyprogesterone acetate has a protective effect against endometrial cancer that is at least as strong as for combined oral contraceptives, but that, based on the limited available evidence, there is no association with ovarian cancer (32). Regarding cervical neoplasia, studies of depot medroxyprogesterone acetate do not show a strong adverse effect, but as with combined oral contraceptives it is uncertain whether there is no association or a slightly increased risk (33).

Second-Generation Effects

Fertility

Return of fertility may be delayed for several months after withdrawal of medroxyprogesterone acetate. The length of the delay is not related to the duration of use. There is no evidence of permanent impairment of fertility (2,34).

Teratogenicity

If a breakthrough pregnancy occurs during the use of depot medroxyprogesterone acetate, the developing embryo and fetus will continue to be exposed to it for months, and an adverse effect cannot be entirely excluded, but little concrete information has emerged. Clitoral hypertrophy has been described in three infants exposed to medroxyprogesterone in utero. In view of the hormonal spectrum of medroxyprogesterone, this is a conceivable adverse effect, but there is no confirmation, nor is it clear whether the drug harms the fetus in any other way (25).

Lactation

Many studies have shown that lactation is not adversely affected by depot medroxyprogesterone acetate and that breast-milk production may even be increased (35). Because of the low binding affinity of medroxyprogesterone to sex hormone binding globulin, the concentration of steroids in the milk is close to that in the maternal plasma, unlike the 19-nortestosterone derivatives.

Children whose mothers used depot medroxyprogesterone acetate while breastfeeding have been followed up in Thailand for 17 years and in Chile for 4.5 years, with no documented effect on growth or development (36). In undernourished lactating women the metabolic effects seem to be more pronounced than among healthy users (17).

Susceptibility Factors

Depot medroxyprogesterone acetate should not be used in women with breast cancer, genital cancer, undiagnosed uterine bleeding, or suspected pregnancy (37), but these are merely logical precautions.

The only study of depot medroxyprogesterone acetate and HIV infection, conducted among Thai prostitutes, showed an increased risk after adjustment for other variables (38).

Drug Administration

Drug administration route

An injection of medroxyprogesterone acetate 150 mg provides contraception for some 3 months. Peak concentrations in the blood are reached on around the 10th day after injection, but the drug is still detectable in the blood at the 90th day, although with wide interindividual variation.

References

1. World Health Organization. Injectable Hormonal Contraceptives. Technical and Safety Aspects. Geneva: WHO Publication, 1982:65.
2. Kaunitz AM. Long-acting injectable contraception with depot medroxyprogesterone acetate Am J Obstet Gynecol 1994;170(5 Pt 2):1543–9.
3. Landgren BM. Gestagen Methods (Depo-Provera, Mini-pill and Norplant). Uppsala: Swedish Medical Products Agency, 1994:2.
4. American College of Obstetricians and Gynecologists (ACOG). Hormonal Contraception. Washington, DC: ACOG Technical Bulletin, 1994:198.
5. Onu PE. Depot medroxyprogesterone in the management of benign prostatic hyperplasia. Eur Urol 1995; 28(3):229–35.
6. Tatro DS. Drug interaction facts. In: Facts and Comparisons. St Louis, Missouri, 1999:908–10.
7. Anonymous. Medroxyprogesterone and palliative care: new indication. No impact on quality of life. Prescrire Int 2001;10(51):3–4.
8. Lelli G, Angelelli B, Zanichelli L, Strocchi E, Mondini F, Monetti N, Piana E, Pannuti F. The effect of high dose medroxyprogesterone acetate on water and salt metabolism in advanced cancer patients. Chemioterapia 1984; 3(5):327–9.
9. Harvey PJ, Molloy D, Upton J, Wing LM. Dose response effect of cyclical medroxyprogesterone on blood pressure in postmenopausal women. J Hum Hypertens 2001; 15(5):313–21.
10. Black HR, Leppert P, DeCherney A. The effect of medroxyprogesterone acetate on blood pressure. Int J Gynaecol Obstet 1978;17(1):83–7.
11. Mattson RH, Rebar RW. Contraceptive methods for women with neurologic disorders. Am J Obstet Gynecol 1993;168(6 Pt 2):2027–32.
12. Wander HE, Nagel GA, Blossey HC, Kleeberg U. Aminoglutethimide and medroxyprogesterone acetate in the treatment of patients with advanced breast cancer. A phase II study of the Association of Medical Oncology of the German Cancer Society (AIO). Cancer 1986; 58(9):1985–9.
13. Simon S, Schiffer M, Glick SM, Schwartz E. Effect of medroxyprogesterone acetate upon stimulated release of growth hormone in men. J Clin Endocrinol Metab 1967;27(11):1633 6.
14. Gershberg H, Zorrilla E, Hernandez A, Hulse M. Effects of medroxyprogesterone acetate on serum insulin and growth hormone levels in diabetics and potential diabetics. Obstet Gynecol 1969;33(3):383–9.
15. Teichmann AT, Cremer P, Wieland H, Kuhn W, Seidel D. Lipid metabolic changes during hormonal treatment of endometriosis. Maturitas 1988;10(1):27–33.
16. Kongsayreepong R, Chutivongse S, George P, Joyce S, McCone JM, Garza-Flores J, Valles de Bourges V, de La Cruz DL, Perez-Palacios G, Rosseneu M, et al. A multicentre comparative study of serum lipids and apolipoproteins in long-term users of DMPA and a control group of IUD users. World Health Organization. Task Force on Long-Acting Systemic Agents for Fertility Regulation Special Programme of Research, Development and Research Training in Human Reproduction. Contraception 1993;47(2):177–91.
17. Joshi UM, Virkar KD, Amatayakul K, Singkamani R, Bamji MS, Prema K, Whitehead TP, Belsey MA, Hall P, Parker RA. Metabolic side-effects of injectable depot-medroxyprogesterone acetate, 150 mg three-monthly, in undernourished lactating women. WHO Task Force on Long-acting Agents for Fertility Regulation. Bull World Health Organ 1986;64(4):587–94.
18. Kamau RK, Maina FW, Kigondu C, Mati JK. The effect of low-oestrogen combined pill, progestogen-only pill and medroxyprogesterone acetate on oral glucose tolerance test. East Afr Med J 1990;67(8):550–5.
19. Kim C, Seidel KW, Begier EA, Kwok YS. Diabetes and depot medroxyprogesterone contraception in Navajo women. Arch Intern Med 2001;161(14):1766–71.
20. Mahlke M, Grill HJ, Knapstein P, Wiegand U, Pollow K. Oral high-dose medroxyprogesterone acetate (MPA)

liver, acarbose reduces the absorption of glucose from the gut, and the thiazolidinediones reduce insulin resistance in fat. It is not necessary to wait until the maximal dose of one drug has been reached before starting another. However, sulfonylureas and meglitinides should no longer be used when endogenous insulin production is minimal. Combinations of insulin with sulfonylureas or meglitinides should only be used while the patient is changing to insulin, except when long-acting insulin is given at night in order to give the islets a rest and to stimulate daytime insulin secretion.

Large studies of the effects of lifestyle changes, the effects of drugs in preventing or postponing the complications of diabetes, or the usefulness of various combinations are regularly published. The different mechanisms of action of the various classes give different metabolic effects and different adverse effects profiles (27). Comparative costs of the various therapies in the USA have been presented (28).

This subject has been reviewed in relation to combined oral therapy. In a systematic review of 63 studies with a duration of at least 3 months and involving at least 10 patients at the end of the study, and in which HbA_{1c} was reported, five different classes of oral drugs were almost equally effective in lowering blood glucose concentrations (29). HbA_{1c} was reduced by about 1–2% in all cases. Combination therapy gave additive effects. However, long-term vascular risk reduction was demonstrated only with sulfonylureas and metformin.

The adverse effects of combined drug therapy are attributable to the adverse effects of the single drugs. Increased adverse effects or new adverse effects in patients taking combinations have not been reported.

Meglitinides + biguanides

Patients with type 2 diabetes, with unsatisfactory control after taking metformin for 6 months, were randomized to metformin alone, repaglinide alone, or metformin + repaglinide (each 27 patients) (30). Combined therapy reduced HbA_{1c} after 3 months by 1.4% and fasting glucose by 2.2 mmol/l. Repaglinide alone or in combination with metformin increased insulin concentrations. The most common adverse effects were hypoglycemia, diarrhea, and headache. Gastrointestinal adverse effects were common in those taking metformin alone and body weight increased in both groups taking repaglinide.

In 12 patients with type 2 diabetes, a combination of nateglinide 120 mg or placebo with metformin 500 mg before each meal on two separate days was well tolerated (31). One patient taking nateglinide had a headache. One patient was withdrawn because of a myocardial infarction and had multivessel coronary artery disease on catheterization.

In a prospective, randomized, double-blind, placebo-controlled study for 24 weeks, 701 patients took nateglinide 120 mg before the three main meals, or metformin 500 mg tds, or the combination of the two, or placebo (32). The most frequent adverse effect was hypoglycemia, and it was most common in the combination group. There were no differences between those who took nateglinide only or metformin only and there were no episodes of serious hypoglycemia. Diarrhea was more frequent in those taking metformin or the combination, but infection, nausea, headache, and abdominal pain were comparable in the two groups.

Of 82 patients insufficiently controlled by metformin, 27 continued to take metformin with placebo, 28 took titrated repaglinide with placebo, and 27 took metformin with titrated repaglinide for 4–5 months (33). There were no serious adverse effects. Nine patients taking metformin + repaglinide reported 30 hypoglycemic events and three patients taking repaglinide reported nine events.

Meglitinides + sulfonylureas

Glipizide, nateglinide, and their combination have been compared in a double-blind, randomized, placebo-controlled study in 20 patients with type 2 diabetes not requiring insulin (34). Before a standardized breakfast, they took glipizide 10 mg, nateglinide 120 mg, both, or placebo; 4 hours after the meal, blood glucose concentrations were significantly higher after nateglinide, but peak and integrated glucose concentrations did not differ. Integrated insulin concentrations were higher with glipizide. There were three episodes of hypoglycemia in the glipizide alone group and three in the combined group; three required treatment with glucose.

Meglitinides + thiazolidinediones

In 585 patients in a double-blind, randomized, placebo-controlled, multicenter study lasting 16 weeks nateglinide 40 mg tds alone, troglitazone 200 mg/day alone, and the combination were compared (35). The combination was most effective in lowering HbA_{1c}. The most frequent adverse effects were mild hypoglycemia, most often in the combination group. Three patients (two in the combination group and one in the troglitazone alone group) withdrew because of hypoglycemia. Most of the withdrawals were related to increased liver enzymes and weight gain, known adverse effects of troglitazone. Twelve patients withdrew because of predefined changes from baseline (transaminases more than 200% and alkaline phosphatase and bilirubin more than 100% over baseline); seven were taking troglitazone alone, four combined therapy, and one placebo.

In an open trial, 256 patients with type 2 diabetes with inadequate hypoglycemic control (HbA_{1c} over 7.0% during previous therapy) took repaglinide (0.5–4 mg at meals), troglitazone (200–600 mg/day), or a combination of the two for 22 weeks (36). Combination therapy was most effective. Repaglinide only was more effective than troglitazone only. Mean body weight increased in both groups. Serious adverse events were chest pain, cerebrovascular disorders, malignancies, dysrhythmias, electrocardiographic changes suggesting myocardial infarction, and increased aspartate transaminase activity (in one patient taking troglitazone). The serious adverse effects were similar in the different groups. Hypoglycemia occurred in 4% of the patients taking combined therapy, in 16% of those taking troglitazone only, and in 27% of those taking repaglinide only; none needed assistance. There were changes in liver function tests in three patients in the combined group and in one patient each in the two other groups; the drugs were withdrawn in the affected patients and liver function normalized. There were no differences in adverse effects in the different groups. Hypoglycemia occurred in 11 patients taking repaglinide, in seven taking combination therapy, and in one taking troglitazone. Anemia occurred in four patients taking combined therapy and in two taking troglitazone only.

Insulin + meglitinides

In 80 patients taking metformin 850 or 1000 mg tds plus NPH insulin at bedtime, metformin was withdrawn and repaglinide 4 mg tds added in half of the patients for 16 weeks (37). In the repaglinide group the dose of insulin increased slightly and weight gain was 1.8 kg more. Mild hypoglycemia occurred more often in the metformin group; nightly episodes of hypoglycemia occurred only with repaglinide. One patient taking repaglinide had a myocardial infarction, and one had three separate hospitalizations for chest pain (myocardial infarction was excluded). No specific data were presented about gastrointestinal adverse effects or infections.

General adverse effects

The most frequent adverse effect of meglitinides is hypoglycemia. The overall incidence of hypoglycemia with repaglinide is similar to that reported with sulfonylureas, but the incidence of serious hypoglycemia is lower. Other adverse effects are respiratory tract infections and headache. Cardiovascular events and cardiovascular mortality are not different from those in users of sulfonylureas. In Europe, repaglinide is contraindicated in patients with severe liver dysfunction and it is not recommended in people over 75 years old; in America the advice is to use repaglinide cautiously in patients with impaired liver function and there is no restriction on its use in elderly patients. In renal impairment, the half-life of repaglinide is prolonged. Reasons for withdrawal are hyperglycemia, hypoglycemia, and myocardial infarction (38).

Organs and Systems

Metabolism

Repaglinide has a short duration of action and improves postprandial hyperglycemia, a potential risk factor for cardiovascular changes (39). In a double-blind, multiple-dose, parallel-group study repaglinide stimulated mealtime insulin secretion (40). Bouts of hypoglycemia were equally frequent with placebo and repaglinide. When repaglinide was added to NPH monotherapy in patients with HbA_{1c} over 7.1% for 3 months, 38% of the patients had an HbA_{1c} below 7.1% (41). The incidence of hypoglycemia did not change.

When glipizide was compared with repaglinide in 75 patients there were no major hypoglycemic events; minor events were the same in both groups, but after the start of therapy the events occurred much later with repaglinide than glipizide (42).

The effect of a missed meal during repaglinide and glibenclamide therapy has been compared in 83 randomized patients (43). During two meals there were six separate hypoglycemic events in those taking glibenclamide. Blood glucose fell from 4.3 mmol/l to 3.4 mmol/l in those taking glibenclamide when lunch was omitted. There were no changes in blood glucose in those taking repaglinide.

Factitious hypoglycemia has been attributed to repaglinide in an 18-year-old man who had bouts of hypoglycemia for 2 months (44). After glucose administration he recovered promptly and was sent home, but the next night his glucose was 1 mmol/l with high concentrations of insulin (395 pmol/l), C-peptide (2966 pmol/l), and proinsulin (81 pmol/l). The plasma concentrations of repaglinide in three specimens were 4.8–21 ng/ml. Metformin was below the detection limit. He finally admitted to taking repaglinide 4 mg regularly.

Immunologic

- A 62-year-old woman with type 2 diabetes, hypertension, and chronic hepatitis C virus infection developed palpable purpura over her legs and buttocks 3 weeks after starting to take repaglinide 500 mg qds (45). The purpura ulcerated and became infected. Repaglinide was withdrawn and the purpura resolved. A biopsy showed leukocytoclastic vasculitis.

Repaglinide, which is metabolized in the liver, is cleared more slowly in people with liver disease, and hepatitis C may have played a part in this case. Although hepatitis C can cause a leukocytoclastic vasculitis, the clinical correlation and the rapid disappearance of the purpura after the withdrawal of repaglinide makes it likely that this was an adverse effect of the drug. Caution with repaglinide in liver disease is important.

Susceptibility Factors

Renal disease

In renal impairment the half-life of repaglinide is prolonged. Patients with severe renal impairment (creatinine clearance 20–40 ml/minute) had excess accumulation of the drug after taking multiple doses for 5 days (46).

In 235 patients with normal renal function or moderate to severe renal impairment switched from their original therapy to repaglinide (titrated to 0.5–4 mg tds within 4 weeks and continued for 3 months), the number of episodes of hypoglycemia increased with increasing severity of renal impairment during the run-in period but not during treatment (47). The final dose tended to be lower in patients with severe renal impairment. Although the concentrations of repaglinide in the patients with renal impairment were higher, they did not exceed the effective concentrations in people without renal impairment.

Patients with mild to moderate impairment can be treated with repaglinide. However, patients with severe renal impairment have other problems, and it is wise not to use repaglinide in patients with severe renal disease, or at least to adjust the dosage (46).

Hepatic disease

The clearance of repaglinide is reduced and the half-life prolonged (2.5-fold) in patients with chronic liver disease (48).

Drug–Drug Interactions

Clarithromycin

Clarithromycin, an inhibitor of CYP3A4, increases the plasma concentrations and the effect of repaglinide; this can enhance the blood glucose lowering effect and increase the risk of hypoglycemia (49).

Gemfibrozil

In 12 healthy subjects gemfibrozil raised the AUC of repaglinide 8-fold and itraconazole raised it 1.4-fold; however, the combination increased it nearly 20-fold (50).

Ketoconazole

In healthy subjects, ketoconazole increased mean AUC of repaglinide by 15% and mean C_{max} by 7% (51).

Nifedipine

Concomitant treatment with the CYP3A4 substrate nifedipine altered the mean AUC and mean C_{max} of repaglinide by 11 and 3% respectively (51).

Oral contraceptives

Concomitant treatment with ethinylestradiol + levonorgestrel altered the mean AUC and mean C_{max} of repaglinide by 1 and 17% respectively (51).

Rifampicin

Rifampicin 600 mg reduced the AUC of repaglinide by 57% and shortened its half-life from 1.5 to 1.1 hours in nine healthy volunteers after 5 days (52). The effect may even be greater when rifampicin is used for a longer period. In another study in healthy volunteers, rifampicin reduced the mean AUC of repaglinide by 31% and the mean C_{max} by 26%.

Simvastatin

Concomitant treatment with the CYP3A4 substrate simvastatin altered the mean AUC and mean C_{max} of repaglinide by 2 and 27% respectively (51).

References

1. Dabrowski M, Wahl P, Holmes WE, Ashcroft FM. Effect of repaglinide on cloned beta cell, cardiac and smooth muscle types of ATP-sensitive potassium channels. Diabetologia 2001;44(6):747–56.
2. Lindsay JR, McKillop AM, Mooney MH, O'Harte FP, Flatt PR, Bell PM. Effects of nateglinide on the secretion of glycated insulin and glucose tolerance in type 2 diabetes. Diabetes Res Clin Pract 2003;61(3):167–73.
3. Hu S, Boettcher BR, Dunning BE. The mechanisms underlying the unique pharmacodynamics of nateglinide. Diabetologia 2003;46(Suppl 1):M37–43.
4. Cohen RM, Ramlo-Halsted BA. How do the new insulin secretagogues compare? Diabetes Care 2002;25(8):1472–3.
5. Kahn SE, Montgomery B, Howell W, Ligueros-Saylan M, Hsu CH, Devineni D, McLeod JF, Horowitz A, Foley JE. Importance of early phase insulin secretion to intravenous glucose tolerance in subjects with type 2 diabetes mellitus. J Clin Endocrinol Metab 2001;86(12):5824–9.
6. Parulkar AA, Fonseca VA. Recent advances in pharmacological treatment of type 2 diabetes mellitus. Compr Ther 1999;25(8–10):418–26.
7. Ratner RE. Repaglinide therapy in the treatment of type 2 diabetes. Today's Ther Trends 1999;17:57–66.
8. Culy CR, Jarvis B. Repaglinide: a review of its therapeutic use in type 2 diabetes mellitus. Drugs 2001;61(11):1625–60.
9. Juhl CB, Porksen N, Hollingdal M, Sturis J, Pincus S, Veldhuis JD, Dejgaard A, Schmitz O. Repaglinide acutely amplifies pulsatile insulin secretion by augmentation of burst mass with no effect on burst frequency. Diabetes Care 2000;23(5):675–81.
10. Hatorp V, Huang WC, Strange P. Repaglinide pharmacokinetics in healthy young adult and elderly subjects. Clin Ther 1999;21(4):702–10.
11. Gomis R. Repaglinide as monotherapy in Type 2 diabetes. Exp Clin Endocrinol Diabetes 1999;107(Suppl 4):S133–5.
12. Damsbo P, Marbury TC, Hatorp V, Clauson P, Muller PG. Flexible prandial glucose regulation with repaglinide in patients with type 2 diabetes. Diabetes Res Clin Pract 1999;45(1):31–9.
13. Moses RG, Gomis R, Frandsen KB, Schlienger JL, Dedov I. Flexible meal-related dosing with repaglinide facilitates glycemic control in therapy-naive type 2 diabetes. Diabetes Care 2001;24(1):11–15.
14. Hatorp V, Huang WC, Strange P. Pharmacokinetic profiles of repaglinide in elderly subjects with type 2 diabetes. J Clin Endocrinol Metab 1999;84(4):1475–8.
15. Massi-Benedetti M, Damsbo P. Pharmacology and clinical experience with repaglinide. Expert Opin Investig Drugs 2000;9(4):885–98.
16. Bouhanick B, Barbosa SS. Repaglinide: Novonorm, une alternative chez le diabétique de type 2. [Rapaglinide: Novonorm, an alternative in type 2 diabetes.] Presse Méd 2000;29(19):1059–61.
17. Gribble FM, Manley SE, Levy JC. Randomized dose ranging study of the reduction of fasting and postprandial glucose in type 2 diabetes by nateglinide (A-4166). Diabetes Care 2001;24(7):1221–5.
18. Wolffenbuttel BH, Landgraf R. A 1-year multicenter randomized double-blind comparison of repaglinide and glyburide for the treatment of type 2 diabetes. Dutch and German Repaglinide Study Group. Diabetes Care 1999;22(3):463–7.
19. Marbury T, Huang WC, Strange P, Lebovitz H. Repaglinide versus glyburide: a one-year comparison trial. Diabetes Res Clin Pract 1999;43(3):155–66.
20. Landgraf R, Bilo HJ, Muller PG. A comparison of repaglinide and glibenclamide in the treatment of type 2 diabetic patients previously treated with sulphonylureas. Eur J Clin Pharmacol 1999;55(3):165–71.
21. Mafauzy M. Repaglinide versus glibenclamide treatment of type 2 diabetes during Ramadan fasting. Diabetes Res Clin Pract 2002;58(1):45–53.
22. Moran A, Phillips J, Milla C. Insulin and glucose excursion following premeal insulin lispro or repaglinide in cystic fibrosis-related diabetes. Diabetes Care 2001;24(10):1706–10.
23. Hanefeld M, Bouter KP, Dickinson S, Guitard C. Rapid and short-acting mealtime insulin secretion with nateglinide controls both prandial and mean glycemia. Diabetes Care 2000;23(2):202–7.
24. Kalbag JB, Walter YH, Nedelman JR, McLeod JF. Mealtime glucose regulation with nateglinide in healthy volunteers: comparison with repaglinide and placebo. Diabetes Care 2001;24(1):73–7.
25. Hollander PA, Schwartz SL, Gatlin MR, Haas SJ, Zheng H, Foley JE, Dunning BE. Importance of early insulin secretion: comparison of nateglinide and glyburide in previously

diet-treated patients with type 2 diabetes. Diabetes Care 2001;24(6):983–8.
26. Jovanovic L, Dailey G 3rd, Huang WC, Strange P, Goldstein BJ. Repaglinide in type 2 diabetes: a 24-week, fixed-dose efficacy and safety study. J Clin Pharmacol 2000;40(1):49–57.
27. Inzucchi SE. Oral antihyperglycemic therapy for type 2 diabetes: scientific review. JAMA 2002;287(3):360–72.
28. Holmboe ES. Oral antihyperglycemic therapy for type 2 diabetes: clinical applications. JAMA 2002;287(3):373–6.
29. Van Gaal LF, De Leeuw IH. Rationale and options for combination therapy in the treatment of Type 2 diabetes. Diabetologia 2003;46(Suppl 1):M44–50.
30. Moses R, Slobodniuk R, Boyages S, Colagiuri S, Kidson W, Carter J, Donnelly T, Moffitt P, Hopkins H. Effect of repaglinide addition to metformin monotherapy on glycemic control in patients with type 2 diabetes. Diabetes Care 1999;22(1):119–24.
31. Hirschberg Y, Karara AH, Pietri AO, McLeod JF. Improved control of mealtime glucose excursions with coadministration of nateglinide and metformin. Diabetes Care 2000;23(3):349–53.
32. Horton ES, Clinkingbeard C, Gatlin M, Foley J, Mallows S, Shen S. Nateglinide alone and in combination with metformin improves glycemic control by reducing mealtime glucose levels in type 2 diabetes. Diabetes Care 2000;23(11):1660–5.
33. Moses R. Repaglinide in combination therapy with metformin in Type 2 diabetes. Exp Clin Endocrinol Diabetes 1999;107(Suppl 4):S136–9.
34. Carroll MF, Izard A, Riboni K, Burge MR, Schade DS. Control of postprandial hyperglycemia: optimal use of short-acting insulin secretagogues. Diabetes Care 2002;25(12):2147–52.
35. Rosenstock J, Shen SG, Gatlin MR, Foley JE. Combination therapy with nateglinide and a thiazolidinedione improves glycemic control in type 2 diabetes. Diabetes Care 2002;25(9):1529–33.
36. Raskin P, Jovanovic L, Berger S, Schwartz S, Woo V, Ratner R. Repaglinide/troglitazone combination therapy: improved glycemic control in type 2 diabetes. Diabetes Care 2000;23(7):979–83.
37. Furlong NJ, Hulme SA, O'Brien SV, Hardy KJ. Repaglinide versus metformin in combination with bedtime NPH insulin in patients with type 2 diabetes established on insulin/metformin combination therapy. Diabetes Care 2002;25(10):1685–90.
38. Schatz H. Preclinical and clinical studies on safety and tolerability of repaglinide. Exp Clin Endocrinol Diabetes 1999;107(Suppl 4):S144–8.
39. Schmitz O, Lund S, Andersen PH, Jonler M, Porksen N. Optimizing insulin secretagogue therapy in patients with type 2 diabetes: a randomized double-blind study with repaglinide. Diabetes Care 2002;25(2):342–6.
40. Van Gaal LF, Van Acker KL, De Leeuw IH. Repaglinide improves blood glucose control in sulphonylurea-naive type 2 diabetes. Diabetes Res Clin Pract 2001;53(3):141–8.
41. de Luis DA, Aller R, Cuellar L, Terroba C, Ovalle H, Izaola O, Romero E. Effect of repaglinide addition to NPH insulin monotherapy on glycemic control in patients with type 2 diabetes. Diabetes Care 2001;24(10):1844–5.
42. Madsbad S, Kilhovd B, Lager I, Mustajoki P, Dejgaard A; Scandinavian Repaglinide Group. Comparison between repaglinide and glipizide in Type 2 diabetes mellitus: a 1-year multicentre study. Diabet Med 2001;18(5):395–401.
43. Damsbo P, Clauson P, Marbury TC, Windfeld K. A double-blind randomized comparison of meal-related glycemic control by repaglinide and glyburide in well-controlled type 2 diabetic patients. Diabetes Care 1999;22(5):789–94.
44. Hirshberg B, Skarulis MC, Pucino F, Csako G, Brennan R, Gorden P. Repaglinide-induced factitious hypoglycemia. J Clin Endocrinol Metab 2001;86(2):475–7.
45. Margolin N. Severe leucocytoclastic vasculitis induced by repaglinide in a patient with chronic hepatitis C. Clin Drug Invest 2002;22:795–6.
46. Schumacher S, Abbasi I, Weise D, Hatorp V, Sattler K, Sieber J, Hasslacher C. Single- and multiple-dose pharmacokinetics of repaglinide in patients with type 2 diabetes and renal impairment. Eur J Clin Pharmacol 2001;57(2):147–52.
47. Hasslacher C; Multinational Repaglinide Renal Study Group. Safety and efficacy of repaglinide in type 2 diabetic patients with and without impaired renal function. Diabetes Care 2003;26(3):886–91.
48. Anonymous. Clinical news. Interactions and pharmacokinetics of repaglinide. Pharm J 2000;264:503.
49. Niemi M, Neuvonen PJ, Kivisto KT. The cytochrome P4503A4 inhibitor clarithromycin increases the plasma concentrations and effects of repaglinide. Clin Pharmacol Ther 2001;70(1):58–65.
50. Niemi M, Backman JT, Neuvonen M, Neuvonen PJ. Effects of gemfibrozil, itraconazole, and their combination on the pharmacokinetics and pharmacodynamics of repaglinide: potentially hazardous interaction between gemfibrozil and repaglinide. Diabetologia 2003;46(3):347–51.
51. Hatorp V, Hansen KT, Thomsen MS. Influence of drugs interacting with CYP3A4 on the pharmacokinetics, pharmacodynamics, and safety of the prandial glucose regulator repaglinide. J Clin Pharmacol 2003;43(6):649–60.
52. Niemi M, Backman JT, Neuvonen M, Neuvonen PJ, Kivisto KT. Rifampin decreases the plasma concentrations and effects of repaglinide. Clin Pharmacol Ther 2000;68(5):495–500.

Melarsoprol

General Information

Melarsoprol is a trivalent arsenical with activity against East African and West African trypanosomiasis. It is the drug of choice in the case of *Trypanosoma rhodesiense* infection with nervous system involvement (stage II disease) and in stage I patients refractory or intolerant to suramin and pentamidine. Melarsoprol administered intravenously can cause a reactive encephalopathy, with a clinical picture consisting of high fever, headache, tremor, convulsions, and on occasion coma and death. The incidence of arsenic encephalopathy varies from 3 to 18% in various series (SEDA-12, 708) (1).

In a case-control study of physical growth, sexual maturity, and academic performance in 100 young subjects (aged 6–20 years) with and without a past history of sleeping sickness, melarsoprol-treated patients weighed less, were shorter, and had sexual maturity ratings significantly different from the corresponding controls (2).

The efficacy and safety of two regimens of melarsoprol have been compared in patients with nervous system involvement from *Trypanosoma brucei gambiense*: a conventional regimen lasting 26 days, starting at 1.2 mg/kg and rising to 3.6 mg/kg ($n = 259$), and a regimen of 2.2 mg/kg for 10 days ($n = 250$) (3). Parasitological cure

24 hours after treatment was 100% in both groups. Disappointingly, the rates of encephalopathy were no better (in fact marginally worse) with the new schedule, despite using 30% less drug overall, and there were six drug-related deaths in each arm. However, the new schedule is quicker and cheaper, and treatment deviations were significantly fewer in the new schedule arm. In a further detailed prospective study of the drug in eight patients with advanced leukaemia, three developed seizures attributable to the drug at doses broadly comparable to those used in trypanosomiasis.

In 42 patients with late-stage *Trypanosoma brucei gambiense* trypanosomiasis, who relapsed after initial treatment with melarsoprol, a sequential combination of intravenous eflornithine (100 mg/kg every 6 hours for 4 days) followed by three daily injections of melarsoprol (3.6 mg/kg, up to 180 mg) was used (4). They were followed for 24 months. In one case the administration of eflornithine had to be interrupted for 48 hours because of convulsions, but treatment was then resumed without recurrence. Other adverse effects during treatment were abdominal pain or vomiting ($n = 4$ each), diarrhea ($n = 1$), and loss of hearing ($n = 1$). Two patients died during treatment:

- A 37-year-old man died of an acute cholera-like syndrome, with severe diarrhea, vomiting, and dehydration, after the last dose of eflornithine but before receiving his first dose of melarsoprol;
- A 34-year-old man died of an unknown cause after having received all 16 doses of eflornithine as well as the first injection of melarsoprol.

In a randomized trial in 500 patients infected with *Trypanosoma brucei gambiense* treated with 10 daily consecutive doses of melarsoprol 2.2 mg/kg, the adverse effects were: encephalopathic syndrome 5.6%, death from encephalopathy 2.4%, polyneuropathy less than 1%, severe bullous dermatitis 1.2%, severe maculopapular rash 3.2%, severe pruritus 3.2% (5). Milder reactions were fever, headache, and diarrhea.

Organs and Systems

Nervous system

Melarsoprol given intravenously in patients with trypanosomiasis can cause a peripheral neuropathy within 2–5 weeks (SEDA-14, 243). It also causes a reactive arsenical encephalopathy in 3–5% of patients with trypanosomiasis (SEDA-13, 834) (6).

- Myalgia, distal paresthesia, and rapidly progressive weakness in all limbs developed in a young woman treated for 38 days with melarsoprol; there was massive distal Wallerian degeneration in the peripheral nerve, and abnormalities in the dorsal ganglia and spinal cord. Very high concentrations of arsenic were found in the spinal cord. All the findings were typical of toxic arsenic accumulation; in this case, renal dysfunction was probably at the root of the arsenic poisoning (SEDA-16, 316).

In patients with *Trypanosoma gambiense* sleeping sickness, the incidence of drug-induced encephalopathy was increased in patients with trypanosomes present in the nervous system, in patients with high CSF lymphocyte counts, and among those in whom no trypanosomes were found in either the blood or a lymph node aspirate. The authors of this report considered that aggressive therapeutic schemes may result in greater toxicity, especially in patients with impaired blood–brain barrier (SEDA-16, 316). Without data on dosage, renal function, and cerebral involvement before therapy it is impossible to assess this conclusion.

In a large-scale review it was estimated that encephalopathic syndromes occur in 5–10% of patients, and that 10–50% of these die as a result (7).

Encephalopathic syndromes complicating treatment of stage II human African trypanosomiasis with melarsoprol in 588 patients have been reviewed (8). The overall rate of encephalopathy was 5.8% and presented in three ways: coma, convulsions, and psychotic reactions. The overall death rate was 38%. Comatose patients had a death rate of 52% and were commonly co-infected with malaria (14/16). Symptoms during treatment of fever (RR = 11.5), headache (RR = 2.5), bullous eruptions (RR = 4.5), and systolic hypotension (RR = 2.6) were associated with an increased risk of encephalopathic syndromes, especially coma.

In 56 patients with African trypanosomiasis, one treated with melarsoprol (total dose 26 mg/kg) developed a reactive arsenical encephalopathy (9).

References

1. Pepin J, Milord F. The treatment of human African trypanosomiasis. Adv Parasitol 1994;33:1–47.
2. Aroke AH, Asonganyi T, Mbonda E. Influence of a past history of Gambian sleeping sickness on physical growth, sexual maturity and academic performance of children in Fontem, Cameroon. Ann Trop Med Parasitol 1998; 92(8):829–35.
3. Burri C, Nkunku S, Merolle A, Smith T, Blum J, Brun R. Efficacy of new, concise schedule for melarsoprol in treatment of sleeping sickness caused by *Trypanosoma brucei gambiense*: a randomised trial. Lancet 2000; 355(9213):1419–25.
4. Mpia B, Pepin J. Combination of eflornithine and melarsoprol for melarsoprol-resistant Gambian trypanosomiasis. Trop Med Int Health 2002;7(9):775–9.
5. Blum J, Burri C. Treatment of late stage sleeping sickness caused by *T.b. gambiense*: a new approach to the use of an old drug. Swiss Med Wkly 2002;132(5–6):51–6.
6. Nkanga NG, Mutombo L, Kazadi K, Kazyumba GL. Neuropathies arsénicales après traitement de la trypanosomiase humaine au mélarsoprol. Med Afr Noire 1988;35:73.
7. Anonymous. WHO Control and surveillance of African trypanosomiasis. WHO Tech Rep Ser 1998;881:1–114.
8. Blum J, Nkunku S, Burri C. Clinical description of encephalopathic syndromes and risk factors for their occurrence and outcome during melarsoprol treatment of human African trypanosomiasis. Trop Med Int Health 2001;6(5):390–400.
9. Ruiz JA, Simarro PP, Josenando T. Control of human African trypanosomiasis in the Quicama focus, Angola. Bull World Health Organ 2002;80(9):738–45.

Melatonin

General Information

Melatonin (*N*-acetyl-5-methoxytryptamine) is a neurohormone secreted by the pineal gland from the amino acid precursor L-tryptophan. Its endogenous secretion is photosensitive and has a circadian rhythm—plasma melatonin concentrations are highest at night in both diurnal and nocturnal animals, and fall with age (1). The nocturnal melatonin peak coincides with a drop in body temperature and increased sleepiness in healthy humans. Oral melatonin has a short half-life (30–50 minutes) and extensive first-pass metabolism. Its clearance is reduced in severe liver disease (2).

Uses

Melatonin has been promoted as a treatment for conditions ranging from jet lag to cancer (1,3–5) and is sometimes used for sleep induction (1). Because melatonin is present in small amounts in some foods, it is licensed as a nutritional supplement in the USA.

General adverse effects

Acute exogenous administration of melatonin causes sedation, fatigue, self-reported vigor, confusion, and a reduction in body temperature in healthy subjects. The effects of chronic treatment have not been studied, and adverse effects have not been systematically reported.

Timing is critical for melatonin to be effective: if it is given at the wrong time for sleep disorders or jet lag, it can cause increased daytime sleepiness (5,6) and worsened mental performance (7). Drowsiness and a small fall in body temperature are commonly reported effects (8), particularly after daytime administration, when endogenous concentrations of melatonin are low.

Organs and Systems

Cardiovascular

There was an increase in blood pressure throughout 24 hours in a double-blind, placebo-controlled, crossover study in 47 hypertensive patients who were also taking nifedipine (9). This finding differs from other studies in which melatonin had a mild hypotensive effect (10) and may indicate an interaction between melatonin and nifedipine. Tachycardia, chest pain, and cardiac dysrhythmias have also been reported, although the relation to melatonin was not clearly established (5).

Nervous system

Four of six children with pre-existing severe neurological disorders had increased seizure activity within 2 weeks of starting oral melatonin 5 mg at bedtime (11). Seizure frequency returned to baseline after treatment was stopped, and increased again after rechallenge with melatonin 1 mg. A convulsion during melatonin treatment, which recurred when medication was continued, has been reported to the WHO database but not published (5). Headache, which recovered after melatonin was withdrawn, has also been reported in a few cases (5).

Dyskinesia and akathisia have been reported after withdrawal of long-term melatonin (12).

- A 22-year-old woman of Ashkenazi origin, with spastic diplegia resulting from cerebral palsy and severe mental retardation, had insomnia for 6 years. She had taken melatonin 5 mg each night at 8 p.m. for the past year, with a good response. However, 1 week after melatonin was stopped, because of repeated vomiting, she gradually developed involuntary lip-smacking movements and tongue protrusion, with extreme restlessness, moaning, and shouting. These symptoms continued for 2 weeks, accompanied by marked worsening of insomnia. She was restless, could not sit still, and was shouting, moaning, and grunting. Melatonin was reintroduced in gradually increasing doses, and 2 days after a dose of 5 mg was reached, the involuntary movements disappeared and her agitated state and insomnia improved. A month later, another episode of abdominal pain and vomiting made her discontinue melatonin again. Within 2 days she developed identical involuntary lip and tongue movements and akathisia. Melatonin 5 mg was re-administered and all her symptoms disappeared by the next day. No antiemetic drugs were given during these episodes.

This case raises an important question regarding the dopamine-blocking effect of melatonin. Like dopamine receptor antagonists, melatonin should be used with care, because of the risk of tardive dyskinesia, which has serious morbidity and a low remission rate. Melatonin should be used with special caution in patients with organic brain damage.

Sensory systems

- Loss of visual acuity, reduced color vision, and altered light adaptation developed in a 42-year-old woman 2 weeks after she started to take a high protein diet and melatonin 1 mg/day (13). She had also been taking sertraline for the past 4 years. Her vision improved within 2 months of stopping the melatonin and the high protein diet.

This patient's retinal melatonin concentration may have been boosted by increased serotonin (a melatonin precursor) from the effect of sertraline, the high protein intake, and the exogenous melatonin.

Retinal damage has been briefly reported as an adverse effect of melatonin (8).

Psychological, psychiatric

A severely depressed woman developed a mixed affective state after taking melatonin for 7 days in a clinical trial (14). Confusion, hallucinations, and paranoia temporally related to melatonin have also been described (5).

Endocrine

There was suppression of endogenous melatonin secretion in two of five patients with bipolar disorder after 12 weeks of treatment with high-dose melatonin (10 mg/day) (15).

Table 1 The genera of Meliaceae

Aglaia (Chinese rice flower)
Azadirachta (azadirachta)
Carapa (carapa)
Cedrela (cedrela)
Dysoxylum (mahogany)
Guarea (guarea)
Khaya (African mahogany)
Lansium (lansium)
Melia (melia)
Swietenia (mahogany)
Toona (redcedar)
Trichilia (trichilia)
Xylocarpus (mangrove)

potential cause of Reye's syndrome in 13 infants who developed vomiting, drowsiness, metabolic acidosis, a polymorphonuclear leukocytosis, and encephalopathy within hours of taking margosa oil; liver biopsy in one infant showed pronounced fatty infiltration of the liver (1). In experimental animals given margosa oil there was also fatty infiltration of the proximal renal tubules and cerebral edema. Electron microscopy showed mitochondrial damage.

Reference

1. Sinniah D, Baskaran G. Margosa oil poisoning as a cause of Reye's syndrome. Lancet 1981;1(8218):487–9.

Melitracen

See also Tricyclic antidepressants

General Information

Melitracen is structurally and pharmacologically related to imipramine, with two methyl groups attached to the central ring. It has similar efficacy to amitriptyline, with a somewhat more rapid effect and similar adverse effects (1).

Reference

1. Francesconi G, LoCascio A, Mellina S, et al. Controlled comparison of melitracen and amitriptyline in depressed patients. Curr Ther Res Clin Exp 1976;20:529.

Meloxicam

See also Non-steroidal anti-inflammatory drugs

General Information

Meloxicam, a COX-2 inhibitor, has been marketed in some countries and promoted as having an improved safety profile over current NSAIDs. It has a long half-life, is highly protein-bound, is metabolized to inactive compounds, and is excreted in the urine and feces. Neither hepatic insufficiency nor moderate renal dysfunction affects its pharmacokinetics, but in one study meloxicam plasma concentrations were 26% higher in patients over 65 than in younger patients.

Changes have been made to the Summary of Product Characteristics by the manufacturers of meloxicam (1), in agreement with the type of adverse drug reaction reports received by the Committee on Safety of Medicine in the UK. Warnings about gastrointestinal reactions (perforation, ulceration, and/or bleeding) and skin reactions (including erythema multiforme and Stevens–Johnson syndrome) have been strengthened (2).

Organs and Systems

Nervous system

About 7% of patients have dizziness and headache (3).

Gastrointestinal

Gastrointestinal adverse effects were the most frequently reported (in about 15–20% of patients), but their incidence was lower with meloxicam than with piroxicam, naproxen, and diclofenac in long-term double-blind studies. They were more frequent with a dosage of 15 mg/day than with 7.5 mg/day, were judged to be severe in 1.7%, and led to withdrawal in about 4% of patients. The most frequent symptoms were abdominal pain, dyspepsia, eructation, nausea, and vomiting. Upper gastrointestinal perforation, ulceration, and bleeding occurred rarely with meloxicam; the incidence was dose related and lower than with the comparators (4,5). A double-blind endoscopic microbleeding comparison of meloxicam and piroxicam in healthy volunteers showed better gastrointestinal tolerability with meloxicam. Fecal blood loss and endoscopy scores were higher in piroxicam-treated patients, and six piroxicam volunteers versus one treated with meloxicam withdrew because of severe gastrointestinal toxicity; colitis was reported in one case (6). In a few patients meloxicam suppositories can cause abdominal pain and rectal bleeding.

A large prospective comparison of meloxicam 7.5 mg/day with piroxicam 20 mg/day for a median of 28 days suggested that meloxicam has a lower propensity to cause gastroduodenal adverse events. However, serious gastrointestinal events (that is, ulceration, perforation, or bleeding), albeit rare, had similar frequencies in meloxicam and piroxicam recipients, and furthermore the difference in the incidence of adverse gastrointestinal events, although statistically significant, was clinically less relevant (7). Reports received by the Swedish Adverse Drug Reaction Advisory Committee (SADRAC) have suggested that meloxicam has a similar adverse drug reactions profile to other NSAIDs (8) and reports of gastrointestinal hemorrhage have started to appear (9).

Colitis has been described as an adverse effect of meloxicam (SEDA-20, 94).

- Ischemic colitis occurred in a 49-year-old woman 10 days after she started to take meloxicam 15 mg/day for osteoarthritis; meloxicam was withdrawn and her symptoms completely resolved within 1 week (10).

Although meloxicam is considered to be a preferential COX-2 inhibitor, its safety profile is not much different from other traditional NSAIDs, especially in high doses (11).

Liver

Acute cytolytic hepatitis has been described in a 46-year-old woman who took meloxicam for 4 days (12).

Urinary tract

Deterioration in renal function, reversible on withdrawal, was rare (0.4%) (3).

Skin

Rash, pruritus, and other skin problems occurred in about 6.5% of patients (3).

The manufacturers of meloxicam have recently included a warning about the possible occurrence of life-threatening skin reactions in the Summary of Product Characteristics (SEDA-23, 120).

- Erythema multiforme has been reported in a 19-year-old man 8 days after he started to take meloxicam for tendonitis; withdrawal and therapy with corticosteroids resulted in complete recovery (13).

Immunologic

Meloxicam may be relatively safe when given to patients with NSAID-induced urticaria/angioedema (14,15). Of 148 NSAID-sensitive subjects with an unequivocal history of urticaria with or without angioedema, who were challenged with increasing oral doses of meloxicam (1–7 mg/day) in a single-blind placebo-controlled trial, only two had a positive test (urticaria in one and urticaria/angioedema in the other); both had chronic idiopathic urticaria (16).

Drug Administration

Drug administration route

Local tolerability with intramuscular administration is reportedly good (17). Serum creatine kinase activity can increase slightly. Gastrointestinal disorders, central nervous system adverse events, and skin rashes have been reported with intramuscular administration.

Drug–Drug Interactions

Methotrexate

In 13 patients with rheumatoid arthritis, oral meloxicam for 1 week had no effect on the pharmacokinetics of a single dose of intravenous methotrexate 15 mg (18).

References

1. Anonymous. BI strengthens meloxicam warnings. Scrip 1998;31:2368.
2. Committee on Safety of Medicines/Medicines Control Agency. Meloxicam (Mobic): gastrointestinal and skin reactions. Curr Probl Pharmacovig 1998;24:13.
3. Auvinet B, Ziller R, Appelboom T, Velicitat P. Comparison of the onset and intensity of action of intramuscular meloxicam and oral meloxicam in patients with acute sciatica. Clin Ther 1995;17(6):1078–98.
4. Huskisson EC, Ghozlan R, Kurthen R, Degner FL, Bluhmki E. A long-term study to evaluate the safety and efficacy of meloxicam therapy in patients with rheumatoid arthritis. Br J Rheumatol 1996;35(Suppl 1):29–34.
5. Hosie J, Distel M, Bluhmki E. Meloxicam in osteoarthritis: a 6-month, double-blind comparison with diclofenac sodium. Br J Rheumatol 1996;35(Suppl 1):39–43.
6. Patoia L, Santucci L, Furno P, Dionisi MS, Dell'Orso S, Romagnoli M, Sattarinia A, Marini MG. A 4-week, double-blind, parallel-group study to compare the gastrointestinal effects of meloxicam 7.5 mg, meloxicam 15 mg, piroxicam 20 mg and placebo by means of faecal blood loss, endoscopy and symptom evaluation in healthy volunteers Br J Rheumatol 1996;35(Suppl 1): 61–7.
7. Dequeker J, Hawkey C, Kahan A, Steinbruck K, Alegre C, Baumelou E, Begaud B, Isomaki H, Littlejohn G, Mau J, Papazoglou S. Improvement in gastrointestinal tolerability of the selective cyclooxygenase (COX)-2 inhibitor, meloxicam, compared with piroxicam: results of the Safety and Efficacy Large-scale Evaluation of COX-inhibiting Therapies (SELECT) trial in osteoarthritis. Br J Rheumatol 1998;37(9):946–51.
8. Anonymous. Meloxicam safety similar to other NSAIDs. WHO Drug Inf 1998;12:147.
9. del Val A, Llorente MJ, Tenias JM, Lluch A. Hemorragia digestiva alta causada por meloxicam. [Upper digestive hemorrhage caused by meloxicam.] Rev Esp Enferm Dig 1998;90(6):461–2.
10. Garcia B, Ramaholimihaso F, Diebold MD, Cadiot G, Thiefin G. Ischaemic colitis in a patient taking meloxicam. Lancet 2001;357(9257):690.
11. Degner F, Richardson B. Review of gastrointestinal tolerability and safety of meloxicam. Inflammopharmacology 2001;9:71–80.
12. Staerkel P, Horsmans Y. Meloxicam-induced liver toxicity. Acta Gastroenterol Belg 1999;62(2):255–6.
13. Nikas SN, Kittas G, Karamaounas N, Drosos AA. Meloxicam-induced erythema multiforme. Am J Med 1999;107(5):532–4.
14. Kosnik M, Music E, Matjaz F, Suskovic S. Relative safety of meloxicam in NSAID-intolerant patients. Allergy 1998; 53(12):1231–3.
15. Quaratino D, Romano A, Di Fonso M, Papa G, Perrone MR, D'Ambrosio FP, Venuti A. Tolerability of meloxicam in patients with histories of adverse reactions to nonsteroidal anti-inflammatory drugs. Ann Allergy Asthma Immunol 2000;84(6):613–17.
16. Nettis E, Di Paola R, Ferrannini A, Tursi A. Meloxicam in hypersensitivity to NSAIDs. Allergy 2001;56(8):803–4.
17. Euller-Ziegler L, Velicitat P, Bluhmki E, Turck D, Scheuerer S, Combe B. Meloxicam: a review of its pharmacokinetics, efficacy and tolerability following intramuscular administration. Inflamm Res 2001; 50(Suppl 1):S5–9.
18. Hubner G, Sander O, Degner FL, Turck D, Rau R. Lack of pharmacokinetic interaction of meloxicam with methotrexate in patients with rheumatoid arthritis. J Rheumatol 1997;24(5):845–51.

Melphalan

See also Cytostatic and immunosuppressant drugs

General Information

Melphalan (L-phenylalanine mustard) is an alkylating agent that has been used to treat a wide variety of solid malignancies, including cancers of the breast and ovary, and multiple myeloma. Intravenous melphalan has been used to treat rhabdomyosarcoma, lymphomas, multiple myeloma, and neuroblastoma (1).

The adverse effects of high-dose intravenous melphalan have been reviewed (2). Two patients who received less than 100 mg/m^2 recovered from marrow aplasia within 3 weeks without major complications. A third patient died 6 days after injection of 290 mg/m^2, probably because of a cardiac dysrhythmia before complete marrow failure had become established. After intravenous administration of more than 125 mg/m^2, gastrointestinal adverse effects, such as hemorrhagic diarrhea, or bowel perforation, can occur. These, together with reduced ADH secretion and electrolyte disturbances are the predominant clinical problems and the reasons for early death before the occurrence of infectious or bleeding complications from prolonged marrow aplasia.

Organs and Systems

Respiratory

Melphalan can cause an acute interstitial pneumonia with hypoxemia (3). This is probably due to a hypersensitivity mechanism and should be distinguished from fibrosing pneumonitis, which melphalan can also cause (4).

Fatal pulmonary fibrosis and atypical epithelial proliferation has been reported in patients with multiple myeloma treated with melphalan (4).

Urinary tract

Acute renal insufficiency has been attributed to melphalan in a patient with third stage ovarian cancer (5).

Reproductive system

Primary ovarian failure has been recognized in adults after intermittent low-dose melphalan, and has also been reported in three adolescents after high-dose melphalan (6).

Drug–Drug Interactions

Busulfan

The possibility that melphalan and busulfan may cause additive lung damage has been discussed in the light of a 59-year-old patient with chronic myeloid leukemia who developed severe interstitial lung fibrosis after short-term sequential treatment with the two drugs (7).

References

1. Sarosy G, Leyland-Jones B, Soochan P, Cheson BD. The systemic administration of intravenous melphalan. J Clin Oncol 1988;6(11):1768–82.
2. Jost LM. Uberdosierung von Melphalan (Alkeran): Symptome und Behandlung. [Overdose with melphalan (Alkeran): symptoms and treatment. A review.] Onkologie 1990;13(2):96–101.
3. Liote H, Gauthier JF, Prier A, Gauthier-Rahman S, Kaplan G, Akoun G. Pneumopathie interstitielle, aiguë, reversible, induite par le melphalan. [Acute, reversible, interstitial pneumopathy induced by melphalan.] Rev Mal Respir 1989;6(5):461–4.
4. Taetle R, Dickman PS, Feldman PS. Pulmonary histopathologic changes associated with melphalan therapy. Cancer 1978;42(3):1239–45.
5. Kashimura M, Kondo M, Abe T, Shinohara M, Baba S. [A case report of acute renal failure induced by melphalan in a patient with ovarian cancer.] Gan No Rinsho 1988;34(14):2015–18.
6. Kellie SJ, Kingston JE. Ovarian failure after high-dose melphalan in adolescents. Lancet 1987;1(8547):1425.
7. Schallier D, Impens N, Warson F, Van Belle S, De Wasch G. Additive pulmonary toxicity with melphalan and busulfan therapy. Chest 1983;84(4):492–3.

Memantine

General Information

Memantine is an amantadine derivative that has been studied in patients with Parkinson's disease. Its adverse effects include agitation, restlessness, insomnia, pronounced delirious states, and muscular hypotonia. All were reversible after dosage reduction or withdrawal.

Organs and Systems

Psychological, psychiatric

A toxic psychosis was reported in two patients taking memantine (1).

Reference

1. Riederer P, Lange KW, Kornhuber J, Danielczyk W. Pharmacotoxic psychosis after memantine in Parkinson's disease. Lancet 1991;338(8773):1022–3.

Meningococcal vaccine

See also Vaccines

General Information

Meningococcal vaccines have been comprehensively reviewed, distinguishing conventional polysaccharide vaccines, non-polysaccharide group B meningococcal vaccines, and conjugated meningococcal vaccines (1).

Reports of clinical trials in children, adults, and asplenic individuals have been provided (2) and surveyed (SEDA-11, 288) (SEDA-16, 379) (SEDA-17, 370) (SED-12, 813).

Polysaccharide vaccines

Polysaccharide meningococcal vaccines in various combinations against meningococcal disease caused by meningococci of groups A, C, W135, and Y have been commercially available for many years. Studies mostly using a bivalent serogroup A + C vaccine carried out in about 15 countries, including some millions of people, have shown efficacy of 61–99%. Meningococcal group A vaccine is more immunogenic than group C vaccine in infants and small children. However, infants below 6 months of age produce a weak response, and meningococcal group C vaccine should not be used before the age of 2 years. Meningococcal group B polysaccharide vaccine is poorly immunogenic in humans and is therefore not available commercially.

Adverse reactions are infrequent and mild, consisting of local soreness or localized erythema at the injection site, and systemic reactions (transient fever, headache, fatigue), lasting 1–2 days (3,4). With the quadrivalent vaccine used in Canada, fever was reported in less than 1%, local reactions in 6.3%, and rash in 1.6% among those aged 11 years or older. Local reactions were also the most reported adverse effect in other reports.

Non-polysaccharide group B meningococcal vaccines

Considering the poor immunogenicity of polysaccharide group B vaccines, different vaccines have been developed—a Norwegian outer membrane complex group B vaccine and a Cuban vaccine in which the group C polysaccharide is added to a mixture of high molecular weight B outer membrane proteins and proteoliposomes. Both vaccines have been used in clinical trials, mainly in Latin America, but more conclusive studies with these two products are awaited. Adverse reactions with the Cuban vaccine have been studied. Among 16 700 vaccinees, mostly older than 4 years, local reactions were observed in 62%, and systemic reactions in 4.3%.

From studies in 370 infants and children and 171 adults aged 18–30 years, who received three doses of outer membrane protein meningococcal vaccine developed in either Cuba or Norway or a control vaccine (Hib vaccine), the vaccines are promising candidates for the control of epidemics caused by homologous epidemic strains (5). However, the vaccines would not confer protection during a heterologous epidemic. All vaccinees had more pain, induration, and erythema at the injection site than did Hib vaccine recipients; there were no serious adverse events, and 95% of individuals who reported symptoms said that the symptoms did not interfere with their normal activities.

A genetically engineered vaccine containing six meningococcal class I (PorA) outer membrane proteins, representing 80% of group B meningococcal strains prevalent in the UK, has been assessed in 103 infants who received the vaccine at ages 2, 3, and 4 months with routine infant immunization, and a fourth dose at 12–18 months (6). The vaccine was well tolerated, and after the fourth dose there were larger bactericidal responses to all six strains.

Conjugated meningococcal vaccines

Success with the protein-conjugate formulations of *Hemophilus influenzae* vaccines has facilitated research and development on conjugated meningococcal vaccines with preference for monovalent group C or bivalent group A/group C vaccines. Conjugated meningococcal vaccines of serogroup C made by various manufacturers were first licensed in 1999 in the UK and then (at the end of 2000) in many other countries, including some other member states of the European Union (Belgium, Germany, Greece, Luxembourg, Ireland, Portugal, Spain).

Field trials in the UK and the Gambia have shown immunogenicity not only in adults but also in toddlers and even infants. Except for local tenderness in 30–75% of vaccinees, no conjugate vaccine evaluated to date has been associated with significant adverse effects (1).

Vaccine containing oligosaccharides derived from group C meningococcal capsular polysaccharide coupled to CRM197, a non-toxic mutant diphtheria toxin (manufactured by Wyeth Lederle Vaccines and Pediatrics, Pearl River, NY) was given to 114 infants at 2, 3, and 4 months of age; 57 received a vaccine containing 2 μg of oligosaccharide and 5 μg of CRM197, and 57 received a vaccine containing 10 μg of oligosaccharide and 25 μg of CRM197 (7). The infants received DTP and Hib vaccine at the same time. In each group, 25 infants received a polysaccharide vaccine booster at median age of 83 weeks. Antibody concentrations required for protection are estimated to be 1–2 μg/ml. All the infants achieved a concentration of 2 μg/ml by age 4 months after two doses of conjugated meningococcal vaccine, and concentrations of bactericidal antibodies were much higher than after meningococcal polysaccharide vaccines. Antibody concentrations fell significantly by age 14 months. After boosting with polysaccharide vaccine all the children achieved antibody concentrations over 2 μg/ml. Local and systemic reactions were rare after meningococcal conjugate vaccines and were significantly less common at the site of DTP/Hib immunization for all three doses. The high-dose cohort had more systemic reactions than the low-dose cohort (Table 1). One infant required hospitalization for a viral illness soon after the second injection.

The results of a randomized, double-blind trial of safety, immunogenicity, and induction of immunological memory in 182 healthy infants has been published (8). The infants received either conjugated meningococcal vaccine (conjugated to CRM197, a non-toxic mutant of diphtheria toxin) of lot 1 (60 infants) or lot 2 (60 infants) or hepatitis B vaccine as a control vaccine. Diphtheria and tetanus toxoids and whole cell pertussis (DTP) vaccine reconstituted with Hib-tetanus conjugate was co-administered in the other leg. Polio vaccine was given orally. According to the UK immunization schedule, these vaccines were given at 2, 3, and 4 months of age. At 12 months the children received either meningococcal A and C polysaccharide vaccine or conjugated meningococcal serogroup C vaccine. The conjugated meningococcal vaccines were

Mercaptamine

General Information

Mercaptamine (cysteamine), an aminothiol, is used to reduce tissue cystine content in patients with nephropathic cystinosis, an autosomal recessive lysosomal storage disorder in which intracellular cystine accumulates due to impaired transport out of lysosomes (1). The clinical manifestations include renal tubular Fanconi syndrome in the first year of life, with hypophosphatemic rickets, hypokalemia, polyuria, dehydration and acidosis, growth retardation, hypothyroidism, photophobia, renal glomerular deterioration by 10 years of age, and late complications such as myopathy, pancreatic insufficiency, and retinal blindness. The cystinosis gene, CTNS, codes for cystinosin, a 367 amino acid protein with seven transmembrane domains. More than 50 CTNS mutations have been identified, but about 50% of Northern European patients have a 57257-bp deletion which removes the first nine exons of CTNS. The mainstay of cystinosis therapy is oral mercaptamine, 60–90 mg/kg/day qds every 6 hours, and generally achieves about 90% depletion of cellular cystine, as measured in circulating leucocytes. This delays renal glomerular deterioration, enhancing growth, preventing hypothyroidism, and lowering muscle cystine content. In one study, for every month of treatment before 3 years of age, 14 months' worth of later renal function were preserved.

Mercaptamine is available for oral administration as hydrochloride and bitartrate salts and as sodium phosphomercaptamine. Topical mercaptamine prepared from the oral formulation has been used to treat severe photophobia from corneal crystal deposition in cystinosis (2).

- An 8-year-old boy with nephropathic cystinosis had debilitating and worsening photophobia from corneal crystal deposition (3). After 8 months of topical application of mercaptamine, he has marked improvement, both subjectively and objectively.

Mercaptamine has also been used to treat paracetamol overdose (4).

Adverse effects include lethargy, hyperthermia, and rash (5), and nausea and vomiting (6). The risk of vomiting correlates inversely with body weight (7).

Organs and Systems

Sensory systems

In 93 children with nephropathic cystinosis oral mercaptamine 51 mg/kg for up to 73 months produced 82% cystine depletion from leukocytes and improved creatinine clearance and growth (8). However, 14% of the patients could not tolerate the taste and smell of mercaptamine, which is excreted in the breath.

Hematologic

In a phase I trial myelosuppression was the main adverse effect of mercaptamine in five of 24 patients (9). One had grade 4 thrombocytopenia and two had grade 3 thrombocytopenia; anemia and leukopenia were milder (grade 1 to 2).

Gastrointestinal

In four children with nephropathic cystinosis receiving mercaptamine 14.35 mg/kg qds serum gastrin concentrations up to 90 minutes later rose as did gastric acid output (10). Two of the four subjects had visual and histological evidence of gastric inflammation. The clinical effect of this acid production is unknown.

Skin

Mercaptamine hydrochloride contained in "neutral" permanent-wave preparations has been used in American beauty salons since 1993 and can cause contact dermatitis (11).

- A hairdresser, allergic to mercaptamine hydrochloride, had positive patch-test reactions to mercaptamine hydrochloride, glyceryl thioglycolate, diglyceryl thioglycolate, and *p*-phenylenediamine.

There were negative results with mercaptamine hydrochloride (1.0% in petrolatum) in 64 controls. People whose hair had been waved with mercaptamine hydrochloride were not allergic.

References

1. Gahl WA. Early oral cysteamine therapy for nephropathic cystinosis. Eur J Pediatr 2003;162(Suppl 1):S38–41.
2. Tsilou ET, Thompson D, Lindblad AS, Reed GF, Rubin B, Gahl W, Thoene J, Del Monte M, Schneider JA, Granet DB, Kaiser-Kupfer MI. A multicentre randomised double masked clinical trial of a new formulation of topical cysteamine for the treatment of corneal cystine crystals in cystinosis. Br J Ophthalmol 2003;87(1):28–31.
3. Khan AO, Latimer B. Successful use of topical cysteamine formulated from the oral preparation in a child with keratopathy secondary to cystinosis. Am J Ophthalmol 2004;138 (4):674–5.
4. Smith JM, Roberts WO, Hall SM, White TA, Gilbertson AA. Late treatment of paracetamol poisoning with mercaptamine. BMJ 1978;1(6109):331–3.
5. Corden BJ, Schulman JD, Schneider JA, Thoene JG. Adverse reactions to oral cysteamine use in nephropathic cystinosis. Dev Pharmacol Ther 1981;3(1):25–30.
6. Gahl WA, Ingelfinger J, Mohan P, Bernardini I, Hyman PE, Tangerman A. Intravenous cysteamine therapy for nephropathic cystinosis. Pediatr Res 1995;38(4):579–84.
7. Tenneze L, Daurat V, Tibi A, Chaumet-Riffaud P, Funck-Brentano C. A study of the relative bioavailability of cysteamine hydrochloride, cysteamine bitartrate and phosphocysteamine in healthy adult male volunteers. Br J Clin Pharmacol 1999;47(1):49–52.
8. Gahl WA, Reed GF, Thoene JG, Schulman JD, Rizzo WB, Jonas AJ, Denman DW, Schlesselman JJ, Corden BJ, Schneider JA. Cysteamine therapy for children with nephropathic cystinosis. N Engl J Med 1987;316(16):971–7.
9. Kim-Triana B, Misset JL, Madelmont JC, Godeneche D, Musset M, Mathe G. Phase I trial of Perrimustine, a new cysteamine (2-chloroethyl) nitrosourea: an intrapatient escalation scheme. Anticancer Drugs 1992;3(3):225–31.

10. Wenner WJ, Murphy JL. The effects of cysteamine on the upper gastrointestinal tract of children with cystinosis. Pediatr Nephrol 1997;11(5):600–3.
11. Landers MC, Law S, Storrs FJ. Permanent-wave dermatitis: contact allergy to cysteamine hydrochloride. Am J Contact Dermat 2003;14(3):157–60.

Mercury and mercurial salts

General Information

Mercury is a silver-colored metallic element in fluid form (symbol Hg; atomic no. 80). Its symbol derives from the Greek name for the element hydrargyros. It is found as the sulfide salt in cinnabar, the source of the pigment vermilion.

With a few exceptions, the use of metallic mercury in medicine is considered to be outdated; the few exceptions include its use in certain preservatives and in dental amalgam. The radioactive nuclides ^{197}Hg and ^{203}Hg have been used diagnostically, but the amount of mercury involved is very small. Even the mercury thermometer is rapidly being replaced by safer alternative devices. The use of mercury in dermatological therapy should be abandoned because of the risk of mercury intoxication (1).

Aryl mercurials that have been used medicinally include phenylmercuric acetate, phenylmercuric nitrate, nitromersol, thiomersal, merbromin (mercurochrome), and mercurobutol. These compounds are variously used as preservatives in drugs, including vaccines, for skin disinfestation, the treatment of infections of the skin and mucosa, and in contraceptive jellies and hemorrhoidal remedies; they have also been used in some cosmetics. The aryl mercurials are better absorbed across the mucous membranes than most inorganic mercury salts.

Regrettably, some therapeutic exposure to mercury continues, more particularly generally outside the Western world. Non-prescription laxatives containing mercurial compounds are still sold in some countries. The presence of mercury may not always be divulged on the label. Mercury poisoning can also occur through consumption of fish that have swum in waters that have been contaminated with methyl mercury from industrial waste (Minamata disease) (2). When it was first described, in May 1956, the marine products in Minamata Bay contained high concentrations of mercury (6–36 ppm). Mercury was also found in the hair of patients, their families, and the inhabitants of the Shiranui Sea coastline (maximum 705 ppm). Typical symptoms include sensory disturbances (glove and stocking type), ataxia, dysarthria, constriction of the visual fields, auditory disturbances, and tremor. Mercury poisoning has also been seen in the children of mothers who have eaten contaminated marine life (congenital Minamata disease).

Acute and chronic mercury poisoning

The characteristic clinical picture of acute mercury poisoning includes sudden profound circulatory collapse with tachycardia, hypotension and peripheral vasoconstriction, vomiting, and bloody diarrhea due to hemorrhagic colitis. Renal insufficiency usually develops within 24 hours and is associated with albuminuria, epithelial cell casts, and red cells in the urine, glycosuria, and aminoaciduria. Oliguria can proceed to complete anuric failure. There is also neutrophilic leukocytosis due to tissue necrosis (SED-11, 483) (3).

Symptoms of chronic mercury poisoning have been reviewed (4–6). The symptoms are listed in Table 1. The urinary tract is very sensitive to poisoning by all forms of mercury, a sensitive indicator of early injury being a rise in the urinary excretion of *N*-acetyl-beta-D-glucosaminidase (NAG) (7).

In 70 patients with psoriasis treated with an ointment containing ammoniated mercury, symptoms and signs of mercury poisoning were detected in 33 (8): albuminuria, headache, gingivitis, erythroderma, nausea, dizziness, precordial pain, contact dermatitis, conjunctivitis, epistaxis, keratitis, tremor, neuritis, hematological changes, metallic taste in mouth, and purpura.

Acrodynia ("pink disease") is thought to be a particular form of mercury hypersensitivity, which can be caused by organic or inorganic mercury; it formerly occurred in young children exposed to teething formulations containing mercury compounds. Typical signs include pink scaling palms and soles, flushed cheeks, pruritus, photophobia, profuse irritability, and insomnia. A modern case of acrodynia involved a patient with congenital agammaglobulinemia who had received merthiolate-containing gammaglobulin injections for 15 years (SEDA-6, 225).

Mercury poisoning has been reported in a child who took a Chinese herbal medicine (9).

- A 5-year-old Chinese boy developed oral ulceration, mainly affecting the left lateral aspect of his tongue, and 5 weeks later motor and vocal tics. Herpetic ulceration was diagnosed and confirmed by the isolation of

Table 1 The symptoms of chronic mercury poisoning

System	Symptom
Cardiovascular	Hypertension, hypotension
Nervous system	Emotional disturbances, irritability, hypochondria, psychosis, impaired memory, insomnia, tremor, dysarthria, involuntary movements, vertigo, polyneuropathy, paresthesia, headache
Sensory systems	Corneal opacities and ulcers, conjunctivitis, hypacusis
Endocrine	Hyperthyroidism
Hematologic	Hypochromic anemia, erythrocytosis, lymphocytosis, neutropenia, aplastic anemia
Mouth	Loose teeth, discoloration of the gums and oral mucosa, mouth ulcers, fetor
Gastrointestinal	Anorexia, nausea, vomiting, epigastric pain, diarrhea, constipation
Urinary tract	Nephrotic syndrome
Skin	Tylotic eczema, dry skin, skin ulcers, erythroderma
Musculoskeletal	Acrodynia, arthritis in the legs
Reproductive system	Dysmenorrhea

patients, thiomersal-induced adverse effects due to immunization has not been shown to be a severe risk, and a positive patch test to thiomersal does not represent a contraindication to immunization with thiomersal-containing vaccines. Many of the reactions seen in patch tests with 0.1% thiomersal are probably caused by the irritant nature of thiomersal. It has been pointed out that only half of a series of subjects tested with a solution of 0.1% thiomersal had a positive reaction in patch tests with concentrations of 0.05 and 0.01% (36).

Thiomersal included in patch-test series has given varying frequencies of positive reactions. Cross-reactions occur to a few organic mercurials, but not to inorganic or metallic mercury. The allergic determinant seems to be the ethyl mercury radical in thiomersal.

Frequencies of positive reactions have been reported in the following countries:

- USA: 13.4% in 1967 (37) and 8% in 1972 (38)
- Japan: 5.6 (39) and 16.3% (40)
- Finland: 2.0% (41)
- Denmark: 1.3% (42)
- GDR: 6.9% (43)
- Czechoslovakia: 5.3% in infant inpatients (44)
- France and Belgium: 2.3% in a multicenter study in 200 adult patients submitted to routine patch-testing (45)
- Italy: 5.3% (46)
- Poland: 5.7% (13.8% of all medicinal personnel, tested in this study) (47).

There was a very high peak frequency of positive patch tests in the 20–30 years age group in Sweden (48): 16% of male recruits and 10% of other healthy subjects in nursing schools and among medical students. A common reason for sensitization to thiomersal in the younger generation in Sweden arises from intracutaneous testing with tuberculin containing thiomersal as a preservative. It was shown experimentally that tuberculin could act as adjuvant during sensitization to thiomersal. The iatrogenic occurrence of thiomersal allergy in the Swedish population does not result in eczematous reactions, but merely in false-positive skin tests.

Thiomersal takes second place, after nickel, as a contact allergen in Austria. As in Sweden this high incidence is probably due also to frequent immunization with vaccines containing thiomersal (49).

- A generalized allergic reaction occurred in a 50-year-old nurse with a documented allergy to thiomersal, who received 10 ml of human euglobulin with thiomersal as a preservative.
- A 38-year-old man treated a mild sore throat himself with a thiomersal spray, and about 30 hours after the second application developed a severe laryngeal obstruction, for which emergency tracheotomy was necessary. A subsequent patch test produced a severe disseminated allergic reaction to thiomersal (SED-11, 484) (50).

Serious allergic reactions were reported in 18 patients after the use of a Japanese encephalitis vaccine containing thiomersal (51). Reactions in 15 patients were thought to be related to the product; 13 had urticaria affecting the whole body, one had erythema multiforme, and one had a rash. Fourteen reactions arose after the second immunization. Seven of the 13 urticarial reactions began within 24 hours of vaccination, and the other six within 72 hours. In five patients encephalitis vaccine was the only vaccine given. The thiomersal concentration had been increased from 0.0005% in previous vaccine batches, to 0.0067% in the batch used. However, the concentration of thiomersal was that used in most vaccines.

In topical formulations thiomersal can lead to an allergic contact dermatitis. There was a high incidence of thiomersal allergy in patients with pompholyx, that is vesicular eruptions on the palms and soles (48).

Thiomersal is more soluble and stable than the older mercurials. It does not influence tear-film wetting of cornea or contact lenses, or the stability of the tear film itself. Thiomersal has been known to cause both a blepharoconjunctivitis and a punctate keratitis in contact lens wearers. Thiomersal keratoconjunctivitis accounted for 32 of 312 consecutive referrals to an outpatient department for problems related to contact lenses (52). The typical appearances included non-specific conjunctival changes, limbal follicles, superficial punctate keratopathy, and superior corneal epithelial opacities. Atypical cases presented with superior limbitis, coarse punctate keratopathy, severe keratopathy with visual loss, pseudodendritic corneal lesions, or acute conjunctival hyperemia without keratopathy. In atypical cases, the diagnosis can be difficult but can be aided by the use of topical challenge with thiomersal. The condition can be incorrectly attributed to allergy. However, a large number of cases of allergic conjunctivitis have been attributed to thiomersal as a constituent of a solution for preserving soft contact lenses (SED-11, 484) (53).

- A 26-year-old man with a 2-year history of repeated episodes of dermatitis, swelling of the eyelids, and burning eyes was thought to have delayed contact allergy (54). The original diagnosis was of occupational allergy, but patch tests confirmed that the conjunctivitis was due to thiomersal-containing eye-drops, which had been used to treat the condition.

In an effort to reduce exposure to mercury the FDA have recommended that vaccine manufacturers phase out its use. In response to this, some blood products are also being manufactured free of thiomersal (55). In July 1999 the American Academy of Pediatrics and the US Public Health Service issued a joint statement calling for the removal of thiomersal, a mercury-containing preservative, from vaccines. This action was prompted partly by a risk assessment by the FDA, which consisted of hazard identification, dose–response assessment, exposure assessment, and risk characterization (56). The review showed no evidence of harm caused by the doses of thiomersal in vaccines, except for local hypersensitivity reactions. However, it was noted that some infants may be exposed to cumulative doses of mercury during the first 6 months of life that exceed the Environmental Protection Agency recommendations. In the UK the Committee on Safety of Medicines and the Department of Health reviewed the available data relating to thiomersal in vaccines and possible neurodevelopmental disorders, including autism, an issue that has gained media attention (57). There was no evidence of neurodevelopmental harm, a known effect of acute intoxication with mercury, caused by the amounts of thiomersal that are found in vaccines.

The amounts of thiomersal in the UK schedule of childhood vaccination are lower than in the USA. No specific action has been recommended in the vaccination program. European and American regulatory authorities have recommended that vaccine manufacturers should phase out their use of thiomersal whenever possible as a precaution (SEDA-25, 278).

Inorganic salts

Chronic mercurialism with nervous system involvement, renal insufficiency, and progressive colitis has been described after the long-term use of remedies containing inorganic mercury. Such remedies may also explain the persistence of other unexplained disorders, such as pink disease. Inorganic and organic mercury compounds may cause allergic dermatitis (SEDA-22, 247) (28). Frank poisoning from these sources, although uncommon today, is still possible, and occasional case reports appear (SEDA-13, 195); in one instance, injudicious chronic use of an ammoniated mercury ointment led to a peripheral polyneuropathy, which was only partly reversible (SEDA-22, 247). As with other metals, reactions to mercury can occur after occupational or environmental exposure; in one case, a child already known to be hypersensitive to mercurochrome developed a severe rash after wearing plastic boots which were found to contain mercurous chloride (58).

Despite several warnings over many years, the use of mercuric chloride solutions during operations in an attempt to kill cancer cells implanted in healthy tissues persists in some countries. Intraperitoneal administration, when seeding of a visceral cancer is feared, carries the risk of mercury absorption and nephrotoxicity. Death from intoxication after peritoneal lavage with a mercuric chloride solution has been reported (3).

Health authorities in Canada have warned consumers not to use Diana Cream (Diana de Beauté), a product that is used for skin lightening, mainly by Afro-Caribbean communities. The Directorate General of Pharmaceutical Affairs & Drug Control has prohibited the registration, import, and sale of the product, which is manufactured in Lebanon and is being illegally imported. It contains ammoniated mercury, bismuth subnitrate, and salicylic acid. The mercury content poses a high risk of mercury poisoning in adults and a serious health hazard to unborn and nursing infants of women who use the product (59).

Peripheral polyneuropathy as a result of chronic ammoniated mercury poisoning has been studied and followed over 2 years (60).

- A 36-year-old man developed peripheral polyneuropathy after chronic perianal use of an ammoniated mercury ointment. He had very high blood and urine mercury concentrations. Sural nerve biopsy showed mixed axonal degeneration/demyelination. His symptoms improved progressively over 2 years after withdrawal of the ointment, but neurophysiological recovery was incomplete.
- A 4-month-old boy was hospitalized with a weeping eczema covering more than the half of the body surface and complicated by skin hemorrhage and infection by *Klebsiella pneumoniae* and *Proteus mirabilis*. Apart from general therapy, a compound zinc oxide ointment containing, among other ingredients, yellow mercuric oxide 2 g per 40 g of base was applied daily. After 12 days, he rapidly developed cardiovascular collapse, acute pulmonary edema, and coma Stage II, with right hemiparesis, generalized hypertonia, and muscular tremor. The mercury concentrations in blood, urine, and CSF were respectively 120 ng/ml (normal <10 ng/ml), creatinine 260 micrograms/g (normal <5 micrograms/g), and 4.8 ng/ml (normal <0.1 ng/ml). Despite therapy with dimercaprol and vigorous supportive measures, the child's condition deteriorated, he developed *Klebsiella aerogenes* septicemia, and died 6 weeks later (61).

Organs and Systems

Sensory systems

Topical treatment with phenylmercuryl acetate can cause band-shaped corneal opacities (62). Long-term use of eye-drops containing phenylmercuric nitrate as a preservative can cause pigmentation of the anterior lens capsule. In 31 patients who used eye-drops containing phenylmercuric nitrate as a preservative for 3–15 years, a brownish pigmentation of the anterior capsule of the pupillary area developed. Light and electron microscopic studies on two lenses showed deposits of dense particulate material resembling melanin pigment on and in the anterior capsule of the lens in the area of the pupil (63). Electron microprobe analysis and neutron activation analysis established the presence of mercury. However, the pigmentation does not seem to be associated with visual impairment.

The use of mercurials in the eye can lead to a bluish-gray deposit of mercuric oxide on the eyelids, conjunctivae, and Descemet's layer. Phenylmercuric nitrate used in a 0.004% concentration can cause mercuria lentis. Mercurial compounds have been found in the aqueous humor, having penetrated the eye from hydrophilic-gel contact lenses preserved with thiomersal. Although it remains to be established whether deposition of mercury in the eye is clinically important, the concentrations found are similar to those reported in cases of systemic poisoning by organic mercurials (64).

Psychological, psychiatric

There is continuing debate that there is an association between autism and thiomersal-containing vaccines. Some authors believe that review of the literature supports the hypothesis that mercury in vaccines may be a factor in the pathogenesis of autism (65). The World Health Organization's Global Advisory Committee on Vaccine Safety (GACvS) has also kept this issue under review and concluded in November 2002 that there is no evidence of toxicity in infants, children, or adults who have been exposed to thiomersal in vaccines. The CSM is also keeping the issue under close review and studies of the possible toxicology of thiomersal continue to appear (66).

The usual dose of ethyl mercury in pediatric vaccines is small (about 12.5–25 micrograms of mercury). However, the metabolism of ethyl mercury in infants who receive vaccines containing thiomersal is unknown. The mean doses of mercury in 40 full-term infants exposed to thiomersal-containing vaccines were 46 (range 38–63) micrograms in 2-month-old children and 111 (range 88–175) micrograms in 6-month-old children. Blood mercury concentrations in the thiomersal-exposed 2-month-old children ranged from less than 3.8 to 21 nmol/l; in 6-month-old children all the concentrations were below 7.5 nmol/l. Only one of 15 blood samples from 21 controls contained measurable concentrations of mercury. Urine concentrations of mercury were low after vaccination, but stool concentrations were high in thiomersal-exposed 2-month-old children (mean 82 ng/g dry weight). The mean half life of ethyl mercury was 7 days.

This study was not designed as a formal assessment of the pharmacokinetics of mercury. However, it showed that the administration of vaccines containing thiomersal did not seem to raise blood concentrations of mercury above safe values in infants. Ethyl mercury seems to be eliminated from the blood rapidly via the stools. The authors concluded that the thiomersal in routine vaccines poses very little risk in full-term infants.

Urinary tract

Membranous glomerulonephritis has been attributed to mercury in a patient with diabetes mellitus.

- A 21-year-old man with a 16-year history of diabetes mellitus, who had been using an ointment containing 10% mercuric ammonium chloride for eczema for about 3 weeks, became tired, with fasciculation in the limbs and poor control of his diabetes (67). Nephrotic syndrome and hypertension were diagnosed 1 month later, and at 2 months he was very weak with tremor of the hands, was almost unable to walk, and had lost 20 kg. His behavior suggested an acute psychosis. The urine mercury concentration was 250 micrograms/l. He was treated with sodium 2,3-dimercaptopropane-1-sulfonate (Dimaval) capsules for 12 days (total dose 6.3 g). The highest urine mercury excretion during antidote treatment was 2336 micrograms/day. He had proteinuria of up to 11 g/day and renal biopsy showed diffuse membranous glomerulonephritis without diabetic nephropathy. Similarly, his neuropathy did not have typical features of diabetic neuropathy. He improved over the next year.

Immunologic

Merthiolate was tested as a matter of routine in an extended standard series of skin tests in patients with different subtypes of eczema and varicose complex (68). Of 880 patients 53% responded positively to one or more allergens, 3.9% to merthiolate. The latest results of skin tests in adults have confirmed the persistence of contact allergy to merthiolate and justify further follow-up and systematic screening.

Attention has been given to mercury as a cause of autoimmune responses, especially in the kidney (69). Exposure to mercury can cause immune responses to various auto-antigens and autoimmune disease of the kidney and other tissues. Although epidemiological studies have shown that occupational exposure to mercury does not usually result in autoimmunity, mercury can cause the formation of antinuclear antibodies, scleroderma-like disease, lichen planus, or membranous nephropathy in some individuals. In experimental animals mercury causes autoimmune disease similar to that observed in humans, with emphasis on the importance of immunogenetic and pharmacogenetic factors.

Homeopathic medicines can cause mercury allergy (baboon syndrome).

- A 5-year-old girl developed an itchy erythematous macular rash, symmetrically distributed in the anogenital area and thighs (70). The lesions developed into a widespread maculopapular vesicular rash in 48 hours, sparing the face, palms, and soles. The eruption cleared after systemic corticosteroids and antihistamines, with scaling and post-inflammatory hypopigmentation. She had had neonatal periumbilical dermatitis associated with the application of merbromin to the cord, and 24 hours before the onset of the rash had taken a single homeopathic tablet (Mercurius Heel), which contained soluble mercury. Allergy tests to a standard series of foods and respiratory allergens were negative and total IgE was normal. Patch-testing to allergens showed positive reactions to thiomersal and metallic mercury.

Previous sensitization and the subsequent development of an allergic contact dermatitis from vaccines that contain thiomersal has received more attention than before (71). Cross-reactivity, exposure factors, and tolerance to vaccines containing thiomersal have been studied in 125 patients sensitized to mercury derivatives in a cross-sectional study (71). Childhood vaccinations, merbromin used as an antiseptic, broken thermometers, and the use of drops were the main sources of previous exposure. There was sensitization to thiomersal in 57 patients and 24 had a positive intradermal reaction. Ammoniated mercury elicited positive reactions in 78% of all patients and merbromin in 66%. In most cases (100/125) there was cross-reactivity among different mercury derivatives. Intramuscular thiomersal caused a mild local reaction in only five patients (4% of the total, 9% of thiomersal positive reactions). Most of the patients had positive tests to both organic and inorganic mercury derivatives. Vaccination with thiomersal is relatively safe, even for individuals with delayed type hypersensitivity, since more than 90% of allergic patients tolerated intramuscular challenge tests with thiomersal. However, in such patients it would be advisable to restrict the use of mercurial antiseptics and mercury thermometers.

Drug Administration

Drug administration route

Mercury toxicity has resulted from the use of an ointment containing mercuric ammonium chloride (67).

References

1. Kern F, Roberts N, Ostlere L, Langtry J, Staughton RC. Ammoniated mercury ointment as a cause of peripheral neuropathy. Dermatologica 1991;183(4):280–2.
2. Harada M. Minamata disease: methylmercury poisoning in Japan caused by environmental pollution. Crit Rev Toxicol 1995;25(1):1–24.

3. Laundy T, Adam AE, Kershaw JB, Rainford DJ. Deaths after peritoneal lavage with mercuric chloride solutions: case report and review of the literature. BMJ (Clin Res Ed) 1984;289(6437):96–8.
4. LeClercq A, Melennec J, Proteau J. Intoxication mercurielle. Concours Med 1973;95:6055.
5. Ciaccio EI. Mercury: therapeutic and toxic aspects. Semin Drug Treat 1971;1(2):177–94.
6. Ward OC, Hingerty D. Pink Disease from cutaneous absorption of mercury. J Ir Med Assoc 1967;60(357):94–5.
7. Boogaard PJ, Houtsma AT, Journee HL, Van Sittert NJ. Effects of exposure to elemental mercury on the nervous system and the kidneys of workers producing natural gas. Arch Environ Health 1996;51(2):108–15.
8. Young E. Ammoniated mercury poisoning. Br J Dermatol 1960;72:449–55.
9. Li AM, Chan MH, Leung TF, Cheung RC, Lam CW, Fok TF. Mercury intoxication presenting with tics. Arch Dis Child 2000;83(2):174–5.
10. Matsumoto J, Natsuaki M. Three cases of mercury allergy. Skin Res 1997;39:48–52.
11. Schwarz S, Husstedt I, Bertram HP, Kuchelmeister K. Amyotrophic lateral sclerosis after accidental injection of mercury. J Neurol Neurosurg Psychiatry 1996; 60(6):698.
12. Hohage H, Otte B, Westermann G, Witta J, Welling U, Zidek W, Heidenreich S. Elemental mercurial poisoning. South Med J 1997;90(10):1033–6.
13. Torres-Alanis O, Garza-Ocanas L, Pineyro-Lopez A. Intravenous self-administration of metallic mercury: report of a case with a 5-year follow-up. J Toxicol Clin Toxicol 1997;35(1):83–7.
14. Lorscheider FL, Vimy MJ. Mercury exposure from "silver" fillings. Lancet 1991;337(8749):1103.
15. Lorscheider FL, Vimy MJ, Summers AO. Mercury exposure from "silver" tooth fillings: emerging evidence questions a traditional dental paradigm. FASEB J 1995; 9(7):504–8.
16. Kupsinel R. Mercury amalgam toxicity: a major common denominator of degenerative disease. J Orthomol Psychiatr 1984;13:240.
17. Dodes JE. The amalgam controversy. An evidence-based analysis. J Am Dent Assoc 2001;132(3):348–56.
18. Staehle HJ. Gesundheitsstörungen durch Amalgam? [Illnesses caused by amalgam?] Med Klin (Munich) 1998;93(2):99–106.
19. Osborne JW, Albino JE. Psychological and medical effects of mercury intake from dental amalgam. A status report for the American Journal of Dentistry. Am J Dent 1999;12(3):151–6.
20. Adachi A, Horikawa T, Takashima T, Ichihashi M. Mercury-induced nummular dermatitis. J Am Acad Dermatol 2000;43(2 Pt 2):383–5.
21. McGivern B, Pemberton M, Theaker ED, Buchanan JA, Thornhill MH. Delayed and immediate hypersensitivity reactions associated with the use of amalgam. Br Dent J 2000;188(2):73–6.
22. Vena GA, Foti C, Grandolfo M, Angelini G. Mercury exanthem. Contact Dermatitis 1994;31(4):214–16.
23. Unni M. Exfoliative dermatitis due to topical mercury application. Indan J Dermatol Venereol Leprol 1994;60: 56–7.
24. Moszczynski P, Rutowski J, Slowinski S, Bem S, Jakus-Stoga D. Effects of occupational exposure to mercury vapors on T cell and NK-cell populations. Arch Med Res 1996;27(4):503–7.
25. Slee PH, den Ottolander GJ, de Wolff FA. A case of merbromin (Mercurochrome) intoxication possibly resulting in aplastic anemia. Acta Med Scand 1979;205(6):463–6.
26. Weber G. Todliche Intoxikation nach Grobscher Drei-Phasen-Gerbung. [Fatal intoxication following Grob's triple-phase tanning.] MMW Munch Med Wochenschr 1977;119(44):1437–8.
27. Camarasa G. Contact dermatitis from mercurochrome. Contact Dermatitis 1976;2(2):120–1.
28. Kanerva L, Tarvainen K, Estlander T, Jolanki R. Occupational allegic contact dermatitis caused by mercury and benzoyl peroxide. Eur J Dermatol 1994;4:359–61.
29. Lohiya G. Asthma and urticaria after hepatitis B vaccination. West J Med 1987;147(3):341.
30. Clements CJ, Ball LK, Ball R, Pratt RD. Thiomersal in vaccines: is removal warranted? Drug Saf 2001;24(8): 567–74.
31. van't Veen AJ. Vaccines without thiomersal: why so necessary, why so long coming? Drugs 2001;61(5):565–72.
32. Magos L. Review on the toxicity of ethylmercury, including its presence as a preservative in biological and pharmaceutical products. J Appl Toxicol 2001;21(1):1–5.
33. Rohyans J, Walson PD, Wood GA, MacDonald WA. Mercury toxicity following merthiolate ear irrigations. J Pediatr 1984;104(2):311–13.
34. Hodgkinson DJ, Irons GB, Williams TJ. Chemical burns and skin preparation solutions. Surg Gynecol Obstet 1978;147(4):534–6.
35. Gille J, Goerz G. Thiomersal: Ein häufiges Kontaktallergen. Z Hautkr 1992;67:1049–54.
36. l'Allemand D, Gruters A, Heidemann P, Schurnbrand P. Iodine-induced alterations of thyroid function in newborn infants after prenatal and perinatal exposure to povidone iodine. J Pediatr 1983;102(6):935–8.
37. Epstein S. Sensitivity to merthiolat: a cause of false delayed intradermal reactions: clinical and histological investigations. J Allergy Clin Immunol 1963;34:225.
38. Rudner EJ, Clendenning WE, Epstein E. Epidemiology of contact dermatitis in North America: 1972. Arch Dermatol 1973;108(4):537–40.
39. Massuda T, Honda S, Nakauchi Y, et al. Patch test: the data at the Allergy Clinic of Department of Dermatology of Tokyo University Hospital for the past three years. Jpn J Dermatol Ser B 1970;80:133.
40. Osawa J, Kitamura K, Ikezawa Z, Nakajima H. A probable role for vaccines containing thimerosal in thimerosal hypersensitivity. Contact Dermatitis 1991;24(3):178–82.
41. Hannuksela M, Kousa M, Pirila V. Allergy to ingredients of vehicles. Contact Dermatitis 1976;2(2):105–10.
42. Hjorth N. Sensitivity to organic mercury compounds. Contact Dermatitits Newsletter 1976;1:15.
43. Loechel I, Zschunke E. Zur Aktualität der Quecksilberallergie. [Mercury allergy.] Dermatol Monatsschr 1971;157(8):570–8.
44. Novak M, Kvicalova E, Friedlanderova B. Reactions to merthiolate in infants. Contact Dermatitis 1986;15(5):309–10.
45. Lachapelle JM, Chabeau G, Ducombs G, Lacroix M, Martin P, Reuter G, Marot L. Enquête multicentrique relative à la fréquence des tests épicutanés positifs au mercure et au thiomersal. [Multicenter survey related to the frequency of positive patch tests with mercury and thiomersal.] Ann Dermatol Venereol 1988;115(8):793–6.
46. Lisi P, Perno P, Ottaviani M, Morelli P. Minimum eliciting patch test concentration of thimerosal. Contact Dermatitis 1991;24(1):22–6.
47. Kiec-Swierczynska M. Uczulajace dzialanie mertiolatu (preparat odkzzajacy) na podstawie materialu Instytutu Medycyny Pracy w Lodzi. [Allergic reaction to merthiolate (a disinfectant) based on material from the Occupational Medicine Institute in Lodz.] Med Pr 1996;47(2):125–31.
48. Moller H. Merthiolate allergy: a nationwide iatrogenic sensitization. Acta Derm Venereol 1977;57(6):509–17.
49. Aberer W. Vaccination despite thimerosal sensitivity. Contact Dermatitis 1991;24(1):6–10.

50. Maibach H. Acute laryngeal obstruction presumed secondary to thiomersal (merthiolate) delayed hypersensitivity. Contact Dermatitis 1975;1(4):221–2.
51. Andersen MM, Ronne T. Side-effects with Japanese encephalitis vaccine. Lancet 1991;337(8748):1044.
52. Wilson-Holt N, Dart JK. Thiomersal keratoconjunctivitis, frequency, clinical spectrum and diagnosis. Eye 1989;3(Pt 5): 581–7.
53. Rietschel RL, Wilson LA. Ocular inflammation in patients using soft contact lenses. Arch Dermatol 1982;118(3):147–9.
54. Iliev D, Wuthrich B. Conjunctivitis to thimerosal mistaken as hay fever. Allergy 1998;53(3):333–4.
55. Sawyer LA. Antibodies for the prevention and treatment of viral diseases. Antiviral Res 2000;47(2):57–77.
56. Ball LK, Ball R, Pratt RD. An assessment of thimerosal use in childhood vaccines. Pediatrics 2001;107(5):1147–54.
57. Current Vaccine and Immunisation Issues. London: Department of Health, 15 Oct 2001. PL/CMO/2001/5.
58. Koch P, Nickolaus G. Allergic contact dermatitis and mercury exanthem due to mercury chloride in plastic boots. Contact Dermatitis 1996;34(6):405–9.
59. Anonymous. Ammoniated mercury in skin lightening cream-warning against use and prohibition. WHO Pharm Newslett 1998;5/6:1.
60. Deleu D, Hanssens Y, al-Salmy HS, Hastie I. Peripheral polyneuropathy due to chronic use of topical ammoniated mercury. J Toxicol Clin Toxicol 1998;36(3):233–7.
61. De Bont B, Lauwerys R, Govaerts H, Moulin D. Yellow mercuric oxide ointment and mercury intoxication. Eur J Pediatr 1986;145(3):217–18.
62. Hugues FC, Le Jeunne C. Systemic and local tolerability of ophthalmic drug formulations. An update. Drug Saf 1993;8(5):365–80.
63. Garron LK, Wood IS, Spencer WH, Hayes TL. A clinical pathologic study of mercurialentis medicamentosus. Trans Am Ophthalmol Soc 1976;74:295–320.
64. Burstein NL. Corneal cytotoxicity of topically applied drugs, vehicles and preservatives. Surv Ophthalmol 1980; 25(1):15–30.
65. Novak M, Klezlova V. [Allergy to merthiolate (Thimerosalum) in a set of standard epicutaneous tests in patients with eczematous diseases and leg ulcer during three periods between 1979 and 1999.] Cesko-Slov Dermatol 2000;75:3–10.
66. Bigazzi PE. Metals and kidney autoimmunity. Environ Health Perspect 1999;107(Suppl 5):753–65.
67. Audicana M, Bernedo N, Gonzalez I, Munoz D, Fernandez E, Gastaminza G. An unusual case of baboon syndrome due to mercury present in a homeopathic medicine. Contact Dermatitis 2001;45(3):185.
68. Audicana MT, Munoz D, del Pozo MD, Fernandez E, Gastaminza G, Fernandez de Corres L. Allergic contact dermatitis from mercury antiseptics and derivatives: study protocol of tolerance to intramuscular injections of thimerosal. Am J Contact Dermat 2002;13(1):3–9.
69. Pelclova D, Lukas E, Urban P, Preiss J, Rysava R, Lebenhart P, Okrouhlik B, Fenclova Z, Lebedova J, Stejskalova A, Ridzon P. Mercury intoxication from skin ointment containing mercuric ammonium chloride. Int Arch Occup Environ Health 2002;75(Suppl):S54–9.
70. Bernard S, Enayati A, Roger H, Binstock T, Redwood L. The role of mercury in the pathogenesis of autism. Mol Psychiatry 2002;7(Suppl 2):S42–3.
71. Pichichero ME, Cernichiari E, Lopreiato J, Treanor J. Mercury concentrations and metabolism in infants receiving vaccines containing thiomersal: a descriptive study. Lancet 2002;360(9347):1737–41.

Mescaline

General Information

Mescaline is one of eight hallucinogenic alkaloids derived from the peyote cactus, slices of which ("peyote buttons") have been used in religious rites by North and South American Indian tribes. Mescaline itself is only one of the alkaloids present in peyote, but it produces the same effects as the crude preparation. Chemically, it is related to amfetamine. In doses of some 300–500 mg it depresses nervous system activity and produces visual and occasionally auditory hallucinations, illusions, depersonalization, and depressive symptoms. The total picture can closely resemble that caused by lysergic acid diethylamide. Its physical effects include nausea, tremor, and sweating.

Organs and Systems

Psychological, psychiatric

The effects of mescaline have been investigated in a psychiatric research study (1). Psychosis induced during the experiment was measured with the Brief Psychiatric Rating Scale and the Paranoid Depression Scale. During use of mescaline neuropsychological measures showed reduced functioning of the right hemisphere. Single photon emission computed tomography (SPECT) studies showed a hyperfrontal pattern, with an emphasis on the right hemisphere. The authors discussed the possible educational value of experimentally induced psychosis in understanding the psychotic state.

Reference

1. Hermle L, Funfgeld M, Oepen G, Botsch H, Borchardt D, Gouzoulis E, Fehrenbach RA, Spitzer M. Mescaline-induced psychopathological, neuropsychological, and neurometabolic effects in normal subjects: experimental psychosis as a tool for psychiatric research. Biol Psychiatry 1992;32(11):976–91.

Mesna

General Information

Mesna is used to prevent or ameliorate hemorrhagic cystitis produced by the anticancer drugs cyclophosphamide and ifosfamide. It is excreted by the kidney and binds and detoxifies acrolein in the urine; mesna also prevents the breakdown of acrolein precursors. It is also used as a mucolytic.

Endotracheal instillation of mesna was compared with instillation of saline in mechanically ventilated patients. Following instillation of mesna, there was a significant increase in maximal airway resistance and impairment of oxygenation with a slight increase in $PaCO_2$ (SEDA-20, 183). A single episode of bronchorrhea occurred 10 minutes after the instillation of mesna.

In a randomized, crossover study, 25 volunteers received single doses of intravenous mesna and four different formulations of oral mesna (1). One subject withdrew from the study because of ocular inflammation followed by loss of appetite, nausea, and vomiting. Another developed a rash during the period in which three of his four oral doses were given. Two further subjects developed loose stools after one of the oral doses. Another reported dizziness after an oral dose. One reported pain at the site of the intravenous infusion. The adverse effects were all considered to be mild or moderate and resolved spontaneously without treatment.

Organs and Systems

Respiratory

Bronchorrhea due to inhaled mesna may be the result of mucolysis, but could also be caused by stimulation of bronchial secretions. Application by aerosol or nebulizer is occasionally followed by bronchospasm, but mesna is usually well tolerated by people with asthma (SEDA-20, 183).

Drug–Drug Interactions

Platinum cytotoxic agents

Platinum agents are now combined with ifosfamide in the treatment of cancer. The possibility that mesna may interfere with the anticancer effects of platinum has been investigated using cultured malignant glioma cells (2). Mesna protected tumor cell lines from the cytotoxic effect of the platinum agents. This in vitro study emphasizes the importance of specifying in detail the infusion schedules of mesna and platinum agents.

References

1. Cudmore MA, Silva J Jr, Fekety R, Liepman MK, Kim KH. Clostridium difficile colitis associated with cancer chemotherapy. Arch Intern Med 1982;142(2):333–5.
2. Abe H, Tsunaga N, Yamashita S, Ishiguro K, Mitani I. [Anticancer drug-induced colitis—case report and review of the literature.] Gan To Kagaku Ryoho 1997;24(5):619–24.

Mesulergine

General Information

Mesulergine is an 8-alpha-aminoergoline derivative that acts as a dopamine receptor agonist. In a blind, crossover study in six patients with hyperprolactinemia, mesulergine 0.5 mg caused fewer adverse effects than bromocriptine 2.5 mg, while the prolactin release-inhibitory effect of the two was of the same order (1).

The most frequent adverse effect of mesulergine is dyskinesia, mostly in patients who have had similar reactions with levodopa. Orthostatic light-headedness and visual hallucinations are also common. Other adverse effects include anorexia, nausea, drowsiness, ankle swelling, insomnia, confusion, irritability, visual disturbance, chest pain, rash, and augmented body odor.

In one study of 17 patients with mild Parkinson's disease who were given either mesulergine or pergolide, mesulergine impaired the quality of life; frequent adverse effects were vomiting, lassitude, abdominal discomfort, depression, right bundle-branch block, fuzzy-headedness, and increasing insulin requirements in a patient with diabetes (SEDA-13, 113).

Reference

1. Lamberts SW, Klyn JG, Oosterom R. Mechanism of action and tolerance of mesulergine. Clin Pharmacol Ther 1984;36(5):620–7.

Mesuximide

See also Antiepileptic drugs

General Information

Mesuximide (*N*,2-dimethyl-2-phenylsuccinimide) is a succinimide anticonvulsant with actions similar to those of ethosuximide. Its activity is mostly due to its main metabolite, *N*-desmethylmesuximide, which has a half-life of about 48 hours (1).

Mesuximide has been used in 112 children with intractable epilepsy taking other anticonvulsants (2). There was a 50% or greater reduction in seizure frequency in 40 patients after 9 weeks. After a mean of 3.7 years, 39 patients were still taking mesuximide and 22 of them had derived long-term benefit. In patients with good seizure control, fasting plasma concentrations of desmethylmesuximide were 25–45 μg/mg. Of the 112 patients 41 developed adverse effects while taking mesuximide treatment, but none was serious or irreversible.

Of 26 patients with complex partial seizures refractory to phenytoin, carbamazepine, phenobarbital, or primidone, mesuximide produced a 50% or greater reduction in seizure frequency in eight after 8 weeks, and five of those continued to benefit after 3–34 months (1). Drowsiness, gastrointestinal disturbances, hiccups, irritability, and headache were the common adverse effects.

Drug Administration

Drug overdose

Mesuximide can cause profound nervous system depression (3). In one patient this responded to charcoal hemoperfusion (1).

Methadone

General Information

Methadone is an OP_3 (μ) receptor agonist with pharmacological properties similar to those of morphine. It is an attractive alternative OP_3 opioid receptor analgesic, because of its lack of neuroactive metabolites, a clearance that is independent of renal function, good oral systemic availability, a longer half-life with fewer doses needed per day, and extremely low cost. It is mainly metabolized by CYP3A4.

Drug studies

Pain relief

Experience with methadone in cancer pain is limited. Its long half-life tends to produce delayed toxicity, especially in older patients, but in chronic renal insufficiency and stable liver disease methadone is safe, unlike morphine.

Methadone is being used increasingly for treating chronic pain and cancer pain (neuropathic and somatic) that is non-responsive or has lost responsiveness because of tolerance to high-dose μ opioid receptor agonists (for example morphine, fentanyl, oxycodone) (1). There are several protocols for converting from morphine to methadone and for initiating and stabilizing maintenance dosages.

In a prospective uncontrolled study, 45 patients with advanced cancer were given 0.1% methadone 2–3 times a day as required (2). Ten had nausea and vomiting, none had drowsiness, and 17 had constipation. In another study, nine of 29 patients in a tertiary level cancer pain clinic could not take opioid analgesics owing to uncomfortable adverse effects: nausea, vomiting, and drowsiness in four and other adverse effects in five (3). The average daily dose of methadone at the end of the titration phase (range 1–79 days) was 208 (range 15–1520) mg. Twenty patients had methadone toxicity during titration. In 12 patients mild drowsiness was a problem, six patients had nausea, and one patient each had confusion and severe headaches. In a third cross-sectional prospective study, 24 patients with advanced cancer pain were rapidly switched form oral morphine to oral methadone using a fixed ratio of 1:5 (4). There was a significant reduction in pain intensity and adverse effects intensity within 24 hours of substitution, although five patients required alternative treatments.

In a prospective, open, uncontrolled study 50 patients with a history of cancer taking daily oral morphine (90–800 mg) but with uncontrolled pain with or without severe opioid adverse effects were switched to oral 8-hourly methadone in a dose ratio of 1:4 for patients receiving less than 90 mg of morphine daily, 1:8 for patients receiving 90–300 mg daily, and 1:12 for patients receiving more than 300 mg daily (5). Methadone was effective in 80% of the patients when comparing analgesic response with opioid-related adverse effects. Ten patients were switched because of uncontrolled pain, eight because of moderate or severe adverse effects in the presence of acceptable pain control, and 32 because of uncontrolled pain with morphine-related adverse effects. In the last 32 there were significant improvements in pain intensity, nausea and vomiting, constipation, and drowsiness, with a 20% increase in methadone dose over and above the recommended starting dose.

In a prospective uncontrolled study of intrathecal methadone in 24 patients with a history of intractable chronic non-malignant pain, methadone was a better analgesic than morphine, with improved quality of life and no adverse effects in 13 patients (6). The final rates of methadone infusion were 20% higher than the preceding morphine rates.

Opioid dependence

An analysis of the balance of benefit to harm during methadone maintenance treatment for diamorphine dependence has shown lower mortality and morbidity with improvement in quality of life (7). The risks of methadone treatment include an increased risk of opiate overdosage during induction into treatment, and adverse effects of methadone in some patients. However, with careful management the benefits of prescribing methadone outweigh the risks.

The validity of self-reported opiate and cocaine use has been studied in 175 veterans enrolled in a methadone treatment program (8). Urine analysis showed higher rates of substance use than the patients themselves reported. The authors encouraged the development of more objective measures for assessing patient progress and the performance of the methadone program.

Organs and Systems

Cardiovascular

A variety of complications following parenteral self-administration of oral methadone were noted, including regional thrombosis, often associated with shock and multiorgan failure (9).

The use of methadone/dihydrocodeine has been linked to an acute myocardial infarction (10).

- A 22-year-old man with a 6-year history of intravenous heroin use was maintained on methadone 60 mg/day and dihydrocodeine 0.5 g/day. He had an extensive anterior myocardial infarction as a result of occlusion of the left anterior descending coronary artery, which was reopened by percutaneous transluminal coronary angioplasty.

This case presents circumstantial evidence only, and the association was probably not a true one.

There has been a report of five cases of episodes of syncope and an electrocardiogram showing ventricular tachydysrhythmias with prolonged QT intervals and episodes of torsade de pointes; all the patients were taking high doses of methadone (270–660 mg/day) with no previous history of cardiac disease (11). Torsade de pointes also occurred when high doses (3 mg/kg) of the long-acting methadone derivative, levomethadyl acetate HCl (LAAM), were given to a 41-year-old woman with a history of heroin dependence (12). She was also taking fluoxetine and intravenous cocaine, which can prolong the QT interval, and fluoxetine and marijuana, which inhibit the activity of CYP3A4, which is responsible for the metabolism of LAAM and its active metabolite.

In a retrospective case study in methadone maintenance treatment programs in the USA and a pain management center in Canada, 17 methadone-treated patients developed torsade de pointes during 5 years (13). The dose of methadone was 65–1000 mg/day. Six patients had had an increase in methadone dose in the months just before the onset of torsade de pointes. One patient had taken nelfinavir, a potent inhibitor of CYP3A4, begun just before the development of torsade de pointes. The above two risk factors (increased drug dosage and drug interactions) are important when eliciting the cause of torsade de pointes in patients taking methadone.

Respiratory

In 10 stable methadone-maintained patients (50–120 mg/day) and nine healthy subjects assessed using polysomnography, the methadone-maintained patients had more abnormalities of sleep architecture, with a higher prevalence of central sleep apnea (14). Methadone depresses respiration, probably by acting on μ opioid receptors in the ventral surface of the medulla and possibly on other receptor sites in the lung and spinal cord. All the patients taking methadone also used benzodiazepines and cannabis, which may have influenced the above findings.

Nervous system

Reversible choreic movements of the upper limbs, torso, and speech mechanism developed in a 25-year-old man taking methadone as a heroin substitute (15).

Spastic paraparesis has been attributed to methadone (16).

- A 43-year-old patient taking methadone for pain secondary to a squamous cell carcinoma of the larynx, which progressed despite surgery and radiation therapy, developed reversible spastic paraparesis with prominent extensor spasms in the legs while receiving an infusion of high-dose intravenous methadone 100 mg/hour. On the second day, after 5 hours on 100 mg/hour, he noted weakness in both legs, uncontrollable trembling, bilateral tinnitus, and generalized anxiety. Dexamethasone 6 mg intravenously every 6 hours was started and the methadone was reduced to 60 mg/hour. Dexamethasone was withdrawn when an MRI scan confirmed the absence of metastases in the thoracic and cervical spinal cord. Because of persistent spastic paraparesis, methadone was switched to levorphanol 40 mg/hour intravenously, and there was complete resolution of symptoms 24 hours later.

Methadone can cause movement disorders characterized by tremor, choreiform movements, and a gait abnormality (17).

- A 41-year-old woman with a 15-year history of chronic neuropathic pain was given methadone 5 mg tds and then qds. One month after the final increase she had bilateral tremor spreading from her arm up to her neck, followed by choreiform movements of the torso, a broad-based gait, and staccato-like speech. She was switched from methadone to modified-release oxycodone 60 mg/day, with complete resolution after 3 weeks.

Psychological, psychiatric

In a randomized, double-blind, crossover study of 20 patients on a stable methadone regimen, a single dose of methadone caused episodic memory deficits (18). This was significant in patients with a history of diamorphine use averaging more than 10 years duration. Such deficits can be avoided by giving methadone in divided doses.

Psychomotor and cognitive performance has been studied in 18 opioid-dependent methadone maintenance patients and 21 non-substance abusers (19). Abstinence from heroin and cocaine for the previous 24 hours was verified by urine testing. The methadone maintenance patients had a wide range of impaired functions, including psychomotor speed, working memory, decision making, and metamemory. There was also possible impairment of inhibitory mechanisms. In the areas of time estimation, conceptual flexibility, and long-term memory, the groups performed similarly.

Endocrine

Prolonged therapy with methadone causes increases in serum thyroid hormone-binding globulin, triiodothyronine, and thyroxine, as well as albumin, globulin, and prolactin, and these must be monitored (SEDA-15, 71) (SEDA-17, 81).

Fluid balance

Methadone-induced edema soon after start of treatment is recognized, and distal leg edema after 7 years of treatment has been described (SEDA-17, 81).

Gastrointestinal

In a randomized, double-blind, placebo-controlled trial of the efficacy of intravenous methylnaltrexone (0.015–0.095 mg/kg) in treating chronic methadone-induced constipation in 22 patients attending a methadone maintenance program (oral methadone linctus 30–100 mg/day), methylnaltrexone induced immediate bowel movements in all subjects (20). There were no opioid withdrawal symptoms or significant adverse effects.

Skin

Subcutaneous administration can cause skin erythema and induration at the injection site (SEDA-16, 81).

Parenteral self-administration of oral methadone can cause cellulitis, abscess formation, and necrosis of the skin and deeper tissues (9).

Death

There has been a cross-sectional survey of 238 patients in New South Wales who died during a methadone maintenance program in a 5-year period (21). There were 50 deaths (21%) in the first week of methadone maintenance treatment, 88% of which were drug-related. These findings reinforce the importance of a thorough drug and alcohol assessment of people seeking methadone maintenance treatment, cautious prescribing of methadone, frequent clinical review of patients, and tolerance to methadone during stabilization.

In a retrospective study of cases from the Jefferson County Coroner/Medical Examiners Office, Alabama, USA between January 1982 and December 2000 there were 101 deaths in patients in whom methadone was detected in the blood (22). Methadone was the sole intoxicant in 15 cases, with a mean concentration of 0.27 μg/ml. A benzodiazepine was the most frequently detected co-intoxicant in 60 of the 101 cases and the only co-intoxicant in another 30 cases. In 26 cases methadone had been taken with a range of non-benzodiazepine substances, including antidepressants, antipsychotic drugs, antiepileptic drugs, and cocaine. The high incidence of benzodiazepine + methadone related deaths can be explained by synergistic respiratory depression. Higher concentrations of methadone can occur with chronic abuse of methadone plus benzodiazepines, because over time benzodiazepines inhibit the hepatic enzymes that metabolize methadone. This might explain why the mean methadone concentration in the 30 deaths attributed to methadone plus a benzodiazepine was only 0.6 μg/ml.

Long-Term Effects

Drug tolerance

Several methadone studies have focused on opioid-dependent or opioid-abusing subjects. For example, six opioid-dependent individuals maintained on methadone subsequently developed cancer and continued to use methadone, but in a higher dose as an analgesic (16,23). The first five were partly refractory to the analgesic effects of opioids other than methadone, but all six achieved adequate analgesia without sedation or respiratory depression from aggressive upward intravenous methadone titration using an infusion of 100 mg/hour. Methadone was given in divided doses every 6–12 hours rather than once daily, as is customary in maintenance therapy for opioid dependence. The reasons for increasing the methadone dosage and frequency of administration are cross-tolerance to other opioids and the presence in methadone-maintained individuals of hyperalgesia to pain (a low pain tolerance to pain detection ratio) (24). These issues are also relevant to determining whether other drugs are more effective than morphine in managing acute pain in these patients.

Drug withdrawal

Four patients with methadone withdrawal psychosis have been described (SEDA-20, 79).

Second-Generation Effects

Pregnancy

Methadone is extensively used in opioid withdrawal and maintenance programs (see Drug tolerance in this monograph), and has been safely used for this purpose in pregnancy, with only mild effects on the offspring (25). However, fetal exposure to methadone in utero can cause a neonatal abstinence syndrome after delivery.

The outcomes in 100 chronic opiate-dependent pregnant women who received levomethadone substitution treatment have been reported (26). The average gestational age at delivery was 38 weeks and the mean birth weight was 2869 g. The rate of premature labor was 19% and the risk of premature delivery 11%. There were withdrawal symptoms in 74% of the neonates at a mean of 39 hours and all responded well to levomethadone.

Fetotoxicity

A newborn girl born of an HIV-positive mother who took antiretroviral drugs and methadone during pregnancy developed a methadone abstinence syndrome at day 7 (27). She was HIV-negative and was treated symptomatically for 15 days with chlorpromazine. The platelet count was 1049×10^9/l on day 17 and fell progressively to 290×10^9/l at 8 weeks. The authors suggested that the thrombocytosis had been secondary to intrauterine methadone exposure.

Susceptibility Factors

From a literature search and subsequent analysis of data on the relation between methadone prescribing and mortality, it was concluded that (28):

(a) 69% of deaths attributed to methadone occurred in subjects who had not previously received methadone;
(b) 51% of deaths attributed to methadone occurred during the dose-stabilizing period of methadone maintenance treatment;
(c) the dose of illicit methadone exceeded that prescribed for methadone maintenance therapy;
(d) deaths were attributed to discharge from prison and immediate intravenous injection of methadone in people who had lost their tolerance to high doses of methadone when incarcerated.

Subsequent advice related to the above identifiable susceptibility factors included:

(a) restriction of take-home prescriptions with daily supervised consumption of methadone in pharmacy premises;
(b) meticulous evaluation of substance abuse history;
(c) slowing down of increases and tolerance testing during the stabilization period of methadone maintenance; enhanced psychosocial assistance during the first months out of prison;
(d) use of naloxone as an adjunct to methadone syrup.

Drug Administration

Drug dosage regimens

The role of opioid rotation in cancer pain management has been described, highlighting the limitations of equianalgesic tablets and the need for monitoring and individualization of dose. This is particularly important when methadone is used as the opioid for conversion. The authors referred to a greater than expected potency of methadone, with excessive sedation and opioid-related adverse effects, if the switch is done on a one-to-one basis. They suggested that the calculated equianalgesic dose of methadone should be reduced by 75–90% and the dose then titrated upwards if necessary (29,30).

Drug administration route

Methadone has been used for intrathecal administration. Although this route can provide prolonged analgesia, the adverse effects have been reported to be unacceptable (SEDA-16, 81).

Of 90 patients undergoing abdominal or lower limb surgery randomly assigned double-blind to two groups, 60 received racemic methadone in initial doses of 3–6 mg followed by 6–12 mg by continuous infusion over 24 hours, and 30 received repeated boluses of 3–6 mg every 8 hours (31). In both groups the highest visual analogue score occurred 2 hours after surgery. From then on the pain diminished gradually and significantly at each recording. Opioid-related adverse effects were not different between the two groups, except for miosis, which was significantly more common in the bolus group. The results suggested that both epidural methadone protocols used in this study provide effective and safe postoperative analgesia. However, the infusion method should be preferred, as the doses of methadone can be reduced after the first day of treatment.

Drug–Drug Interactions

Antiretroviral drugs

Methadone is often used for opioid replacement therapy in intravenous drug abusers. The incidence of HIV infection is significantly higher in this population than in the general public, and interactions with drugs used for the treatment of AIDS are therefore important.

Methadone is predominantly metabolized by CYP3A4. Antiretroviral therapy with a non-nucleoside reverse transcriptase inhibitor (for example efavirenz, abacavir, and nevirapine) and/or a protease inhibitor (for example amprenavir) will induce the metabolism of methadone. This therapeutic combination is becoming increasingly common in HIV-positive substance misusers. Two studies have explicitly shown a significant reduction of methadone concentration by 28–87%. In the first study, 11 patients taking methadone maintenance therapy were given efavirenz and had a mean increase in methadone dosage requirement of 22% (32). In the second study, five methadone-maintained opioid-dependent individuals were given a combination of abacavir and amprenavir; the methadone concentration fell to 35% of the original concentration within 14 days (33).

In a prospective study of 54 patients taking antiretroviral drugs who also took methadone and a further 154 patients who did not take methadone there were similar clinical, virological, and immunological outcomes after 12 months (34). These results support the usefulness of methadone in the management of intravenous drug users with HIV infection.

Ritonavir, indinavir, saquinavir

In an in vitro study of the effects of the HIV-1 protease inhibitors, ritonavir, indinavir, and saquinavir, which are metabolized by the liver CYP3A4, all three protease inhibitors inhibited methadone demethylation and buprenorphine dealkylation in rank order of potency ritonavir > indinavir > saquinavir (35). Clinical studies are required to establish the further relevance of these observations.

Zidovudine

The metabolism of the antiviral nucleoside zidovudine to the inactive glucuronide form in vitro was inhibited by methadone (36). The concentration of methadone required for 50% inhibition was over 8 μg/ml, a supratherapeutic concentration, thus raising questions about the clinical significance of the effect. However, in eight recently detoxified heroin addicts, acute methadone treatment increased the AUC of oral zidovudine by 41% and of intravenous zidovudine by 19%, following the start of oral methadone (50 mg/day) (37). These effects resulted primarily from inhibition of zidovudine glucuronidation, but also from reduced renal clearance of zidovudine, and methadone concentrations remained in the target range throughout. It is recommended that increased toxicity surveillance, and possibly reduction in zidovudine dose, are indicated when the two drugs are co-administered.

Cimetidine

Cimetidine increases the effects of methadone, probably by inhibition of methadone metabolism (38).

Enzyme inducers

Enzyme-inducing drugs, such as carbamazepine, phenobarbital, phenytoin, and rifampicin, enhance the metabolism of methadone, leading to lower serum methadone concentrations (39).

Fluconazole

In a randomized, double-blind, placebo-controlled trial, oral fluconazole increased the serum methadone AUC by 35% (40). Although renal clearance was not significantly affected, mean serum methadone peak and trough concentrations rose significantly, while renal clearance was not significantly altered.

Phenytoin

Phenytoin enhances the metabolism of methadone (40).

Rifampicin

Enzyme-inducing drugs, such as rifampicin, enhance the metabolism of methadone, leading to lower serum methadone concentrations (40). This interaction is thought to have caused acute methadone withdrawal symptoms in two patients with AIDS (SEDA-16, 81).

Selective serotonin re-uptake inhibitors

Fluvoxamine

Fluvoxamine increases the effects of methadone, probably by inhibition of methadone metabolism (41).

Paroxetine

Paroxetine 20 mg/day, a selective CYP2D6 inhibitor, was given for 12 days to 10 patients on methadone maintenance (42). Eight were genotyped as CYP2D6 homozygous extensive metabolizers and two as poor metabolizers. Paroxetine increased the steady-state concentrations of *R*-methadone and *S*-methadone, especially in the extensive metabolizers.

Use of methadone in opioid withdrawal

A widely used technique for opioid detoxification, pioneered by Isbell and Vogel (43), involves the substitution of methadone for the illicit opioid, followed by a gradual reduction in the amount of methadone taken.

Methadone maintenance treatment was established in 1964 in New York City by Vincent Dole and Marie Nyswander. In the initial studies, subjects who were heavily addicted to heroin were evaluated and stabilized on daily methadone doses as inpatients before transfer to an outpatient clinic for continued treatment. With further experience, it was feasible to drop the inpatient phase (44).

Methadone is used to substitute for a variety of opioid drugs. It is well absorbed after oral ingestion, with peak blood concentrations after about 4 hours. Steady-state concentrations are reached after about 5 days. By virtue of its long duration of action (the half-life with regular dosing is about 22 hours), methadone suppresses opioid withdrawal symptoms for 24–36 hours. In the early stages of treatment patients may report problems such as drowsiness, insomnia, nausea, euphoria, difficulty in micturition, and excessive sweating. With the exception of chronic constipation and excessive sweating, these effects do not generally persist.

Methadone maintenance treatment is considered to be a medically safe treatment with relatively few and minimal adverse effects. However, the danger of serious adverse effects and death with the increasing use of methadone as maintenance therapy in drug addicts has been highlighted. It must be emphasized that a daily maintenance dose of 50–100 mg is toxic in a non-tolerant adult and as little as 10 mg can be fatal in a child. There is an increasing number of reports of the deaths of children of mothers on maintenance therapy from inadvertent ingestion.

British studies have shown that, using methadone, about 80% of inpatients, but only 17% of outpatients, were successfully withdrawn (45,46). However, the technique is not without problems, one being that the methadone reduces but does not eliminate withdrawal symptoms. The withdrawal response has been described as being akin to a mild case of influenza, objectively mild but subjectively severe (47). The fear of withdrawal symptoms expressed by those dependent on drugs should not be underestimated: these factors are associated with the subsequent severity of withdrawal symptoms, and they are more closely related to symptom severity than drug dosage (48). Methadone substitution can result in a protracted withdrawal response, with patients still experiencing significantly more symptoms than controls 2 weeks after withdrawal (49).

In a study of methadone withdrawal, patients who were withdrawn over 10 days had a withdrawal syndrome that began to increase in severity from day 3, with peak severity of symptoms on day 13; in those who were withdrawn over 21 days, symptoms began to increase about day 10 with a peak on day 20 and abated thereafter, although some patients did not recover fully until 40 days after starting withdrawal (50). Thus, the duration of the withdrawal syndrome is much the same for both treatments in terms of symptom severity. It is possible that an exponential rather than linear reduction in dosage may improve the withdrawal response. These results may be of clinical significance, in that patients may feel it important that they recover from withdrawal as quickly as possible, in order to participate fully in other aspects of drug withdrawal programs. However, although there was no difference between the 10-day and 21-day programs regarding completion rates for detoxification (70 and 79% respectively), the dropout rates after detoxification were significantly different. During the 10 days after the last dose of methadone, the dropout rate in the 21-day group was 18% compared with 30% in the 10-day group. These results may also have financial implications in respect of the number of subjects who can be admitted to treatment programs.

In some treatment programs, total abstinence is not considered to be a practical objective and treatment may involve the use of drugs such as methadone as maintenance therapy with the expectation of reducing illicit drug consumption (51). Well-organized methadone maintenance treatment can reduce the intake of illicit opioids in many injecting drug users (52,53).

Outcome studies of methadone maintenance treatment have reported favorable results. High rates of patient retention, reduced criminality, and improved social rehabilitation are reported. Despite its proved effectiveness, it remains a controversial approach among substance abuse treatment providers, public officials, policy makers, the medical profession, and the public at large. Nevertheless, almost every nation with a significant narcotic addiction problem has established a methadone maintenance treatment program.

For patients entering treatment from an institution where they have been drug-free, initial daily methadone doses should be no more than 20 mg. Otherwise initial daily doses of 30–40 mg should be sufficient to obtain the necessary balance between withdrawal and narcotic symptoms. Thereafter, stabilization is achieved by gradually increasing the dose. When methadone is given in adequate oral doses (usually 60 mg/day or more), a single dose in a stabilized patient lasts 24–36 hours, without creating euphoria and sedation. Tolerance to methadone seems to remain steady, and patients can be maintained on the same dose, in some cases for more than 20 years. The methadone dose must be determined individually, owing to individual variability in pharmacokinetics and pharmacodynamics. Maintenance of appropriate methadone blood concentrations is recommended.

Tolerance to the narcotic properties of methadone develops within 4–6 weeks, but tolerance to the autonomic effects (for example constipation and sweating) develops more slowly.

The major adverse effects during treatment occur during the initial stabilization phase. In addition to constipation and sweating, the most frequently reported adverse effects are transient skin rash, weight gain, and fluid retention. Since the main metabolic pathway of methadone is CYP3A4, numerous drug interactions can be expected. Drugs that interact with methadone are listed in the table in the monograph on opioids.

References

1. Ayonrinde OT, Bridge DT. The rediscovery of methadone for cancer pain management. Med J Aust 2000;173(10):536–40.
2. Mercadante S, Casuccio A, Agnello A, Barresi L. Methadone response in advanced cancer patients with pain followed at home. J Pain Symptom Manage 1999;18(3):188–92.
3. Hagen NA, Wasylenko E. Methadone: outpatient titration and monitoring strategies in cancer patients. J Pain Symptom Manage 1999;18(5):369–75.
4. Mercadante S, Casuccio A, Calderone L. Rapid switching from morphine to methadone in cancer patients with poor response to morphine. J Clin Oncol 1999;17(10):3307–12.
5. Mercadante S, Casuccio A, Fulfaro F, Groff L, Boffi R, Villari P, Gebbia V, Ripamonti C. Switching from morphine to methadone to improve analgesia and tolerability in cancer patients: a prospective study. J Clin Oncol 2001;19(11):2898–904.
6. Mironer YE, Tollison CD. Methadone in the intrathecal treatment of chronic nonmalignant pain resistant to other neuraxial agents: the first experience. Neuromodulation 2001;4:25–31.
7. Bell J, Zador D. A risk-benefit analysis of methadone maintenance treatment. Drug Saf 2000;22(3):179–90.
8. Chermack ST, Roll J, Reilly M, Davis L, Kilaru U, Grabowski J. Comparison of patient self-reports and urinalysis results obtained under naturalistic methadone treatment conditions. Drug Alcohol Depend 2000;59(1):43–9.
9. Nathan HJ. Narcotics and myocardial performance in patients with coronary artery disease. Can J Anaesth 1988;35(3 Pt 1):209–13.
10. Backmund M, Meyer K, Zwehl W, Nagengast O, Eichenlaub D. Myocardial Infarction associated with methadone and/or dihydrocodeine. Eur Addict Res 2001;7(1):37–9.
11. Hays H, Woodroffe MA. High dosing methadone and a possible relationship to serious cardia arrhythmias. Pain Res Manag 2001;6(2):64.
12. Deamer RL, Wilson DR, Clark DS, Prichard JG. Torsades de pointes associated with high dose levomethadyl acetate (ORLAAM). J Addict Dis 2001;20(4):7–14.
13. Krantz MJ, Lewkowiez L, Hays H, Woodroffe MA, Robertson AD, Mehler PS. Torsade de pointes associated with very-high-dose methadone. Ann Intern Med 2002;137(6):501–4.
14. Teichtahl H, Prodromidis A, Miller B, Cherry G, Kronborg I. Sleep-disordered breathing in stable methadone programme patients: a pilot study. Addiction 2001;96(3):395–403.
15. Wasserman S, Yahr MD. Choreic movements induced by the use of methadone. Arch Neurol 1980;37(11):727–8.
16. Manfredi PL, Gonzales GR, Payne R. Reversible spastic paraparesis induced by high-dose intravenous methadone. J Pain 2001;2(1):77–9.
17. Clark JD, Elliott J. A case of a methadone-induced movement disorder. Clin J Pain 2001;17(4):375–7.
18. Curran HV, Kleckham J, Bearn J, Strang J, Wanigaratne S. Effects of methadone on cognition, mood and craving in detoxifying opiate addicts: a dose-response study. Psychopharmacology (Berl) 2001;154(2):153–60.
19. Mintzer MZ, Stitzer ML. Cognitive impairment in methadone maintenance patients. Drug Alcohol Depend 2002;67(1):41–51.
20. Yuan CS, Foss JF, O'Connor M, Osinski J, Karrison T, Moss J, Roizen MF. Methylnaltrexone for reversal of constipation due to chronic methadone use: a randomized controlled trial. JAMA 2000;283(3):367–72.
21. Zador D, Sunjic S. Deaths in methadone maintenance treatment in New South Wales, Australia 1990–1995. Addiction 2000;95(1):77–84.
22. Mikolaenko I, Robinson CA Jr, Davis GG. A review of methadone deaths in Jefferson County, Alabama. Am J Forensic Med Pathol 2002;23(3):299–304.
23. Manfredi PL, Gonzales GR, Cheville AL, Kornick C, Payne R. Methadone analgesia in cancer pain patients on chronic methadone maintenance therapy. J Pain Symptom Manage 2001;21(2):169–74.
24. Doverty M, Somogyi AA, White JM, Bochner F, Beare CH, Menelaou A, Ling W. Methadone maintenance patients are cross-tolerant to the antinociceptive effects of morphine. Pain 2001;93(2):155–63.
25. Pinto F, Torrioli MG, Casella G, Tempesta E, Fundaro C. Sleep in babies born to chronically heroin addicted mothers. A follow up study. Drug Alcohol Depend 1988;21(1):43–7.
26. Kastner R, Hartl K, Lieber A, Hahlweg BC, Knobbe A, Grubert T. Substitutionsbehandlung von opiatabhängigen schwangeren'—Analyse der Behandlungverläufe an der 1. Ufk München. [Maintenance therapy in opiate-dependent pregnant patients—analysis of the course of therapy at the clinic of the University of Munich.] Geburtschilfe Frauenheilkd 2002;62:32–6.
27. Garcia-Algar O, Brichs LF, Garcia ES, Fabrega DM, Torne EE, Sierra AM. Methadone and neonatal thrombocytosis. Pediatr Hematol Oncol 2002;19(3):193–5.
28. Vormfelde SV, Poser W. Death attributed to methadone. Pharmacopsychiatry 2001;34(6):217–22.
29. Indelicato RA, Portenoy RK. Opioid rotation in the management of refractory cancer pain. J Clin Oncol 2002;20(1):348–52.
30. Watanabe S, Tarumi Y, Oneschuk D, Lawlor P. Opioid rotation to methadone: proceed with caution. J Clin Oncol 2002;20(9):2409–10.
31. Prieto-Alvarez P, Tello-Galindo I, Cuenca-Pena J, Rull-Bartomeu M, Gomar-Sancho C. Continuous epidural infusion of racemic methadone results in effective postoperative analgesia and low plasma concentrations. Can J Anaesth 2002;49(1):25–31.
32. Bart PA, Rizzardi PG, Gallant S, Golay KP, Baumann P, Pantaleo G, Eap CB. Methadone blood concentrations are decreased by the administration of abacavir plus amprenavir. Ther Drug Monit 2001;23(5):553–5.
33. Clarke SM, Mulcahy FM, Tjia J, Reynolds HE, Gibbons SE, Barry MG, Back DJ. The pharmacokinetics of methadone in HIV-positive patients receiving the non-nucleoside reverse transcriptase inhibitor efavirenz. Br J Clin Pharmacol 2001;51(3):213–17.
34. Moreno A, Perez-Elias MJ, Casado JL, Munoz V, Antela A, Dronda F, Navas E, Moreno S. Long-term outcomes of protease inhibitor-based therapy in antiretroviral treatment-naive HIV-infected injection drug users on methadone maintenance programmes. AIDS 2001;15(8):1068–70.
35. Iribarne C, Berthou F, Carlhant D, Dreano Y, Picart D, Lohezic F, Riche C. Inhibition of methadone and

buprenorphine N-dealkylations by three HIV-1 protease inhibitors. Drug Metab Dispos 1998;26(3):257–60.
36. Trapnell CB, Klecker RW, Jamis-Dow C, Collins JM. Glucuronidation of 3′-azido-3′-deoxythymidine (zidovudine) by human liver microsomes: relevance to clinical pharmacokinetic interactions with atovaquone, fluconazole, methadone, and valproic acid. Antimicrob Agents Chemother 1998;42(7):1592–6.
37. McCance-Katz EF, Rainey PM, Jatlow P, Friedland G. Methadone effects on zidovudine disposition (AIDS Clinical Trials Group 262). J Acquir Immune Defic Syndr Hum Retrovirol 1998;18(5):435–43.
38. Dawson GW, Vestal RE. Cimetidine inhibits the in vitro N-demethylation of methadone. Res Commun Chem Pathol Pharmacol 1984;46(2):301–4.
39. Finelli PF. Letter: Phenytoin and methadone tolerance. N Engl J Med 1976;294(4):227.
40. Cobb MN, Desai J, Brown LS Jr, Zannikos PN, Rainey PM. The effect of fluconazole on the clinical pharmacokinetics of methadone. Clin Pharmacol Ther 1998;63(6):655–62.
41. Iribarne C, Picart D, Dreano Y, Berthou F. In vitro interactions between fluoxetine or fluvoxamine and methadone or buprenorphine. Fundam Clin Pharmacol 1998;12(2):194–9.
42. Begre S, von Bardeleben U, Ladewig D, Jaquet-Rochat S, Cosendai-Savary L, Golay KP, Kosel M, Baumann P, Eap CB. Paroxetine increases steady-state concentrations of (R)-methadone in CYP2D6 extensive but not poor metabolizers. J Clin Psychopharmacol 2002;22(2):211–15.
43. Isbell H, Vogel VH, Chapman KW. Present status of narcotic addiction with particular reference to medical indications and comparative addiction liability of the newer and older analgesic drugs. JAMA 1948;138:1019.
44. Dole VP, Nyswander M. A medical treatment for diacetylmorphine (heroin) addiction. A clinical trial with methadone hydrochloride. JAMA 1965;193:646–50.
45. Glossop M, Johns A, Green L. Opiate withdrawal: in-patient vs out-patient programmes and preferred vs random assignment to treatment. BMJ (Clin Res Ed) 1986;293:103.
46. Gossop M, Green L, Phillips G, Bradley B. What happens to opiate addicts immediately after treatment: a prospective follow up study. BMJ (Clin Res Ed) 1987;294(6584):1377–80.
47. Kleber HD. Detoxification from narcotics. In: Lowinson L, Ruiz P, editors. Substance Abuse. Baltimore: Williams and Wilkins, 1981:317.
48. Phillips GT, Gossop M, Bradley B. The influence of psychological factors on the opiate withdrawal syndrome. Br J Psychiatry 1986;149:235–8.
49. Gossop M, Bradley B, Phillips GT. An investigation of withdrawal symptoms shown by opiate addicts during and subsequent to a 21-day in-patient methadone detoxification procedure. Addict Behav 1987;12(1):1–6.
50. Gossop M, Griffiths P, Bradley B, Strang J. Opiate withdrawal symptoms in response to 10-day and 21-day methadone withdrawal programmes. Br J Psychiatry 1989;154:360–3.
51. Newman RG, Whitehill WB. Double-blind comparison of methadone and placebo maintenance treatments of narcotic addicts in Hong Kong. Lancet 1979;2(8141):485–8.
52. Lowinson JH, Marion IJ, Joseph H, Dole VP. Methadone maintenance. In: Lowinson JH, Ruiz P, Millman RB, editors. Substance Abuse. A Comprehensive Textbook. 2nd ed. Baltimore: Williams and Wilkins, 1992:550.
53. Ball JC, Ross A. The Effectiveness of Methadone Maintenance Treatment. New York: Springer-Verlag, 1991.

Methanthelinium

General Information

Oral doses of 25–100 mg methanthelinium have typical anticholinergic adverse effects. Methanthelinium is considered to be more toxic than propantheline, mainly because its ganglion-blocking activity is relatively more marked than its antimuscarinic effect. Perhaps for this reason, impotence (1) has appeared to be a greater problem with this drug; central nervous adverse reactions, even including psychosis, have been reported in the past.

Reference

1. schwartz NH, Robinson BD. Impotence due to methantheline bromide. NY State J Med 1952;52(12):1530.

Methapyrilene

See also Antihistamines

General Information

Methapyrilene is a first-generation antihistamine with a relatively strong sedative effect. It is therefore a constituent of many sedative and sleep-inducing over-the-counter formulations.

Long-Term Effects

Drug abuse

Owing to easy access and abuse, intoxication with a fatal outcome has been reported with methapyrilene (1).

Reference

1. Winek CL, Fochtman FW, Trogus WJ Jr, Fusia EP, Shanor SP. Methapyrilene toxicity. Clin Toxicol 1977;11(3):287–94.

Methohexital

See also General anesthetics

General Information

Methohexital is an ultrashort-acting barbiturate that is widely used in dental anesthesia because of its rapid onset and short duration of action.

Of 4379 dental patients who received methohexital, 6.7% experienced restlessness, 5.5% respiratory disorders (respiratory obstruction, hiccuping, laryngeal spasm, apnea, or sneezing), 1.1% venous complications, 1.0%

delayed recovery, 0.5% excitation, 0.27% nausea and vomiting, and 0.2% other mild reactions (1). Pain at the site of injection occurs in up to 64% of patients; the addition of lidocaine 10 mg significantly reduced the incidence to 22% (2).

A selective inhibitor of neuronal nitric oxide synthase, 7-nitroindazole, prolonged the duration of methohexital-induced narcosis in rats (3). This finding is consistent with previous work showing potentiation of anesthetic agents by non-specific nitric oxide synthase inhibitors.

Organs and Systems

Cardiovascular

Vasodilatation and depressed myocardial contractility are possible hemodynamic consequences of high-dose methohexital anesthesia (4).

Respiratory

Rectal administration of methohexital, sometimes used for children with needle-phobia, can cause apnea, particularly if there are pre-existing nervous system abnormalities (SED-12, 242) (5).

Nervous system

Seizures are a possible but rare complication of methohexital (6); it is inadvisable to use it in a patient with a history of epilepsy.

References

1. McDonald D. Methohexitone in dentistry. Aust Dent J 1980;25(6):335–42.
2. Millar JM, Barr AM. The prevention of pain on injection. A study of the effect of intravenous lignocaine before methohexitone. Anaesthesia 1981;36(9):878–80.
3. Motzko D, Glade U, Tober C, Flohr H. 7-Nitro indazole enhances methohexital anesthesia. Brain Res 1998;788(1–2):353–5.
4. Todd MM, Drummond JC, Sang H. The hemodynamic consequences of high-dose methohexital anesthesia in humans. Anesthesiology 1984;61(5):495–501.
5. Yemen TA, Pullerits J, Stillman R, Hershey M. Rectal methohexital causing apnea in two patients with meningomyeloceles. Anesthesiology 1991;74(6):1139–41.
6. Rockoff MA, Goudsouzian NG. Seizures induced by methohexital. Anesthesiology 1981;54(4):333–5.

Methotrexate

General Information

Methotrexate is a folic acid antagonist that acts by inhibiting dihydrofolate reductase. Owing to its immunosuppressive and anti-inflammatory properties, low-dosage methotrexate (7.5–15 mg/week) has been extensively investigated for other therapeutic purposes characterized by inflammation or cellular proliferation. Since the mid-1980s, methotrexate has become one of the most widely used disease-modifying anti-rheumatic drugs (DMARDs) in rheumatoid arthritis. It also has a significant degree of efficacy in psoriasis, asthma, and inflammatory bowel disease, and may also be effective in systemic lupus erythematosus, giant cell arteritis, and Wegener's granulomatosis. The exact mechanisms by which methotrexate affects these diseases are still uncertain, and its clinical effects probably result from multiple biochemical events at a variety of cellular sites (1).

General adverse effects

Most of the experience regarding the adverse effects of low-dose methotrexate has accumulated in patients with rheumatoid arthritis. Adverse effects are very common during the first year of treatment and reach an incidence of 60–70%. However, they are rarely severe enough to require permanent drug withdrawal, even after very long-term treatment. Based on a cohort study of 152 patients with rheumatoid arthritis, the probability of methotrexate continuation was 30% at 10 years, and adverse effects were the most frequent reason (50%) for drug withdrawal (2). Even though the overall withdrawal rate for methotrexate-induced adverse effects is 7–16%, long-term methotrexate treatment required drug withdrawal because of adverse effects less often than several other second-line DMARDs (SEDA-22, 416). In a retrospective analysis of 437 rheumatoid arthritis patients treated for 3–106 months (mean = 35 months), the most common adverse effects were gastrointestinal disorders (20%), raised liver function tests (13%), respiratory disorders (6.4%), hematological abnormalities (4.4%), weakness (3.4%), central nervous system disorders (2.8%), infections (2.3%), mucocutaneous disorders (2.3%), and arthralgia (1.8%) (3). A Ritchie's index of 10 or less, a low polymorphonuclear leukocyte count, and the absence of rheumatoid factor predicted the occurrence of adverse effects.

In one study, 10 patients (of an original 29) were still taking methotrexate after a mean of 13 years and a mean cumulative dose of 9.7 g (4). The overall drug withdrawal rate was 48%, and the rate of adverse effects, particularly on the gut and central nervous system, fell with time (85% at baseline, 90% at 90 months, 62% at 160 months). It was felt that routine folate supplementation might have contributed to the observed reduction in toxicity, except for mouth ulcers or soreness. Very similar findings were found in another long-term (132 months) prospective study (5).

Raised methotrexate serum concentrations (over 100 nmol/l at 36–42 hours after ingestion) are expected to increase the likelihood of several adverse effects, that is, gastrointestinal and hematological effects, but similar adverse effects can be found even with low methotrexate serum concentrations. Reduced red cell folate concentrations during methotrexate treatment also related to adverse effects and rises in liver enzymes, and red cell folate concentrations above 800 nmol/l protected against common adverse effects and treatment withdrawal (6). Several investigators now advocate the concomitant use of folic acid (5–7 mg/week and up to 27.5 mg/week) to reduce some of methotrexate-associated adverse effects without reducing its efficacy (7).

Prevention of adverse effects

It is possible to reduce the incidence of several adverse effects of methotrexate by using folic or folinic acid. The usual practice is to give weekly folic acid in patients who are taking weekly methotrexate (on a different day) and daily folinic acid in those who are taking daily methotrexate. Folic acid supplementation is now commonly given to reduce the adverse effects of methotrexate, in particular its mucosal and gastrointestinal toxic effects (SED-14, 1297) (SEDA-23, 406), but less is known about how long this should be continued in patients taking long-term treatment.

In a meta-analysis of 307 patients with rheumatoid arthritis from seven randomized clinical trials, of whom 147 took folate supplementation, hematological adverse effects were not significantly reduced in the folate group (8). However, there was a 79% reduction in mucosal and gastrointestinal adverse effects in patients taking folic acid and a non-significant trend toward a reduction (42%) in patients taking folinic acid. Disease activity was not modified by low doses of folate. Finally, the authors noted that folinic acid is more expensive.

In 75 patients with rheumatoid arthritis taking methotrexate (up to 20 mg/week) and folic acid (5 mg/day), folic acid was withdrawn and the patients were randomized to restart folic acid ($n = 38$) or to take placebo ($n = 37$) double-blind, and were regularly assessed for 1 year (9). There were more withdrawals with placebo (46%) than with folic acid (21%) and more nausea. There were no obvious differences in efficacy. This suggests that folic acid supplementation is still helpful in the long term.

Organs and Systems

Cardiovascular

Cardiovascular adverse effects of methotrexate are extremely rare.

- There has been one detailed report of ventricular dysrhythmias and myocardial infarction, with recurrence of frequent ventricular extra beats on each readministration of methotrexate in a 36-year-old man (10).

It has been suggested that methotrexate increases mortality in patients with rheumatoid arthritis with cardiovascular co-morbidity (11). This assumption was based on a retrospective analysis of 632 patients with rheumatoid arthritis, of whom 73 died. The simultaneous presence of methotrexate and evidence of cardiovascular disease was an independent predictor of mortality. There was no such association with other DMARDs. The authors suggested that this effect may result from a methotrexate-induced increase in serum homocysteine, encouraging atherosclerosis.

Respiratory

Isolated and sustained cough is an unusual adverse effect of methotrexate. Among 13 patients who had a cough, only three met the criteria for methotrexate-induced pneumonitis (12). An irritant effect of methotrexate on the airways was therefore suggested.

Pneumonitis

Acute or subacute interstitial pneumonitis is an important but unpredictable and potentially life-threatening adverse effect of low-dose methotrexate (13–16).

Presentation

In patients with definite or probable methotrexate-induced lung injury, the predominant clinical features include shortness of breath, cough, and fever (13). Pathological examination usually shows an interstitial inflammatory cell infiltrate (sometimes granulomatous or with alveolar damage), and variable degrees of interstitial fibrosis. Unfortunately, confirmatory evidence is sometimes hard to obtain, particularly in patients with rheumatoid arthritis in whom rheumatoid interstitial lung disease can also occur. Infectious pneumonias, particularly viral or *Pneumocystis jiroveci* pneumonia, which resemble methotrexate pneumonitis and can occur as a result of immunosuppression, should also be carefully excluded.

- Pulmonary endoalveolar hemorrhage was a possible complication of pneumonitis in a 57-year-old woman who voluntarily increased her dosage of methotrexate from 7.5 mg once a week to 7.5 mg/day for 15 days (17).

The potential severity of methotrexate pneumonitis was finally exemplified in a careful retrospective multicenter study of 29 patients with definite or probable criteria for methotrexate-induced lung injury (13). Overall, five patients (17%) died, two of them after methotrexate rechallenge.

Frequency

The prevalence of methotrexate pneumonitis has been variably estimated from 0.3 to 18%, with a mean estimated prevalence of 3.3% (14,16). In a review of the respiratory complications of methotrexate, the authors concluded that pneumonitis occurs in 7% of patients, in 25% of whom it is fatal as a result of respiratory failure (18). This can occur with any dose of methotrexate, given via any route; it has occurred after the intrathecal administration of 12 mg given for central nervous system prophylaxis (19). In a review of 194 patients with rheumatoid arthritis and 38 with psoriatic arthritis, the prevalences of pneumonitis were 2.1 and 0.03% respectively (14), which is similar to the 3.2% incidence in a prospective study of 124 patients with rheumatoid arthritis (20). Another analysis performed over 5 years showed that the estimated prevalence of definite or probable pneumonitis was only 0.86% in 1162 patients (10 patients, of whom three died), but this conclusion was based on a limited retrospective identification of cases (21).

Mechanism

Even though methotrexate pneumonitis was first described about 30 years ago, very little is known about the mechanism, and whether it is due to direct cumulative toxicity, hypersensitivity, or an idiosyncratic reaction. In one case, interleukin-8 was speculated to play an important role in the pathogenesis (22).

Susceptibility factors

Susceptibility factors for methotrexate pneumonitis are still poorly understood. In one study, no risk factors were identified and periodic pulmonary function tests were not predictive (20). In contrast, advanced age, diabetes, pre-existing rheumatoid pleuropulmonary involvement or previous lung disease, previous use of DMARDs, and hypoalbuminemia were suggested as the most reliable predictors of methotrexate-induced pneumonitis in a large historical case-control study (15,23). The weekly dose, the cumulative dose, and the duration of treatment were not related to its occurrence. A history of drug-induced pulmonary disorders was also thought to favor methotrexate pneumonitis, but this was based on a single case report in a patient who previously had aminorex-induced primary pulmonary hypertension (SEDA-22, 416).

Management

The management of methotrexate pneumonitis primarily requires methotrexate withdrawal and supportive care. Although glucocorticoids are commonly used, there is as yet no evidence that they positively influence the outcome. Any readministration of methotrexate is dangerous, and four of six patients treated again with methotrexate developed recurrent lung toxicity, of whom two died (13).

Based on a report of 9 cases and a careful reanalysis of 123 previously published cases, the clinical spectrum and histopathology of methotrexate-induced pneumonitis have been reviewed (24). The authors stressed that methotrexate pneumonitis should be promptly recognized to avoid a severe outcome, although no specific features could be identified compared with other drug-induced adverse lung effects and no definite pathological findings compared with rheumatoid lung. Diagnostic criteria therefore mostly included a history of exposure, the exclusion of other pulmonary diseases, especially infections, and the presence of pulmonary infiltrates on the chest X-ray. Once methotrexate pneumonitis developed, 13% of the patients died from respiratory failure, clearly underlining the fact that methotrexate pneumonitis is potentially life-threatening. Methotrexate reintroduction should also be strongly discouraged in such cases, because about 25% of patients experience recurrence.

Nervous system

Reports of necrotizing leukoencephalopathy in association with methotrexate have been verified by biopsy or autopsy (25,26). Serial electroencephalography can predict this, since slow-wave activity develops during the administration of high-dose methotrexate. Autopsy has shown widespread necrosis and spongiosis in the cerebral and cerebellar white matter in such cases (25).

Chronic brain edema, multifocal white matter necrosis, and deep brain atrophy have been reported in patients who received high-dose methotrexate therapy, with an incidence of 4% (27). All patients received methotrexate 8–9 g/m^2 intravenously over 4 hours. The encephalopathy began abruptly, an average of 6 days after the second or third weekly treatment, presenting with behavioral abnormalities. These ranged from laughter to lethargy or unresponsiveness. In some patients, there were focal sensorimotor or reflex signs and generalized seizures. The disorder lasted from 15 minutes to 72 hours, and it disappeared as abruptly as it began, without specific treatment.

A rare case of a reversible neurological disturbance associated with focal subcortical white matter pathology has been described after administration of methotrexate 3 g/m^2. In patients who received 8–12.5 g/m^2, the incidence of neurological abnormalities was 4%. All of these patients were also receiving methotrexate intrathecally as well, but the relevance of this is not known (28).

In one case, low-dose methotrexate was implicated in leukoencephalopathy (29).

Treatment with intrathecal methotrexate of children under 5 years of age with acute lymphoblastic leukemia (irrespective of other drugs) has structural and functional effects on the developing neocerebellar–frontal subsystem (30).

Acute dysarthria has been attributed to methotrexate (31).

- A 71-year-old man was given oral methotrexate (15 mg/week) for a cutaneous T cell lymphoma. Within 3 weeks he developed progressive dysarthria and incoordination, and neurological examination showed mild buccofacial dyskinesia. Complete examination was otherwise normal, and he fully recovered 6–8 weeks after methotrexate withdrawal.

This case is reminiscent of other previously reported neurological abnormalities with low-dose methotrexate.

Psychological, psychiatric

There was a significantly higher risk of late cognitive impairment (concentration and memory) in patients ($n = 39$) taking adjuvant cyclophosphamide, fluorouracil, and methotrexate than in controls matched for age, disease, surgery, and radiation dose (32).

In studies of the neurotoxic effects of low-dose methotrexate treatment, dizziness, headache, visual disturbances or hallucinations, lack of concentration, cognitive dysfunction, and depression-like symptoms were detected in 1–35% of patients (33,34). Advanced age and mild renal insufficiency were possible susceptibility factors (34).

Nutrition

Of patients receiving high-dose methotrexate (5–8 g/m^2), 95% developed a significant increase in serum phenylalanine concentrations, probably due to inhibition of dihydropteridine reductase (35). The clinical significance of this is not obvious, although it is possible that it may contribute to the transient neurological disturbance observed in some patients taking high-dose methotrexate.

Hematologic

Significant hematological abnormalities occur in 10–24% of patients who take methotrexate. Mild to moderate leukopenia is the most frequent, followed by thrombocytopenia. Isolated thrombocytopenia and anemia are uncommon (SEDA-22, 416) (36). In a retrospective study in 315 patients, 13 had thrombocytopenia, two of whom also had pancytopenia (37). Thrombocytopenia correlated with the weekly dosage of methotrexate administered on the same day as NSAIDs, and methotrexate was safely reintroduced in patients who developed thrombocytopenia as a result of concomitant administration of both drugs, provided that NSAIDs were withheld at least on the day of methotrexate administration.

Pancytopenia is a rare but potentially fatal complication, and numerous reports have been published. The characteristics and incidence of pancytopenia have been carefully re-evaluated from case reports and clinical trials published from 1980 to 1995 (38). Of 70 reported cases, 12 patients died (17%). Impaired renal function was the most important contributing factor (54%), particularly in fatal cases (10/12). Other important susceptibility factors included advanced age (over 65 years), hypoalbuminemia, concurrent infection, and/or concomitant multiple medications (particularly co-trimoxazole). The mean cumulative dosage was 675 (10–4800) mg, and the minimal cumulative methotrexate dose leading to fatal pancytopenia was 10 mg. This confirms that pancytopenia can occur at any time during treatment, even in the absence of known susceptibility factors. Bone marrow biopsy showed megaloblastosis and hypocellularity. Eosinophilia and increased mean corpuscular volume were rarely observed. In an overall review of five long-term prospective studies (511 patients), the calculated incidence of methotrexate-induced pancytopenia was 1.4%. Although severe myelosuppression sometimes required folinic acid, there are as yet no data to determine whether prophylactic folate supplementation can reduce the incidence of pancytopenia.

In a double-blind, placebo-controlled study of the safety and efficacy of methotrexate therapy combined with glucocorticoids in patients with giant cell arteritis over 24 months, adverse events were defined as a new diagnosis of any condition during treatment (39). The combination of methotrexate plus prednisolone reduced the number of relapses and improved the course of the disease. Methotrexate was withdrawn in three patients who had adverse events that were clearly drug-related. One had leukopenia, anemia, and mucositis, one developed pancytopenia, and one oral ulcers. These patients were not taking folic acid or folinic acid supplements.

Gastrointestinal

Gastrointestinal adverse effects (stomatitis, anorexia, abdominal pain, dyspepsia, nausea, vomiting, diarrhea, and weight loss) are very common, particularly after oral administration of methotrexate (up to 50%), and often require dosage adjustment (3). Folic acid supplementation reduces the incidence of several gastrointestinal adverse effects.

Stomatitis can sometimes be particularly harmful and has been reported as the cause of transient or permanent treatment withdrawal in 4.5 and 1.1% of 1539 patients respectively (40). However, one study did not show significant differences in the number of oral lesions or the duration or frequency of stomatitis between patients with rheumatoid arthritis taking methotrexate and those not taking methotrexate (19/51 versus 9/46), although the prevalence of ulceration was higher in the methotrexate group (41).

Liver

Cytolytic hepatitis has been reported in a 58-year-old man being treated with intramuscular methotrexate 10 mg/week (total dose over the previous 4 years 2.3 g); it resolved within 2 weeks of stopping therapy (42).

Hepatic fibrosis and cirrhosis

The main concern over long-term treatment with methotrexate is hepatic fibrosis and cirrhosis. Methotrexate hepatotoxicity was initially reported in children given high daily dose methotrexate for leukemia. After its introduction for the treatment of psoriasis, several papers published in the late 1960s pointed out the possible risk of severe hepatic fibrosis and cirrhosis in patients taking moderate daily doses. Since then many studies have focused on the extent of long-term methotrexate hepatotoxicity in patients taking low-dose methotrexate for psoriasis and rheumatoid arthritis. However, the evidence on the frequency and severity of severe liver disease in these patients is still highly controversial, since there may be liver histological changes before methotrexate treatment, particularly in patients with psoriasis. Furthermore, there are numerous confounding factors (Table 1) which can contribute to histological liver changes, leading several authors to suggest as early as 1990 that methotrexate-induced hepatic fibrosis and cirrhosis is uncommon and only occurs in patients with other susceptibility factors (43).

Frequency

The incidence of liver cirrhosis after a mean dose of 2 g is 7–10%. Once 1.5 g has been administered (44), or 2 years after starting long-term treatment, biopsy should be discussed (45).

Liver failure or cirrhosis were identified among 24 patients in a retrospective survey of more than 16 600 patients with rheumatoid arthritis who had taken

Table 1 Susceptibility factors for hepatotoxicity of methotrexate

Strong association	Previous or concurrent heavy alcohol use
	Pre-existing liver disease
	Daily methotrexate administration
	Renal insufficiency
Probable association	Duration of methotrexate treatment (over 2 years)
	Cumulative methotrexate dose (over 1500 mg)
	Prior treatment with arsenicals
	Obesity with diabetes mellitus
Possible or potential association	Maximum weekly dose over 25 mg
	Obesity alone
	Diabetes mellitus alone
	Heterozygous $alpha_1$ -antitrypsin deficiency
	Felty's syndrome
	Prior treatment with vitamin A
	Concurrent NSAID use
	Concurrent treatment with ciclosporin
	Concurrent PUVA treatment
No association	Sex
	HLA phenotype
	Extent of psoriatic skin involvement
	Duration of rheumatoid arthritis
	Glucocorticoid therapy
Negative association	Concurrent folate supplementation
	Concurrent hydroxychloroquine use

methotrexate for at least 5 years, giving an estimated 5-year frequency of one in 1000 (46).

No morphological features of methotrexate hepatotoxicity were demonstrated after 2 years of methotrexate treatment in 48 patients with primary biliary cirrhosis (47).

Collectively, the available data suggest that methotrexate rarely causes significant serious liver damage in patients who have been otherwise carefully selected, who present no risk factors for methotrexate-induced hepatotoxicity, and who have received lower weekly dosages with strict monitoring of liver function (for example transaminases) in order to reduce methotrexate doses when liver enzymes are persistently raised (48).

Diagnosis and monitoring

Routine liver function tests do not reliably indicate liver damage, and they may not become abnormal until there is already considerable liver damage. It is therefore common practice to monitor patients by conducting annual liver biopsies. Measurement of the serum amino-terminal propeptide of type III procollagen (PIII PI) has been used as an alternative to liver biopsy; high concentrations correlate with fibrosis on liver biopsy (49). No patient with a normal serum concentration had an abnormal biopsy. An increase in the plasma phenylalanine/tyrosine ratio in children and adolescents can provide clinical evidence of liver damage before the appearance of symptoms in patients who have taken high doses of methotrexate (50).

Methods of monitoring patients for possible methotrexate hepatotoxicity and guidelines have been reviewed (48,51,52). It should be mentioned that the frequent rise in serum transaminases (involving 30–80% of patients) after the start of treatment is transient and does not predict liver damage; only persistently abnormal transaminases are potential indicators of methotrexate hepatotoxicity.

Mechanism

Folate depletion may be a factor in the pathogenesis of methotrexate-induced liver disease. In 30 patients on long-term methotrexate therapy, aimed at determining whether erythrocyte concentrations of folate and methotrexate might provide an indication for liver biopsy, there was no difference between red cell folate concentrations in patients with cirrhosis or progressive liver fibrosis and patients without fibrosis or with non-progressive hepatic fibrosis. Erythrocyte methotrexate concentrations were higher in patients with progressive hepatic disease, but cumulative dose and length of treatment were stronger predictors. In individual cases, erythrocyte folate and methotrexate concentrations were not a reliable guide (53).

Pathology

In patients with rheumatoid arthritis, baseline histological liver abnormalities were less common, with mild fibrosis only in 0–15% of patients. In retrospective studies with no pre-methotrexate liver biopsies, mild fibrosis was found in 3–35% of patients taking methotrexate, moderate or severe fibrosis in 0–10%, and cirrhosis in 0–2%. However, no case of cirrhosis was identified in studies which compared pre- and postmethotrexate biopsies or sequential biopsies while on long-term methotrexate, that is, a mean cumulative dose of 1200–5000 mg (52). Again, both worsening and improvement of histological lesions occurred. The application of guidelines to prevent methotrexate hepatotoxicity may account for these reassuring results. Liver biopsy changes were moderate or absent in patients with juvenile rheumatoid arthritis who took a cumulative dose of over 3000 mg (SEDA-21, 388) (52).

In 22 of 29 patients (76%) who were treated with low-pulse doses of methotrexate for rheumatoid arthritis, liver biopsy specimens showed variability in liver cell nuclear size, glycogenated nuclei, and fatty change. Occasionally there was mild portal infiltration with lymphocytes. There were no significant differences in age, duration of treatment, or cumulative dose amongst the cases. Serial increases in serum transaminases and/or alkaline phosphatase activity and development of hypoalbuminemia during treatment were indicators of development of liver disease (54).

In another study, the pathological lesions found in liver biopsies from patients treated with methotrexate were non-specific, consisting usually of macrovesicular steatosis, nuclear pleomorphism, chronic inflammatory infiltrates in the portal tracts, focal liver cell necrosis, fibrosis, and cirrhosis (52).

The pathological features of methotrexate-induced liver damage have been comprehensively reviewed (52). In patients with psoriasis, baseline liver biopsies were often abnormal, with mild fibrosis, moderate or severe fibrosis, and cirrhosis in 0–30, 0–7, and 0–1.5% respectively. These figures increased after methotrexate use, with fibrosis and cirrhosis in 14–34 and 0–21% respectively.

Ultrastructural studies have sometimes identified Ito cell prominence and collagen deposition in the perisinusoidal space of Disse during the first months of treatment and before the appearance of any signs of fibrosis, but these findings have been disputed in rheumatoid arthritis patients. Using immunohistochemical quantification, increased matrix proteins, collagen and transforming growth factor alpha were also found as possible early markers of methotrexate hepatotoxicity (55).

Susceptibility factors

The susceptibility factors for methotrexate-induced hepatotoxicity are listed in Table 1.

In a meta-analysis of 636 patients from 15 studies, who took chronic low-dose methotrexate for rheumatoid arthritis or psoriasis, the risk of liver toxicity increased with cumulative dose and heavy alcohol intake (56).

In one study, the risk of developing cirrhosis progressively increased with the total cumulative dose of methotrexate, from 13% at 2200 mg to 26% at 4000 mg (57). However, studies that compared sequential liver biopsies in patients on treatment and included specific recommendations for patient selection and the monitoring of methotrexate hepatotoxicity, gave contrasting results, with a lower incidence of cirrhosis even after high cumulative methotrexate doses (up to 5100 mg) (52). In addition, although histological lesions can worsen during treatment, improvement or absence of progression of prior fibrosis/cirrhosis has been found in very long-term follow-up of patients still taking methotrexate after 10 years (58).

The incidence and susceptibility factors of rises in serum transaminases have been detailed from a retrospective analysis of 66 patients with rheumatoid arthritis (59). There was an asymptomatic increase in serum transaminases in 42 and 49% of patients respectively, an incidence 4–5 times greater than that found in 21 patients taking other DMARDs. Although most of the rises in transaminases were transient and spontaneously reversible, 14 patients had sustained rises. There was a close relation between the incidence of high transaminases and the weight-adjusted dose of methotrexate. In a multivariate regression analysis, only obesity, methotrexate dose (over 0.15 mg/kg/week), and the concomitant presence of gastrointestinal adverse effects were significantly and independently associated with the likelihood of a rise in alanine transaminase. In the 14 patients who had persistently high transaminases, weekly folic acid 5 mg produced a sustained fall in serum alanine transaminase within 3 months, but three patients had to be withdrawn because of exacerbation of rheumatoid arthritis.

Urinary tract

Low-dose methotrexate is usually not regarded as nephrotoxic, and one report of nephrotic syndrome with minimal change disease on renal biopsy should be regarded with caution, since there was recovery after glucocorticoid treatment and withdrawal of concomitant NSAIDs (SEDA-22, 416).

However, renal toxicity occurs with high-dose methotrexate and more likely to occur with concomitant administration of other nephrotoxic agents, such as aminoglycosides, cephalosporins, NSAIDs, and diuretics (60).

The pathogenesis of methotrexate-induced nephrotoxicity is not understood, but it is thought to result from crystallization of methotrexate in the renal tubules. Adequate hydration and urinary alkalinization are necessary to minimize this effect (61). Urinary beta$_2$ microglobulin may be a useful marker of methotrexate nephrotoxicity (62).

When serum methotrexate concentrations are high, leucovorin (folinic acid) rescue may protect against renal damage. Methotrexate concentrations are only transiently lowered by hemoperfusion, and they are unaffected by peritoneal dialysis once there is acute renal insufficiency. Sustained reductions in drug concentrations and recovery of renal function have been reported after charcoal hemoperfusion followed by hemodialysis (63,64).

Co-administration of methotrexate and procarbazine in the treatment of medulloblastomas increases the risk of methotrexate nephrotoxicity. Delayed administration of methotrexate until 72 hours after procarbazine therapy has been given may reduce this risk (65).

Skin

Since the first descriptions of the rapid development of a large number of nodules, also termed "accelerated nodulosis," in methotrexate-treated patients, a number of such reports have accumulated in patients with rheumatoid arthritis or, more rarely, psoriatic arthritis (66–68). Nodulosis is characterized by the development of small, painful, multiple nodules, sometimes disseminated; pulmonary, meningeal, or pericardial nodulosis has also been reported in a few patients (SEDA-21, 387) (67,69,70). Four cases of nodulosis and four of cutaneous vasculitis were noted during a long-term follow-up of 437 rheumatoid arthritis patients (3), but the estimated incidence of accelerated nodulosis was found to be higher in other studies: that is, 8–12% (5,66,70).

The nodules can appear at any time during treatment, with or without concomitant cutaneous vasculitis, and are usually found in patients with erosive disease and a high titer of rheumatoid factor. This has raised the question as to whether they are a reason to modify treatment, and whether they are rheumatic or represent a true adverse effect of methotrexate; certainly, methotrexate-associated nodulosis is very similar to idiopathic rheumatoid arthritis nodulosis and sometimes disappears despite continuation of methotrexate. However, prompt regression on methotrexate withdrawal and recurrence on rechallenge in several patients strongly argue for a causal drug-related effect.

There was a characteristic clinical and histopathological spectrum of skin lesions, distinct from rheumatoid papules, in four patients who took low-dose methotrexate for acute flares of collagen vascular disease (71). These so-called methotrexate-induced rheumatoid papules developed shortly after methotrexate administration consisted of erythematous indurated papules mostly affecting the proximal limbs, and disappeared after methotrexate was withdrawn or tapered. Histology showed inflammatory infiltrates of interstitially arranged histiocytes and a few neutrophils, but no features of leukocytoclastic vasculitis.

Isolated cutaneous leukocytoclastic vasculitis occurs infrequently in patients taking methotrexate, and an immediate-type hypersensitivity reaction has been thought to be involved, in view of prompt recurrence after drug readministration or a positive mast cell degranulation test as recorded in several patients (SEDA-21, 388) (SEDA-22, 417) (72).

Other isolated reports included the occurrence of skin ulceration (SEDA-22, 388) and one fatal case of toxic epidermal necrolysis (SEDA-21, 388).

Persistent hyperpigmentation is an unusual manifestation of weekly administration of methotrexate (73).

- Severely ulcerated psoriatic plaques and acute extensive exfoliative dermatitis occurred in a 37-year-old man who had taken methotrexate for 5 years for psoriasis (74).

In the context of a case of severe reactivation of recent sunburn after a single injection of methotrexate for ectopic pregnancy in a 40-year-old woman, the authors reviewed the literature on methotrexate photosensitivity (75). Photodermatitis reactivation is the only well-documented type of photosensitivity associated with methotrexate. It can occur if methotrexate is given at 2–5 days after excessive exposure to ultraviolet or X-radiation.

A previously unreported skin reaction mimicking Stevens–Johnson syndrome has been reported (76).

- A 61-year-old woman inadvertently took a high dose of methotrexate (10 mg/day) for psoriasis, and developed mucosal ulcers after 3 months. One month later, methotrexate (20 mg/week) was restarted, but she developed painful oral ulceration and burning skin lesions 3 days later. She had an erythema multiform-like rash and several buccal ulcers. There was a moderate pancytopenia. Histological examination of the skin showed features consistent with an acute graft-versus-host reaction. All medications except aspirin were withdrawn, and she recovered fully after treatment with calcium folinate and prednisolone.

The authors speculated that concomitant aspirin may have contributed to this severe reaction.

Hair

Mild alopecia is common in patients taking methotrexate (77,78).

Nails

Yellow nail pigmentation without paronychia has been noted in a patient with psoriasis taking methotrexate (79).

Musculoskeletal

Arthralgia and myalgia sometimes occur within 24 hours of methotrexate injections in patients with rheumatoid arthritis. These transient effects, which can be accompanied by fatigue, malaise, and various neuropsychological disorders, have escaped recognition, but they occurred in 10% of patients over 18 months and sometimes resulted in treatment withdrawal (80).

Leg pain and spontaneous fractures attributed to prolonged high-dose methotrexate therapy in pediatric oncology have been recognized since the 1970s, but there have been some cases in patients taking low-dose methotrexate (81,82). All the same, it is still controversial as to whether methotrexate can actually cause changes in bone metabolism (83). There was a significant reduction in bone mineral density in 11 postmenopausal women taking methotrexate for primary biliary cirrhosis compared with 11 matched controls not taking methotrexate (84). Among 133 patients with rheumatoid arthritis, methotrexate without glucocorticoids was not associated with changes in the bone mineral density after 3 years of treatment, but methotrexate plus prednisone (over 5 mg/day) produced greater bone loss than prednisone alone (85). In contrast, another study failed to show accelerated bone loss in methotrexate users compared with non-users, but the study was limited to 10 patients in each group (86).

The possible effects of methotrexate on bone metabolism and bone loss have been discussed in the context of two adults (87) and in relation to a study in children with juvenile rheumatoid arthritis (88) who had delayed bone healing after surgery. The two adults, aged 52 and 62 years, had been taking methotrexate (7.5 and 15 mg/week) for 14 and 15 months when they underwent metatarsal and tibial osteotomy. Because X-ray examination 5 and 6 months after surgery showed non-union, methotrexate was withdrawn; the bone healed promptly in both patients within 2 months. The authors thought that the outcome in these patients without risk factors for bone fragility suggested that temporary methotrexate withdrawal should be considered in cases of delayed bone healing after surgery.

In contrast, in a longitudinal study of 32 patients with juvenile rheumatoid arthritis, there was no evidence of deleterious effects of long-term, low-dose methotrexate on bone mass density (88). The cumulative dose of glucocorticoids, weight, and height were the main determinants of bone mass changes.

Furthermore, there is evidence that it is disease activity rather than methotrexate that accounts for changes in bone mass (89). This 2-year longitudinal study involved 22 patients taking methotrexate and 18 patients taking other DMARDs; it was strictly controlled for the use of glucocorticoids. There were significant and equal reductions in trabecular bone mineral density in both groups. Bone loss was most marked in patients with active disease.

Sexual function

Impotence has very rarely been attributed to methotrexate (90).

Reproductive system

Although the occurrence of gynecomastia requiring surgical excision in two patients might have been coincidental (91), in another patient it disappeared after methotrexate withdrawal and recurred on rechallenge (92).

Immunologic

Immediate hypersensitivity reactions are rare after low-dose methotrexate.

- A 53-year-old woman had three episodes of angioedema while taking methotrexate, with no recurrence after withdrawal (93).

Vasculitis has been infrequently reported in patients taking low-dose methotrexate (SEDA-21, 388) (SEDA-22, 417) (94). Although most cases have been observed in patients with rheumatoid arthritis, suggesting that the underlying disease plays a part, vasculitis has also been described in a patient with ankylosing spondylitis (95). Methotrexate was also reported to have exacerbated pre-existing urticarial vasculitis in a 32-year-old woman; the lesions recurred after rechallenge (96).

Infection risk

Methotrexate-related immunosuppression can be expected to increase the likelihood of infections. The infection rate reported in patients taking low-dose methotrexate has varied from one study to another. In a literature review focusing on patients with rheumatoid arthritis taking methotrexate, the mean infection rate was 1.8% in retrospective studies, 4.6% in open studies, and 11.6% in double-blind studies (97). Infections usually occurred within 1.5 years of starting treatment and mostly comprised common respiratory or cutaneous bacterial infections, *Herpes zoster*, and, more rarely, opportunistic infections. In one comparative study, the overall risk of infections was considered to be low and similar in patients taking methotrexate and azathioprine (97), but others have found a higher prevalence of infections and an increase in antibiotic use in patients with rheumatoid arthritis taking methotrexate as compared to other DMARDs, except cyclophosphamide (98,99).

NSAIDs

Theoretically, NSAIDs can increase methotrexate serum concentrations by competition for renal tubular secretion (140). Since the publication of case histories reporting severe toxic effects in patients taking methotrexate and NSAIDs, there has been much concern among patients taking low-dose methotrexate (SEDA-20, 89) (SEDA-21, 100). However, most of the reports related to patients taking doses of methotrexate higher than those recommended in rheumatoid arthritis. From often mutually contradictory data, it appears that co-administration of most NSAIDs and stable low-dose methotrexate is relatively safe and that the supposed risks have little clinical significance in patients with normal renal function who are regularly monitored for hepatic, hematological, and renal toxicity (141).

In one study there was a significant reduction in renal methotrexate clearance and creatinine clearance in patients who took NSAIDs plus a high maintenance dose of methotrexate (16.6 mg/week), but no change in either variable in patients taking a stable maintenance dose of 7.5 mg/week (142). This suggests that patients taking higher doses should be more closely monitored for early signs of renal impairment that could predispose them to methotrexate toxicity.

Penicillin

Concomitant penicillin administration has been reported to exacerbate the hematological toxicity of low-dose methotrexate (143). This could have been due to inhibition of the tubular secretion of methotrexate.

Probenecid

Probenecid competes with methotrexate for renal tubular secretion, and can cause severe hematological toxicity.

- Severe pancytopenia occurred in an elderly patient taking low-dose methotrexate and probenecid (144).

Triamterene

Drugs that inhibit folate metabolism increase the likelihood of serious adverse reactions to methotrexate, particularly hematological toxicity. Bone marrow suppression and reduced plasma folate concentrations resulted from the concomitant administration of triamterene with methotrexate (145).

References

1. Cronstein BN. Molecular therapeutics. Methotrexate and its mechanism of action. Arthritis Rheum 1996; 39(12):1951–60.
2. Alarcon GS, Tracy IC, Strand GM, Singh K, Macaluso M. Survival and drug discontinuation analyses in a large cohort of methotrexate treated rheumatoid arthritis patients. Ann Rheum Dis 1995;54(9):708–12.
3. Bologna C, Viu P, Picot MC, Jorgensen C, Sany J. Long-term follow-up of 453 rheumatoid arthritis patients treated with methotrexate: an open, retrospective, observational study. Br J Rheumatol 1997;36(5):535–40.
4. Kremer JM. Safety, efficacy, and mortality in a long-term cohort of patients with rheumatoid arthritis taking methotrexate: followup after a mean of 13.3 years. Arthritis Rheum 1997;40(5):984–5.
5. Weinblatt ME, Maier AL, Fraser PA, Coblyn JS. Longterm prospective study of methotrexate in rheumatoid arthritis: conclusion after 132 months of therapy. J Rheumatol 1998;25(2):238–42.
6. Andersen LS, Hansen EL, Knudsen JB, Wester JU, Hansen GV, Hansen TM. Prospectively measured red cell folate levels in methotrexate treated patients with rheumatoid arthritis: relation to withdrawal and side effects. J Rheumatol 1997;24(5):830–7.
7. Morgan SL, Baggott JE, Vaughn WH, Austin JS, Veitch TA, Lee JY, Koopman WJ, Krumdieck CL, Alarcon GS. Supplementation with folic acid during methotrexate therapy for rheumatoid arthritis. A double-blind, placebo-controlled trial. Ann Intern Med 1994; 121(11):833–41.
8. Ortiz Z, Shea B, Suarez-Almazor ME, Moher D, Wells GA, Tugwell P. The efficacy of folic acid and folinic acid in reducing methotrexate gastrointestinal toxicity in rheumatoid arthritis. A metaanalysis of randomized controlled trials. J Rheumatol 1998;25(1):36–43.
9. Griffith SM, Fisher J, Clarke S, Montgomery B, Jones PW, Saklatvala J, Dawes PT, Shadforth MF, Hothersall TE, Hassell AB, Hay EM. Do patients with rheumatoid arthritis established on methotrexate and folic acid 5 mg daily need to continue folic acid supplements long term? Rheumatology (Oxford) 2000;39(10):1102–9.
10. Kettunen R, Huikuri HV, Oikarinen A, Takkunen JT. Methotrexate-linked ventricular arrhythmias. Acta Derm Venereol 1995;75(5):391–2.
11. Landewe RB, van den Borne BE, Breedveld FC, Dijkmans BA. Methotrexate effects in patients with rheumatoid arthritis with cardiovascular comorbidity. Lancet 2000;355(9215):1616–7.
12. Schnabel A, Dalhoff K, Bauerfeind S, Barth J, Gross WL. Sustained cough in methotrexate therapy for rheumatoid arthritis. Clin Rheumatol 1996;15(3):277–82.
13. Kremer JM, Alarcon GS, Weinblatt ME, Kaymakcian MV, Macaluso M, Cannon GW, Palmer WR, Sundy JS, St Clair EW, Alexander RW, Smith GJ, Axiotis CA. Clinical, laboratory, radiographic, and histopathologic features of methotrexate-associated lung injury in patients with rheumatoid arthritis: a multicenter study with literature review. Arthritis Rheum 1997;40(10):1829–37.
14. Salaffi F, Manganelli P, Carotti M, Subiaco S, Lamanna G, Cervini C. Methotrexate-induced pneumonitis in patients with rheumatoid arthritis and psoriatic arthritis: report of five cases and review of the literature. Clin Rheumatol 1997;16(3):296–304.
15. Golden MR, Katz RS, Balk RA, Golden HE. The relationship of pre-existing lung disease to the development of methotrexate pneumonitis in patients with rheumatoid arthritis. J Rheumatol 1995;22(6):1043–7.
16. Barrera P, Laan RF, van Riel PL, Dekhuijzen PN, Boerbooms AM, van de Putte LB. Methotrexate-related pulmonary complications in rheumatoid arthritis. Ann Rheum Dis 1994;53(7):434–9.
17. Kokelj F, Plozzer C, Muzzi A, Ciani F. Endoalveolar haemorrhage due to methotrexate overdosage in a patient treated for psoriatic arthritis. J Dermatol Treat 1999;10:67–9.
18. Massin F, Coudert B, Marot JP, Foucher P, Camus P, Jeannin L. La pneumopathie du methotrexate. [Pneumopathy caused by methotrexate.] Rev Mal Respir 1990;7(1):5–15.
19. Martins da Cunha AC, Bartsch CH, Gadner H. Acute respiratory failure after intrathecal methotrexate administration. Pediatr Hematol Oncol 1990;7(2):189–92.

20. Cottin V, Tebib J, Massonnet B, Souquet PJ, Bernard JP. Pulmonary function in patients receiving long-term low-dose methotrexate. Chest 1996;109(4):933–8.
21. Bartram SA. Experience with methotrexate-associated pneumonitis in northeastern England: comment on the article by Kremer et al. Arthritis Rheum 1998;41(7):1327–8.
22. Yoshida S, Onuma K, Akahori K, Sakamoto H, Yamawaki Y, Shoji T, Nakagawa H, Hasegawa H, Amayasu H. Elevated levels of IL-8 in interstitial pneumonia induced by low-dose methotrexate. J Allergy Clin Immunol 1999;103(5 Pt 1):952–4.
23. Alarcon GS, Kremer JM, Macaluso M, Weinblatt ME, Cannon GW, Palmer WR, St Clair EW, Sundy JS, Alexander RW, Smith GJ, Axiotis CA. Risk factors for methotrexate-induced lung injury in patients with rheumatoid arthritis. A multicenter, case-control study. Methotrexate-Lung Study Group. Ann Intern Med 1997;127(5):356–64.
24. Imokawa S, Colby TV, Leslie KO, Helmers RA. Methotrexate pneumonitis: review of the literature and histopathological findings in nine patients. Eur Respir J 2000;15(2):373–81.
25. Fujii Y, Mizuno Y, Hongo T, Igarashi Y, Arai T, Kino I, Okamoto K. [Serial spectral EEG analysis in a patient with non-Hodgkin's lymphoma complicated by leukoencephalopathy induced by high-dose methotrexate.] Gan To Kagaku Ryoho 1988;15(4 Pt 1):713–17.
26. Poskitt KJ, Steinbok P, Flodmark O. Methotrexate leukoencephalopathy mimicking cerebral abscess on CT brain scan. Childs Nerv Syst 1988;4(2):119–21.
27. Ebner F, Ranner G, Slavc I, Urban C, Kleinert R, Radner H, Einspieler R, Justich E. MR findings in methotrexate-induced CNS abnormalities. Am J Neuroradiol 1989;10(5):959–64.
28. Borgna-Pignatti C, Battisti L, Marradi P, Balter R, Caudana R. Transient neurologic disturbances in a child treated with moderate-dose methotrexate. Br J Haematol 1992;81(3):448.
29. Worthley SG, McNeil JD. Leukoencephalopathy in a patient taking low dose oral methotrexate therapy for rheumatoid arthritis. J Rheumatol 1995;22(2):335–7.
30. Lesnik PG, Ciesielski KT, Hart BL, Benzel EC, Sanders JA. Evidence for cerebellar–frontal subsystem changes in children treated with intrathecal chemotherapy for leukemia: enhanced data analysis using an effect size model. Arch Neurol 1998;55(12):1561–8.
31. Aplin CG, Russell-Jones R. Acute dysarthria induced by low dose methotrexate therapy in a patient with erythrodermic cutaneous T cell lymphoma: an unusual manifestation of neurotoxicity. Clin Exp Dermatol 1999;24(1):23–4.
32. Schagen SB, van Dam FS, Muller MJ, Boogerd W, Lindeboom J, Bruning PF. Cognitive deficits after postoperative adjuvant chemotherapy for breast carcinoma. Cancer 1999;85(3):640–50.
33. Rau R, Schleusser B, Herborn G, Karger T. Longterm combination therapy of refractory and destructive rheumatoid arthritis with methotrexate (MTX) and intramuscular gold or other disease modifying antirheumatic drugs compared to MTX monotherapy. J Rheumatol 1998;25(8):1485–92.
34. Wernick R, Smith DL. Central nervous system toxicity associated with weekly low-dose methotrexate treatment. Arthritis Rheum 1989;32(6):770–5.
35. Dhondt JL, Farriaux JP, Millot F, Taret S, Hayte JM, Mazingue F. Methotrexate a haute close et hyperphenylalaninennie. [High-dose methotrexate and hyperphenylalaninemia.] Arch Fr Pediatr 1991;48(4):249–51.
36. Lapadula G, De Bari C, Acquista CA, Dell'Accio F, Covelli M, Iannone F. Isolated thrombocytopenia associated with low dose methotrexate therapy. Clin Rheumatol 1997;16(4):429–30.
37. Franck H, Rau R, Herborn G. Thrombocytopenia in patients with rheumatoid arthritis on long-term treatment with low dose methotrexate. Clin Rheumatol 1996;15(3):266–70.
38. Gutierrez-Urena S, Molina JF, Garcia CO, Cuellar ML, Espinoza LR. Pancytopenia secondary to methotrexate therapy in rheumatoid arthritis. Arthritis Rheum 1996;39(2):272–6.
39. Jover JA, Hernandez-Garcia C, Morado IC, Vargas E, Banares A, Fernandez-Gutierrez B. Combined treatment of giant-cell arteritis with methotrexate and prednisone. a randomized, double-blind, placebo-controlled trial. Ann Intern Med 2001;134(2):106–14.
40. Carpenter EH, Plant MJ, Hassell AB, Shadforth MF, Fisher J, Clarke S, Hothersall TE, Dawes PT. Management of oral complications of disease-modifying drugs in rheumatoid arthritis. Br J Rheumatol 1997;36(4):473–8.
41. Ince A, Yazici Y, Hamuryudan V, Yazici H. The frequency and clinical characteristics of methotrexate (MTX) oral toxicity in rheumatoid arthritis (RA): a masked and controlled study. Clin Rheumatol 1996;15(5):491–4.
42. Fisher A, Mor E, Hytiroglou P, Emre S, Boccagni P, Chodoff L, Sheiner P, Schwartz M, Thung SN, Miller C. FK506 hepatotoxicity in liver allograft recipients. Transplantation 1995;59(11):1631–2.
43. Kaplan MM. Methotrexate hepatotoxicity and the premature reporting of Mark Twain's death: both greatly exaggerated. Hepatology 1990;12(4 Pt 1):784–6.
44. Lin Y, Huang Y, Lee S, Wu J, Chang C, Chen C, Hwang S. [Clinical study of methotrexate-induced hepatic injury in patients with psoriasis.] Chin J Gastroenterol 1991;8:277–81.
45. Cunliffe RN, Scott BB. Review article: monitoring for drug side-effects in inflammatory bowel disease. Aliment Pharmacol Ther 2002;16(4):647–62.
46. Walker AM, Funch D, Dreyer NA, Tolman KG, Kremer JM, Alarcon GS, Lee RG, Weinblatt ME. Determinants of serious liver disease among patients receiving low-dose methotrexate for rheumatoid arthritis. Arthritis Rheum 1993;36(3):329–35.
47. Bach N, Thung SN, Schaffner F. The histologic effects of low-dose methotrexate therapy for primary biliary cirrhosis. Arch Pathol Lab Med 1998;122(4):342–5.
48. Kremer JM, Alarcon GS, Lightfoot RW Jr, Willkens RF, Furst DE, Williams HJ, Dent PB, Weinblatt ME. Methotrexate for rheumatoid arthritis. Suggested guidelines for monitoring liver toxicity. American College of Rheumatology. Arthritis Rheum 1994;37(3):316–28.
49. Risteli J, Sogaard H, Oikarinen A, Risteli L, Karvonen J, Zachariae H. Aminoterminal propeptide of type III procollagen in methotrexate-induced liver fibrosis and cirrhosis. Br J Dermatol 1988;119(3):321–5.
50. Hilton MA, Bertolone S, Patel CC. Daily profiles of plasma phenylalanine and tyrosine in patients with osteogenic sarcoma during treatment with high-dose methotrexate-citrovorum rescue. Med Pediatr Oncol 1989;17(4):265–70.
51. Roenigk HH Jr, Auerbach R, Maibach HI, Weinstein GD. Methotrexate in psoriasis: revised guidelines. J Am Acad Dermatol 1988;19(1 Pt 1):145–56.
52. West SG. Methotrexate hepatotoxicity. Rheum Dis Clin North Am 1997;23(4):883–915.
53. Zachariae H, Schroder H, Foged E, Sogaard H. Methotrexate hepatotoxicity and concentrations of methotrexate and folate in erythrocytes—relation to liver fibrosis and cirrhosis. Acta Dermatol Venereol 1987;67(4):336–40.

Immunologic

Lupus-like syndrome has been attributed to methyldopa, causing hemolytic anemia, arthritis, photosensitivity, and high titers of antinuclear antibody (1:256) and of IgG antibodies to class I histones in a 55-year-old man who took methyldopa 250 mg bd for 13 months; the syndrome resolved spontaneously when methyldopa was withdrawn (11).

Long-Term Effects

Drug withdrawal

A withdrawal syndrome with rebound hypertension has been reported with methyldopa (12). Although it is similar to that associated with clonidine, it is less well defined, less severe, and less frequent.

- Withdrawal of methyldopa has been associated with the development of an acute manic syndrome in a 62-year-old man who had had methyldopa withdrawn 4 weeks before; there had been no previous history of psychiatric disorder (13).

Drug–Drug Interactions

Mianserin

Mianserin has alpha-adrenoceptor activity and so might interact with methyldopa (14). In 11 patients with essential hypertension, the addition of mianserin 60 mg/day (in divided doses) for 2 weeks did not reduce the hypotensive effect of methyldopa. In patients treated with methyldopa, there were additive hypotensive effects after the first dose of mianserin, but these were not significant after 1 or 2 weeks of combined treatment. The results of this study appear to have justified the authors' conclusion that adding mianserin to treatment with methyldopa will not result in loss of blood pressure control.

References

1. Webster J, Koch HF. Aspects of tolerability of centrally acting antihypertensive drugs. J Cardiovasc Pharmacol 1996;27(Suppl 3):S49–54.
2. Rosen B, Ovsyshcher IA, Zimlichman R. Complete atrioventricular block induced by methyldopa. Pacing Clin Electrophysiol 1988;11(11 Pt 1):1555–8.
3. Rosenblum AM, Montgomery EB. Exacerbation of parkinsonism by methyldopa. JAMA 1980;244(24):2727–8.
4. Arze RS, Ramos JM, Rashid HU, Kerr DN. Amenorrhoea, galactorrhoea, and hyperprolactinaemia induced by methyldopa. BMJ (Clin Res Ed) 1981;283(6285):194.
5. Egbert D, Hendricksen DK. Congestive heart failure and respiratory arrest secondary to methyldopa-induced hemolytic anemia. Ann Emerg Med 1988;17(5):526–8.
6. Glazer N, Goldstein RJ, Lief PD. A double blind, randomized, crossover study of adverse experiences among hypertensive patients treated with atenolol and methyldopa. Curr Ther Res 1989;45:782.
7. Gloth FM 3rd, Busby MJ. Methyldopa-induced diarrhea: a case of iatrogenic diarrhea leading to request for nursing home placement. Am J Med 1989;87(4):480–1.
8. Troster M, Sullivan SN. Acute colitis due to methyldopa. Can J Gastroenterol 1989;3:182.
9. Picaud A, Walter P, de Preville G, Nicolas P. Hépatite toxique mortelle au cours de la grossesse. [Fatal toxic hepatitis in pregnancy. A discussion of the role of methyldopa.] J Gynecol Obstet Biol Reprod (Paris) 1990;19(2):192–6.
10. Arranto AJ, Sotaniemi EA. Morphologic alterations in patients with alpha-methyldopa-induced liver damage after short- and long-term exposure. Scand J Gastroenterol 1981;16(7):853–63.
11. Nordstrom DM, West SG, Rubin RL. Methyldopa-induced systemic lupus erythematosus. Arthritis Rheum 1989;32(2):205–8.
12. Burden AC, Alexander CP. Rebound hypertension after acute methyldopa withdrawal. BMJ 1976;1(6017):1056–7.
13. Labbate LA, Holzgang AJ. Manic syndrome after discontinuation of methyldopa. Am J Psychiatry 1989;146(8):1075–6.
14. Elliott HL, Whiting B, Reid JL. Assessment of the interaction between mianserin and centrally-acting antihypertensive drugs. Br J Clin Pharmacol 1983;15(Suppl 2):S323–8.

Methylenedioxymetamfetamine

See also Amphetamines

General Information

Methylenedioxymetamfetamine (MDMA, ecstasy) is a recreational drug with actions like those of amphetamine. It is the usual and expected constituent of the tablets that are known as ecstasy, although adulteration with other substances is not uncommon (see the section on Drug contamination in this monograph). MDMA and other drugs, such as its *N*-demethylated derivative (MDA), 3,4-methylenedioxyamfetamine (MDA), 3,4-methylenedioxyethylamfetamine (MDEA), *N*-methylbenzodioxazolylbutamine (MBDB), and 4-bromo-2,5-dimethoxyphenylethylamine (2-CB or Nexus), are often grouped together as "ecstasy". Some have used the term "enactogen", meaning "touching within", to describe ecstasy.

In low doses MDMA produces a pleasant altered state of mind, with enhanced emotional closeness, but it is also used in high doses and settings in which toxicity is often reported (1). In the UK, considerable adverse effects have been reported from its use at rave dances. In the 1970s and 1980s its mind-altering effect caused some clinicians to advocate its use as an adjunct to psychotherapy (2).

Concern has been raised about the increasing use of ecstasy in Europe (3), particularly the UK and the Netherlands. The patterns and trends of substance use among college students have been evaluated over a 30-year period (4). Alcohol use remained stable, but illicit drug use peaked in 1978 and fell sharply over the next 20 years. Ecstasy was the exception: its use rose from 4.1% in 1989 to 10% in 1999. Ecstasy was the second most frequently tried illicit drug after marijuana.

Associated with increased physical activity and altered thermoregulation, ecstasy has been reported to cause unconsciousness, seizures, hyperthermia, tachycardia, hypotension, disseminated intravascular coagulation, and acute renal insufficiency, as well as death.

Ecstasy has a mild stimulant effect and is modestly hallucinogenic. The results of one study suggested that tolerance to its effects develops, but that adverse effects can increase with continued use (5). Recent reports have highlighted some disturbing effects, particularly when it is used while dancing vigorously at rave parties (6). In this setting, with increased physical activity, ecstasy can cause unconsciousness, seizures, hyperthermia, tachycardia, hypotension, disseminated intravascular coagulation, rhabdomyolysis, and acute renal insufficiency (7). Severe complications are also linked to uncontrolled fluid intake, hemodilution, and salt-losing syndromes. Deaths after the use of ecstasy in such settings have been described (8). It has been suggested that severe toxicity from ecstasy can result from altered thermoregulation in the face of excessive activity in warm environments (9).

Deaths related to ecstasy and MDEA in seven young white men, two of whom had hyperthermia, have been reviewed (10). In all cases, autopsy showed striking liver damage with necrosis; five patients had heart damage (contraction band necrosis and cell necrosis with inflammation), and others had brain damage, including focal bleeding, gross edema, and hypoxic changes. In one patient, who died of acute water intoxication, the pituitary gland was necrotic and there was accompanying cerebral edema. The authors proposed that the spectrum of pathological findings suggested more than one mechanism of damage, injury being caused by hyperthermia in some cases and a toxic effect (directly accountable for damage to liver and other organs) in others.

Ecstasy that is sold on the streets is a heterogeneous substancer, with enormous variations in its main active ingredients. It most often contains derivatives of MDMA and 3,4-methylenedioxy-*N*-ethylamfetamine (MDEA). Other amphetamine derivatives that it can contain include 3,4-MDA, *N*-methyl-1-(1,3-benzodioxol-5-yl)-2-butanamine (MBDB), and 2,5-dimethoxy-4-bromamfetamine (DOB). The amount of active ingredient in street ecstasy ranges from none to very high. In addition, other amphetamines or hallucinogens can be mixed in. A survey of 3021 young adults (14–24 years old) in Germany showed that regular use of ecstasy by itself is uncommon (2.6%). Among lifetime users, 97% have also used cannabinoids, 59% cocaine, 48% other substances, 46% hallucinogens, and 26% opiates. However, the interviews revealed that the use of ecstasy and hallucinogens is increasing, especially in young people. The authors observed that a large number of first-time users are at risk of regular use (11).

As recreational use of ecstasy has dramatically increased in recent years, deaths related to its use have been reported. In a retrospective review of all violent deaths from 1992 to 1997 in South Australia, six deaths were associated with ecstasy abuse; all occurred after September 1995. Three victims had documented hyperthermia and there was evidence of hyperthermia in another. The authors suggested that individual susceptibility to MDMA may be caused by impaired metabolism by CYP2D6 or through genetically poor metabolism (seen in 5–9% of Caucasians). One woman, who died with a cerebral hemorrhage, had fluoxetine (a CYP2D6 inhibitor) present in her blood. Furthermore, toxicology identified paramethoxyamfetamine (PMA) in all the cases, amfetamine/metamfetamine in four cases, and MDMA in only two cases. PMA, which is sold as an MDMA substitute or is present as a contaminant, is associated with a high rate of lethal complications (12).

- A 35-year-old male criminal died under suspicious circumstances (13). The police had seen him alive about 1.5 hours before the alleged time of death during a patrol visit to his home. Evaluation of the corpse showed an obvious head injury and the body was in an advanced stage of rigor mortis, despite the fact that the alleged time of death had been less than 4 hours earlier. The body temperature was significantly raised (42°C). A witness testified that the deceased had taken ecstasy at various times during the night, after which he had been groaning, before taking off his clothes and thrashing on the floor while hitting his head and bumping into things. When resuscitation had been attempted, his jaw had been locked. Toxicology detected amfetamine, metamfetamine, and PMA in the blood.

The authors suggested that in a subgroup of amfetamine abusers, a triad of amfetamine use, prolonged exertion, and hyperthermia can be potentially lethal. Any temperature above 42°C requires active cooling (to below 38.5°C) and carries a poor prognosis. In this case rigor mortis may have started almost at the time of death. An ecstasy tablet that was allegedly from the same batch contained 50 mg of PMA.

The pharmacological and pharmacokinetic effects of ecstasy have been studied in healthy volunteers (14). In the pilot phase, two subjects each took ecstasy 50, 100, and 150 mg. In the second phase, eight subjects took ecstasy 75 and 125 mg. All were CYP2D6 extensive metabolizers. The ecstasy plasma concentrations were not proportional to dose, probably indicating non-linear kinetics in the dosage range usually taken recreationally. While the results were not conclusive (owing to problems in the study design) and require further exploration, the finding that relatively small increases in the dose of ecstasy ingested can translate to disproportionate rises in ecstasy plasma concentrations, if confirmed, would be important.

Organs and Systems

Cardiovascular

Cardiotoxicity following ecstasy use has been reported (15).

- A 16-year-old boy took three tablets of ecstasy and amfetamine 0.3 g and several hours later had convulsions and a temperature of 40.9°C. His heart rate was 210/minute and his blood pressure 100/75 mmHg. His creatine kinase activity was raised and he had myoglobinuria, renal impairment, hyperkalemia, and hypocalcemia. An electrocardiogram showed ventricular and supraventricular tachycardias but no myocardial ischemia. A diagnosis of serotonin syndrome due to ecstasy ingestion with associated hyperpyrexia and rhabdomyolysis was made. Following active treatment, his condition stabilized, with restoration of sinus rhythm and normal urine output. However, 12 hours later he developed jaundice, raised liver enzymes, and coagulopathy, suggesting acute liver failure due to ecstasy. With supportive treatment, his liver function improved. However, another 12 hours later, he developed neurons and can cause lasting changes in neuronal responses to dopamine (32). They further stated that although parkinsonism has not been reported after MDMA, the possibility that such an association exists cannot be excluded. They raised the possibility that clinical evidence of parkinsonism can be missed, particularly when the disorder is mild and, as in their patient, when tremor is absent. They pointed out that with valproate the first full report of parkinsonism did not appear until 18 years after its introduction into the USA, even though those who commonly prescribe it (neurologists and psychiatrists) should have noticed it earlier. The authors clarified that they had mentioned MPTP as an example of a substance that may have a delayed neurotoxic effect on monoaminergic neurons, without intending to suggest that MDMA acts chemically in the same manner as MPTP. They agreed that a contaminant could have played a role, and raised a concern that contaminants also put MDMA users at risks of adverse effects. They countered the argument that all idiosyncratic responses have to be immediate, by quoting examples from the literature to suggest that the course of a reaction depends on the underlying mechanism.

The patient discussed in the case report also responded, alleging that his permission had not been obtained before publication (33). Contradicting the original published report, he stated that he had never used marijuana; the authors defended their data by stating that when the patient's friend, who had accompanied him to the clinic, mentioned cannabis use the patient did not deny it. He also reported using creatine, ephedrine, caffeine, and aspirin, none of which, the authors noted, has previously been associated with parkinsonian symptoms.

Other neurological adverse effects have been reported in a first-time ecstasy user (34).

- A 19-year-old man, an occasional user of benzodiazepines and heroin, developed dizziness and loss of consciousness the morning after taking ecstasy for the first time. He was intubated and ventilated. He had a monocular hematoma, pulmonary edema, and cutaneous emphysema, without focal neurological deficits. There was rhabdomyolysis with renal insufficiency but no rise in temperature. Body fluid toxicological analysis showed only benzodiazepines and amphetamines. After he was weaned from the respirator, although awake, he did not react to noxious stimuli and showed no spontaneous movements. A CT scan of the brain had been normal on admission, but 2 and 3 weeks later it showed multiple hypodense lesions in the white matter. One month after admission, he was in a vegetative state, with marked spasticity, intermittent non-specific reactions to noise, and sustained generalized myoclonus. An electroencephalogram showed generalized slowing with intermittent theta wave activity. An MRI scan showed bilateral severe white matter damage.

Brain damage in this patient was restricted to the white matter. Although hypoxia was present at the time of admission, the authors did not believe that it was the only causative factor. By a process of elimination, they concluded that ecstasy might have caused the toxic encephalopathy, although it was not detected by toxicological analysis. They suggested that myelin damage might be an indirect sequel of MDMA-related metabolic oxidative stress and multiorgan failure due to individual susceptibility. They also entertained the idea of a lipophilic toxic contaminant rather than MDMA as the causative toxic agent.

An unusual case of bilateral sixth nerve palsy associated with ecstasy has been reported (35).

- A 17-year-old man developed horizontal diplopia in all directions of gaze while using ecstasy tablets every 5–7 days for 2 months. A diagnosis of bilateral sixth nerve palsy was confirmed. Ocular motility returned to normal within 5 days without treatment. There was no evidence of inflammation or degenerative disease of the central nervous system.

The authors speculated that the most likely cause of the lesion was either an interaction of ecstasy with serotonergic neurons or cerebral edema (albeit not detected by MRI) secondary to ecstasy.

Psychological, psychiatric

Concerns have been raised about the long-term nervous system effects of MDMA use from animal data, which suggest that the dose of MDMA used for recreational purposes by humans can cause toxic effects in non-human primates, especially involving the serotonin system. In a case-control study, 10 long-term MDMA users were compared with 10 controls who had not used MDMA but were drug abusers and were matched for age, sex, education, and premorbid intellect (36). All participated in a single photon emission computed tomography (SPECT) study with a serotonin transporter (SERT) ligand. Dopamine transporter binding was determined from scans acquired 23 hours after injection of the tracer. Hair analysis, which covers about the last 4 weeks of drug use, generally confirmed the drug use history, although two ecstasy users tested negative for both amfetamine and metamfetamine. On neuropsychological testing, both groups showed comparable performances in tests of verbal and spatial memory, psychomotor speed, attention, and executive function. Larger lifetime doses of ecstasy were associated with reduced verbal memory performance on the California Verbal Learning Test and more errors in the Spatial Working Memory Test. Ecstasy users showed a cortical reduction of SERT binding prominently in primary sensorimotor cortex, with normal dopamine transporter binding in the lenticular nuclei. There was also an association between the length of the MDMA-free period (mean 18 days) before the scan and ligand binding in the cingulate. Spatial working memory performance and SERT binding in the left calcarine cortex were negatively correlated with the estimated lifetime dose of MDMA in the ecstasy users. While these results could be coincidental, or reduced SERT binding could be the imaging correlate of a psychobiological predisposition to heavy use of ecstasy, the authors suggested that this study provided evidence for specific albeit temporary serotonergic neurotoxicity of MDMA in humans. If confirmed, these effects on the serotonergic system could underlie psychiatric morbidity in ecstasy users.

The neurotransmitter systems involved in the psychological and information processing effects of ecstasy have been studied in 16 ecstasy-naïve subjects (37). Ecstasy produced a state of enhanced mood, well-being, increased emotional sensitiveness, little anxiety, moderate thought disturbances, but no hallucinations or panic reactions. It caused thought disturbances, such as difficulty in concentrating, thought blocking, and difficulty in reaching decisions. Women had greater subjective responses to ecstasy than men. For instance, they scored higher on ratings of anxiety, adverse effects, and thought disturbances, suggesting differences in the metabolism of ecstasy. Prepulse inhibition of the startle response was used to measure physiological changes. Prepulse inhibition and startle habituation have been used as operational measures of sensorimotor gating and habituation functions, respectively, in investigations of attention. Moreover, some studies have associated prepulse inhibition with endogenous serotonin release. Ecstasy 1.7 mg/kg increased prepulse inhibition, suggesting that the overflow of endogenous serotonin caused by ecstasy may interfere with the startle response and cause a breakdown of cognitive integrity. This effect further suggests serotonin dysregulation in response to ecstasy.

Reports of adverse neuropsychiatric effects of MDMA have included descriptions of flashbacks, anxiety, insomnia (38), panic attacks (25,39), and psychosis (40). Subacute adverse effects that have been reported following MDMA use include drowsiness, depression, anxiety, and irritability (41). Prolonged or chronic effects have also been reported, including panic disorder (42,43), psychosis (40,44,45), flashbacks (40), major depressive disorder (25,46), and memory disturbance (25). The observation that only certain individuals develop neuropsychiatric disturbances after using ecstasy suggests that certain predisposing psychiatric factors (or high-dose regimens) may make some individuals more vulnerable to these untoward effects.

With increasing use of ecstasy, there is considerable interest in its effects on psychopathology and cognition. The residual effects of ecstasy on psychopathology and cognition have been examined in 18 current regular users, 15 ex-users with an average abstinence of 2 years, 16 ecstasy-naïve polydrug users, and 15 non-drug users (47). Both current and previous users had significantly worse psychopathology than the controls and polydrug users. Ecstasy users had higher scores on the Symptoms Check List SCL-90-R Global Severity Index and the Positive Symptom Distress Index. They also scored significantly higher on eight specific factors on the SCL-90-R: somatization, obsessive-compulsive disorder, anxiety, phobic anxiety, interpersonal sensitivity, depression, paranoid ideation, and altered appetite/restless sleep. Current users had higher scores across more categories, but the values were not significantly different from ex-users. Current and ex-users had lower working memory and verbal learning abilities than the controls and polydrug users, but there were no significant differences between the two groups. Using regression analyses, the investigators found that the best indicator of increased psychopathology was a high consumption of cannabis, while cognitive deficits were best predicted by the amount of previous ecstasy use. Thus, the investigators suggested that ecstasy-induced cognitive impairment may not be reversible over time and with abstinence, suggesting that ecstasy is a potent neurotoxin.

The neuropsychological effects of ecstasy have been studied in 20 polydrug users (48). Various functions and processes throughout the brain, such as verbal fluency, spatial working memory, and attention, were assessed. Ecstasy users showed a significant deficit in complex visual pattern recognition and spatial working memory compared with the polydrug abusers who were not taking ecstasy. Since these tests are sensitive to temporal lobe functioning, the authors suggested that there is a selective temporal lobe deficit in ecstasy users, with relative sparing of executive functioning. Based on previous studies, they postulated that serotonin dysfunction in the temporal lobe may be associated with impaired visuospatial working memory. However, they did not study a drug-free control group and the ecstasy group used higher amounts of drugs in general. In addition, the sample size was small.

Some reports have suggested that the relation between the dose of ecstasy and its complications may not be straightforward (49). Some people have problems with very small amounts.

- A 21-year-old woman developed a protracted psychotic depersonalization disorder with suicidal tendency after taking two tablets of ecstasy for the first time (50).
- A 23-year-old man with no prior psychiatric history developed panic disorder after taking a single dose of ecstasy (42).
- A psychosis occurred in an 18-year-old man who had used ecstasy on an occasional recreational basis (51).

The acute and short-term effects of a recreational dose of MDMA (1.7 mg/kg) given to 13 MDMA-naïve healthy volunteers in a double-blind, placebo-controlled study have been reported (52). MDMA produced a state of enhanced mood, well-being, and enhanced emotional responsiveness, with mild depersonalization, derealization, thought disorder, and anxiety. The subjects also had changes in their sense of space and time, heightened sensory awareness, and increased psychomotor drive. MDMA increased blood pressure moderately, except in one case of a transient hypertensive reaction. The most frequent somatic adverse effects were jaw clenching, poor appetite, restlessness, and insomnia. Lack of energy, difficulty in concentrating, fatigue, and feelings of restlessness during the next day were also described. The authors suggested that MDMA produces a psychological profile different from classic hallucinogens or psychostimulants. The potential risk of hypertensive effects of recreational dosages of ecstasy should also be considered in the safety profile.

Using PET with a radioligand that selectively labels the serotonin (5-HT) transporter, 14 MDMA users who were currently abstaining (for 3 weeks) from use and 15 MDMA-naïve controls were studied (53). MDMA users showed a reduction in global and regional brain 5-HT transporter binding, a measure of the number of 5-HT neurons, compared with controls. Deficiency in SERT correlated positively with the extent of previous drug use. The authors suggested that ecstasy users are susceptible to MDMA-induced serotonin neural injury.

usually associated with rapid deterioration and a poor prognosis.

Skin

Two cases of facial papules have been reported (78).

- A 20-year-old woman developed diarrhea and a pruritic yellowish skin 7 days after she had taken half a tablet of ecstasy. Her liver was enlarged and tender. Her urine was positive for MDMA. A diagnosis of acute hepatotoxicity after MDMA was made. She rapidly developed reddish papules over the face with a perioral and acne-like distribution.
- A 21-year-old-man developed similar skin lesions after using ecstasy, without hepatotoxicity.

Both patients responded to a low fat diet and 1% metronidazole ointment. The authors suggested that serotonin indirectly affects the nerve endings of the eccrine glands via other peptides, and that the interaction of MDMA with serotonin may have caused the rapid development of pimples in these abusers.

Immunologic

Four healthy male MDMA users volunteered for a randomized, double-blind, double-dummy, crossover pilot study in which they took single oral doses of MDMA 75 mg ($n = 2$) or 100 mg ($n = 2$), alcohol (0.8 mg/kg), MDMA plus alcohol, or placebo to study the effects on their immune system. The doses of MDMA were compatible with those used for recreational use (79). The baseline immunological parameters were within the reference ranges. Acute MDMA use produced time-dependent immune dysfunction, which paralleled MDMA plasma concentrations and MDMA-induced cortisol stimulation kinetics. The changes in the immune system after MDMA peaked at 1–2 hours. Although the total leukocyte count remained unchanged, there was a fall in the ratio of CD4 to CD8 T cells and in the percentage of mature T lymphocytes (CD3 cells), probably because of a fall in both the percentage and the absolute number of T helper cells. The fall in CD4 cell count and in the functional responsiveness of lymphocytes to mitogenic stimulation with phytohemagglutinin A was MDMA dose-dependent. Alcohol produced a decrease in T helper cells, B lymphocytes, and mitogen-induced lymphocyte proliferation. Combined MDMA and alcohol use produced the greatest suppressive effect on CD4 cell count and mitogen-stimulated lymphoproliferation. Immune function was partially restored at 24 hours. According to the authors, these results provided the first evidence that recreational use of MDMA alone or in combination with alcohol alters immunological status. The reaction of the immune system to MDMA appears to be an alteration of physiological homeostasis, similar to that seen in volunteers exposed to acute physiologic stress, suggesting that MDMA could be a "chemical stressor". Moreover, combined MDMA and alcohol use produced additive effects. This is an important finding, since in the general population alcohol and MDMA are commonly taken together.

Because other drugs of abuse can cause immune dysfunction in regular users, the effects of acute administration of ecstasy on the immune system have been studied in both controlled and natural settings (80). In the controlled study, 18 male ecstasy users were given two doses of ecstasy 100 mg at intervals of 4 or 24 hours. There were significant reductions in CD4 T helper cells (30%) and the lymphoproliferative response to phytohemagglutinin mitogenic stimulation (68%) 1.5 hours after the first dose, and a 103% increase in the number of natural killer cells. At 4 hours, CD4 T helper cells and lymphocyte proliferative responses were reduced by 40% and 87%, but natural killer cell numbers increased to 141%. At 24 hours, the second dose augmented the alterations in the numbers of CD4 T helper cells and natural killer cells about threefold. The authors suggested that this large effect after repeated administration of ecstasy increases the interval during which the immune response is compromised, leading to a higher risk of illness and infection in ecstasy abusers.

In the uncontrolled study, 30 recreational users of ecstasy (mean age 24 years) were observed for 2 years and had lymphocyte counts at yearly intervals. The ecstasy users tended to have lower white blood cell counts over time. Lymphocyte counts were significantly lower than in healthy controls by year 1 and significantly lower than that the following year. CD4 and CD19 cell numbers fell significantly from basal to year 1 and from year 1 to year 2. Natural killer cell numbers were always lower than in healthy controls but did not fall with time. The authors extended these results to suggest a possible role of serotonin dysregulation caused by ecstasy in compromising immune function. These findings suggest that ecstasy abusers may be at a significantly higher risk of infectious diseases.

Death

MDMA and MDEA, or "eve," have rapidly become popular drugs of abuse in recent years in Europe and to some extent in other developed countries as well. Over the years, reports of deaths following their use at "rave" parties have generated considerable public concern.

In a study of all ecstasy-positive deaths (22 of 19 366 deaths) in New York City from January 1997 to June 2000, 18 were men, average age 27 years (81). The deaths fell into three categories: acute drug intoxication ($n = 13$), mechanical injury ($n = 7$), and a combination of natural causes and acute drug intoxication ($n = 2$). Only two of the deaths due to acute drug intoxication were caused by ecstasy alone, and one death was caused by a combination of ecstasy and coronary artery disease. Seven deaths were caused by a combination of cocaine/opiates and ecstasy. Acute ecstasy poisoning includes symptoms such as hypertension, hyperthermia, and delirium, and can progress to intracranial hemorrhage, status epilepticus, and death. Based on reports from harm-reduction organizations and previous studies, the authors discussed the lack of standardization of ecstasy tablets and the danger of harmful additives that could react with other drugs to cause life-threatening symptoms.

Death rate

In a report from the UK it was noted that the annual death rate from ecstasy use is uncertain (82). A meta-analysis of surveys of illegal drug use by 15–24-year-old individuals in the UK in 1996 showed that 7% had used ecstasy in the previous year and 3% in the previous month, a rate 44% higher than in 1993–1995. But the actual numbers of ecstasy-related deaths are more difficult to ascertain. In Scotland, ecstasy-related deaths are defined as "ecstasy found in the body"; in England, on the other hand, it is defined as "ecstasy written on the death certificate." Using these disparate definitions, 11 deaths were reported in Scotland and 18 in England in the 15–24-year-old category. Based on all available data, the author of the report suggested a 26-fold range (0.2–5.3) of possible ecstasy-related deaths per 10 000 within this age group. To make death estimates more reliable, the author recommended that the definition of "ecstasy-related-death" should be unified, and that surveys should ask directly about regular, sporadic, and first-time drug use, so as to determine which group is at most risk. The author expressed concern that these data (poor as they are) may be used by the courts and policy makers as if they were more valid, citing the example of Switzerland, which has recently liberalized the guidelines on sentencing people who supply ecstasy tablets, in contrast to suppliers of heroin, based on their interpretation of the data that the death rate in ecstasy users is at the lower end of the range.

This report generated two responses. One group felt that estimating such death rates is even more complex than noted (83). They asked whether, if someone purchased ecstasy but instead got a contaminated or a very different compound, causing death, the death would be classified as ecstasy-related or as something else? Furthermore, they wondered if the definition of ecstasy-related death is based on the detection of MDMA (or its metabolites) in the blood or on detection of other compounds (consumed under the presumption of its being ecstasy). Citing their own experience, they suggested that criteria for inclusion should include: "Would the deceased still be alive if (s)he had not abused the substance?" Thus, even deaths from causes such as traffic accidents, when the death was secondary to intoxication with the compound, should be included.

The second group, while agreeing with the original report, raised the concern that surveys that are more frequent would be economically prohibitive (84). They noted that in 1997 The National Program on Substance Abuse Deaths (NPSAD) was established to monitor drug-related deaths in the UK. It uses a "cause of death ratio," which looks at the number of drug-related deaths in specific categories (for example 15–24-year-olds) and the drugs implicated in these deaths. According to the authors, this method allows rapid surveillance of the pattern of deaths over time.

Pathology

Three deaths have been reported after the ingestion of MDMA/MDEA, in which immunohistological studies further elucidated the causes of the deaths (85). One death was caused by MDMA intoxication, one was from MDEA, and the third was from combined intoxication. One case had been reported previously (SEDA-22, 31).

- A 19-year-old man consumed ecstasy for the entire duration of a discotheque party (lasting until morning) and had respiratory difficulty, uncoordinated movements, generalized hypertonia, and hyperpyrexia (40.6°C). The diagnosis was disseminated intravascular coagulation and was treated with heparin but suffered severe blood loss from the oral cavity and injection wounds. He subsequently had a cardiac arrest.
- A 20-year-old man took many ecstasy tablets at a discotheque, returned home complaining of feeling feverish (axillary temperature 40°C), went to bed, and was found dead 10 hours later, his pillow soaked with blood.
- A 19-year-old man was found unconscious near a discotheque. His course progressively worsened, with the appearance of diffuse subcutaneous petechiae. While being treated for hypotension, he developed sustained convulsions and uremia and later died.

In all cases, amphetamines were detected in the urine. The pathological findings showed diffuse subserous petechiae and polyvisceral stasis. The brains showed massive edema and signs of neuronal hypoxia. In two cases, the heart showed coagulative myocytolysis, while one had areas of subendocardial hemorrhage. The lungs showed subpleural and intra-alveolar hemorrhages with severe edema, and in two cases microthrombotic formations inside lung capillaries. In two cases, the liver showed evidence of microvesicular steatosis and in one case centrilobular necrosis. Liver cells in the central zones showed coagulation necrosis with precipitation of fibrin in the whole area affected by necrosis. In the kidney, fibrin thrombi in the renal glomeruli were observed in two of the cases, while acute tubular necrosis was observed in one.

The findings in these three cases were similar to those seen in deaths from hyperthermia and disseminated intravascular coagulation. The myocardial necrosis (coagulative myocytolysis) without infarct necrosis suggested adrenergic overdrive. In two cases the muscle showed the typical pathological changes observed in deaths due to malignant hyperpyrexia. Myoglobin was detected in the proximal tubules in all three cases. The authors interpreted the clinical, histopathological, and toxicological data as indicative of an idiosyncratic response to ecstasy.

Long-Term Effects

Drug dependence

There are few preclinical or clinical data to suggest that repeated use of MDMA is associated with increased tolerance or dependence. However, anecdotal reports suggest that in some individuals, increasing amounts of MDMA are used in order to achieve the same reinforcing psychoactive effects (44,86).

Second-Generation Effects

Pregnancy

Workers in Canada have tried to characterize women who reported gestational exposure to ecstasy (87). The Motherisk Program is a large Teratogen Information Service based in Toronto and receives over 150 calls daily about exposure to various agents during pregnancy. The authors reviewed the data from 1998 to 2000. The study group consisted of all pregnant women who had been exposed to ecstasy. The control group was randomly selected pregnant women who visited the Motherisk Clinic during the same week as the subject who called about ecstasy. The 132 ecstasy-exposed women were significantly younger, earlier in gestational age, and weighed less than the non-exposed controls. The ecstasy users had had significantly fewer pregnancies and live births and had a higher rate of therapeutic abortions but not spontaneous abortions. Significantly more ecstasy users reported unplanned pregnancies and were more likely to be single and white. The ecstasy users were more likely than controls to have had alcohol exposure in pregnancy, and significantly more drank heavily. The ecstasy-exposed women were more likely to binge-drink and smoke cigarettes during pregnancy, and more were significantly heavy smokers. Ecstasy users also had a greater tendency to use marijuana, cocaine, amphetamines, ketamine, gamma-hydroxybutyrate, and psilocybin.

Of the 132 women who reported ecstasy use, 129 had used it during pregnancy, of whom 101 reported previous use of ecstasy before their pregnancy, but had discontinued it. The mean gestational age of last ecstasy exposure was 5.0 weeks (range 1–24 weeks). All but three used tablets: two snorted and one used a liquid formulation. The mean dose taken on one occasion was 1.24 tablets. Of the 122 patients whose data were included in the analysis, most (57%) had only one exposure to ecstasy during pregnancy; 10 women had more than five exposures. One 15-year-old girl did not realize she was pregnant until 24 weeks gestation and had used two tablets of ecstasy four times a day. Only seven of the ecstasy group reported exposure to ecstasy alone. Ecstasy-associated adverse events were reported by 33 of 77 respondents. The physical adverse effect most commonly reported was vomiting (23%). The authors raised significant concerns about the potential teratogenic effects in these women, due to clustering of risk factors.

Drug Administration

Drug formulations

In New Zealand, "herbal ecstasy" is a term used for many different herbal formulations, none of which contains ecstasy. Some of the names for these herbs (which can be sold in stores) include "The Bomb", "Reds", and "Sublime". Analysis of "The Bomb" showed substantial amounts of ephedrine; the Ministry of Health in New Zealand removed it from the market. Some symptoms associated with herbal ecstasy include headache, dizziness, palpitation, tachycardia, and raised blood pressure. Thus, in countries where the term "herbal ecstasy" is commonly used, it is important that those who see patients who have taken herbal ecstasy should not confuse it with ecstasy, as toxicity and medical management may be quite different (88).

Drug contamination

It is not uncommon for people to be deceived into consuming other substances, believing them to be MDMA. At dance parties and "raves" for young adults, compounds passed as ecstasy may be more lethal than MDMA, either because they contain more potent amphetamines than MDMA or because of adulteration with other substances. In three fatal cases reported in the USA, the victims (two men aged 19 and 24 and a woman aged 18) believed that they were using MDMA but had in fact taken PMA, a more potent central stimulant with structural and pharmacological similarities to MDMA (89). They became agitated and developed bruxism, severe hyperthermia, convulsions, and hemorrhages. The presence of PMA was confirmed by enzyme immunoassay, and MDMA was not detected. PMA is not a contaminant of MDMA.

Drug–Drug Interactions

Alcohol

The pharmacokinetic and pharmacodynamic interactions of single doses of ecstasy 100 mg and alcohol 0.8 g/kg have been investigated in nine healthy men (mean age 23 years) in a double-blind, double-dummy, randomized, placebo-controlled crossover design (90). Each underwent four 10-hour experimental sessions, including blood sampling, with 1 week between each. For the task used to test the recognition and recording of visual information, the conditions involving ethanol yielded significantly more errors and fewer responses than ecstasy alone or placebo alone. The combination of ecstasy with ethanol reversed the subjective effect of sedation caused by alcohol alone. In addition, the combination extended the sense of euphoria caused by ecstasy to 5.25 hours. The addition of ethanol caused plasma ecstasy concentrations to rise by 13%. These results show that the combination of ecstasy with alcohol potentiates the euphoria of ecstasy and reduces perceived sedation. However, psychomotor impairment of visual processing caused by alcohol is not reversed. This is a concern for road safety, as people who take both drugs would feel sober, but their driving would still be compromised, although the extent of driving impairment under these conditions is not known. The increase in plasma concentrations of ecstasy caused by alcohol could exacerbate the adverse effects of ecstasy.

Ritonavir

An important consideration in the use of all HIV-1 protease inhibitors, but of ritonavir in particular, is their potential for drug interactions through their effects on cytochrome P450 isozymes. The various interactions of ritonavir with other antiretroviral drugs have been reviewed (91). Ritonavir, which inhibits CYP2D6, the principal pathway by which MDMA is metabolized, can also produce clinically relevant interactions with recreational drugs (92).

- A 32-year-old HIV-positive man, who added ritonavir 600 mg bd to his antiretroviral regimen of zidovudine and lamivudine, became unwell within hours after having taken two and a half tablets of ecstasy, estimated to contain 180 mg of MDMA. He was hypertonic, sweating profusely, tachypneic, tachycardic, and cyanosed. Shortly after he had a tonic-clonic seizure and a cardiorespiratory arrest. Attempts at resuscitation were unsuccessful. Blood concentrations obtained post-mortem showed an MDMA concentration of 4.56 mg/l, in the range of that reported in a patient with a life-threatening illness and symptoms similar to this patient after an overdose of 18 tablets of MDMA.

A patient infected with HIV-1 who was taking ritonavir and saquinavir had a prolonged effect from a small dose of MDMA and a near-fatal reaction from a small dose of gamma-hydroxybutyrate (93).

Selective serotonin re-uptake inhibitors (SSRIs)

An MDMA-related psychiatric adverse effect may have been enhanced by an SSRI (94).

- A 52-year-old prisoner, who was taking the SSRI citalopram 60 mg/day, suddenly became aggressive, agitated, and grandiose after using ecstasy. He carried out peculiar compulsive movements and had extreme motor restlessness, but no fever or rigidity. He was given chlordiazepoxide and 2 days later was asymptomatic. Citalopram was reintroduced, and 2 days later he reported visual hallucinations of little bugs in the cell. Promazine was substituted for citalopram and his condition improved 2 days later.

The authors suggested that SSRIs such as citalopram can potentiate the neurochemical and behavioral effects of MDMA.

References

1. Solowij N, Hall W, Lee N. Recreational MDMA use in Sydney: a profile of "Ecstacy" users and their experiences with the drug. Br J Addict 1992;87(8):1161–72.
2. Liester MB, Grob CS, Bravo GL, Walsh RN. Phenomenology and sequelae of 3,4-methylenedioxy-methamphetamine use. J Nerv Ment Dis 1992;180(6):345–52.
3. Vaiva G, Boss V, Bailly D, Thomas P, Lestavel P, Goudemand M. An "accidental" acute psychosis with ecstasy use. J Psychoactive Drugs 2001;33(1):95–8.
4. Pope HG Jr, Ionescu-Pioggia M, Pope KW. Drug use and life style among college undergraduates: a 30-year longitudinal study. Am J Psychiatry 2001;158(9):1519–21.
5. Lessick M, Vasa R, Israel J. Severe manifestations of oculoauriculovertebral spectrum in a cocaine exposed infant. J Med Genet 1991;28(11):803–4.
6. Henry JA. Ecstasy and the dance of death. BMJ 1992;305(6844):5–6.
7. Gelenberg AJ. One man's ecstasy. Biol Ther Psychiatry Newslett 1992;15:45–7.
8. Screaton GR, Singer M, Cairns HS, Thrasher A, Sarner M, Cohen SL. Hyperpyrexia and rhabdomyolysis after MDMA ("ecstasy") abuse. Lancet 1992;339(8794):677–8.
9. Henry JA, Jeffreys KJ, Dawling S. Toxicity and deaths from 3,4-methylenedioxymethamphetamine ("ecstasy"). Lancet 1992;340(8816):384–7.
10. Campkin NT, Davies UM. Another death from Ecstacy. J R Soc Med 1992;85(1):61.
11. Schuster P, Lieb R, Lamertz C, Wittchen HU. Is the use of ecstasy and hallucinogens increasing? Results from a community study. Eur Addict Res 1998;4(1-2):75–82.
12. Byard RW, Gilbert J, James R, Lokan RJ. Amphetamine derivative fatalities in South Australia–is "Ecstasy" the culprit? Am J Forensic Med Pathol 1998;19(3):261–5.
13. James RA, Dinan A. Hyperpyrexia associated with fatal paramethoxyamphetamine (PMA) abuse. Med Sci Law 1998;38(1):83–5.
14. de la Torre R, Farre M, Ortuno J, Mas M, Brenneisen R, Roset PN, Segura J, Cami J. Non-linear pharmacokinetics of MDMA ("ecstasy") in humans. Br J Clin Pharmacol 2000;49(2):104–9.
15. Barrett PJ, Taylor GT. "Ecstasy" ingestion: a case report of severe complications. J R Soc Med 1993;86(4):233–4.
16. McCann UD, Ricaurte GA. Lasting neuropsychiatric sequelae of (+-)methylenedioxymethamphetamine ("ecstasy") in recreational users. J Clin Psychopharmacol 1991;11(5):302–5.
17. Duxbury AJ. Ecstasy—dental implications. Br Dent J 1993;175(1):38.
18. Ames D, Wirshing WC. Ecstasy, the serotonin syndrome, and neuroleptic malignant syndrome—a possible link? JAMA 1993;269(7):869–70.
19. Campkin NJ, Davies UM. Treatment of "ecstasy" overdose with dantrolene. Anaesthesia 1993;48(1):82–3.
20. Mintzer S, Hickenbottom S, Gilman S. Parkinsonism after taking ecstasy. N Engl J Med 1999;340(18):1443.
21. Sewell RA, Cozzi NV. More about parkinsonism after taking ecstasy. N Engl J Med 1999;341(18):1400.
22. Baggott M, Mendelson J, Jones R. More about parkinsonism after taking ecstasy. N Engl J Med 1999;341(18):1400–1.
23. Mintzer S, Hickenbottom S, Gilman S. More about parkinsonism after taking Ecstasy. N Engl J Med 1999;341:1401.
24. Borg GJ. More about parkinsonism after taking ecstasy. N Engl J Med 1999;341(18):1400.
25. Bertram M, Egelhoff T, Schwarz S, Schwab S. Toxic leukencephalopathy following "ecstasy" ingestion. J Neurol 1999;246(7):617–18.
26. Schroeder B, Brieden S. Bilateral sixth nerve palsy associated with MDMA ("ecstasy") abuse. Am J Ophthalmol 2000;129(3):408–9.
27. Semple DM, Ebmeier KP, Glabus MF, O'Carroll RE, Johnstone EC. Reduced in vivo binding to the serotonin transporter in the cerebral cortex of MDMA ("ecstasy") users. Br J Psychiatry 1999;175:63–9.
28. Vollenweider FX, Liechti ME, Gamma A, Greer G, Geyer M. Acute psychological and neurophysiological effects of MDMA in humans. J Psychoactive Drugs 2002;34(2):171–84.
29. Greer G, Strassman RJ. Information on "Ecstasy". Am J Psychiatry 1985;142(11):1391.
30. Whitaker-Azmitia PM, Aronson TA. "Ecstasy" (MDMA)-induced panic. Am J Psychiatry 1989;146(1):119.
31. Creighton FJ, Black DL, Hyde CE. "Ecstasy" psychosis and flashbacks. Br J Psychiatry 1991;159:713–15.
32. Peroutka SJ, Newman H, Harris H. Subjective effects of 3,4-methylenedioxymethamphetamine in recreational users. Neuropsychopharmacology 1988;1(4):273–7.
33. McCann UD, Ricaurte GA. MDMA ("ecstasy") and panic disorder: induction by a single dose. Biol Psychiatry 1992;32(10):950–3.
34. Pallanti S, Mazzi D. MDMA (Ecstasy) precipitation of panic disorder. Biol Psychiatry 1992;32(1):91–5.
35. McGuire P, Fahy T. Chronic paranoid psychosis after misuse of MDMA ("ecstasy"). BMJ 1991;302(6778):697.
36. Schifano F. Chronic atypical psychosis associated with MDMA ("ecstasy") abuse. Lancet 1991;338(8778):1335.
37. Benazzi F, Mazzoli M. Psychiatric illness associated with "ecstasy". Lancet 1991;338(8781):1520.
38. Morgan MJ, McFie L, Fleetwood H, Robinson JA. Ecstasy (MDMA): are the psychological problems associated with its use reversed by prolonged abstinence? Psychopharmacology (Berl) 2002;159(3):294–303.
39. Fox HC, McLean A, Turner JJ, Parrott AC, Rogers R, Sahakian BJ. Neuropsychological evidence of a relatively

selective profile of temporal dysfunction in drug-free MDMA ("ecstasy") polydrug users. Psychopharmacology (Berl) 2002;162(2):203–14.
40. Barrett PJ. "Ecstasy" misuse—overdose or normal dose? Anaesthesia 1993;48(1):83.
41. Wodarz N, Boning J. "Ecstasy"-induziertes psychotisches Depersonalisationssyndrom. ["Ecstasy"-induced psychotic depersonalization syndrome.] Nervenarzt 1993;64(7):478–80.
42. Williams H, Meagher D, Galligan P. M.D.M.A. ("Ecstasy"); a case of possible drug-induced psychosis. Ir J Med Sci 1993;162(2):43–4.
43. Vollenweider FX, Gamma A, Liechti M, Huber T. Psychological and cardiovascular effects and short-term sequelae of MDMA ("ecstasy") in MDMA-naive healthy volunteers. Neuropsychopharmacology 1998;19(4):241–51.
44. McCann UD, Szabo Z, Scheffel U, Dannals RF, Ricaurte GA. Positron emission tomographic evidence of toxic effect of MDMA ("Ecstasy") on brain serotonin neurons in human beings. Lancet 1998;352(9138):1433–7.
45. Windhaber J, Maierhofer D, Dantendorfer K. Panic disorder induced by large doses of 3,4-methylenedioxymethamphetamine resolved by paroxetine. J Clin Psychopharmacol 1998;18(1):95–6.
46. Winstock AR. Chronic paranoid psychosis after misuse of MDMA. BMJ 1991;302(6785):1150–1.
47. MacInnes N, Handley SL, Harding GF. Former chronic methylenedioxymethamphetamine (MDMA or ecstasy) users report mild depressive symptoms. J Psychopharmacol 2001;15(3):181–6.
48. Ricaurte GA, McCann UD. Experimental studies on 3,4-methylenedioxymethamphetamine (MDA, "ecstasy") and its potential to damage brain serotonin neurons. Neurotox Res 2001;3(1):85–99.
49. Heffernan TM, Ling J, Scholey AB. Subjective ratings of prospective memory deficits in MDMA ("ecstasy") users. Hum Psychopharmacol 2001;16(4):339–44.
50. Verkes RJ, Gijsman HJ, Pieters MS, Schoemaker RC, de Visser S, Kuijpers M, Pennings EJ, de Bruin D, Van de Wijngaart G, Van Gerven JM, Cohen AF. Cognitive performance and serotonergic function in users of ecstasy. Psychopharmacology (Berl) 2001;153(2):196–202.
51. Reneman L, Lavalaye J, Schmand B, de Wolff FA, van den Brink W, den Heeten GJ, Booij J. Cortical serotonin transporter density and verbal memory in individuals who stopped using 3,4-methylenedioxymethamphetamine (MDMA or "ecstasy"): preliminary findings. Arch Gen Psychiatry 2001;58(10):901–6.
52. Reneman L, Majoie CB, Schmand B, van den Brink W, den Heeten GJ. Prefrontal N-acetylaspartate is strongly associated with memory performance in (abstinent) ecstasy users: preliminary report. Biol Psychiatry 2001;50(7):550–4.
53. Bhattachary S, Powell JH. Recreational use of 3,4-methylenedioxymethamphetamine (MDMA) or "ecstasy": evidence for cognitive impairment. Psychol Med 2001;31(4):647–58.
54. Croft RJ, Mackay AJ, Mills AT, Gruzelier JG. The relative contributions of ecstasy and cannabis to cognitive impairment. Psychopharmacology (Berl) 2001;153(3):373–9.
55. Liechti ME, Gamma A, Vollenweider FX. Gender differences in the subjective effects of MDMA. Psychopharmacology (Berl) 2001;154(2):161–8.
56. Harry RA, Sherwood R, Wendon J. Detection of myocardial damage and cardiac dysfunction following ecstasy ingestion. Clin Intensive Care 2001;12:85–7.
57. D'Costa DF. Transient myocardial ischaemia associated with accidental Ecstasy ingestion. Br J Cardiol 1998;5:290–1.
58. Brody S, Krause C, Veit R, Rau H. Cardiovascular autonomic dysregulation in users of MDMA ("Ecstasy"). Psychopharmacology (Berl) 1998;136(4):390–3.
59. Duflou J, Mark A. Aortic dissection after ingestion of "ecstasy" (MDMA). Am J Forensic Med Pathol 2000;21(3):261–3.
60. Lester SJ, Baggott M, Welm S, Schiller NB, Jones RT, Foster E, Mendelson J. Cardiovascular effects of 3,4-methylenedioxymethamphetamine. A double-blind, placebo-controlled trial. Ann Intern Med 2000;133(12):969–73.
61. Levine AJ, Drew S, Rees GM. "Ecstasy" induced pneumomediastinum. J R Soc Med 1993;86(4):232–3.
62. Ryan J, Banerjee A, Bong A. Pneumomediastinum in association with MDMA ingestion. J Emerg Med 2001; 20(3):305–6.
63. Rejali D, Glen P, Odom N. Pneumomediastinum following Ecstasy (methylenedioxymetamphetamine, MDMA) ingestion in two people at the same 'rave'. J Laryngol Otol 2002;116(1):75–6.
64. Ahmed JM, Salame MY, Oakley GD. Chest pain in a young girl. Postgrad Med J 1998;74(868):115–16.
65. Ajaelo I, Koenig K, Snoey E. Severe hyponatremia and inappropriate antidiuretic hormone secretion following ecstasy use. Acad Emerg Med 1998;5(8):839–40.
66. Gomez-Balaguer M, Pena H, Morillas C, Hernandez A. Syndrome of inappropriate antidiuretic hormone secretion and "designer drugs" (ecstasy). J Pediatr Endocrinol Metab 2000;13(4):437–8.
67. Roques V, Perney P, Beaufort P, Hanslik B, Ramos J, Durand L, Le Bricquir Y, Blanc F. Hepatite aiguë a l'ecstasy. [Acute hepatitis due to ecstasy.] Presse Méd 1998;27(10):468–70.
68. Jonas MM. Case records of the Massachusetts General Hospital. Weekly clinicopathological exercises. Case 6-2001. A 17-year-old girl with marked jaundice and weight loss. N Engl J Med 2001;344(8):591–9.
69. Hwang I, Daniels AM, Holtzmuller KC. "Ecstasy"-induced hepatitis in an active duty soldier. Mil Med 2002;167(2):155–6.
70. Garbino J, Henry JA, Mentha G, Romand JA. Ecstasy ingestion and fulminant hepatic failure: liver transplantation to be considered as a last therapeutic option. Vet Hum Toxicol 2001;43(2):99–102.
71. De Carlis L, De Gasperi A, Slim AO, Giacomoni A, Corti A, Mazza E, Di Benedetto F, Lauterio A, Arcieri K, Maione G, Rondinara GF, Forti D. Liver transplantation for ecstasy-induced fulminant hepatic failure. Transplant Proc 2001;33(5):2743–4.
72. Caballero F, Lopez-Navidad A, Cotorruelo J, Txoperena G. Ecstasy-induced brain death and acute hepatocellular failure: multiorgan donor and liver transplantation. Transplantation 2002;74(4):532–7.
73. Wollina U, Kammler HJ, Hesselbarth N, Mock B, Bosseckert H. Ecstasy pimples—a new facial dermatosis. Dermatology 1998;197(2):171–3.
74. Gill JR, Hayes JA, deSouza IS, Marker E, Stajic M. Ecstasy (MDMA) deaths in New York City: a case series and review of the literature. J Forensic Sci 2002;47(1):121–6.
75. Gore SM. Fatal uncertainty: death-rate from use of ecstasy or heroin. Lancet 1999;354(9186):1265–6.
76. Ramsey JD, Johnston A, Holt DW. Death rate from use of ecstasy or heroin. Lancet 1999;354(9196):2166.
77. Lind J, Oyefeso A, Pollard M, Baldacchino A, Ghodse H. Death rate from use of ecstasy or heroin. Lancet 1999;354(9196):2167.
78. Fineschi V, Centini F, Mazzeo E, Turillazzi E. Adam (MDMA) and Eve (MDEA) misuse: an immunohistochemical study on three fatal cases. Forensic Sci Int 1999;104(1):65–74.
79. O'Connor A, Cluroe A, Couch R, Galler L, Lawrence J, Synek B. Death from hyponatraemia-induced cerebral oedema associated with MDMA ("Ecstasy") use. NZ Med J 1999;112(1091):255–6.

80. Hartung TK, Schofield E, Short AI, Parr MJ, Henry JA. Hyponatraemic states following 3,4-methylenedioxy-methamphetamine (MDMA, "ecstasy") ingestion. Quart J Med 2002;95(7):431–7.
81. Cherney DZ, Davids MR, Halperin ML. Acute hyponatraemia and 'ecstasy': insights from a quantitative and integrative analysis. Quart J Med 2002;95(7):475–83.
82. Pacifici R, Zuccaro P, Farre M, Pichini S, Di Carlo S, Roset PN, Ortuno J, Segura J, de la Torre R. Immunomodulating properties of MDMA alone and in combination with alcohol: a pilot study. Life Sci 1999;65(26):PL309–16.
83. Pacifici R, Zuccaro P, Farre M, Pichini S, Di Carlo S, Roset PN, Palmi I, Ortuno J, Menoyo E, Segura J, de la Torre R. Cell-mediated immune response in MDMA users after repeated dose administration: studies in controlled versus noncontrolled settings. Ann NY Acad Sci 2002;965:421–33.
84. Murray MO, Wilson NH. Ecstasy related tooth wear. Br Dent J 1998;185(6):264.
85. Goorney BP, Scholes P. Transient haemolytic anaemia due to ecstasy in a patient on HAART. Int J STD AIDS 2002;13(9):651.
86. McCann UD, Ricaurte GA. Major metabolites of (+/-)3,4-methylenedioxyamphetamine (MDA) do not mediate its toxic effects on brain serotonin neurons. Brain Res 1991;545(1–2):279–82.
87. Ho E, Karimi-Tabesh L, Koren G. Characteristics of pregnant women who use ecstasy (3, 4-methylenedioxymethamphetamine). Neurotoxicol Teratol 2001;23(6):561–7.
88. Yates KM, O'Connor A, Horsley CA. "Herbal Ecstasy": a case series of adverse reactions. NZ Med J 2000; 113(1114):315–17.
89. Kraner JC, McCoy DJ, Evans MA, Evans LE, Sweeney BJ. Fatalities caused by the MDMA-related drug paramethoxyamphetamine (PMA). J Anal Toxicol 2001;25(7):645–8.
90. Hsu A, Granneman GR, Bertz RJ. Ritonavir. Clinical pharmacokinetics and interactions with other anti-HIV agents. Clin Pharmacokinet 1998;35(4):275–91.
91. Henry JA, Hill IR. Fatal interaction between ritonavir and MDMA. Lancet 1998;352(9142):1751–2.
92. Harrington RD, Woodward JA, Hooton TM, Horn JR. Life-threatening interactions between HIV-1 protease inhibitors and the illicit drugs MDMA and gamma-hydroxybutyrate. Arch Intern Med 1999;159(18):2221–4.
93. Lauerma H, Wuorela M, Halme M. Interaction of serotonin reuptake inhibitor and 3,4-methylenedioxymethamphetamine? Biol Psychiatry 1998;43(12):929.
94. Hernandez-Lopez C, Farre M, Roset PN, Menoyo E, Pizarro N, Ortuno J, Torrens M, Cami J, de La Torre R. 3,4-Methylenedioxymethamphetamine (ecstasy) and alcohol interactions in humans: psychomotor performance, subjective effects, and pharmacokinetics. J Pharmacol Exp Ther 2002;300(1):236–44.

Methylnaltrexone

See also Opioid antagonists

General Information

Methylnaltrexone is an opioid receptor antagonist that acts peripherally and can be of value in preventing the unwanted effects of opioids while maintaining their central analgesic effects (SEDA-21, 92) (1).

Reference

1. Yuan CS. Clinical status of methylnaltrexone, a new agent to prevent and manage opioid-induced side effects. J Support Oncol 2004;2(2):111–17.

Methylphenidate

See also Anorectic drugs

General Information

Methylphenidate is a piperidine derivative, structurally related to amphetamine, but a milder central nervous system stimulant. However, large doses produce symptoms of generalized central nervous system stimulation and convulsions. It is more active than amphetamine as an antidepressant, as a treatment for overdosage of depressant drugs, and in exacerbating schizophrenic symptoms. Occasionally, anorexia, nausea, dry mouth, nervousness, insomnia, dizziness, and palpitation have been recorded.

Considerable concern surrounds the use of methylphenidate, and to a lesser extent amphetamine and pemoline, in hyperactive children or those with attention deficit hyperactivity disorder (ADHD), because of possible detrimental effects on general physical and emotional growth and central nervous system development. The Psychopharmacology Pediatric Subcommittee of the FDA in the USA has reviewed the literature relevant to growth suppression by stimulants in the treatment of hyperkinesia. There is clear evidence of temporary retardation in weight increase and a suggestion of temporary slowing of height increase related to dose and absence of drug holidays during the prepubertal period (1–3). Drug holidays allow growth rebound in children who require higher doses.

At an NIH Consensus Conference, one of the conclusions was that "... careful therapeutic use of stimulants is effective in treating the core symptoms of ADHD as long as a child is taking the medication" (4). However, the panel identified "... the need to study the benefits and risk of long-term use of such medications. Although behavioral treatments produced positive short-term results it remains unclear what combinations of these strategies are most effective... Although little information exists concerning the long-term effects of psychostimulants, there is no conclusive evidence that careful therapeutic use is harmful. When adverse drug reactions do occur, they are usually related to dose. It is well known that psychostimulants have abuse potential ...". However, drugs used for ADHD, other than psychostimulants, have their own adverse reaction patterns: "tricyclic antidepressants may induce cardiac arrhythmias, bupropion at high doses can cause seizures, and pemoline is associated with liver damage." Effects associated with moderate doses include reduced appetite and insomnia. These effects occur early in treatment and may abate with continued dosing. There may be negative effects on growth rate, but final height does not appear to be affected. Rarely, children and adults who take high doses have hallucinogenic responses. The need for long-term follow-up looking for potential adverse effects was highlighted by the conference.

The short-term and long-term efficacy and safety of pharmacological and nonpharmacological interventions in patients with ADHD have been discussed in a systematic review of 92 reports of 78 randomized clinical trials (5). There was substantial heterogeneity in the data, and so a meta-analysis was not performed. In 22 comparisons of stimulants, the drugs did not generally differ in efficacy. The evidence was too limited for a reliable assessment of the effectiveness of stimulant drugs compared with tricyclic antidepressants. Of six comparisons of drugs and non-drug interventions, five showed that stimulants were more effective. In 20 trials of combined interventions there was no compelling evidence to support combination treatment. Of nine comparisons of tricyclic antidepressants with placebo, six showed benefit with desipramine, whereas the effect of imipramine (three trials) was inconsistent. The study with the highest methodological score showed greater benefit with methylphenidate than placebo. Adverse effects, such as sleep disorders, headache, tics, reduced appetite, abdominal pain, irritability, nausea, and fatigue, were assessed in 29 trials. No evidence was available for more severe, long-term adverse effects, such as the risk of addiction with stimulants, liver toxicity with pemoline, or cardiac dysrhythmias with antidepressants. The authors concluded that in patients with ADHD published studies of treatment regimens provide limited information of effectiveness because of small sample sizes, flawed methods, and heterogeneity across outcomes. Thus, pharmacological interventions in ADHD are consistently more effective than nonpharmacological interventions. Combined interventions are not more beneficial than single interventions.

Two reviews have addressed the diagnosis and management of ADHD and have summarized the effects of stimulants, including those of methylphenidate and Adderall® (a mixture of equal components of D-amfetamine saccharate, D,L-amfetamine aspartate, D-amfetamine sulfate, and D,L-amfetamine sulfate, which seems to be gaining popularity in the treatment of ADHD) (6,7).

The results of the National Institute of Mental Health Collaborative Multimodal Treatment Study of children with attention deficit hyperkinetic disorder have been analysed (8). This double-blind, placebo-controlled methylphenidate titration trial identified the optimum dose and replicated previously reported methylphenidate response rates and dose-related adverse events. For parent ratings, the severity of the following adverse events increased as the dose was raised: appetite suppression, dull/listless appearance, stomachache, tearfulness, and trouble sleeping. For teacher ratings, the only significant drug-related adverse event that had a dose-related trend was reduced appetite. Other adverse events reported by teachers were dull/listless appearance, crabbiness, and buccal movement or chewing. However, these teacher-reported adverse events improved with increased methylphenidate dosage. The authors also emphasized that parents report more dose-related adverse events than teachers do, making them better reporters of safety during dosage titration.

As more adults with ADHD are being treated with methylphenidate, the possibility of drug interactions with methylphenidate increases (9). However, based on a study in extensive and poor CYP2D6 metabolizers, it has been suggested that CYP2D6 is not involved in the metabolism of methylphenidate, and that drugs that are inhibitors of CYP2D6 should not affect methylphenidate plasma concentrations (10).

Organs and Systems

Cardiovascular

Significant increases in blood pressure and/or pulse rate after methylphenidate are more frequent when it is given parenterally (11) (SEDA-4, 9).

Cardiac dysrhythmias, shock, cardiac muscle pathology, and liver pathology have all been reported (12).

Ambulatory blood pressure monitoring showed changes in blood pressure and heart rate in boys aged 7–11 years taking stimulant therapy (13). This preliminary study with chronic methylphenidate or Adderall® (dexamfetamine + levamfetamine) for ADHD showed alterations in awake and asleep blood pressures, with profound nocturnal dipping. Modified-release formulations of methylphenidate and Adderall® now allow more sustained blood concentrations in children. The effects of these newer formulations on cardiovascular indices should be evaluated.

Nervous system

A first case of neuroleptic malignant syndrome probably caused by methylphenidate has been reported in a child with multicystic encephalomalacia due to severe perinatal hypoxic/ischemic encephalopathy (14). At 1.5 years of age, because her circadian rhythm was irregular or reversed, methylphenidate (3 mg/day) was given for its antihypnotic effect. The diagnostic criteria of neuroleptic malignant syndrome (15) were fulfilled in this case, including three major manifestations (fever, rigidity, and raised creatine kinase activity) and six minor ones (tachycardia, abnormal blood pressure, tachypnea, altered consciousness, sweating, and leukocytosis). Other predisposing factors, such as pre-existing severe brain damage suggestive of organic fragility and infection, may have contributed.

There is continuing concern about the potential for methylphenidate to precipitate tics or Tourette's syndrome, in subjects with and without pre-existing tics. However, in a placebo-controlled crossover study in 91 children with ADHD, the usual doses of methylphenidate did not produce significantly more tics than placebo in children with or without pre-existing tics (16). This study had limitations of sample size and statistical power. Moreover, these conclusions cannot be generalized to patients who use higher doses of methylphenidate, because a dose-dependent relation between methylphenidate and tics has been proposed (17). Until the effect of methylphenidate in larger populations has been studied with more exacting measures of tics, it would be wise to monitor for tics, especially if higher doses (0.5–1.3 mg/kg) of methylphenidate are required.

The risk of using methylphenidate for long periods has been highlighted by a case of a stroke in a child (18).

- An 8-year-old boy, who had taken methylphenidate (20 mg/day) for 18 months, suddenly developed paresthesia in his left arm, with spontaneous resolution after a few days. Two months later he had intense paresthesia in the left arm, spreading to the left side of the face; 48 hours later he developed weakness of the arm that extended to the whole of the left side of the body. He remained lucid. The episode resolved spontaneously within 24 hours. After a symptom-free period of 2 months, he had a third episode, similar to the previous ones, but more severe and leaving a residual deficit. Methylphenidate was withdrawn and he did not subsequently relapse. A CT scan showed a hypodense area in the left thalamus, and an MRI scan showed multiple lesions in both thalami. A cerebral angiogram showed enlargement of the basilar artery and the proximal segment of both posterior cerebral arteries.

The authors suggested that in this case the stroke was due to a vasculitis, which has previously been reported with methylphenidate (19).

Episodes of explosive behavior, apparently due to methylphenidate, masquerading as unmanageable ADHD, have been reported (20).

- A 10-year-old boy developed motor and vocal tics and severe obsessive-compulsive symptoms, predominantly about symmetry. These were not evident before he started taking methylphenidate. At 7 years of age he had begun a regimen of methylphenidate 20 mg/day in divided doses. Paradoxically, his impulsive behavior increased and he began to have explosions of aggressive and violent behavior, during which he would lash out at his family or destroy things. After a year of methylphenidate therapy, the tics subsided spontaneously but other symptoms remained. Eventually, because of severe impairment resulting from obsessive-compulsive symptoms, his parents stopped giving him methylphenidate. A few months later there were no further obsessive-compulsive preoccupations and no tics, and he did not have any explosive behavior.

It is well recognized that in vulnerable individuals, methylphenidate can induce or aggravate Tourette's syndrome, most often characterized by motor tics and occasionally vocal tics (21). Moreover, obsessive-compulsive symptoms caused by methylphenidate have also been reported (22,23). However, it is not clear whether explosive episodes associated with Tourette's syndrome are an integral part of the disorder or occur as part of a co-morbid disorder, predominantly ADHD or obsessive-compulsive disorder. In this case the explosive episodes coincided with a period of treatment with methylphenidate. In view of the extreme, sudden, discrete nature of the outbursts and the temporal relation to treatment, it was concluded that the episodes were behavioral problems caused by methylphenidate, rather than a feature of the underlying ADHD.

As with other stimulants, chorea (24) and choreoathetosis (25) can be precipitated in children and adults at methylphenidate doses ranging from therapeutic to abuse levels. These symptoms respond to drug withdrawal or neuroleptic drugs.

Psychological, psychiatric

Methylphenidate-induced obsessive-compulsive symptoms are very rare (26); a second case has been reported (22).

- An 8-year-old boy had unusual difficulties in completing a trial of methylphenidate for ADHD. Methylphenidate 10 mg/day initially improved his school performance, but by the end of the second week of treatment severe obsessive-compulsive behavior began to emerge, requiring drug withdrawal. He eventually refused to eat because he suspected that his food was being poisoned. His parents reported that he became more sensitive and easily upset, appearing increasingly tense and fearful. He continued to have intrusive distressing contamination worries. He had repetitive tic-like movements of his head and neck, frequently rubbed his face with his shirtsleeves, and avoided touching his face directly with his fingers for fear of contamination. His symptoms gradually and completely dissipated over 2–3 months without specific intervention. While very mild symptoms of ADHD persisted, he remained entirely free of symptoms at 1 year. Medication was not restarted.

This case lends further support to existing anecdotal evidence associating methylphenidate with obsessive-compulsive disorder of acute onset. However, rechallenge was not attempted, and causality should be viewed as being uncertain.

In a small percentage of hyperactive children, there were gross behavioral changes with hallucinations after brief administration of modest doses of methylphenidate; the reaction subsided after withdrawal (27).

Endocrine

Methylphenidate has been reported to cause stunting of growth by impairing growth hormone secretion (28).

- A 10-year-old boy with ADHD and chronic asthma, who was using inhaled corticosteroids, developed almost complete growth arrest during methylphenidate treatment. Growth hormone stimulation tests and measurement of growth hormone-dependent growth factors suggested that methylphenidate had altered growth hormone secretion and had impaired growth. Determination of growth velocity was a sensitive marker for the evaluation of growth.

Metabolism

The association between childhood treatment with methylphenidate and adult height and weight has been investigated in 97 boys, aged 4–12 years, who were referred to a child psychiatry out-patients clinic and took methylphenidate for an average of 36 months (29). They were re-evaluated between ages 21 and 23 years. Hierarchical analysis predicted adult height and weight from sets of both nonmedication-related and medication-related variables. Medicated individuals who had attained their final stature did not differ in average height or weight from family, community, or nonmedicated

4 Anonymous. Diagnosis and treatment of attention deficit hyperactivity disorder (ADHD). NIH Consensus Statement 1998;16(2):1–37.
5 Jadad AR, Boyle M, Cunningham C. Treatment of attention deficit/hyperactivity disorder. Evid Based Med 2000;5:179.
6 Perrin JM, Stein MT, Amler RW, Blondis TA, Feldman HM, Meyer BP. American Academy of Pediatrics. Subcommittee on Attention-Deficit/Hyperactivity Disorder and Committee on Quality Improvement. Clinical practice guideline: treatment of the school-aged child with attention-deficit/hyperactivity disorder. Pediatrics 2001;108(4):1033–44.
7 Kirby K, Floriani V, Bernstein H. Diagnosis and management of attention-deficit/hyperactivity disorder in children. Curr Opin Pediatr 2001;13(2):190–9.
8 Greenhill LL, Swanson JM, Vitiello B, Davies M, Clevenger W, Wu M, Arnold LE, Abikoff HB, Bukstein OG, Conners CK, Elliott GR, Hechtman L, Hinshaw SP, Hoza B, Jensen PS, Kraemer HC, March JS, Newcorn JH, Severe JB, Wells K, Wigal T. Impairment and deportment responses to different methylphenidate doses in children with ADHD: the MTA titration trial. J Am Acad Child Adolesc Psychiatry 2001;40(2):180–7.
9 Markowitz JS, Morrison SD, DeVane CL. Drug interactions with psychostimulants. Int Clin Psychopharmacol 1999;14(1):1–18.
10 DeVane CL, Markowitz JS, Carson SW, Boulton DW, Gill HS, Nahas Z, Risch SC. Single-dose pharmacokinetics of methylphenidate in CYP2D6 extensive and poor metabolizers. J Clin Psychopharmacol 2000;20(3):347–9.
11 Witton K. On the use of parenteral methylphenidate: a follow-up report. Am J Psychiatry 1964;121:267–8.
12 Chernoff RW, Wallen MH, Muller OF. Cardiac toxicity of methylphenidate: report of two cases. Nord Hyg Tidskr 1962;266:400–1.
13 Stowe CD, Gardner SF, Gist CC, Schulz EG, Wells TG, Felin JF. 24-hour ambulatory blood pressure monitoring in male children receiving stimulant therapy. Ann Pharmacother 2002;36(7–8):1142–9.
14 Ehara H, Maegaki Y, Takeshita K. Neuroleptic malignant syndrome and methylphenidate. Pediatr Neurol 1998;19(4):299–301.
15 Levenson JL. Neuroleptic malignant syndrome. Am J Psychiatry 1985;142(10):1137–45.
16 Law SF, Schachar RJ. Do typical clinical doses of methylphenidate cause tics in children treated for attention-deficit hyperactivity disorder? J Am Acad Child Adolesc Psychiatry 1999;38(8):944–51.
17 Castellanos FX, Giedd JN, Elia J, Marsh WL, Ritchie GF, Hamburger SD, Rapoport JL. Controlled stimulant treatment of ADHD and comorbid Tourette's syndrome: effects of stimulant and dose. J Am Acad Child Adolesc Psychiatry 1997;36(5):589–96.
18 Schteinschnaider A, Plaghos LL, Garbugino S, Riveros D, Lazarowski A, Intruvini S, Massaro M. Cerebral arteritis following methylphenidate use. J Child Neurol 2000;15(4):265–7.
19 Trugman JM. Cerebral arteritis and oral methylphenidate. Lancet 1988;1(8585):584–5.
20 Adrian N. Explosive outbursts associated with methylphenidate. J Am Acad Child Adolesc Psychiatry 2001; 40(6):618–19.
21 Budman CL, Bruun RD, Park KS, Lesser M, Olson M. Explosive outbursts in children with Tourette's disorder. J Am Acad Child Adolesc Psychiatry 2000;39(10):1270–6.
22 Kouris S. Methylphenidate-induced obsessive-compulsiveness. J Am Acad Child Adolesc Psychiatry 1998;37(2):135.
23 Kotsopoulos S, Spivak M. Obsessive-compulsive symptoms secondary to methylphenidate treatment. Can J Psychiatry 2001;46(1):89.
24 Extein I. Methylphenidate-induced choreoathetosis. Am J Psychiatry 1978;135(2):252–3.
25 Weiner WJ, Nausieda PA, Klawans HL. Methylphenidate-induced chorea: case report and pharmacologic implications. Neurology 1978;28(10):1041–4.
26 Koizumi HM. Obsessive-compulsive symptoms following stimulants. Biol Psychiatry 1985;20(12):1332–3.
27 Janowsky DS, el-Yousel MK, Davis JM, Sekerke HJ. Provocation of schizophrenic symptoms by intravenous administration of methylphenidate. Arch Gen Psychiatry 1973;28(2):185–91.
28 Holtkamp K, Peters-Wallraf B, Wuller S, Pfaaffle R, Herpertz-Dahlmann B. Methylphenidate-related growth impairment. J Child Adolesc Psychopharmacol 2002;12(1):55–61.
29 Kramer JR, Loney J, Ponto LB, Roberts MA, Grossman S. Predictors of adult height and weight in boys treated with methylphenidate for childhood behavior problems. J Am Acad Child Adolesc Psychiatry 2000;39(4):517–24.
30 Greenhill LL, Findling RL, Swanson JM; ADHD, Study Group. A double-blind, placebo-controlled study of modified-release methylphenidate in children with attention-deficit/hyperactivity disorder. Pediatrics 2002; 109(3):E39.
31 Lopez F, Silva R, Pestreich L, Muniz R. Comparative efficacy of two once daily methylphenidate formulations (Ritalin LA and Concerta) and placebo in children with attention deficit hyperactivity disorder across the school day. Paediatr Drugs 2003;5(8):545–55.
32 Goodman CR. Hepatotoxicity due to methylphenidate hydrochloride. NY State J Med 1972;72(18):2339–40.
33 Wilens TE, Biederman J, Mick E, Faraone SV, Spencer T. Attention deficit hyperactivity disorder (ADHD) is associated with early onset substance use disorders. J Nerv Ment Dis 1997;185(8):475–82.
34 Hechtman L, Weiss G. Controlled prospective fifteen year follow-up of hyperactives as adults: non-medical drug and alcohol use and anti-social behaviour. Can J Psychiatry 1986;31(6):557–67.
35 Schain RJ, Reynard CL. Observations on effects of a central stimulant drug (methylphenidate) in children with hyperactive behavior. Pediatrics 1975;55(5):709–16.
36 Biederman J, Wilens T, Mick E, Spencer T, Faraone SV. Pharmacotherapy of attention-deficit/hyperactivity disorder reduces risk for substance use disorder. Pediatrics 1999;104(2):e20.
37 Wolraich ML, Greenhill LL, Pelham W, Swanson J, Wilens T, Palumbo D, Atkins M, McBurnett K, Bukstein O, August G. Randomized, controlled trial of oros methylphenidate once a day in children with attention-deficit/hyperactivity disorder. Pediatrics 2001;108(4):883–92.
38 Massello W 3rd, Carpenter DA. A fatality due to the intranasal abuse of methylphenidate (Ritalin). J Forensic Sci 1999;44(1):220–1.
39 Hong R, Matsuyama E, Nur K. Cardiomyopathy associated with the smoking of crystal methamphetamine. JAMA 1991;265(9):1152–4.
40 Rajs J, Falconer B. Cardiac lesions in intravenous drug addicts. Forensic Sci Int 1979;13(3):193–209.
41 White SR, Yadao CM. Characterization of methylphenidate exposures reported to a regional poison control center. Arch Pediatr Adolesc Med 2000;154(12):1199–203.
42 Schaller JL, Behar D. Carbamazepine and methylphenidate in ADHD. J Am Acad Child Adolesc Psychiatry 1999; 38(2):112–13.
43 Lewis BR, Aoun SL, Bernstein GA, Crow SJ. Pharmacokinetic interactions between cyclosporine and bupropion or methylphenidate. J Child Adolesc Psychopharmacol 2001;11(2):193–8.

44 Jansen IH, Olde Rikkert MG, Hulsbos HA, Hoefnagels WH. Toward individualized evidence-based medicine: five "N of 1" trials of methylphenidate in geriatric patients J Am Geriatr Soc 2001;49(4):474–6.
45 Lavretsky H, Kumar A. Methylphenidate augmentation of citalopram in elderly depressed patients. Am J Geriatr Psychiatry 2001;9(3):298–303.
46 Wilens TE, Spencer TJ, Swanson JM, Connor DF, Cantwell D. Combining methylphenidate and clonidine: a clinically sound medication option. J Am Acad Child Adolesc Psychiatry 1999;38(5):614–19.
47 Fenichel RF. Combining methylphenidate and clonidine: the role of post-marketing surveillance. J Child Adolesc Psychopharmacol 1995;5:155–6.
48 Cantwell DP, Swanson J, Connor DF. Case study: adverse response to clonidine. J Am Acad Child Adolesc Psychiatry 1997;36(4):539–44.
49 Markowitz JS, Logan BK, Diamond F, Patrick KS. Detection of the novel metabolite ethylphenidate after methylphenidate overdose with alcohol coingestion. J Clin Psychopharmacol 1999;19(4):362–6.
50 McCance EF, Price LH, Kosten TR, Jatlow PI. Cocaethylene: pharmacology, physiology and behavioral effects in humans. J Pharmacol Exp Ther 1995;274(1):215–23.
51 Bourland JA, Martin DK, Mayersohn M. Carboxylesterase-mediated transesterification of meperidine (Demerol) and methylphenidate (Ritalin) in the presence of [^{2}H6]ethanol: preliminary in vitro findings using a rat liver preparation J Pharm Sci 1997;86(12):1494–6.
52 Camicioli R, Lea E, Nutt JG, Sexton G, Oken BS. Methylphenidate increases the motor effects of L-dopa in Parkinson's disease: a pilot study. Clin Neuropharmacol 2001;24(4):208–13.
53 Garrettson LK, Perel JM, Dayton PG. Methylphenidate interaction with both anticonvulsants and ethyl biscoumacetate. JAMA 1969;207(11):2053–6.
54 Kupferberg HJ, Jeffery W, Hunninghake DB. Effect of methylphenidate on plasma anticonvulsant levels. Clin Pharmacol Ther 1972;13(2):201–4.
55 Flemenbaum A. Hypertensive episodes after adding methylphenidate (Ritalin) to tricyclic antidepressants. (Report of three cases and review of clinical advantages.) Psychosomatics 1972;13(4):265–8.
56 Gara L, Roberts W. Adverse response to methylphenidate in combination with valproic acid. J Child Adolesc Psychopharmacol 2000;10(1):39–43.

Methylphenobarbital

See also Antiepileptic drugs

General Information

The adverse effects of methylphenobarbital are similar to those of phenobarbital, to which methylphenobarbital is metabolized.

Organs and Systems

Immunologic

Giant cell myocarditis has been reported in a patient taking phenytoin, phenobarbital, and methylphenobarbital, and in one taking primidone (1).

Second-Generation Effects

Teratogenicity

There is an association of methylphenobarbital with oral clefts and cardiac malformations (2).

References

1. Daniels PR, Berry GJ, Tazelaar HD, Cooper LT. Giant cell myocarditis as a manifestation of drug hypersensitivity. Cardiovasc Pathol 2000;9(5):287–91.
2. Arpino C, Brescianini S, Robert E, Castilla EE, Cocchi G, Cornel MC, de Vigan C, Lancaster PA, Merlob P, Sumiyoshi Y, Zampino G, Renzi C, Rosano A, Mastroiacovo P. Teratogenic effects of antiepileptic drugs: use of an International Database on Malformations and Drug Exposure (MADRE). Epilepsia 2000;41(11):1436–43.

Methyl-tert-butylether and monoctanoin

General Information

Methyl-tert-butylether and monoctanoin are solvents that are used for the rapid dissolution of cholesterol gallstones in patients who are not considered suitable for surgery. They are given by direct infusion into the gallbladder (1). However, they are suitable only for cholesterol stones, take too long to act, are often not successful, and have high rates of adverse effects (2).

The results of contact dissolution of gallstones using infusions of methyl-tert-butylether by percutaneous transhepatic gallbladder puncture have been assessed in 803 patients (3). Stones were dissolved in 724 of 761 patients in whom gallbladder puncture was successful. The 30-day mortality was 0.4%. Common complications were biliary leak, fever, leukocytosis, abdominal pain, and mild increases in transaminases. Toxic effects due to ether were not reported.

Fever, abdominal pain, nausea, vomiting, and diarrhea all occur frequently with methyl-tert-butylether and monoctanoin. Activities of serum amylase or liver enzymes can be slightly raised.

In 343 patients treated with monoctanoin there were adverse effects in 67% (4). Abdominal pain was the commonest (in 40%), followed by nausea (25%), vomiting (15%), diarrhea (16%), and fever (5%). One patient with hepatic cirrhosis developed an acidosis and encephalopathy. The adverse effects were usually dose-related and responded to reduction in infusion rate. The effects were life threatening in 12 patients (5%), but there were no permanent sequelae and no deaths.

Of 42 patients, 19 of whom received methyl tert-butylether alone and 23 with bile acid-ethylenediaminetetraacetate, there were mild complications in 40: vomiting in 12, pain at the start of treatment in 32, raised liver enzymes in six, and fever and leukocytosis in five (5). In those given methyl tert-butylether alone, there were two serious complications (gallbladder wall necrosis with perforation in one and catheter dislocation in the other). In those given combination therapy there were five serious complications: pericystic extravasation in two and catheter dislocation, sterile perihepatic abscess, and perihepatic biloma in one each. A CT scan with intravenous contrast after treatment was performed in 27 patients and showed gallbladder mural hyperemia and edematous swelling of the pericystic tissue layer in 26 cases.

Organs and Systems

Respiratory

Non-cardiogenic pulmonary edema has been reported with monoctanoin after appropriate intra-biliary use (6). If monoctanoin is injected intravenously in error, fatal respiratory and cardiac arrest can occur (7).

Biliary tract

Cholecystitis can be induced, at least when methyl-tert-butylether is used alongside ethylenediaminetetra-acetic acid (SEDA-16, 428). Most such effects are probably attributable to over-rapid infusion.

Necrotizing choledochomalacia has also been described with monoctanoin (8). Gallstone impaction has been described.

References

1. LaFerla G, McCulloch A, Murray WR. In-vivo chemical choledocholitholysis using MTBE. Br J Hosp Med 1987;37(2):163–4.
2. Sauerbruch T. Non-surgical management of bile duct stones refractory to routine endoscopic measures. Baillières Clin Gastroenterol 1992;6(4):799–817.
3. Hellstern A, Leuschner U, Benjaminov A, Ackermann H, Heine T, Festi D, Orsini M, Roda E, Northfield TC, Jazrawi R, Kurtz W, Schmeck-Lindenau HJ, Stumpf J, Eidsvoll BE, Aadland E, Lux G, Boehnke E, Wurbs D, Delhaye M, Cremer M, Sinn I, Horing E, v Gaisberg U, Neubrand M, Paul F, et al. Dissolution of gallbladder stones with methyl tert-butyl ether and stone recurrence: a European survey. Dig Dis Sci 1998;43(5):911–20.
4. Palmer KR, Hofmann AF. Intraductal mono-octanoin for the direct dissolution of bile duct stones: experience in 343 patients. Gut 1986;27(2):196–202.
5. Janowitz P, Schumacher KA, Kratzer W, Tudyka J, Wechsler JG. Transhepatic topical dissolution of gallbladder stones with MTBE and EDTA. Results, side effects, and correlation with CT imaging. Dig Dis Sci 1993;38(11):2121–9.
6. Shustack A, Noseworthy TW, Johnston RG, Anderson BJ, Johnston D, Bailey RJ. Noncardiogenic pulmonary edema during intrabiliary infusion of mono-octanoin. Crit Care Med 1986;14(7):659–60.
7. Hejka AG, Poquette M, Wiebe DA, Huntington RW 3rd. Fatal intravenous injection of monooctanoin. Am J Forensic Med Pathol 1990;11(2):165–70.
8. Crabtree TS, Dykstra R, Kelly J, Preshaw RM. Necrotizing choledochomalacia after use of monooctanoin to dissolve bile-duct stones. Can J Surg 1982;25(6):644–6.

Methylthioninium chloride

General Information

Methylthioninium chloride (methylene blue) has been used for a variety of purposes, including marking of polyps, identification of sinus and fistula tracts, localizing islet cell tumors (1), marking of skin incisions in plastic surgery (2), labelling of vascular malformations, and the treatment of methemoglobinemia. Transient burning and blue discoloration can occur (3).

Organs and Systems

Hematologic

Severe hemolytic reactions have been attributed to methylthioninium chloride (4).

Immunologic

Methylthioninium chloride marking of a colonic polyp resulted in an inflammatory mass with small arteries showing both segmental and circumferential fibrinoid necrosis with thrombosis (5).

- A 68-year-old Hispanic woman had multiple polyps associated with recurrent episodes of hematochezia over several years. All but a single polyp were removed endoscopically. The region of the remaining polyp was labelled with 2 ml of methylthioninium chloride injected in divided doses to aid operative localization. Because surgery was postponed, methylthioninium chloride was again injected. At surgery the polyp and a 5 cm perirectal indurated mass were identified, and there was a blue track from the submucosal to the outer portions of muscularis propria into the adjacent fat. Microscopically, the mucosa was intact and the submucosa was edematous. There were acute inflammatory cells in the submucosa and muscularis propria. Inflammation (acute and chronic), fibroblastic proliferation, and fat necrosis were seen in areas outside the muscularis propria and extending to the connective tissue margin. A prominent finding was fibrinoid necrosis of small arteries, in some cases segmental and in others circumferential. The internal elastic lamina was destroyed and there were thromboses and vessel wall inflammation. There was no evidence of infiltrating carcinoma in the adenomatous polyp or the adjacent colon. The inflammation and vascular changes were only in the mass defined grossly by induration; sections away from this area were unremarkable. The blue track contained blue–black pigment within macrophages.

The mechanisms of the tissue damage and vascular changes in this case were unclear.

Anaphylactic shock has been attributed to methylthioninium chloride (SEDA-22, 526).

Second-Generation Effects

Pregnancy

Significant neonatal morbidity can occur after transabdominal infusion of methylthioninium chloride to diagnose premature rupture of fetal membranes, to stain the amniotic fluid in twin pregnancies, or after postpartum administration of methylthioninium chloride. Toxic manifestations include hyperbilirubinemia, Heinz body hemolytic anemia, and possible desquamation of the skin. In most cases it appears that toxicity was the result of an overdose of methylthioninium chloride (6–9).

Fetotoxicity

Multiple ileal occlusions have been reported in babies born to mothers who had twin pregnancies and who had received methylthioninium chloride administered during amniocentesis (10–12). In a number of cases it was found that methylthioninium chloride had been injected into the amniotic sac of the affected twins.

Methylthioninium chloride phototoxicity may also be related to the high prenatal dose of the dye relative to patient's small size and young gestational age (13).

The fetal death rate appears to increase after the use of methylthioninium chloride during pregnancy. In a retrospective cohort study of all women who had an amniocentesis during twin pregnancy from 1980 to 1991 in New South Wales in Australia, women who were exposed to methylthioninium chloride dye during the procedure were compared with women who had amniocentesis without dye exposure (14). Fetal death occurred in 32% of pregnancies that had exposure to a high concentration of methylthioninium chloride, compared with 15% of pregnancies exposed to a low concentration and 4.3% of pregnancies with no exposure to dye. It was concluded that methylthioninium chloride dye use during mid-trimester amniocentesis in twin pregnancy increases the risk of fetal death.

Drug Administration

Drug administration route

Methylthioninium chloride is sometimes given intrathecally to track the source of a cerebrospinal fluid leak. This procedure involves considerable risk of spinal cord damage, with its attendant neurological consequences (15–17).

- A 59-year-old man had 6 ml of unbuffered methylthioninium chloride injected into the lumbar theca in an attempt to localize the source of cerebrospinal fluid rhinorrhea (18). After injection of the dye he became shocked, and within the next few days developed a mild paraparesis, which subsequently progressed to total paraplegia.

Drug overdose

Overdosage of methylthioninium chloride given intravenously, which has happened inadvertently during urinary tract surgery, can cause shock and pseudocyanosis. The latter is due to the blue tinge of methylthioninium chloride, and it can create confusion as to the patient's circulatory status. Patients receiving methylthioninium chloride should be examined for unstable hemoglobins or an abnormal hexose monophosphate pathway if the risk of methemoglobinemia is to be minimized; this has been described with a normal dose (19).

References

1. Ko TC, Flisak M, Prinz RA. Selective intra-arterial methylene blue injection: a novel method of localizing gastrinoma. Gastroenterology 1992;102(3):1062–4.
2. Granick MS, Heckler FR, Jones EW. Surgical skin-marking techniques. Plast Reconstr Surg 1987;79(4):573–80.
3. Martinez Portillo F, Hoang-Boehm J, Weiss J, Alken P, Junemann K. Methylene blue as a successful treatment alternative for pharmacologically induced priapism. Eur Urol 2001;39(1):20–3.
4. Gauthier TW. Methylene blue-induced hyperbilirubinemia in neonatal glucose-6-phosphate dehydrogenase (G6PD) deficiency. J Matern Fetal Med 2000;9(4):252–4.
5. Borczuk AC, Petterino B, Alt E. Inflammatory mass with fibrinoid necrosis of vessels caused by methylene blue marking of a colonic polyp. Cardiovasc Pathol 1998;7:267–9.
6. Sills MR, Zinkham WH. Methylene blue-induced Heinz body hemolytic anemia. Arch Pediatr Adolesc Med 1994;148(3):306–10.
7. Elias S, Gerbie AB, Simpson JL, Nadler HL, Sabbagha RE, Shkolnik A. Genetic amniocentesis in twin gestations. Am J Obstet Gynecol 1980;138(2):169–74.
8. Kirsch IR, Cohen HJ. Heinz body hemolytic anemia from the use of methylene blue in neonates. J Pediatr 1980;96(2):276–8.
9. Serota FT, Bernbaum JC, Schwartz E. The methylene-blue baby. Lancet 1979;2(8152):1142–3.
10. Nicolini U, Monni G. Intestinal obstruction in babies exposed in utero to methylene blue. Lancet 1990; 336(8725):1258–9.
11. Dolk H. Methylene blue and atresia or stenosis of ileum and jejunum. EUROCAT Working Group. Lancet 1991; 338(8773):1021–2.
12. Cragan JD, Martin ML, Khoury MJ, Fernhoff PM. Dye use during amniocentesis and birth defects. Lancet 1993; 341(8856):1352.
13. Porat R, Gilbert S, Magilner D. Methylene blue-induced phototoxicity: an unrecognized complication. Pediatrics 1996;97(5):717–21.
14. Kidd SA, Lancaster PA, Anderson JC, Boogert A, Fisher CC, Robertson R, Wass DM. Fetal death after exposure to methylene blue dye during mid-trimester amniocentesis in twin pregnancy. Prenat Diagn 1996; 16(1):39–47.
15. Gross SW. Neurological deficits resulting from intrathecal administration of methylene blue. Neuroradiology 1974; 7(2):117.
16. Schultz P, Schwarz GA. Radiculomyelopathy following intrathecal instillation of methylene blue. A hazard reaffirmed. Arch Neurol 1970;22(3):240–4.
17. Arieff AJ, Pyzik SW. Quadriplegia after intrathecal injection of methylene blue. JAMA 1960;173:794–6.
18. Sharr MM, Weller RO, Brice JG. Spinal cord necrosis after intrathecal injection of methylene blue. J Neurol Neurosurg Psychiatry 1978;41(4):384–6.
19. Whitwam JG, Taylor AR, White JM. Potential hazard of methylene blue. Anaesthesia 1979;34(2):181–2.

taking the drug. The prominent clinical effect was an oculogyric crisis in all cases, while children who took higher doses also became drowsy. All extrapyramidal symptoms were treated successfully with a single intravenous dose of procyclidine hydrochloride 0.1 mg/kg.

Severe parkinsonism has been reported in a 73-year-old woman with tuberculosis of the large intestine who had taken metoclopramide for nausea; she recovered on withdrawal of the drug and treatment with biperiden (7).

The "blue tongue" sign, in which the tongue is blue and swollen and obstructs the upper airway, is an unusual but dangerous manifestation of the same group of adverse effects (SED-12, 940) (8).

Acute dystonia has been reported in three men with AIDS who had received metoclopramide; they recovered on withdrawal and treatment with biperiden or diazepam (9). Dystonic reactions seem to be particularly problematic in the very young and the very old, but the frequency is disputed (10). In one overview acute movement disorders were thought to have occurred in about one in 80 young adults (SEDA-17, 414). When metoclopramide is given by intravenous injection, for example as an aid to gastric emptying imaging, akathisia seems to occur mainly in women or young men, and more often if the injection is more rapid.

The fact that the neurological reactions can be difficult or impossible to distinguish from spontaneous parkinsonism perhaps explains reports of apparently irreversible effects; almost certainly in such cases the disorders were not exclusively due to the drug.

A lengthy withdrawal reaction has also been described after 6 months of treatment, characterized by an alternation of an akinetic state and akathisia reminiscent of the restlessness seen in parkinsonism (11); even after a year of symptomatic treatment the effects had not fully subsided.

Psychological, psychiatric

Supersensitivity psychosis has been reported in two men, aged 74 and 65 years, who had taken metoclopramide 5 mg qds for 6 and 3 months respectively (12). Hallucinations and delusions developed 12 hours after the drug was withdrawn in one patient and 3 days after withdrawal in the other. Both recovered after treatment with risperidone.

Endocrine

Hyperprolactinemia and galactorrhea, sometimes with gynecomastia, are classic complications of metoclopramide that can equally well occur in adults, children, or neonates (13) (SEDA-22, 390).

Vasopressin release has been claimed to be enhanced by metoclopramide, while aldosterone release is impaired (SED-12, 940).

Hematologic

Effects of metoclopramide on the blood are very uncommon, but neutropenia has been reported in circumstances suggesting that a causal link is likely (SEDA-13, 329).

Methemoglobinemia has been reported following gross accidental overdosage of metoclopramide in an infant (SEDA-15, 392).

Liver

Complex liver disorders very occasionally occur with metoclopramide, with cholestasis and opening of arteriovenous shunts in the liver (SEDA-16, 419). In two cases a condition resembling Reye's syndrome has been seen (14).

Susceptibility Factors

Hepatic disease

If there is impaired liver function, metoclopramide can accumulate. In eight patients with severe alcoholic cirrhosis there was a 50% lower clearance than in eight healthy volunteers; the apparent volume of distribution and absolute systemic availability were similar in the two groups (15).

Other features of the patient

Metoclopramide is contraindicated when stimulation of gastrointestinal motility could be dangerous, for example when there is hemorrhage, obstruction, or a risk of perforation.

Patients with pre-existing dyskinesias should not be given metoclopramide, and both the very young and the very old have a greater risk of adverse reactions, as do patients with cardiac disorders or asthma.

Drug Administration

Drug formulations

In a four-way crossover study in 16 healthy men a modified-release formulation of metoclopramide (30 mg) administered fasting and after a high-fat meal, an immediate-release formulation (30 mg) and a short intravenous infusion of 30 mg have been compared (16). The absolute systemic availability of the modified-release formulation was about 17% lower than that of the immediate-release formulation. Food had no significant effect on absorption. Uniform absorption of the drug from modified-release formulations supports their use in long-term treatment.

Seven patients from Peru developed extrapyramidal symptoms when supposedly taking lincomycin: in fact each capsule contained no less than 500 mg of metoclopramide (17).

Drug–Drug Interactions

Alcohol

Intravenous metoclopramide 20 mg accelerated gastric emptying and increased the rate of absorption of alcohol in seven subjects (18). In another similar study the sedative effects of alcohol were enhanced (19).

Ciclosporin

It has been suggested that metoclopramide increases the systemic availability of ciclosporin (SED-11, 783) (20).

Cisplatin

Metoclopramide reduces renal plasma flow, suggesting that concurrent use could increase the nephrotoxicity of cisplatin (21), an important observation in view of the specific usefulness of metoclopramide to treat cytotoxic drug-induced emesis.

Digoxin

When digoxin is given in a slowly dissolving form, the plasma concentrations achieved are reduced by about one-third if metoclopramide is given at the same time (22); liquid or readily dissolvable solid forms of digoxin are unlikely to be affected.

Paracetamol

In five health subjects intravenous metoclopramide increased the rate of absorption of a single dose of paracetamol 1.5 g (23).

Quinidine

Metoclopramide increases the serum concentrations of quinidine by up to 20% (24).

Theophylline

Metoclopramide reduces serum concentrations of theophylline (25).

References

1. Vidal Company A, Rodriguez Martin A, Barrio Merino A, Lorente Garcia-Maurino A, Garcia Llop LA. Bloqueo A-V por intoxicación con metoclopramida. [Atrioventricular block caused by metoclopramide poisoning.] An Esp Pediatr 1991;34(4):313–14.
2. Bevacqua BK. Supraventricular tachycardia associated with postpartum metoclopramide administration. Anesthesiology 1988;68(1):124–5.
3. Huerta Blanco R, Hernandez Cabrera M, Quinones Morales I, Cardenes Santana MA. Bloqueo cardiaco completo inducido por metoclopramida intravenosa. [Complete heart block induced by intravenous metoclopramide.] An Med Interna 2000;17(4):222–3.
4. Sheridan C, Chandra P, Jacinto M, Greenwald ES. Transient hypertension after high doses of metoclopramide. N Engl J Med 1982;307(21):1346.
5. Brower RD, Dreyer CF, Kent TA. Neuroleptic malignant syndrome in a child treated with metoclopramide for chemotherapy-related nausea. J Child Neurol 1989; 4(3):230–2.
6. Lifshitz M, Gavrilov V. Adverse reactions to metoclopramide in young children: a 6-year retrospective study and review of the literature. J Pharm Technol 2002;18:125–7.
7. Hoogendam A, Hofmeijer J, Frijns CJ, Heeringa M, Schouten-Tjin a Tsoi SL, Jansen PA. Ernstig parkinsonisme ten gevolge van metoclopramide bij een patiente met polyfarmacie. [Severe parkinsonism due to metoclopramide in a patient with polypharmacy.] Ned Tijdschr Geneeskd 2002;146(4):175–7.
8. Alroe C, Bowen P. Metoclopramide and prochlorperazine: "the blue-tongue sign". Med J Aust 1989;150(12):724–5.
9. van Der Kleij FG, de Vries PA, Stassen PM, Sprenger HG, Gans RO. Acute dystonia due to metoclopramide: increased risk in AIDS. Arch Intern Med 2002;162(3):358–9.
10. Bateman DN, Darling WM, Boys R, Rawlins MD. Extrapyramidal reactions to metoclopramide and prochlorperazine. Q J Med 1989;71(264):307–11.
11. Noll AM, Pinsky D. Withdrawal effects of metoclopramide. West J Med 1991;154(6):726–8.
12. Lu ML, Pan JJ, Teng HW, Su KP, Shen WW. Metoclopramide-induced supersensitivity psychosis. Ann Pharmacother 2002;36(9):1387–90.
13. Madani S, Tolia V. Gynecomastia with metoclopramide use in pediatric patients. J Clin Gastroenterol 1997;24(2):79–81.
14. Casteels-Van Daele M. Reye syndrome or side-effects of anti-emetics? Eur J Pediatr 1991;150(7):456–9.
15. Magueur E, Hagege H, Attali P, Singlas E, Etienne JP, Taburet AM. Pharmacokinetics of metoclopramide in patients with liver cirrhosis. Br J Clin Pharmacol 1991;31(2):185–7.
16. Vergin H, Fisch U, Mahr G, Winterhalter B. Analysis of formulation and food effect on the absorption of metoclopramide. Int J Clin Pharmacol Ther 2002;40(4):169–74.
17. Cosentino C, Torres L, Scorticati MC, Micheli F. Movement disorders secondary to adulterated medication. Neurology 2000;55(4):598–9.
18. Bateman DN, Kahn C, Mashiter K, Davies DS. Pharmacokinetic and concentration-effect studies with intravenous metoclopramide. Br J Clin Pharmacol 1978;6(5):401–7.
19. Gibbons DO, Lant AF. Effects of intravenous and oral propantheline and metoclopramide on ethanol absorption. Clin Pharmacol Ther 1975;17(5):578–84.
20. Wadhwa NK, Schroeder TJ, O'Flaherty E, Pesce AJ, Myre SA, First MR. The effect of oral metoclopramide on the absorption of cyclosporine. Transplantation 1987; 43(2):211–13.
21. Israel R, O'Mara V, Austin B, Bellucci A, Meyer BR. Metoclopramide decreases renal plasma flow. Clin Pharmacol Ther 1986;39(3):261–4.
22. Manninen V, Apajalahti A, Melin J, Karesoja M. Altered absorption of digoxin in patients given propantheline and metoclopramide. Lancet 1973;1(7800):398–400.
23. Nimmo J, Heading RC, Tothill P, Prescott LF. Pharmacological modification of gastric emptying: effects of propantheline and metoclopromide on paracetamol absorption. BMJ 1973;1(5853):587–9.
24. Guckenbiehl W, Gilfrich HJ, Just H. Einfluss von Laxantien und Metoclopramid auf die Chinidin-Plasma-konzentration wahrend Langzeittherapie bei Patienten mit Herzrhythmusstorungen. [Effect of laxatives and metoclopramide on plasma quinidine concentration during prolonged administration in patients with heart rhythm disorders.] Med Welt 1976;27(26):1273–6.
25. Janisch HD, Tonnesmann U, et al. Untersuchung zum Einfluss von Metoclopramid auf die Bioverfugbarkeit und den Blutspiegelverlauf von Theophyllin. Therapiewoche 1958;36:2758.

Metocurine

See also Neuromuscular blocking drugs

General Information

Metocurine is a non-depolarizing neuromuscular blocker, a synthetic derivative of D-tubocurarine. No metabolites have been detected and it depends almost entirely on renal function for its excretion; 40–50% of the drug is

In a case of fixed drug eruption, a provocation test showed cross-reactivity with tinidazole but not with secnidazole (24).

Reproductive system

A genital mucosal erosion occurred in a 38-year-old woman who had taken metronidazole 400 mg tds for 10 days for bacterial vaginitis (SEDA-16, 310).

Long-Term Effects

Drug tolerance

Resistance of *H. pylori* to metronidazole was found in 30% of isolates in the Lebanon (25), 42% in Brazil (26), and 80–90% in Africa (27).

Mutagenicity

Mutagenicity of metronidazole has been demonstrated in some bacterial systems (SEDA-13, 832). Studies on breakages in single-stranded DNA in the lymphocytes of patients treated with metronidazole for *Trichomonas* vaginitis have suggested that such breakages were repaired after withdrawal. Another study reported chromosomal aberrations in the lymphocytes of ten volunteers taking metronidazole (SEDA-21, 301). A mutagenic effect would theoretically be possible in patients with a DNA repair defect (SEDA-16, 310).

There has been concern that metronidazole may be genotoxic, as there have been reports of mutagenicity in several bacterial species. The genotoxic effects of metronidazole (250 mg bd for 10 days) and nalidixic acid (400 mg bd for 10 days) have been assessed in women with *Trichomonas vaginalis* infections (28). The genotoxic potential of these drugs was evaluated using a sister chromatid exchange test in peripheral blood lymphocytes. Metronidazole had no effect but nalidixic acid caused an increase in sister chromatid exchange frequency. This result confirms that there is little evidence of genotoxicity with metronidazole.

Tumorigenicity

Prolonged high-dose exposure of mice to metronidazole leads to an increased incidence of lung tumors, and in one study there was an increase in lymphoreticular neoplasia in female animals. These results, which caused much concern when first published, are probably non-specific and not relevant to humans; these and other neoplasms have also been induced in mice merely by varying the diet. Several long-term follow-up studies in man have failed to demonstrate an excess cancer risk (SEDA-13, 831). There has been a single report of cancers in three patients with Crohn's disease who had taken metronidazole for years (SEDA-11, 595) (29), but they had also taken sulfasalazine and glucocorticoids, and this cannot be regarded as constituting reasonable evidence of a causal link.

Second-Generation Effects

Teratogenicity

Tests for embryotoxicity and teratogenicity in different animal species have been negative, and there have been no reports of adverse effects on the fetus in pregnant women given metronidazole for trichomoniasis. Despite this, it is still wise to avoid metronidazole during the first trimester of pregnancy.

In a retrospective cohort study using the national birth registry in Denmark, comparing 124 women who took the drug with 13 327 who did not, there was no evidence of any increased risk to the unborn child (30).

In a prospective case-control study in Israel of 857 pregnant women seeking telephone advice regarding gestational exposure to prescribed drugs, 228 women who had taken metronidazole were compared with 629 controls exposed to non-teratogenic agents (31). The mean daily dose of metronidazole was 973 mg for a mean duration of 7.9 days; 90% had used the medication orally, 6% by suppository, and 4% intravenously. Most (86%) had been exposed to metronidazole in the first trimester of pregnancy. There was no difference in the rate of major congenital malformations between the groups (1.6 versus 1.4%), even after accounting for terminations due to prenatally diagnosed malformations. Neonatal birth weight was reduced in the metronidazole group (3.2 versus 3.3 kg) and this was not explained by an earlier gestational age at delivery or a higher prematurity rate but may have been due to the underlying conditions for which metronidazole was prescribed. These findings agree with previous meta-analyses showing that the use of metronidazole in pregnancy is not associated with an increased risk of fetal abnormality, despite in vitro evidence of mutagenesis and inconsistent animal evidence of fetal abnormalities caused by metronidazole.

Lactation

Metronidazole is excreted in the breast milk. There were no adverse effects in nursing infants (SEDA-13, 832), but one should still be cautious in using metronidazole in nursing mothers (SEDA-18, 295).

Susceptibility Factors

Age

In a randomized trial in 100 Iranian children, mebendazole (200 mg tds for 5 days, $n = 50$) was compared with metronidazole (5 mg/kg tds for 7 days, $n = 50$) in giardiasis (32). The two drugs were equally effective (over 85% cure rates). There were no adverse effects of mebendazole, whereas nausea, anorexia, and metallic taste were respectively observed in 4.9, 6, and 24% of those taking metronidazole.

Drug–Drug Interactions

Alcohol

Metronidazole has a disulfiram-like effect in users of alcohol, sufficient to justify a warning (SEDA-13, 833).

An unusual Antabuse-type reaction reported on one occasion seems to have been due to an interaction of metronidazole with the alcohol present in X-Prep (SEDA-15, 398).

Antibiotics

In vitro, the combination of metronidazole with antibiotics has an additive effect against anaerobic bacteria (SEDA-13, 833).

Carbamazepine

Metronidazole can increase the toxicity of carbamazepine (33) by inhibiting its metabolism.

Cephalosporins

The use of high doses of metronidazole in combination with cefamandole and clindamycin has been associated with encephalopathy (SEDA-12, 705).

Ciclosporin

An interaction with metronidazole and ciclosporin, in which ciclosporin blood concentrations rise, has been suggested, though only in isolated case histories (SEDA-19, 351) (34).

It has been confirmed that metronidazole can produce a two-fold increase in blood concentrations of ciclosporin and tacrolimus, with a subsequent increase in serum creatinine in both cases (35).

The interaction of metronidazole with ciclosporin significantly increased blood ciclosporin and tacrolimus concentrations in two patients (35). Since both of these immunosuppressive drugs are toxic in overdosage, and since patients taking them are prone to infections, this is potentially a serious interaction.

Fluorouracil

Pretreatment with metronidazole increased the toxicity of fluorouracil given by a daily bolus dose (36). The clinical significance of this is yet to be determined.

Gentamicin

In guinea pigs, metronidazole augmented gentamicin-induced ototoxicity, determined by the measurement of compound action potentials (37).

Lithium

Metronidazole can increase the toxicity of lithium (38).

Phenytoin

In a patient taking phenytoin, there was a disproportionate increase in the serum concentration of the hydroxylated metabolite of metronidazole, suggesting that phenytoin induces metronidazole-metabolizing enzymes (SEDA-12, 706) (39).

Quinidine

Serum quinidine concentrations rose during concomitant administration of metronidazole (40). The authors speculated that the mechanism was inhibition of cytochrome P_{450}.

Tacrolimus

A possible interaction with metronidazole recently reported is that it significantly increased blood ciclosporin and tacrolimus concentrations in two patients (35). Since both of these immunosuppressive drugs are toxic in overdosage, and since patients taking them are susceptible to infections, this is potentially a serious interaction.

Vecuronium bromide

Metronidazole can potentiate the effects of non-depolarizing muscle relaxants (41).

Serum concentrations of metronidazole rose during concomitant administration of ciprofloxacin and metronidazole (42). The authors speculated that the mechanism was inhibition of cytochrome P_{450} by ciprofloxacin.

Warfarin and other coumarins

The effect of warfarin is potentiated by metronidazole (43,44). The mechanism is stereoselective inhibition by metronidazole of the metabolism of *S*-warfarin, the more potent isomer (43). There is a similar interaction with acenocoumarol (45,46).

References

1. Wain AM. Metronidazole vaginal gel 0.75% (MetroGel-Vaginal): a brief review. Infect Dis Obstet Gynecol 1998;6(1):3–7.
2. Stranz MH, Bradley WE. Metronidazole (Flagyl IV, Searle). Drug Intell Clin Pharm 1981;15(11):838–46.
3. Freedman B, Shah S, Lau A. Metronidazole-induced peripheral neuropathy. J Appl Ther Res 2000;3:49–54.
4. Urtasun RC, Rabin HR, Partington J. Human pharmacokinetics and toxicity of high-dose metronidazole administered orally and intravenously. Surgery 1983;93(1 Pt 2):145–8.
5. Roe FJ. Toxicologic evaluation of metronidazole with particular reference to carcinogenic, mutagenic, and teratogenic potential. Surgery 1983;93(1 Pt 2):158–64.
6. Alston TA. Neurotoxicity of metronidazole. Ann Intern Med 1985;103(1):161.
7. Dreger LM, Gleason PP, Chowdhry TK, Gazzuolo DJ. Intermittent-dose metronidazole-induced peripheral neuropathy. Ann Pharmacother 1998;32(2):267–8.
8. Zivkovic SA, Lacomis DL, Giuliani MJ. Sensory neuropathy associated with metronidazole: report of four cases and review of the literature. J Clin Neuromuscular Dis 2001;3:8–12.
9. Corson AP, Chretien JH. Metronidazole-associated aseptic meningitis. Clin Infect Dis 1994;19(5):974.
10. Allroggen H, Abbott RJ, Bibby K. Acute visual loss following administration of metronidazole: a case report. Neuro-Ophthalmology 2000;23:89–94.
11. Beloosesky Y, Grosman B, Marmelstein V, Grinblat J. Convulsions induced by metronidazole treatment for Clostridium difficile-associated disease in chronic renal failure. Am J Med Sci 2000;319(5):338–9.
12. Arik N, Cengiz N, Bilge A. Metronidazole-induced encephalopathy in a uremic patient: a case report. Nephron 2001;89(1):108–9.
13. Iqbal SM, Murthy JG, Banerjee PK, Vishwanathan KA. Metronidazole ototoxicity—report of two cases. J Laryngol Otol 1999;113(4):355–7.

Organs and Systems

Cardiovascular

Prodysrhythmic effects of mexiletine have been reported in up to 29% of patients, although it has been suggested that on average the incidence is lower than has been reported with other antidysrhythmic drugs (20).

Mexiletine can have major hemodynamic effects in patients with pre-existing impairment of left ventricular dysfunction (21). Circulatory depression with bradycardia and hypotension have been reported (17,22,23).

Other cardiovascular effects include widening of the QRS complex, atrioventricular dissociation, heart block, sinus arrest, and cardiac arrest (23,24).

Respiratory

Mexiletine has been associated with pulmonary fibrosis and eventual respiratory failure (25).

Nervous system

The commonest adverse effects of mexiletine are on the nervous system, and include centrally mediated gastrointestinal distress (38%), light-headedness (20%), tremor (12%), and coordination difficulties (11%). The figures in parentheses are quoted from a study in which mexiletine was compared with quinidine (26). Other reported adverse effects include changes in sleep habit, weakness, headache, visual problems, and nervousness. Slurred speech, dysarthria, diplopia, and ataxia have also been reported (18).

Mexiletine 300–400 mg/day has been used to treat some of the symptoms of multiple sclerosis in 30 patients with painful tonic seizures, attacks of neuralgia, paroxysmal itching, and Lhermitte's sign (27). Mexiletine produced similar therapeutic effects to lidocaine. In one patient, weakness worsened during the administration of mexiletine. In two patients when mexiletine was replaced by placebo there was a suggestion of some rebound in painful tonic seizures.

In three patients with neuropathic pain, mexiletine added to the analgesic regimen caused some improvement in visual analogue scores for pain (10). All three had some symptoms of nausea, and two became depressed. One patient also reported feeling "trembly and shaky" on occasion, but there was no objective evidence of tremor.

Sensory systems

In two patients with neuropathic pain and pre-existing ocular disease, mexiletine caused persistent ophthalmic changes (28).

- A 39-year-old woman took mexiletine 300 mg tds for 3 days and developed transient blindness with residual reduced visual acuity due to an acute pigmentary retinopathy. Her vision improved markedly after withdrawal of mexiletine, but when she restarted it she developed clouding of the vision, which resolved again on withdrawal. The pigmentary changes persisted.
- A man with a history of glaucoma took mexiletine 300 mg tds and developed worsening visual acuity. Mexiletine was withdrawn and he took carbamazepine 200 mg/day instead. However, he started to see red and green spots. The serum carbamazepine concentration was below that usually associated with visual disturbances. No structural abnormalities were detected.

Hematologic

Mexiletine can cause a spuriously low platelet count as a result of clumping of platelets due to antibodies (29); however, it can also cause a true thrombocytopenia (30,31).

Eosinophilia and atypical lymphocytosis associated with liver dysfunction have also been described (32).

Gastrointestinal

Nausea and vomiting are common and probably central in origin, since they occur with intravenous as well as oral therapy (17).

Mexiletine affects the esophagus, and can cause heartburn (1) and esophageal spasm and ulceration (1,33).

Liver

Changes in liver function tests, resolving on withdrawal, have been reported (34). In one case there was histological evidence of cholestasis.

Skin

Mexiletine can occasionally cause generalized rashes (SEDA-17, 224) (26,32), pseudolymphomatous change with erythroderma (35), and contact urticaria (36).

- Exfoliative dermatitis has been reported in a 68-year-old man who had taken mexiletine and diltiazem for 3 weeks (37). Patch tests with 1, 10, and 30% mexiletine and diltiazem in petrolatum were positive, but a lymphocyte stimulation test was negative.
- Drug eruptions occurred in a 56-year-old woman, a 50-year-old man, and a 66-year-old woman, who developed disseminated maculopapular eruptions with high fever after oral mexiletine (38). In all cases the liver transaminase activities were raised and there was an eosinophilia with atypical lymphocytes; in two cases there was a lymphadenopathy. In all cases patch tests were positive.
- An acute exanthematous pustular eruption has been reported in a 56-year-old man who had taken mexiletine 300 mg/day for 1 month (39). There was mild liver dysfunction. Patch tests with mexiletine 10 and 20% were subsequently positive, but a lymphocyte stimulation test was negative.

In addition to these cases, 37 cases of drug eruption due to mexiletine have been reported in Japan, with several common clinical features (37). The interval between initial drug therapy and the start of the eruption was relatively long (48–88 days); there was a high proportion of positive patch tests (86–97%) but a low incidence of positive lymphocyte stimulation tests (23–27%); there were frequent systemic symptoms, such as fever (93–94%) and liver dysfunction (43–78%); finally, some patients had multiple drug eruptions.

Immunologic

Mexiletine caused an increased incidence of positive antinuclear antibody (ANA) titers in some studies (8,40), but not in others (41,42). The clinical significance of this effect is not clear. For example, there have been no reports of a lupus-like syndrome attributable to mexiletine.

Mexiletine caused increases in the serum activities of aspartate transaminase, alanine transaminase, and alkaline phosphatase in a few patients (8).

Susceptibility Factors

Renal disease

Mexiletine is mainly cleared polymorphically by CYP2D6 in the liver, and poor metabolizers and the slower among the extensive metabolizers have a higher incidence of mild adverse effects (nausea and light-headedness) (43). However, renal insufficiency can also be associated with an increase in plasma mexiletine concentrations (44).

Hepatic disease

Mexiletine is mainly cleared polymorphically by CYP2D6 in the liver, and poor metabolizers and the slower among the extensive metabolizers have a higher incidence of mild adverse effects (nausea and light-headedness) (43).

Drug Administration

Drug overdose

Overdosage with mexiletine resulted in death in two cases due to cardiovascular effects (45,46).

- Status epilepticus was the chief presenting feature in a 17-year-old boy who took an unspecified amount of mexiletine (47). The seizures responded to intravenous diazepam and phenytoin, but he also had agitation and hallucinations, which took 24 hours to abate. A urine specimen was positive for both benzodiazepines and amphetamines, but this was subsequently found to be a false positive result, because of the presence of large amounts of mexiletine, confirmed by thin-layer chromatography. The serum mexiletine concentration was 44 μmol/l, the usual target range being about 4–11 μmol/l.

Drug–Drug Interactions

Antacids

Mexiletine interacts with antacids, but the interaction is unlikely to be clinically important (48).

Antidysrhythmic drugs

Interactions of mexiletine with other cardioactive drugs have been reviewed (48). The most important are beneficial interactions with beta-adrenoceptor antagonists, quinidine, and amiodarone in the suppression of ventricular tachydysrhythmias. During these interactions the adverse effects of mexiletine may also be less common, although this effect is inconsistent (17).

Fluvoxamine

Mexiletine is metabolized by CYP2D6, CYP1A2, and CYP3A4; fluvoxamine inhibits CYP1A2. It is not surprising therefore that fluvoxamine 50 mg bd for 7 days increased the C_{max} and AUC of a single oral dose of mexiletine 200 mg in six healthy Japanese men (49).

Omeprazole

Mexiletine is metabolized mainly by CYP2D6 and CYP1A2. Omeprazole is an inducer of CYP1A2 and might therefore be expected to interact with mexiletine. However, in a study in nine healthy men there was no evidence of an effect of steady-state omeprazole 40 mg/day on the single-dose kinetics of mexiletine 200 mg (50).

Phenytoin

Mexiletine interacts with phenytoin, but the interaction is unlikely to be clinically important (48).

Propafenone

Mexiletine and propafenone are metabolized by the same enzymes, CYP2D6, CYP1A2, and CYP3A4. In 15 healthy volunteers, eight of whom were extensive metabolizers of CYP2D6, administration of oral mexiletine 100 mg bd on days 1–8 and oral propafenone 1 mg bd on days 5–12 significantly reduced the clearance of R(−) mexiletine from 41 to 28 l/hour and of S(+) mexiletine from 43 to 29 l/hour in the extensive metabolizers (51). The new values were no different from the clearance values in the poor metabolizers. Propafenone also reduced the partial metabolic clearances of mexiletine to hydroxymethylmexiletine, parahydroxymexiletine, and metahydroxymexiletine by about 70% in the extensive metabolizers. Propafenone had no effect on the kinetics of mexiletine in the poor metabolizers. There were no electrocardiographic changes during this interaction. Smokers had higher clearance rates than non-smokers, but the effects of propafenone were similar in the two groups. In contrast, mexiletine had little effect on the disposition of propafenone. The authors proposed that these effects could explain at least in part the increased efficacy that sometimes occurs when mexiletine and propafenone are combined in patients in whom a single drug was not effective. They also recommended that the dosages of the drugs should be titrated slowly when they are used together, in order to reduce the risk of adverse effects.

Rifampicin

Mexiletine interacts with rifampicin, but the interaction is unlikely to be clinically important (48).

Sevoflurane

- A 79-year-old woman was given mexiletine 125 mg intravenously over 10 minutes during anesthesia after

Hematologic

In 1979 the first case of leukopenia due to mianserin was reported (6), followed by another soon after (7). In July 1980, the Australian Drug Evaluation Committee issued a preliminary caution concerning further cases that had been reported to its National Monitoring Centres and 6 months later published detailed reports of four other cases (8), all of which had occurred within 1 year of marketing in Australia, despite 6 years of use in Europe. Inquiries unearthed reports of seven similar episodes held by drug surveillance organizations in other countries, and the Committee expressed its concern that "if a causal relationship between mianserin and these blood disorders is subsequently confirmed, the incidence of disorders due to mianserin may be significantly greater than that of disorders due either to the phenothiazines or the tricyclic antidepressants" (9). In 1985 the UK Committee on Safety of Medicines issued a statement concerning 15 reports that the Committee had received during 5 years (10). Three of the patients subsequently died, one with aplastic anemia, one with granulocytopenia, and one with both erythrocyte and leukocyte hypoplasia. The New Zealand Department of Health's Clinical Services Letter mentioned three cases of agranulocytosis that occurred in New Zealand in 1982 (11). Another report (12) described thrombocytopenia and leukopenia based on an immune mechanism without generalized marrow depression. A high rate of agranulocytosis has been reported by the IMMP in New Zealand: one case out of 1822 and one fatal case out of 11 537 (12).

Mouth and teeth

The lack of anticholinergic effects reported in clinical studies has been supported by a double blind, placebo-controlled comparison of mianserin (10–60 mg/day) and amitriptyline (25–150 mg/day) in healthy volunteers (13). Mianserin tended to increase saliva flow, while amitriptyline significantly reduced it. However, a further experiment in healthy volunteers showed that single doses of mianserin (50–70 mg) produced a significant 29% reduction of salivation compared with placebo (14). This may account for the glossitis that has previously been reported (SEDA-9, 23).

Liver

Hepatotoxicity from mianserin has been reported in eight cases (SEDA-17, 22).

Musculoskeletal

Mianserin can cause joint symptoms and arthritis (SEDA-16, 11).

Drug Administration

Drug overdose

One of the putative benefits of mianserin is its alleged safety in overdose, which may be related to a reduced risk of cardiovascular adverse effects and convulsions. Data from the UK Committee on Safety of Medicines suggest that mianserin accounts for 11% of reported convulsions and 5.8% of use, putting it intermediate between amitriptyline and maprotiline (15). On the other hand, in the London Poisons Unit survey, involving 84 patients who took mianserin alone (up to 1000 mg), there were no deaths and no patients with convulsions, although this could represent a frequency of up to 3.6% (12).

A survey of 100 cases of overdose with mianserin reported to the London Centre of the UK Poisons Information Service included 54 patients who took mianserin alone in amounts up to and in three cases in excess of 1000 mg (12). Plasma mianserin concentrations were 70–665 ng/l (the usual mean target concentration is 50 ng/l). There were no reports of convulsions, cardiac dysrhythmias, or profound coma in any patient taking mianserin alone, but there were two deaths in patients who took multiple drugs. The authors concluded that in acute overdosage mianserin is less toxic than tricyclic antidepressants.

Drug–Drug Interactions

Clonidine and methyldopa

Mianserin lacks potential for peripheral adrenergic interactions, but since it has α-adrenoceptor activity, it might interact with the centrally acting α-adrenoceptor agonists clonidine and methyldopa. In healthy volunteers, pretreatment with mianserin 60 mg/day for 3 days did not modify the hypotensive effects of a single 300 mg dose of clonidine, and in 11 patients with essential hypertension, the addition of mianserin 60 mg/day (in divided doses) for 2 weeks did not reduce the hypotensive effects of clonidine or methyldopa (16). In patients taking methyldopa, there were additive hypotensive effects after the first dose of mianserin, but these were not significant after 1 or 2 weeks of combined treatment. The results of this study appear to have justified the authors' conclusion that combining mianserin with centrally-acting hypotensive agents will not result in loss of blood pressure control.

References

1. Brogden RN, Heel RC, Speight TM, Avery GS. Mianserin: a review of its pharmacological properties and therapeutic efficacy in depressive illness. Drugs 1978;16(4):273–301.
2. Kopera H, Klein W, Schenk H. Psychotropic drugs and the heart: clinical implications. Prog Neuropsychopharmacol 1980;4(4–5):527–35.
3. Goldie A, Edwards JG. Electrocardiographic changes during treatment with maprotiline and mianserin. Neuropharmacology 1984;23(2B):273–5.
4. Whiteford H, Klug P, Evans L. Disturbed cardiac function possibly associated with mianserin therapy. Med J Aust 1984;140(3):166–7.
5. Edwards JG, Glen-Bott M. Mianserin and convulsive seizures. Br J Clin Pharmacol 1983;15(Suppl 2):299S–311S.
6. Curson DA, Hale AS. Mianserin and agranulocytosis. BMJ 1979;1(6160):378–9.
7. McHarg AM, McHarg JF. Leucopenia in association with mianserin treatment. BMJ 1979;1(6163):623–4.
8. Anonymous. Mianserin: a possible cause of neutropenia and agranulocytosis. Adverse Drug Reactions Advisory Committee. Med J Aust 1980;2(12):673–4.

9. Anonymous. Side effects associated with mianserin. Scrip 1982;707:11.
10. Stricker BH, Barendregt JN, Claas FH. Thrombocytopenia and leucopenia with mianserin-dependent antibodies. Br J Clin Pharmacol 1985;19(1):102–4.
11. Coulter DM, Edwards IR. Mianserin and agranulocytosis in New Zealand. Lancet 1990;336(8718):785–7.
12. Shaw WL. The comparative safety of mianserin in overdose. Curr Med Res Opin 1980;6(Suppl 7):44.
13. Kopera H. Anticholinergic effects of mianserin. Curr Med Res Opin 1980;6(Suppl 7):132.
14. Clemmesen L, Jensen E, Min SK, Bolwig TG, Rafaelsen OJ. Salivation after single-doses of the new antidepressants femoxetine, mianserin and citalopram. A cross-over study. Pharmacopsychiatry 1984;17(4):126–32.
15. Edwards JG. Antidepressants and convulsions. Lancet 1979;2(8156–8157):1368–9.
16. Elliott HL, Whiting B, Reid JL. Assessment of the interaction between mianserin and centrally-acting antihypertensive drugs. Br J Clin Pharmacol 1983; 15(Suppl 2):323S–8S.

Mibefradil

See also Calcium channel blockers

General Information

Mibefradil is a member of a class of calcium antagonists that specifically block the T-type calcium channel. It was marketed as an antihypertensive and antianginal drug with an adverse effects profile similar to that of placebo (1) and a favorable pharmacokinetic profile, allowing once-a-day dosage (2).

Owing to its attractive pharmacological profile, namely an anti-ischemic action with little or no negative inotropism, mibefradil was tested in a large-scale mortality trial in heart failure (MACH-I, Mortality Assessment in Congestive Heart Failure Trial). However, early in June 1998, only a few months after its launch, Roche Laboratories withdrew mibefradil from the market, after several dangerous interactions with at least 25 drugs had been reported (3,4) associated with rhabdomyolysis and life-threatening cardiac dysrhythmias; these problems were detected by postmarketing surveillance (4). The FDA stated that: "since [mibefradil] has not been shown to offer special benefits (such as treating patients who do not respond to other anti-hypertensive and antianginal drugs), the drug's problems are viewed as an unreasonable risk to consumers."

In the MACH-1 (Mortality Assessment in Congestive Heart Failure) trial, 2590 patients with moderate to severe congestive heart failure were randomized to mibefradil or placebo (5). Mibefradil given for a maximum of 3 years did not affect mortality or morbidity. However, a subgroup analysis by concomitant drugs showed that digoxin, class I antidysrhythmic drugs, amiodarone, and other drugs associated with torsade de pointes increased the risk of death with mibefradil. These worrisome drug–drug interactions were consistent with the results of postmarketing surveillance, which prompted withdrawal of mibefradil from the market by its manufacturers in June 1998, even before complete results of the trial became available.

The safety and efficacy of mibefradil in association with beta-blockers was assessed in 205 patients with chronic stable angina, randomized to placebo or mibefradil 25 or 50 mg/day for 2 weeks (6). Besides an improvement in angina with mibefradil, it dose-dependently reduced heart rate and increased the PR interval. One patient taking mibefradil had an escape junctional rhythm 26 hours after the last dose of 50 mg. The nodal rhythm disappeared on withdrawal of mibefradil, but based on the overall results it was concluded that mibefradil was safe and effective when given for a short time with beta-blockers.

In a Prescription-Event Monitoring study in 3085 patients, mean age 65 years, the commonest reported adverse events and reasons for stopping were malaise/lassitude, dizziness, edema, and headache (7).

Organs and Systems

Cardiovascular

Mibefradil causes slight bradycardia associated with its hypotensive effect. In a Prescription-Event Monitoring study in 3085 patients, mean age 65 years, there were seven reports of serious bradycardia/collapse thought to be possible adverse drug reactions to mibefradil (7). All were in patients over 65 years and six were thought to have resulted from a drug interaction. In all, there were 11 possible drug interactions. Nine (eight reports of bradycardia and one of syncope) involved beta-blockers. Collapse and severe bradycardia occurred in a patient who had started to take a dihydropyridine calcium channel blocker within 24 hours of stopping mibefradil. Palpitation and dyspnea occurred in a patient taking digoxin and sotalol. None of the 53 deaths during the study was attributed to mibefradil.

Abrupt switch of therapy from mibefradil to other dihydropyridine calcium antagonist was reported to cause shock, fatal in one case, in four patients also taking beta-blockers (8).

Drug–Drug Interactions

General

Mibefradil inhibits CYP3A4 (2). Other drugs that are metabolized by this pathway accumulate as a result. Drugs that were commonly affected included amiodarone, astemizole, ciclosporin, cisapride, erythromycin, imipramine, lovastatin, propafenone, quinidine, simvastatin (9), tacrolimus (10), tamoxifen, terfenadine, thioridazine, and drugs that impair sinoatrial node function (for example beta-blockers) (6).

- Severe rhabdomyolysis occurred in an 83-year-old woman who developed progressive immobilizing myopathy, low back pain, and oliguria; she was taking simvastatin and mibefradil (9). The symptoms disappeared completely after 4 weeks of withdrawal.

Mibefradil was probably responsible for raising plasma concentrations of simvastatin to toxic concentrations.

Beta-blockers

In a Prescription-Event Monitoring study in 3085 patients, mean age 65 years, there were 11 possible drug interactions. Nine involved beta-blockers, with eight reports of bradycardia and one of syncope. One patient developed palpitation and dyspnea while also taking digoxin and sotalol.

Calcium channel blockers

In a Prescription-Event Monitoring study in 3085 patients, mean age 65 years, one patient developed collapse and severe bradycardia after starting to take a dihydropyridine calcium channel blocker within 24 hours of stopping mibefradil (7).

References

1. Braun S, van der Wall EE, Emanuelsson H, Kobrin I. Effects of a new calcium antagonist, mibefradil (Ro 40-5967), on silent ischemia in patients with stable chronic angina pectoris: a multicenter placebo-controlled study. The Mibefradil International Study Group. J Am Coll Cardiol 1996;27(2):317–22.
2. Billups SJ, Carter BL. Mibefradil: a new class of calcium-channel antagonists. Ann Pharmacother 1998; 32(6):659–71.
3. SoRelle R. Withdrawal of Posicor from market. Circulation 1998;98(9):831–2.
4. Po AL, Zhang WY. What lessons can be learnt from withdrawal of mibefradil from the market? Lancet 1998;351(9119):1829–30.
5. Levine TB, Bernink PJ, Caspi A, Elkayam U, Geltman EM, Greenberg B, McKenna WJ, Ghali JK, Giles TD, Marmor A, Reisin LH, Ammon S, Lindberg E. Effect of mibefradil, a T-type calcium channel blocker, on morbidity and mortality in moderate to severe congestive heart failure: the MACH-1 study. Mortality Assessment in Congestive Heart Failure Trial. Circulation 2000; 101(7):758–64.
6. Alpert JS, Kobrin I, DeQuattro V, Friedman R, Shepherd A, Fenster PE, Thadani U. Additional antianginal and anti-ischemic efficacy of mibefradil in patients pretreated with a beta blocker for chronic stable angina pectoris. Am J Cardiol 1997;79(8):1025–30.
7. Riley J, Wilton LV, Shakir SA. A post-marketing observational study to assess the safety of mibefradil in the community in England. Int J Clin Pharmacol Ther 2002;40(6):241–8.
8. Mullins ME, Horowitz BZ, Linden DH, Smith GW, Norton RL, Stump J. Life-threatening interaction of mibefradil and beta-blockers with dihydropyridine calcium channel blockers. JAMA 1998;280(2):157–8.
9. Schmassmann-Suhijar D, Bullingham R, Gasser R, Schmutz J, Haefeli WE. Rhabdomyolysis due to interaction of simvastatin with mibefradil. Lancet 1998; 351(9120):1929–30.
10. Krahenbuhl S, Menafoglio A, Giostra E, Gallino A. Serious interaction between mibefradil and tacrolimus. Transplantation 1998;66(8):1113–15.

Miconazole

See also Antifungal azoles

General Information

Miconazole has been evaluated as a topical, oral, and intravenous agent. Its absorption is slightly better than that of clotrimazole, but is still insufficient for use as a systemic agent, particularly in view of its relatively short half-life of around 8–9 hours (1). Miconazole has also been given intravenously and intrathecally. It is highly protein-bound and does not diffuse well into the CSF; however, it does penetrate readily into synovial and vitreous fluids (2).

The indications for miconazole have diminished with the advent of newer antifungal azoles (3) and it has largely been superseded by other azoles; infection with *Pseudallescheria boydii* remains one of the few indications (4).

General adverse effects

Topical miconazole is well tolerated. Parenteral administration carries a higher frequency of adverse effects, some probably being caused by Cremophor (polyethoxylated castor oil, the carrier). Adverse effects include fever, chills, pruritus, rash, nausea, vomiting, diarrhea, hyponatremia, cardiac toxicity, phlebitis, hyperlipidemia, and central nervous system disturbances. Hypersensitivity reactions can occur. Tumor-inducing effects have not been reported.

Organs and Systems

Cardiovascular

Local phlebitis is not uncommon after intravenous miconazole (5); the type of intravenous solution used is of importance.

Collapse after rapid intravenous injection has been described, as have some cases of tachycardia, ventricular tachycardia, and even, in a few instances, cardiorespiratory arrest, attributable to the histamine-releasing properties of Cremophor (SED-12, 679) (2).

Nervous system

Arachnoiditis has been described after intrathecal injection (6).

Psychological, psychiatric

Acute toxic psychosis is a rare consequence of miconazole (SED-12, 679) (7).

Endocrine

Hyperlipidemia has been described in many patients given miconazole; this may be caused by the solvent (SED-12, 679) (2).

Skin

Pruritus and rashes have been reported with miconazole but do not seem to be frequent (5).

Drug–Drug Interactions

Anticoagulants

Miconazole can potentiate the effects of coumarin anticoagulants (SED-12, 679) (2). Potentiation of the anticoagulatory effects of acenocoumarol was noted after vaginal administration of miconazole capsules to two postmenopausal patients (8) and after oral administration of miconazole gel in three elderly patients with oral candidiasis (9). In both instances there were no major bleeding complications. However, it appears prudent to consider the use of non-azole topical antifungal agents in patients who are taking CYP3A4 metabolized drugs with a narrow therapeutic index.

Phenytoin

Miconazole can increase serum concentrations of phenytoin (SED-12, 679) (10).

Sulfonylureas

Enhancement of the effects of hypoglycemic sulfonamides has been reported (SED-12, 679) (2).

References

1. Mikamo H, Kawazoe K, Sato Y, Ito K, Tamaya T. Pharmacokinetics of miconazole in serum and exudate of pelvic retroperitoneal space after radical hysterectomy and pelvic lymphadenectomy. Int J Antimicrob Agents 1997;9(3):207–11.
2. Drouhet E, Dupont B. Evolution of antifungal agents: past, present, and future. Rev Infect Dis 1987;9(Suppl 1):S4–S14.
3. Walsh TJ, Pizzo A. Treatment of systemic fungal infections: recent progress and current problems. Eur J Clin Microbiol Infect Dis 1988;7(4):460–75.
4. Walsh TJ, Peter J, McGough DA, Fothergill AW, Rinaldi MG, Pizzo PA. Activities of amphotericin B and antifungal azoles alone and in combination against *Pseudallescheria boydii*. Antimicrob Agents Chemother 1995;39(6):1361–4.
5. Stevens DA. Miconazole in the treatment of coccidioidomycosis. Drugs 1983;26(4):347–54.
6. Sung JP, Campbell GD, Grendahl JG. Miconazole therapy for fungal meningitis. Arch Neurol 1978;35(7):443–7.
7. Cohen J. Antifungal chemotherapy. Lancet 1982;2(8297):532–7.
8. Lansdorp D, Bressers HP, Dekens-Konter JA, Meyboom RH. Potentiation of acenocoumarol during vaginal administration of miconazole. Br J Clin Pharmacol 1999;47(2):225–6.
9. Ortin M, Olalla JI, Muruzabal MJ, Peralta FG, Gutierrez MA. Miconazole oral gel enhances acenocoumarol anticoagulant activity: a report of three cases. Ann Pharmacother 1999;33(2):175–7.
10. Rolan PE, Somogyi AA, Drew MJ, Cobain WG, South D, Bochner F. Phenytoin intoxication during treatment with parenteral miconazole. BMJ (Clin Res Ed) 1983;287(6407):1760.

Midazolam

See also Benzodiazepines

General Information

Midazolam is used mainly in parenteral form in anesthesia, as a sedative adjunct to medical and dental procedures, and in status epilepticus (1). Its pharmacology and therapeutics have been extensively reviewed (2). It produces greater amnesia than diazepam, useful in terms of its anesthetic use, but carries a risk of cardiorespiratory depression and death (SED-12, 99), particularly at the extremes of age and when combined with the opioid fentanyl (SEDA-22, 42), which can cause accumulation of midazolam (see Drug–Drug Interactions in this monograph). Vomiting has been reported in 10% of children having midazolam sedation before radiology (SEDA-22, 41). Behavioral disinhibition (SEDA-18, 44), acute withdrawal, and hiccups appear to be relatively common (SEDA-22, 41); hallucinations, flumazenil-reversible dystonia, and hypersensitivity have all been observed (SED-12, 99) (SEDA-17, 44).

Clinical electrophysiological procedures can be very complex and prolonged, requiring safe and effective conscious sedation. A study in 700 patients has shown that intermittent midazolam plus fentanyl in electrophysiological procedures is safe and efficacious (3). All the staff were ACLS-certified and had successfully completed conscious sedation training courses, but none was an anesthetist; one team member was dedicated to monitoring conscious sedation and providing rescue defibrillation if required.

The pharmacology and adverse effects of midazolam in infants and children have been reviewed (4).

Midazolam has been carefully evaluated for adverse effects when used in critically ill infants and children; several difficulties, including prolonged obtundation and paradoxical behavioral and withdrawal reactions, have been noted (SEDA-19, 35) (5). Midazolam by the buccal route has been evaluated in children with persistent seizures; it was both effective and well tolerated (6), offering obvious practical advantages to rectal or parenteral administration. The availability of flumazenil, a specific benzodiazepine antagonist, to correct any adverse or overdose effects from injected midazolam should not encourage laxity in its use. Recent reports have highlighted kinetic interactions between midazolam and a variety of other drugs (see Drug–Drug Interactions in this monograph), and its effects can be magnified or prolonged in patients with hepatic or renal insufficiency (SEDA-20, 32).

Midazolam was used in a wide range of doses (0.03–0.6 mg/kg) in 91 children undergoing diagnostic or minor operative procedures with intravenous midazolam sedation (7). Opioids were co-administered in 84% and oxygen desaturation occurred in 32%, most of whom had received high doses of opioids in addition to the midazolam. Other adverse events included airway obstruction ($n = 3$) and vomiting ($n = 1$). The presence of independent appropriate trained personnel not directly involved in performing the procedure, appropriate resuscitation equipment, and monitoring were recommended whenever midazolam and opioids are co-administered for intravenous sedation.

A cherry-flavored midazolam syrup was evaluated for premedication in 85 children requiring general anesthesia (8). The patients received a randomly assigned dose of 0.25, 0.5, or 1 mg/kg. All clinicians and observers were blinded to the treatment group. There was satisfactory dose-related sedation in 81%, and 83% had satisfactory non-dose-related anxiolysis at separation from parents and at anesthetic induction. One or more adverse events occurred in 36%, but only 31% of these were judged as possibly related to midazolam (hiccups 6%, hypoxemia 6%, vomiting 5%, hallucinations 4%, drooling 4%, agitation 2%, coughing 2%, diplopia 2%, dizziness 2%, and hypotension 2%). The authors suggested that although adverse effects were common, they were minor.

Intranasal midazolam 0.2 mg/kg and intravenous diazepam 0.3 mg/kg have been compared in a prospective randomized study in 47 children (aged 6 months to 5 years) with febrile seizures that lasted over 10 minutes (9). Intranasal midazolam controlled seizures significantly earlier than intravenous diazepam. None of the children had respiratory distress, bradycardia, or other adverse effects. Electrocardiography, blood pressure, and pulse oximetry were normal in all children during seizure activity and after cessation of seizures.

In a Canadian multicenter, open, randomized trial in 156 patients to determine whether sedation with propofol would lead to shorter times to tracheal extubation and length of stay in ICU than sedation with midazolam, the patients who received propofol spent longer at the target sedation level than those who received midazolam (60 versus 44% respectively) (10). Propofol allowed clinically significantly earlier tracheal extubation than midazolam (6.7 versus 25 hours). However, this did not result in earlier discharge from the ICU.

In a double-blind, randomized, placebo-controlled study during coronary angiography in 90 patients, midazolam with or without fentanyl and local anesthesia provided better hemodynamic stability than placebo (11).

In a randomized study in 301 agitated or aggressive patients, intramuscular midazolam was more rapidly sedating than a mixture of haloperidol + promethazine (12). There was only one important adverse event, transient respiratory depression, in one of the 151 patients who were given midazolam.

Organs and Systems

Cardiovascular

The incidence of hypotension with the use of midazolam for pre-hospital rapid-sequence intubation of the trachea has been assessed in a retrospective chart review of two aeromedical crews (13). The rapid-sequence protocols were identical, except for the dose of midazolam. Both crews used 0.1 mg/kg, but one crew had a maximum dose of 5 mg imposed. This meant that patients over 50 kg received lower doses of midazolam; they also had a higher incidence of hypotension. This relation was also present in patients with traumatic brain injury, implying that cerebral perfusion could be compromised at a critical time in those without dosage restriction.

Midazolam depresses both cardiovascular and respiratory function, especially in elderly patients (14). As little as 0.01 mg/kg can obtund the response to hypoxia and hypercapnia (15). The simultaneous use of opiates (such as fentanyl) commonly produces hypoxia (16).

Hypertension and tachycardia during coronary angiography can cause significant problems. In a double-blind, randomized, placebo-controlled study during coronary angiography in 90 patients, midazolam with or without fentanyl under local anesthesia provided better hemodynamic stability than placebo (11).

Respiratory

Intranasal midazolam is a successful route of administration for sedating children. However, it can cause nasal burning, irritation, and lacrimation (17). In a study of an alternative route of administration, namely inhalation via a nebulizer, bronchospasm developed in two of the 10 patients studied. This formulation of midazolam has a pH of 3.0, and this was thought to be the reason it caused bronchospasm.

Nervous system

Two premature neonates, who already had epileptic manifestations related to severe hypoxic ischemic encephalopathy, developed seizures (one tonic and the other tonic-clonic) within a few seconds of receiving intravenous midazolam (0.15 μg/kg) for sedation (18). In one, the seizure recurred after rechallenge on the same day. Benzodiazepines occasionally cause tonic seizures, especially after intravenous administration to children with Lennox–Gastaut syndrome. This seems to be the first report related to midazolam in newborns.

Involuntary epileptiform movements have been described in three of six premature infants given midazolam for sedation (19). The infants had been born at 24–26 weeks gestation, were aged 23–32 days, and weighed on average 671 g. They were given midazolam 100 μg/kg by slow bolus injection for sedation and then had accentuated myoclonic jerks resembling clonic seizures within 5 minutes. In all cases it was the first dose of midazolam and the cardiorespiratory parameters remained normal. The abnormal movements resolved within 5–10 minutes. There has also been a report of convulsions caused by midazolam in two preterm infants (20). They were of 26 and 28 weeks gestation and were given midazolam 100 and 150 μg/kg intravenously before tracheal intubation. Both were successfully treated with flumazenil 10 μg/kg.

The safety of midazolam in very low birth-weight neonates is being questioned. In 200 children weighing 3–15 kg premedicated with rectal midazolam 0.5 or 1.0 mg/kg before minor surgery, the incidence of hiccups was 22% and 26% respectively (21). The mean age of children with hiccups was 6 months and of children without hiccups 20 months. Intranasal ethyl chloride spray was 100% successful in treating the hiccups. The incidence of hiccups was related to age but not dose. The effectiveness of ethyl chloride was postulated to be via cold nasopharyngeal stimulation.

The effects of sevoflurane and halothane anesthesia, including the effect of midazolam 0.5 mg/kg premedication, on recovery characteristics have been studied in 100 children aged 6 months to 6 years undergoing myringotomy (22). Children who received sevoflurane had about 50% faster recovery times and discharge-home times than those who received halothane. However, sevoflurane without midazolam premedication was associated with 67% postoperative agitation compared with 40% in the premedicated group. Midazolam delayed early recovery times by about 5 minutes, but had no effect on discharge times. In view of the very high incidence of postoperative agitation in the control group midazolam was seen as an effective premedicant.

Midazolam can cause paradoxical reactions, including increased agitation and poor cooperation (23,24). Often other drugs are required to continue the procedure successfully. Reversal of these reactions by flumazenil, a benzodiazepine antagonist, has been reported.

Sevoflurane often causes postoperative delirium and agitation in children, and this may be severe. The effect of intravenous clonidine 2 μg/kg on the incidence and severity of postoperative agitation has been assessed in a double-blind, randomized, placebo-controlled trial in 40 boys who had anesthetic induction with sevoflurane after oral midazolam premedication (25). There was agitation in 16 of those who received placebo and two of those who received clonidine; the agitation was severe in six of those given placebo and none of those given clonidine.

The effect of a single bolus dose of midazolam before the end of sevoflurane anesthesia has been investigated in a double-blind, randomized, placebo-controlled trial in 40 children aged 2–7 years (26). Midazolam significantly reduced the incidence of delirium after anesthesia. However, when it was used for severe agitation, midazolam only reduced the severity of agitation without abolishing it.

In the presence of acute neurological injuries, midazolam produces a high risk of raised intracranial pressure (27), and the risk of airway obstruction (28) is a further concern.

Recovery after propofol or midazolam has been compared in two studies (29,30). Memory was significantly impaired by midazolam, an effect that was reminiscent of the problems experienced with short-acting oral benzodiazepine hypnotics, such as triazolam.

Psychological, psychiatric

Midazolam can cause an unpleasant state of dysphoria if surgical stimuli are applied to the patient, who may nevertheless appear calm and untroubled. Amnesia is also routinely produced and can be beneficial. Delayed recovery of cognitive function occurs after the use of benzodiazepines as premedication (31).

There was a variety of significant nervous system adverse effects in six of 104 patients who underwent transesophageal echocardiography, including aggression, euphoria, depression, and intense hiccups (32). These effects occurred despite careful titration and relatively low doses of intravenous midazolam (mean 4.8 mg), and were generally reversible with intravenous flumazenil 0.25–0.5 mg.

Hematologic

Fat emulsions affect coagulation and fibrinolysis (33). In 36 patients undergoing aortocoronary bypass operations with midazolam/fentanyl- or propofol/alfentanil-based anesthesia, factor XIIa concentrations and kallikrein-like activity were about 30% higher in the propofol group. The authors suggested that there had been stronger activation of the contact phase at the start of recirculation and stronger fibrinolysis in the propofol group. They also found more hypotension in the propofol group, which they assumed to be due to release of kallikrein, resulting in release of bradykinin. Propofol has not been proven to cause increased perioperative bleeding.

In a 40-month-old boy a withdrawal syndrome with neurological symptoms was accompanied by thrombocytosis, which peaked at 1230 $\times$ 10^9/l (34). Recovery from the withdrawal syndrome was accompanied by normalization of the platelet count. The relevance of this change in platelet count was not clear. The boy had also been given fentanyl, and the authors suggested that the combination of midazolam with fentanyl should be used with caution.

Urinary tract

The conjugates of the main metabolite of midazolam, α-hydroxymidazolam, accumulate in renal insufficiency. In five patients with severe renal insufficiency (creatinine clearance 7 ml/minute or less), in whom prolonged sedation after midazolam was immediately reversed by flumazenil, there were high serum concentrations of glucuronidated α-hydroxymidazolam, even at times when the concentrations of the unconjugated metabolite and midazolam itself were low (35). Glucuronidated α-hydroxymidazolam is about one-tenth as potent as midazolam and unconjugated α-hydroxymidazolam, and accumulation of the conjugated metabolite in renal insufficiency may be important.

Body temperature

Midazolam premedication causes exaggerated perioperative hypothermia in 15 elderly surgical patients compared with 15 young patients (36). The same group also showed that atropine prevents midazolam-induced core hypothermia in 40 elderly patients (37). The thermoregulatory effects of benzodiazepine agonists and cholinergic inhibitors oppose each other, and the combination leaves core temperature unchanged.

Long-Term Effects

Drug withdrawal

The withdrawal of an infusion of midazolam, used as sedation in intensive care units, is associated with occasional severe and bizarre behavioral disturbances, particularly in children (38). These are similar in nature to the withdrawal effects seen with other short-acting benzodiazepines.

Susceptibility Factors

Age

The pharmacology and adverse effects of midazolam in infants and children have been reviewed (4). The optimal dose of intramuscular midazolam for preoperative sedation has been studied in a double-blind prospective study of 600 patients who were age-stratified (39). The patients received intramuscular atropine 0.6 mg and one of five doses of midazolam 15 minutes before induction of anesthesia. For the age groups 20–39, 40–59, and 60–79 years, the optimal sedative and amnesic effects of midazolam were 0.10, 0.08, and 0.04 mg/kg respectively. The frequency with which the undesirable adverse effects of reduced blood pressure, oxygen desaturation, oversedation, loss of eyelash reflex, and tongue root depression occurred increased with age, and optimal doses for a low incidence of adverse effects were 0.08, 0.06, and 0.04 mg/kg in the same age groups respectively.

Drug Administration

Drug administration route

Midazolam nasal spray 2 mg/kg has been compared with a citric acid placebo for conscious sedation in children undergoing painful procedures (40). Citric acid was added to the placebo, so that the sensation of nasal burning caused by midazolam did not unblind the observers. Parents and nurses judged the procedure to be more comfortable with midazolam, but the children rated the discomfort of the procedure similar in the two groups. Anxiety was significantly reduced by midazolam. There was nasal discomfort in 43% of the midazolam group. The authors concluded that midazolam intranasal spray effectively reduces anxiety, but that its use may be limited by nasal discomfort.

Drug–Drug Interactions

Antifungal azole derivatives

The pharmacokinetics and pharmacodynamics of midazolam are significantly affected by antifungal azoles. The effects of fluconazole (400 mg loading dose followed by 200 mg/day) on the kinetics of midazolam have been studied in 10 mechanically ventilated adults receiving a stable infusion of midazolam (41). Concentrations of midazolam were increased up to fourfold after the start of fluconazole therapy; these changes were most marked in patients with renal insufficiency. During the study, the ratio of α-hydroxymidazolam to midazolam progressively fell. The authors concluded that in ICU patients receiving fluconazole, reduction of the dose of midazolam should be considered if the degree of sedation is increasing.

In a study of the effects of itraconazole 200 mg/day and rifampicin 600 mg/day on the pharmacokinetics and pharmacodynamics of oral midazolam 7.5–15 mg during and 4 days after the end of the treatment, switching from inhibition to induction of metabolism caused an up to 400-fold change in the AUC of oral midazolam (42).

In an in vitro study of midazolam biotransformation using human liver microsomes, midazolam metabolism was competitively inhibited by the antifungal azoles ketoconazole, itraconazole, and fluconazole, and the antidepressant fluoxetine and its metabolite norfluoxetine (43). The degree of inhibition was consistent with the inhibition reported in pharmacokinetic studies, and suggests that in vitro assay is useful for predicting significant interactions.

Diltiazem

Diltiazem caused a 43% mean increase in the half-life of midazolam in 30 patients who underwent coronary artery bypass grafting (44). Similar effects were observed with alfentanil. The proposed mechanism was diltiazem-induced inhibition of benzodiazepine metabolism by CYP3A. Patients taking diltiazem had delayed early postoperative recovery as a result.

Drugs that influence CYP3A

Midazolam is selectively metabolized by CYP3A4, with which several drugs interact, influencing its pharmacokinetics and pharmacodynamics.

Itraconazole, an inhibitor of CYP3A, and rifampicin, an inducer of CYP3A, altered the pharmacokinetics and pharmacodynamics of oral midazolam in nine healthy volunteers (42). The half-life was prolonged from 2.7 to 7.6 hours by itraconazole and reduced to 1.0 hour by rifampicin. These effects were still present, although less marked, at 4 days after withdrawal of itraconazole and rifampicin. Similarly, after acute administration, the period of drowsiness was increased from 76 to 201 minutes with itraconazole and fell to 35 minutes with rifampicin; the effects were again less marked 4 days after withdrawal.

The protease inhibitor saquinavir, propofol, and fluconazole (41,45,46) increased the systemic availability and peak plasma concentrations and prolonged the half-life of midazolam, thus increasing its sedative effects. The dosage of midazolam should be reduced in patients taking these drugs.

Grapefruit juice reduced the metabolism of midazolam; prolonged sedation can be expected in some circumstances (47).

Chronic administration of glucocorticoids, which induce CYP3A4, reduces the sedative effect of midazolam by increasing its clearance; higher doses are therefore required for sedation (48).

Fentanyl

Several adverse effects have been reported with the combined use of fentanyl and midazolam, including chest wall rigidity, making ventilation with a bag and mask impossible (SEDA-16, 79). In neonates, hypotension can occur (SEDA-16, 80), and respiratory arrest in a child and sudden cardiac arrest have been reported (SEDA-16, 80). However, in one study there were no cardiac electrophysiological effects of midazolam combined with fentanyl in subjects undergoing cardiac electrophysiological studies (SEDA-18, 80).

Glucocorticoids

Chronic administration of glucocorticoids, which induce CYP3A4, reduces the sedative effect of midazolam by increasing its clearance; higher doses are therefore required for sedation (48).

Grapefruit juice

Grapefruit juice reduced the metabolism of midazolam; prolonged sedation can be expected in some circumstances (47).

Halothane

Midazolam produced marked reduction of the MAC of halothane in humans at lower serum concentrations than required to cause sleep (49).

Isoflurane

The effects of the combination of midazolam and isoflurane on memory were studied in a randomized, double-blind study in 28 volunteers (50). Midazolam 0.03 mg/kg or 0.06 mg/kg combined with isoflurane 0.2% almost completely abolished explicit and implicit memory, but there were more variable effects on the level of sedation. The duration of the deficit averaged 45 minutes. The study was remarkable for the very low doses required to abolish memory, owing to synergy of the combination of midazolam and isoflurane and abolition of memory at subhypnotic doses with this combination. However, the subjects did not undergo surgery, so caution must be exercised in extrapolating the result to surgical patients, because painful stimuli increase the dosage required to abolish memory.

Macrolides

Interactions of macrolide antibiotics with midazolam are clinically important. Increases in serum concentration, AUC, and half-life, and a reduction in clearance have been documented (51). These changes can result in clinical effects, such as prolonged psychomotor impairment, amnesia, or loss of consciousness (52).

Erythromycin potentiates the effects of oral midazolam (SEDA-17, 125). Either midazolam should be avoided in patients taking erythromycin or the dose should be reduced by 50–75% (53,54).

Nitrous oxide

The combination of midazolam with nitrous oxide produced retrograde amnesia in 21 women undergoing elective cesarean section (55). All had spinal anesthesia. After delivery the patients received intravenous midazolam, average dose 94 μg/kg, and inhaled nitrous oxide 50%. At the end of surgery, flumazenil was given in 0.1 mg increments until the patient awoke. Another nine women were given only nitrous oxide inhalation after delivery. Of the women who received midazolam and nitrous oxide, 33% could not recall their baby's face, while all of the women not given midazolam could. The results suggest that midazolam plus nitrous oxide can produce retrograde amnesia not reversed by flumazenil.

Pethidine

Rectal pethidine is not advised in children, owing to enormous variability in systemic availability (SEDA-18, 82). When used for sedation in children undergoing esophagogastroduodenoscopy, hypoxia with dysrhythmias was more likely to occur with a combination of pethidine and diazepam than with pethidine and midazolam (SEDA-18, 81).

Rifampicin

In a study of the effects of itraconazole 200 mg/day and rifampicin 600 mg/day on the pharmacokinetics and pharmacodynamics of oral midazolam 7.5–15 mg during and 4 days after the end of the treatment, switching from inhibition to induction of metabolism caused an up to 400-fold change in the AUC of oral midazolam (42).

Saquinavir

Saquinavir substantially potentiates the effects of midazolam by raising its blood concentrations, and this suggests that a parallel interaction could occur with other protease inhibitors (and no doubt certain other benzodiazepines) in similar combinations (46).

References

1. Parent JM, Lowenstein DH. Treatment of refractory generalized status epilepticus with continuous infusion of midazolam. Neurology 1994;44(10):1837–40.
2. Lauven PM. Pharmacology of drugs for conscious sedation. Scand J Gastroenterol Suppl 1990;179:1–6.
3. Pachulski RT, Adkins DC, Mirza H. Conscious sedation with intermittent midazolam and fentanyl in electrophysiology procedures. J Interv Cardiol 2001;14(2):143–6.
4. Blumer JL. Clinical pharmacology of midazolam in infants and children. Clin Pharmacokinet 1998;35(1):37–47.
5. Hughes J, Gill A, Leach HJ, Nunn AJ, Billingham I, Ratcliffe J, Thornington R, Choonara I. A prospective study of the adverse effects of midazolam on withdrawal in critically ill children. Acta Paediatr 1994;83(11):1194–9.
6. Scott RC, Besag FM, Neville BG. Buccal midazolam and rectal diazepam for treatment of prolonged seizures in childhood and adolescence: a randomised trial. Lancet 1999;353(9153):623–6.
7. Karl HW, Cote CJ, McCubbin MM, Kelley M, Liebelt E, Kaufman S, Burkhart K, Albers G, Wasserman G. Intravenous midazolam for sedation of children undergoing procedures: an analysis of age- and procedure-related factors. Pediatr Emerg Care 1999;15(3):167–72.
8. Marshall J, Rodarte A, Blumer J, Khoo KC, Akbari B, Kearns G. Pediatric pharmacodynamics of midazolam oral syrup. Pediatric Pharmacology Research Unit Network. J Clin Pharmacol 2000;40(6):578–89.
9. Wassner E, Morris B, Fernando L, Rao M, Whitehouse WP. Intranasal midazolam for treating febrile seizures in children. Buccal midazolam for childhood seizures at home preferred to rectal diazepam. BMJ 2001;322(7278):108.
10. Hall RI, Sandham D, Cardinal P, Tweeddale M, Moher D, Wang X, Anis AH. Propofol vs midazolam for ICU sedation: a Canadian multicenter randomized trial. Chest 2001;119(4):1151–9.
11. Baris S, Karakaya D, Aykent R, Kirdar K, Sagkan O, Tur A. Comparison of midazolam with or without

22 mmHg and improved the following symptoms of orthostatic hypotension compared to placebo: dizziness/light-headedness, weakness/fatigue, syncope, low energy, impaired ability to stand, and feelings of depression. The overall adverse effects were mainly mild to moderate. One or more adverse effects were reported by 22% of the placebo group compared with 27% of the midodrine-treated group. Scalp pruritus/tingling, which was reported by 10 of 74 (13.5%) of those given midodrine, was most frequent. Other reported adverse effects included supine hypertension (8%) and feelings of urinary urgency (4%).

Organs and Systems

Cardiovascular

Supine hypertension occurs in up to 3% of subjects, although it is not clear how the underlying pathology of the hypotension influences the likelihood of this reaction.

Nervous system

- A 33-year-old schizophrenic woman took midodrine 4 mg/day because of postural hypotension due to risperidone 6 mg/day (13). She developed an acute dystonic reaction, which recurred several times on rechallenge, and the dose of risperidone had to be halved to minimize the hypotension.

References

1. Mauro VF. Focus on midodrine: an oral peripheral-acting alpha-agonist for the treatment of orthostatic hypotension. Formulary 1997;32:225–31.
2. Low PA, Gilden JL, Freeman R, Sheng KN, McElligott MA; Efficacy of midodrine vs placebo in neurogenic orthostatic hypotension. A randomized, double-blind multicenter study. Midodrine Study Group. JAMA 1997;277(13):1046–51.
3. Fouad-Tarazi FM, Okabe M, Goren H. Alpha sympathomimetic treatment of autonomic insufficiency with orthostatic hypotension. Am J Med 1995;99(6):604–10.
4. Ward CR, Gray JC, Gilroy JJ, Kenny RA. Midodrine: a role in the management of neurocardiogenic syncope. Heart 1998;79(1):45–9.
5. Jankovic J, Gilden JL, Hiner BC, Kaufmann H, Brown DC, Coghlan CH, Rubin M, Fouad-Tarazi FM. Neurogenic orthostatic hypotension: a double-blind, placebo-controlled study with midodrine. Am J Med 1993;95(1):38–48.
6. Sra J, Maglio C, Biehl M, Dhala A, Blanck Z, Deshpande S, Jazayeri MR, Akhtar M. Efficacy of midodrine hydrochloride in neurocardiogenic syncope refractory to standard therapy. J Cardiovasc Electrophysiol 1997;8(1):42–6.
7. Calkins H. Pharmacologic approaches to therapy for vasovagal syncope. Am J Cardiol 1999;84(8A):Q20–5.
8. Perez-Lugones A, Schweikert R, Pavia S, Sra J, Akhtar M, Jaeger F, Tomassoni GF, Saliba W, Leonelli FM, Bash D, Beheiry S, Shewchik J, Tchou PJ, Natale A. Usefulness of midodrine in patients with severely symptomatic neurocardiogenic syncope: a randomized control study. J Cardiovasc Electrophysiol 2001;12(8):935–8.
9. Rowe PC, Calkins H. Neurally mediated hypotension and chronic fatigue syndrome. Am J Med 1998;105(3A):S15–21.
10. Karas B, Grubb BP, Boehm K, Kip K. The postural orthostatic tachycardia syndrome: a potentially treatable cause of chronic fatigue, exercise intolerance, and cognitive impairment in adolescents. Pacing Clin Electrophysiol 2000;23(3):344–51.
11. Perazella MA. Pharmacologic options available to treat symptomatic intradialytic hypotension. Am J Kidney Dis 2001;38(4 Suppl 4):S26–36.
12. Gairard AC, Cordonnier AL, Charles A, Viala A, Patri E, Germain C, Lafay N, Gury C. Recherche de la dose efficace de la midodrine dans l'hypertension orthostatique iatrogène à partir d'une étude pilote. J Pharm Clin 2000;19:256–9.
13. Takahashi H. Acute dystonia induced by adding midodrine, a selective alpha 1 agonist, to risperidone in a patient with catatonic schizophrenia. J Neuropsychiatry Clin Neurosci 2000;12(2):285–6.

Mifepristone

General Information

Mifepristone (RU-486) has become best known as an abortifacient. It is a potent antagonist at progesterone receptors and glucocorticoid receptors. The abortifacient effect is thought to be primarily due to blockade of endometrial progesterone receptors, but mifepristone also impedes the production of human chorionic gonadotropin and progesterone in the placenta. When given in a single dose of 10 mg/kg by mouth to induce menses, heavy bleeding was reported in some cases (1).

Whatever the adverse effects of mifepristone, the risks have to be looked at realistically and compared with those of the alternatives available to a particular woman in particular circumstances. Particularly in rural areas in developing countries, the risks of surgical and non-professional abortion are high, whereas, as has been shown in a study in rural India, a regimen of mifepristone plus misoprostol can be used as effectively and safely, through family planning clinics and country hospitals, as in a European environment (2).

Observational studies

The effective oral doses of mifepristone are 100–600 mg, and at any dose the bulk of recipients abort. Of 150 healthy women who received the higher dose, 131 attained a complete abortion. Three women reported bleeding for more than 2 weeks after abortion; 16 women had a reduced hemoglobin concentration of under 11 g/dl, justifying iron therapy. Other adverse effects were uterine contractions and pelvic pain ($n = 4$), transient asthenia ($n = 3$), and nausea ($n = 2$) (3). These findings seem to be typical, even though dosage schemes have varied; as little as 100 mg orally has been used successfully with similar adverse effects (SED-12, 1037) (4).

Placebo-controlled studies

In a double-blind, randomized, controlled trial, 896 healthy women requesting a medical abortion (57–63 days gestation, mean age 25 years) were randomized to a single oral dose of mifepristone 200 mg or 600 mg, both followed in 48 hours by gemeprost 1 mg vaginally (5). The complete abortion rates were similar with the lower and higher doses of mifepristone (92 versus 92%). The incidences of adverse effects were similar, with the exception of nausea at 1 week, which was less frequent in the low-dose group (3.6 versus 7.6%).

Organs and Systems

Electrolyte balance

Severe hypokalemia has been attributed to long-term mifepristone (6).

- An extremely ill 51-year-old man with Cushing's syndrome, due to an ACTH-secreting pituitary macroadenoma, which had failed to respond to conventional surgical, medical, and radiotherapeutic approaches, responded dramatically in the short-term and long-term to high-dose mifepristone (up to 25 mg/kg/day) for 18 months. However, she developed severe hypokalemia, attributed to excessive cortisol activation of mineralocorticoid receptors; it responded to spironolactone.

This case shows the potential need for concomitant mineralocorticoid receptor blockade when mifepristone is used to treat Cushing's syndrome, since mineralocorticoid concentrations can rise markedly, reflecting corticotropin disinhibition.

Reproductive system

Long-term mifepristone is primarily used as a means of treating uterine myomas, endometriosis (25–100 mg/day), and possibly inoperable meningiomas (200 mg/day) or inoperable Cushing's syndrome. While it is primarily regarded as an antiprogestogen, some of these uses reflect its antiglucocorticoid and antiproliferative effects. However, there are also data to suggest that, acting as an antiprogestogen, mifepristone can promote an unopposed estrogen milieu, and can thus have a proliferative effect on the endometrium.

- An adolescent girl with Cushingoid features and osteoporosis took mifepristone 400 mg/day for its antiglucocorticoid effect in an attempt to prevent further bone loss (7). Her striae, weight gain, and buffalo hump markedly improved, and further bone loss was halted. However, with each of the two 6-month courses of mifepristone (9 months apart) she developed massive simple endometrial hyperplasia and a markedly enlarged uterus. This reverted to normal after withdrawal of mifepristone.

The authors suggested that interval pelvic imaging may be advisable in women who take long-term mifepristone.

Drug Administration

Drug dosage regimens

There has sometimes been reluctance to use higher doses of mifepristone, because of a supposedly greater risk of severe adverse effects. However, in a randomized comparison of a single oral dose of mifepristone (either 200 mg or 600 mg) followed 48 hours later by oral misoprostol 400 μg the two regimens produced identical results as regards the induction of abortion and the incidence of adverse effects (8).

The optimal dose of mifepristone to secure an abortion without excessive adverse effects is not known. In a study in nearly 900 women there was no appreciable difference between oral doses of 200 or 600 mg, followed after 48 hours by gemeprost 1 mg vaginally (5). The similarity of adverse reactions with the lower and higher doses of mifepristone has been confirmed by others (9). However, in another study mifepristone 0.5 mg, which has sometimes been recommended on supposed safety grounds, was not sufficient to induce abortion (10). The frequencies of various adverse effects of mifepristone in effective doses have emerged from various studies. In one study nausea, vomiting, or diarrhea in women using a standard regimen occurred in 68%, 36%, and 20% respectively (11); these risks are not considered to be problematic. The combination of oral mifepristone and vaginal misoprostol is also effective and safe, has few serious adverse effects, and is well accepted by women (12).

References

1. Nieman LK, Choate TM, Chrousos GP, Healy DL, Morin M, Renquist D, Merriam GR, Spitz IM, Bardin CW, Baulieu EE, et al. The progesterone antagonist RU 486. A potential new contraceptive agent. N Engl J Med 1987;316(4):187–91.
2. Coyaji K, Elul B, Krishna U, Otiv S, Ambardekar S, Bopardikar A, Raote V, Ellertson C, Winikoff B. Mifepristone abortion outside the urban research hospital setting in India. Lancet 2001;357(9250):120–2.
3. Maria B, Stampf F, Goepp A, Ulmann A. Termination of early pregnancy by a single dose of mifepristone (RU 486), a progesterone antagonist. Eur J Obstet Gynecol Reprod Biol 1988;28(3):249–55.
4. Mishell DR Jr, Shoupe D, Brenner PF, Lacarra M, Horenstein J, Lahteenmaki P, Spitz IM. Termination of early gestation with the anti-progestin steroid RU 486: medium versus low dose. Contraception 1987;35(4):307–21.
5. Dhall GI, Calder A, Gomez-Alzugaray M, Ho PC, Pretnar Darovec A, Chen JK, Bygdeman M, Kovacs L, Albert SG, Kavkasidze G, Song LJ, Van Look PFA, Von Hertzen H, Noonan E, Ali M, Peregoudov A, Laperriere N, Grimes D. World Health Organization Task Force on Post-ovulatory Methods of Fertility Regulation. Medical abortion at 57 to 63 days' gestation with a lower dose of mifepristone and gemeprost. A randomized controlled trial. Acta Obstet Gynecol Scand 2001;80(5):447–51.
6. Chu JW, Matthias DF, Belanoff J, Schatzberg A, Hoffman AR, Feldman D. Successful long-term treatment of refractory Cushing's disease with high-dose mifepristone (RU 486). J Clin Endocrinol Metab 2001;86(8):3568–73.
7. Newfield RS, Spitz IM, Isacson C, New MI. Long-term mifepristone (RU486) therapy resulting in massive benign endometrial hyperplasia. Clin Endocrinol (Oxf) 2001;54(3):399–404.
8. Wu YM, Gomez-Alzugaray M, Haukkamaa M, Ngoc NTN, Ho PC, Pretnar-Darovec A, Healy DL, Sotnikova E, Shah RS, Pavlova NG, Chen JK, Song S, Bygdeman M, Kovacs L, Khomasuridze A, Song LJ, Hamzaoui R, Alexaniants S, Von Hertzen H. Comparison of two doses of mifepristone in combination with misoprostol for early medical abortion: a randomised trial. World Health Organisation Task Force on Post-ovulatory Methods of Fertility Regulation. BJOG 2000;107(4):524–30.

distal fusion of the proximal finger stumps by thin strands of tissue; the index finger was normal. The left leg had an amputation deformity at the mid-tibial/fibular level. There was an omphalocele. Histological examination of the placenta showed an absence of amnion on the chorionic surface, with reactive changes in the superficial chorionic stroma and "vernix granulomas" on the chorionic surface. These findings are diagnostic of early amnion rupture. There were no features of *Varicella* embryopathy.

Möbius' syndrome in association with congenital central alveolar hypoventilation has been described in Brazil (32).

Misoprostol-induced arthrogryposis has been reported in 15 Brazilian patients (33).

References

1. el-Refaey H, Rajasekar D, Abdalla M, Calder L, Templeton A. Induction of abortion with mifepristone (RU 486) and oral or vaginal misoprostol. N Engl J Med 1995;332(15):983–7.
2. Jain JK, Mishell DR Jr. A comparison of misoprostol with and without laminaria tents for induction of second-trimester abortion. Am J Obstet Gynecol 1996;175(1):173–7.
3. Phillips K, Berry C, Mathers AM. Uterine rupture during second trimester termination of pregnancy using mifepristone and a prostaglandin. Eur J Obstet Gynecol Reprod Biol 1996;65(2):175–6.
4. Creinin MD, Vittinghoff E, Keder L, Darney PD, Tiller G. Methotrexate and misoprostol for early abortion: a multicenter trial. I. Safety and efficacy. Contraception 1996;53(6):321–7.
5. Bugalho A, Mocumbi S, Faundes A, David E. Termination of pregnancies of <6 weeks gestation with a single dose of 800 microg of vaginal misoprostol. Contraception 2000;61(1):47–50.
6. Schaff EA, Fielding SL, Westhoff C, Ellertson C, Eisinger SH, Stadalius LS, Fuller L. Vaginal misoprostol administered 1, 2, or 3 days after mifepristone for early medical abortion: A randomized trial. JAMA 2000;284(15):1948–53.
7. Acharya G, Al-Sammarai MT, Patel N, Al-Habib A, Kiserud T. A randomized, controlled trial comparing effect of oral misoprostol and intravenous syntocinon on intra-operative blood loss during cesarean section. Acta Obstet Gynecol Scand 2001;80(3):245–50.
8. Tang OS, Miao BY, Lee SW, Ho PC. Pilot study on the use of repeated doses of sublingual misoprostol in termination of pregnancy up to 12 weeks gestation: efficacy and acceptability. Hum Reprod 2002;17(3):654–8.
9. Ghorab MN, El Helw BA. Second-trimester termination of pregnancy by extra-amniotic prostaglandin F2alpha or endocervical misoprostol. A comparative study. Acta Obstet Gynecol Scand 1998;77(4):429–32.
10. Ng PS, Chan AS, Sin WK, Tang LC, Cheung KB, Yuen PM. A multicentre randomized controlled trial of oral misoprostol and i.m. syntometrine in the management of the third stage of labour. Hum Reprod 2001;16(1):31–5.
11. Oyelese Y, Landy HJ, Collea JV. Cervical laceration associated with misoprostol induction. Int J Gynaecol Obstet 2001;73(2):161–2.
12. Al-Hussaini TK. Uterine rupture in second trimester abortion in a grand multiparous woman. A complication of misoprostol and oxytocin. Eur J Obstet Gynecol Reprod Biol 2001;96(2):218–19.
13. Hofmeyr GJ, Nikodem VC, de Jager M, Gelbart BR. A randomised placebo controlled trial of oral misoprostol in the third stage of labour. Br J Obstet Gynaecol 1998;105(9):971–5.
14. Hofmeyr GJ, Gulmezoglu AM, Alfirevic Z. Misoprostol for induction of labour: a systematic review. Br J Obstet Gynaecol 1999;106(8):798–803.
15. Fong YF, Singh K, Prasad RN. Severe hyperthermia following use of vaginal misoprostol for pre-operative cervical priming. Int J Gynaecol Obstet 1999;64(1):73–4.
16. Gherman RB, McBrayer S, Browning J. Uterine rupture associated with vaginal birth after cesarean section: a complication of intravaginal misoprostol? Gynecol Obstet Invest 2000;50(3):212–13.
17. Jwarah E, Greenhalf JO. Rupture of the uterus after 800 micrograms misoprostol given vaginally for termination of pregnancy. BJOG 2000;107(6):807.
18. Hill DA, Chez RA, Quinlan J, Fuentes A, LaCombe J. Uterine rupture and dehiscence associated with intravaginal misoprostol cervical ripening. J Reprod Med 2000;45(10):823–6.
19. Sciscione AC, Nguyen L, Manley JS, Shlossman PA, Colmorgen GH. Uterine rupture during preinduction cervical ripening with misoprostol in a patient with a previous Caesarean delivery. Aust NZ J Obstet Gynaecol 1998;38(1):96–7.
20. Wing DA, Lovett K, Paul RH. Disruption of prior uterine incision following misoprostol for labor induction in women with previous cesarean delivery. Obstet Gynecol 1998;91(5 Pt 2):828–30.
21. Fletcher H, McCaw-Binns A. Rupture of the uterus with misoprostol (prostaglandin El) used for induction of labour. J Obstet Gynaecol 1998;18(2):184–5.
22. Plaut MM, Schwartz ML, Lubarsky SL. Uterine rupture associated with the use of misoprostol in the gravid patient with a previous cesarean section. Am J Obstet Gynecol 1999;180(6 Pt 1):1535–42.
23. Mathews JE, Mathai M, George A. Uterine rupture in a multiparous woman during labor induction with oral misoprostol. Int J Gynaecol Obstet 2000;68(1):43–4.
24. Searle GD. Important drug warning concerning unapproved use of intravaginal or oral misoprostol in pregnant women for induction of labor or abortion. Media Release, 23 August 2000.
25. Gonzalez CH, Marques-Dias MJ, Kim CA, Sugayama SM, Da Paz JA, Huson SM, Holmes LB. Congenital abnormalities in Brazilian children associated with misoprostol misuse in first trimester of pregnancy. Lancet 1998;351(9116):1624–7.
26. Sitruk-Ware R, Davey A, Sakiz E. Fetal malformation and failed medical termination of pregnancy. Lancet 1998;352(9124):323.
27. Pastuszak AL, Schuler L, Speck-Martins CE, Coelho KE, Cordello SM, Vargas F, Brunoni D, Schwarz IV, Larrandaburu M, Safattle H, Meloni VF, Koren G. Use of misoprostol during pregnancy and Möbius' syndrome in infants. N Engl J Med 1998;338(26):1881–5.
28. Vargas FR, Schuler-Faccini L, Brunoni D, Kim C, Meloni VF, Sugayama SM, Albano L, Llerena JC Jr, Almeida JC, Duarte A, Cavalcanti DP, Goloni-Bertollo E, Conte A, Koren G, Addis A. Prenatal exposure to misoprostol and vascular disruption defects: a case-control study. Am J Med Genet 2000;95(4):302–6.
29. Orioli IM, Castilla EE. Epidemiological assessment of misoprostol teratogenicity. BJOG 2000;107(4):519–23.
30. Brasil R, Coelho HL, D'Avanzo B, La Vecchia C. Misoprostol and congenital anomalies. Pharmacoepidemiol Drug Saf 2000;9:401–3.
31. Genest DR, Di Salvo D, Rosenblatt MJ, Holmes LB. Terminal transverse limb defects with tethering and

omphalocele in a 17 week fetus following first trimester misoprostol exposure. Clin Dysmorphol 1999;8(1):53–8.
32. Nunes ML, Friedrich MA, Loch LF. Association of misoprostol, Moebius syndrome and congenital central alveolar hypoventilation. Case report. Arq Neuropsiquiatr 1999;57(1):88–91.
33. Coelho KE, Sarmento MF, Veiga CM, Speck-Martins CE, Safatle HP, Castro CV, Niikawa N. Misoprostol embryotoxicity: clinical evaluation of fifteen patients with arthrogryposis. Am J Med Genet 2000;95(4):297–301.

Mitomycin

See also Cytostatic and immunosuppressant drugs

General Information

Mitomycin is an alkylating agent that is used intravenously to treat upper gastrointestinal and breast cancers and by direct instillation to treat superficial bladder tumors. Its main adverse effects are thrombocytopenia and leukopenia. Rare but severe adverse effects are hemolytic–uremic syndrome, pneumonitis, and cardiac failure.

Organs and Systems

Respiratory

Biopsy-proven mitomycin pneumonitis occurred in five of 44 patients who were given mitomycin in conjunction with low-dose doxorubicin 20 mg/week (1). The picture was of pulmonary infiltrates clinically and radiologically, progressive dyspnea, and hypoxia, and improvement with glucocorticoids. The mean total dose of mitomycin that had been given in the five patients was 89 mg. Mitomycin-induced interstitial pneumonitis occurs in 2–38% of cases (2,3) and at cumulative doses of 20 mg/m^2 or greater, although doses up to 30 mg/m^2 have been used safely. It is characteristically of slow-onset (3).

A fatal case of mitomycin C-induced pneumonitis has been reported in a radiotherapy/chemotherapy trial in 43 patients (4). The dose was 8 mg/m^2 on days 1 and 29, radiotherapy and vindesine being given on the intervening days.

Urinary tract

Hemolytic–uremic syndrome has often been described in patients treated with mitomycin (5–7). Up to 1990 the United States National Cancer Registry received 85 reports of cancer-associated hemolytic–uremic syndrome and 84 had received a cumulative dose of 60 mg mitomycin or more as part of their treatment (8).

Hemolytic–uremic syndrome presents as a Coombs-negative microangiopathic hemolytic anemia, thrombocytopenia, and renal insufficiency, and the outcome is often fatal. The underlying pathology is thought to be vascular endothelial damage. It occurs 4–7 months after the start of chemotherapy. Blood transfusion can cause clinical deterioration in those affected (9). Histology of the kidney in the hemolytic–uremic syndrome caused by mitomycin shows mesangial proliferative glomerulonephritis with partial thickening and/or splitting of the basement membrane. On electron microscopy there is accumulation of non-homogeneous material in the subendothelial spaces. Neither immunoglobulin nor complement deposition is found (10). Treatment with hemodialysis and immunosuppressive drugs is not always successful. Plasmapheresis is commonly used (11). Prophylactic glucocorticoids can reduce the severity and prevent hemolytic–uremic syndrome in patients receiving mitomycin (12). Erythropoietin is also reportedly beneficial (13).

Mitomycin when administered intravesically causes cystitis of variable severity, which can lead to mucosal ulceration in the worst cases. However, there has also been a report of bladder fibrosis and loss of function in a 74-year-old man who had received 20 mg/week for 8 weeks (14).

Ten cases of bladder wall calcification have been reported after intravesicular administration of mitomycin. These lesions can resemble tumor recurrence in the bladder, and biopsy is advocated to distinguish between the two (15).

Skin

There have been several reports of erythematous blistering skin eruption of the palms and soles affecting patients treated with intravesical mitomycin. This has been attributed to contact dermatitis, but more widespread skin involvement and an association with eosinophilic interstitial cystitis suggest that it may be a more generalized allergic reaction (16–20).

Local extravasation of mitomycin causes inflammation and ulceration, starting within 7–10 days and lasting several weeks. In four cases the onset of tissue necrosis was delayed several weeks or months after exposure (21,22). In one case, ulceration seemed to have been precipitated by drinking ethanol, and in another by exposure to the sun.

Three cases of allergic dermatitis have been described after intravesical mitomycin (23). A type IV hypersensitivity reaction was demonstrated on patch-testing. Six cases of purpuric allergic drug eruption from intravesicular mitomycin have been reported (24).

References

1. Colozza M, Tonato M, Grignani F, Davis S. Low-dose mitomycin and weekly low-dose doxorubicin combination chemotherapy for patients with metastatic breast carcinoma previously treated with cyclophosphamide, methotrexate, and 5-fluorouracil. Cancer 1988;62(2):262–5.
2. Verweij J, van Zanten T, Souren T, Golding R, Pinedo HM. Prospective study on the dose relationship of mitomycin C-induced interstitial pneumonitis. Cancer 1987;60(4):756–61.
3. Linette DC, McGee KH, McFarland JA. Mitomycin-induced pulmonary toxicity: case report and review of the literature. Ann Pharmacother 1992;26(4):481–4.
4. Furuse K, Kubota K, Kawahara M, Kodama N, Ogawara M, Akira M, Nakajima S, Takada M, Kusunoki Y, Negoro S, et al. Phase II study of concurrent radiotherapy and chemotherapy for unresectable stage III non-small-cell lung cancer. Southern Osaka Lung Cancer Study Group. J Clin Oncol 1995;13(4):869–75.
5. Mackintosh J, Tattersal M. Mitomycin-C induced hemolytic–uraemic syndrome. Aust NZ J Med 1988;18:182.

SSRIs

The combination of conventional MAO inhibitors with serotonin-potentiating agents, such as SSRIs, is contraindicated, because of the risk of the serotonin syndrome. Moclobemide may be less likely to cause this interaction, although both case reports and clinical series have suggested that some patients have suffered significant adverse effects consistent with serotonin toxicity (SEDA-20, 6) (SEDA-21, 10). After steady-state therapy with the SSRI fluoxetine (20–40 mg/day for 23 days), 12 subjects took fluoxetine plus moclobemide (600 mg/day) and 6 took fluoxetine and placebo (31). There was no difference in the rates of adverse effects between the two groups and no evidence of serotonin toxicity, although fluoxetine inhibited the metabolism of moclobemide. The authors suggested that patients can be safely switched from fluoxetine to moclobemide without the need for the currently advised 5-week washout (which is necessary to allow the long-acting fluoxetine metabolite, norfluoxetine, to be eliminated). However, case reports have suggested that some patients can develop serotonin toxicity when moclobemide is combined with SSRIs (23,25,28) or clomipramine (26), so great caution is still needed in clinical practice. Overdoses of moclobemide and SSRIs can cause serious and sometimes fatal serotonin toxicity (SEDA-18, 16).

Tyramine

Moclobemide in conventional doses (300–600 mg/day) does not significantly potentiate the pressor effects of oral tyramine, and special dietary restrictions are therefore not usually necessary. However, higher doses of moclobemide are sometimes used to treat patients with resistant depression. Moclobemide 900 mg/day and 1200 mg/day have been compared with placebo in 12 healthy volunteers (32). Neither dose of moclobemide significantly potentiated the pressor effect of 50 mg of tyramine, which has been estimated to be the upper limit of dietary tyramine content, even of large meals containing substantial amounts of cheese. However, one subject taking moclobemide 1200 mg/day had an increase in systolic blood pressure of over 30 mmHg. Individuals have rather different sensitivities to the pressor effects of oral tyramine challenge, and the number studied in this series was small. Accordingly, clinical extrapolation might not be straightforward. Patients taking conventional doses of moclobemide are sometimes advised to restrict their intake of cheese or other tyramine-containing foods, and this advice is clearly prudent if subjects take higher doses.

Venlafaxine

Interactions of moclobemide with venlafaxine, a potent serotonin re-uptake inhibitor, have been reported (25,33).

- A 34-year-old man took 2.625 g of venlafaxine (therapeutic dose 75–375 mg/day) and 3 g of moclobemide, plus an unknown amount of alcohol 1 hour before being admitted to hospital. Within 20 minutes of arrival his conscious level deteriorated and he had increased muscle tone, with clonus in all limbs. He was treated with intubation, paralysis, and ventilation, and sedated with midazolam and morphine. He regained consciousness after 2 days.

This case report confirms the serious consequences of combined overdosage of moclobemide with drugs that potentiate brain serotonin function (see also the monograph on SSRIs).

References

1. Amrein R, Allen SR, Guentert TW, Hartmann D, Lorscheid T, Schoerlin MP, Vranesic D. The pharmacology of reversible monoamine oxidase inhibitors. Br J Psychiatry Suppl 1989;6:66–71.
2. Simpson GM, de Leon J. Tyramine and new monoamine oxidase inhibitor drugs. Br J Psychiatry Suppl 1989;6:32–7.
3. Versiani M, Oggero U, Alterwain P, Capponi R, Dajas F, Heinze-Martin G, Marquez CA, Poleo MA, Rivero-Almanzor LE, Rossel L, et al. A double-blind comparative trial of moclobemide v. imipramine and placebo in major depressive episodes. Br J Psychiatry Suppl 1989;6:72–7.
4. Realini R, Mascetti R, Calanchini C. Efficacité et tolerance du moclobemide (Ro 11-1163 *Aurorix*) en comparaison avec la maprotiline chez des patients ambulatoires présentant un épisode dépressif majeur. [Effectiveness and tolerance of moclobemide (Ro 11-1163 Aurorix) in comparison with maprotiline in ambulatory patients presenting with a major depressive episode.] Psychol Med 1989;21:1689.
5. Laux G. Moclobemid in der Depressionsbehandlung – eine Übersicht. [Moclobemide in the treatment of depression – an overview.] Psychiatr Prax 1989;16(Suppl 1):37–40.
6. Koczkas C, Holm P, Karlsson A, Nagy A, Ose E, Petursson H, Ulveras L, Wenedikter O. Moclobemide and clomipramine in endogenous depression. A randomized clinical trial. Acta Psychiatr Scand 1989;79(6):523–9.
7. Larsen JK, Holm P, Hoyer E, Mejlhede A, Mikkelsen PL, Olesen A, Schaumburg E. Moclobemide and clomipramine in reactive depression. A placebo-controlled randomized clinical trial. Acta Psychiatr Scand 1989;79(6):530–6.
8. Baumhackl U, Biziere K, Fischbach R, Geretsegger C, Hebenstreit G, Radmayr E, Stabl M. Efficacy and tolerability of moclobemide compared with imipramine in depressive disorder (DSM-III): an Austrian double-blind, multicentre study. Br J Psychiatry Suppl 1989;6:78–83.
9. Burner M. Antidépresseur inhibiteur reversible et sélectif de la MAO-A. [Reversible Inhibitory antidepressant, selective for MAO-A.] Med Hyg 1990;48:2245.
10. Bakish D, Bradwejn J, Nair N, McClure J, Remick R, Bulger L. A comparison of moclobemide, amitriptyline and placebo in depression: a Canadian multicentre study. Psychopharmacology (Berl) 1992;106(Suppl):S98–S101.
11. Delini-Stula A, Baier D, Kohnen R, Laux G, Philipp M, Scholz HJ. Undesirable blood pressure changes under naturalistic treatment with moclobemide, a reversible MAO-A inhibitor – results of the drug utilization observation studies. Pharmacopsychiatry 1999;32(2):61–7.
12. Dunn NR, Freemantle SN, Pearce GL, Mann RD. Galactorrhoea with moclobemide. Lancet 1998;351(9105):802.
13. Timmings P, Lamont D. Intrahepatic cholestasis associated with moclobemide leading to death. Lancet 1996; 347(9003):762–3.
14. Korpelainen JT, Hiltunen P, Myllyla VV. Moclobemide-induced hypersexuality in patients with stroke and Parkinson's disease. Clin Neuropharmacol 1998;21(4):251–4.
15. Montejo AL, Llorca G, Izquierdo JA, Rico-Villademoros F. Incidence of sexual dysfunction associated with antidepressant agents: a prospective multicenter study of 1022 outpatients. Spanish Working Group for the Study of Psychotropic-Related Sexual Dysfunction. J Clin Psychiatry 2001;62(Suppl 3):10–21.
16. Pons G, Schoerlin MP, Tam YK, Moran C, Pfefen JP, Francoual C, Pedarriosse AM, Chavinie J, Olive G.

Moclobemide excretion in human breast milk. Br J Clin Pharmacol 1990;29(1):27–31.
17. Vine R, Norman TR, Burrows GD. A case of moclobemide overdose. Int Clin Psychopharmacol 1988;3(4):325–6.
18. Heinze G, Sanchez A. Overdose with moclobemide. J Clin Psychiatry 1986;47(8):438.
19. Camaris C, Little D. A fatality due to moclobemide. J Forensic Sci 1997;42(5):954–5.
20. Butzkueven H. A case of serotonin syndrome induced by moclobemide during an extreme heatwave. Aust NZ J Med 1997;27(5):603–4.
21. Ferrer-Dufol A, Perez-Aradros C, Murillo EC, Marques-Alamo JM. Fatal serotonin syndrome caused by moclobemide–clomipramine overdose. J Toxicol Clin Toxicol 1998;36(1–2):31–2.
22. Gillman PK. Serotonin syndrome—clomipramine too soon after moclobemide? Int Clin Psychopharmacol 1997;12(6):339–42.
23. Singer PP, Jones GR. An uncommon fatality due to moclobemide and paroxetine. J Anal Toxicol 1997;21(6):518–20.
24. Francois B, Marquet P, Desachy A, Roustan J, Lachatre G, Gastinne H. Serotonin syndrome due to an overdose of moclobemide and clomipramine. A potentially life-threatening association. Intensive Care Med 1997;23(1):122–4.
25. Roxanas MG, Machado JF. Serotonin syndrome in combined moclobemide and venlafaxine ingestion. Med J Aust 1998;168(10):523–4.
26. Chan BS, Graudins A, Whyte IM, Dawson AH, Braitberg G, Duggin GG. Serotonin syndrome resulting from drug interactions. Med J Aust 1998;169(10):523–5.
27. Dardennes RM, Even C, Ballon N, Bange F. Serotonin syndrome caused by a clomipramine–moclobemide interaction. J Clin Psychiatry 1998;59(7):382–3.
28. Benazzi F. Serotonin syndrome with molobemide–fluoxetine combination. Pharmacopsychiatry 1996;29(4):162.
29. Hartter S, Dingemanse J, Baier D, Ziegler G, Hiemke C. Inhibition of dextromethorphan metabolism by moclobemide. Psychopharmacology (Berl) 1998;135(1):22–6.
30. Van Haarst AD, Van Gerven JM, Cohen AF, De Smet M, Sterrett A, Birk KL, Fisher AL, De Puy ME, Goldberg MR, Musson DG. The effects of moclobemide on the pharmacokinetics of the 5-$HT_{1B/1D}$ agonist rizatriptan in healthy volunteers. Br J Clin Pharmacol 1999;48(2):190–6.
31. Dingemanse J, Wallnofer A, Gieschke R, Guentert T, Amrein R. Pharmacokinetic and pharmacodynamic interactions between fluoxetine and moclobemide in the investigation of development of the "serotonin syndrome". Clin Pharmacol Ther 1998;63(4):403–13.
32. Dingemanse J, Wood N, Guentert T, Oie S, Ouwerkerk M, Amrein R. Clinical pharmacology of moclobemide during chronic administration of high doses to healthy subjects. Psychopharmacology (Berl) 1998;140(2):164–72.
33. Coorey AN, Wenck DJ. Venlafaxine overdose. Med J Aust 1998;168(10):523.

Modafinil

General Information

Modafinil is a benzhydrylsulfinylacetamide wake-promoting agent for oral administration (1). It selectively targets neuronal pathways in the sleep/wake centers of the brain. It is well absorbed and its half-life is about 12–15 hours, which largely reflects the half-life of its levorotatory enantiomer. It is metabolized, mainly in the liver, by amide hydrolysis with lesser contributions from CYP-mediated oxidation, and. less than 10% of the dose is excreted as unchanged drug.

In controlled clinical trials, modafinil reduced excessive daytime sleepiness in patients with narcolepsy (2).

In an open, randomized, crossover study in healthy men, concomitant administration of single oral doses of modafinil (200 mg) and dexamfetamine (10 mg), each given separately, produced a slight increase in blood pressure and the cardiovascular effects were more pronounced after concomitant administration (3). These changes were considered not to be clinically relevant and would not necessarily preclude short-term administration of the two drugs together. The most frequent adverse events with modafinil or dexamfetamine were headache, dizziness, insomnia, and dry mouth.

Modafinil was effective in narcolepsy in a 9-week, randomized, placebo-controlled, double-blind, 21-center trial in 271 patients (4). During treatment withdrawal, the patients did not have symptoms associated with amphetamine withdrawal. Nausea and rhinitis were significantly more common in the treatment group; in contrast, in a previous multicenter study in the USA there was a higher incidence of headache (5). Modafinil was also effective in the treatment of somnolence due to pramipexole in a patient with Parkinson's disease (6).

Once-daily modafinil for an average of 4.6 weeks has been evaluated in an open trial in 11 children aged 5–15 years with ADHD (7). This pilot study, with non-blinded ratings, a small number of subjects, and a short duration of treatment, showed significant improvement. Adverse events were responsible for drug withdrawal in one child. The most common adverse event was delayed onset of sleep or sleep disruption, which, in two of three cases, responded to a reduction in dosage. No patient taking modafinil lost weight or had a reduced appetite. A larger-scale, double-blind, placebo-controlled study will be needed to further substantiate the efficacy and safety of modafinil.

In a 9-week, single-blind, placebo-controlled pilot study in 72 patients with multiple sclerosis who took modafinil 200 mg/day for 2 weeks, there was significant improvement in fatigue compared with placebo run-in treatment (8). The most frequent adverse effects were headache, nausea, and anxiety, and these were rated as either mild or moderate.

Long-Term Effects

Drug dependence

The abuse potential of modafinil is very low and differs from that of methylphenidate (9). The data suggest that the subjective effects of modafinil may be similar to those of drugs such as phenylpropanolamine or caffeine, although a direct comparison with these drugs would be required to draw adequate conclusions. Furthermore, modafinil cannot be injected intravenously or smoked, and its once-daily dosing in the management of excessive daytime sleepiness in patients with narcolepsy suggests that it does not carry the same public health or safety concerns for abuse as amphetamines, since drugs that have a long half-life have less of a tendency to produce a "rush" and hence are less likely to be abused. However, the effects of social responses to the availability of modafinil can only be determined by post-marketing surveillance.

Drug–Drug Interactions

General

In vitro, modafinil caused reversible inhibition of CYP2C19 in human liver microsomes (1). It also caused a small, but concentration-dependent, induction of CYP1A2, CYP2B6, and CYP3A4 and inhibition of CYP2C9 activity in primary cultures of human hepatocytes. In clinical studies of interactions of modafinil with methylphenidate, dexamfetamine, warfarin, ethinylestradiol, and triazolam, the only substantive interactions were with ethinylestradiol and triazolam, apparently through induction of CYP3A4, primarily in the gastrointestinal tract (1). The results suggested that modafinil can affect the pharmacokinetics of drugs that are metabolized by certain CYP isozymes. Compounds that induce or inhibit CYP activity are unlikely to have major effects on the pharmacokinetics of modafinil.

Clozapine

Clozapine toxicity occurred after modafinil administration to reverse sedation associated with clozapine (10).

- A 42-year-old man with schizophrenia, taking haloperidol, quetiapine, divalproex, gabapentin, benzatropine, and lorazepam, was given clozapine 25 mg at bedtime titrated to 400 mg/day over 13 days. His non-psychotropic medications included levothyroxine, furosemide, potassium, and docusate sodium. All other psychotropic drugs were tapered and withdrawn by day 69. On day 70 the serum clozapine concentration was 761ng/mL. Because of persistent psychotic symptoms, the dose of clozapine was increased to 450 mg/day on day 77, but this resulted in severe sedation. He was given modafinil 100 mg/day on day 82, titrated to 300 mg/day by day 101; this produced slight improvement in sedation. On day 116 he complained of dizziness, had an unsteady gait, and fell twice. He was afebrile and tachycardic but had a normal blood pressure; his blood oxygen saturation was 86%. His serum clozapine concentration on day 112 was 1400 ng/ml. Clozapine and modafinil were withdrawn. His gait disturbance and hypoxemia resolved. Clozapine 100 mg/day was restarted on day 121 and increased to 300 mg/day by day 122. The clozapine concentration 21 days later was 1236 ng/ml and 5 weeks later 960 ng/ml.

It is possible that inhibition of CYP2C19 by modafinil interfered with clozapine clearance in this case (11). Despite the potential of modafinil for reversing clozapine-associated sedation (12), caution is required when prescribing this drug combination.

Dexamfetamine

The potential for an interaction of modafinil with dexamfetamine, each at steady state, has been investigated in an open, randomized study in 32 healthy subjects (13). All took modafinil orally once daily for 28 days (200 mg on days 1–7 and 400 mg on days 8–28). On days 22–28, half of them also took dexamfetamine 20 mg orally 7 hours after modafinil. The steady-state pharmacokinetics of modafinil and its metabolites, modafinil acid and modafinil sulfone, were unaltered by low-dose dexamfetamine. Adverse events (abdominal pain, headache, and insomnia) were similar in the two groups and mild or moderate in nature. In another open, randomized, crossover study in healthy men, concomitant administration of single oral doses of modafinil (200 mg) and dexamfetamine (10 mg) showed no clinically significant pharmacokinetic interaction (3). Some patients with narcolepsy may require a change from dexamfetamine to modafinil, and arguably such a transition can be made without any washout period.

References

1. Robertson P Jr, Hellriegel ET. Clinical pharmacokinetic profile of modafinil. Clin Pharmacokinet 2003;42(2):123–37.
2. Jasinski DR, Kovacevic-Ristanovic R. Evaluation of the abuse liability of modafinil and other drugs for excessive daytime sleepiness associated with narcolepsy. Clin Neuropharmacol 2000;23(3):149–56.
3. Wong YN, Wang L, Hartman L, Simcoe D, Chen Y, Laughton W, Eldon R, Markland C, Grebow P. Comparison of the single-dose pharmacokinetics and tolerability of modafinil and dextroamphetamine administered alone or in combination in healthy male volunteers. J Clin Pharmacol 1998;38(10):971–8.
4. Becker PM, Jamieson AO, Jewel CE, Bogan RK, James DS. Randomized trial of modafinil as a treatment for the excessive daytime somnolence of narcolepsy: US Modafinil Narcolepsy Multicenter Study Group. Neurol 2000;54(5):1166–75.
5. Anonymous. Randomized trial of modafinil for the treatment of pathological somnolence in narcolepsy. US Modafinil Narcolepsy Multicenter Study Group. Ann Neurol 1998;43(1):88–97.
6. Hauser RA, Wahba MN, Zesiewicz TA, McDowell Anderson W. Modafinil treatment of pramipexole-associated somnolence. Mov Disord 2000;15(6):1269–71.
7. Rugino TA, Copley TC. Effects of modafinil in children with attention-deficit/hyperactivity disorder: an open-label study. J Am Acad Child Adolesc Psychiatry 2001;40(2):230–5.
8. Rammohan KW, Rosenberg JH, Lynn DJ, Blumenfeld AM, Pollak CP, Nagaraja HN. Efficacy and safety of modafinil (provigil) for the treatment of fatigue in multiple sclerosis: a two centre phase 2 study. J Neurol Neurosurg Psychiatry 2002;72(2):179–83.
9. Jasinski DR. An evaluation of the abuse potential of modafinil using methylphenidate as a reference. J Psychopharmacol 2000;14(1):53–60.
10. Dequardo JR. Modafinil-associated clozapine toxicity. Am J Psychiatry 2002;159(7):1243–4.
11. Robertson P, DeCory HH, Madan A, Parkinson A. In vitro inhibition and induction of human hepatic cytochrome P450 enzymes by modafinil. Drug Metab Dispos 2000;28(6):664–71.
12. Teitelman E. Off-label uses of modafinil. Am J Psychiatry 2001;158(8):1341.
13. Hellriegel ET, Arora S, Nelson M, Robertson P Jr. Steady-state pharmacokinetics and tolerability of modafinil administered alone or in combination with dextroamphetamine in healthy volunteers. J Clin Pharmacol 2002;42(4):450–60.

Mofebutazone

See also Non-steroidal anti-inflammatory drugs

General Information

Adverse reactions to mofebutazone are similar to those of the parent drug, phenylbutazone, and include skin reactions, including epidermal necrolysis and bullous drug eruption (1). Gastrotoxicity, hepatotoxicity, nephrotoxicity, edema, headache, and hematological adverse effects (SED-9, 145) (2) have been described.

References

1. Walchner M, Rueff F, Przybilla B. Delayed-type hypersensitivity to mofebutazone underlying a severe drug reaction. Contact Dermatitis 1997;36(1):54–5.
2. Kimura S, Shorota N. [A case report of massive bleeding from conjunctiva due to drug-induced thrombocytopenia.] Nippon Ganka Kiyo 1971;22(11):954–8.

Molsidomine

See also Antianginal drugs

General Information

Molsidomine is a vasodilator that acts as a nitric oxide donor and has been used in angina pectoris, heart failure, and after myocardial infarction.

In a multicenter, randomized, double-blind, crossover, placebo-controlled study of the efficacy of two regimens of molsidomine in 90 patients with stable angina, beneficial effects on exercise load did not seem to be reduced by 6 weeks of continuous therapy, suggesting lack of tolerance (1). The most frequently reported adverse effect of molsidomine was headache, as for all other nitric oxide donors.

Reference

1. Messin R, Karpov Y, Baikova N, Bruhwyler J, Monseu MJ, Guns C, Geczy J. Short- and long-term effects of molsidomine retard and molsidomine nonretard on exercise capacity and clinical status in patients with stable angina: a multicenter randomized double-blind crossover placebo-controlled trial. J Cardiovasc Pharmacol 1998;31(2):271–6.

Monoamine oxidase inhibitors

General Information

All available monoamine oxidase (MAO) inhibitors (excepting moclobemide, toloxatone, brofaromine, and selegiline) act via a "suicide" mechanism, by causing long-lasting, irreversible, competitive inhibition of mitochondrial MAO, which persists until new enzyme is manufactured (1). Most of these drugs also produce a non-specific reduction in the activity of hepatic drug-metabolizing enzymes.

Table 1 lists the MAO inhibitors that are already available or under investigation. These compounds fall into different chemical categories, including compounds that have the following properties: antidepressant (moclobemide), antihypertensive (pargyline), antineoplastic (procarbazine), and antimicrobial (furazolidone).

Antidepressant drugs of various classes (tricyclics, MAO inhibitors, SSRIs) have broad efficacy in generalized anxiety and in panic disorder, but SSRIs are now the treatments of choice (2,3). Selegiline has been used to treat Parkinson's disease. Other drugs that have MAO inhibitory activity, but are not used as such, include debrisoquine, linezolid, and isoniazid.

The monoamine oxidase inhibitors epitomize cyclical fashions in drug use and the impact of adverse effects. They were the first psychotropic drugs for which a clear biochemical action was defined. Early excitement was quickly tempered by reports of liver toxicity with the hydrazine derivatives, leading to synthesis of the cyclopropylamine drug, tranylcypromine, which in turn elicited the food and drug interactions that led to an overall decline in popularity.

Then in the 1980s there was a reappraisal of the benefit-to-harm balance of the MAO inhibitors. This spawned both a search for safer and more selective or rapidly reversible enzyme inhibitors (including moclobemide, toloxatone, and brofaromine), as well as a review and retrial of the older compounds.

The scientific underpinnings of this renaissance have been reviewed (4). Much of the earlier work was conducted using inadequate doses of phenelzine, whose efficacy was later validated using adequate drug concentrations (to produce 85% or more enzyme inhibition) (5). A review of eleven studies conducted in 1963–1982 that compared MAO inhibitors and tricyclic compounds showed that in three studies there was no difference, four favored tricyclic antidepressants, and in three MAO inhibitors were superior (6). The three studies that favored MAO inhibitors were among the four most recently conducted (all since 1979). An article in 1985 entitled "Should the use of MAO be abandoned?" (7) was accompanied by commentaries from six British and US experts in psychopharmacology. The consensus was clearly in favor of continued use, with the recognition that even if a specific responder is difficult to define there are individuals who respond when all other drugs have failed. No clear-cut clinical or metabolic features distinguish such individuals; an earlier claim that the clinical response and susceptibility to adverse effects might be influenced by genetically determined rapid or slow acetylation of phenelzine was not confirmed by a review of seven studies (8).

There have been many studies of the efficacy and toxicity of selective inhibitors of MAO type A (SEDA-16, 7) (SEDA-17, 16) (SEDA-18, 16).

The adverse effects of the MAO inhibitors include hepatocellular damage, similar to that which led to the withdrawal of the earlier hydrazine derivatives, hypotension, often a pronounced adverse effect (possibly due to the accumulation of a pseudotransmitter normally protein food that contains decarboxylating bacteria can convert amino acids to amines such as tyramine, phenylethylamine, and histamine, and the amine composition of foodstuffs is variable and unpredictable; for example, identical-looking pieces of cheese can vary 100-fold in tyramine content. The diversity and number of substances (listed in Table 2) and unpredictability in the occurrence of adverse effects have contributed to the unpopularity of the MAO inhibitors as therapeutic agents.

Two facts simplify the understanding and use of these drugs.

(1) The interactions listed in Table 2 fall into three categories:

 (a) hypertensive crisis due to the release and potentiation of catecholamines similar to that experienced in pheochromocytoma;
 (b) a serotonin syndrome, caused by excess serotonin availability in the nervous system;
 (c) exacerbation or prolongation of the normal actions of the object drug (sedation or coma due to alcohol, anesthetics, or opioid analgesics; atropine-like central toxicity due to tricyclic antidepressants).

 The consequences of the hypertensive interaction are variable. Many individuals remain unaware of relatively minor increases in blood pressure. However, if the rise is large and rapid (an increase of 30 mmHg or more in systolic pressure within 20 minutes), the patient experiences a sudden severe occipital headache and palpitation, which may be associated in rare instances with subarachnoid hemorrhage or cardiac failure, if the cerebral vasculature or cardiac musculature are already weakened.

 The serotonin syndrome is characterized by three or more of the following symptoms: confusion, hypomania, agitation, myoclonus, hyper-reflexia, hyperthermia, shivering, sweating, ataxia, and diarrhea (47). It is most often seen in patients taking a combination of drugs that increase serotonin availability by different mechanisms. Drug combinations that have been reported to cause the serotonin syndrome have been reviewed and the pathophysiology of the syndrome discussed (45). It is probably mediated by stimulation of 5-HT_2 receptors. In most reported cases the drug combination associated with the syndrome included a MAO inhibitor (see Table 2). The syndrome is rare, although it has been reported more often during the past few years, and is often due to a combination of a MAO inhibitor and a selective serotonin re-uptake inhibitor. In most cases the symptoms are mild and resolve rapidly after drug withdrawal and supportive therapy. It must, however, be borne in mind that this syndrome can be fatal, and if combinations of serotonergic drugs are used they should be used with great caution.

(2) A second factor that can improve the use of these drugs is adequate patient education. Patients must be aware of the name and nature of the drug they are taking and its potential to interact with proscribed foods and prescribed or over-the-counter medications. In addition, patients should understand what symptoms to expect when an interaction occurs, such as unexpected drowsiness (after alcohol or other drugs) or a sudden severe headache (within 2 hours of a meal or medication). Because of the many variables involved, foods or medications that are taken with impunity on one occasion can interact dangerously on another. The director of a British counselling service has reported that of 119 patients taking MAO inhibitors who experienced problems, 35 reported hypertensive crises, 4 fatal (48). Despite warnings, these patients had eaten amine-containing foodstuffs or taken over-the-counter cold remedies. MAO inhibitors should not be prescribed unless the patient is able to understand such instructions and repeat them after explanation; compliance can be confirmed at subsequent inquiry. Those who take multiple medications, who have difficulty with comprehension or compliance (such as the elderly), or who are frightened by such explanations should not be given these drugs.

 The management of a patient who experiences these drug interactions depends on their nature. For symptoms due to exacerbation or prolongation of drug effects, specific or supportive measures (cardiovascular or respiratory) may be indicated. In the case of a hypertensive crisis, symptoms usually abate within 1–2 hours, as the blood pressure falls. If hypertension is seen early, or if it persists or recurs, it can be treated with parenteral phentolamine or chlorpromazine, but the danger of causing hypotension should be weighed carefully.

 The combination of central nervous system stimulants with MAO inhibitors in treatment-resistant depressed patients has been reported (49). However, this use should be restricted to patients in whom there is careful monitoring by specialists, because of the potential for hypertensive crisis.

Buspirone

The combination of buspirone with a MAO inhibitor can cause the serotonin syndrome (50).

Etamivan

Etamivan is contraindicated in patients taking MAO inhibitors (51).

Fenfluramine

Fenfluramine can produce an acute confusional state if it is given together with a MAO inhibitor (SED-9, 9).

Fluoxetine

The problem of the long half-life of fluoxetine, which leads to interactions with MAO inhibitors, even after withdrawal, has been discussed previously (SEDA-13, 12), and caused the manufacturer to circulate a warning to that effect.

Ginseng

Interactions of antidepressants with herbal medicines have been reported (52). Herbal medicines are widely used for their psychotropic properties and patients sometimes take herbal formulations in addition to conventional psychotropic drugs, such as antidepressants. Ginseng has been reported to cause mania, tremor, and headache in combination with conventional MAO inhibitors.

Isoniazid

Isoniazid inhibits MAO, and during isoniazid treatment the ingestion of several kinds of cheese can cause flushing, palpitation, tachycardia, and increased blood pressure (53). Similar symptoms occur with isoniazid after the ingestion of skipjack fish (*Thunnidae*) (53). The symptoms, notably headache, palpitation, erythema, redness of the eyes, itching, diarrhea, and wheezing, are thought to be caused mainly by the high histamine content of this fish. The undesirable effects that occur when MAO inhibitors are taken together with isoniazid resemble the symptoms seen after the simultaneous ingestion of these foods.

Lithium

Interactions of lithium with antidepressants have been reviewed: tricyclic antidepressants and MAO inhibitors—no serious problems; SSRIs—a few reports of the serotonin syndrome (54).

Nefazodone

Co-administration of nefazodone with a MAO inhibitor or SSRI can cause the serotonin syndrome (55).

Neuroleptic drugs

Additive hypotensive effects can occur when a MAO inhibitor is combined with an antipsychotic drug (56). However, the combination can be beneficial in treating the negative symptoms of schizophrenia (57).

Opioids

The interactions of MAO inhibitors with opioids, which can lead to sudden and fatal reactions, have been reviewed (SEDA-18, 14).

Dextromethorphan is metabolized by CYP2D6 to dextrorphan, which binds to phencyclidine receptors and is thought to account for the toxic effects of hallucinations, tachycardia, hypertension, ataxia, and nystagmus. Individuals who are slow metabolizers, those who take long-acting dextromethorphan formulations, and those who take serotonin re-uptake inhibitors or MAO inhibitors are at increased risk of adverse effects.

Phenylephrine

Patients taking medications with pressor effects, such as MAO inhibitors, tricyclic antidepressants, and anticholinergic agents, should be monitored closely if phenylephrine is used (SEDA-16, 542).

Sumatriptan

On theoretical grounds sumatriptan should not be used with a MAO inhibitor (58).

Trazodone

Trazodone is related to nefazodone but probably potentiates 5-HT neurotransmission less. Trazodone is often added to MAO inhibitors and SSRIs at low doses (50–150 mg/day) as a hypnotic, but such combinations can rarely provoke the serotonin syndrome.

- The serotonin syndrome occurred in a 60-year-old woman when the addition of trazodone 50 mg/day to nefazodone 500 mg/day caused confusion, restlessness, sweating, and nausea after the third day of treatment (59). The symptoms settled quickly on withdrawal of both antidepressants.

References

1. Youdim MBH, Finberg JPM. Monoamine oxidase inhibitor antidepressants. In: Grahame-Smith DG, Cohen PJ, editors. Preclinical Psychopharmacology. Amsterdam: Excerpta Medica, 1983:38.
2. Lader M. Psychiatric disorders. In: Speight T, Holford N, editors. Avery's Drug Treatment. 4th ed. Auckland: ADIS Internation Press, 1997:1437.
3. Menkes DB. Antidepressant drugs. New Ethicals 1994;31:101.
4. Murphy DL, Sunderland T, Cohen RM. Monoamine oxidase-inhibiting antidepressants. A clinical update. Psychiatr Clin North Am 1984;7(3):549–62.
5. Paykel ES, Parker RR, Penrose RJ, Rassaby ER. Depressive classification and prediction of response to phenelzine. Br J Psychiatry 1979;134:572–81.
6. Liebowitz MR, Quitkin FM, Stewart JW, McGrath PJ, Harrison W, Rabkin J, Tricamo E, Markowitz JS, Klein DF. Phenelzine vs imipramine in atypical depression. A preliminary report. Arch Gen Psychiatry 1984;41(7):669–77.
7. White K, Simpson G. Should the use of MAO inhibitors be abandoned? Integrat Psychiatry 1985;3:34.
8. Rose S. The relationship of acetylation phenotype to treatment with MAOIs: a review. J Clin Psychopharmacol 1982;2(3):161–4.
9. Rabkin J, Quitkin F, Harrison W, Tricamo E, McGrath P. Adverse reactions to monoamine oxidase inhibitors. Part I. A comparative study. J Clin Psychopharmacol 1984;4(5):270–8.
10. Rabkin JG, Quitkin FM, McGrath P, Harrison W, Tricamo E. Adverse reactions to monoamine oxidase inhibitors. Part II. Treatment correlates and clinical management. J Clin Psychopharmacol 1985;5(1):2–9.
11. Razani J, White KL, White J, Simpson G, Sloane RB, Rebal R, Palmer R. The safety and efficacy of combined amitriptyline and tranylcypromine antidepressant treatment. A controlled trial. Arch Gen Psychiatry 1983;40(6):657–61.
12. Kronig MH, Roose SP, Walsh BT, Woodring S, Glassman AH. Blood pressure effects of phenelzine. J Clin Psychopharmacol 1983;3(5):307–10.
13. Linet LS. Mysterious MAOI hypertensive episodes. J Clin Psychiatry 1986;47(11):563–5.
14. Blackwell B. Clinical and pharmacological observations of the interactions of monoamine oxidase inhibitors, amines and foodstuffs. Cambridge University: MD Thesis, 1966.
15. Evans DL, Davidson J, Raft D. Early and late side effects of phenelzine. J Clin Psychopharmacol 1982;2(3):208–10.
16. Reiderer P, Reynolds GP. Deprenyl is a selective inhibitor of brain MAO-B in the long-term treatment of Parkinsons's disease. Br J Clin Pharmacol 1980;9(1):98–9.

Morphine

See also Opioid analgesics

General Information

Morphine and its two glucuronides may have neuroexcitatory effects and affinity for non-opioid receptors (glycine and/or *N*-methyl-D-aspartate), effects that will not be antagonized by naloxone. Furthermore, these other opioid effects may be related to the mechanism of some adverse effects, including hyperalgesia, allodynia, and myoclonus, which are increasingly being reported after high doses of morphine, but which do not seem to occur after methadone, fentanyl, sufentanil, or ketobemidone (1).

Morphine is the benchmark "step 3" opioid analgesic based on the WHO's concept of an analgesic ladder (2). Revised recommendations for the use of morphine in cancer pain have been published by the European Association for Palliative Care's Expert Working Group on Opioid Analgesics (3). In summary, oral morphine is still the opioid of first choice for moderate to severe cancer pain, every 4 hours for normal-release morphine and 12- or 24-hourly for modified-release morphine. If patients are not able to take morphine orally the preferred alternative is subcutaneous infusion, especially in patients who require continuous parenteral morphine. A small proportion of patients develop intolerable adverse effects with oral morphine, and a change to an alternative opioid (for example hydromorphone, oxycodone, methadone, transdermal fentanyl) or a change in the rate of administration should be considered. If despite optimal use of systemic opioids and non-opioids a patient still has intolerable adverse effects or inadequate analgesia, spinal (epidural or intrathecal) administration of an opioid analgesic in combination with a local anesthetic or clonidine should be considered.

In a randomized, double-blind study in 94 patients with acute renal colic, morphine had equal analgesic efficacy to pethidine and a similar adverse effects profile (4).

Managing the adverse effects of morphine

The strategies used in managing the adverse effects of oral morphine have been reassessed in another special article compiled by the Expert Working Group of the European Association of Palliative Care Network (5). Factors that predict opioid adverse effects include:

(1) *Drug-related factors* There is little evidence suggesting that any one opioid agonist has a substantially better adverse effects profile than any other.
(2) *Route-related factors* There is limited evidence to suggest differences in adverse effects associated with specific routes of systemic administration.
(3) *Patient-related factors* There is evidence to suggest that there is interindividual variability in sensitivity to opioid-related adverse effects; the variables include genetic susceptibility, the presence of co-morbidity, and age.
(4) *Dose-related factors* A dose-response relation is most evident with the CNS adverse effects of sedation, cognitive impairment, hallucinations, myoclonus, and respiratory depression, although there is still interindividual variability in dose responsiveness to these effects; nausea and vomiting are common at the start of therapy but are then unpredictable.
(5) *Starting doses and escalation* The adverse effects of morphine, especially cognitive impairment, occur transiently and abate spontaneously; there are no reports of a relation between the starting dose of morphine or dose escalation and the occurrence of nausea, vomiting, or delirium.
(6) *Drug interactions* Adverse effects of concurrent medications may be synergistic or cumulative with those associated with opioids.

The reviewers also stressed the importance of differentiating opioid-related adverse effects from other causes of co-morbidity that might mimic opioid-induced adverse effects. Examples include cerebral metastases, stroke, metabolic changes, septicemia, bowel obstruction, and iatrogenic factors (other drugs or radiotherapy).

Four different approaches to the management of opioid adverse effects were described in the review:

(1) *Dosage reduction* A reduction in the dosage of the systemic opioid is usually enough to relieve adverse effects. If dosage reduction is accompanied by loss of pain control, a non-opioid analgesic (for example an NSAID) can be added. Specific therapy, such as radiotherapy, chemotherapy, or surgery, that targets the cause of the pain can be helpful, as can a regional anesthetic or neuroablative intervention (for example celiac plexus blockade in patients with pancreatic cancer).
(2) *Symptomatic management of the adverse effects.*
(3) *Opioid rotation.*
(4) *Switching the route of administration.*

The reviewers also examined the symptomatic management of specific adverse effects and commented that most approaches are based on cumulative anecdotal evidence and that there have been few prospective evaluations of the efficacy and toxicity of these approaches over a long period of use. Polypharmacy adds to the burden of adverse effects and drug interactions.

Nausea and vomiting

The authors of two related double-blind, randomized, placebo-controlled studies of the use of dexamethasone prophylaxis for nausea and vomiting after epidural morphine for postcesarean or posthysterectomy analgesia concluded that 5 mg of dexamethasone is an effective dose (6,7). Meanwhile, ADL 8-2698, a trans-3-4-dimethyl-4 piperidine that is a novel opioid antagonist, produced improved gastrointestinal transit time (peripherally mediated opioid activity) without affecting centrally mediated opioid analgesia (8). This contrasts with naloxone or nalmefene, which tend to antagonize central opioid effects, resulting in withdrawal symptoms in up to 50% of patients when used to treat constipation.

Intravenous droperidol 1.25 mg and intravenous dexamethasone 8 mg, given at the end of cesarean section, have been compared in reducing the incidence of nausea and vomiting caused by epidural morphine 3 mg in 120 women in a randomized, double-blind, placebo-controlled study (9). The incidence of nausea and vomiting was 18% with dexamethasone, 21% with droperidol, and 51% with saline. About 11–13% of the women who were given dexamethasone or droperidol required rescue antiemetic therapy compared with 41% in the saline group. The incidence of pruritus was similar among the three groups (26–42%). Six women (16%) given droperidol reported restlessness compared with none in the other two groups.

Pruritus

The effectiveness of intravenous ondansetron in preventing intrathecal morphine-induced pruritus has been investigated in a randomized, double-blind, placebo-controlled study in 60 consecutive women undergoing cesarean section (10). All were given spinal anesthesia with bupivacaine and intrathecal morphine 0.15 mg and then randomly divided into three groups. Group 1 received intravenous saline injections as placebo, group 2 received diphenhydramine 30 mg intravenously, and group 3 received ondansetron 0.1 mg/kg intravenously. Group 3 had a significantly lower incidence of pruritus (25%) than both group 1 (85%) and group 2 (80%), with no difference in postoperative pain scores between the groups.

In another randomized, double-blind study, 140 patients undergoing cesarean section had anesthesia with epidural bupivacaine 100 mg and adrenaline to which was added morphine 2 mg and droperidol 0, 1.25, 2.5, or 5.0 mg (11). Previous evidence had suggested that intravenous droperidol reduces morphine-induced pruritus, but that the effect disappeared when the dose was increased from 2.5 mg to 5.0 mg (12). However, in this study, epidural droperidol caused a dose-dependent reduction in morphine-induced pruritus even at a dose of 5 mg.

Myoclonus

Gabapentin has been used to treat morphine-induced myoclonus in a 54-year-old patient with gallbladder cancer (13). Effective pain control was maintained with morphine 300 mg, but after 24 hours the patient developed generalized muscular movements while asleep. Gabapentin 300 mg bd produced complete resolution of symptoms after 12 hours. In another case gabapentin 600 mg/day was used to treat a 1-month history of spontaneous jerking of both wrists after an increase in the dose of morphine to 120 mg/day; the myoclonus disappeared over the next 24 hours (8,13).

Organs and Systems

Cardiovascular

Adverse cardiac effects due to morphine are rare. They comprise inappropriate heart rate responses to hypotension, rather than conduction defects. They are not especially associated with inferior myocardial infarction, as was previously thought (SED-11, 142) (14).

Respiratory

Non-cardiogenic pulmonary edema occurred in three cancer patients, all of whom had received rapidly escalating doses of morphine over a short period (15).

Nervous system

A patient with Guillain–Barré syndrome experienced shock with morphine sulfate (16).

- A 69-year-old woman developed interscapular pain after a mild respiratory infection. Non-opioid analgesics were ineffective, so she was given modified-release morphine 10 mg. On day 4 she had rapidly progressive weakness in her legs and on day 5 she was found unconscious with no detectable blood pressure. She recovered with naloxone 0.8 intravenously. Her paralysis persisted. Nerve conduction studies confirmed slowed neurotransmission. Further investigation excluded other potential causes and Guillain–Barré syndrome was diagnosed.

The episode of unconsciousness was attributed to opioid toxicity in a patient in whom autonomic dysfunction may already have been present. It was suggested that opioid analgesics should be used with caution in patients with Guillain–Barré syndrome, because of the risk of hypotension consequent on autonomic dysfunction.

High doses of chronic morphine can cause hyperalgesia or allodynia (pain caused by a stimulus that does not normally provoke pain) (17).

- A 9-month-old girl with an inoperable and partially resected astrocytoma of the hypothalamus had morphine-induced allodynia, and became extremely distressed during routine care, such as nappy changing, feeding, and washing. The allodynia resolved after the dosage of morphine was reduced from 6950 μg/kg/hour to 280 μg/kg/hour.

Intravenous patient-controlled administration of morphine (total 56 mg in 9 hours) was associated with downbeat nystagmus in a 61-year-old man with a Grade 3 adenocarcinoma of the gastro-esophageal junction and a previous small cerebellar infarct (18). Withdrawal of the analgesia led to complete resolution of all signs and symptoms within 12 hours.

Psychological, psychiatric

Hallucinations have been described after the use of morphine in various dosage forms; in one series, patients experienced adequate pain relief and no further hallucinations or nightmares when changed to oxycodone (19). Delusions and hallucinations have been reported in a patient who was also taking dosulepin (20). Restlessness, vomiting, and disorientation were described in two male patients over 60 years of age taking modified-release morphine for relief of pain in advanced cancer (21).

Endocrine

Morphine can cause prolactin release (22); this effect is not antagonized by naloxone.

Mouth and teeth

There is a clear association between the administration of morphine and dry mouth (23).

Gastrointestinal

Nausea and vomiting are frequent adverse effects associated with the use of PCA opioids. Droperidol and tropisetron may reduce the incidence and severity of nausea and vomiting caused by morphine (SEDA-19, 84).

Morphine reduces the rate of transient lower esophageal sphincter relaxation in patients with reflux disease, thus reducing the number of reflux episodes; the effect was reversed by naloxone (SEDA-22, 12).

Biliary tract

Morphine can cause choledochal sphincter spasm, especially if there is a previous history of cholecystectomy (24).

- A 60-year-old man received intramuscular morphine 10 mg with scopolamine 0.4 mg as premedication and 40 minutes later complained of sharp right upper quadrant pain radiating to the back. The symptoms were identical to the gallbladder pain he had experienced in the past and for which he had had a cholecystectomy 25 years before. He had complete relief from intravenous naloxone 0.9 mg.

Skin

A purpuric rash has been reported in a patient taking morphine (25).

Death

- A 14-year-old boy with infectious mononucleosis was given intravenous morphine 10 mg for pain relief with good effect, but 2 hours later was found unresponsive, lying on his back, and not breathing (26). An autopsy showed marked bilateral tonsillar enlargement with considerable narrowing of the upper airway. The blood morphine concentration was 0.08 μg/ml.

The coroner concluded that the morphine had contributed to respiratory compromise and death.

Long-Term Effects

Drug withdrawal

Acute opioid withdrawal syndrome apparently precipitated by naloxone following epidural morphine has been reported (27).

- A 28-year-old nulliparous woman with no history of opioid exposure underwent elective cesarean section with epidural anesthesia. On delivery she received morphine 2 mg epidurally. At 8 hours after delivery she complained of pruritus and received naloxone 0.14 mg intravenously in fractional doses. After 2 minutes she felt warm in her legs, trunk, and face. Pruritus resolved and analgesia was maintained. After 5 minutes she began to shiver in a waxing and waning pattern every 2 minutes. She was restless and agitated and had tachypnea, lacrimation, and rhinorrhea. Her symptoms resolved in 40 minutes.

Previous reports of opioid withdrawal on single exposure have been described after the administration of intramuscular morphine in healthy individuals. This case suggests that opioid dependence can occur after acute exposure to morphine by the epidural route too. An alternative explanation (28) is that the stress of labor may have led to increased endogenous opioid activity, particularly B-endorphin, and that the antagonistic effect of naloxone on the endogenous opioid system contributed to the clinical effects in this patient. Moreover, the authors pointed out that many symptoms characteristic of the classic opioid withdrawal syndrome were not present in the patient.

Second-Generation Effects

Pregnancy

In a double-blind, randomized, controlled study of analgesia in labor, the addition of morphine 150 μg to an intrathecal combination of fentanyl (25 μg) and bupivacaine (2.5 mg) significantly prolonged analgesia to more than 4 hours without increasing opioid-related adverse effects (29).

Susceptibility Factors

Genetic factors

Accumulation of morphine-6-glucuronide is a risk factor for opioid toxicity during morphine treatment. However, it does not occur in all patients with renal insufficiency, which is the most common reason for accumulation of morphine-6-glucuronide; this suggests that other risk factors can contribute to morphine-6-glucuronide toxicity.

- Two men, aged 87 and 65 years, both with renal insufficiency, took oral morphine 30 mg/day for pain management (30). While the 65-year-old tolerated morphine well despite a high plasma morphine-6-glucuronide concentration of 1735 nmol/l, the 87-year-old had severe sleepiness and drowsiness, even though the plasma morphine-6-glucuronide concentration was only 941 nmol/l.

The patients were screened for genetic polymorphisms in the OPRM1-gene (coding for μ opioid receptors), P glycoprotein, and other candidate genes that code for transporters that may play an important role in determining the central nervous system concentration of morphine or morphine-6-glucuronide. The 65-year-old patient was a homozygous carrier of the mutated G118 allele of the μ opioid receptor gene, which has previously been related to reduced glucuromorphine potency (a protector gene). In contrast, the 87-year-old patient was a homozygous carrier of the wild-type allele A118. This observation implies that a single nucleotide polymorphism, the G118 allele, has a protective effect against morphine-6-glucuronide toxicity.

Age

Children

Of 44 children undergoing major genitourinary or lower abdominal surgery in a randomized, single-blind study, 24 were given morphine 0.1 mg/kg epidurally and 20 were given the same dose intravenously immediately after intubation (31). Postoperatively PCA boluses were administered to both groups. Both techniques provided sufficient pain relief. Of the children given epidural morphine, one required treatment for pruritus and seven vomited more than once, compared to none in those given intravenous morphine.

A study of PCA in children suggested that the pharmacokinetics of morphine are similar to those in adults, with the exception of young infants (32).

Neonates with reduced capacity for glucuronidation may have reduced efficacy of morphine, because of reduced renal excretion of morphine-6-glucuronide.

In a 7-year, retrospective, multicenter, observational study, 95 children aged 1–19 years with cancer pain and treated with long-acting morphine were investigated for adverse effects and age-dependent analgesic effects (33). The adverse effects most frequently reported were constipation (10 patients at the beginning of treatment, 20 patients during the course of therapy, and 3 patients at the end of data collection), followed by vomiting (five, eight, and two patients), and nausea (two, six, and three patients), especially in children aged 7 years or more. Some of the children repeatedly complained of pruritus (five, eleven, and two patients). There were no cases of respiratory depression. Oral long-acting morphine proved to be safe and effective, even in very young patients with a history of malignancy.

There have been another two studies of the analgesic effect of intrathecal morphine in children (34,35). In a prospective, double-blind study, 30 children (aged 9–19 years) scheduled for spinal fusion were randomly allocated to a single dose of saline or intrathecal morphine 2 or 5 μg/kg; after surgery, a PCA device provided access to additional intravenous morphine (34). The doses of 2 and 5 μg/kg had similar analgesic effectiveness and adverse effects profiles (nausea, vomiting, pruritus). There were no episodes of severe respiratory depression. Low-dose intrathecal morphine supplemented with PCA morphine provides better analgesia than PCA morphine alone.

In a smaller prospective, open, uncontrolled study, 12 children (3–6 years of age) were given either intermittent intrathecal morphine 5 μg/kg qds or a continuous infusion of a mixture of bupivacaine (40 μg/kg/hour) and morphine (0.6 μg/kg/hour) for intense postoperative pain after selective dorsal rhizotomy (35). The bupivacaine/morphine mixture provided better analgesia with fewer adverse effects. The incidence of pruritus was 83% with morphine compared with 33% with bupivacaine/morphine. Otherwise the adverse effects were similar.

Elderly people

Morphine, as an intravenous bolus of 2 or 3 mg every 5 minutes until pain relief or adverse effects occurred, was given to 875 patients who were under 70 years old and 175 patients who were over 70 years old in a prospective, uncontrolled, non-blinded study (36). The total dose of morphine was not significantly different between the groups. There was no significant difference in the incidence of morphine-related adverse effects, the number of sedated patients, and the number of patients in whom dose titration had to be stopped. The results only applied to the immediate and short-term postoperative periods and the patients studied had a variety of surgical procedures unrelated to age. The results suggested that intravenous morphine can be safely given to elderly patients using the same protocol that is used in younger ones. The generalizability of this study is limited because the sample size was small.

Renal disease

There was a higher incidence of adverse effects of morphine in patients with renal insufficiency who receive opioids for some time (37), and in patients with hemolytic uremic syndrome who were given ketamine with subcutaneous morphine postoperatively (38).

Patients with renal insufficiency may experience a stronger and more prolonged effect, because of reduced renal excretion of morphine-6-glucuronide.

Hepatic disease

Morphine is extensively metabolized. Its main metabolite, morphine-3-glucuronide is without analgesic effects, while morphine-6-glucuronide (also called morphine glucuronide) is supposed to be more potent than morphine. In patients with cirrhosis, morphine clearance may be reduced and the half-life prolonged, and dosages should be reduced (SEDA 22, 101).

Other features of the patient

Myoclonus is more likely in patients taking psychotropic or non-steroidal anti-inflammatory drugs as adjunct analgesia (39).

Drug Administration

Drug additives

Low-dose intrathecal morphine (0.3 mg) plus 0.5% spinal bupivacaine and patient-controlled intravenous morphine (given as a 1 mg bolus with a 5-minute lockout period) has been compared with patient-controlled intravenous morphine alone in 38 patients undergoing knee surgery in a randomized, double-blind study (40). The former combination provided effective analgesia with a low and non-significant incidence of emesis, pruritus, and respiratory depression.

Drug dosage regimens

Oral morphine is more effective after repeated rather than single doses. This is probably due to penetration into the central nervous system of morphine-6-glucuronide, the active metabolite (41).

In a dose-response study of the effects of epidural morphine after cesarean section the quality of analgesia increased with the dose of morphine to a ceiling dose of 3.75 mg (42). Adverse effects were not dose-related.

recipients who received muromonab prophylaxis, intragraft thromboses were found in 13 (5.6%), and the use of very high-dose methylprednisolone (30 mg/kg) was suggested to be a major risk factor (22). In contrast, and despite the evidence of procoagulant activity, some investigators have failed to identify evidence that muromonab increases the risk of thromboembolic complications (20,23).

Respiratory

Dyspnea and pulmonary edema sometimes develop during the cytokine-release syndrome. Pulmonary toxicity was mostly observed in patients who had fluid retention and weight gain before receiving muromonab. The incidence has been markedly reduced by the formulation of guidelines for management (3). Cytokine release and complement activation with further neutrophil activation and pulmonary vascular endothelium damage were suggested to be involved (24).

Nervous system

Self-limiting and benign central nervous system manifestations mimicking those of aseptic meningitis, that is fever, headache, nuchal rigidity, cognitive disorders, and photophobia, were observed in 3–10% of patients who received muromonab (3). The symptoms were usually delayed for 2–3 days and resolved spontaneously despite continuation of treatment. More severe neurological disorders requiring withdrawal have been observed in up to 7% of patients (25). The various reported symptoms consisted of slowly reversible diffuse encephalopathy with mental changes, neurosensory hallucinations, tinnitus with reversible hearing loss, transient hemiparesis, cerebral infarction, generalized or focal seizures, cortical blindness, psychotic symptoms, obtundation, and coma (SED-13, 1132) (SEDA-21, 380) (25). Diabetes and severely impaired renal function were possibly significant risk factors (SEDA-19, 353) (SEDA-21, 380). Neurotoxic symptoms were supposedly mediated by cytokine release and potentiated by uremic toxins. Raised concentrations of tumor necrosis factor alfa in the cerebrospinal fluid were suggested to play a major role in muromonab-induced aseptic meningitis and encephalopathy (26).

Muromonab-induced aseptic meningitis is relatively common and is usually benign, with prompt recovery despite continuation of treatment.

- In a 28-year-old man the clinical features of aseptic meningitis were prolonged over 1 month after the administration of muromonab, and persistent severe headaches resolved only after several aspirations of cerebrospinal fluid (27).

This case was described as a syndrome of headache with neurological deficits and CSF lymphocytosis (HaNDL syndrome).

Sensory systems

Eyes

Spontaneously reversible mild conjunctivitis and episcleritis have been noted in 75 and 10% of patients respectively.

Diffuse anterior scleritis responding to an increased dosage of prednisone was mentioned in one patient (28).

Isolated visual loss (persistent in one patient) shortly after muromonab administration is rare (SEDA-20, 340) (29).

Ears

Ototoxicity from muromonab has been described, but the incidence is unknown (SEDA-21, 380). Audiograms performed before and 48–72 hours after administration of muromonab showed sensorineural hearing loss of at least 15 db in five of seven renal transplant patients (30). A third audiogram 2 weeks after muromonab treatment showed amelioration or complete recovery in all four of the patients who were tested.

Hematologic

Acute thrombocytopenia has been reported in one patient (SEDA-21, 380).

Liver

Hepatitis has been attributed to cytokine release from muromonab (31).

- A 31-year-old man underwent renal transplantation for end-stage renal disease secondary to hypertension. He was given basiliximab for induction immunosuppression. At 13 months after transplantation he had evidence of transplant rejection. His creatinine concentration rose acutely from 83 to 165 μmol/l over 1 week. This was his first rejection episode (Banff IIa). There was no evidence of viral infection. He received muromonab with conventional prophylaxis (antihistamines, paracetamol, and corticosteroids) to reduce the severity of cytokine release. This was his first exposure to muromonab. Initially he complained of fever and nausea, and the following day he was somnolent and had right upper quadrant tenderness. Liver function tests, which had been normal on the day of admission, were abnormal. Hepatitis serology showed positive hepatitis B core antibody (IgM and IgG), positive hepatitis A antibody, negative hepatitis surface antigen, and negative hepatitis C antibody. The hepatitis B core antibody (IgM and IgG) had been positive before transplantation 16 months before. Muromonab was withdrawn and he showed signs of clinical and chemical improvement. Rejection was successfully treated with glucocorticoids and antithymocyte globulin.

Urinary tract

Spontaneously reversible increases in serum creatinine concentrations occurred in 8–18% of muromonab-treated patients, and were thought to have resulted from inhibition of renal prostaglandin synthesis and release of cytokines (32,33). There were no adverse consequences on short-term graft survival or graft function (32).

Isolated cases of hemolytic-uremic syndrome have been reported (SED-13, 1133) (SEDA-21, 380).

Immunologic

An antibody response to muromonab has been detected in 40% of patients undergoing a 14-day induction regimen of muromonab 5 mg/day (10). It has been suggested that the incidence of antimuromonab antibodies depended on the immunosuppressive regimen, but this was based on a retrospective study in a limited number of patients (SEDA-22, 409). Furthermore, sensitization was not relevant in most patients. Only raised IgG anti-idiotypic antibodies in high enough titers (over 1:1000) significantly neutralize the binding of muromonab to the CD3 receptor and reduce clinical efficacy, thus precluding further muromonab administration.

Antimuromonab IgE antibodies have been identified after 10–25 days of treatment in six of 181 patients, and only in those with high titers of antimuromonab IgG antibodies (34). Immediate IgE-mediated anaphylactic reactions, namely anaphylactic shock, bronchospasm, urticaria, have been rarely reported and have sometimes been difficult to differentiate from the cytokine-release syndrome (35,36). Late-onset reactions after the first week of treatment, including cutaneous erythema, a fall in blood pressure, or serum sickness-like reactions, are infrequent (37).

Rare anaphylactic reactions with antimuromonab IgE antibodies have been reported (SED-14, 1309). Anaphylactoid reactions to muromonab can also occur (38).

- A 15-year-old girl underwent uneventful renal transplantation. On the third postoperative day she received her first dose of muromonab for a presumptive diagnosis of graft rejection. Despite premedication with diphenhydramine, paracetamol, and high-dose methylprednisolone, within 20 seconds after intravenous muromonab, she developed shortness of breath, digital paresthesia, facial edema, laryngeal stridor, reduced oxygen saturation, and a fall in blood pressure. She recovered after intubation and appropriate vasopressor administration, but required transplant nephrectomy for hemorrhagic and coagulative necrosis of the transplanted kidney.

This acute reaction was supposedly mediated by nonimmunologic mast cell degranulation, as screening for IgE antimuromonab antibodies was negative.

As with other potent immunosuppressive drugs, muromonab has been suspected to increase the risk of infections. Multiple possible biases in studies of the incidence of muromonab-associated infections have been discussed (3); there were no differences among patients who received muromonab compared with those who received other immunosuppressive regimens. Since then, several other investigators have reported their findings, indicating that this debate continues.

In patients with renal transplants, the overall incidence of infections during the first three posttransplantation months was significantly higher in one trial of patients treated with prophylactic muromonab or ciclosporin (39), but there was no significant difference in the severity of infections in another similar trial (40). Both studies failed to identify any adverse impact of infectious episodes on patient survival. In a comparison of prophylactic ATG-Fresenius with muromonab there were more common minor infections (for example, cutaneous mycosis, *Herpes simplex* virus infections) in the muromonab arm, but a similar incidence of life-threatening or severe infections (41). In contrast to these findings, a large retrospective study showed a significantly higher incidence of infection-related deaths among patients who received muromonab for induction therapy compared with those who did not receive muromonab (42). However, renal graft survival was significantly improved in patients treated with muromonab, and there were no subsequent viral deaths after the routine use of appropriate anti-infectious prophylaxis.

In patient with liver transplants (43,44) or heart transplants (45), retrospective studies have shown that muromonab treatment is an additional or independent risk factor for symptomatic cytomegalovirus infections in cytomegalovirus-seropositive patients or in recipients of cytomegalovirus-seropositive donors, suggesting that cytomegalovirus prophylaxis should be implemented in these patients. It has also been suggested that early muromonab administration in the posttransplant period increases the likelihood of invasive cytomegalovirus disease after liver transplantation (46). In contrast, other investigators failed to show an increased incidence of cytomegalovirus infections after muromonab versus triple drug therapy in heart transplant patients (47). Based on a retrospective study of 154 liver transplant patients, muromonab was suggested as a risk factor for *Pneumocystis jiroveci* pneumonia (48).

These results suggest that the incidence and severity of infections is more likely to be related to the degree of immunosuppression than to the effect of an individual drug.

Long-Term Effects

Tumorigenicity

As expected from its pronounced immunosuppressive activity, muromonab is a significant risk factor for secondary neoplasia, especially when high doses, increased treatment duration, sequential courses, or early retreatment are used (49). Whether the increased risk of neoplasia after muromonab-based immunosuppression is due to the drug itself or reflects the overall degree of immunosuppression is a matter of debate, and conflicting results have emerged. Several retrospective or controlled studies did not show more frequent malignancies after muromonab compared with other immunosuppressive regimens (50–52). On the other hand, the rate of non-Hodgkin's lymphomas was higher in kidney and heart transplant recipients who received muromonab prophylaxis rather than antithymocyte/antilymphocyte globulin (53). Using data from the manufacturers and the literature, the rate of malignancies after muromonab was estimated to be 0.57% (54), but potential under-reporting strongly limited the validity of this estimation. Although the roles of high cumulative doses or repeated courses as risk factors are not definitely proven, it is usually recommended not to exceed 14 days of treatment with cumulative doses of 70 mg (3).

An analysis of the Australia and New Zealand Dialysis and Transplant Registry (7953 patients with 9460 renal transplants) has confirmed that immunosuppression with polyclonal and monoclonal muromonab antibodies independently increases the risk of virus-mediated cancer (55). The increased risk was about 60% for non-Hodgkin's lymphoma and 75% for non-Hodgkin's lymphoma plus, in women, carcinoma of the cervix, vagina, and vulva.

References

1. Wilde MI, Goa KL. Muromonab CD3: a reappraisal of its pharmacology and use as prophylaxis of solid organ transplant rejection. Drugs 1996;51(5):865–94.
2. Abramowicz D, Norman DJ, Goldman M, De Pauw L, Kinnaert P, Kahana L, Thistlethwaite JR, Shield CF, Monaco AP, Vanherweghem JL, et al. OKT3 prophylaxis improves long-term renal graft survival in high-risk patients as compared to cyclosporine: combined results from the prospective, randomized Belgian and US studies. Transplant Proc 1995;27(1):852–3.
3. Kreis H. Adverse events associated with OKT3 immunosuppression in the prevention or treatment of allograft rejection. Clin Transplant 1993;7:431–46.
4. Jeyarajah DR, Thistlethwaite JR Jr. General aspects of cytokine-release syndrome: timing and incidence of symptoms. Transplant Proc 1993;25(2 Suppl 1):16–20.
5. Brown M, Korb S, Light JA, Light T, Jonsson J, Aquino A. Low-dose OKT3 induction therapy following renal transplantation leads to improved graft function and decreased adverse effects. Transplant Proc 1993;25(1 Pt 1):553–5.
6. Norman DJ, Kimball JA, Bennett WM, Shihab F, Batiuk TD, Meyer MM, Barry JM. A prospective, double-blind, randomized study of high-versus low-dose OKT3 induction immunosuppression in cadaveric renal transplantation. Transpl Int 1994;7(5):356–61.
7. Parlevliet KJ, Bemelman FJ, Yong SL, Hack CE, Surachno J, Wilmink JM, ten Berge IJ, Schellekens PT. Toxicity of OKT3 increases with dosage: a controlled study in renal transplant recipients. Transpl Int 1995;8(2):141–6.
8. Vasquez EM, Fabrega AJ, Pollak R. OKT3-induced cytokine-release syndrome: occurrence beyond the second dose and association with rejection severity. Transplant Proc 1995;27(1):873–4.
9. Buysmann S, Hack CE, van Diepen FN, Surachno J, ten Berge IJ. Administration of OKT3 as a two-hour infusion attenuates first-dose side effects. Transplantation 1997;64(11):1620–3.
10. Norman DJ, Chatenoud L, Cohen D, Goldman M, Shield CF 3rd. Consensus statement regarding OKT3-induced cytokine-release syndrome and human antimouse antibodies. Transplant Proc 1993;25(2 Suppl 1):89–92.
11. Bemelman FJ, Buysmann S, Wilmink JM, Surachno S, Hack CE, Schellekens PT, ten Berge RJ. Effects of divided doses of steroids on side effects, cytokines, and activation of complement and granulocytes, coagulation and fibrinolysis after OKT3. Transplant Proc 1994;26(6):3096–7.
12. Abramowicz D, De Pauw L, Le Moine A, Sermon F, Surquin M, Doutrelepont JM, Ickx B, Depierreux M, Vanherweghem JL, Kinnaert P, Goldman M, Vereerstraeten P. Prevention of OKT3 nephrotoxicity after kidney transplantation. Kidney Int Suppl 1996;53:S39–43.
13. Gaughan WJ, Francos BB, Dunn SR, Francos GC, Burke JF. A retrospective analysis of the effect of indomethacin on adverse reactions to orthoclone OKT3 in the therapy of acute renal allograft rejection. Am J Kidney Dis 1994;24(3):486–90.
14. Vincenti F, Danovitch GM, Neylan JF, Steiner RW, Everson MP, Gaston RS. Pentoxifylline does not prevent the cytokine-induced first dose reaction following OKT3—a randomized, double-blind placebo-controlled study. Transplantation 1996;61(4):573–7.
15. Chatenoud L. OKT3-induced cytokine-release syndrome: prevention effect of anti-tumor necrosis factor monoclonal antibody. Transplant Proc 1993;25(2 Suppl 1):47–51.
16. Friend PJ, Hale G, Chatenoud L, Rebello P, Bradley J, Thiru S, Phillips JM, Waldmann H. Phase I study of an engineered aglycosylated humanized CD3 antibody in renal transplant rejection. Transplantation 1999;68(11): 1632–7.
17. Woodle ES, Xu D, Zivin RA, Auger J, Charette J, O'Laughlin R, Peace D, Jollife LK, Haverty T, Bluestone JA, Thistlethwaite JR Jr. Phase I trial of a humanized, Fc receptor nonbinding OKT3 antibody, huOKT3gamma1(Ala-Ala) in the treatment of acute renal allograft rejection. Transplantation 1999;68(5):608–16.
18. Hall KA, Dole EJ, Hunter GC, Zukoski CF, Putnam CW. Hyperpyrexia-related ventricular tachycardia during OKT3 induction therapy. Transplantation 1992;54(6):1112–13.
19. Abramowicz D, Pradier O, Marchant A, Florquin S, De Pauw L, Vereerstraeten P, Kinnaert P, Vanherweghem JL, Goldman M. Induction of thromboses within renal grafts by high-dose prophylactic OKT3. Lancet 1992;339 (8796):777–8.
20. Raasveld MH, Hack CE, ten Berge IJ. Activation of coagulation and fibrinolysis following OKT3 administration to renal transplant recipients: association with distinct mediators. Thromb Haemost 1992;68(3):264–7.
21. Gomez E, Aguado S, Gago E, Escalada P, Alvarez-Grande J. Main graft vessels thromboses due to conventional-dose OKT3 in renal transplantation. Lancet 1992;339(8809):1612–13.
22. Abramowicz D, Pradier O, De Pauw L, Kinnaert P, Mat O, Surquin M, Doutrelepont JM, Vanherweghem JL, Capel P, Vereerstraeten P, et al. High-dose glucocorticosteroids increase the procoagulant effects of OKT3. Kidney Int 1994;46(6):1596–602.
23. Hollenbeck M, Westhoff A, Bach D, Grabensee B, Kolvenbach R, Kniemeyer HW. Doppler sonography and renal graft vessel thromboses after OKT3 treatment. Lancet 1992;340(8819):619–20.
24. Raasveld MH, Bemelman FJ, Schellekens PT, van Diepen FN, van Dongen A, van Royen EA, Hack CE, ten Berge IJ. Complement activation during OKT3 treatment: a possible explanation for respiratory side effects. Kidney Int 1993;43(5):1140–9.
25. Shihab F, Barry JM, Bennett WM, Meyer MM, Norman DJ. Cytokine-related encephalopathy induced by OKT3: incidence and predisposing factors Transplant Proc 1993; 25(1 Pt 1):564–5.
26. Reiss R, Makoff D, Rodriguez H, Graham S, Mittleman J, Jordan S. Encephalopathy and cerebral infarction in OKT3-treated patients with concomitant elevation of cerebrospinal fluid tumour necrosis factor alpha. Nephrol Dial Transplant 1993;8(5):464–8.
27. Thomas MC, Walker R, Wright A. HaNDL syndrome after "benign" OKT3-induced meningitis. Transplantation 1999;67(10):1384–5.
28. McCarthy JM, Sullivan K, Keown PA, Rollins DT. Diffuse anterior scleritis during OKT3 monoclonal antibody therapy for renal transplant rejection. Can J Ophthalmol 1992;27(1):22–4.
29. Dukar O, Barr CC. Visual loss complicating OKT3 monoclonal antibody therapy. Am J Ophthalmol 1993;115(6):781–5.
30. Hartnick CJ, Smith RV, Tellis V, Greenstein S, Ruben RJ. Reversible sensorineural hearing loss following

administration of muromonab-CD3 (OKT3) for cadaveric renal transplant immunosuppression. Ann Otol Rhinol Laryngol 2000;109(1):45–7.
31. Go MR, Bumgardner GL. OKT3 (muromonab-CD3) associated hepatitis in a kidney transplant recipient. Transplantation 2002;73(12):1957–9.
32. Batiuk TD, Bennett WM, Norman DJ. Cytokine nephropathy during antilymphocyte therapy. Transplant Proc 1993;25(2 Suppl 1):27–30.
33. First MR, Schroeder TJ, Hariharan S. OKT3-induced cytokine-release syndrome: renal effects (cytokine nephropathy). Transplant Proc 1993;25(2 Suppl 1):25–6.
34. Abramowicz D, Crusiaux A, Niaudet P, Kreis H, Chatenoud L, Goldman M. The IgE humoral response in OKT3-treated patients. Incidence and fine specificity. Transplantation 1996;61(4):577–81.
35. Abramowicz D, Crusiaux A, Goldman M. Anaphylactic shock after retreatment with OKT3 monoclonal antibody. N Engl J Med 1992;327(10):736.
36. Georgitis JW, Browning MC, Steiner D, Lorentz WB. Anaphylaxis and desensitization to the murine monoclonal antibody used for renal graft rejection. Ann Allergy 1991;66(4):343–7.
37. Turner M, Holman J. Late reactions during initial OKT3-treatment. Clin Transplant 1993;7:1–3.
38. Berkowitz RJ, Possidente CJ, McPherson BR, Guillot A, Braun SV, Reese JC. Anaphylactoid reaction to muromonab-CD3 in a pediatric renal transplant recipient. Pharmacotherapy 2000;20(1):100–4.
39. Abramowicz D, Goldman M, De Pauw L, Vanherweghem JL, Kinnaert P, Vereerstraeten P. The long-term effects of prophylactic OKT3 monoclonal antibody in cadaver kidney transplantation—a single-center, prospective, randomized study. Transplantation 1992;54(3):433–7.
40. Norman DJ, Kahana L, Stuart FP Jr, Thistlethwaite JR Jr, Shield CF 3rd, Monaco A, Dehlinger J, Wu SC, Van Horn A, Haverty TP. A randomized clinical trial of induction therapy with OKT3 in kidney transplantation. Transplantation 1993;55(1):44–50.
41. Bock HA, Gallati H, Zurcher RM, Bachofen M, Mihatsch MJ, Landmann J, Thiel G. A randomized prospective trial of prophylactic immunosuppression with ATG-fresenius versus OKT3 after renal transplantation. Transplantation 1995;59(6):830–40.
42. Petrie JJ, Rigby RJ, Hawley CM, Suranyi MG, Whitby M, Wall D, Hardie IR. Effect of OKT3 in steroid-resistant renal transplant rejection. Transplantation 1995;59(3):347–52.
43. Hadley S, Samore MH, Lewis WD, Jenkins RL, Karchmer AW, Hammer SM. Major infectious complications after orthotopic liver transplantation and comparison of outcomes in patients receiving cyclosporine or FK506 as primary immunosuppression. Transplantation 1995;59 (6):851–9.
44. Portela D, Patel R, Larson-Keller JJ, Ilstrup DM, Wiesner RH, Steers JL, Krom RA, Paya CV. OKT3 treatment for allograft rejection is a risk factor for cytomegalovirus disease in liver transplantation. J Infect Dis 1995;171 (4):1014–18.
45. Wechsler ME, Giardina EG, Sciacca RR, Rose EA, Barr ML. Increased early mortality in women undergoing cardiac transplantation. Circulation 1995;91(4):1029–35.
46. Hooks MA, Perlino CA, Henderson JM, Millikan WJ Jr, Kutner MH. Prevalence of invasive cytomegalovirus disease with administration of muromonab CD-3 in patients undergoing orthotopic liver transplantation. Ann Pharmacother 1992;26(5):617–20.
47. Lake K, Anderson D, Milfred S, Love K, Pritzker M, Emery R. The incidence of cytomegalovirus disease is not increased after OKT3 induction therapy. J Heart Lung Transplant 1993;12(3):537–8.
48. Hayes MJ, Torzillo PJ, Sheil AG, McCaughan GW. *Pneumocystis carinii* pneumonia after liver transplantation in adults. Clin Transplant 1994;8(6):499–503.
49. Swinnen LJ, Costanzo-Nordin MR, Fisher SG, O'Sullivan EJ, Johnson MR, Heroux AL, Dizikes GJ, Pifarre R, Fisher RI. Increased incidence of lymphoproliferative disorder after immunosuppression with the monoclonal antibody OKT3 in cardiac-transplant recipients. N Engl J Med 1990;323(25):1723–8.
50. Anderson P, Schroeder T, Hariharan S, First M. Incidence of posttransplant lymphoproliferative disease in OKT-3 treated renal transplant recipients. Clin Transplant 1993;7:582–5.
51. Batiuk TD, Barry JM, Bennett WM, Meyer MM, Tolzman D, Norman DJ. Incidence and type of cancer following the use of OKT3: a single center experience with 557 organ transplants. Transplant Proc 1993;25(1 Pt 2):1391.
52. McAlister V, Grant D, Roy A, Yilmaz Z, Ghent C, Wall W. Posttransplant lymphoproliferative disorders in liver recipients treated with OKT3 or ALG induction immunosuppression. Transplant Proc 1993;25(1 Pt 2):1400–1.
53. Opelz G, Henderson R. Incidence of non-Hodgkin lymphoma in kidney and heart transplant recipients. Lancet 1993;342(8886–8887):1514–16.
54. Bertin D, Haverty T, Sanders M, et al. Posttransplant development of lymphoproliferative disroders and other malignancies following orthoclone OKT3 therapy. In: Lieberman R, Mukherjee A, editors. Principles of Drug Development in Transplantation and Autoimmunity, 1996:633–41.
55. Hibberd AD, Trevillian PR, Wlodarzcyk JH, Gillies AH, Stein AM, Sheil AG, Disney AP. Cancer risk associated with ATG/OKT3 in renal transplantation. Transplant Proc 1999;31(1–2):1271–2.

Muzolimine

See also Diuretics

General Information

Muzolimine is a diuretic with a long duration of action, slightly more effective than furosemide. In Germany muzolimine was withdrawn 2 years after its introduction.

Organs and Systems

Nervous system

Of 29 patients with chronic renal insufficiency treated with high doses of muzolimine, five developed a neurological syndrome very similar to multiple sclerosis (1). Other reports of severe neurotoxicity with muzolimine have appeared (SEDA-16, 225).

Reference

1. Gilli M, Papurello D, Chiado Cutin I, Bradac GB, Delsedime M, Dettoni E, Giangrandi C, Fidelio T, Rocci E, Riccio A. Azione neurotossica della muzolimina ad alte dosi in pazienti uremica. Osservazione su un gruppo di 29 soggetti. [Neurotoxic action of muzolimine at high doses in uremic patients. Observation of a group of 29 subjects.] Minerva Urol Nefrol 1989;41(3):215–18.

MW-2884

See also Non-steroidal anti-inflammatory drugs

General Information

MW-2884 (10-methoxy-4*H*-benzo-(4,5)-cycloheptathiophene-4-glindene acetic acid) is an inhibitor of monokine release. In 12 patients with rheumatoid arthritis it caused gastrointestinal disturbances, temporary liver function impairment, and allergic skin reactions. One patient stopped taking it because of severe urticaria (1).

Reference

1. Seibel MJ, Bruckle W, Respondek M, Beveridge T, Schnyder J, Muller W. Erste klinische Erfahrungen in der Behandlung chronischer Polyarthritiden mit einem neuen Monokin-Release-Inhibitor. [Initial clinical experiences in the treatment of chronic polyarthritis with a new monokine release inhibitor.] Z Rheumatol 1989;48(3):147–51.

Mycophenolate mofetil

General Information

Mycophenolate mofetil, the morpholinoethyl ester of mycophenolic acid (rINN), is an antimetabolite that interferes with the synthesis of nucleic acids and selectively inhibits the proliferation of T and B lymphocytes. It has been used to treat psoriasis and to prevent acute renal allograft rejection in combination with ciclosporin and glucocorticoids.

Uses

In 16 renal transplant patients with suspected ciclosporin nephrotoxicity, the addition of mycophenolate allowed safe reduction in the dosage of ciclosporin, with subsequent improvement in renal function and arterial blood pressure over 6 months (1). It might allow the rapid withdrawal of glucocorticoids in patients taking ciclosporin or tacrolimus, and therefore reduce the incidence of glucocorticoid-induced post-transplant diabetes, hypercholesterolemia, and hypertension (2). There have been several reports of patients with ciclosporin-associated thrombotic microangiopathy/hemolytic-uremic syndrome in whom mycophenolate was successfully substituted (3,4).

When mycophenolate replaced ciclosporin in 17 renal transplant patients with ciclosporin nephropathy, serum creatinine concentrations fell by a mean of 26% (5). There were no cases of acute allograft rejection. Adverse effects of mycophenolate were not mentioned.

There were beneficial effects on blood pressure, lipid profile, and glomerular hemodynamics by switching from ciclosporin to mycophenolate in an open study in 17 renal transplant patients with stable renal function who took ciclosporin and prednisone in two steps (6). In step I mycophenolate was added and the dose of ciclosporin was progressively reduced to produce one-third of the original trough concentration; this took about 20 weeks. In step II, ciclosporin was gradually withdrawn over 6 weeks. During step I, two patients dropped out, one with severe diarrhea which reversed after mycophenolate withdrawal and one with biopsy-proven acute rejection, with recovery after mycophenolate withdrawal and an increase in the dose of ciclosporin. During step II there was no acute rejection. At 1 year after the end of the study, two patients had stopped taking mycophenolate, one because of recurrent upper airway infections (probably not related to mycophenolate) and one because of Kaposi's sarcoma of the leg. In the last case a possible role of mycophenolate could not be ruled out (SEDA-24, 429).

Mycophenolate has also been studied in various chronic inflammatory disorders, such as rheumatoid arthritis, pemphigus vulgaris, and psoriasis. In 70 patients with chronic active Crohn's disease, mycophenolate plus glucocorticoids produced benefit on disease activity comparable to azathioprine plus glucocorticoids (7). Two of the 35 patients randomized to mycophenolate had significant adverse effects that required drug withdrawal, namely rashes and vomiting.

General adverse effects

In three pivotal clinical trials of mycophenolate mofetil in kidney transplant recipients, adverse effects were in accordance with the known antiproliferative effect of mycophenolate, namely gastrointestinal disorders, leukopenia, and opportunistic infections, in particular cytomegalovirus tissue invasive disease (SED-13, 1130) (SEDA-20, 346). Nephrotoxicity was not observed in clinical trials, and renal function significantly improved in six patients converted to mycophenolate for ciclosporin nephrotoxicity (8).

In one patient, mycophenolate mofetil was putatively involved in a constellation of symptoms that included fever, exudative pharyngitis, adynamic ileus, electrolytic abnormalities, and myocardial dysfunction, which resolved on withdrawal (SEDA-20, 346).

Organs and Systems

Respiratory

Interstitial pneumonitis with severe respiratory failure has been reported in two patients (SEDA-21, 389) (SEDA-22, 418). One patient improved after mycophenolate mofetil was withdrawn, but interstitial fibrosis was found on serial lung biopsies. The other patient died from respiratory failure 3 months later. Although other drugs may have been involved in these two patients, one other reported case with recurrence of respiratory failure on each rechallenge of mycophenolate is particularly convincing.

There was a dry cough in five of 45 patients taking mycophenolate, associated with dyspnea and hypoxia in one patient and asthma exacerbation in another (9). As the symptoms reversed only after mycophenolate mofetil withdrawal, the authors suggested that dry cough and dyspnea should be considered as early symptoms of pulmonary toxicity.

Hematologic

There was a dose-related increase in the incidence of leukopenia in the three pivotal trials.

Abnormalities of neutrophil morphology have been reported with mycophenolate.

- In two transplant patients, changes in circulating neutrophils (nuclear hypolobulation and abnormal clumping of nuclear chromatin) were identified after 4–5 months of treatment with mycophenolate (10). A bone marrow aspirate in one patient showed hypocellularity, abnormal clumping of chromatin beyond the promyelocyte stage, and almost no segmented neutrophils. These morphological abnormalities preceded the appearance of peripheral neutropenia in both patients and normalized after mycophenolate withdrawal.

The authors suggested that neutrophil dysplasia had resulted from inhibition of guanosine nucleoside synthesis.

Gastrointestinal

Mycophenolate mofetil often causes gastrointestinal disorders, most commonly a dose-related diarrhea and more rarely esophagitis, gastritis, duodenal or colonic ulceration, and gastrointestinal hemorrhage (SEDA-22, 418). Diarrhea can be extremely severe for various reasons, such as inappropriate dosage in low-weight patients, renal insufficiency, drug interactions (for example with sulfinpyrazone) interfering with the renal tubular excretion of mycophenolate metabolites. That was the case in two patients who had frequent diarrhea with significant weight loss and electrolyte disturbances requiring parenteral nutrition (SEDA-21, 389).

Pooled data from the tricontinental and the US studies in kidney transplant patients showed incidences of diarrhea of 31 and 36% in patients taking 2 and 3 g/day respectively (11). In a retrospective study, 29% of 109 mycophenolate-treated patients had diarrhea that required hospitalization and 12% developed upper intestinal symptoms (gastritis, esophagitis) (12). Frequent dosage reduction was necessary and only 28% of patients were still taking full doses after 1 year.

Gastrointestinal toxicity was confirmed to be the most frequent adverse effect (53%) in 120 pancreas transplant patients who received a triple immunosuppressive regimen consisting of mycophenolate, tacrolimus, and prednisone (13). As a result, conversion from mycophenolate to azathioprine at 1 year was mostly due to gastrointestinal toxicity, which was significantly more frequent in recipients of pancreas transplantation alone (49%) compared with recipients of pancreas transplantation after previous kidney transplantation (26%) or recipients of simultaneous pancreas and kidney transplants (14%). In another study in 120 kidney transplant patients randomized to receive tacrolimus and prednisone with or without mycophenolate, there was a high rate of mycophenolate withdrawal (43%) during the first 6 months, mostly because of gastrointestinal toxicity (14). In both of these studies, the withdrawal rate was higher than in the pivotal trials in kidney transplant patients (4–10% after 6 months) (11). As both studies used a combination of tacrolimus plus mycophenolate rather than mycophenolate plus ciclosporin, a synergistic effect on the gastrointestinal tract, or more probably higher serum concentrations of mycophenolic acid due to an interaction with tacrolimus, could have contributed (SEDA-21, 390) (SEDA-22, 421).

The mechanism of gastrointestinal toxicity is not well understood.

- A 42-year-old woman with a renal transplant taking triple immunosuppression (azathioprine, ciclosporin, and glucocorticoids) was converted after 7 years from azathioprine plus ciclosporin to mycophenolate (2 g/day) because of ciclosporin nephrotoxicity (15). Within 2 months she had developed severe persistent watery diarrhea (5–10 stools/day) and lost 7 kg over 2 months. Investigations ruled out an infectious cause and there were features of duodenal villous atrophy on histological examination. Diarrhea disappeared after mycophenolate withdrawal and two subsequent duodenal biopsies showed improvement 2 months later and further complete recovery 6 months later.

This report suggests that loss of normal villous structure is one of the possible mechanisms of mycophenolate-induced severe diarrhea.

Diarrhea is the most commonly reported adverse effect in patients with transplants taking mycophenolate. In 26 renal transplant recipients with persistent afebrile diarrhea (daily fecal output over 200 g), prospectively investigated for infections and morphological and functional integrity of the gastrointestinal tract, all but one had an erosive enterocolitis; 70% had malabsorption of nutrients, which contributed to the diarrhea (16). In about 60% an infectious origin was demonstrated and successfully treated with antimicrobial drugs without changing the immunosuppressive regimen. In about 40% there was no infection but a Crohn's disease-like pattern of inflammation. These patients also had less pronounced malabsorption of bile acids but a significantly faster colonic transit time, which correlated with trough concentrations of mycophenolic acid. Withdrawal of mycophenolate was associated with allograft rejection in one-third of these patients.

Ischemic colitis has also been attributed to mycophenolate (17).

- A 49-year-old woman taking ciclosporin, prednisolone, and mycophenolate developed acute refractory rejection 4 days after renal transplantation. After an unsuccessful glucocorticoid pulse, her immunosuppressive regimen was successively changed to muromonab and tacrolimus with mycophenolate maintenance. Twelve days after transplantation she had abdominal pain and watery/bloody diarrhea. Colonoscopy showed multiple ulcers with mucosal injection and colon edema. A biopsy suggested ischemic colitis and cytomegalovirus infection was ruled out. Her symptoms persisted until mycophenolate was withdrawn and further colonoscopy showed complete resolution.

Patients with inflammatory bowel disease unresponsive to azathioprine or intolerant of it may benefit from mycophenolate mofetil. Of 12 patients so treated, three had minor adverse effects (headache, nausea, arthralgia). Three with ulcerative colitis developed rectal bleeding while taking mycophenolate mofetil. Histological features of the mucosa were highly suggestive of drug-induced bleeding. Enterohepatic recycling results in high colonic concentrations of mycophenolic acids, which may have a direct toxic effect on the epithelium (18).

Liver

In two renal transplant patients, serum bilirubin concentrations increased to 46 and 63 μmol/l within 3–7 days of mycophenolate treatment, and further increased to 98 μmol/l in one patient after the dose was increased (19). The bilirubin concentration returned to normal or pretreatment values after withdrawal or dosage reduction. Although both patients also received ciclosporin, which has been associated with hyperbilirubinemia, the temporal relation and a possible dose-dependent effect favored a causative role of mycophenolate.

Skin

Mycophenolate-induced eczema has been reported (20).

- A 45-year-old woman with a liver transplant began to take mycophenolate mofetil (2 g/day) before planned ciclosporin withdrawal. After 3 days she developed pruritus and a bullous eruption on her hands and feet. The lesions improved after mycophenolate was withdrawn, but soon reappeared after readministration of a lower dose (500 mg/day). A skin biopsy showed dyshidrotic eczema and a skin test with mycophenolate mofetil produced recurrence.

Hair

Alopecia has been noted in two patients converted from ciclosporin to mycophenolate (SEDA-22, 418).

- Onycholysis with blisters and loose toenails has been observed in a 45-year-old man who took tacrolimus, prednisone, and mycophenolate for 3 weeks after renal transplantation (21). The lesions improved after withdrawal and recurred after two subsequent re-exposures.

Immunologic

Transplant rejection

In a randomized study, 14 patients with liver transplants were given calcineurin inhibitors and 14 were given mycophenolate mofetil monotherapy (22). Those who were given mycophenolate had reversible episodes of acute graft rejection and there were no such episodes in those who were given calcineurin inhibitors.

In 11 patients with orthotopic liver transplants who had adverse effects from ciclosporin or tacrolimus, mycophenolate mofetil monotherapy for 1 year was successful. This was followed by a randomized, controlled trial in 18 patients, of whom nine were given mycophenolate mofetil (23). Five patients completed the 3 month trial. Of these, two had an episode of acute rejection, one after 2 months and one after 3 months, which did not respond to the reintroduction of tacrolimus and intravenous glucocorticoids. One had a glucocorticoid-responsive episode of severe acute rejection after 3 weeks. The other two patients had normal liver function tests after 2 weeks and 2 months respectively, when the trial was stopped. Mycophenolate mofetil allows a reduction of the dose of calcineurin inhibitor, with a low risk of rejection and improvement in renal function. However, it is associated with an unacceptable risk of acute rejection.

Infection risk

The role of mycophenolate in the occurrence of opportunistic infections is debated. In a retrospective comparison of 358 simultaneous pancreas plus kidney transplant patients who received a ciclosporin-based immunosuppressive regimen, the rate of opportunistic infections was similar in patients treated with mycophenolate ($n = 109$) and azathioprine ($n = 249$) (12). However, very few patients taking mycophenolate were available for long-term comparison. In contrast, another retrospective comparison of 135 renal transplant patients (69 for prophylactic treatment and 66 for rescue therapy) showed that the combination of mycophenolate, tacrolimus, and prednisone ($n = 49$) produced fewer rejection episodes, but a significantly higher incidence of infectious episodes than the combination of mycophenolate, ciclosporin, and prednisone (24). In another randomized trial of 120 renal transplant patients, there was a significantly higher rate of asymptomatic or symptomatic cytomegalovirus infection in patients who took mycophenolate, tacrolimus, and prednisone than in patients who took tacrolimus plus prednisone (20 versus 5%) (14). Overall, both of these studies suggest that mycophenolate plus tacrolimus has a more potent immunosuppressive effect, with an increased risk of infections (and theoretically lymphoproliferative disorders), as the counterpart of a possible greater effect on acute rejection prophylaxis.

Bacterial infections

- Staphylococcal septicemia complicated by endocarditis has been reported in a 50-year-old woman after 5 months of treatment with mycophenolate for atopic dermatitis (25).

As the skin of most patients with atopic dermatitis can be colonized with *Staphylococcus aureus*, the authors suggested caution in using mycophenolate, which can also cause leukopenia. This patient had previously taken ciclosporin and azathioprine, which were ineffective, but without apparent infectious complications. A specific role of mycophenolate is therefore debatable and the occurrence of bacterial septicemia may have been purely coincidental.

Mycobacterium hemophilum is a pathogen that is found in immunosuppressed patients, such as those with malignancy, AIDS, and organ transplants. Systemic lupus erythematosus can make patients more susceptible to infection.

- A 25-year-old Chinese woman with systemic lupus erythematosus had a disease course characterized by multiple flares involving the kidneys, central nervous system, and gastrointestinal tract (26). She was given mycophenolate mofetil and multiple courses of antibiotics, with a poor response. After about 9 months she developed a recurrent right leg cellulitis. Two initial skin biopsies yielded negative bacterial and mycobacterial cultures, but histopathology of the muscle of her right thigh showed acid-fast bacilli and culture subsequently grew *M. hemophilum*.

The authors concluded that this complication had been due to late diagnosis, multiple antibiotics, and immunocompromise. These points must be taken into consideration when treating a patient with mycophenolate mofetil.

Virus infections

Cytomegalovirus

The role of mycophenolate in the rate and severity of cytomegalovirus infection in transplant patients has been debated (SEDA-23, 407) and is difficult to evaluate in otherwise immunosuppressed patients. Whereas there was a dose-related increase in the incidence of cytomegalovirus disease in the three pivotal trials, a later analysis did not confirm that mycophenolate mofetil is specifically associated with an increased risk of cytomegalovirus infection, and suggested that over-immunosuppression rather than mycophenolate mofetil per se was the main contributing factor (SEDA-22, 418) (27–29).

- Severe cytomegalovirus pancolitis has been reported in a 59-year-old man taking only mycophenolate and prednisone for Wegener's granulomatosis (30).

In a retrospective study of 84 cytomegalovirus-seronegative renal transplant patients who received a kidney from a cytomegalovirus-seropositive donor without cytomegalovirus prophylaxis, the incidence of primary cytomegalovirus infection was similar in the 24 patients who took mycophenolate plus ciclosporin and prednisone, compared with the 60 patients who took ciclosporin and prednisone alone (31). However, the incidence of cytomegalovirus disease was nearly twice as high in the mycophenolate group (67 versus 30%), but with no difference in the severity of the disease. The authors speculated that the more frequent incidence of symptomatic cytomegalovirus disease might have been due to some specific effects of mycophenolate on the primary immune response to cytomegalovirus.

Mycophenolate mofetil has been compared with azathioprine in combination with ciclosporin and glucocorticoids in 65 children after kidney transplantation (32). The main adverse effects of this treatment were infections of the urinary tract and the upper respiratory tract, abdominal pain, and diarrhea. Opportunistic infections with cytomegalovirus or cytomegalovirus syndrome occurred in 20% within the first 6 months and tissue-invasive cytomegalovirus disease in 3.1%. These results were similar to those in adults.

Varicella

A retrospective study in 19 children with renal transplants identified three who developed disseminated varicella, despite a prior history of chickenpox in two and pretransplant varicella vaccination in one (33). The clinical disease was mild and responded promptly to oral aciclovir. Although this was based on very few patients, the incidence of 16% was thought to be unexpectedly higher than that reported in historic controls (0.7–1.9%), and might have resulted from the higher degree of immunosuppression achieved with mycophenolate mofetil.

Herpes simplex

To evaluate whether mycophenolate mofetil is effective in treating moderate to severe atopic dermatitis, an open pilot study was conducted in 10 patients (34). There were no serious adverse effects, but one patient had to discontinue treatment because he developed *Herpes simplex* retinitis, which resolved after treatment with aciclovir. Although there is no direct evidence that mycophenolate mofetil is a major cause of *Herpes* retinitis, in this patient it seems likely that it was due to immunosuppression. In contrast, in vivo and in vitro mycophenolate mofetil strongly potentiates the antiherpetic effects of aciclovir, ganciclovir, and penciclovir (35). It is probably therefore enough to give antiviral therapy only when clinical signs of *Herpes* infection occur.

Fungal infections

There have been two cases of intestinal microsporidiosis (36) and one case of *Nocardia asteroides* brain abscess (37) in adults taking mycophenolate mofetil.

Body temperature

- Isolated and intermittent drug fever with a spiking pattern has been attributed to mycophenolate in a 41-year-old man with a renal transplant (38). The relation to treatment was confirmed by the exclusion of numerous infectious causes, the persistence of fever despite ciclosporin withdrawal, subsidence of fever after mycophenolate withdrawal, and the absence of further episodes of fever during follow-up.

Long-Term Effects

Tumorigenicity

- Kaposi's sarcoma recurred 4 months after starting mycophenolate in a 58-year-old renal transplant patient who 7 years before had had similar lesions that reversed on withdrawal of ciclosporin (39).
- Kaposi's sarcoma has been reported after a mean of 7 months of treatment in three renal transplant patients whose immunosuppressive regimen included mycophenolate mofetil (40).

The investigators of the second case found that the incidence of Kaposi's sarcoma in patients taking regimens containing mycophenolate mofetil was 0.8% (3/371 patients) compared with 0.1% in patients not taking it (2/1464). It was suggested that mycophenolate mofetil might increase the susceptibility to Kaposi's sarcoma.

Second-Generation Effects

Pregnancy

- A 33-year-old woman was given a living related donor kidney transplantation during the first trimester, followed by mycophenolate mofetil, tacrolimus, and prednisone (41). The mother did well, except for mild pre-eclampsia and mild renal insufficiency. The child was born prematurely during the 36th week. The only teratogenic effects detected were hypoplastic nails and a short fifth finger.

Susceptibility Factors

Age

The adverse effects of mycophenolate mofetil in children have been reviewed retrospectively in 24 renal transplant patients (mean age 14 years) switched from azathioprine to mycophenolate mofetil a mean of 4.8 years after transplantation (42). The mean dose of mycophenolate mofetil was 560 mg/m^2. After a mean of 9.6 months, 13 had to discontinue treatment because of adverse effects, namely severe and partially reversible anemia (10 patients, of whom three required transfusions), neutropenia ($n = 1$), and diarrhea ($n = 2$). The anemia was normocytic and normochromic in nine patients, and such a high incidence of severe anemia was unexpected from the available adult data. Although patients who discontinued treatment had a lower pretreatment-calculated creatinine clearance, this was not significant and probably not the major cause of anemia. The author speculated that the anemia resulted from a disproportionately high unbound plasma concentration of mycophenolate mofetil, due to reduced protein binding and impaired renal clearance.

Drug–Drug Interactions

Ciclosporin

In 52 patients taking mycophenolate mofetil 1 g bd, prednisone, and ciclosporin to a target blood concentration of 125–175 ng/ml for 6 months after transplantation, withdrawal of ciclosporin resulted in almost a doubling of mycophenolic acid trough concentrations (43).

Tacrolimus

Patients taking tacrolimus have higher mycophenolate mofetil plasma trough concentrations than patients taking ciclosporin (44). Compared with the combination of ciclosporin plus mycophenolate mofetil, tacrolimus plus similar doses of mycophenolate produced significantly higher serum concentrations of mycophenolic acid, resulting in a greater degree of in vitro immunosuppression (SEDA-21, 390).

References

1. Hueso M, Bover J, Seron D, Gil-Vernet S, Sabate I, Fulladosa X, Ramos R, Coll O, Alsina J, Grinyo JM. Low-dose cyclosporine and mycophenolate mofetil in renal allograft recipients with suboptimal renal function. Transplantation 1998;66(12):1727–31.
2. Stegall MD, Wachs ME, Everson G, Steinberg T, Bilir B, Shrestha R, Karrer F, Kam I. Prednisone withdrawal 14 days after liver transplantation with mycophenolate: a prospective trial of cyclosporine and tacrolimus. Transplantation 1997;64(12):1755–60.
3. Lecornu-Heuze L, Ducloux D, Rebibou JM, Martin L, Billerey C, Chalopin JM. Mycophenolate mofetil in cyclosporin-associated thrombotic microangiopathy. Nephrol Dial Transplant 1998;13(12):3212–13.
4. McGregor DO, Robson RA, Lynn KL. Haemolytic–uraemic syndrome in a renal transplant recipient treated by conversion to mycophenolate mofetil. Nephron 1998;80(3):365–6.
5. Houde I, Isenring P, Boucher D, Noel R, Lachanche JG. Mycophenolate mofetil, an alternative to cyclosporine A for long-term immunosuppression in kidney transplantation? Transplantation 2000;70(8):1251–3.
6. Schrama YC, Joles JA, van Tol A, Boer P, Koomans HA, Hene RJ. Conversion to mycophenolate mofetil in conjunction with stepwise withdrawal of cyclosporine in stable renal transplant recipients. Transplantation 2000;69(3):376–83.
7. Neurath MF, Wanitschke R, Peters M, Krummenauer F, Meyer zum Buschenfelde KH, Schlaak JF. Randomised trial of mycophenolate mofetil versus azathioprine for treatment of chronic active Crohn's disease. Gut 1999;44(5):625–8.
8. Ducloux D, Fournier V, Bresson-Vautrin C, Rebibou JM, Billerey C, Saint-Hillier Y, Chalopin JM. Mycophenolate mofetil in renal transplant recipients with cyclosporine-associated nephrotoxicity: a preliminary report. Transplantation 1998;65(11):1504–6.
9. Elli A, Aroldi A, Montagnino G, Tarantino A, Ponticelli C. Mycophenolate mofetil and cough. Transplantation 1998;66(3):409.
10. Banerjee R, Halil O, Bain BJ, Cummins D, Banner NR. Neutrophil dysplasia caused by mycophenolate mofetil. Transplantation 2000;70(11):1608–10.
11. Simmons WD, Rayhill SC, Sollinger HW. Preliminary risk-benefit assessment of mycophenolate mofetil in transplant rejection. Drug Saf 1997;17(2):75–92.
12. Odorico JS, Pirsch JD, Knechtle SJ, D'Alessandro AM, Sollinger HW. A study comparing mycophenolate mofetil to azathioprine in simultaneous pancreas–kidney transplantation. Transplantation 1998;66(12):1751–9.
13. Gruessner RW, Sutherland DE, Drangstveit MB, Wrenshall L, Humar A, Gruessner AC. Mycophenolate mofetil in pancreas transplantation. Transplantation 1998;66(3):318–23.
14. Shapiro R, Jordan ML, Scantlebury VP, Vivas C, Gritsch HA, Casavilla FA, McCauley J, Johnston JR, Randhawa P, Irish W, Hakala TR, Fung JJ, Starzl TE. A prospective, randomized trial to compare tacrolimus and prednisone with and without mycophenolate mofetil in patients undergoing renal transplantation: first report. J Urol 1998;160(6 Pt 1):1982–6.
15. Ducloux D, Ottignon Y, Semhoun-Ducloux S, Labbe S, Saint-Hillier Y, Miguet JP, Carayon P, Chalopin JM. Mycophenolate mofetil-induced villous atrophy. Transplantation 1998;66(8):1115–16.
16. Maes BD, Dalle I, Geboes K, Oellerich M, Armstrong VW, Evenepoel P, Geypens B, Kuypers D, Shipkova M, Geboes K, Vanrenterghem YF. Erosive enterocolitis in mycophenolate mofetil-treated renal-transplant recipients with persistent afebrile diarrhea. Transplantation 2003;75(5):665–72.
17. Kim HC, Park SB. Mycophenolate mofetil-induced ischemic colitis. Transplant Proc 2000;32(7):1896–7.
18. Skelly MM, Logan RF, Jenkins D, Mahida YR, Hawkey CJ. Toxicity of mycophenolate mofetil in patients with inflammatory bowel disease. Inflamm Bowel Dis 2002;8(2):93–7.
19. Chueh SC, Huang CY, Lai MK. Mycophenolate mofetil-induced hyperbilirubinemia in renal transplant recipients. Transplant Proc 2000;32(7):1901–2.
20. Semhoun-Ducloux S, Ducloux D, Miguet JP. Mycophenolate mofetil-induced dyshidrotic eczema. Ann Intern Med 2000;132(5):417.
21. Rault R. Mycophenolate-associated onycholysis. Ann Intern Med 2000;133(11):921–2.
22. Schlitt HJ, Barkmann A, Boker KH, Schmidt HH, Emmanouilidis N, Rosenau J, Bahr MJ, Tusch G, Manns MP, Nashan B, Klempnauer J. Replacement of calcineurin inhibitors with mycophenolate mofetil in liver-transplant patients with renal dysfunction: a randomised controlled study. Lancet 2001;357(9256):587–91.

23. Stewart SF, Hudson M, Talbot D, Manas D, Day CP. Mycophenolate mofetil monotherapy in liver transplantation. Lancet 2001;357(9256):609–10.
24. Daoud AJ, Schroeder TJ, Shah M, Hariharan S, Peddi VR, Weiskittel P, First MR. A comparison of the safety and efficacy of mycophenolate mofetil, prednisone and cyclosporine and mycophenolate mofetil, and prednisone and tacrolimus. Transplant Proc 1998;30(8):4079–81.
25. Satchell AC, Barnetson RS. Staphylococcal septicaemia complicating treatment of atopic dermatitis with mycophenolate. Br J Dermatol 2000;143(1):202–3.
26. Teh CL, Kong KO, Chong AP, Badsha H. *Mycobacterium haemophilum* infection in an SLE patient on mycophenolate mofetil Lupus 2002;11(4):249–52.
27. Moreso F, Seron D, Morales JM, Cruzado JM, Gil-Vernet S, Perez JL, Fulladosa X, Andres A, Grinyo JM. Incidence of leukopenia and cytomegalovirus disease in kidney transplants treated with mycophenolate mofetil combined with low cyclosporine and steroid doses. Clin Transplant 1998;12(3):198–205.
28. Sarmiento JM, Munn SR, Paya CV, Velosa JA, Nguyen JH. Is cytomegalovirus infection related to mycophenolate mofetil after kidney transplantation? A case-control study. Clin Transplant 1998;12(5):371–4.
29. Paterson DL, Singh N, Panebianco A, Wannstedt CF, Wagener MM, Gayowski T, Marino IR. Infectious complications occurring in liver transplant recipients receiving mycophenolate mofetil. Transplantation 1998;66(5):593–8.
30. Woywodt A, Choi M, Schneider W, Kettritz R, Gobel U. Cytomegalovirus colitis during mycophenolate mofetil therapy for Wegener's granulomatosis. Am J Nephrol 2000;20(6):468–72.
31. ter Meulen CG, Wetzels JF, Hilbrands LB. The influence of mycophenolate mofetil on the incidence and severity of primary cytomegalovirus infections and disease after renal transplantation. Nephrol Dial Transplant 2000;15(5):711–14.
32. Staskewitz A, Kirste G, Tonshoff B, Weber LT, Boswald M, Burghard R, Helmchen U, Brandis M, Zimmerhackl LB. Mycophenolate mofetil in pediatric renal transplantation without induction therapy: results after 12 months of treatment. German Pediatric Renal Transplantation Study Group. Transplantation 2001;71(5):638–44.
33. Rothwell WS, Gloor JM, Morgenstern BZ, Milliner DS. Disseminated varicella infection in pediatric renal transplant recipients treated with mycophenolate mofetil. Transplantation 1999;68(1):158–61.
34. Grundmann-Kollmann M, Podda M, Ochsendorf F, Boehncke WH, Kaufmann R, Zollner TM. Mycophenolate mofetil is effective in the treatment of atopic dermatitis. Arch Dermatol 2001;137(7):870–3.
35. Neyts J, Andrei G, De Clercq E. The novel immunosuppressive agent mycophenolate mofetil markedly potentiates the antiherpesvirus activities of acyclovir, ganciclovir, and penciclovir in vitro and in vivo. Antimicrob Agents Chemother 1998;42(2):216–22.
36. Guerard A, Rabodonirina M, Cotte L, Liguory O, Piens MA, Daoud S, Picot S, Touraine JL. Intestinal microsporidiosis occurring in two renal transplant recipients treated with mycophenolate mofetil. Transplantation 1999;68(5):699–707.
37. Magee CC, Halligan RD, Milford EL, Sayegh MH. Nocardial infection in a renal transplant recipient on tacrolimus and mycophenolate mofetil. Clin Nephrol 1999;52(1):44–6.
38. Chueh SC, Hong JC, Huang CY, Lai MK. Drug fever caused by mycophenolate mofetil in a renal transplant recipient—a case report. Transplant Proc 2000;32(7):1925–6.
39. Gomez E, Aguado S, Rodriguez M, Alvarez-Grande J. Kaposi's sarcoma after renal transplantation—disappearance after reduction of immunosuppression and reappearance 7 years later after start of mycophenolate mofetil treatment. Nephrol Dial Transplant 1998;13(12):3279–80.
40. Eberhard OK, Kliem V, Brunkhorst R. Five cases of Kaposi's sarcoma in kidney graft recipients: possible influence of the immunosuppressive therapy. Transplantation 1999;67(1):180–4.
41. Pergola PE, Kancharla A, Riley DJ. Kidney transplantation during the first trimester of pregnancy: immunosuppression with mycophenolate mofetil, tacrolimus, and prednisone. Transplantation 2001;71(7):994–7.
42. Butani L, Palmer J, Baluarte HJ, Polinsky MS. Adverse effects of mycophenolate mofetil in pediatric renal transplant recipients with presumed chronic rejection. Transplantation 1999;68(1):83–6.
43. Gregoor PJ, de Sevaux RG, Hene RJ, Hesse CJ, Hilbrands LB, Vos P, van Gelder T, Hoitsma AJ, Weimar W. Effect of cyclosporine on mycophenolic acid trough levels in kidney transplant recipients. Transplantation 1999;68(10):1603–6.
44. Hubner GI, Eismann R, Sziegoleit W. Drug interaction between mycophenolate mofetil and tacrolimus detectable within therapeutic mycophenolic acid monitoring in renal transplant patients. Ther Drug Monit 1999;21(5):536–9.

Myeloid colony-stimulating factors

See also Individual agents

General Information

Around 10 glycoprotein myeloid hemopoietic growth factors or colony-stimulating factors (CSFs) have so far been identified and purified; their genes have been cloned and active recombinant proteins have been produced. Recombinant factors produced by yeast or mammalian cells are glycosylated, as they are in their native state, whereas those expressed in bacterial systems are not. Glycosylation may be clinically relevant with regard to the efficacy and antigenicity of the molecule, although antibody formation has not been observed, even after prolonged therapy (1). Most clinical studies with CSFs have hitherto been performed with granulocyte-macrophage colony-stimulating factor (GM-CSF) and granulocyte colony-stimulating factor (G-CSF), although clinical trials of other colony-stimulating factors have also been initiated in a number of centers. GM-CSF leads to a dose-related sustained increase in peripheral neutrophil numbers, with a delayed increase in circulating monocytes and eosinophils. The effect of G-CSF appears to be more restricted to neutrophils. Multi-CSF (IL-3) stimulates the production of all types of leukocytes, as well as platelets and reticulocytes (2).

Both granulocyte colony-stimulating factor (G-CSF) and granulocyte-macrophage colony-stimulating factor (GM-CSF) have been extensively investigated for the treatment of chemotherapy-induced neutropenia, reducing the duration of neutropenia after bone marrow transplantation, or mobilizing peripheral blood progenitor cells after myelosuppressive chemotherapy (3). Other clinical uses are indicated in the monographs on the individual growth factors.

Two reviews have examined the available data on the effects of hemopoietic growth factors on the duration of neutropenia and mortality in drug-induced agranulocytosis, which mostly consists of isolated case reports or small series of patients (4,5). The authors reached contrasting opinions, suggesting that hemopoietic growth factors might or might not be of interest in patients with severe drug-induced agranulocytosis. Adverse effects were noted in 13 of 118 case reports (4). Although most of them were benign, pulmonary toxicity or acute respiratory distress syndrome occurred in a few patients.

Comparative studies

There were no major differences in the adverse effect profiles in 42 patients with breast cancer randomized to filgrastim (G-CSF) or molgramostim (GM-CSF) (SEDA-22, 407). There were no significant differences in the adverse effects profiles and severity of adverse effects in 181 patients with cancers randomized to receive filgrastim (G-CSF) or sargramostim (GM-CSF) for chemotherapy-induced myelosuppression (6).

The effects and the safety of a 5-day regimen of G-CSF ($n = 9$) or GM-CSF ($n = 8$) have been compared (7). Most patients complained of flu-like symptoms in both groups (six and seven respectively), but rash at the injection site was observed only in four patients treated with GM-CSF. In the G-CSF group, there was a fall in platelet count (below $150 \times 10^9/l$) in five patients, raised serum lactic dehydrogenase activity, and raised uric acid concentrations; three patients required transient treatment with allopurinol.

The frequency and severity of adverse effects associated with the prophylactic use of filgrastim or sargramostim have been assessed in a retrospective review of the medical records of 490 cancer patients from ten centers (8). Sargramostim-treated patients had significantly more frequent non-infectious fever, fatigue, diarrhea, injection site reactions, edema, and dermatological adverse effects, whereas skeletal pain was more frequent with filgrastim. In addition, switching to the alternative treatment was more frequent in the sargramostim group (18% of patients) than in the filgrastim group (none of the patients). The authors tried to minimize selection bias, but the strength of the results was limited by the retrospective nature of the study.

Susceptibility Factors

Age

Guidelines for the appropriate use of hemopoietic growth factors in children have been proposed by a panel of European experts, who carefully summarized the potential indications and recommendations, and concluded that adult guidelines are applicable to children in most cases (9). The authors considered that growth factors should be used in children for only a limited number of circumstances: prophylaxis or treatment in low-risk patients treated with chemotherapy, routine use in aplastic anemia, and mobilization of peripheral blood progenitor cells in healthy pediatric donors.

References

1. Sieff CA. Haemopoietic growth factors: in vitro and in vivo studies. In: Hoffbrand AV, editor. Recent Advances in Haematology 1. London: Churchill Livingstone, 1988:1.
2. Klingemann HG, Shepherd JD, Eaves CJ, Eaves AC. The role of erythropoietin and other growth factors in transfusion medicine. Transfus Med Rev 1991;5(1):33–47.
3. Vose JM, Armitage JO. Clinical applications of hematopoietic growth factors. J Clin Oncol 1995;13(4):1023–35.
4. Beauchesne MF, Shalansky SJ. Nonchemotherapy drug-induced agranulocytosis: a review of 118 patients treated with colony-stimulating factors. Pharmacotherapy 1999;19(3):299–305.
5. Vial T, Gallant C, Choquet-Kastylevsky G, Descotes J. Treatment of drug-induced agranulocytosis with haematopoietic growth factors. A review of the clinical experience. BioDrugs 1999;11:185–200.
6. Beveridge RA, Miller JA, Kales AN, Binder RA, Robert NJ, Harvey JH, Windsor K, Gore I, Cantrell J, Thompson KA, Taylor WR, Barnes HM, Schiff SA, Shields JA, Cambareri RJ, Butler TP, Meister RJ, Feigert JM, Norgard MJ, Moraes MA, Helvie WW, Patton GA, Mundy LJ, Henry D, Sheridan MJ, et al. A comparison of efficacy of sargramostim (yeast-derived RhuGM-CSF) and filgrastim (bacteria-derived RhuG-CSF) in the therapeutic setting of chemotherapy-induced myelosuppression. Cancer Invest 1998;16(6):366–73.
7. Fischmeister G, Kurz M, Haas OA, Micksche M, Buchinger P, Printz D, Ressmann G, Stroebel T, Peters C, Fritsch G, Gadner H. G-CSF versus GM-CSF for stimulation of peripheral blood progenitor cells (PBPC) and leukocytes in healthy volunteers: comparison of efficacy and tolerability. Ann Hematol 1999;78(3):117–23.
8. Milkovich G, Moleski RJ, Reitan JF, Dunning DM, Gibson GA, Paivanas TA, Wyant S, Jacobs RJ. Comparative safety of filgrastim versus sargramostim in patients receiving myelosuppressive chemotherapy. Pharmacotherapy 2000;20(12):1432–40.
9. Schaison G, Eden OB, Henze G, Kamps WA, Locatelli F, Ninane J, Ortega J, Riikonen P, Wagner HP. Recommendations on the use of colony-stimulating factors in children: conclusions of a European panel. Eur J Pediatr 1998;157(12):955–66.

Myristicaceae

See also Herbal medicines

General Information

There are three genera of the family of Myristicaceae:

- *Horsfieldia*
- *Myristica* (nutmeg)
- *Virola* (virola).

Myristica fragrans

Myristica fragrans (nutmeg) has long been a highly desired spice. In the seventeenth century physicians claimed that a nutmeg pomander was a cure for the bloody flux and the sweating sickness, later called the black plague, and nutmeg was also supposed to have aphrodisiac properties (1). Mace, the dried shell of the nutmeg, is used as a spice; it should not be confused with chemical Mace, which is a form of tear gas containing 1% chloracetophenone (CN) gas in a solvent of sec-butanol, propylene glycol, cyclohexene, and dipropylene glycol methyl ether; some formulations also include oleoresin *Capsicum* (from peppers).

Myristicin is methoxysafrole, the principal aromatic constituent of the volatile oil of nutmeg. Myristicin is also found in several members of the carrot family (Apiaceae, formerly Umbelliferae), such as *Petroselinum crispum* (parsley) (2). Safrole is a mutagenic and animal carcinogenic monoterpenoid. It is the major component of oil of sassafras, and lesser quantities occur in essential oils from cinnamon, mace, nutmeg, and star anise. Some of its known or possible metabolites have mutagenic activity in bacteria and it has weak hepatocarcinogenic effects in rodents. Experiments in mice have suggested the possibility of transplacental and lactational carcinogenesis. The carcinogenic effect is primarily mediated by the formation of 1′-hydroxysafrole, followed by sulfonation to an unstable sulfate that reacts to form DNA adducts; these metabolites are formed by CYP2C9 and CYP2E1, the latter contributing three-fold more to the metabolic clearance than the former (3).

Adverse effects

Asthma has been attributed to nutmeg (4).

- A 27-year-old man developed rhinitis and asthma 1 year after starting to prepare a certain kind of sausage, having a previous allergy to coconut, banana, and kiwi and allergic rhinitis to horses, cats, dogs, and cows. There was a positive immediate skin prick test with paprika (dry powder of *Capsicum annuum*), coriander (*Coriandrum sativum*), and mace (shell of *M. fragrans*) at concentrations of 10%. There were specific IgE antibodies to paprika, coriander, and mace.

Large doses of nutmeg seed can cause nausea, vomiting, flushing, dry mouth, tachycardia, nervous system stimulation possibly with epileptiform convulsions, miosis, mydriasis, euphoria, and hallucinations (5).

- A 16-year-old youth who had taken nutmeg for recreational purposes developed a number of neurological symptoms and signs along with non-specific electrocardiographic changes and anticholinergic-type symptoms (6).

Among 55 patients with suspected contact dermatitis, skin patch tests that were positive at concentrations of both 10% and 25% were most common with ginger ($n = 7$), nutmeg ($n = 5$), and oregano ($n = 4$); other spices produced no responses or one positive response (7). Positive reactions at only one concentration were more likely at 25%: nutmeg ($n = 5$), ginger and cayenne ($n = 4$), curry, cumin, and cinnamon ($n = 3$), turmeric, coriander, and sage ($n = 2$), oregano ($n = 1$), and basil and clove ($n = 0$).

Contact allergy has been reported with mace (8).

Nutmeg is sometimes abused for its hallucinogenic potential; less than one tablespoon can be enough to produce severe symptoms similar to those seen in anticholinergic poisoning (9,10). It can also cause psychosis, both acute (11,12) and chronic (13).

- A 13-year-old girl took 15–24 g of nutmeg in gelatin capsules over 3 hours and smoked two joints of marijuana (14). She developed bizarre behavior and visual, auditory, and tactile hallucinations, nausea, gagging, hot/cold sensations, and blurred vision, followed by numbness, double, and "triple" vision, headache, and drowsiness. There was nystagmus, muscle weakness, and ataxia. She received activated charcoal 50 g and recovered within 2 days.

Deaths from acute poisoning have been reported (15).

References

1. Milton G. Nathaniel's Nutmeg. Hodder and Stoughton: London, 1999.
2. Hallstrom H, Thuvander A. Toxicological evaluation of myristicin. Nat Toxins 1997;5(5):186–92.
3. Ueng YF, Hsieh CH, Don MJ, Chi CW, Ho LK. Identification of the main human cytochrome P450 enzymes involved in safrole 1′-hydroxylation. Chem Res Toxicol 2004;17(8):1151–6.
4. Sastre J, Olmo M, Novalvos A, Ibanez D, Lahoz C. Occupational asthma due to different spices. Allergy 1996;51(2):117 20.
5. Servan J, Chochon F, Duclos H. Hallucinations apres ingestion volontaire de noix de muscade: une toxicomanie méconnue. [Hallucinations after voluntary ingestion of nutmeg: an unrecognized drug abuse.] Rev Neurol (Paris) 1998;154(10):708.
6. McKenna A, Nordt SP, Ryan J. Acute nutmeg poisoning. Eur J Emerg Med 2004;11(4):240–1.
7. Futrell JM, Rietschel RL. Spice allergy evaluated by results of patch tests. Cutis 1993;52(5):288–90.
8. Frazier CA. Contact allergy to mace. JAMA 1976;236(22):2526.
9. Lavy G. Nutmeg intoxication in pregnancy. A case report. J Reprod Med 1987;32(1):63–4.
10. Abernethy MK, Becker LB. Acute nutmeg intoxication. Am J Emerg Med 1992;10(5):429–30.
11. Kelly BD, Gavin BE, Clarke M, Lane A, Larkin C. Nutmeg and psychosis. Schizophr Res 2003;60(1):95–6.
12. Dinakar HS. Acute psychosis associated with nutmeg toxicity. Med Times 1977;105(12):63–4.
13. Brenner N, Frank OS, Knight E. Chronic nutmeg psychosis. J R Soc Med 1993;86(3):179–80.
14. Sangalli BC, Chiang W. Toxicology of nutmeg abuse. J Toxicol Clin Toxicol 2000;38(6):671–8.
15. Stein U, Greyer H, Hentschel H. Nutmeg (myristicin) poisoning—report on a fatal case and a series of cases recorded by a poison information centre. Forensic Sci Int 2001;118(1):87–90.

Myrrh

General Information

Myrrh is an oleo gum resin obtained from the stem of *Commiphora molmol*, a tree that grows in north-east Africa and the Arabian Peninsula. In mice, myrrh showed no mutagenic effects and was a potent cytotoxic drug against solid tumor cells (1). The antitumor potential of *Commiphora molmol* was comparable with that of cyclophosphamide. Studies in hamsters suggested an antischistosomal activity of myrrh (2).

Observational studies

Facioliasis

The efficacy of myrrh has been studied in seven patients aged 10–41 years (five men, two women) with fascioliasis and 10 age- and sex-matched healthy volunteers (3). Myrrh was given orally in the morning on an empty stomach in a dosage of 12 mg/kg/day for 6 days. All the patients were passing *Fasciola* eggs in their stools (mean 36 eggs per gram of stool). The symptoms and signs of fascioliasis resolved during treatment with myrrh, and *Fasciola* eggs could not be demonstrated in the stools 3 weeks and 3 months after treatment. Antifasciola antibody titers became negative in six of the seven patients. There were no adverse effects.

Schistosomiasis

The efficacy and adverse effects of myrrh and the most effective dosage schedule have been studied in 204 patients (169 men and 35 women) with schistosomiasis aged 12–68 years and 20 healthy non-infected age- and sex-matched volunteers (2). The patients were divided into two groups: 86 patients with schistosomal colitis and 118 with hepatosplenic schistosomiasis, further divided into two subgroups—77 patients with compensated disease and 41 with decompensated disease. All but 12 had received one or more courses of praziquantel. The dosage of myrrh was 10 mg/kg/day for 3 days on an empty stomach 1 hour before breakfast. A second course of 10 mg/kg/day for 6 days was given to patients who still had living ova in rectal or colonic biopsy specimens. The response rate to a single course of myrrh was 92% in 187 patients. The cure rates were 91, 94, and 90% in patients with schistosomal colitis, compensated hepatosplenic schistosomiasis, and decompensated hepatosplenic schistosomiasis respectively. The cure rate was less in patients who had previously taken praziquantel and in patients with impaired liver function. *Schistosoma hematobium* infection was the most responsive ($n = 4$, cure rate 100%), followed by mixed infections ($n = 29$, cure rate 93%). Those infected with *Schistosoma mansoni* had the lowest cure rate ($n = 171$, cure rate 91%). There was no impairment of liver function after treatment with myrrh. In contrast, liver function tests significantly improved in patients with impaired liver function. There were no significant effects of myrrh on the electrocardiogram. Adverse effects of myrrh were reported in 24 of the 204 patients. Giddiness, somnolence, or mild fatigue were the most common (2.5%), and all other adverse effects were minor and less frequent. None of the healthy volunteers reported any adverse effects, nor were there any significant changes in liver or kidney function. A second course of myrrh resulted in a cure in 13 of the 17 patients who did not respond to a single course.

References

1. al-Harbi MM, Qureshi S, Ahmed MM, Rafatullah S, Shah AH. Effect of *Commiphora molmol* (oleo-gum-resin) on the cytological and biochemical changes induced by cyclophosphamide in mice. Am J Chin Med 1994;22(1):77–82.
2. Sheir Z, Nasr AA, Massoud A, Salama O, Badra GA, El-Shennawy H, Hassan N, Hammad SM. A safe, effective, herbal antischistosomal therapy derived from myrrh. Am J Trop Med Hyg 2001;65(6):700–4.
3. Massoud A, El Sisi S, Salama O, Massoud A. Preliminary study of therapeutic efficacy of a new fasciolicidal drug derived from *Commiphora molmol* (myrrh). Am J Trop Med Hyg 2001;65(2):96–9.

Myrtaceae

See also Herbal medicines

General Information

The family of Myrtaceae (Table 1) includes guava and various types of gums.

Eucalyptus species

Eucalyptus oil has been used in different medications to relieve symptoms of asthma and rhinitis and is a constituent of cold remedies and ointments designed to be rubbed on to the chest or applied around and even into the nostrils (Vicks Vaporub, Obat Madjan, etc.). Applied to the skin it acts as a rubefacient and counterirritant, but substantial concentrations of volatile oil can be inhaled from the skin. Eucalyptus oil has also been used systemically to treat asthma.

Adverse effects

Fever and headache occurred in a heavy consumer of eucalyptus extract (1).

Table 1 The genera of Myrtaceae

Baeckea (baeckea)
Callistemon (bottle brush)
Calothamnus (net bush)
Calyptranthes (mountain bay)
Chamelaucium (chamelaucium)
Corymbia (corymbia)
Eucalyptus (gum)
Eugenia (stopper)
Feijoa (feijoa)
Gomidesia (gomidesia)
Leptospermum (tea tree)
Lophostemon (lophostemon)
Marlierea (marlierea)
Melaleuca (melaleuca)
Metrosideros (lehua)
Myrcia (rodwood)
Myrcianthes (myrcianthes)
Myrciaria (guava berry)
Myrtus (myrtus)
Pimenta (pimenta)
Pseudanamomis (pseudanamomis)
Psidium (guava)
Rhodomyrtus (rhodomyrtus)
Siphoneugena (siphoneugena)
Syncarpia (turpentine tree)
Syzygium (syzygium)
Tristaniopsis (tristaniopsis)

Respiratory
Asthma can be exacerbated by eucalyptus (2).

- In a 30-year-old woman the symptoms of asthma and rhinoconjunctivitis were exacerbated by eucalyptus pollens and by ingestion of an infusion containing eucalyptus. There were specific IgE antibodies to eucalyptus pollens but not to common aeroallergens.

Eucalyptus oil has been reported to cause vocal cord dysfunction (3).

- A 46-year-old woman with vocal cord dysfunction associated with exposure to eucalyptus underwent inhalation challenges consisting of water, ammonia, pine oil, and a combination of eucalyptus (dried leaves) and ammonia. Vocal cord dysfunction occurred within minutes of exposure to eucalyptus.

Skin
Contact urticaria has been ascribed to eucalyptus pollen (4).

Drug overdose
Eucalyptus oil has caused death in doses of up to 560 ml in adults and 15 ml in children.

- A 73-year-old woman who deliberately took 200–250 ml of eucalyptus oil was found unconscious in her home after she had vomited and had been incontinent of urine and feces. Despite intensive treatment she developed pneumonitis and aspiration pneumonia to which she ultimately succumbed (5).

In a telephone survey of 109 parents or guardians of children under 5 years who had been involved in actual or suspected ingestion of eucalyptus oil, 90 incidents had involved vaporizer solutions, 15 eucalyptus oil formulations, and the remainder other medicinal products containing eucalyptus oil (6).

In a retrospective analysis of case histories of 109 children admitted to the Royal Children's Hospital, Melbourne, between 1 January 1981 and 31 December 1992 with a diagnosis of eucalyptus oil poisoning, there were clinical effects in 59%; 31 had depression of consciousness, 27 were drowsy, three were unconscious after taking known or estimated volumes of 5–10 ml, and one was unconscious with hypoventilation after taking an estimated 75 ml (7). Vomiting occurred in 37%, ataxia in 15%, and pulmonary disease in 11%. No treatment was given to 12%; ipecac or oral activated charcoal was given to 21%, nasogastric charcoal to 57%, and gastric lavage without anesthesia to 4% and under anesthesia to 6%. All recovered.

Of 42 children with oral eucalyptus oil poisoning, 33 were entirely asymptomatic (8). This group included all of the four children who were reported to have taken more than 30 ml of eucalyptus oil. Only two of the others had symptoms or clinical signs on presentation to hospital. No child required advanced life support. There was no correlation between the amount of eucalyptus oil taken and the presence of symptoms.

Systemic eucalyptus oil toxicity can result from topical application.

- A 6-year-old girl presented with slurred speech, ataxia and muscle weakness progressing to unconsciousness following the widespread application of a home remedy for urticaria containing eucalyptus oil. Six hours after removal of the topical preparation her symptoms had resolved and there were no long-term sequelae (9).

Administrative route
Systemic effects of eucalyptus oil applied locally have been reported (9).

- A 6-year-old girl was treated with a home-made concoction mainly containing 50 ml of eucalyptus oil (consisting of 80–85% cineole oil) for pruritus. As the mixture seemed to relieve her symptoms, the parents applied it more and more generously to the girl's skin. She subsequently developed symptoms of intoxication: slurred speech, unsteady gait, and drowsiness. Eventually she lost consciousness and was unrousable. She was admitted to hospital, where several tests were negative, but her urine sample contained components of eucalyptus oil. She made a full recovery within 24 hours after withdrawal of the external herbal treatment.

Melaleuca species

The undiluted essential oil from the leaves of *Melaleuca alternifolia* (tea tree), which contains the sesquiterpene viridiflorene and the monoterpenoids eucalyptol, limonene, and terpinen-4-ol, has been used as a topical natural cure for bacterial and fungal skin infections.

Adverse effects
Nervous system

- A 23-month-old boy became confused and was unable to walk 30 minutes after ingesting less than 10 ml of T36-C7, a commercial product containing 100% tea tree oil (10). His condition improved and he was asymptomatic within 5 hours of ingestion.

Skin
Tea tree oil can have adverse effects on the skin (11). Several patients developed an allergic contact dermatitis (12), which was most commonly caused by the constituent d-limonene (13). Internal use of half a teaspoonful of the oil can result in a dramatic rash (14), whereas half a teacup can induce coma followed by a semiconscious state with hallucinations (15). Less than 10 ml is sufficient to produce serious signs of toxicity in small children.

- In one case, allergic contact dermatitis to tea tree oil presented with an extensive erythema multiforme-like reaction (16). However, a skin biopsy from a target-like lesion showed a spongiotic dermatitis without the features of erythema multiforme. Five months after treatment with systemic and topical glucocorticoids, patch testing elicited a 3+ reaction to old, oxidized tea tree oil, a 2+ reaction to fresh tea tree oil, a 2+ reaction to colophony, a 1+ reaction to abitol, and a 1+ reaction to balsam of Peru.

Of 1216 patients who were patch tested, 14 with eczema had used products (creams, hair products, and essential oils) containing tea tree oil (17). They were patch tested for a standard panel of allergens, topical emulgents, perfumes, plants, topical medications, metal, gloves, topical

Nabumetone

See also Non-steroidal anti-inflammatory drugs

General Information

Nabumetone is a naproxen derivative, whose efficacy is related to its active metabolite, 6-methoxy-2-naphthylacetic acid. Not unexpectedly, a study in 2000 patients, mostly treated for more than 6 months, elicited an adverse events pattern similar to the other derivatives of this class of NSAIDs (SEDA-13, 81). Adverse effects were reported in 18% of patients and 10% stopped taking the drug because of adverse reactions. Diarrhea was the most common problem (13%) followed by abdominal pain (9.9%), dyspepsia (9.3%), nausea (7.8%), and flatulence (4.7%). Ten ulcers were detected. Nervous system reactions, skin rashes, edema, unspecified eye disorders, and liver function test abnormalities all occur (1).

A postmarketing surveillance study in 10 800 patients with osteoarthritis and rheumatoid arthritis, who were followed up at 12 months, reported that 12% of patients discontinued the drug because of adverse events; 11 serious events may have been related to nabumetone and seven of these were gastrointestinal hemorrhage (2). In 6148 patients treated with nabumetone in long term trials, the 3-month cumulative incidence of clinically detected perforations, ulcers, and bleeding was 0.1% and the 6-month incidence was 0.2% (3).

Organs and Systems

Metabolism

Nabumetone-induced pseudoporphyria has been described (SEDA-16, 11) (SEDA 22, 117), and a further five cases in four adults and a child have been reported (4–6).

Gastrointestinal

Being a non-acidic compound and a weak inhibitor of prostaglandin synthesis, nabumetone was designed as a prodrug that could be administered without causing gastric damage. This theoretical advantage still awaits confirmation. Although there was no gastrointestinal toxicity in animals, in humans gastric problems with NSAIDs are not primarily a local effect but are exerted systemically, so a metabolite formed after gastric passage could still cause gastric problems. Again, although radiochromium evaluation of gastrointestinal blood loss in healthy volunteers and endoscopic studies in patients with rheumatoid arthritis showed that nabumetone provokes less gastric damage than naproxen, the usual defects of such studies limit their clinical relevance (SEDA-13, 81). The same applies to the preliminary results of a long-term study in patients with osteoarthritis and rheumatoid arthritis, which also showed that nabumetone is less gastrotoxic than naproxen, but it was not possible to exclude the possibility that the dosage was lower than was needed for optimal efficacy (7).

Susceptibility Factors

Age

After repeated once-daily doses, nabumetone accumulates in elderly patients but not in others; it is therefore wise to reduce the dose in elderly patients.

Drug–Drug Interactions

Warfarin

Concomitant therapy with warfarin and NSAIDs is of concern, owing to the potential for increasing bleeding.

- In a 72-year-old man the concomitant use of nabumetone and warfarin led to an increased international normalized ratio and hemarthrosis (8).

Previous reports suggested a lack of interaction of nabumetone with warfarin, but close monitoring is advisable when these two drugs are co-administered.

References

1. Jenner PN, Johnson ES. Review of the experience with nabumetone in clinical trials outside of the United States. Am J Med 1987;83(4B):110–14.
2. Jenner PN. A 12-month postmarketing surveillance study of nabumetone. A preliminary report. Drugs 1990;40(Suppl 5):80–6.
3. Lipani JA, Poland M. Clinical update of the relative safety of nabumetone in long-term clinical trials. Inflammopharmacology 1995;3:351–61.
4. Antony F, Layton AM. Nabumetone-associated pseudoporphyria. Br J Dermatol 2000;142(5):1067–9.
5. Checketts SR, Morgan GJ Jr. Two cases of nabumetone induced pseudoporphyria. J Rheumatol 1999;26(12):2703–5.
6. Cron RQ, Finkel TH. Nabumetone induced pseudoporphyria in childhood. J Rheumatol 2000;27(7):1817–18.
7. Roth SH. New understandings of NSAID gastropathy. Scand J Rheumatol Suppl 1989;78:24–9.
8. Dennis VC, Thomas BK, Hanlon JE. Potentiation of oral anticoagulation and hemarthrosis associated with nabumetone. Clin Reumatol 2000;75:967–70.

Naftidrofuryl

General Information

Naftidrofuryl is a complex acid ester of diethylaminoethanol, with direct vasodilatory properties and antagonistic effects on 5-HT (via 5-HT_2 receptors) and bradykinin. It also causes an intracellular increase in ATP concentrations, improves cellular oxidative metabolism (by activating succinate dehydrogenase), and reduces blood and plasma viscosity and fibrinogen concentrations.

Naftidrofuryl has been marketed in Europe for over 20 years for the treatment of peripheral and cerebrovascular diseases and for senile dementia (1). A few placebo-controlled studies have reported increases in drinking and improving alcohol abstinence in the short term, considering that the studies lasted for only 12 weeks. Additional long-term follow-up studies, with the possibility of studying outcomes of naltrexone treatment programs after stopping the drug and with suitable comparison groups, are necessary. Similar results with similar conclusions were seen in a 12-week randomized controlled trial in 55 alcohol-dependent men treated with naltrexone 50 mg or placebo (2).

To examine the relation between adverse effects profiles, study retention, and treatment outcomes in alcohol-dependent individuals receiving naltrexone for relapse prevention, 92 subjects had their adverse effects monitored weekly and categorized as either neuropsychiatric or gastrointestinal (3). The neuropsychiatric adverse effects had little effect on medication compliance but reduced the length of study retention. In contrast, the gastrointestinal adverse effects significantly affected medication compliance but not study retention.

In an open, single-blind, randomized study, naltrexone (50 mg/day) and acamprosate (1665–1998 mg/day) were used for 1 year by 157 recently detoxified alcohol-dependent men with moderate dependence (4). The time to first relapse was 63 days (naltrexone) and 42 days (acamprosate); after 1 year, 41% of those given naltrexone and 17% of those given acamprosate had not relapsed. Adverse effects were more common with naltrexone and were worse during the first 2 weeks of treatment. They included nausea (25 versus 4%), abdominal pain (23 versus 4%), drowsiness (35 versus 2%), headache (13 versus 6%), and nasal congestion (23 versus 7%).

The Health Technology Board of Scotland has concluded that in people with alcohol dependence, naltrexone reduces drinking (5). In a multicenter, double-blind, placebo-controlled, 12-week study of naltrexone 50 mg/day in 202 patients with alcohol dependence naltrexone was well tolerated, with few adverse effects: abdominal pain (8.6%), headache (7.5%), nausea (6.5%), and dizziness (5.4%); there were no changes in liver function tests (6). However, those who took naltrexone did not have significant improvements in drinking history or fewer relapses.

Pruritus

Naltrexone 50 mg/day has been used to relieve pruritus in cholestatic liver disease in five patients (7). Pruritus scores fell, but two patients developed severe nausea, vomiting, light-headedness, or tremor, requiring withdrawal of treatment. The reviewers commented that these reactions may or may not have been related to opioid withdrawal and that the trial had had several design limitations. They pointed out that one concern relating to the chronic use of high-dose naltrexone is an asymptomatic rise in serum transaminases, although the doses used in this study have not been reported to produce liver function abnormalities.

Organs and Systems

Nervous system

Headache occurred in two children, and an opioid withdrawal syndrome occurred in one child during the first 3 days of treatment when naltrexone was given for protracted apnea in children with increased beta-endorphin concentrations in the cerebrospinal fluid (8).

Psychological, psychiatric

Panic attacks precipitated by naltrexone have been reported (9).

- A 29-year-old woman with bulimia nervosa and a family history of anxiety was enrolled in a trial of naltrexone (100 mg/day). She had no history of opioid use. Within hours of her first dose she experienced alarm, anxiety, chest discomfort, shortness of breath, a fear of dying, sweating, nausea, and derealization. She was unable to remain at home or to go out alone. For 3 days she continued to take naltrexone, with an increasing frequency of panic attacks. On day 4 she was treated with alprazolam (0.5 mg) but relapsed after further naltrexone. Withdrawal of naltrexone led to complete remission of symptoms.

This effect was attributed to an action of naltrexone in removing the endogenous opioid effect at OP_3 (μ) opioid receptors in the locus ceruleus and thus resulting in unchecked noradrenergic hyperactivity.

Acute psychosis secondary to the use of naltrexone has been reported (10).

- A 44-year-old physically healthy woman developed auditory and visual hallucinations and persecutory delusions. She had been given naltrexone hydrochloride 50 mg/day 3 days before the acute psychotic incident in order to prevent relapse of alcohol dependence. Her psychotic symptoms completely resolved 48 hours after withdrawal of naltrexone.

In studies of its use in treating alcohol, opioid, and nicotine dependence, naltrexone has not been reported to cause depression or dysphoria. Patients who complain of naltrexone-associated dysphoria often have co-morbid depressive disorders or depression resulting from opioid or alcohol withdrawal states (11). Co-morbid depression is not a contraindication to naltrexone. Small pilot studies have supported the use of naltrexone in combination with antidepressants for the treatment of patients with co-morbid depression. The risk of non-fatal overdose is significantly increased after naltrexone treatment, as a result of reduced tolerance, compared with patients taking substitution methadone (12).

Hematologic

Idiopathic thrombocytopenic purpura has been attributed to naltrexone (13).

Gastrointestinal

The risk factors for naltrexone-induced nausea have been studied in 120 alcohol-dependent patients in an open trial (14). After 5–30 days of abstinence, they received a bolus dose of naltrexone 25 mg followed by 50 mg/day for 10 weeks. Moderate to severe nausea was reported in 15%. The risk of nausea was significantly predicted by poor medication compliance, intensity of drinking during treatment, short duration of abstinence, young age, and female sex.

Gastrointestinal adverse effects of naltrexone were also observed in 183 alcohol-dependent individuals who received either naltrexone or nefazodone (15). These adverse effects predicated early termination of naltrexone used to treat alcohol dependence (16).

Liver

Reversible hepatocellular injury has been reported with naltrexone in doses of up to 300 mg/day, which is five times that usually used for opioid blockade (SED-11, 147) (17). Five of twenty-six patients treated with naltrexone for obesity developed raised serum transaminase activities after 3–8 weeks of treatment. In another study in which 60 obese subjects received naltrexone for 8 weeks, there were abnormal liver function tests in six patients. Three patients failed to complete the course. Nausea and vomiting occurred within the first 24 hours of treatment but responded to a reduction in dose. There were also changes in mentation such as decreased mental acuity, depression, and anxiety, all of which resolved after withdrawal. This is significant, as adverse effects from naltrexone have previously been attributed to mild physical withdrawal syndromes.

Biliary tract

A woman with chronic cholestasis and disabling pruritus had severe but transient opioid withdrawal-like reactions after oral naltrexone 12.5 mg and 2 mg (18). This observation suggests the hypothesis that increased central opioidergic tone is a component of the pathophysiology of cholestasis.

Skin

Skin rashes have been attributed to naltrexone (SEDA-21, 92).

Musculoskeletal

Rhabdomyolysis has been attributed to naltrexone (19).

- A 28-year-old alcoholic was given naltrexone 50 mg/day on the eighth day of a detoxification regimen. On day 17 there was a marked rise in creatine kinase activity (2654 U/l) but no accompanying symptoms of myalgia, weakness, or chest pain. Naltrexone was withheld immediately. The creatine kinase peaked at over 18 000 U/l on day 19 and then fell to within the reference range by day 25. A diagnosis of rhabdomyolysis without accompanying renal insufficiency was suggested.

Long-Term Effects

Drug abuse

Three opiate-dependent individuals abused intravenous naltrexone, believing it to be diamorphine, and developed acute opiate withdrawal symptoms; they were managed with a combined regimen of diazepam, prochlorperazine, and hyoscine (20,21).

Drug Administration

Drug administration route

Six cases of complications loosely related to the use of naltrexone pellet implantation during the highly controversial rapid and ultra-rapid opioid detoxification procedures have been reported (22). These included pulmonary edema, prolonged opioid withdrawal states, drug toxicity, withdrawal from cross-dependence to alcohol and benzodiazepines, aspiration pneumonia, and death. The risk of these controversial procedures and of naltrexone in this novel delivery system are high; a robust scientifically validated program of research is needed to justify such treatment packages.

Drug–Drug Interactions

Clonidine

When naltrexone was given to a group of clonidine-detoxified opioid-dependent subjects, several complained of anorexia and weight loss (23).

Diazepam

The effects of naltrexone on diazepam intoxication were investigated in 26 non-drug-abusing subjects who received either naltrexone 50 mg or placebo and 90 minutes later oral diazepam 10 mg in a double-blind crossover trial (24). Naltrexone was significantly associated with negative mood states, such as sedation, fatigue, and anxiety, compared with placebo, while positive states (friendliness, vigor, liking the effects of diazepam, feeling high from diazepam) were significantly more common with placebo. Naltrexone significantly delayed the time to peak diazepam concentrations (135 minutes) compared with placebo (75 minutes), but there were no significant differences in the concentrations of nordiazepam, the main metabolite of diazepam, at any stage in the study.

References

1. Streeton C, Whelan G. Naltrexone, a relapse prevention maintenance treatment of alcohol dependence: a meta-analysis of randomized controlled trials. Alcohol Alcohol 2001;36(6):544–52.
2. Morris PL, Hopwood M, Whelan G, Gardiner J, Drummond E. Naltrexone for alcohol dependence: a randomized controlled trial. Addiction 2001;96(11):1565–73.
3. Oncken C, Van Kirk J, Kranzler HR. Adverse effects of oral naltrexone: analysis of data from two clinical trials. Psychopharmacology (Berl) 2001;154(4):397–402.
4. Rubio G, Jimenez-Arriero MA, Ponce G, Palomo T. Naltrexone versus acamprosate: one year follow-up of alcohol dependence treatment. Alcohol Alcohol 2001;36(5):419–25.
5. Slattery J, Chick J, Cochrane M, Craig J, Godfrey C, Macpherson K, Parrott S, Quinn S, Tochel C, Watson H. Prevention of relapse in alcohol dependence. Health Technology Assessment Report 3. Glasgow: Health Technology Board for Scotland, 2003.

200 mg/day was added in an attempt to improve persistent negative symptoms, and after a week the dosage was increased to 300 mg/day. One week later, he reported anxiety and dizziness and was hypotensive. The combined concentrations of clozapine and its active metabolite norclozapine had increased from 309 ng/ml before nefazodone to 566 ng/ml. The nefazodone dosage was reduced to 200 mg/day and the anxiety, dizziness, and hypotension resolved over the next 7 days. At the same time plasma concentrations of clozapine and norclozapine fell to 370 ng/ml.

These results suggest that in some individuals CYP3A4 plays a significant role in the metabolism of clozapine and that the combination of nefazodone and clozapine should therefore be used with caution. It is possible that in this case concomitant treatment with risperidone may have increased the effect of nefazodone to reduce the clearance of clozapine.

Selective serotonin re-uptake inhibitors (SSRIs)

Concentrations of nefazodone and its metabolites can be increased by fluoxetine and paroxetine (SEDA-20, 9). Combinations of serotonin agents produce serotonin toxicity, and a case of serotonin syndrome occurred when nefazodone (200 mg/day) was combined with fluoxetine (40 mg/day) in a 50-year-old man (24). The toxic symptoms settled 3 days after withdrawal of both antidepressants.

Statins

Nefazodone can cause myositis and rhabdomyolysis in patients taking pravastatin and simvastatin (25). The postulated mechanism involves inhibition of CYP3A4, leading to reduced clearance of the HMG-CoA reductase inhibitors and muscle toxicity.

Substrates of CYP3A4

Nefazodone is a weak inhibitor of CYP2D6, but a potent inhibitor of CYP3A4, and increases plasma concentrations of drugs that are substrates of CYP3A4, such as triazolam, alprazolam, ciclosporin, astemizole, cisapride, terfenadine, and carbamazepine (26). Co-administration with terfenadine, astemizole, or cisapride should be avoided, because of the risk of cardiac dysrhythmias (SEDA-20, 9).

Terfenadine

Drugs that inhibit CYP3A4 inhibit the clearance of terfenadine, an antihistamine that can prolong the QT_c interval. This can cause potentially dangerous interactions. In a double-blind, placebo-controlled study of the effect of nefazodone (600 mg/day for 1 week) on the pharmacokinetics of terfenadine (120 mg/day for 14 days) and another antihistamine, loratadine (20 mg/day for 14 days), in 67 healthy volunteers, nefazodone significantly reduced the clearance of terfenadine and prolonged the mean QT_c interval (27). In addition, nefazodone produced a similar but smaller decrease in the clearance of loratadine and combined treatment also significantly increased the QT_c interval. This effect of nefazodone on the clearance of terfenadine is predictable, as is the increase in QT_c interval. Loratadine is also partly metabolized by CYP2D6, which probably explains the lesser effect of nefazodone on loratadine clearance. Loratadine by itself does not increase the QT_c interval significantly, but cardiotoxicity may be a possibility when it is combined with nefazodone.

References

1. Fontaine R. Novel serotonergic mechanisms and clinical experience with nefazodone. Clin Neuropharmacol 1992;15(Suppl 1:Part A):99A.
2. Nemeroff CB. Evolutionary trends in the pharmacotherapeutic management of depression. J Clin Psychiatry 1994;55(Suppl):3–15.
3. Rush AJ, Armitage R, Gillin JC, Yonkers KA, Winokur A, Moldofsky H, Vogel GW, Kaplita SB, Fleming JB, Montplaisir J, Erman MK, Albala BJ, McQuade RD. Comparative effects of nefazodone and fluoxetine on sleep in outpatients with major depressive disorder. Biol Psychiatry 1998;44(1):3–14.
4. Lerner V, Matar MA, Polyakova I. Nefazodone-associated subjective complaints of burning sensations. J Clin Psychiatry 2000;61(3):216–17.
5. Dubin H, Spier S, Giannandrea P. Nefazodone-induced mania. Am J Psychiatry 1997;154(4):578–9.
6. Warnock JK, Biggs F. Nefazodone-induced hypoglycemia in a diabetic patient with major depression. Am J Psychiatry 1997;154(2):288–9.
7. Schrader GD, Roberts-Thompson IC. Adverse effect of nefazodone: hepatitis. Med J Aust 1999;170(9):452.
8. Lucena MI, Andrade RJ, Gomez-Outes A, Rubio M, Cabello MR. Acute liver failure after treatment with nefazodone. Dig Dis Sci 1999;44(12):2577–9.
9. Aranda-Michel J, Koehler A, Bejarano PA, Poulos JE, Luxon BA, Khan CM, Ee LC, Balistreri WF, Weber FL Jr. Nefazodone-induced liver failure: report of three cases. Ann Intern Med 1999;130(4 Part 1):285–8.
10. Schirren CA, Baretton G. Nefazodone-induced acute liver failure. Am J Gastroenterol 2000;95(6):1596–7.
11. Eloubeidi MA, Gaede JT, Swaim MW. Reversible nefazodone-induced liver failure. Dig Dis Sci 2000;45(5):1036–8.
12. Khan AY, Preskorn SH. Increase in plasma levels of clozapine and norclozapine after administration of nefazodone. J Clin Psychiatry 2001;62(5):375–6.
13. Gupta S, Gilroy WR. Hair loss associated with nefazodone. J Fam Pract 1997;44:20–1.
14. Brodie-Meijer CC, Diemont WL, Buijs PJ. Nefazodone-induced clitoral priapism. Int Clin Psychopharmacol 1999;14(4):257–8.
15. Benazzi F. Nefazodone withdrawal symptoms. Can J Psychiatry 1998;43(2):194–5.
16. Rajagopalan M, Little J. Discontinuation symptoms with nefazodone. Aust NZ J Psychiatry 1999;33(4):594–7.
17. Lauber C. Nefazodone withdrawal syndrome. Can J Psychiatry 1999;44(3):285–6.
18. Kotlyar M, Golding M, Brewer ER, Carson SW. Possible nefazodone withdrawal syndrome. Am J Psychiatry 1999;156(7):1117.
19. Yapp P, Ilett KF, Kristensen JH, Hackett LP, Paech MJ, Rampono J. Drowsiness and poor feeding in a breast-fed infant: association with nefazodone and its metabolites. Ann Pharmacother 2000;34(11):1269–72.
20. Benson BE, Mathiason M, Dahl B, Smith K, Foley MM, Easom LA, Butler AY. Toxicities and outcomes associated with nefazodone poisoning. An analysis of 1,338 exposures. Am J Emerg Med 2000;18(5):587–92.

21. Laroudie C, Salazar DE, Cosson JP, Cheuvart B, Istin B, Girault J, Ingrand I, Decourt JP. Carbamazepine–nefazodone interaction in healthy subjects. J Clin Psychopharmacol 2000;20(1):46–53.
22. Taylor D, Bodani M, Hubbeling A, Murray R. The effect of nefazodone on clozapine plasma concentrations. Int Clin Psychopharmacol 1999;14(3):185–7.
23. Khan AY, Preskorn SH. Increase in plasma levels of clozapine and norclozapine after administration of nefazodone. J Clin Psychiatry 2001;62:375–6.
24. Smith DL, Wenegrat BG. A case report of serotonin syndrome associated with combined nefazodone and fluoxetine. J Clin Psychiatry 2000;61(2):146.
25. Alderman CP. Possible interaction between nefazodone and pravastatin. Ann Pharmacother 1999;33(7–8):871.
26. Wright DH, Lake KD, Bruhn PS, Emery RW Jr. Nefazodone and cyclosporine drug–drug interaction. J Heart Lung Transplant 1999;18(9):913–15.
27. Abernethy DR, Barbey JT, Franc J, Brown KS, Feirrera I, Ford N, Salazar DE. Loratadine and terfenadine interaction with nefazodone: both antihistamines are associated with QTc prolongation. Clin Pharmacol Ther 2001;69(3):96–103.

Nefopam

General Information

Nefopam, an orphenadrine derivative, is a centrally acting non-opioid analgesic. Various adverse effects have been reported, including nausea, vomiting, epigastric pain, dizziness, drowsiness and mental confusion, hypotension, tachycardia, skin rashes, xerostomia, and urinary retention; some of these may be related to its anticholinergic properties (SEDA-11, 100). Its unsatisfactory adverse effects profile was confirmed in two studies of pain control in cancer and rheumatoid arthritis (SEDA-15, 104)

In one study, five of 33 patients (15%) stopped treatment because of the severity of adverse effects attributed to nefopam (1).

In an open trial 120 patients undergoing elective hepatic resection were randomized to receive postoperative intravenous patient-controlled analgesia with morphine either alone or in combination with nefopam (20 mg 4-hourly) or propacetamol (2 g 6-hourly) (2). Nefopam plus morphine was the most effective treatment. Adverse effects, especially sedation, were comparable in the three groups, but there was significantly more nausea in the morphine group and more sweating in the nefopam group (requiring early drug withdrawal in three cases). Tachycardia was seen more often in the nefopam group but did not reach significance.

Organs and Systems

Urinary tract

There have been 53 cases of reversible urinary retention, hesitancy, a poor stream, or dribbling reported to the UK Committee on Safety of Medicines.

Long-Term Effects

Drug abuse

Three cases of nefopam abuse have been reported (3). The patients had the same pattern of a history of chronic pain, concomitant anxiolytic and antidepressant drug therapy, and abuse of nefopam due to its primarily psychostimulant-like symptoms. The recommended dose of nefopam is 20 mg intramuscularly every 6 hours, with a maximum recommended dose of 120 mg/day. Daily consumption in the three patients was 120–1840 mg/day.

Susceptibility Factors

The UK Committee on Safety of Medicines received 12 reports of confusion and 22 of hallucinations and recommended that nefopam be used with caution in the elderly, in patients with symptoms of urinary retention, or in conjunction with other drugs that have anticholinergic activity (4).

References

1. Minotti V, Patoia L, Roila F, Basurto C, Tonato M, Pasqualucci V, Maresca V, Del Favero A. Double-blind evaluation of analgesic efficacy of orally administered diclofenac, nefopam, and acetylsalicylic acid (ASA) plus codeine in chronic cancer pain. Pain 1989;36(2):177–83.
2. Mimoz O, Incagnoli P, Josse C, Gillon MC, Kuhlman L, Mirand A, Soilleux H, Fletcher D. Analgesic efficacy and safety of nefopam vs. propacetamol following hepatic resection. Anaesthesia 2001;56(6):520–5.
3. Villier C, Mallaret MP. Nefopam abuse. Ann Pharmacother 2002;36(10):1564–6.
4. D'Arcy PF. Drug reactions and interactions. Int Pharm J 1989;3:91.

Nelfinavir

See also Protease inhibitors

General Information

Nelfinavir is a non-peptidic inhibitor of the HIV protease. Its most prominent adverse effect is diarrhea, which occurs in up to one-third of individuals. However, the diarrhea is usually mild and can be controlled, if necessary, by antidiarrheal agents (1). Other adverse effects, including rash, nausea, headache, and weakness, are reported in under 5%.

Observational studies

In a multicenter, open, uncontrolled trial of protease inhibitors in conjunction with NRTIs for at least 96 weeks in 32 children, the pharmacokinetics of nelfinavir showed large interindividual differences (2). In all, 17 children suffered adverse events, most of which were mild and occurred early in treatment. The rate of drug-related adverse effects was 0.16 per patient-year in those taking nelfinavir.

neuroleptic drugs, the pooled results of a total of 14 trials suggested that amisulpride was more effective in improving global state ($n = 651$), general mental state ($n = 695$), and the negative symptoms of schizophrenia ($n = 506$). Amisulpride was as effective as typical neuroleptic drugs in relieving positive symptoms. It was less likely to cause at least one general adverse event ($n = 751$), to cause one extrapyramidal symptom ($n = 771$), or to require the use of antiparkinsonian drugs ($n = 851$). There were no clear differences in other adverse events compared with typical drugs. Amisulpride also seemed to be more acceptable than typical drugs, as measured by early withdrawal ($n = 1512$) than typical drugs, but this result may have been overestimated owing to publication bias, which could not be excluded with certainty.

A further meta-analysis of 10 randomized controlled clinical trials of amisulpride in "acutely ill patients" ($n = 1654$) was supported in part by a grant from Sanofi-Synthélabo, the marketing authorization holder (20). Amisulpride was significantly better than typical neuroleptic drugs by about 11% on the BPRS. In four studies in patients with "persistent negative symptoms," amisulpride was significantly better than placebo ($n = 514$), but there was no significant difference between amisulpride and typical drugs (only three studies; $n = 130$). Low doses of amisulpride (50–300 mg/day) were not associated with significantly more use of antiparkinsonian drugs than placebo ($n = 507$), and usual doses caused fewer extrapyramidal adverse effects than typical neuroleptic drugs ($n = 1599$). In four studies in acutely ill patients, significantly fewer patients taking amisulpride dropped out compared with patients taking typical drugs, mainly because of fewer adverse events; in three small studies with conventional neuroleptic drugs as comparators there was only a trend in favor of amisulpride in this regard.

Amisulpride versus flupenthixol

In a randomized, double-blind, multicenter comparison of amisulpride 1000 mg/day ($n = 70$) and flupenthixol 25 mg/day ($n = 62$) for 6 weeks, the two drugs significantly improved the acute psychotic symptoms to a similar extent (21). The total numbers of dropouts were 19 with amisulpride and 25 with flupenthixol. Adverse effects accounted for 8.6 and 18% respectively of the totals. Amisulpride caused significantly fewer extrapyramidal adverse effects. Apart from the extrapyramidal adverse effects, there were treatment-related adverse events in 87% of the patients given amisulpride and 92% of those given flupenthixol. Prolactin concentrations were higher with amisulpride.

Amisulpride versus haloperidol

Fixed doses of amisulpride (100, 400, 800, and 1200 mg/day) and haloperidol (16 mg/day) have been compared in a 4-week, double-blind, randomized trial in 319 patients with acute exacerbations of schizophrenia (22). Amisulpride 400 mg/day and 800 mg/day was effective in treating the positive symptoms of schizophrenia, with fewer extrapyramidal adverse effects than haloperidol, which was associated with the highest proportion of extrapyramidal symptoms. The incidence of extrapyramidal symptoms in patients treated with amisulpride increased with increasing dose (31%, 42%, 45%, and 55% for 100, 400, 800, and 1200 mg/day respectively). The rate of withdrawals due to adverse events was higher with haloperidol (16%) than with amisulpride (0%, 5%, 3%, and 5% respectively).

The long-term safety and efficacy of amisulpride in subchronic and chronic schizophrenia have been assessed in an open, multicenter study in 489 patients randomly allocated to amisulpride (mean dose 605 mg/day; $n = 370$) or haloperidol (mean dose 14.6 mg/day; $n = 119$) for 12 months (23). Improvement in mean total score on the BPRS was significantly greater with amisulpride than with haloperidol. The proportion of patients with at least one treatment-emergent adverse event was similar in the two groups, 69% with amisulpride and 70% with haloperidol, but extrapyramidal symptoms occurred more often with haloperidol (41%) than with amisulpride (26%); endocrine disorders occurred in 4% of those taking amisulpride and 3% of those taking haloperidol. Amenorrhea (6 versus 0%) and weight increase (11 versus 4%) were more frequent with amisulpride. There were serious adverse events in 10% of the patients taking amisulpride and 7% of those taking haloperidol.

Atypical versus typical drugs

There is no clear evidence that atypical neuroleptic drugs are more effective or better tolerated than typical neuroleptic drugs. It has therefore been suggested that typical neuroleptic drugs can be used in the initial treatment of schizophrenia, unless the patient has previously not responded to these drugs or has unacceptable extrapyramidal adverse effects, based on a meta-analysis of 52 randomized comparisons of atypical neuroleptic drugs with typical neuroleptic drugs (12 649 patients) or alternative atypical neuroleptic drugs (24). After correction for the higher than recommended doses of typical neuroleptic drugs that are used in some trials, there was a modest advantage of atypical neuroleptic drugs in terms of extrapyramidal adverse effects, but the differences in efficacy and overall tolerability disappeared, suggesting that many of the perceived benefits of atypical neuroleptic drugs are really due to excessive doses of the comparator drugs used in trials. Other reviews of atypical neuroleptic drugs have not added anything new (25,26). Both types of neuroleptic drugs have serious shortcomings, particularly their adverse effects on the extrapyramidal and endocrine systems. However, quality of life is said to be superior with atypical neuroleptic drugs, from an analysis of seven controlled trials and eight open trials (27).

An independent cross-sectional survey, not sponsored by the pharmaceutical industry, in schizophrenic outpatients clinically stabilized on a neuroleptic drug for a period of 6 months showed that quality-of-life measures and Global Assessment of Functioning did not differ significantly in patients taking typical neuroleptic drugs ($n = 44$) and novel ones (risperidone, $n = 50$; olanzapine, $n = 48$; quetiapine, $n = 42$; clozapine, $n = 46$) (28).

Adverse effects have been studied in people with mental retardation treated with atypical neuroleptic drugs ($n = 17$), typical neuroleptic drugs ($n = 17$), or no drugs ($n = 17$) (29). The patients taking atypical neuroleptic drugs did not have different overall adverse events from those taking no medications, and both had significantly fewer overall adverse effects than those taking typical neuroleptic drugs. However, the study had some important flaws: patients taking typical neuroleptic drugs were on average 7 years older than those taking atypical drugs; they had also taken medication for longer and had more stereotypic movement disorders at baseline. This jeopardizes the conclusions.

Atypical drugs versus haloperidol

In a randomized double-blind trial in 157 inpatients with chronic schizophrenia, clozapine ($n = 40$), olanzapine ($n = 39$), and risperidone ($n = 41$), but not haloperidol ($n = 37$), produced statistically significant improvements in total scores on the Positive and Negative Syndrome Scale after 14 weeks (30). Patients who had failed to respond to any typical neuroleptic drug were eligible, including patients who had previously failed to respond to haloperidol. High doses were used (the mean daily doses achieved during the last period of study were: clozapine 525 mg, olanzapine 30 mg, risperidone 12 mg, and haloperidol 26 mg). There was a significant fall in the Extrapyramidal Symptom Rating Score with the three atypical drugs at the end of the study and no change with haloperidol. One patient developed agranulocytosis, two had hypertensive episodes, and four had seizures while taking clozapine.

The results of 11 studies in 1933 patients with schizophrenia, who were randomly assigned to amisulpride ($n = 1247$), haloperidol ($n = 309$), risperidone ($n = 113$), flupenthixol ($n = 62$), or placebo ($n = 202$) have been reviewed (31). Extrapyramidal signs occurred in 15% of those given amisulpride ($n = 579$), 12% of those given risperidone ($n = 113$), and 31% of those given haloperidol ($n = 214$). In contrast, endocrine disorders were more frequent with amisulpride (4%) and risperidone (6%) than with haloperidol (1%). In a subgroup of patients with predominant negative schizophrenia who had at least one electrocardiogram recorded during treatment, there was a relative prolongation of the QT_c interval of at least 60 ms in three of 296 patients treated with amisulpride compared with no cases with both haloperidol ($n = 80$) and risperidone ($n = 91$); however, there were no ventricular dysrhythmias.

Clozapine versus typical neuroleptic drugs

A meta-analysis of 30 randomized controlled comparisons of clozapine with typical neuroleptic drugs ($n = 2530$) has been published (32). Clozapine was more effective in reducing symptoms in patients with both treatment-resistant and non-resistant schizophrenia. In a subset of 13 trials hematological problems tended to be more frequent in patients taking clozapine (OR = 1.93, CI = 0.96, 3.87); hypersalivation was also more frequent (OR = 5.50, CI = 4.26, 7.10), as were fever (OR = 1.89, CI = 1.38, 2.60) and sedation (OR = 1.94, CI = 1.50, 2.50). Xerostomia (OR = 0.29, CI = 0.20, 0.42) and extrapyramidal symptoms (OR = 0.46, CI = 0.28–0.75) were more frequent in the patients treated with typical neuroleptic drugs. There was no difference between the two groups in weight gain (OR = 1.07, CI = 0.37, 3.10), hypotension or dizziness (OR = 1.66, CI = 0.74, 3.71), or seizures (OR = 1.60, CI = 0.84, 3.04). Although there were fewer deaths in the clozapine group, statistical significance was not reached (OR = 0.50, CI = 0.11, 2.30). One of the flaws of this meta-analysis was that there was no information on dropouts.

Clozapine versus chlorpromazine

In 42 elderly patients (mean age 67 years) with schizophrenia randomly assigned to clozapine, titrated to 300 mg/day ($n = 24$), or chlorpromazine, titrated to a maximum of 600 mg/day ($n = 18$), the two medications were equally effective at 5 weeks (33). In each group there was one patient with a serious and potentially fatal adverse effect: agranulocytosis in the clozapine group and paralytic ileus in the chlorpromazine group; both drugs significantly lowered the white cell count.

Clozapine versus chlorpromazine and haloperidol

Clozapine has been compared with typical neuroleptic drugs in seven studies in patients with chronic refractory schizophrenia (34) ($n = 1124$). Of the 10 comparisons of second-generation versus typical neuroleptic drugs ($n = 1801$), there was a significant difference in six favoring second-generation neuroleptic drugs on measures of treatment efficacy; in the other four there was no significant difference between treatments. ANCOVA with the baseline score as a co-variate was performed to compare the efficacy of clozapine with that of typical neuroleptic drugs in terms of BPRS total score; there was a significant reduction in psychopathology in those who took clozapine, and the reduction was greater among those with higher BPRS scores. When the assessment was performed with other scales (BPRS positive symptom subscale, SANS) there were no significant treatment effects for clozapine over typical neuroleptic drugs. The subjects who took clozapine had significantly fewer extrapyramidal effects; tardive dyskinesia occurred equally in the two groups. Weight gain was reported in patients who took chlorpromazine (1%) and clozapine (7.1%), but in none of those who took haloperidol. Patients taking chlorpromazine (3.4%) or clozapine (2.9%) had difficulty in concentrating, but none of those taking haloperidol did. Other adverse events reported in patients taking clozapine included neutropenia (2.0%), enuresis (1.0%), and seizures (0.4%); neuroleptic malignant syndrome developed in 0.5% of the patients who took chlorpromazine. Completion rates were higher for clozapine (70%; $n = 400$) than for the typical neuroleptic drugs (56%; $n = 398$). Despite the superior efficacy of clozapine in the treatment of resistant patients, the extent of this in terms of scope (symptoms improved) and magnitude (effect size) was variable. Using what might be regarded as a non-stringent criterion of a 20–30% reduction in total psychopathology scores, under half of the patients responded in most of the studies.

Clozapine versus haloperidol

Clozapine and haloperidol have been compared in 75 schizophrenic outpatients, who met criteria for residual positive or negative symptoms after being treated for at least 6 weeks with typical neuroleptic drugs, in a 10-week randomized, double-blind, parallel-group comparison (35). There was no evidence of any superior efficacy or chlorpromazine equivalents resulted in a 6% increase in the hazard of presumptive tardive dyskinesia (224). Furthermore, a positive correlation between tardive dyskinesia and circulating neuroleptic drug concentrations has been reported (247); however, in one study there was no significant difference in serum concentrations of thioridazine, its metabolites, or radio-receptor activity between patients with and without tardive dyskinesia (248). Histories of more and longer drug-free periods were more common in moderate and severe tardive dyskinesia than in mild forms (249). There was a positive association between neuroleptic drug-free periods and persistent tardive dyskinesia (250).

In one study, previous neuroleptic drug use at study entry was the only significant predictor of tardive dyskinesia (251). Psychiatric outpatients aged over 45 years, who had taken neuroleptic drugs for 0–30 days ($n = 176$), were compared with 131 who had taken neuroleptic drugs for more than 30 days. The cumulative incidences of tardive dyskinesia were 23% and 37% at the end of 12 months. In the patients who had never used neuroleptic drugs before ($n = 87$), the mean cumulative incidence of tardive dyskinesia after the use of typical neuroleptic drugs (median dose 68 mg/day of chlorpromazine equivalents) was 3.4% at baseline and 5.9% at 1 and 3 months.

The relation between handedness and tardive dyskinesia has been studied. The estimated rate ratio, comparing left-handers and mixed-handers with pure right-handers, adjusted for confounders, was 0.25. The handedness effect was stronger for men than for women (252).

There are various other possible risk factors, for example diabetes mellitus (SEDA-16, 47) (253), organicity, affective disorder, and a history of ECT or alcohol abuse (254).

Mechanism

Pharmacogenetic assessments of neuroleptic drug-induced tardive dyskinesia have been reviewed (255). The dopamine D_3 receptor (DRD3) gene has a single nucleotide polymorphism that results in a serine to glycine amino acid substitution (Ser9Gly) in the N terminal and gives rise to allelic differences in dopamine affinity; autosomal inheritance of two polymorphic Ser9Gly alleles (2–2 genotype), but not homozygosity for the wild-type allele (1–1 genotype), was a susceptibility factor (256). The severity of tardive dyskinesia was greater in homozygotes for the glycine variant of DRD3 than in serine/serine homozygotes or serine/glycine heterozygotes.

Another polymorphism has been identified in intron 1 of the CYP1A2 gene; similarly, there is an association between the severity of tardive dyskinesia and one of the corresponding genotypes. It is said that CYP1A2 may be important in neuroleptic drug metabolism after CYP2D6 saturation during long-term treatment.

The hypothesis of oxidative damage to striatal neurons mediated by neuroleptic drug enhancement of glutamatergic neurotransmission has been tested in a case-control study (257). Several markers of excitatory neurotransmission (*N*-acetylaspartylglutamate, *N*-acetylaspartate, aspartate, and glutamate) and of oxidative damage (superoxide dismutase, protein carbonyl content, and lipid hydroperoxides) were measured in the CSF of patients with schizophrenia who had taken neuroleptic drugs chronically, and who had ($n = 11$) or had not ($n = 9$) developed tardive dyskinesia. There was an inverse correlation between CSF concentrations of aspartate and superoxide dismutase activity in tardive dyskinesia, what suggests a causative relation between enhanced excitatory amino acid neurotransmission and the oxidative damage associated with tardive dyskinesia. Another plausible model for the development of tardive dyskinesia is that lower activity of superoxide dismutase renders the striatal neurons more vulnerable to excitatory neurotransmission that is exacerbated by neuroleptic drugs, as shown in a subgroup of patients with schizophrenia.

There are conflicting results on the possible relation between plasma iron concentrations and movement disorders (SEDA-19, 45). A significant correlation between serum ferritin concentrations and the severity of choreoathetoid movements has been observed (258). All 30 subjects had a minimum lifetime cumulative exposure to typical neuroleptic drugs of 3 years. Nevertheless, and as was stated by the authors, it is unclear whether higher body iron stores exacerbate the symptoms of tardive dyskinesia or predispose to its development.

Reversibility

The rate of reversibility of tardive dyskinesia after drug withdrawal is 0–90% (225). Since patients with tardive dyskinesia rarely have subjective complaints (259), periodic assessment of dyskinetic movements is essential in making an early diagnosis and can increase the chance of reversing the disorder. Some reports are relatively encouraging regarding reversibility (260,261); the characteristics of reversible and irreversible forms have been reviewed, but no firm conclusion can be drawn (262). However, the prognosis of tardive dyskinesia was better in patients treated for a shorter duration and in those treated with lower doses (263).

Prevention and treatment

In dealing with the whole problem of dyskinesia, the preeminent role of prevention must be emphasized (254), particularly because treatment is so unrewarding. Various agents have been studied, including agonists and antagonists at various CNS neurotransmitters, and newer dopamine receptor antagonists, which supposedly act only at dopamine D_2 receptors (sites that are not linked to adenyl cyclase). The few supposedly positive results that have been claimed for a number of drugs must be interpreted with great caution (SEDA-18, 49) (264).

Treatment of tardive dyskinesia is often unsatisfactory, especially in severe cases. A large number of treatments have been proposed (SEDA-20, 40), including antiparkinsonian drugs, benzodiazepines, baclofen, hormones, calcium channel blockers, valproate, propranolol, opiates, cyproheptadine, tryptophan, lithium, manganese, niacin, botulinum toxin, ECT, dietary control, and biofeedback training. In an open study, 20 patients (mean age 65 years) with severe unresponsive tardive dyskinesia (mean duration 44 months, mean exposure 52 months) were treated with tetrabenazine (mean dose 58 mg/day) (265). The mean score on the AIMS motor subset, determined from videotapes, improved by 54%. Sedation was the only subjective complaint.

Abnormal lipid peroxidation and low lipid-corrected plasma concentrations of vitamin E are associated with tardive dyskinesia (266).Vitamin E has therefore been used for its antioxidant properties (SEDA-21, 47) (267–270). A meta-analysis has summarized eight double-blind, placebo-controlled studies of vitamin E in the treatment of tardive dyskinesia in 221 patients (271). Overall, vitamin E had a better effect than placebo; 28% of those who took vitamin E had a 33% or greater reduction in AIMS scores, compared with only 4.6% in the placebo arm. The number of patients included in any study was very small, never more than 28. The rationale for using vitamin E and for finding a better indicator of vitamin E deficiency has been explored (266). Since much of the vitamin E in plasma is carried in the low-density lipoprotein fraction, relating vitamin E content to the sum of cholesterol and triglycerides in the plasma could produce a high degree of specificity and sensitivity in defining vitamin E deficiency. Patients with tardive dyskinesia had lower concentrations of lipid-corrected vitamin E. However, the authors admitted that the lower concentration of vitamin E could have resulted from, predisposed to, or served as a marker of the susceptibility to tardive dyskinesia. The possible involvement of free radicals and treatment with vitamin E has been extensively reviewed (272). A further study has concluded that the addition of vitamin E to neuroleptic drug medication at the start of treatment can reduce the severity of acute neuroleptic drug-induced parkinsonism (273). This has been observed by comparing two groups of randomly allocated patients treated with neuroleptic drugs ($n = 20$) or with neuroleptic drugs plus vitamin E 600 IU/day ($n = 19$). From days 0–14, there was a mean reduction in SARS scores of 10% in those treated with vitamin E versus an increase of 78% in the comparison group. More recently, vitamin E (alpha-tocopherol), with its antioxidant properties, has been reported to be effective.

A beneficial effect of pyridoxine has been reported (274).

- A 22-year-old man with chronic organic persecutory paranoid ideation and recurrent explosive attacks had received neuroleptic drugs since the age of 7. While taking haloperidol, up to 25 mg/day, and trihexyphenidyl, up to 4 mg/day, he developed involuntary movements that were diagnosed as tardive dyskinesia: blinking, movements of the forehead and eyebrows, tongue-thrusting, licking of the lips, smacking, and chewing. He scored 27 on items 1–7 of the AIMS. He began to take pyridoxine, 200 mg/day, and after 5 days had a drastic reduction in the severity of all his movement disorders.
- A 41-year-old man had dramatic relief from tardive dyskinesia and akathisia with high-dose piracetam (275).

Reserpine has been used with apparent improvement in symptoms, but deterioration followed withdrawal (276), and reserpine has also been reported to cause the condition.

A double-blind study of propranolol showed short-term improvement, and two of four subjects responded to long-term propranolol (277); unfortunately this study has not been replicated.

Tetrahydroisoxazoylpyridinol (THIP), an analogue of gamma-aminobutyric acid (GABA), which is a GABA receptor antagonist, produced no change in tardive dyskinesia, in either a dose-finding study or a 4-week placebo-controlled study, but pre-existing parkinsonism increased significantly and eye-blinking rates fell (278); these are preliminary findings, more than a decade old, and hard to interpret.

Tardive akathisia

Akathisia can occur relatively early, within days or weeks, but sometimes occurs later. A 1986 review (279) considered 24 cases of tardive akathisia seen over a long period; in three of these the condition had appeared after only 1 or 2 months of neuroleptic drug therapy, but the remainder had been treated for at least 1 year, and seven had been treated with neuroleptic drugs for at least 5 years. Whereas tardive dyskinesia most often starts in the bucco-oral region and extends to the fingers and occasionally to the lower limbs and trunk, tardive akathisia most often affects the legs or is described as a generalized sensation throughout the limbs and trunk. Moreover, while a reduction in dosage can induce a temporary worsening of masked tardive dyskinesia and an increased dosage an improvement, the effects of dosage changes on akathisia are less certain.

Tardive Tourette's syndrome

There have been at least seven published cases of Tourette's syndrome ascribed to neuroleptic drugs and emerging either during treatment or after withdrawal. Some authors believe that a tardive Tourette-like syndrome may be a subtype of the more frequent tardive dyskinesia, because it can be masked by an increase in neuroleptic drug dosage and exacerbated by withdrawal. However, the symptoms can readily be confused with exacerbation of the underlying psychosis; misdiagnosis of the condition, at least in some of the published case reports, cannot be completely ruled out.

Tardive dystonia

Tardive dystonia is a rare, late-onset, persistent dystonia associated with neuroleptic drugs, which usually affects young men. It tends to affect the muscles of the neck, shoulder girdle, and trunk, causing opisthotonos. Sometimes, patients can become incapacitated (280,281). The incidence is 1–2% (282). Once developed, it is a very persistent disorder, with a low remission rate of only 14%; withdrawal of neuroleptic drugs increases the chances of remission.

Tardive dystonia has sometimes been thought to be a subtype of tardive dyskinesia (SED-13, 123). However, some features of this condition are clearly different from those of tardive dyskinesia (SEDA-20, 41). The diagnosis of tardive dystonia should meet the following criteria: (a) the presence of chronic dystonia; (b) a history of neuroleptic drug treatment preceding (less than 2 months) or

Despite similar mean body weights (olanzapine 84 kg versus risperidone 81 kg), 32% of those who took olanzapine were characterized by the atherogenic metabolic triad (hyperinsulinemia and raised apolipoprotein B and small-density LDL concentrations) compared with only 5% of those who took risperidone.

Diabetes mellitus

Several cases of de novo onset or exacerbation of existing diabetes mellitus in patients treated with neuroleptic drugs have been reported and were not significantly related to weight gain. These included eight patients treated with clozapine (387,388) and two patients treated with olanzapine (388).

Neuroleptic drug treatment of non-diabetic patients with schizophrenia can be associated with adverse effects on glucose regulation, as has been suggested by the results of a study in which modified oral glucose tolerance tests were performed in 48 patients with schizophrenia taking clozapine, olanzapine, risperidone, or typical neuroleptic drugs, and 31 untreated healthy control subjects (389). Newer neuroleptic drugs, such as clozapine and olanzapine, compared with typical agents, were associated with adverse effects on blood glucose regulation, which can vary in severity regardless of adiposity and age.

Weight gain

Shortly after the typical neuroleptic drugs were introduced in the 1950s, marked increases in body weight were observed, and excessive weight gain has been reported in up to 50% of patients receiving long-term neuroleptic drug treatment (390–396).

However, changes in weight during psychosis are also related to the condition; Kraepelin wrote, "The taking of food fluctuates from complete refusal to the greatest voracity... Sometimes, in quite short periods, very considerable differences in the body weight are noticed ..." (397). It was observed early on that food intake and weight often fell as psychosis worsened, but eating and weight returned to normal or increased when an acute psychotic episode abated. However, since the start of the neuroleptic drug era in the 1950s, a new pattern of sustained increased weight has commonly been detected. The question of whether weight gain is associated with efficacy is important; in one study there was no obvious relation between the magnitude of weight gain and therapeutic efficacy (398).

The association between clozapine-related weight gain and increased mean arterial blood pressure has been examined in 61 patients who were randomly assigned to either clozapine or haloperidol in a 10-week parallel group, double-blind study, and in 55 patients who chose to continue to take clozapine in a subsequent 1-year, open, prospective study (399). Clozapine was associated with significant weight gain in both the double-blind trial (mean 4.2 kg) and the open trial (mean 5.8 kg), but haloperidol was not associated with significant weight gain (mean 0.4 kg). There were no significant correlations between change in weight and change in mean arterial blood pressure for clozapine or haloperidol.

Serum leptin, a peripheral hormone secreted by fat, correlates inversely with body weight; in 22 patients taking clozapine who gained weight, those who had the most pronounced 2-week increase in leptin had the least gain in body weight after 6 and 8 months (400).

Epidemiology

Several reviews have addressed the issue of weight gain (401–405). Comparison of different studies of weight gain during treatment with atypical neuroleptic drugs is hampered by problems with study design, recruitment procedures, patient characteristics, measurement of body weight, co-medications, and duration of therapy. These problems have to be considered when assessing this type of information, particularly figures collected in accordance with the last-observation-carried-forward technique, which is one of the most common approaches taken; this type of analysis can produce marked underestimates of the magnitude of weight gain.

There has been one comprehensive meta-analysis including over 80 studies and over 30 000 patients (406). A meta-analysis of trials of neuroleptic drugs showed the following mean weight gains in kg after 10 weeks of treatment: clozapine, 4.5; olanzapine, 4.2; thioridazine, 3.2; sertindole, 2.9; chlorpromazine, 2.6; risperidone, 2.1; haloperidol, 1.1; fluphenazine, 0.43; ziprasidone 0.04; molindone, −0.39; placebo, −0.74 (407,408). In one study, excessive appetite was a more frequent adverse event in patients treated with olanzapine versus haloperidol (24 versus 12%) (152). Loss of weight has been observed after withdrawal of neuroleptic drugs (409).

The percentages of patients who gain more than 7% of their baseline body weight are highest for olanzapine (29%) and lowest for ziprasidone (9.8%). Although these figures are useful for comparing different drugs, they do not illustrate how weight increases over time, nor the total gain. Body weight tends to increase at first but reaches a plateau by about 1 year; with olanzapine 12.5–17.5 mg/day, patients gained, on average, 12 kg (410).

Risperidone and olanzapine, the two most commonly used atypical drugs, have been compared in trials; patients who took olanzapine gained almost twice as much weight (4.1 kg) as those who took risperidone (2.3 kg) (81). In two groups of inpatients, who took either risperidone ($n = 50$) or olanzapine ($n = 50$) for schizophrenia the mean body weight at baseline was 83 kg in the risperidone group and 85 kg in the olanzapine group; after 4 months of treatment, the mean body weights were 83 and 87 kg respectively (411). The increase in body weight with olanzapine was statistically significant.

In a retrospective chart review of 91 patients with schizophrenia (120 treatment episodes; mean age 38 years), there was weight gain with zotepine (4.3 kg), clozapine (3.1 kg), sulpiride (1.9 kg), and risperidone (1.5 kg), but not in patients treated with typical neuroleptic drugs (mean gain 0.0–0.5 kg) (412). The mean duration of treatment was 28–34 days, the maximum weight gain being in the first 3–5 weeks. The mean increases in weight were 4.3% in the patients with normal weight, 3.0% in those with mild obesity, and 1.9% in those with severe obesity (BMI over 30).

In another retrospective study, 65 patients with schizophrenia who gained weight while taking clozapine for 6 months were followed (413). After that they were switched to a combination of clozapine with quetiapine for 10 months: clozapine was tapered to 25% of the current dose and quetiapine was added proportionately. During clozapine monotherapy the mean weight gain was 6.5 kg and 13 patients developed diabetes. At the end of the combination period, the mean weight loss was 9.4 kg; patients who developed diabetes showed significant improvement, resulting in a rapid fall in insulin requirements and/or withdrawal of insulin and replacement with an oral hypoglycemic agent. The mechanism of clozapine-associated weight gain is uncertain.

Mechanism

The mechanisms of weight gain are not known. Olanzapine, for example, affects at least 19 different receptor sites, may have reuptake inhibition properties, and may affect hormones such as prolactin. Animal models do not help to elucidate mechanisms, since they have not shown clear results: some studies have shown weight gain with neuroleptic drugs in rats and others have not.

However, a serotonergic mechanism has been proposed (414). Most of the atypical drugs, which most commonly cause weight gain, interact with 5-HT_{2C} receptors; however, ziprasidone also binds to 5-HT_{2C} receptors with high affinity and does not cause weight gain or does so to a lesser extent. In 152 patients treated with clozapine, Cys23Ser polymorphism of the 5-HT_{2C} receptor did not explain the weight gain that occurred (415), nor was there an association between specific alleles of the dopamine D_4 receptor gene (416). In contrast, in 19-year-old monozygotic twins who gained around 40 kg after taking mainly clozapine, weight gain was related to an unspecified genotype (417). An association between weight gain and a 5-HT_{2C} receptor gene polymorphism has been identified in 123 Chinese Han patients with schizophrenia taking chlorpromazine ($n = 69$), risperidone ($n = 46$), clozapine ($n = 4$), fluphenazine ($n = 3$), or sulpiride ($n = 1$) (418). Weight gain was substantially greater in the patients with the wild-type genotype than in those with a variant genotype (–759C/T), at both 6 and 10 weeks; this effect was seen in men and women.

Susceptibility factors

In general, people with schizophrenia have a greater tendency to be overweight and obese than those who do not have schizophrenia (419). The evidence suggests that weight gain will progress most rapidly during the first 3–20 weeks of treatment with second-generation neuroleptic drugs; there is little evidence that dose affects weight gain. There are no sex differences, but there is a positive correlation between weight gain and age. Smokers treated with neuroleptic drugs may gain less weight than non-smokers (412,420). Patients in hospital are more likely to gain weight than those in the community, perhaps because they have an unrestricted diet and limited physical activity; there is some evidence that those with a lower baseline BMI are likely to gain more weight (402).

However, in the USA, data from a large health and nutrition survey ($n = 17\,689$) and from patients with schizophrenia to be enrolled in a clinical trial ($n = 420$) showed no differences; the mean BMIs were high and a substantial proportion of the population was obese (419).

The genetic basis of some reactions associated with neuroleptic drugs is of particular interest. An important association between weight gain and a 5-HT_{2C} receptor gene polymorphism has now been identified in 123 Chinese Han schizophrenic patients taking chlorpromazine ($n = 69$), risperidone ($n = 46$), clozapine ($n = 4$), fluphenazine ($n = 3$), or sulpiride ($n = 1$) (418). Weight gain was substantially greater in the patients with the wild-type genotype than in those with a variant genotype (–759C/T), at both 6 and 10 weeks; this effect was seen in men and women. In addition, a homozygous non-functional genotype, CYP2D6*4, was found in a 17-year-old schizophrenic patient who developed severe akathisia, parkinsonism, and drowsiness after taking risperidone 6 mg/day for 3 months; he had a high plasma concentration of risperidone and an active metabolite (421).

Clinical features

Obesity is associated with increased risks of dyslipidemia, hypertension, type 2 diabetes mellitus, cardiovascular disease, osteoarthritis, sleep apnea, and numerous other disorders; all these conditions have been associated with increased mortality. In the EUFAMI (European Federation of Associations of Families of Mentally Ill People) Patient Survey undertaken in 2001 across four countries and involving 441 patients, treatment-induced adverse effects were a fundamental problem; of the 91% of patients who had adverse effects, 60% had weight gain, and of these more than half (54%) rated weight gain as the most difficult problem to cope with (422). Furthermore, weight gain can adversely affect patients' adherence to medication, undermining the success of drug treatment for schizophrenia.

A report has illustrated how extreme the problem of weight gain associated with neuroleptic drugs can be (423).

- A 32-year-old man with schizophrenia taking neuroleptic drugs was switched to olanzapine 20 mg/day for better control. He weighed 101 kg and his BMI was 31 kg/m^2. After 6 months he had gained 4.5 kg and after 1 year 17 kg. Because of poor control, risperidone 4 mg/day was added and 16 months later he had had a 34.6 kg increase from baseline and had a BMI of 42 kg/m^2 (that is in the range of severe obesity). He had both increased appetite and impaired satiety. His serum triglycerides were 4.0 mmol/l, and his fasting blood glucose was 6.7 mmol/l. He and his physician agreed on a goal of losing 12 kg over 12 months and he was referred to a dietician. Over the next 5 weeks, he lost 2.7 kg and after 2 years his BMI was 38 kg/m^2 and 1 year later 39 kg/m^2. He was given nizatidine 300 mg bd and 1 year later his weight was 95 kg (BMI 29 kg/m^2). His triglycerides and fasting blood glucose concentrations were within the reference ranges.

Comparative studies

The charts of 94 long-term inpatients have been reviewed retrospectively to examine the changes in weight, fasting glucose, and fasting lipids in those taking either risperidone ($n = 47$) or olanzapine ($n = 47$)

(385). The patients had increased weight, triglycerides, and cholesterol, and the changes were significantly higher with olanzapine; olanzapine but not risperidone considerably increased glucose concentrations. One case of new-onset diabetes mellitus occurred in a patient taking olanzapine. Weight should be monitored in patients taking maintenance atypical neuroleptic drugs, especially dibenzodiazepines.

Management

Behavioral treatment of obesity has given good results in patients taking neuroleptic drugs (424). More dubious is the use of antiobesity drugs, as some of them can cause psychotic reactions.

Good results have been reported with amantadine, which increases dopamine release (425). In 12 patients with a mean weight gain of 7.3 kg during olanzapine treatment, amantadine 100–300 mg/day over 3–6 months produced an average weight loss of 3.5 kg without adverse effects. In contrast, calorie restriction did not lead to weight loss in 39 patients with mental retardation who were taking risperidone, 37 of whom gained weight, the mean gain being 8.3 kg over 26 months (426).

Electrolyte balance

Care should be taken when treating hyponatremic patients with neuroleptic drugs (427).

Mineral balance

In one controlled study, 12 patients who were receiving various neuroleptic drugs had significantly increased urinary calcium and hydroxyproline concentrations and reduced urinary alkaline phosphatase compared with five controls (428). The possibility of a reduction in bone mineralization (429) may contribute to the increased risk of hip fracture associated with neuroleptic drug treatment in the elderly.

Hematologic

Rarely reported hematological reactions to various neuroleptic drugs include agranulocytosis, thrombocytopenic purpura, hemolytic anemia, leukopenia, and eosinophilia. These are thought to represent allergic or hypersensitivity reactions, although this has been questioned in one detailed case report of chlorpromazine-induced agranulocytosis (430).

The reported incidence of agranulocytosis is variable, ranging from 1 in 3000 to 1 in 250 000. Most cases are seen within the first 2 months after the start of treatment, but there have been a few reports in which agranulocytosis occurred only after many years. Frequent white cell counts are of limited value in monitoring, since counts fall rapidly and abruptly. Careful attention should be given to possible early warning signs, such as fever, sore throat, and lymphadenopathy. Treatment requires immediate withdrawal and preventive measures against infection. Granulocyte colony-stimulating factor (GCSF) has been used to treat neuroleptic drug-induced agranulocytosis (431).

In view of the association of agranulocytosis with clozapine and of aplastic anemia with remoxipride, hemopoietic disorders have been studied using information from the UK monitoring system (432). The Committee on Safety of Medicines and the erstwhile Medicines Control Agency in the UK received 999 reports of hemopoietic disorders related to neuroleptic drugs between 1963 and 1996; there were 65 deaths. There were 182 reports of agranulocytosis; chlorpromazine and thioridazine were associated with the highest number of deaths—27 of 56 and 9 of 24 respectively. The much lower mortality with clozapine-induced agranulocytosis—two of 91 (2.2%)—was explained as a function of the stringent monitoring requirements for this drug, which allow early detection and treatment.

There is greater variability in the reference ranges for all white blood cell indices in patients with schizophrenia than in the healthy population (433). This suggests that abnormal hematological findings in patients with schizophrenia should be assessed in the context of a reference range specifically determined in patients with schizophrenia.

Gastrointestinal

The possibility of fatal intestinal dilatation, although very rare, warrants careful evaluation of persistent complaints of constipation, particularly in patients who also have vomiting and abdominal pain, distension, or tenderness (434). Acute intestinal pseudo-obstruction (Ogilvie's syndrome) has been reported in a patient taking haloperidol plus benzatropine (435).

- A 64-year-old woman started to take oral haloperidol 0.5 mg tds, and 3 days later was given intravenous benzatropine 2 mg for dystonia plus a second dose 1 hour later because she had not responded to the first dose. Her dystonia improved, but she started to develop abdominal distension and discomfort, and within the next 3–4 hours her whole abdomen had become significantly distended. Haloperidol and benzatropine were withdrawn and she was treated with hydration, nasogastric suction, a rectal tube, and frequent change of position. With this conservative therapy, her abdominal distension resolved completely in 24 hour.

Liver

When a neuroleptic drug causes jaundice it generally occurs within 2–4 weeks and has many characteristics of an allergic reaction, being accompanied by fever, rashes, and eosinophilia, although a direct toxic mechanism has also been implicated. Symptoms generally subside rapidly after withdrawal, but cholestasis may be prolonged.

Liver damage due to atypical neuroleptic drugs generally occurs within the first weeks of treatment, but the delay is highly variable, being 1–8 weeks for clozapine, 12 days to 5 months for olanzapine, and 1 day to 17 months for risperidone (436).

There is evidence of a significant hepatotoxic effect of the phenothiazines and in persons under age 50, but not over 50 (437).

Hepatotoxicity may be as frequent with piperidine and piperazine phenothiazines as with chlorpromazine, despite previous suggestions that the toxicity of these compounds is less.

More common are minor dose-related abnormalities in liver function tests with various neuroleptic drugs.

Urinary tract

Urinary retention, incontinence, or dysuria can occasionally occur with neuroleptic drugs that have marked anticholinergic effects.

Skin

Many skin reactions have been reported with neuroleptic drugs, including urticaria, abscesses after intramuscular injection, rashes, photosensitivity or exaggerated sunburn, contact dermatitis, and melanosis or blue-gray skin discoloration. Skin rashes are usually benign. Chlorpromazine is most often implicated (incidence 5–10%).

Non-phenothiazines, such as haloperidol and loxitane, cause fewer urticarial reactions. As with any other class of drug, patients may be allergic to excipients in various tablet or capsule forms, or to preservatives, for example methylparabens in liquid dosage forms (438).

Abnormal skin pigmentation (SEDA-19, 49) is more common in women and generally occurs on the exposed parts of the body. This reaction may be due to deposition of melanin-drug complexes. It was commonly seen in the decade after the introduction of the phenothiazines, but rarely today (438).

- A 45-year-old schizophrenic woman with blue eyes and blond hair who had received a lifetime exposure of at least 1748 g of chlorpromazine had blue discoloration of the skin by age 36 (439). Chlorpromazine was withdrawn and clozapine substituted (up to a maximum of 600 mg/day). The skin pigmentation resolved over 4 years.

Complications at the site of injection of depot neuroleptic drugs, including pain, bleeding or hematoma, leakage of drug from the injection site, acute inflammatory induration, and transient nodules, have been reported (SEDA-20, 43).

Seborrheic dermatitis has been observed in patients receiving long-term neuroleptic drugs (SEDA-17, 57), and this adverse effect appears to be highly associated with drug-induced parkinsonism.

More serious types of skin reactions are rare, but angioedema, non-thrombocytopenic purpura, exfoliative dermatitis, and Stevens–Johnson syndrome have been reported.

Potentially serious skin reactions are best treated by withdrawing the offending agent and switching to a structurally unrelated neuroleptic drug. When the offending agent is a phenothiazine, non-phenothiazines such as haloperidol or molindone may be preferable to the more closely related thioxanthenes.

Musculoskeletal

Rhabdomyolysis has been described in a handicapped child without other symptoms of neuroleptic malignant syndrome (440).

- A 6-year-old boy who was taking clonazepam 2.6 mg/day, diazepam 10 mg/day, and phenobarbital 50 mg/day was given oral haloperidol (0.3 mg/day) plus biperiden (0.3 mg/day) for choreoathetosis. After haloperidol had been introduced, his mother noticed that his urine sometimes became dark brown. He had myoglobinuria (660 ng/ml; reference range below 10 ng/ml) but no renal insufficiency. Haloperidol and biperiden were withdrawn and 2 days later his urine was normal.

A marked increase in creatine kinase activity without neuroleptic malignant syndrome has been previously described (SEDA-21, 48) and, another report has further emphasized this possibility (441).

- A 19-year-old schizophrenic patient taking risperidone 6 mg/day and olanzapine 20 mg/day had a creatine kinase activity of 6940 U/l without clinical manifestations of neuroleptic malignant syndrome; when he switched to clozapine (dose not stated) the creatine kinase fell to about 300 U/l. Because he developed granulocytopenia, he was given quetiapine instead, and the creatine kinase again rose to 3942 U/l but fell after 4 days to 389 U/l without withdrawal of quetiapine.

The authors concluded that the mechanism by which creatine kinase increases is not comparable for olanzapine, quetiapine, and clozapine, and that the increase can be self-limiting.

Sexual function

The frequency and course of sexual disturbances associated with neuroleptic drugs have been studied in a prospective open study of clozapine 261 mg/day (in 75 men and 25 women, mean age 29 years) and haloperidol 16 mg/day (41 men and 12 women, mean age 26 years) (442). There were no statistically significant differences between those taking haloperidol and those taking clozapine. During 1–6 weeks of treatment with clozapine, the most frequent sexual disturbances among women were diminished sexual desire (28%) and amenorrhea (12%), while among men they were diminished sexual desire (57%), erectile dysfunction (24%), orgasmic dysfunction (23%), ejaculatory dysfunction (21%), and increased sexual desire (15%).

Neuroleptic drug-induced sexual dysfunction, including erectile and ejaculatory dysfunction and changes in libido and the quality of orgasm, appear to be reversible on withdrawal.

Male dysfunction

Although the mechanism involved in neuroleptic drug-induced male sexual dysfunction is not entirely understood, it can occur at several levels, including the cortex, hypothalamus, pituitary gland, and the gonads, involving, for example, gonadotrophins and testosterone. Another mechanism involves the sympathetic and parasympathetic nervous systems and may explain why thioridazine and other highly anticholinergic drugs are mainly responsible for male sexual dysfunction, including impotence and retrograde ejaculation (443,444).

The first report of spontaneous ejaculation associated with the therapeutic use of neuroleptic drugs was described in 1983 (445).

One study showed a reduction in the strength of erection in men with schizophrenia, further accentuated in those who are taking neuroleptic drugs (SEDA-20, 44).

In 12 men with schizophrenia (mean age 36 years) receiving neuroleptic drugs, amantadine 100 mg/day for 6 weeks improved sexual function (446). All 12 patients, who had a sustained relationship with a female partner, had reported sexual dysfunction. Four areas of sexual function were assessed: desire, erection, ejaculation, and satisfaction; there was an improvement in all but ejaculation. Amantadine had no effect on the symptoms of schizophrenia.

Priapism

Neurotropic drug-induced priapism has been reviewed (447). It is said that neuroleptic drugs are most commonly implicated. A prior history of prolonged erections can be identified in as many as 50% of patients presenting with priapism who are using neuroleptic drugs. According to another review, the frequency of priapism with neuroleptic drugs may be increased by the fact that schizophrenia is said to be accompanied by an increase in sexual activity (448).

In one case, priapism followed the use of first risperidone and then ziprasidone (449).

- A 22-year-old African-American with chronic undifferentiated schizophrenia developed priapism after taking risperidone 4 mg bd, clonazepam 0.5 mg bd, vitamin E 400 IU bd, and a multivitamin for over 6 months. He did not respond to subcutaneous terbutaline 0.25 mg. Irrigation of the corpora with phenylephrine 200 μ resulted in detumescence; risperidone was withdrawn. A few months later he took ziprasidone 20 mg bd for 1 week, clonazepam 1 mg bd, and vitamin E 400 IU bd. The ziprasidone dosage was increased to 40 mg bd, but early the next morning he developed a firm erection with some discomfort that lasted about 2 hour and resolved when he urinated; the next morning he had a similar erection that also lasted 2 hour and resolved.

Priapism in twins suggests a hereditary predisposition (450).

- Identical twin brothers, aged 37 years, had both suffered from bipolar disorder since their early twenties and had been treated with chlorpromazine, haloperidol, lithium, and carbamazepine before developing priapism. One of them developed priapism after taking trazodone 400 mg/day, and in the 2 years after the initial episode he suffered recurrent painless erections. Initially they occurred daily and lasted 4–5 hours. During a relapse of mania at age 37, he was given oral zuclopenthixol 40 mg/day. On the tenth day he presented with priapism of 4 days duration, which persisted despite zuclopenthixol withdrawal, needle aspiration, and phenylephrine instillation, but subsided 2 weeks later with conservative management. The other twin presented with priapism of 75 hour duration and hypomania at age 31 years. He had been taking lithium and chlorpromazine for the preceding 2 years.

Priapism necessitates prompt urological consultation and sometimes even surgical intervention (443,451,452).

Female dysfunction

Female orgasm is inhibited by some central depressant and psychotropic drugs, including neuroleptic drugs, antidepressants, and anxiolytic benzodiazepines (165).

Immunologic

Hypogammaglobulinemia in a 22-year-old woman with brief psychotic disorder has been attributed to neuroleptic drug therapy (453). About 4 months after she had started to receive neuroleptic drugs, her serum concentrations of total protein had fallen to 58 g/l, with an IgG concentration of 3.49 g/l, an IgA concentration of 0.54 g/l, and an IgM concentration of 0.34 g/l.

Antiphospholipid syndrome is a disorder of recurrent arterial or venous thrombosis, thrombocytopenia, hemolytic anemia, or a positive Coombs' test, and in women recurrent idiopathic fetal loss, associated with raised concentrations of antiphospholipid antibodies. In systemic lupus erythematosus, the risk of this syndrome is about 40%, compared with a risk of 15% in the absence of antiphospholipid antibodies (454). However, only half of those with antiphospholipid antibodies have systemic lupus erythematosus, and the overall risk of the syndrome is about 30%. In patients who have antiphospholipid antibodies associated with chlorpromazine, there appears to be no increased risk of the syndrome. In contrast, in the primary antiphospholipid syndrome, the only clinical manifestations are the features of this syndrome.

- Symptomatic antiphospholipid syndrome has been described in a 42-year-old woman treated with chlorpromazine 260 mg/day (455). She presented with sudden right-sided weakness, numbness, and headache. Examination confirmed upper motor neuron signs affecting the right arm, leg, and face, with hemiplegia and hemiparesthesia. Autoantibody screening showed positive antinuclear antibodies, with an IgG titer of 50 and an IgM titer of 1600. Anticardiolipin antibody was positive with a raised IgM titer of 24 (normal less than 9). The symptoms and the serological findings resolved after withdrawal of the phenothiazine.

Drug-induced lupus erythematosus has been reviewed (456,457). Neuroleptic drugs, particularly chlorpromazine and chlorprothixene, have often been associated with this autoimmune disorder. It is recommended that several diagnostic criteria for this condition should be met: (1) exposure to a drug suspected to cause lupus erythematosus; (2) no previous history of the condition; (3) detection of positive antinuclear antibodies; and (4) rapid improvement and a gradual fall in the antinuclear antibodies and other serological findings on drug withdrawal. Rare disorders of connective tissue resembling systemic lupus erythematosus have been reported with chlorpromazine, perphenazine, and chlorprothixene (458).

Body temperature

Neuroleptic drugs interfere with the temperature regulatory function of the hypothalamus and peripherally with the sweating mechanism, resulting in poikilothermy. This can result in either hyperthermia or hypothermia, depending on the environmental temperature.

Hyperthermia
A series of cases has been reported in which heat stroke occurred during hot weather, probably due to impaired heat adaptation in patients taking benzatropine and ethylbenzatropine (459); this can occur with other anticholinergic and neuroleptic drugs as well.

Hypothermia
Reduced body temperature has been observed in a study of 14 drug-free and 7 patients with schizophrenia taking different neuroleptic drugs (460). The temperature fell by about 0.36°C at 24 hours after the drug-free subjects started to take neuroleptic drugs.

Hypothermia, defined as a body temperature lower than 35°C, has been observed in individual cases.

- A 73-year-old woman with diabetes mellitus and schizophrenia was given haloperidol 8 mg/day instead of zuclopenthixol; she also took levomepromazine 75 mg at night; 10 days later she was found unconscious with a rectal temperature of 31.5°C (461). A few weeks later, she had two further episodes, first with olanzapine 10 mg/day (rectal temperature 31.7°C) and then with thioridazine 40 mg/day (rectal temperature 34°C). She was therefore given dixyrazine 150 mg/day and alimemazine 20 mg at night, and had no more episodes of hypothermia.
- An 83-year-old woman developed a rectal temperature of 33.1°C 3 weeks after starting to take olanzapine 5 mg/day (462).
- A 68-year-old schizophrenic woman with type 1 diabetes mellitus developed a body temperature of 33.4°C 1 week after starting to take quetiapine 100 mg bd (462).

In the two last cases, the most common causes of hypothermia, such as hypothyroidism, infection, and cold exposure, were ruled out.

Death

The role of neuroleptic drugs in sudden death is controversial (SEDA-18, 47) (SEDA-20, 26) (SEDA-20, 36). Cardiac dysrhythmias may be involved, but there may also be multiple non-cardiac causes, including asphyxia, convulsions, or hyperpyrexia.

Long-Term Effects

Drug withdrawal

Various somatic complaints have been reported in patients in whom neuroleptic drugs are abruptly withdrawn (SEDA-20, 44). The incidence of these complaints varies widely in different reports, from 0 to 75%. Common complaints include headache, vomiting, nausea, diarrhea, insomnia, abdominal pain, rhinorrhea, and muscle aches. On rare occasions, the symptoms resemble those of benzodiazepine withdrawal (appetite change, dizziness, tremulousness, numbness, nightmares, a bad taste in the mouth, fever, sweating, vertigo, tachycardia, and anxiety), but it is possible that in some of the reported cases there was actually benzodiazepine withdrawal. Some of these symptoms may also have been linked to the simultaneous withdrawal of anticholinergic drugs (SED-11, 113) (463). Parkinsonism, not explained by withdrawal of anticholinergic drugs, has also been reported as an unusual withdrawal effect of neuroleptic drugs (464).

Worsening of psychotic symptoms and/or dyskinetic movements can occur when dosages are lowered or a neuroleptic drug is withdrawn. A functional increase in mesolimbic and striatal dopaminergic sensitivity has been suggested as an explanation (465). Psychotic relapse is rarely seen in the first 2 weeks after withdrawal, but physical withdrawal symptoms generally begin within 48 hours of the last dose (SEDA-14, 54).

Withdrawal emergent syndrome has been described in children (466,467) and consists of nausea, vomiting, ataxia, and choreiform dyskinesia primarily affecting the extremities, trunk, and head after sudden withdrawal of neuroleptic drugs (468). In one study, there were withdrawal symptoms in 51% of children, twice as many being affected by the withdrawal of low-dose, high-potency compounds compared with other drugs. Symptoms usually appear within a few days to 2 weeks after drug withdrawal; spontaneous remission is likely within the next 8–12 weeks.

The Omnibus Budget Reconciliation Act of 1987 (OBRA '87) regulations (www.elderlibrary.org) specify when neuroleptic drugs can and cannot be used to treat behavioral disturbances in nursing home residents in the USA. Accordingly, neuroleptic drugs can legally be used in patients with delirium or dementia only if there are psychotic or agitated features that present a danger to the patient or others. Preventable causes of agitation must be excluded and the nature and frequency of these behaviors must be documented. Non-dangerous agitation, uncooperativeness, wandering, restlessness, insomnia, and impaired memory are insufficient in isolation to justify the use of neuroleptic drugs. With this in mind, the effects of withdrawing haloperidol, thioridazine, and lorazepam have been examined in a double-blind, crossover study in 58 nursing home residents (43 women and 15 men, mean age 86 years), half of whom continued to take the psychotropic drugs that had been prescribed, while the other half were tapered to placebo (469). After 6 weeks, the patients were tapered to the reverse schedule and took it for another 6 weeks. There were no differences between drug and placebo in functioning, adverse effects, and global impression. Cognitive functioning improved during placebo. The authors concluded that gradual dosage reductions of psychoactive medications must be attempted, unless clinically contraindicated, when trying to withdraw these drugs. Similar conclusions have been reached in other studies (SEDA-22, 54).

There has been a randomized controlled study of the factors that affect neuroleptic drug withdrawal or dosage reduction among people with learning disabilities, who were being treated for behavioral problems with typical neuroleptic drugs (470). Of 36 patients, 12 completed full withdrawal and a further 7 achieved and maintained at least a 50% reduction. Drug withdrawal or dosage reduction was not associated with increased maladaptive behavior. This result reinforces concerns that neuroleptic drug treatment for maladaptive behavior reduction is often ineffective and inappropriate.

not to worsen peripheral or central autonomic toxicity. Other serious, but less frequent, complications include paralytic ileus and hypothermia. Acute renal insufficiency has been very rarely reported, but is apparently reversible and can occur secondary to severe hypotension or other causes after acute ingestion (502).

Of 524 inquiries received by the National Poisons Information Service concerning new neuroleptic drugs over 9 months, only 45 cases involved overdose with a single agent (olanzapine, $n = 10$; clozapine, $n = 8$; risperidone, $n = 10$; sulpiride, $n = 16$) (503). There were no deaths or cases of convulsions. Cardiac dysrhythmias occurred only with sulpiride. Symptoms were most marked with clozapine: most patients had agitation, dystonia, central nervous system depression, and tachycardia. Most of the patients who had taken risperidone were asymptomatic.

Neuroleptic drug poisoning in 86 children has been retrospectively studied in two pediatric hospitals in the USA (1987–1997), with about 9000 and 11 000 annual admissions (504). Most (70%) occurred in children under 6 years of age; over two-thirds of the cases (78%) were unintentional. The owner of the medication, when identified (85% of cases), was the grandmother (22%), another family member (21%), the patient (13%), or a non-family caregiver (8%); the most common places where ingestion occurred were the patient's home (64%) or a relative's home (22%). There was a depressed level of consciousness in 91% and a dystonic reaction in 51%; there were no deaths.

- A 46-year-old woman took amisulpride (12 g), alprazolam (40 mg), and sertraline (1 g) with suicidal intent, and 3 hours later was still unconscious and was intubated (505). Her body temperature rose from 37.1°C on admission to 38°C soon after. She was discharged on the third day.
- A 50-year-old man who took an overdose of ziprasidone 3120 mg (52 tablets) had no serious effects; he was a little drowsy and his speech was slightly slurred (506). Ziprasidone blood concentrations were not measured.

Fatal intoxication has been reported with melperone (507).

- A 36-year-old woman was found dead in her flat about 2 days after her last contact with one of her relatives. Besides melperone, she was known to take diazepam and carbamazepine. The police found four empty containers of 100 melperone tablets (100 mg per tablet). Post-mortem blood concentration analysis showed melperone, diazepam, nordiazepam, and carbamazepine; the melperone concentration in venous blood was very high (17.1 μg/ml).

Drug–Drug Interactions

Adrenoceptor agonists

Neuroleptic drugs can reduce or block the pressor effects of alpha-adrenoceptor agonists. When using drugs with both alpha- and beta-adrenoceptor activity, neuroleptic drug blockade of alpha-adrenoceptors can lead to unopposed beta predominance, resulting in severe hypotension (508).

A neuroleptic malignant-like syndrome occurred when norephedrine was combined with neuroleptic drugs (338).

Alcohol

Alcohol-induced CNS and respiratory depression is enhanced by neuroleptic drugs (509), but enhancement can be slight if both are used in reasonable amounts (510).

Alpha-adrenoceptor antagonists

Neuroleptic drugs can intensify the effects of alpha-adrenoceptor antagonists, for example phentolamine, causing severe hypotension (467).

Amfebutamone (bupropion)

Bupropion has about the same seizure potential as tricyclic antidepressants (SEDA-8, 30), but the manufacturers noted an increased risk of seizures in patients taking over 600 mg/day in combination with lithium or neuroleptic drugs (SEDA-10, 20).

Antacids

Antacids containing aluminium and magnesium reduce the gastrointestinal absorption of chlorpromazine and other phenothiazines by forming complexes (511). The clinical significance of this is unknown.

Antihistamines

Drugs with a CNS depressant effect (antihistamines, hypnotics, sedatives, narcotic analgesics, alcohol, etc.) will have an increase in effect caused by interaction with neuroleptic drugs.

Benzatropine

Benzatropine and ethylbenzatropine are particularly likely to interact additively with other drugs with both anticholinergic and antihistaminic activity, such as neuroleptic drugs; complications such as hyperpyrexia, coma, and toxic psychosis have been reported several times when such combinations were used (512–514).

Benzodiazepines

Neuroleptic drugs can potentiate the sedative effects of benzodiazepines pharmacodynamically.

In a brief review, emphasis has been placed on pharmacokinetic interactions between neuroleptic drugs and benzodiazepines, as much information on their metabolic pathways is emerging (515). Thus, CYP3A4, which plays a dominant role in the metabolism of benzodiazepines, also contributes to the metabolism of clozapine, haloperidol, and quetiapine, and plasma neuroleptic drug concentrations can rise.

Intramuscular levomepromazine in combination with an intravenous benzodiazepine has been said to increase the risk of airways obstruction, on the basis of five cases of respiratory impairment in patients who received injections of psychotropic drugs (516). The doses of levomepromazine were higher in the five cases that had accompanying airways obstruction than in another 95 patients who did not.

Beta-adrenoceptor antagonists

The cardiac effects of neuroleptic drugs can be potentiated by propranolol (517).

In general, concurrent use of neuroleptic and antihypertensive drugs merits close patient monitoring (518).

Bromocriptine

The dopamine-blocking activity of neuroleptic drugs can antagonize the effects of dopamine receptor agonists, such as bromocriptine. Conversely, bromocriptine has been reported to cause exacerbation of schizophrenic symptoms (519).

Caffeine

Neuroleptic drugs can precipitate from solution when mixed with coffee or tea (520), but the clinical significance of this physicochemical interaction is unknown (521).

Caffeine can alter blood concentrations of neuroleptic drugs (SEDA-5, 6).

Excess caffeine can stimulate the CNS, which can worsen psychosis and thus interfere with the effects of neuroleptic drugs (522).

Cannabis

In 10 patients, schizophrenia was acutely worsened after cannabis use, despite verified adequate depot treatment with neuroleptic drugs (523).

Carbamazepine

Plasma concentrations of neuroleptic drugs can be lowered by carbamazepine, and patients should be monitored for reduced efficacy (524).

- A 54-year-old man who had been taking neuroleptic drugs for about 30 years developed neuroleptic malignant syndrome within 3 days of taking add-on carbamazepine (400 mg/day) (525).

This syndrome does not appear to have been described with carbamazepine alone, and it was speculated that its pathogenesis could involve rebound cholinergic activity after a reduction in plasma neuroleptic drug concentrations by carbamazepine.

Cocaine

In a retrospective study of 116 patients taking neuroleptic drugs, 42% of cocaine users versus 14% of non-users developed dystonic reactions (526). This suggests that the use of cocaine may be a major risk factor for acute dystonic reactions secondary to the use of neuroleptic drugs.

This has been confirmed in a 2-year study on the island of Curaçao in the Netherlands Antilles, where cocaine and cannabis are often abused (168). The sample consisted of 29 men with neuroleptic-induced acute dystonias aged 17–45 years who had received high potency neuroleptic drugs in the month before admission; 9 were cocaine users and 20 non-users. Cocaine use was a major risk factor for neuroleptic-induced acute dystonia and should be added to the list of well-known risk factors such as male sex, younger age, neuroleptic dose and potency, and a history of neuroleptic-induced acute dystonias. The authors suggested that high-risk cocaine-using psychiatric patients who start to take neuroleptic drugs should be provided with a prophylactic anticholinergic drug to prevent neuroleptic drug-induced acute dystonias.

Corticosteroids

By reducing gastrointestinal motility, neuroleptic drugs enhance the absorption of corticosteroids (509).

Digoxin

By reducing gastrointestinal motility, neuroleptic drugs increase the systemic availability of digoxin and other inotropic drugs and thereby increase the potential for toxicity (510).

Guanethidine

Phenothiazines may inhibit the hypotensive action of guanethidine (510). This antagonism does not occur with molindone (508).

Hypoglycemic drugs

Because phenothiazines affect carbohydrate metabolism, they can interfere with the control of blood glucose in diabetes mellitus (387,509).

Levodopa

Levodopa and neuroleptic drugs can interfere with the effects of each other at dopamine receptors; the patient should be monitored for deterioration in both parkinsonism and mental state. If an antiemetic is required in a patient taking levodopa, one that does not affect central dopamine receptors should be chosen.

Lithium

Neuroleptic drugs are often used in mood stabilizer combinations. However, there have been few controlled studies of the use of such combinations, and interactions are potentially dangerous. The advantages and disadvantages of all currently used mood stabilizer combinations have been extensively reviewed (527). Some effects are well known: neurotoxicity, hypotension, somnambulistic-like events, and cardiac and respiratory arrest associated with the combination of lithium and traditional neuroleptic drugs considered as a first-line treatment for classic euphoric mania with psychotic features.

Several cases of neurotoxicity have been reported when lithium was combined with thioridazine, and patients should be carefully monitored (528–530).

Occasionally, long-term use of lithium is associated with cogwheel rigidity and a parkinsonian tremor. More often than not, concurrent or past treatment with a neuroleptic drug is involved. Neuroleptic malignant syndrome has also been reported in patients taking lithium and a neuroleptic drug, such as amoxapine (531), clozapine (532), haloperidol (533), olanzapine, (534), and risperidone (535). However, a causal interaction has not been established (536), and it should also be remembered that lithium toxicity itself can cause neuroleptic malignant syndrome (537).

Vitiello B, Ritz L, Davies M, Robinson J, McMahon D. Research Units on Pediatric Psychopharmacology Autism Network. Risperidone in children with autism and serious behavioral problems. N Engl J Med 2002;347(5):314–21.
96. Carlsson C, Dencker SJ, Grimby G, Häggendal J. Noradrenaline in blood-plasma and urine during chlorpromazine treatment. Lancet 1966;1:1208.
97. Chatterton R. Eosinophilia after commencement of clozapine treatment. Aust NZ J Psychiatry 1997;31(6):874–6.
98. Leo RJ, Kreeger JL, Kim KY. Cardiomyopathy associated with clozapine. Ann Pharmacother 1996;30(6):603–5.
99. Juul Povlsen U, Noring U, Fog R, Gerlach J. Tolerability and therapeutic effect of clozapine. A retrospective investigation of 216 patients treated with clozapine for up to 12 years. Acta Psychiatr Scand 1985;71(2):176–85.
100. Petrie WM, Ban TA, Berney S, Fujimori M, Guy W, Ragheb M, Wilson WH, Schaffer JD. Loxapine in psychogeriatrics: a placebo- and standard-controlled clinical investigation. J Clin Psychopharmacol 1982;2(2):122–6.
101. Mandelstam JP. An inquiry into the use of Innovar for pediatric premedication. Anesth Analg 1970;49(5):746–50.
102. Yanovski A, Kron RE, Townsend RR, Ford V. The clinical utility of ambulatory blood pressure and heart rate monitoring in psychiatric inpatients. Am J Hypertens 1998;11(3 Pt 1):309–15.
103. Branchey MH, Lee JH, Amin R, Simpson GM. High- and low-potency neuroleptics in elderly psychiatric patients. JAMA 1978;239(18):1860–2.
104. Haddad PM, Anderson IM. Antipsychotic-related QT_c prolongation, torsade de pointes and sudden death. Drugs 2002;62(11):1649–71.
105. Warner JP, Barnes TR, Henry JA. Electrocardiographic changes in patients receiving neuroleptic medication. Acta Psychiatr Scand 1996;93(4):311–13.
106. FDA Psychopharmacological Drugs Advisory Committee, 19 July 2000. Briefing Document of Zeldox Capsules (Ziprasidone HCI). www.fda.gov/ohrms/dockets/ac00/backgrd/361b1a.pdf, 19/07/2000.
107. Dessertenne F. La tachycardie ventriculaire a deux foyers opposés variables. [Ventricular tachycardia with 2 variable opposing foci.] Arch Mal Coeur Vaiss 1966;59(2]:263–72.
108. Buckley NA, Sanders P. Cardiovascular adverse effects of antipsychotic drugs. Drug Saf 2000;23(3):215–28.
109. Moss AJ. The QT interval and torsade de pointes. Drug Saf 1999;21(Suppl 1):5–10.
110. Viskin S. Long QT syndromes torsade de pointes. Lancet 1999;354(9190):1625–33.
111. Glassman AH, Bigger JT Jr. Antipsychotic drugs: prolonged QT_c interval, torsade de pointes, and sudden death. Am J Psychiatry 2001;158(11):1774–82.
112. Yap YG, Camm J. Risk of torsades de pointes with non-cardiac drugs. Doctors need to be aware that many drugs can cause qt prolongation. BMJ 2000; 320(7243):1158–9.
113. Kiriike N, Maeda Y, Nishiwaki S, Izumiya Y, Katahara S, Mui K, Kawakita Y, Nishikimi T, Takeuchi K, Takeda T. Iatrogenic torsade de pointes induced by thioridazine. Biol Psychiatry 1987;22(1):99–103.
114. Connolly MJ, Evemy KL, Snow MH. Torsade de pointes ventricular tachycardia in association with thioridazine therapy: report of two cases. New Trends Arrhythmias 1985;1:157.
115. Sharma ND, Rosman HS, Padhi ID, Tisdale JE. Torsades de pointes associated with intravenous haloperidol in critically ill patients. Am J Cardiol 1998;81(2):238–40.
116. Michalets EL, Smith LK, Van Tassel ED. Torsade de pointes resulting from the addition of droperidol to an existing cytochrome P450 drug interaction. Ann Pharmacother 1998;32(7–8):761–5.
117. Barber JM. Risk of sudden death on high-dose antipsychotic medication: QT_c dispersion. Br J Psychiatry 1998;173:86–7.
118. Reilly JG, Ayis SA, Ferrier IN, Jones SJ, Thomas SH. QT_c-interval abnormalities and psychotropic drug therapy in psychiatric patients. Lancet 2000;355(9209):1048–52.
119. Iwahashi K. Significantly higher plasma haloperidol level during cotreatment with carbamazepine may herald cardiac change. Clin Neuropharmacol 1996;19(3):267–70.
120. Tzivoni D, Banai S, Schuger C, Benhorin J, Keren A, Gottlieb S, Stern S. Treatment of torsade de pointes with magnesium sulfate. Circulation 1988;77(2):392–7.
121. O'Brien JM, Rockwood RP, Suh KI. Haloperidol-induced torsade de pointes. Ann Pharmacother 1999;33(10):1046–50.
122. Coulter DM, Bate A, Meyboom RH, Lindquist M, Edwards IR. Antipsychotic drugs and heart muscle disorder in international pharmacovigilance: data mining study. BMJ 2001;322(7296):1207–9.
123. Zornberg GL, Jick H. Antipsychotic drug use and risk of first-time idiopathic venous thromboembolism: a case-control study. Lancet 2000;356(9237):1219–23.
124. Cronqvist M, Pierot L, Boulin A, Cognard C, Castaings L, Moret J. Local intraarterial fibrinolysis of thromboemboli occurring during endovascular treatment of intracerebral aneurysm: a comparison of anatomic results and clinical outcome. AJNR Am J Neuroradiol 1998;19(1):157–65.
125. Hilpert F, Ricome JL, Auzepy P. Insuffisances respiratoires aiguës durant les traitements au long cours par les neuroleptiques. [Acute respiratory failure during long-term treatment with neuroleptic drugs.] Nouv Presse Méd 1980;9(39):2897–900.
126. Flaherty JA, Lahmeyer HW. Laryngeal–pharyngeal dystonia as a possible cause of asphyxia with haloperidol treatment. Am J Psychiatry 1978;135(11):1414–15.
127. Joseph KS. Asthma mortality and antipsychotic or sedative use. What is the link? Drug Saf 1997;16(6):351–4.
128. Faheem AD, Brightwell DR, Burton GC, Struss A. Respiratory dyskinesia and dysarthria from prolonged neuroleptic use: tardive dyskinesia? Am J Psychiatry 1982;139(4):517–18.
129. Portnoy RA. Hyperkinetic dysarthria as an early indicator of impending tardive dyskinesia. J Speech Hear Disord 1979;44(2):214–19.
130. Kumra S, Jacobsen LK, Lenane M, Smith A, Lee P, Malanga CJ, Karp BI, Hamburger S, Rapoport JL. Case series: spectrum of neuroleptic-induced movement disorders and extrapyramidal side effects in childhood-onset schizophrenia. J Am Acad Child Adolesc Psychiatry 1998;37(2):221–7.
131. Ballard C, Grace J, McKeith I, Holmes C. Neuroleptic sensitivity in dementia with Lewy bodies and Alzheimer's disease. Lancet 1998;351(9108):1032–3.
132. Caligiuri MP, Rockwell E, Jeste DV. Extrapyramidal side effects in patients with Alzheimer's disease treated with low-dose neuroleptic medication. Am J Geriatr Psychiatry 1998;6(1):75–82.
133. Mirsattari SM, Power C, Nath A. Parkinsonism with HIV infection. Mov Disord 1998;13(4):684–9.
134. Kompoliti K, Goetz CG. Hyperkinetic movement disorders misdiagnosed as tics in Gilles de la Tourette syndrome. Mov Disord 1998;13(3):477–80.
135. Sriwatanakul K. Minimizing the risk of antipsychotic-associated seizures. Drug Ther 1982;12:65.
136. Simpson GM, Cooper TA. Clozapine plasma levels and convulsions. Am J Psychiatry 1978;135(1):99–100.
137. Itil TM, Polvan N, Ucok A, Eper E, Guven F, Hsu W. Comparison of the clinical and electroencephalographical effects of molindone and trifluoperazine in

acute schizophrenic patients. Behav Neuropsychiatry 1971;3(5):25–32.

138. Baldessarini RJ. Drugs and the treatment of psychiatric disorders. In: Goodman LS, Gilman A, editors. The Pharmacological Basis of Therapeutics. 6th ed. New York: MacMillan, 1980:391.
139. Oliver AP, Luchins DJ, Wyatt RJ. Neuroleptic-induced seizures. An in vitro technique for assessing relative risk. Arch Gen Psychiatry 1982;39(2):206–9.
140. Woolley J, Smith S. Lowered seizure threshold on olanzapine. Br J Psychiatry 2001;178(1):85–6.
141. Simpson GM, Pi EH, Sramek JJ Jr. Adverse effects of antipsychotic agents. Drugs 1981;21(2):138–51.
142. Kane JM. Antipsychotic drug side effects: their relationship to dose. J Clin Psychiatry 1985;46(5 Pt 2):16–21.
143. Armstrong M, Daly AK, Blennerhassett R, Ferrier N, Idle JR. Antipsychotic drug-induced movement disorders in schizophrenics in relation to CYP2D6 genotype. Br J Psychiatry 1997;170:23–6.
144. Maurer I, Zierz S, Moller HJ, Jerusalem F. Neuroleptic associated extrapyramidal symptoms. Br J Psychiatry 1996;167:551–2.
145. Chetty M, Gouws E, Miller R, Moodley SV. The use of a side effect as a qualitative indicator of plasma chlorpromazine levels. Eur Neuropsychopharmacol 1999;9(1–2):77–82.
146. Rapoport A, Stein D, Shamir E, Schwartz M, Levine J, Elizur A, Weizman A. Clinico-tremorgraphic features of neuroleptic-induced tremor. Int Clin Psychopharmacol 1998;13(3):115–20.
147. Van Den Bos H, Rosenbauer C, Goldney RD. The assessment of involuntary movement disturbances in a psychiatric hospital population: an Australian experience. Aust J Psychopharmacol 1999;9:42–3.
148. Farde L, Nordstrom AL, Wiesel FA, Pauli S, Halldin C, Sedvall G. Positron emission tomographic analysis of central D_1 and D_2 dopamine receptor occupancy in patients treated with classical neuroleptics and clozapine. Relation to extrapyramidal side effects. Arch Gen Psychiatry 1992;49(7):538–44.
149. Nordstrom AL, Farde L, Wiesel FA, Forslund K, Pauli S, Halldin C, Uppfeldt G. Central D_2-dopamine receptor occupancy in relation to antipsychotic drug effects: a double-blind PET study of schizophrenic patients. Biol Psychiatry 1993;33(4):227–35.
150. Peuskens J. Risperidone in the treatment of patients with chronic schizophrenia: a multi-national, multi-centre, double-blind, parallel-group study versus haloperidol. Risperidone Study Group. Br J Psychiatry 1995;166(6):712–26.
151. Small JG, Hirsch SR, Arvanitis LA, Miller BG, Link CG. Quetiapine in patients with schizophrenia. A high- and low-dose double-blind comparison with placebo. Seroquel Study Group. Arch Gen Psychiatry 1997;54(6):549–57.
152. Tollefson GD, Beasley CM Jr, Tran PV, Street JS, Krueger JA, Tamura RN, Graffeo KA, Thieme ME. Olanzapine versus haloperidol in the treatment of schizophrenia and schizoaffective and schizophreniform disorders: results of an international collaborative trial. Am J Psychiatry 1997;154(4):457–65.
153. Zimbroff DL, Kane JM, Tamminga CA, Daniel DG, Mack RJ, Wozniak PJ, Sebree TB, Wallin BA, Kashkin KB. Controlled, dose-response study of sertindole and haloperidol in the treatment of schizophrenia. Sertindole Study Group. Am J Psychiatry 1997;154(6):782–91.
154. Brody AL. Acute dystonia induced by rapid increase in risperidone dosage. J Clin Psychopharmacol 1996;16(6):461–2.
155. Jauss M, Schroder J, Pantel J, Bachmann S, Gerdsen I, Mundt C. Severe akathisia during olanzapine treatment of acute schizophrenia. Pharmacopsychiatry 1998;31(4):146–8.
156. Landry P, Cournoyer J. Acute dystonia with olanzapine. J Clin Psychiatry 1998;59(7):384.
157. Caligiuri MR, Jeste DV, Lacro JP. Antipsychotic-induced movement disorders in the elderly: epidemiology and treatment recommendations. Drugs Aging 2000;17(5):363–84.
158. Kapur S, Zipursky R, Jones C, Remington G, Houle S. Relationship between dopamine D(2) occupancy, clinical response, and side effects: a double-blind PET study of first-episode schizophrenia. Am J Psychiatry 2000;157(4):514–20.
159. Mazurek MF, Rosebush PI. Circadian pattern of acute, neuroleptic-induced dystonic reactions. Am J Psychiatry 1996;153(5):708–10.
160. Koek RJ, Pi EH. Acute laryngeal dystonic reactions to neuroleptics. Psychosomatics 1989;30(4):359–64.
161. Sovner R, McGorrill S. Stress as a precipitant of neuroleptic-induced dystonia. Psychosomatics 1982;23(7):707–9.
162. Angus JW, Simpson GM. Hysteria and drug-induced dystonia. Acta Psychiatr Scand Suppl 1970;212:52–8.
163. Iqbal N. Heroin use, diplopia, largactil. Saudi Med J 2000;21(12):1194.
164. Ibrahim ZY, Brooks EF. Neuroleptic-induced bilateral temporomandibular joint dislocation. Am J Psychiatry 1996;153(2):293–4.
165. Ilchef R. Neuroleptic-induced laryngeal dystonia can mimic anaphylaxis. Aust NZ J Psychiatry 1997;31(6):877–9.
166. Fines RE, Brady WJ Jr, Martin ML. Acute laryngeal dystonia related to neuroleptic agents. Am J Emerg Med 1999;17(3):319–20.
167. Bulling M. Drug-induced dysphagia. Aust NZ J Med 1999;29(5):748.
168. van Harten PN, van Trier JC, Horwitz EH, Matroos GE, Hoek HW. Cocaine as a risk factor for neuroleptic-induced acute dystonia. J Clin Psychiatry 1998;59(3):128–30.
169. Lynch G, Green JF, King DJ. Antipsychotic drug-induced dysphoria. Br J Psychiatry 1996;169(4):524.
170. Hollistar LE. Antipsychotic drug-induced dysphoria. Br J Psychiatry 1997;170:387.
171. King DJ. Antipsychotic drug-induced dysphoria. Br J Psychiatry 1996;168:656.
172. Kasantikul D. Drug-induced akathisia and suicidal tendencies in psychotic patients. J Med Assoc Thai 1998;81(7):551–4.
173. Ashleigh EA, Larsen PD. A syndrome of increased affect in response to risperidone among patients with schizophrenia. Psychiatr Serv 1998;49(4):526–8.
174. Perenyi A, Norman T, Hopwood M, Burrows G. Negative symptoms, depression, and parkinsonian symptoms in chronic, hospitalised schizophrenic patients. J Affect Disord 1998;48(2–3):163–9.
175. Tollefson GD, Sanger TM, Lu Y, Thieme ME. Depressive signs and symptoms in schizophrenia: a prospective blinded trial of olanzapine and haloperidol. Arch Gen Psychiatry 1998;55(3):250–8.
176. Miller CH, Hummer M, Oberbauer H, Kurzthaler I, DeCol C, Fleischhacker WW. Risk factors for the development of neuroleptic induced akathisia. Eur Neuropsychopharmacol 1997;7(1):51–5.
177. Brune M. The incidence of akathisia in bipolar affective disorder treated with neuroleptics—a preliminary report. J Affect Disord 1999;53(2):175–7.
178. Drotts DL, Vinson DR. Prochlorperazine induces akathisia in emergency patients. Ann Emerg Med 1999;34(4 Pt 1):469–75.
179. Brune M. Acute neuroleptic-induced akathisia in patients with traumatic paraplegia: two case reports. Gen Hosp Psychiatry 1999;21(5):386–8.
180. Kurzthaler I, Hummer M, Kohl C, Miller C, Fleischhacker WW. Propranolol treatment of olanzapine-induced akathisia. Am J Psychiatry 1997;154(9):1316.
181. Auzou P, Ozsancak C, Hannequin D, Augustin P. Akathisie déclenchée par de faibles doses de

347. Rosebush PI, Stewart TD, Gelenberg AJ. Twenty neuroleptic rechallenges after neuroleptic malignant syndrome in 15 patients. J Clin Psychiatry 1989;50(8):295–8.
348. Hayashi T, Furutani M, Taniyama J, Kiyasu M, Hikasa S, Horiguchi J, Yamawaki S. Neuroleptic-induced Meige's syndrome following akathisia: pharmacologic characteristics. Psychiatry Clin Neurosci 1998;52(4):445–8.
349. Wirz-Justice A, Werth E, Savaskan E, Knoblauch V, Gasio PF, Muller-Spahn F. Haloperidol disrupts, clozapine reinstates the circadian rest-activity cycle in a patient with early-onset Alzheimer disease. Alzheimer Dis Assoc Disord 2000;14(4):212–15.
350. Madsen AL, Keidling N, Karle A, Esbjerg S, Hemmingsen R. Neuroleptics in progressive structural brain abnormalities in psychiatric illness. Lancet 1998; 352(9130):784–5.
351. Shah GK, Auerbach DB, Augsburger JJ, Savino PJ. Acute thioridazine retinopathy. Arch Ophthalmol 1998; 116(6):826–7.
352. Anonymous. Epidemiology of cataract. Lancet 1982; 1(8286):1392–3.
353. Webber SK, Domniz Y, Sutton GL, Rogers CM, Lawless MA. Corneal deposition after high-dose chlorpromazine hydrochloride therapy. Cornea 2001;20(2):217–19.
354. Leung AT, Cheng AC, Chan WM, Lam DS. Chlorpromazine-induced refractile corneal deposits and cataract. Arch Ophthalmol 1999;117(12):1662–3.
355. Weiss EM, Bilder RM, Fleischhacker WW. The effects of second-generation antipsychotics on cognitive functioning and psychosocial outcome in schizophrenia. Psychopharmacology (Berl) 2002;162(1):11–17.
356. Browne S, Garavan J, Gervin M, Roe M, Larkin C, O'Callaghan E. Quality of life in schizophrenia: insight and subjective response to neuroleptics. J Nerv Ment Dis 1998;186(2):74–8.
357. Heinz A, Knable MB, Coppola R, Gorey JG, Jones DW, Lee KS, Weinberger DR. Psychomotor slowing, negative symptoms and dopamine receptor availability—an IBZM SPECT study in neuroleptic-treated and drug-free schizophrenic patients. Schizophr Res 1998; 31(1):19–26.
358. Wistedt B. Neuroleptics and depression. Arch Gen Psychiatry 1982;39(6):745.
359. Wilkins-Ho M, Hollander Y. Toxic delirium with low-dose clozapine. Can J Psychiatry 1997;42(4):429–30.
360. Mahendran R. Obsessional symptoms associated with risperidone treatment. Aust NZ J Psychiatry 1998; 32(2):299–301.
361. Howland RH. Chlorpromazine and obsessive-compulsive symptoms. Am J Psychiatry 1996;153(11):1503.
362. Stip E. Memory impairment in schizophrenia: perspectives from psychopathology and pharmacotherapy. Can J Psychiatry 1996;41(8 Suppl 2):S27–34.
363. Weiser M, Shneider-Beeri M, Nakash N, Brill N, Bawnik O, Reiss S, Hocherman S, Davidson M. Improvement in cognition associated with novel antipsychotic drugs: a direct drug effect or reduction of EPS? Schizophr Res 2000;46(2–3):81–9.
364. Eitan N, Levin Y, Ben-Artzi E, Levy A, Neumann M. Effects of antipsychotic drugs on memory functions of schizophrenic patients. Acta Psychiatr Scand 1992;85(1):74–6.
365. Braff DL, Saccuzzo DP. Effect of antipsychotic medication on speed of information processing in schizophrenic patients. Am J Psychiatry 1982;139(9):1127–30.
366. Van Putten T, May PR, Marder SR, Wittmann LA. Subjective response to antipsychotic drugs. Arch Gen Psychiatry 1981;38(2):187–90.
367. Rifkin A, Quitkin F, Klein DF. Akinesia: a poorly recognized drug-induced extrapyramidal behavior disorder. Arch Gen Psychiatry 1975;32:672.
368. Bilder RM, Goldman RS, Volavka J, Czobor P, Hoptman M, Sheitman B, Lindenmayer JP, Citrome L, McEvoy J, Kunz M, Chakos M, Cooper TB, Horowitz TL, Lieberman JA. Neurocognitive effects of clozapine, olanzapine, risperidone, and haloperidol in patients with chronic schizophrenia or schizoaffective disorder. Am J Psychiatry 2002;159(6):1018–28.
369. Moritz S, Woodward TS, Krausz M, Naber D. PERSIST Study Group. Relationship between neuroleptic dosage and subjective cognitive dysfunction in schizophrenic patients treated with either conventional or atypical neuroleptic medication. Int Clin Psychopharmacol 2002;17(1):41–4.
370. Naber D, Moritz S, Lambert M, Pajonk FG, Holzbach R, Mass R, Andresen B. Improvement of schizophrenic patients' subjective well-being under atypical antipsychotic drugs. Schizophr Res 2001;50(1–2):79–88.
371. Magharious W, Goff DC, Amico E. Relationship of gender and menstrual status to symptoms and medication side effects in patients with schizophrenia. Psychiatry Res 1998;77(3):159–66.
372. Moller HJ, Kissling W, Maurach R. Beziehungen zwischen Haloperidol-Serumspiegel, Prolactin-Serumspiegel, antipsychotischen Effekt und extrapyramidalen Begleitwirkungen. [Relationship between haloperidol blood level, prolactin blood level, antipsychotic effect and extrapyramidal side effects.] Pharmacopsychiatrica 1981;14:27.
373. Zarifian E, Scatton B, Bianchetti G, Cuche H, Loo H, Morselli PL. High doses of haloperidol in schizophrenia. A clinical, biochemical, and pharmacokinetic study. Arch Gen Psychiatry 1982;39(2):212–15.
374. Brown WA, Laughren T. Low serum prolactin and early relapse following neuroleptic withdrawal. Am J Psychiatry 1981;138(2):237–9.
375. Phillips P, Shraberg D, Weitzel WD. Hirsutism associated with long-term phenothiazine neuroleptic therapy. JAMA 1979;241(9):920–1.
376. Atmaca M, Kuloglu M, Tezcan E, Canatan H, Gecici O. Quetiapine is not associated with increase in prolactin secretion in contrast to haloperidol. Arch Med Res 2002;33(6):562–5.
377. Schyve PM, Smithline F, Meltzer HY. Neuroleptic-induced prolactin level elevation and breast cancer: an emerging clinical issue. Arch Gen Psychiatry 1978;35(11):1291–301.
378. Mortensen PB. The incidence of cancer in schizophrenic patients. J Epidemiol Community Health 1989;43(1):43–7.
379. Pollock A, McLaren EH. Serum prolactin concentration in patients taking neuroleptic drugs. Clin Endocrinol (Oxf) 1998;49(4):513–16.
380. Spitzer M, Sajjad R, Benjamin F. Pattern of development of hyperprolactinemia after initiation of haloperidol therapy. Obstet Gynecol 1998;91(5 Pt 1):693–5.
381. Feek CM, Sawers JS, Brown NS, Seth J, Irvine WJ, Toft AD. Influence of thyroid status on dopaminergic inhibition of thyrotropin and prolactin secretion: evidence for an additional feedback mechanism in the control of thyroid hormone secretion. J Clin Endocrinol Metab 1980;51(3):585–9.
382. Melkersson KI, Hulting AL, Rane AJ. Dose requirement and prolactin elevation of antipsychotics in male and female patients with schizophrenia or related psychoses. Br J Clin Pharmacol 2001;51(4):317–24.
383. Kapur S, Roy P, Daskalakis J, Remington G, Zipursky R. Increased dopamine D(2) receptor occupancy and

elevated prolactin level associated with addition of haloperidol to clozapine. Am J Psychiatry 2001;158(2):311–14.
384. Rao KJ, Miller M, Moses A. Water intoxication and thioridazine (Mellaril). Ann Intern Med 1975;82(1):61.
385. Meyer JM. A retrospective comparison of weight, lipid, and glucose changes between risperidone- and olanzapine-treated inpatients: metabolic outcomes after 1 year. J Clin Psychiatry 2002;63(5):425–33.
386. Bouchard RH, Demers MF, Simoneau I, Almeras N, Villeneuve J, Mottard JP, Cadrin C, Lemieux I, Despres JP. Atypical antipsychotics and cardiovascular risk in schizophrenic patients. J Clin Psychopharmacol 2001;21(1):110–11.
387. Popli AP, Konicki PE, Jurjus GJ, Fuller MA, Jaskiw GE. Clozapine and associated diabetes mellitus. J Clin Psychiatry 1997;58(3):108–11.
388. Wirshing DA, Spellberg BJ, Erhart SM, Marder SR, Wirshing WC. Novel antipsychotics and new onset diabetes. Biol Psychiatry 1998;44(8):778–83.
389. Newcomer JW, Haupt DW, Fucetola R, Melson AK, Schweiger JA, Cooper BP, Selke G. Abnormalities in glucose regulation during antipsychotic treatment of schizophrenia. Arch Gen Psychiatry 2002;59(4):337–45.
390. Baptista T. Body weight gain induced by antipsychotic drugs: mechanisms and management. Acta Psychiatr Scand 1999;100(1):3–16.
391. Taylor DM, McAskill R. Atypical antipsychotics and weight gain—a systematic review. Acta Psychiatr Scand 2000;101(6):416–32.
392. Gupta S, Droney T, Al-Samarrai S, Keller P, Frank B. Olanzapine-induced weight gain. Ann Clin Psychiatry 1998;10(1):39
393. Brecher M, Geller W. Weight gain with risperidone. J Clin Psychopharmacol 1997;17(5):435–6.
394. Penn JV, Martini J, Radka D. Weight gain associated with risperidone. J Clin Psychopharmacol 1996;16(3):259–60.
395. Frankenburg FR, Zanarini MC, Kando J, Centorrino F. Clozapine and body mass change. Biol Psychiatry 1998;43(7):520–4.
396. Bustillo JR, Buchanan RW, Irish D, Breier A. Differential effect of clozapine on weight: a controlled study. Am J Psychiatry 1996;153(6):817–19.
397. Kraepelin E. Dementia Praecox and Paraphrenia. Edinburgh: E & S Livingstone, 1919:87.
398. Gupta S, Droney T, Al-Samarrai S, Keller P, Frank B. Olanzapine: weight gain therapeutic efficacy. J Clin Psychopharmacol 1999;19(3):273–5.
399. Baymiller SP, Ball P, McMahon RP, Buchanan RW. Weight and blood pressure change during clozapine treatment. Clin Neuropharmacol 2002;25(4):202–6.
400. Monteleone P, Fabrazzo M, Tortorella A, La Pia S, Maj M. Pronounced early increase in circulating leptin predicts a lower weight gain during clozapine treatment. J Clin Psychopharmacol 2002;22(4):424–6.
401. Wetterling T. Bodyweight gain with atypical antipsychotics. A comparative review. Drug Saf 2001;24(1):59–73.
402. Blin O, Micallef J. Antipsychotic-associated weight gain and clinical outcome parameters. J Clin Psychiatry 2001;62(Suppl 7):11–21.
403. Allison DB, Casey DE. Antipsychotic-induced weight gain: a review of the literature. J Clin Psychiatry 2001;62(Suppl 7):22–31.
404. Kurzthaler I, Fleischhacker WW. The clinical implications of weight gain in schizophrenia. J Clin Psychiatry 2001;62(Suppl 7):32–7.
405. Casey DE, Zorn SH. The pharmacology of weight gain with antipsychotics. J Clin Psychiatry 2001;62(Suppl 7):4–10.
406. Allison DB, Mentore JL, Heo M, Chandler LP, Cappelleri JC, Infante MC, Weiden PJ. Antipsychotic-induced weight gain: a comprehensive research synthesis. Am J Psychiatry 1999;156(11):1686–96.
407. Allison DB, Mentore JL, Heo M, et al. Weight gain associated with conventional and newer antipsychotics: a meta-analysis. Presented at the New Clinical Drug Evaluation Unit 38th Annual Meeting, Boca Raton, Florida, June 10–13, 1998.
408. Kelly DL, Conley RR, Lore RC, et al. Weight gain in adolescents treated with risperidone and conventional antipsychotics over six months. J Child Adolesc Psychopharmacol 1998;813:151–9.
409. Wistedt B. A depot neuroleptic withdrawal study. A controlled study of the clinical effects of the withdrawal of depot fluphenazine decanoate and depot flupenthixol decanoate in chronic schizophrenic patients. Acta Psychiatr Scand 1981;64(1):65–84.
410. Nemeroff CB. Dosing the antipsychotic medication olanzapine. J Clin Psychiatry 1997;58(Suppl 10):45–9.
411. Ganguli R, Brar JS, Ayrton Z. Weight gain over 4 months in schizophrenia patients: a comparison of olanzapine and risperidone. Schizophr Res 2001;49(3):261–7.
412. Wetterling T, Mussigbrodt HE. Weight gain: side effect of atypical neuroleptics? J Clin Psychopharmacol 1999;19(4):316–21.
413. Reinstein MJ, Sirotovskaya LA, Jones LE, Mohan S, Chasanov MA. Effect of clozapine-quetiapine combination therapy on weight and glycaemic control. Clin Drug Invest 1999;18:99–104.
414. Owens DG. Extrapyramidal side effects and tolerability of risperidone: a review. J Clin Psychiatry 1994;55(Suppl 5):29–35.
415. Rietschel M, Naber D, Fimmers R, Moller HJ, Propping P, Nothen MM. Efficacy and side-effects of clozapine not associated with variation in the 5-HT$_{2C}$ receptor. Neuroreport 1997;8(8):1999–2003.
416. Rietschel M, Naber D, Oberlander H, Holzbach R, Fimmers R, Eggermann K, Moller HJ, Propping P, Nothen MM. Efficacy and side-effects of clozapine: testing for association with allelic variation in the dopamine D$_4$ receptor gene. Neuropsychopharmacology 1996;15(5):491–6.
417. Theisen FM, Cichon S, Linden A, Martin M, Remschmidt H, Hebebrand J. Clozapine and weight gain. Am J Psychiatry 2001;158(5):816.
418. Reynolds GP, Zhang ZJ, Zhang XB. Association of antipsychotic drug-induced weight gain with a 5-HT$_{2C}$ receptor gene polymorphism. Lancet 2002;359(9323):2086–7.
419. Allison DB, Fontaine KR, Heo M, Mentore JL, Cappelleri JC, Chandler LP, Weiden PJ, Cheskin LJ. The distribution of body mass index among individuals with and without schizophrenia. J Clin Psychiatry 1999;60(4):215–20.
420. Hummer M, Kemmler G, Kurz M, Kurzthaler I, Oberbauer H, Fleischhacker WW. Weight gain induced by clozapine. Eur Neuropsychopharmacol 1995;5(4):437–40.
421. Kohnke MD, Griese EU, Stosser D, Gaertner I, Barth G. Cytochrome P450 2D6 deficiency and its clinical relevance in a patient treated with risperidone. Pharmacopsychiatry 2002;35(3):116–18.
422. European Federation of Associations of Families of Mentally Ill People. www.eufami.org.
423. O'Keefe C, Noordsy D. Prevention and reversal of weight gain associated with antipsychotic treatment. J Clin Outcomes Manage 2002;9:575–82.
424. Rotatori AF, Fox R, Wicks A. Weight loss with psychiatric residents in a behavioral self control program. Psychol Rep 1980;46(2):483–6.
425. Floris M, Lejeune J, Deberdt W. Effect of amantadine on weight gain during olanzapine treatment. Eur Neuropsychopharmacol 2001;11(2):181–2.

512. Warnes H. Toxic psychosis due to antiparkinsonian drugs. Can Psychiatr Assoc J 1967;12(3):323–6.
513. Dunlap JC, Miller WC. Toxic psychosis following the use of benztropine methanesulfonate (Congentin). J S C Med Assoc 1969;65(6):203–4.
514. el-Yosef MK, Janowsky DS, Davis JM, Sekerke HJ. Reversal of benztropine toxicity by physostigmine. JAMA 1972;220(1):125.
515. Bourin M, Baker GB. Therapeutic and adverse effect considerations when using combinations of neuroleptics and benziodiazepines. Saudi Pharm J 1998;3–4;262–5.
516. Hatta K, Takahashi T, Nakamura H, Yamashiro H, Endo H, Kito K, Saeki T, Masui K, Yonezawa Y. A risk for obstruction of the airways in the parenteral use of levomepromazine with benzodiazepine. Pharmacopsychiatry 1998;31(4):126–30.
517. Ayd FJ Jr. Loxapine update: 1966–1976. Dis Nerv Syst 1977;38(11):883–7.
518. Markowitz JS, Wells BG, Carson WH. Interactions between antipsychotic and antihypertensive drugs. Ann Pharmacother 1995;29(6):603–9.
519. Frye PE, Pariser SF, Kim MH, O'Shaughnessy RW. Bromocriptine associated with symptom exacerbation during neuroleptic treatment of schizoaffective schizophrenia. J Clin Psychiatry 1982;43(6):252–3.
520. Kulhanek F, Linde OK, Meisenberg G. Precipitation of antipsychotic drugs in interaction with coffee or tea. Lancet 1979;2(8152):1130.
521. Bowen S, Taylor KM, Gibb IA. Effect of coffee and tea on blood levels and efficacy of antipsychotic drugs. Lancet 1981;1(8231):1217–18.
522. Bezchlinbnyk KZ, Jeffries JJ. Should psychiatric patients drink coffee? Can Med Assoc 1981;124:357.
523. Knudsen P, Vilmar T. Cannabis and neuroleptic agents in schizophrenia. Acta Psychiatr Scand 1984;69(2):162–74.
524. Fast DK, Jones BD, Kusalic M, Erickson M. Effect of carbamazepine on neuroleptic plasma levels and efficacy. Am J Psychiatry 1986;143(1):117–18.
525. Nisijima K, Kusakabe Y, Ohtuka K, Ishiguro T. Addition of carbamazepine to long-term treatment with neuroleptics may induce neuroleptic malignant syndrome. Biol Psychiatry 1998;44(9):930–1.
526. Hegarty AM, Lipton RG, Merriam AE, Freeman K. Cocaine as a risk factor for acute dystonic reactions. Neurology 1991;41:1670–2.
527. Freeman MP, Stoll AL. Mood stabilizer combinations: a review of safety and efficacy. Am J Psychiatry 1998;155(1):12–21.
528. Jefferson JW, Greist JH, Baudhuin M. Lithium: interactions with other drugs. J Clin Psychopharmacol 1981;1(3):124–34.
529. Waddington JL. Some pharmacological aspects relating to the issue of possible neurotoxic interactions during combined lithium-neuroleptic therapy. Hum Psychopharmacol 1990;5:293–7.
530. Batchelor DH, Lowe MR. Reported neurotoxicity with the lithium/haloperidol combination and other neuroleptics. A literature review. Hum Psychopharmacol 1990; 5:275–80.
531. Gupta S, Racaniello AA. Neuroleptic malignant syndrome associated with amoxapine and lithium in an older adult. Ann Clin Psychiatry 2000;12(2):107–9.
532. Pope HG Jr., Cole JO, Choras PT, Fulwiler CE. Apparent neuroleptic malignant syndrome with clozapine and lithium. J Nerv Ment Dis 1986;174(8):493–5.
533. Spring G, Frankel M. New data on lithium and haloperidol incompatibility. Am J Psychiatry 1981;138(6):818–21.
534. Berry N, Pradhan S, Sagar R, Gupta SK. Neuroleptic malignant syndrome in an adolescent receiving olanzapine–lithium combination therapy. Pharmacotherapy 2003;23(2):255–9.
535. Bourgeois JA, Kahn DR. Neuroleptic malignant syndrome following administration of risperidone and lithium. J Clin Psychopharmacol 2003;23(3):315–17.
536. Deng MZ, Chen GQ, Phillips MR. Neuroleptic malignant syndrome in 12 of 9,792 Chinese inpatients exposed to neuroleptics: a prospective study. Am J Psychiatry 1990;147(9):1149–55.
537. Gill J, Singh H, Nugent K. Acute lithium intoxication and neuroleptic malignant syndrome. Pharmacotherapy 2003;23(6):811–15.
538. Vardy MM, Kay SR. LSD psychosis or LSD-induced schizophrenia? A multimethod inquiry. Arch Gen Psychiatry 1983;40(8):877–83.
539. Robertson GH, Taveras JM, Tadmor R, et al. Computed tomography in metrizamide cisternography: importance of coronal and axial views. J Comput Assist Tomogr 1977;1:241.
540. Hartter S, Dingemanse J, Baier D, Ziegler G, Hiemke C. Inhibition of dextromethorphan metabolism by moclobemide. Psychopharmacology (Berl) 1998;135(1):22–6.
541. Rivera JM, Iriarte LM, Lozano F, Garcia-Bragado F, Salgado V, Grilo A. Possible estrogen-induced NMS. DICP 1989;23(10):811.
542. Houghton GW, Richens A. Inhibition of phenytoin metabolism by other drugs used in epilepsy. Int J Clin Pharmacol Biopharm 1975;12(1–2):210–16.
543. Siris JH, Pippenger CE, Werner WL, Masland RL. Anticonvulsant drug-serum levels in psychiatric patients with seizure disorders. Effects of certain psychotropic drugs. NY State J Med 1974;74(9):1554–6.
544. Sands CD, Robinson JD, Salem RB, Stewart RB, Muniz C. Effect of thioridazine on phenytoin serum concentration: a retrospective study. Drug Intell Clin Pharm 1987; 21(3):267–72.
545. Kutt H, McDowell F. Management of epilepsy with diphenylhydantoin sodium. Dosage regulation for problem patients. JAMA 1968;203(11):969–72.
546. Haidukewych D, Rodin EA. Effect of phenothiazines on serum antiepileptic drug concentrations in psychiatric patients with seizure disorder. Ther Drug Monit 1985;7(4):401–4.
547. Gram LF, Christiansen J, Overo KF. Interaction between neuroleptics and tricyclic antidepressants. In: Morselli PL, Garranttini S, Cohen SN, editors. Drug Interactions. New York: Raven Press, 1974:271.
548. Vincent FM. Phenothiazine-induced phenytoin intoxication. Ann Intern Med 1980;93(1):56–7.
549. Jann MW, Fidone GS, Hernandez JM, Amrung S, Davis CM. Clinical implications of increased antipsychotic plasma concentrations upon anticonvulsant cessation. Psychiatry Res 1989;28(2):153–9.
550. Linnoila M, Viukari M, Vaisanen K, Auvinen J. Effect of anticonvulsants on plasma haloperidol and thioridazine levels. Am J Psychiatry 1980;137(7):819–21.
551. Ereshefsky L, Saklad SR, Watanabe MD, Davis CM, Jann MW. Thiothixene pharmacokinetic interactions: a study of hepatic enzyme inducers, clearance inhibitors, and demographic variables. J Clin Psychopharmacol 1991;11(5):296–301.
552. Miller DD. Effect of phenytoin on plasma clozapine concentrations in two patients. J Clin Psychiatry 1991;52(1):23–5.
553. Sturman G. Interaction between piperazine and chlorpromazine. Br J Pharmacol 1974;50(1):153–5.
554. Bernard JM, Le Roux D, Pereon Y. Acute dystonia during sevoflurane induction. Anesthesiology 1999; 90(4):1215–16.

555. Benazzi F. Urinary retention with sertraline, haloperidol, and clonazepam combination. Can J Psychiatry 1998;43(10):1051–2.
556. Kurlan R. Acute parkinsonism induced by the combination of a serotonin reuptake inhibitor and a neuroleptic in adults with Tourette's syndrome. Mov Disord 1998;13(1):178–9.
557. Lee MS, Kim YK, Lee SK, Suh KY. A double-blind study of adjunctive sertraline in haloperidol-stabilized patients with chronic schizophrenia. J Clin Psychopharmacol 1998;18(5):399–403.
558. Linnoila M, George L, Guthrie S. Interaction between antidepressants and perphenazine in psychiatric inpatients. Am J Psychiatry 1982;139(10):1329–31.
559. Maynard GL, Soni P. Thioridazine interferences with imipramine metabolism and measurement. Ther Drug Monit 1996;18(6):729–31.

Neuromuscular blocking drugs

See also Individual agents

General Information

There are two broad classes of neuromuscular blocking drugs: non-depolarizing agents, of which the prototype is curare (for example, d-tubocurarine, atracurium, metocurine, mivacurium, pancuronium, rocuronium, vecuronium) and depolarizing blockers, such as suxamethonium. This monograph is largely concerned with the former; suxamethonium is the subject of a separate monograph.

Non-depolarizing neuromuscular blocking agents compete with acetylcholine for receptors at the neuromuscular junction and clinical relaxation begins when 80–85% of the receptors on the motor end-plate are blocked. They do not produce depolarization themselves and, by blocking access to the receptors, prevent the normal acetylcholine-induced depolarization. Flaccid paralysis ensues. Their action terminates when acetylcholine again gains access to the receptors, due to diffusion of the relaxant molecules away from the neuromuscular junction. This may be hastened by greatly increasing the number of acetylcholine molecules at the motor end-plate by giving an anticholinesterase such as neostigmine. In contrast, the depolarizing blockers first depolarize the motor end-plate and then prevent further depolarization.

Combining different non-depolarizing neuromuscular blocking agents can result in additive or synergistic effects. When pancuronium is given together with D-tubocurarine or metocurine, the resulting block is greater than would be expected if the effects were purely additive. This potentiation is not seen with the metocurine D-tubocurarine combination (1). Synergism resulting from such combinations is thought to be a postsynaptic effect (2). When different non-depolarizing agents are given consecutively, the neuromuscular blocking action of the second may be considerably modified by the first; the action of vecuronium, for example, lasts longer than expected if pancuronium has been given first (SEDA-11, 124) (3). Caution should therefore be exercised when giving a small dose of a normally short-acting non-depolarizer near the end of an operation when another long-acting agent has been given earlier. The resulting block can be greater than expected and last much longer than desired. Reversal with anticholinesterases can be difficult at the end of surgery if the block is still greater than 90%.

Specialized accounts of adverse effects and interactions in this field are available (4–7), including a review of the older literature (8).

Organs and Systems

Ear, nose, throat

Endotracheal intubation is less traumatic when it is facilitated by a muscle relaxant. Vocal cord hematoma after intubation occurred in six of 36 patients when only fentanyl plus propofol was used, compared with one of 37 when atracurium was added (9).

Nervous system

Drug accumulation will result in paralysis lasting from hours to days. Occasionally, however, paralysis can persist for weeks or even months because of relaxant-associated myopathy (10). Muscle weakness, causing difficulties in the subsequent weaning of such patients from artificial ventilation, has often been described (11–15). This condition has been observed most often after concomitant administration of muscle relaxants and high-dose glucocorticoids, typically in patients with exacerbated asthma requiring mechanical ventilation (16–21). It is not known how these factors combine to produce myopathy; myopathic changes can also occur after either high-dose glucocorticoid therapy or long-term muscle relaxant administration alone. Serial electrophysiological testing, and eventually muscle biopsy, is necessary to diagnose myopathy accurately and to avoid useless trials of weaning the patient from the ventilator. Within some weeks, muscle weakness will resolve sufficiently to allow successful weaning, but extensive rehabilitative measures are required for several months until the patient is independent. In view of the multitude of potential mechanisms of muscle weakness in critically ill patients, it is advisable always to monitor neuromuscular function and to avoid complete paralysis for any length of time in intensive care patients who are treated with muscle relaxants.

Musculoskeletal

Several authors have described heterotopic ossification or myositis ossificans after long-term administration of neuromuscular blocking agents to ICU patients (22–25). However, the causative role of muscle relaxants in the development of this phenomenon has been questioned (26), because of the observation that heterotopic ossification also occurred in critically ill patients not treated with such agents (27). It was suggested that prolonged immobilization is an important factor in the pathogenesis of heterotopic ossification, and that both deep sedation and neuromuscular blockade, by producing complete immobilization, might contribute to the pathophysiology of this severe complication in critical illness, which may require prolonged rehabilitation and surgical removal of ectopic

from 7 to 26%. Clinical doses of these drugs can induce partial curarization in neonates.
(2) Despite reduced plasma cholinesterase activity, the duration of effect of suxamethonium 1 mg/kg is usually not significantly increased in pregnant women.
(3) At clinical doses, transplacental passage of suxamethonium is insufficient to produce paralysis of the neonate.

However, inadequate muscular activity requiring ventilatory support has been reported in babies born to mothers with atypical plasma cholinesterase.

Susceptibility Factors

Age

Children

Neonates are said to be more sensitive to non-depolarizing neuromuscular blocking drugs. Neonates have a lower muscle mass per kilogram body weight, maturation of neuromuscular transmission occurs in the 2 months after full-term birth (88,89), and the "margin of safety" for neuromuscular transmission (that is the fraction of receptors that must be occupied before neuromuscular block can be detected) is reduced in infants under 12 weeks of age (90). Thus, smaller doses should be used in the very young. The greater body water content of neonates, however, tends to mitigate the increased sensitivity, so that several authors recommend similar doses to adults (calculated on a body weight basis). Owing to longer elimination half-lives, recovery is slower in neonates and maintenance doses are needed at longer intervals (91), certainly where most of the older, long-acting relaxants are concerned. There are conflicting data about whether the actions of vecuronium and atracurium (and even pancuronium) are prolonged or not (92).

Most investigators concur that neonates and infants require a larger dose per kilogram of suxamethonium (2–4 mg/kg) to achieve an equivalent effect to that seen in adults. In young children the plasma clearance of non-depolarizing relaxants is quicker and their duration of action shorter (93,94), so that doses may have to be given more often.

Interindividual variation in dose requirements is even more marked in neonates and infants than in adults, so that monitoring of neuromuscular function is essential. Small dysmature babies, especially with temperatures below 36°C, are notoriously unpredictable in their response to relaxants.

Elderly people

In elderly people there is much slower recovery from non-depolarizing relaxants (about 60% in patients over 75 years of age given pancuronium), associated with a decreased rate of elimination (probably through reduced glomerular clearance and, to a lesser extent, reduced hepatic blood flow). The potency of relaxants is not altered. While the initial dose required to produce full relaxation is the same as in young adults, smaller maintenance doses are required at much longer intervals (95,96). The duration of action of atracurium is not increased, since termination of its action does not depend on renal or hepatic function.

Other features of the patient

Acid–base and electrolyte changes

It has long been accepted that respiratory acidosis tends to potentiate the blockade produced by non-depolarizing relaxants and respiratory alkalosis produces resistance to their action. This is true for the monoquaternary agents D-tubocurarine, vecuronium, and rocuronium (possibly by increased conversion to the bisquaternary forms at lower pH), but it may not hold for the bisquaternary relaxants metocurine, pancuronium, and alcuronium (97–99).

Protein binding of muscle relaxants is maximal between pH 8 and 9 and this may account for increased dose requirements in alkalosis.

Alkalosis is often associated with hypokalemia, in which the actions of non-depolarizing agents may be increased and those of depolarizing agents reduced. Hyperkalemia has the opposite effects, probably by lowering muscle transmembrane potential.

Variations in serum sodium affect neuromuscular blocking agents in a similar manner to potassium changes. However, serum concentrations of electrolytes do not always reflect intracellular concentrations or, perhaps more important, the intra/extracellular concentration ratios; in addition, changes in pH and the concentrations of potassium, sodium and other electrolytes are linked and have opposing influences at several sites in the processes of neuromuscular function, so that the expected effect of a change, taken in isolation, may not be found. Nevertheless, it is of practical importance that respiratory acidosis may enhance non-depolarizing block and makes its reversal by neostigmine more difficult. Such a vicious circle in the recovery room is best broken by ventilating the patient until the cause of the respiratory depression is removed or corrected.

Hypermagnesemia enhances the actions of both depolarizing and non-depolarizing neuromuscular blocking agents. Lithium may also do this. Hypercalcemia may be associated with prolongation of suxamethonium blockade and reduced potency of non-depolarizing agents.

Body temperature

In hypothermia, a reduction in blood flow to muscle increases the time to onset of neuromuscular blockade. The actions (depth of block and duration) of depolarizing relaxants are increased. The potency of non-depolarizing neuromuscular blocking agents is reduced according to some investigators, while others maintain that potency is increased and the duration of action prolonged (100–102). Hypothermia produces different changes in the twitch (103) and electromyographic (104) responses to nerve stimulation in the absence of relaxants. The excretion and the metabolism of relaxants are reduced by hypothermia.

Hemodilution

Hemodilution (for example the replacement of 1 liter of blood by dextran-40) increased the potencies and prolonged the actions of suxamethonium, pancuronium, D-tubocurarine, and vecuronium (SEDA-17, 151) (105). To avoid this, blood collection should be carried out before the administration of anesthetic drugs.

Muscle diseases

The neuromuscular blocking effects of muscle relaxants in patients with neuromuscular disorders can differ significantly from those in healthy individuals. This can result in overdose and residual curarization on the one hand or in inadequate muscle relaxation on the other. Patients with Duchenne muscular dystrophy often require surgery for contractures and kyphoscoliosis. The neuromuscular blocking effects of vecuronium in eight children with Duchenne muscular dystrophy (11–15 years old) have been compared with those in eight children (8–18 years old) without this disease (106). After vecuronium 50 microgram/kg, the median train-of-four ratio was 0.14 in the patients versus 0.86 in the controls. The median time for recovery of the train-of-four ratio from 0.1 to 0.25 was 36 minutes in the patients versus 6 minutes in the controls. The authors concluded that patients with Duchenne muscular dystrophy need smaller initial doses of vecuronium. Because of the increased recovery time, patients should be closely observed for signs of residual curarization. Monitoring of neuromuscular transmission is strongly recommended in all patients with neuromuscular disorders who are given neuromuscular blocking agents.

Organ failure

Long-term administration of non-depolarizing muscle relaxants can result in prolonged paralysis, owing to accumulation of the drug itself or of pharmacologically active metabolites (107,108). Patients with renal or hepatic insufficiency are prone to this complication, but prolonged paralysis also has been noted in patients without these risk factors. The incidence of prolonged paralysis can probably be reduced if neuromuscular transmission monitoring is used to guide relaxant administration (109,110). In addition, agents with non-organ-dependent metabolic pathways may be of advantage (111). Residual curarization is only one of the potential reasons for prolonged paralysis after long-term neuromuscular blockade in severely ill patients. The interaction of different agents with other neuromuscular abnormalities, such as relaxant-associated myopathy, critical illness polyneuropathy, or other myopathic changes in the critically ill, still have to be evaluated.

Use in the intensive care unit

In the intensive care unit muscle relaxants are used to facilitate airway management and mechanical ventilation. The duration of administration can range from a single dose to continuous infusions for up to several weeks. Patients in ICU are more likely to have abnormalities of acid–base balance, electrolyte balance, body temperature, and liver and kidney function, predisposing them to the adverse effects of neuromuscular blocking drugs.

The most dangerous adverse effect of muscle relaxants in the ICU is suxamethonium-induced hyperkalemic cardiac arrest (112–117). Prolonged immobilization is believed to result in a spread of immature acetylcholine receptors on the muscle surface, which may mediate massive long-lasting potassium release if suxamethonium is given (118). By this mechanism, cardiac arrest can occur within minutes after suxamethonium administration. Standard resuscitative techniques have often failed, and several patients have died of this complication. Suxamethonium should therefore not be used in patients who are immobilized in the ICU for more than a few days. The shortest period of immobilization reported to be associated with fatal hyperkalemic cardiac arrest after suxamethonium administration was 4 days in a previously healthy young woman with bacterial meningitis (117).

Drug–Drug Interactions

Antibiotics

In very high doses or in sensitive patients (for example in myasthenia), antibiotics can produce paralysis and act additively or synergistically with neuromuscular blocking drugs.

Aminoglycosides

The aminoglycosides have a magnesium-like effect, acting prejunctionally to reduce transmitter release and postjunctionally to increase transmitter release; they also reduce postjunctional sensitivity to acetylcholine. In most cases their effects can be reversed, partly at least by calcium or 4-aminopyridine. Tobramycin is thought also to have a direct effect on muscle.

Beta-lactam antibiotics

Penicillins G and V (119) have been reported to cause neuromuscular block in animal preparations, but only at exceptionally high doses. Calcium is effective in reversal. The acylaminopenicillins augment vecuronium-induced blockade (120). Possible "re-curarization" with piperacillin was successfully reversed by neostigmine (121).

Lincosamides

The lincosamides have prejunctional and postjunctional effects, the principal action probably being on the muscle. This blockade is difficult to reverse with cholinesterase inhibitors or calcium.

Polymixins

The polymyxins probably produce a predominantly postjunctional effect (via ion channel block) and reduce muscle contractility. The block is difficult to reverse, calcium being only partly successful. Neostigmine has been reported to increase blockade produced by polymyxin B and colistin; in such cases 4-aminopyridine might be helpful.

Tetracyclines

The tetracyclines produce a small effect, partly by calcium chelation, thus reducing transmitter release. Reversal is usually, but inconsistently, obtained with calcium or neostigmine.

Peptide antibiotics

An unusually high dose of vancomycin augmented vecuronium-induced block during recovery, thus delaying the detubation of the patient for about 30 minutes (SEDA-16, 7). In another patient vancomycin prolonged the recovery from blockade induced by a suxamethonium infusion for some hours (SEDA-18, 14).

Management

If it is suspected that an antibiotic is contributing to prolonged neuromuscular blockade, the patient should be monitored and the effect of calcium (up to 1 g of calcium chloride slowly) should be observed. If this is unsuccessful, neostigmine (maximum dose 5 mg for an adult) or edrophonium (0.5 mg/kg) can be tried, but these agents may intensify a block due to colistin, lincomycin, or polymyxin B. If the other remedies fail, 4-aminopyridine (maximum dose 0.3 mg/kg) can be successful. Artificial ventilation should be continued until adequate spontaneous efforts are achieved and other possible factors, such as acidosis or electrolyte disturbances, are corrected.

This subject has been reviewed (119,122,123).

General anesthetics

Inhalational anesthetics

The volatile inhalational anesthetic agents and cyclopropane potentiate the actions of neuromuscular blocking drugs. The extent depends on the particular relaxant and inhalational agent used and the concentration of the latter. In comparative studies, isoflurane was the most potent in this respect, enflurane almost as potent, and both were 2–3 times more potent than halothane, which was in turn twice as potent as nitrous oxide, the volatile agents being administered at concentrations of 1.25 MAC (mean alveolar concentration) and the relaxant studied being D-tubocurarine (124). Concerning the older agents, the relaxant dose can be reduced by half with ether anesthesia and by one-fifth or more when cyclopropane is used. The degrees of potentiation by ether and cyclopropane probably lie between those of enflurane and halothane.

The higher the anesthetic concentration, the greater the degree of potentiation and the smaller the dose of relaxant needed (125). The full potentiating effect will only be seen when the tissues are saturated by the inhalational agent. Reducing the concentration of the inhalational agent generally reduces the degree of neuromuscular blockade (126), a desirable feature at the end of an operation. However, this maneuver can take some time to be effective (about half-an-hour for enflurane) and will only diminish the "volatile" contribution to the total block. Nevertheless, there may be occasions, such as in patients with myasthenia or renal or hepatic disease, when the advantages of using higher concentrations of inhalational anesthetic and lower doses of relaxants may outweigh the disadvantages (127).

The potentiation of D-tubocurarine block produced by enflurane slowly continues to increase with time, even after the usual equilibration period has passed (SEDA-5, 132) (128). This does not occur with halothane, and the discrepancy is said to mean that more D-tubocurarine will be required in the first hour of enflurane anesthesia than during equipotent halothane anesthesia, but that thereafter less will be required during enflurane anesthesia. It has been suggested that enflurane, unlike halothane, may produce an effect on muscle that takes time to develop. This may also be part of the mechanism, in addition to the greater potentiating action of enflurane, that explains the report that there is slower spontaneous recovery from pancuronium and a greatly impaired antagonistic effect of neostigmine in patients anesthetized with enflurane 1.3–1.4% compared with halothane 0.55–0.65% (end-tidal, in 70% nitrous oxide) (129). The experimental conditions in this last study, however, were somewhat different from usual clinical practice (130).

It is unfortunately not possible to come to a categorical conclusion on precisely how great the potentiation of a given relaxant will be by a particular inhalational anesthetic, because the effects of inhalational agents are multifactorial and diverse, and the numerous studies done have involved different methods (125,127,131–134). Very approximately, isoflurane and enflurane potentiate the longer-acting relaxants, such as D-tubocurarine and pancuronium, by 50–70% and the shorter-acting agents, vecuronium, atracurium, and mivacurium, by 20–25%. However, the degree of potentiation reported for the shorter-acting relaxants varies greatly (from 0 to 70% for vecuronium), depending on the duration of exposure of the skeletal muscles to the inhalational agent, the mode of nerve stimulation, whether the relaxant is given as a single bolus or by cumulative bolus doses or by infusion (steady-state or not), and the nature of the circulatory changes produced. The potentiation produced by halothane is much less than for isoflurane and enflurane.

Muscle relaxants may also contribute to anesthesia. Pancuronium 0.1 mg/kg has been reported to lower the MAC for halothane by 25% (135). It was conjectured that this could be due to a central effect or peripheral effect, through reduction of afferent input from muscle spindles to the reticular activating system. Recently, however, a similar though not identical study (SEDA-15, 124) (136) failed to confirm that pancuronium, vecuronium, or atracurium lowers the MAC for halothane.

Intravenous anesthetics

Intravenous anesthetic agents have much less influence on the neuromuscular blocking effects of relaxants and most have no clinically significant effect. However, ketamine (SEDA-14, 113) has been reported to significantly potentiate atracurium (137), and also D-tubocurarine but not pancuronium (138) in man. Animal studies suggest that all relaxants will be potentiated by ketamine in a dose-dependent manner (139,140). It has been suggested that had Johnston et al. (138) used a higher dose of ketamine (than 75 mg/m^2), they would have seen potentiation of pancuronium. The main effect of ketamine appears to be a reduction in the sensitivity of the post-junctional membrane to acetylcholine, possibly by ion-channel blockade. Propofol has been reported to potentiate vecuronium-induced and atracurium-induced blocks (141).

Laboratory investigations have shown that some benzodiazepines can produce biphasic effects (142,143), higher doses potentiating neuromuscular blocking agents (142,144); however, several human investigations have failed to show a significant effect (145–147). It has been suggested that agents that are added to commercial formulations of some benzodiazepines to render them more water-soluble may mask the benzodiazepine effect (147).

References

1. Lebowitz PW, Ramsey FM, Savarese JJ, Ali HH. Potentiation of neuromuscular blockade in man produced by combinations of pancuronium and metocurine or pancuronium and d-tubocurarine. Anesth Analg 1980;59(8):604–9.
2. Waud BE, Waud DR. Interaction among agents that block end-plate depolarization competitively. Anesthesiology 1985;63(1):4–15.
3. Rashkovsky OM, Agoston S, Ket JM. Interaction between pancuronium bromide and vecuronium bromide. Br J Anaesth 1985;57(11):1063–6.
4. Bowman WC. Pharmacology of Neuromuscular Function. 2nd ed. London/Boston/Singapore/Sydney/Toronto/ Wellington: Wright, 1990.
5. Muscle Relaxants. In: Agoston S, Bowman WC, editors. Monographs in Anaesthesiology. Amsterdam: Elsevier Science Publishers BV, 1990:19.
6. Lingle CJ, Steinbach JH. Neuromuscular blocking agents. Int Anesthesiol Clin 1988;26(4):288–301.
7. Bowman WC. Non-relaxant properties of neuromuscular blocking drugs. Br J Anaesth 1982;54(2):147–60.
8. Walts LF. Complications of muscle relaxants. In: Katz RL, editor. Muscle Relaxants. Amsterdam: Excerpta Medica, 1975:209.
9. Mencke T, Echternach M, Kleinschmidt S, Lux P, Barth V, Plinkert PK, Fuchs-Buder T. Laryngeal morbidity and quality of tracheal intubation: a randomized controlled trial. Anesthesiology 2003;98(5):1049–56.
10. Gooch JL. Prolonged paralysis after neuromuscular blockade. J Toxicol Clin Toxicol 1995;33(5):419–26.
11. Smith CL, Hunter JM, Jones RS. Vecuronium infusions in patients with renal failure in an ITU. Anaesthesia 1987;42(4):387–93.
12. Op de Coul AA, Lambregts PC, Koeman J, van Puyenbroek MJ, Ter Laak HJ, Gabreels-Festen AA. Neuromuscular complications in patients given Pavulon (pancuronium bromide) during artificial ventilation. Clin Neurol Neurosurg 1985;87(1):17–22.
13. Yate PM, Flynn PJ, Arnold RW, Weatherly BC, Simmonds RJ, Dopson T. Clinical experience and plasma laudanosine concentrations during the infusion of atracurium in the intensive therapy unit. Br J Anaesth 1987;59(2):211–17.
14. Rutledge ML, Hawkins EP, Langston C. Skeletal muscle growth failure induced in premature newborn infants by prolonged pancuronium treatment. J Pediatr 1986;109(5):883–6.
15. Torres CF, Maniscalco WM, Agostinelli T. Muscle weakness and atrophy following prolonged paralysis with pancuronium bromide in neonates. Ann Neurol 1985;18:403.
16. Barohn RJ, Jackson CE, Rogers SJ, Ridings LW, McVey AL. Prolonged paralysis due to nondepolarizing neuromuscular blocking agents and corticosteroids. Muscle Nerve 1994;17(6):647–54.
17. Hirano M, Ott BR, Raps EC, Minetti C, Lennihan L, Libbey NP, Bonilla E, Hays AP. Acute quadriplegic myopathy: a complication of treatment with steroids, nondepolarizing blocking agents, or both. Neurology 1992;42(11):2082–7.
18. Leatherman JW, Fluegel WL, David WS, Davies SF, Iber C. Muscle weakness in mechanically ventilated patients with severe asthma. Am J Respir Crit Care Med 1996;153(5):1686–90.
19. Subramony SH, Carpenter DE, Raju S, Pride M, Evans OB. Myopathy and prolonged neuromuscular blockade after lung transplant. Crit Care Med 1991;19(12):1580–2.
20. Giostra E, Magistris MR, Pizzolato G, Cox J, Chevrolet JC. Neuromuscular disorder in intensive care unit patients treated with pancuronium bromide. Occurrence in a cluster group of seven patients and two sporadic cases, with electrophysiologic and histologic examination. Chest 1994;106(1):210–20.
21. Margolis BD, Khachikian D, Friedman Y, Garrard C. Prolonged reversible quadriparesis in mechanically ventilated patients who received long-term infusions of vecuronium. Chest 1991;100(3):877–8.
22. Ackman JB, Rosenthal DI. Generalized periarticular myositis ossificans as a complication of pharmacologically induced paralysis. Skeletal Radiol 1995;24(5):395–7.
23. Clements NC Jr, Camilli AE. Heterotopic ossification complicating critical illness. Chest 1993;104(5):1526–8.
24. Ray TD, Lowe WD, Anderson LD, Muller AL, Brogdon BG. Periarticular heterotopic ossification following pharmacologically induced paralysis. Skeletal Radiol 1995;24(8):609–12.
25. Goodman TA, Merkel PA, Perlmutter G, Doyle MK, Krane SM, Polisson RP. Heterotopic ossification in the setting of neuromuscular blockade. Arthritis Rheum 1997;40(9):1619–27.
26. Dellestable F, Gaucher A, Voltz C. Heterotopic ossification in critically ill patients: comment on the article by Goodman et al. Arthritis Rheum 1998;41(7):1329–30.
27. Dellestable F, Voltz C, Mariot J, Perrier JF, Gaucher A. Heterotopic ossification complicating long-term sedation. Br J Rheumatol 1996;35(7):700–1.
28. Berg H, Roed J, Viby-Mogensen J, Mortensen CR, Engbaek J, Skovgaard LT, Krintel JJ. Residual neuromuscular block is a risk factor for postoperative pulmonary complications. A prospective, randomised, and blinded study of postoperative pulmonary complications after atracurium, vecuronium and pancuronium. Acta Anaesthesiol Scand 1997;41(9):1095–1103.
29. Debaene B, Plaud B, Dilly MP, Donati F. Residual paralysis in the PACU after a single intubating dose of nondepolarizing muscle relaxant with an intermediate duration of action. Anesthesiology 2003;98(5):1042–8.
30. Appelboam R, Mulder R, Saddler J. Atracurium associated with postoperative residual curarization. Br J Anaesth 2003;90(4):523.
31. Hayes AH, Mirakhur RK, Breslin DS, Reid JE, McCourt KC. Postoperative residual block after intermediate-acting neuromuscular blocking drugs. Anaesthesia 2001;56(4):312–18.
32. Baillard C, Gehan G, Reboul-Marty J, Larmignat P, Samama CM, Cupa M. Residual curarization in the recovery room after vecuronium. Br J Anaesth 2000;84(3):394–5.
33. Fawcett WJ, Dash A, Francis GA, Liban JB, Cashman JN. Recovery from neuromuscular blockade: residual curarisation following atracurium or vecuronium by bolus dosing or infusions. Acta Anaesthesiol Scand 1995;39(3):288–93.
34. Eriksson LI, Sundman E, Olsson R, Nilsson L, Witt H, Ekberg O, Kuylenstierna R. Functional assessment of the pharynx at rest and during swallowing in partially paralyzed humans: simultaneous videomanometry and mechanomyography of awake human volunteers. Anesthesiology 1997;87(5):1035–43.
35. Sundman E, Witt H, Olsson R, Ekberg O, Kuylenstierna R, Eriksson LI. The incidence and mechanisms of pharyngeal and upper esophageal dysfunction in partially paralyzed humans: pharyngeal videoradiography and simultaneous manometry after atracurium. Anesthesiology 2000;92(4):977–84.
36. Payne JP, Hughes R, Al Azawi S. Neuromuscular blockade by neostigmine in anaesthetized man. Br J Anaesth 1980;52(1):69–76.

37. Goldhill DR, Wainwright AP, Stuart CS, Flynn PJ. Neostigmine after spontaneous recovery from neuromuscular blockade. Effect on depth of blockade monitored with train-of-four and tetanic stimuli. Anaesthesia 1989;44(4):293–9.
38. Jones JE, Hunter JM, Utting JE. Use of neostigmine in the antagonism of residual neuromuscular blockade produced by vecuronium. Br J Anaesth 1987;59(11):1454–8.
39. Jones JE, Parker CJ, Hunter JM. Antagonism of blockade produced by atracurium or vecuronium with low doses of neostigmine. Br J Anaesth 1988;61(5):560–4.
40. Tramer MR, Fuchs-Buder T. Omitting antagonism of neuromuscular block: effect on postoperative nausea and vomiting and risk of residual paralysis. A systematic review. Br J Anaesth 1999;82(3):379–86.
41. Krombach J, Hunzelmann N, Koster F, Bischoff A, Hoffmann-Menzel H, Buzello W. Anaphylactoid reactions after cisatracurium administration in six patients. Anesth Analg 2001;93(5):1257–9.
42. Legros CB, Orliaguet GA, Mayer MN, Labbez F, Carli PA. Severe anaphylactic reaction to cisatracurium in a child. Anesth Analg 2001;92(3):648–9.
43. Briassoulis G, Hatzis T, Mammi P, Alikatora A. Persistent anaphylactic reaction after induction with thiopentone and cisatracurium. Paediatr Anaesth 2000;10(4):429–34.
44. Mertes PM, Laxenaire MC. Allergic reactions occurring during anaesthesia. Eur J Anaesthesiol 2002;19(4):240–62.
45. Laxenaire MC, Moneret-Vautrin DA, Watkins J. Diagnosis of the causes of anaphylactoid anaesthetic reactions. A report of the recommendations of the joint Anaesthetic and Immuno-allergological Workshop, Nancy, France: 19 March 1982. Anaesthesia 1983;38(2):147–8.
46. Fisher MM, More DG. The epidemiology and clinical features of anaphylactic reactions in anaesthesia. Anaesth Intensive Care 1981;9(3):226–34.
47. Laxenaire MC. Epidémiologie des réactions anaphylactoïdes peranesthésiques. Quatrième enquête multicentrique (juillet 1994–décembre 1996). [Epidemiology of anesthetic anaphylactoid reactions. Fourth multicenter survey (July 1994–December 1996).] Ann Fr Anesth Reanim 1999;18(7):796–809.
48. Hatton F, Tiret L, Maujol L, N'Doye P, Vourc'h G, Desmonts JM, Otteni JC, Scherpereel P. INSERM. Enquête épidémiologique sur les anesthésies. Premiers résultats. [INSERM. Epidemiological survey of anesthesia. Initial results.] Ann Fr Anesth Reanim 1983;2(5):331–86.
49. Thornton JA, Lorenz W. Histamine and antihistamine in anaesthesia and surgery: report of a symposium. Anaesthesia 1983;38:373.
50. Fisher MM, Munro I. Life-threatening anaphylactoid reactions to muscle relaxants. Anesth Analg 1983;62(6):559–64.
51. Boileau S, Hummer-Sigiel M, Moeller R, Drouet N. Réévaluation des risques respectifs d'anaphylaxie et d'histaminoblitération avec les substances anesthésiologiques. [Reassessment of the respective risks of anaphylaxis and histamine liberation with anesthetic substances.] Ann Fr Anesth Reanim 1985;4(2):195–204.
52. Laxenaire MC. Substances responsables des chocs anaphylactiques peranesthésiques. Troisième enquête multicentrique française (1992–1994). [Substances responsible for peranesthetic anaphylactic shock. A third French multicenter study (1992–94).] Ann Fr Anesth Reanim 1996;15(8):1211–18.
53. Laxenaire MC, Moneret-Vautrin DA, Vervloet D, Alazia M, Francois G. Accidents anaphylactoïdes graves peranesthésiques. [Severe perianesthetic anaphylactic accidents.] Ann Fr Anesth Reanim 1985;4(1):30–46.
54. Laxenaire MC, Moneret-Vautrin DA, Vervloet D. The French experience of anaphylactoid reactions. Int Anesthesiol Clin 1985;23(3):145–60.
55. Galletly DC, Treuren BC. Anaphylactoid reactions during anaesthesia. Seven years' experience of intradermal testing. Anaesthesia 1985;40(4):329–33.
56. Pepys J, Pepys EO, Baldo BA, Whitwam JG. Anaphylactic/anaphylactoid reactions to anaesthetic and associated agents. Skin prick tests in aetiological diagnosis. Anaesthesia 1994;49(6):470–5.
57. Mertes PM, Laxenaire MC, Alla F; Groupe d'Etudes des Réactions Anaphylactoïdes Peranesthésiques. Anaphylactic and anaphylactoid reactions occurring during anesthesia in France in 1999–2000. Anesthesiology 2003;99(3):536–45.
58. Laxenaire MC, Mertes PM; Groupe d'Etudes des Réactions Anaphylactoïdes Peranesthésiques. Anaphylaxis during anaesthesïa. Results of a two-year survey in France. Br J Anaesth 2001;87(4):549–58.
59. Laxenaire M, Mertes P. Anaphylaxis during anaesthesia. Br J Anaesth 2002;88:605–6.
60. Aimone-Gastin I, Gueant JL, Laxenaire MC, Moneret-Vautrin DA. Pathogenesis of allergic reactions to anaesthetic drugs. Int J Immunopathol Pharmacol 1997; 10:193–6.
61. Vervloet D, Nizankowska E, Arnaud A, Senft M, Alazia M, Charpin J. Adverse reactions to suxamethonium and other muscle relaxants under general anesthesia. J Allergy Clin Immunol 1983;71(6):552–9.
62. Vervloet D. Allergy to muscle relaxants and related compounds. Clin Allergy 1985;15(6):501–8.
63. Assem ES. Characteristics of basophil histamine release by neuromuscular blocking drugs in patients with anaphylactoid reactions. Agents Actions 1984;14(3–4):435–40.
64. Watkins J. Heuristic decision-making in diagnosis and management of adverse drug reactions in anaesthesia and surgery: the case of muscle relaxants. Theor Surg 1989;4:212.
65. Harle DG, Baldo BA, Fisher MM. Detection of IgE antibodies to suxamethonium after anaphylactoid reactions during anaesthesia. Lancet 1984;1(8383):930–2.
66. Baldo BA, Harle DG, Fisher MM. In vitro diagnosis and studies on the mechanism(s) of anaphylactoid reactions to muscle relaxant drugs. Ann Fr Anesth Reanim 1985;4(2):139–45.
67. Youngman PR, Taylor KM, Wilson JD. Anaphylactoid reactions to neuromuscular blocking agents: a commonly undiagnosed condition? Lancet 1983;2(8350):597–9.
68. Bird AG. 'Allergic' drug reactions during anaesthesia. Adverse Drug React Bull 1985;110:408.
69. Gueant JL, Aimone-Gastin I, Laroche D, Pitiot V, Gerard P, Moneret-Vautrin DA, Bricard H, Laxenaire MC. Prospective evaluation of cell mediator release in anaphylaxis to anesthetic drugs. Allergy Clin Immunol Int 1996;8:120.
70. Fisher MM, Baldo BA. The diagnosis of fatal anaphylactic reactions during anaesthesia: employment of immunoassays for mast cell tryptase and drug-reactive IgE antibodies. Anaesth Intensive Care 1993;21(3):353–7.
71. Assem ES. Anaphylactic anaesthetic reactions. The value of paper radioallergosorbent tests for IgE antibodies to muscle relaxants and thiopentone. Anaesthesia 1990; 45(12):1032–8.
72. Guilloux L, Ricard-Blum S, Ville G, Motin J. A new radioimmunoassay using a commercially available solid support for the detection of IgE antibodies against muscle relaxants. J Allergy Clin Immunol 1992;90(2):153–9.
73. Moneret-Vautrin DA, Kanny G. Anaphylaxis to muscle relaxants: rational for skin tests. Allerg Immunol (Paris) 2002;34(7):233–40.

74. Fisher M. Intradermal testing after anaphylactoid reaction to anaesthetic drugs: practical aspects of performance and interpretation. Anaesth Intensive Care 1984;12(2):115–20.
75. Mata E, Gueant JL, Moneret-Vautrin DA, Bermejo N, Gerard P, Nicolas JP, Laxenaire MC. Clinical evaluation of in vitro leukocyte histamine release in allergy to muscle relaxant drugs. Allergy 1992;47(5):471–6.
76. Abuaf N, Rajoely B, Ghazouani E, Levy DA, Pecquet C, Chabane H, Leynadier F. Validation of a flow cytometric assay detecting in vitro basophil activation for the diagnosis of muscle relaxant allergy. J Allergy Clin Immunol 1999;104(2 Pt 1):411–18.
77. Monneret G, Benoit Y, Gutowski MC, Bienvenu J. Detection of basophil activation by flow cytometry in patients with allergy to muscle-relaxant drugs. Anesthesiology 2000;92(1):275–7.
78. Monneret G, Benoit Y, Debard AL, Gutowski MC, Topenot I, Bienvenu J. Monitoring of basophil activation using CD63 and CCR3 in allergy to muscle relaxant drugs. Clin Immunol 2002;102(2):192–9.
79. Fisher MM, Baldo BA. Immunoassays in the diagnosis of anaphylaxis to neuromuscular blocking drugs: the value of morphine for the detection of IgE antibodies in allergic subjects. Anaesth Intensive Care 2000;28(2):167–70.
80. Moneret-Vautrin DA, Kanny G, Gueant JL, Widmer S, Laxenaire MC. Prevention by monovalent haptens of IgE-dependent leucocyte histamine release to muscle relaxants. Int Arch Allergy Immunol 1995;107(1–3):172–5.
81. Sage DJ. Management of acute anaphylactoid reactions. Int Anesthesiol Clin 1985;23(3):175–86.
82. Fisher MM. Clinical observations on the pathophysiology and treatment of anaphylactic cardiovascular collapse. Anaesth Intensive Care 1986;14(1):17–21.
83. Harle DG, Baldo BA, Fisher MM. Cross-reactivity of metocurine, atracurium, vecuronium and fazadinium with IgE antibodies from patients unexposed to these drugs but allergic to other myoneural blocking drugs. Br J Anaesth 1985;57(11):1073–6.
84. Leynadier F, Dry J. Anaphylaxis to muscle-relaxant drugs: study of cross-reactivity by skin tests. Int Arch Allergy Appl Immunol 1991;94(1–4):349–53.
85. Fisher MM, Merefield D, Baldo B. Failure to prevent an anaphylactic reaction to a second neuromuscular blocking drug during anaesthesia. Br J Anaesth 1999;82(5):770–3.
86. Thacker MA, Davis FM. Subsequent general anaesthesia in patients with a history of previous anaphylactoid/anaphylactic reaction to muscle relaxant. Anaesth Intensive Care 1999;27(2):190–3.
87. Guay J, Grenier Y, Varin F. Clinical pharmacokinetics of neuromuscular relaxants in pregnancy. Clin Pharmacokinet 1998;34(6):483.
88. Goudsouzian NG. Maturation of neuromuscular transmission in the infant. Br J Anaesth 1980;52(2):205–14.
89. Goudsouzian NG, Standaert FG. The infant and the myoneural junction. Anesth Analg 1986;65(11):1208–17.
90. Crumrine RS, Yodlowski EH. Assessment of neuromuscular function in infants. Anesthesiology 1981;54(1):29–32.
91. Fisher DM, O'Keeffe C, Stanski DR, Cronnelly R, Miller RD, Gregory GA. Pharmacokinetics and pharmacodynamics of d-tubocurarine in infants, children, and adults. Anesthesiology 1982;57(3):203–8.
92. Goudsouzian NG. Muscle relaxants in paediatric anaesthesia. In: Agoston S, Bowman WC, editors. Monographs in Anaesthesiology. Amsterdam: Elsevier Science Publishers BV, 1990;19:285.
93. O'Keeffe C, Gregory GA, Stanski DR, et al. d-Tubocurarine: pharmacodynamics and kinetics in children. Anesthesiology 1979;51:S270.
94. Goudsouzian NG, Liu LM, Cote CJ. Comparison of equipotent doses of non-depolarizing muscle relaxants in children. Anesth Analg 1981;60(12):862–6.
95. Duvaldestin P, Saada J, Berger JL, D'Hollander A, Desmonts JM. Pharmacokinetics, pharmacodynamics, and dose-response relationships of pancuronium in control and elderly subjects. Anesthesiology 1982;56(1):36–40.
96. d'Hollander A, Massaux F, Nevelsteen M, Agoston S. Age-dependent dose-response relationship of ORG NC 45 in anaesthetized patients. Br J Anaesth 1982; 54(6):653–7.
97. Ono K, Ohta Y, Morita K, Kosaka F. The influence of respiratory-induced acid-base changes on the action of non-depolarizing muscle relaxants in rats. Anesthesiology 1988;68(3):357–62.
98. Aziz L, Ono K, Ohta Y, Morita K, Hirakawa M. The effect of CO_2-induced acid-base changes on the potencies of muscle relaxants and antagonism of neuromuscular block by neostigmine in rat in vitro. Anesth Analg 1994;78(2):322–7.
99. Ono K, Nagano O, Ohta Y, Kosaka F. Neuromuscular effects of respiratory and metabolic acid-base changes in vitro with and without nondepolarizing muscle relaxants. Anesthesiology 1990;73(4):710–16.
100. Ham J, Stanski DR, Newfield P, Miller RD. Pharmacokinetics and dynamics of d-tubocurarine during hypothermia in humans. Anesthesiology 1981;55:631.
101. Buzello W, Schluermann D, Schindler M, Spillner G. Hypothermic cardiopulmonary bypass and neuromuscular blockade by pancuronium and vecuronium. Anesthesiology 1985;62(2):201–4.
102. Buzello W, Schluermann D, Pollmaecher T, Spillner G. Unequal effects of cardiopulmonary bypass-induced hypothermia on neuromuscular blockade from constant infusion of alcuronium, d-tubocurarine, pancuronium, and vecuronium. Anesthesiology 1987;66(6):842–6.
103. Heier T, Caldwell JE, Sessler DI, Miller RD. The effect of local surface and central cooling on adductor pollicis twitch tension during nitrous oxide/isoflurane and nitrous oxide/fentanyl anesthesia in humans. Anesthesiology 1990;72(5):807–11.
104. Engbaek J, Skovgaard LT, Friis B, Kann T. The effect of temperature on the evoked EMG response. Anesthesiology 1989;72:A810.
105. Schuh FT. Influence off haemodilution on the potency of neuromuscular blocking drugs. Br J Anaesth 1981;53(3):263–5.
106. Ririe DG, Shapiro F, Sethna NF. The response of patients with Duchenne's muscular dystrophy to neuromuscular blockade with vecuronium. Anesthesiology 1998;88(2):351–4.
107. Segredo V, Caldwell JE, Matthay MA, Sharma ML, Gruenke LD, Miller RD. Persistent paralysis in critically ill patients after long-term administration of vecuronium. N Engl J Med 1992;327(8):524–8.
108. Vandenbrom RH, Wierda JM. Pancuronium bromide in the intensive care unit: a case of overdose. Anesthesiology 1988;69(6):996–7.
109. Frankel H, Jeng J, Tilly E, St Andre A, Champion H. The impact of implementation of neuromuscular blockade monitoring standards in a surgical intensive care unit. Am Surg 1996;62(6):503–6.
110. Rudis MI, Sikora CA, Angus E, Peterson E, Popovich J Jr, Hyzy R, Zarowitz BJ. A prospective, randomized, controlled evaluation of peripheral nerve stimulation versus standard clinical dosing of neuromuscular blocking agents in critically ill patients. Crit Care Med 1997;25(4):575–83.
111. Prielipp RC, Coursin DB, Scuderi PE, Bowton DL, Ford SR, Cardenas VJ Jr, Vender J, Howard D, Casale EJ, Murray MJ. Comparison of the infusion

requirements and recovery profiles of vecuronium and cisatracurium 51W89 in intensive care unit patients. Anesth Analg 1995;81(1):3–12.
112. Horton WA, Fergusson NV. Hyperkalaemia and cardiac arrest after the use of suxamethonium in intensive care. Anaesthesia 1988;43(10):890–1.
113. Hemming AE, Charlton S, Kelly P. Hyperkalaemia, cardiac arrest, suxamethonium and intensive care. Anaesthesia 1990;45(11):990–1.
114. Markewitz BA, Elstad MR. Succinylcholine-induced hyperkalemia following prolonged pharmacologic neuromuscular blockade. Chest 1997;111(1):248–50.
115. Berkahn JM, Sleigh JW. Hyperkalaemic cardiac arrest following succinylcholine in a longterm intensive care patient. Anaesth Intensive Care 1997;25(5):588–9.
116. Lee YM, Fountain SW. Suxamethonium and cardiac arrest. Singapore Med J 1997;38(7):300–1.
117. Hansen D. Suxamethonium-induced cardiac arrest and death following 5 days of immobilization. Eur J Anaesthesiol 1998;15(2):240–1.
118. Martyn JA, White DA, Gronert GA, Jaffe RS, Ward JM. Up-and-down regulation of skeletal muscle acetylcholine receptors. Effects on neuromuscular blockers. Anesthesiology 1992;76(5):822–43.
119. Sokoll MD, Gergis SD. Antibiotics and neuromuscular function. Anesthesiology 1981;55(2):148–59.
120. Tryba M. Wirkungsverstärkung nicht-depolarisierender Muskelrelaxantien durch Acylaminopenicilline. [Potentiation of the effect of non-depolarizing muscle relaxants by acylaminopenicillins. Studies on the example of vecuronium.] Anaesthesist 1985;34(12):651–5.
121. Mackie K, Pavlin EG. Recurrent paralysis following piperacillin administration. Anesthesiology 1990;72(3):561–3.
122. Singh YN, Marshall IG, Harvey AL. The mechanisms of the muscle paralysing actions of antibiotics and their interaction with neuromuscular blocking agents. Rev Drug Metab Drug Interact 1980;3:129.
123. Pittinger C, Adamson R. Antibiotic blockade of neuromuscular function. Annu Rev Pharmacol 1972;12:169–84.
124. Ali HH, Savarese JJ. Monitoring of neuromuscular function. Anesthesiology 1976;45(2):216–49.
125. Miller RD, Way WL, Dolan WM, Stevens WC, Eger EI 2nd. The dependence of pancuronium- and d-tubocurarine-induced neuromuscular blockades on alveolar concentrations of halothane and forane. Anesthesiology 1972;37(6):573–81.
126. Gencarelli PJ, Miller RD, Eger EI 2nd, Newfield P. Decreasing enflurane concentrations and d-tubocurarine neuromuscular blockade. Anesthesiology 1982;56(3):192–4.
127. Eger EI 2nd. Isoflurane: a review. Anesthesiology 1981;55(5):559–76.
128. Stanski DR, Ham J, Miller RD, Sheiner LB. Time-dependent increase in sensitivity to d-tubocurarine during enflurane anesthesia in man. Anesthesiology 1980;52(6):483–7.
129. Delisle S, Bevan DR. Impaired neostigmine antagonism of pancuronium during enflurane anaesthesia in man. Br J Anaesth 1982;54(4):441–5.
130. Hodges RJ, Harkness J. Suxamethonium sensitivity in health and disease; a clinical evaluation of pseudocholinesterase levels. BMJ 1954;4878:18–22.
131. Waud BE. Decrease in dose requirement of d-tubocurarine by volatile anesthetics. Anesthesiology 1979;51(4):298–302.
132. Rupp SM, Miller RD, Gencarelli PJ. Vecuronium-induced neuromuscular blockade during enflurane, isoflurane, and halothane anesthesia in humans. Anesthesiology 1984;60(2):102–5.
133. Cannon JE, Fahey MR, Castagnoli KP, Furuta T, Canfell PC, Sharma M, Miller RD. Continuous infusion of vecuronium: the effect of anesthetic agents. Anesthesiology 1987;67(4):503–6.
134. Swen J, Rashkovsky OM, Ket JM, Koot HW, Hermans J, Agoston S. Interaction between nondepolarizing neuromuscular blocking agents and inhalational anesthetics. Anesth Analg 1989;69(6):752–5.
135. Forbes AR, Cohen NH, Eger EI 2nd. Pancuronium reduces halothane requirement in man. Anesth Analg 1979;58(6):497–9.
136. Fahey MR, Sessler DI, Cannon JE, Brady K, Stoen R, Miller RD. Atracurium, vecuronium, and pancuronium do not alter the minimum alveolar concentration of halothane in humans. Anesthesiology 1989;71(1):53–6.
137. Toft P, Helbo-Hansen S. Interaction of ketamine with atracurium. Br J Anaesth 1989;62(3):319–20.
138. Johnston RR, Miller RD, Way WL. The interaction of ketamine with d-tubocurarine, pancuronium, and succinylcholine in man. Anesth Analg 1974;53(4):496–501.
139. Tsai SK, Lee CM, Tran B. Ketamine enhances phase I and phase II neuromuscular block of succinylcholine. Can J Anaesth 1989;36(2):120–3.
140. Amaki Y, Nagashima H, Radnay PA, Foldes FF. Ketamine interaction with neuromuscular blocking agents in the phrenic nerve-hemidiaphragm preparation of the rat. Anesth Analg 1978;57(2):238–43.
141. Robertson EN, Fragen RJ, Booij LH, van Egmond J, Crul JF. Some effects of diisopropyl phenol (ICI 35 868) on the pharmacodynamics of atracurium and vecuronium in anaesthetized man. Br J Anaesth 1983;55(8):723–8.
142. Driessen JJ, Vree TB, van Egmond J, Booij LH, Crul JF. In vitro interaction of diazepam and oxazepam with pancuronium and suxamethonium. Br J Anaesth 1984;56(10):1131–8.
143. Wali FA. Myorelaxant effect of diazepam. Interactions with neuromuscular blocking agents and cholinergic drugs. Acta Anaesthesiol Scand 1985;29(8):785–9.
144. Driessen JJ, Vree TB, van Egmond J, Booij LH, Crul JF. Interaction of midazolam with two non-depolarizing neuromuscular blocking drugs in the rat in vivo sciatic nerve-tibialis anterior muscle preparation. Br J Anaesth 1985;57(11):1089–94.
145. Asbury AJ, Henderson PD, Brown BH, Turner DJ, Linkens DA. Effect of diazepam on pancuronium-induced neuromuscular blockade maintained by a feedback system. Br J Anaesth 1981;53(8):859–63.
146. Cronnelly R, Morris RB, Miller RD. Comparison of thiopental and midazolam on the neuromuscular responses to succinylcholine or pancuronium in humans. Anesth Analg 1983;62(1):75–7.
147. Driessen JJ, Crul JF, Vree TB, van Egmond J, Booij LH. Benzodiazepines and neuromuscular blocking drugs in patients. Acta Anaesthesiol Scand 1986;30(8):642–6.

Nevirapine

See also Non-nucleoside reverse transcriptase inhibitors (NNRTIs)

General Information

Nevirapine is a non-nucleoside reverse transcriptase inhibitor (1). Concerns about the adverse effects of nevirapine have delayed its implementation in preventing perinatal HIV. Decision analysis has been used to compare three strategies: a single dose of nevirapine, a short course of zidovudine, and no intervention (2). The authors concluded that nevirapine would prevent more deaths than either zidovudine and no intervention, as long as the rate of nevirapine toxicity did not respectively exceed nine and 42 times that observed in an earlier nevirapine clinical trial (HIVNET). Nevirapine would be economically preferable to zidovudine as long as the rate of toxicity did not exceed 22 times that observed in the clinical trial. They thought that implementation of nevirapine should not be delayed by concerns about its adverse effects.

Observational studies

In 77 HIV-positive subjects randomized to switch from protease inhibitors to nevirapine or efavirenz or to continue taking protease inhibitors, quality of life significantly improved among those who switched (3). Lipid profiles improved in those who took nevirapine but gamma-glutamyltransferase and alanine aminotransferase activities increased significantly and one patient interrupted treatment because of hepatotoxicity.

Organs and Systems

Psychological, psychiatric

Various psychiatric abnormalities (delirium, an affective state, and a psychosis) have been described in three patients who took nevirapine for 10–14 days (4):

- cognitive impairment, clouding of consciousness, and a paranoid episode in a 35-year-old man
- delusions of persecutory and depressive thoughts in a 42-year-old woman
- delusions of persecution and infestation and hallucinations in a 36-year-old woman

All three responded to withdrawal of nevirapine.

Metabolism

Lipodystrophy, well recognized with stavudine, has also been reported in nine of 56 patients taking combined HAART therapy including nevirapine, although there must be some doubt as to which drug or combination was responsible (5).

Hematologic

Two patients developed grade 4 thrombocytopenia (under 25×10^9/l) after 42 and 151 days of treatment with nevirapine (6). In the first patient, zidovudine and intravenous immunoglobulin were added to continued nevirapine, and the thrombocytopenia resolved by day 89. In the second, nevirapine was discontinued and alternative antiretroviral therapy was started, whereupon the platelet count returned to normal within 22 days.

Liver

The most frequent laboratory abnormality during nevirapine treatment is an increase in serum gamma-glutamyl transpeptidase activity, usually without changes in other measures of hepatic function. However, in a randomized, placebo-controlled comparison of zidovudine plus nevirapine, zidovudine plus didanosine, and the triple combination of zidovudine plus didanosine and nevirapine in 151 patients, there were abnormal liver function tests in increased frequency in the patients taking nevirapine (19% and 12% versus 6%) (7). Five of 98 patients taking nevirapine had to stop the drug permanently because of raised alanine aminotransferase activity, after which the laboratory abnormalities resolved completely.

Of 70 HIV-infected patients taking nevirapine 33 developed rises in transaminase activities (8). Higher nevirapine concentrations and hepatitis C virus infection were independent predictors of liver toxicity. In those with chronic hepatitis C, nevirapine concentrations over 6 μg/ml were associated with a 92% risk of liver toxicity. The authors concluded that monitoring nevirapine concentrations, especially in individuals with chronic hepatitis C, may be warranted.

In a prospective study of the incidence of severe hepatotoxicity in 312 patients taking nevirapine, hepatitis C and hepatitis B viruses were detected in 43% (9). There was severe hepatotoxicity in 16%, but only 32% of episodes were detected during the first 12 weeks of therapy. The risk was significantly greater among those with chronic viral hepatitis (69% of cases) and those taking concurrent protease inhibitors (82% of cases). However, 84% of patients with chronic hepatitis C or hepatitis B did not have severe hepatotoxicity.

Severe hepatitis has been attributed to nevirapine (10).

- A 36-year-old woman with HIV and hepatitis C infection developed fever, right upper quadrant pain, headache, confusion, and a generalized skin rash. Her antiretroviral treatment included lamivudine (150 mg bd), stavudine (40 mg bd), and nevirapine (200 mg bd). The dose of nevirapine had been doubled 2 weeks before. Her laboratory results were as follows: white cell count 4.1×10^9/l with 18% eosinophils, aspartate aminotransferase 879 U/l, alanine aminotransferase 1424 U/l, lactate dehydrogenase 3268 U/l, activated prothrombin time 14 seconds, partial thromboplastin time 29 seconds. Abdominal ultrasound was normal. Her antiretroviral medications were stopped. She was given intravenous prednisolone (60 mg 6-hourly) and within 8 hours the signs of sepsis had abated and her liver function began to improve and resolved over the next few days. Several weeks later, she was rechallenged with lamivudine and zidovudine, without recurrence of liver toxicity or rash.

The authors argued that, although the syndrome could not be definitively attributed to nevirapine, several factors suggested that nevirapine was the most likely precipitant, including the fact that hepatic failure coincided with a systemic allergic response, which is commonly associated with nevirapine, especially after dose escalation. The rapid improvement with steroid therapy suggested that the hepatic failure was a manifestation of a systemic hypersensitivity reaction. However, since stavudine has also been associated with hepatitis, a causative role of stavudine cannot be excluded. The fact that lamivudine was given again without recurrence of hepatitis renders it an unlikely culprit.

In another case there was severe hepatic failure, which resolved on withdrawal and in which there was no other obvious cause than the use of nevirapine (11).

Significant hepatic deterioration, consistent with cholestasis, occurred 5 months into a HAART regimen including nevirapine (12).

- A 49-year-old man with severe factor VIII deficiency and stable chronic hepatitis C infection took stavudine, didanosine, and nevirapine. After 5 months of well-tolerated therapy, during which his viral load fell from 39 550 cpm to under 50 cpm, he developed anorexia, nausea, vomiting, fatigue, agitation, and biochemical evidence of deteriorating liver function. All drugs were withdrawn. There was no evidence of an infective cause and his hepatitis C status had not changed. Transvenous biopsy of the right hepatic lobe showed profound cholestasis and mild sinusoidal fibrosis, consistent with drug-induced cholestasis.

In four men aged 27, 41, 47, and 49 years, nevirapine was associated with a skin rash, malaise, and icteric hepatitis, 4–6 weeks after the start of therapy; resolution occurred after withdrawal of nevirapine (13).

Two health-care workers exposed to HIV developed severe hypersensitivity reactions to nevirapine; one required orthotopic liver transplantation to overcome the complications of acute hepatic failure and coma (14).

Skin

The principal, dose-limiting, adverse effect of nevirapine in adults is a rash, which occurs in 3–20% of patients, and which progresses to Stevens–Johnson syndrome in 0.5–1% of cases (15). Rash appears to be sex-specific; in 95 women and 263 men, women had a seven-fold higher risk of severe rash and were 3.5 times more likely to discontinue nevirapine than men (16).

In a review of the medical records of HIV-positive patients who had taken nevirapine, delavirdine, or both, the frequency of skin reactions was determined, as were the consequences of rechallenge with the same or the alternative agent (17). The overall incidence of rash attributed to the use of one of the non-nucleoside reverse transcriptase inhibitors (NNRTIs) was 37%. While rash due to delavirdine was more common (8/20 versus 25/69), the rash due to nevirapine was more severe and necessitated more frequent hospitalization. Rash recurred in six of eight patients who were rechallenged with the same agent and in seven of 10 who were switched to the alternative agent. The conclusion was drawn that there is little value in attempting to re-treat patients who have had skin reactions to NNRTIs, except possibly those with limited treatment options.

In a multiple dose study, 21 children aged 3 months to 15 years were treated with nevirapine in dosages of 7.5–400 mg/m^2/day for up to 168 days (18). When it was intended to use dosages over 240 mg/m^2/day they were pretreated with a lower dosage (120 mg/m^2/day) for 28 days to reduce the risk of rash. However, a rash developed in one child after 2 weeks of treatment with nevirapine at a dosage of 240 mg/m^2/day, resolved on withdrawal, and recurred on rechallenge with a single dose of 120 mg/m^2.

An unusually high incidence of nevirapine-associated rash has been reported in Chinese HIV-infected patients (19). Of eight Chinese patients, five developed a rash within 4 weeks of treatment, resolving on withdrawal. Since the total number of patients in this report was small, it remains to be shown whether Chinese are indeed at increased risk of hypersensitivity reactions to nevirapine.

Prevention

While skin reactions to nevirapine cannot be prevented by the use of glucocorticoids (6,20), it is possible to induce tolerance to them, enabling treatment to continue (6). All the same, very severe skin reactions, with characteristics of both Stevens–Johnson syndrome and Lyell's syndrome, have occasionally been reported (21).

A 14-day lead-in period reduces the frequency of rash, and other effective interventions include antihistamines and a longer lead-in period (4 weeks) (22). In an attempt to reduce the rate of nevirapine-associated rash, 469 patients were randomly assigned to different schedules of induction therapy (23). Using a standard procedure, 19% developed a rash compared with 11, 8.6, and 7.7% in subjects assigned to a slowly escalating dose, concomitant administration of prednisone, or both. The rate of drug withdrawal was also reduced by a half using the new approaches.

Drug–Drug Interactions

Methadone

When methadone is used in HIV infection (for pain or treatment of opioid dependence) nevirapine given simultaneously can reduce methadone blood concentrations, the effect being sufficient to cause methadone withdrawal symptoms (24,25).

Oral contraceptives

The mutual pharmacokinetic interaction of nevirapine with ethinylestradiol + norethindrone has been studied in 10 women (26). After a single dose of ethinylestradiol + norethindrone, they took oral nevirapine 200 mg/day (days 2–15), followed by 200 mg bd (days 16–29); on day 30 they took another dose of ethinylestradiol + norethindrone. Steady-state nevirapine reduced the AUC of ethinylestradiol by 29% and significantly reduced its mean residence time and half-life. The AUC of norethindrone was significantly reduced by 18%, but there was no change in C_{max}, mean residence time, or half-life. The kinetics of nevirapine were not affected by the oral contraceptive. The authors attributed this interaction to increased clearance of ethinylestradiol and concluded that oral contraceptives should not be the primary method of birth control in women of child-bearing potential who are taking nevirapine.

Protease inhibitors

Nevirapine induces CYP3A4 and therefore interacts with drugs such as protease inhibitors (27).

St John's wort

St John's wort reduced nevirapine concentrations, because of induction of CYP3A4 (28).

Warfarin

Nevirapine induces the metabolism of warfarin.

- A 38-year-old man with severe primary pulmonary hypertension and AIDS took warfarin 2.5 mg/day while he was taking zidovudine plus didanosine (29). His INR was 2.1–2.4. Later, because of virological failure, he was given a combination of stavudine, lamivudine, and nevirapine, and the INR promptly fell to 1.3. The dosage of warfarin was increased to 5 mg/day and anticoagulant activity was restored. All the antiretroviral drugs were then stopped because of an urticarial eruption, and a few days later stavudine, lamivudine, and saquinavir were given; warfarin 2.5 mg/day produced a stable INR.

References

1. De Wit S, Sternon J, Clumeck N. La nevirapine (viramune): un nouvel inhibiteur du VIH. [Nevirapine (Viramune): a new HIV inhibitor.] Rev Med Brux 1999;20(2):95–9.
2. Stringer JS, Sinkala M, Rouse DJ, Goldenberg RL, Vermund SH. Effect of nevirapine toxicity on choice of perinatal HIV prevention strategies. Am J Public Health 2002;92(3):365–6.
3. Negredo E, Cruz L, Paredes R, Ruiz L, Fumaz CR, Bonjoch A, Gel S, Tuldra A, Balague M, Johnston S, Arno A, Jou A, Tural C, Sirera G, Romeu J, Clotet B. Virological, immunological, and clinical impact of switching from protease inhibitors to nevirapine or to efavirenz in patients with human immunodeficiency virus infection and long-lasting viral suppression. Clin Infect Dis 2002; 34(4):504–10.
4. Wise ME, Mistry K, Reid S. Drug points: Neuropsychiatric complications of nevirapine treatment. BMJ 2002;324(7342):879.
5. Aldeen T, Wells C, Hay P, Davidson F, Lau R. Lipodystrophy associated with nevirapine-containing antiretroviral therapies. AIDS 1999;13(7):865–7.
6. Demoly P, Messaad D, Fabre J, Reynes J, Bousquet J. Nevirapine-induced cutaneous hypersensitivity reactions and successful tolerance induction. J Allergy Clin Immunol 1999;104(2 Pt 1):504–5.
7. Montaner JS, Reiss P, Cooper D, Vella S, Harris M, Conway B, Wainberg MA, Smith D, Robinson P, Hall D, Myers M, Lange JM. A randomized, double-blind trial comparing combinations of nevirapine, didanosine, and zidovudine for HIV-infected patients: the INCAS Trial. Italy, The Netherlands, Canada and Australia Study. JAMA 1998;279(12):930–7.
8. Gonzalez de Requena D, Nunez M, Jimenez-Nacher I, Soriano V. Liver toxicity caused by nevirapine. AIDS 2002;16(2):290–1.
9. Sulkowski MS, Thomas DL, Mehta SH, Chaisson RE, Moore RD. Hepatotoxicity associated with nevirapine or efavirenz-containing antiretroviral therapy: role of hepatitis C and B infections. Hepatology 2002;35(1):182–9.
10. Leitze Z, Nadeem A, Choudhary A, Saul Z, Roberts I, Manthous CA. Nevirapine-induced hepatitis treated with corticosteroids? AIDS 1998;12(9):1115–17.
11. Cattelan AM, Erne E, Salatino A, Trevenzoli M, Carretta G, Meneghetti F, Cadrobbi P. Severe hepatic failure related to nevirapine treatment. Clin Infect Dis 1999;29(2):455–6.
12. Clarke S, Harrington P, Condon C, Kelleher D, Smith OP, Mulcahy F. Late onset hepatitis and prolonged deterioration in hepatic function associated with nevirapine therapy. Int J STD AIDS 2000;11(5):336–7.
13. Prakash M, Poreddy V, Tiyyagura L, Bonacini M. Jaundice and hepatocellular damage associated with nevirapine therapy. Am J Gastroenterol 2001;96(5):1571–4.
14. Johnson S, Baraboutis JG, Sha BE, Proia LA, Kessler HA. Adverse effects associated with use of nevirapine in HIV postexposure prophylaxis for 2 health care workers. JAMA 2000;284(21):2722–3.
15. Metry DW, Lahart CJ, Farmer KL, Hebert AA. Stevens–Johnson syndrome caused by the antiretroviral drug nevirapine. J Am Acad Dermatol 2001;44(Suppl 2):354–7.
16. Bersoff-Matcha SJ, Miller WC, Aberg JA, van Der Horst C, Hamrick Jr HJ, Powderly WG, Mundy LM. Sex differences in nevirapine rash. Clin Infect Dis 2001;32(1):124–9.
17. Gangar M, Arias G, O'Brien JG, Kemper CA. Frequency of cutaneous reactions on rechallenge with nevirapine and delavirdine. Ann Pharmacother 2000;34(7–8):839–42.
18. Luzuriaga K, Bryson Y, McSherry G, Robinson J, Stechenberg B, Scott G, Lamson M, Cort S, Sullivan JL. Pharmacokinetics, safety, and activity of nevirapine in human immunodeficiency virus type 1-infected children. J Infect Dis 1996;174(4):713–21.
19. Ho TT, Wong KH, Chan KC, Lee SS. High incidence of nevirapine-associated rash in HIV-infected Chinese. AIDS 1998;12(15):2082–3.
20. Rey D, Partisani M, Krantz V, Kempf G, Nicolle M, de Mautort E, Priester M, Bernard-Henry C, Lang JM. Prednisolone does not prevent the occurrence of nevirapine-induced rashes. AIDS 1999;13(16):2307.
21. Wetterwald E, Le Cleach L, Michel C, David F, Revuz J. Nevirapine-induced overlap Stevens–Johnson syndrome/ toxic epidermal necrolysis. Br J Dermatol 1999;140(5):980–2.
22. Barreiro P, Soriano V, Gonzalez-Lahoz J, Colebunders R, Schrooten W, Desmet P, De Roo A, Dreezen C. Prevention of nevirapine-associated rash. Lancet 2001;357(9253):392–3.
23. Barreiro P, Soriano V, Casas E, Estrada V, Tellez MJ, Hoetelmans R, de Requena DG, Jimenez-Nacher I, Gonzalez-Lahoz J. Prevention of nevirapine-associated exanthema using slow dose escalation and/or corticosteroids. AIDS 2000;14(14):2153–7.
24. Heelon MW, Meade LB. Methadone withdrawal when starting an antiretroviral regimen including nevirapine. Pharmacotherapy 1999;19(4):471–2.
25. Clarke SM, Mulcahy FM, Tjia J, Reynolds HE, Gibbons SE, Barry MG, Back DJ. Pharmacokinetic interactions of nevirapine and methadone and guidelines for use of nevirapine to treat injection drug users. Clin Infect Dis 2001;33(9):1595–7.
26. Mildvan D, Yarrish R, Marshak A, Hutman HW, McDonough M, Lamson M, Robinson P. Pharmacokinetic interaction between nevirapine and ethinyl estradiol/ norethindrone when administered concurrently to HIV-infected women. J Acquir Immune Defic Syndr 2002;29(5):471–7.
27. Back D, Gibbons S, Khoo S. Pharmacokinetic drug interactions with nevirapine. J Acquir Immune Defic Syndr 2003;34(Suppl 1):S8–14.
28. de Maat MM, Hoetelmans RM, Math t RA, van Gorp EC, Meenhorst PL, Mulder JW, Beijnen JH. Drug interaction between St John's wort and nevirapine. AIDS 2001;15(3):420–1.
29. Dionisio D, Mininni S, Bartolozzi D, Esperti F, Vivarelli A, Leoncini F. Need for increased dose of warfarin in HIV patients taking nevirapine. AIDS 2001;15(2):277–8.

always be doubted (20–22). However, direct transmission of nickel between the hands and the anogenital region has to be taken into account, and food can be a rare source of nickel contact in the anogenital area. In these cases relevance can be proved by oral nickel provocation and a nickel-restricted diet for a limited period may be justified (23).

The therapeutic use of intramuscular chrysotherapy has been limited by the high incidence of skin adverse effects. The pathogenic mechanisms of these are unknown, but could include allergic reactions to gold or to nickel as a contaminant. In order to investigate these mechanisms further, 15 patients who developed skin eruptions after chrysotherapy were assessed using skin biopsy and lymphocyte transformation stimulated by gold and nickel salts in vitro (24). Chrysotherapy caused two main cutaneous eruptions: lichenoid reactions and non-specific dermatitis. Peripheral blood mononuclear cells from patients with lichenoid reactions proliferated in response to gold salts in vitro, while those who developed non-specific dermatitis responded mainly to nickel. Nickel was a significant contaminant of the gold formulation (sodium aurothiomalate, Myocrisin, Rhone-Poulenc Ltd), amounting to a total dose of 650 ng over 6 months. The authors suggested that a significant percentage of skin reactions during chrysotherapy are due to nickel contamination.

- A 79-year-old woman had an abdominal aortic aneurysm repaired with a straight Vanguard R stent, mainly composed of nickel (about 55%) and titanium (about 21%) with a reinforcing thread of platinum (25). Three weeks later she developed severe erythema and eczema on the legs with continuous pruritus and excoriated papules. Patch tests were positive to nickel sulfate and cobalt chloride.

The need for preoperative patch-testing for metals is controversial. Enquiry about metal allergy is recommended before endoluminal surgical procedures.

The mobile-phone culture has spread rapidly and possible effects connected with its use may still be underestimated (26).

- A 36-year-old dermatologist with a history of jewellery intolerance developed dermatitis on the right side of the chin, with red pruritic papules. The dermatitis had worsened after prolonged use of her mobile phone. Patch tests were positive to nickel sulfate. She solved the problem by covering the phone with a plastic case.
- A 32-year-old woman developed dermatitis on her left cheek and suggested that it might have been caused or worsened by her mobile phone. Patch tests showed only positive reaction to nickel sulfate. The dimethylglyoxime test for nickel on the side of her phone was positive. The skin lesion resolved rapidly after she covered the phone with a plastic case.

Long-Term Effects

Tumorigenicity

Carcinogenetic effects of nickel, recognized from occupational medicine, can involve the upper or lower respiratory tract.

Drug Administration

Drug overdose

Nickel poisoning is well defined in occupational medicine and is occasionally experienced as a complication of exposure to nickel (or nickel-plated) medical devices. Use of nickel-plated dialysis equipment gave rise to nickel poisoning in 23 patients in one hemodialysis unit. They developed nausca, vomiting, weakness, headache, and palpitation, all of which remitted 3–13 hours after the end of dialysis (SEDA-6, 225).

References

1. Eliades T, Athanasiou AE. In vivo aging of orthodontic alloys: implications for corrosion potential, nickel release, and biocompatibility. Angle Orthod 2002;72(3):222–37.
2. Shabalovskaya SA. Surface, corrosion and biocompatibility aspects of Nitinol as an implant material. Biomed Mater Eng 2002;12(1):69–109.
3. Savolainen H. Biochemical and clinical aspects of nickel toxicity. Rev Environ Health 1996;11(4):167–73.
4. Barceloux DG. Nickel. J Toxicol Clin Toxicol 1999;37(2): 239–58.
5. Waterman AH, Schrik JJ. Allergy in hip arthroplasty. Contact Dermatitis 1985;13(5):294–301.
6. Kanerva L, Forstrom L. Allergic nickel and chromate hand dermatitis induced by orthopaedic metal implant. Contact Dermatitis 2001;44(2):103–4.
7. Hierholzer S, Hierholzer G. Untersuchungen zur Metalallergie nach Osteosynthesen. [Allergy to metal following osteosynthesis.] Unfallchirurgie 1982;8(6):347–52.
8. Artiunina GP. Toksicheskii pnevmoskleroz i al'veolit u rabochikh gidrometallurgicheskogo proizvodstva nikelia. [Toxic pneumosclerosis and alveolitis in workers of hydrometallurgic production of nickel.] Med Tr Prom Ekol 1996;(3):22–5.
9. Grimaudo NJ. Biocompatibility of nickel and cobalt dental alloys. Gen Dent 2001;49(5):498–503.
10. Budinger L, Hertl M. Immunologic mechanisms in hypersensitivity reactions to metal ions: an overview. Allergy 2000;55(2):108–15.
11. Mancuso G, Berdondini RM. Eyelid dermatitis and conjunctivitis as sole manifestations of allergy to nickel in an orthodontic appliance. Contact Dermatitis 2002; 46(4):245.
12. Kerosuo H, Kullaa A, Kerosuo E, Kanerva L, Hensten-Pettersen A. Nickel allergy in adolescents in relation to orthodontic treatment and piercing of ears. Am J Orthod Dentofacial Orthop 1996;109(2):148–54.
13. Lindsten R, Kurol J. Orthodontic appliances in relation to nickel hypersensitivity. A review. J Orofac Orthop 1997;58(2):100–8.
14. Block GT, Yeung M. Asthma induced by nickel. JAMA 1982;247(11):1600–2.
15. Niordson AM. Nickel sensitivity as a cause of rhinitis. Contact Dermatitis 1981;7(5):273–4.
16. Wahlberg JE. Nickel allergy in hairdressers. Contact Dermatitis 1981;7(6):358–9.
17. Di Gioacchino M, Masci S, Cavallucci E, Pavone G, Andreassi M, Gravante M, Pizzicannella G, Boscolo P. Modificazioni immuno-istopatologiche della mucosa gastro-intestinale in pazient; con allergia da contatto al nichel. [Immuno-histopathologic changes in the gastrointestinal mucosa in patients with nickel contact allergy.] G Ital Med Lav 1995;17(1–6):33–6.

18. Al-Tawil NG, Marcusson JA, Moller E. Lymphocyte transformation test in patients with nickel sensitivity: an aid to diagnosis. Acta Derm Venereol 1981;61(6):511–15.
19. Kapoor-Pillarisetti A, Mowbray JF, Brostoff J, Cronin EA. HLA dependence of sensitivity to nickel and chromium. Tissue Antigens 1981;17(3):261–4.
20. Bauer A, Geier J, Elsner P. Allergic contact dermatitis in patients with anogenital complaints. J Reprod Med 2000;45(8):649–54.
21. Marren P, Wojnarowska F, Powell S. Allergic contact dermatitis and vulvar dermatoses. Br J Dermatol 1992;126(1):52–6.
22. Lucke TW, Fleming CJ, McHenry P, Lever R. Patch testing in vulval dermatoses: how relevant is nickel? Contact Dermatitis 1998;38(2):111–12.
23. Bresser H. Orale Nickelprovokation und nickelarme Diät. Indikation und praktische Durchfuhrung. [Oral nickel provocation and a nickel-free diet. Indications and practical implementation.] Hautarzt 1992;43(10):610–15.
24. Choy EH, Gambling L, Best SL, Jenkins RE, Kondeatis E, Vaughan R, Black MM, Sadler PJ, Panayi GS. Nickel contamination of gold salts: link with gold-induced skin rash. Br J Rheumatol 1997;36(10):1054–8.
25. Gimenez-Arnau A, Riambau V, Serra-Baldrich E, Camarasa JG. Metal-induced generalized pruriginous dermatitis and endovascular surgery. Contact Dermatitis 2000;43(1):35–40.
26. Pazzaglia M, Lucente P, Vincenzi C, Tosti A. Contact dermatitis from nickel in mobile phones. Contact Dermatitis 2000;42(6):362–3.

Niclofolan

General Information

Niclofolan has been used to treat trematode infections, including clonorchiasis, fascioliasis, and paragonimiasis. Sweating, generalized pains, and transient rises in serum transaminase activities have been reported with niclofolan in the treatment of pulmonary infections due to *Paragonimus uterobilaterali* (SEDA-11, 597) (1).

Reference

1. Nwokolo C, Volkmer KJ. Single dose therapy of paragonimiasis with menichlopholan. Am J Trop Med Hyg 1977;26(4):688–92.

Niclosamide

General Information

Niclosamide, widely used in the treatment of tapeworm infestation, is well tolerated in doses of 2 g taken orally before breakfast and is the drug of choice for mass chemotherapy (1). It is has also been used as a molluscicide and in the control of *Schistosoma japonicum* (2).

Niclosamide is not absorbed and reactions consist of mild gastrointestinal disturbances. When treating *Tenia solium* infections an antiemetic is usually given before niclosamide, and patients are subsequently purged to reduce the theoretical risk of cysticercosis, because the dose of niclosamide active against *T. solium* does not destroy ova contained within the tapeworm. Alcohol is usually restricted during treatment, since niclosamide can interfere with its metabolism.

References

1. Sarti E, Rajshekhar V. Measures for the prevention and control of *Taenia solium* taeniosis and cysticercosis. Acta Trop 2003;87(1):137–43.
2. Lowe D, Xi J, Meng X, Wu Z, Qiu D, Spear R. Transport of *Schistosoma japonicum* cercariae and the feasibility of niclosamide for cercariae control. Parasitol Int 2005;54(1):83–9.

Nicorandil

See also Antianginal drugs

General Information

Nicorandil is a potassium channel activator. The potassium channel activators include cromakalim and its levorotatory isomer lemakalim, bimakalim, nicorandil, and pinacidil (1). Older drugs with this property include minoxidil and diazoxide. Nicorandil, a nicotinamide derivative, is the only drug in the group to be specifically designed as one of this fourth class of agents in the management of angina pectoris after organic nitrates, beta-blockers, and calcium antagonists. Apart from being an arterial/coronary vasodilator, through modulation of ATP-sensitive potassium channels, nicorandil also contains a nitrate moiety, giving it properties similar to organic nitrates but lacking the disadvantages of drug tolerance. Thus, nicorandil has two major hemodynamic actions. It causes venodilatation, reducing preload, by its nitrate-like effect, and systemic arterial vasodilatation, reducing systemic vascular resistance and afterload, by its potassium channel opening effect. In the heart it has a selective effect on coronary vasculature compared with myocardial muscle (2), and it does not appear to affect the sinus node or atrioventricular conduction in animals (3). It also has a vasospasmolytic action (4), and in animals is cardioprotective in induced myocardial ischemia (5).

Nicorandil is effective in controlling 69–80% of cases of chronic stable angina when used as monotherapy (6,7). However, clinical experience with nicorandil is still limited, although it has been in general use in Japan for over 8 years. A review of toxicity data has been published (8).

General adverse effects

The arterial and venous vasodilatory properties of nicorandil precipitate postural hypotension, leading to dizziness, syncope, palpitation, and headache, through a mechanism similar to that of organic nitrates. Other minor gastrointestinal symptoms, such as nausea, vomiting, abdominal pain, and diarrhea have been reported, as has flushing lymphocytic infiltrations around the bile ducts, have occasionally been seen.

Rechallenge with crystalline formulations in people in whom liver damage has occurred with the modified-release formulation has been tolerated (33). However, three cases of hepatic dysfunction in patients taking crystalline nicotinic acid 1.5–3.0 g/day have been reported (1). They were all associated with a reduced ratio of esterified cholesterol to free cholesterol in LDL, a reduction in lecithin cholesteryl acyl transferase activity (LCAT), and other evidence of liver dysfunction, including prolonged prothrombin time. Transaminases were in the reference ranges. On reduction of the dosage or withdrawal of nicotinic acid all the abnormalities resolved within 4 weeks. Others have pointed out that some observations suggest that lipid lowering with nicotinic acid is part of a generalized hepatotoxic effect (1).

A "starry sky liver" has been reported in a patient with nicotinic acid-induced hepatitis (34).

- A 50-year-old man developed recurrent sharp lower abdominal pain and nausea, having taken modified-release nicotinic acid 500–2000 mg/day for 8 weeks for hypercholesterolemia. He had a low-grade fever, tachycardia, and hypotension. Abdominal ultrasonography showed a markedly hypoechoic liver of normal size, with relatively echogenic conspicuous portal triads. Aspartate transaminase activity and prothrombin time were raised. Nicotinic acid was withdrawn and the signs and symptoms resolved within several days.

Nicotinic acid can cause hepatic steatosis and clinical hepatic abnormalities that together can simulate the presentation of hepatobiliary neoplasia (35).

- A 52-year-old man with long-standing tetraplegia, who had been taking oral nicotinic acid 2 g/day for several months, developed nausea, vomiting, and fever, raised liver enzymes and total and indirect bilirubin. Ultrasonography showed several hyperechoic intrahepatic lesions and CT scan showed several hypoattenuating lesions, some of which were associated with interrupted vessels and had convex borders, suggestive of a tumor. Other lesions had CT features typical of fatty infiltration of the liver. Niacin was withdrawn. The liver function tests normalized within 4 days and the nausea and vomiting abated. The hepatic lesions on CT scan improved within 1 month and resolved after 9 months.

Skin

Nicotinic acid disturbs the normal cornification of the skin, occasionally leading to reversible ichthyosis and acanthosis nigricans (SEDA-19, 206). Two mechanisms are advanced to explain this effect: insulin resistance induced by nicotinic acid, with compensatory hyperinsulinemia (which in turn leads to increased insulin binding to insulin-like growth factor receptors and stimulation of keratinocytes), or a disturbance of epidermal lipid homeostasis.

Skin problems can be persistent in a proportion of patients, variously estimated at 10–59%, and this can severely limit adherence to therapy. The skin reaction can be ameliorated by concomitant use of non-steroidal anti-inflammatory drugs such as aspirin and indometacin (SEDA-15, 412). Transient exanthems, pruritus, and sometimes wheals are seen, as well as a uniform dryness and scaling of the epidermis, brown pigmentation, and even on occasion an acanthosis nigricans-like dermatosis (15). Persistent rashes can also occur. Doses in excess of 5 g/day are routinely associated with skin manifestations and can on occasion cause liver damage, gout, and ulcer formation. These reactions can be associated with nicotinic acid rather than nicotinamide, which is sometimes recommended as an alternative (36). Increased hair loss has been described.

Musculoskeletal

Nicotinic acid has been associated with the development of myopathy with nocturnal leg aching and cramps, symptoms that can be exacerbated by simultaneous use of other lipid-lowering drugs associated with similar adverse effects, or alcohol, which also has myopathic effects (SEDA-15, 413) (37).

Immunologic

Anaphylactic shock can occur with nicotinic acid (6).

A pseudoallergic reaction has been reported in a patient who took several nicotinic acid-containing formulations (38).

- A previously healthy 40-year-old woman developed a generalized macular erythematous rash associated with palpitation and light-headedness, recurring every few days. The rash started behind the neck and arms, with a sensation of tingling, progressing to a general feeling of heat. She felt ill and had to lie down until the episode subsided after 45–90 minutes, with residual fatigue for several hours. Laboratory findings were all in the reference ranges. She was taking two multivitamin tablets a day, each containing nicotinic acid 20 mg, one B complex tablet containing nicotinic acid 50 mg, and 1–3 tablets of an antiemetic containing nicotinic acid 50 mg. Thus, she had unknowingly taken nicotinic acid up to 240 mg/day. Graded oral challenge with nicotinic acid 20–200 mg reproduced her symptoms.

Drug Administration

Drug formulations

Since nicotinic acid can cause unpleasant flushing and other symptoms of vasodilatation, attempts have been made to develop modified-release formulations. Modified-released nicotinic acid formulations may be better tolerated than the immediate-release formulation, because they reduce the vasodilatory effects of the drug. However, the low frequency of flushing produced by modified-release formulations may be offset by an increased risk of hepatotoxicity. Some reports have suggested a higher frequency of hepatic dysfunction with traditional modified-release nicotinic acid formulations compared with immediate-release products (2,39).

In a double-blind, placebo-controlled study of a modified-release formulation in 128 patients, pruritus was reported in 10 patients taking nicotinic acid and rash in 9 patients; there were no similar effects in those taking placebo (40).

In 517 patients taking a modified-release formulation the most commonly reported adverse events were headache in 92 patients, pain in any part of the body except the abdomen in 46, abdominal pain in 54, diarrhea in 97, dyspepsia in 46, nausea in 72, vomiting in 38, rhinitis in 30, pruritus in 56, and rash in 51 (24).

In a study of the efficacy and tolerability of a modified-release formulation in 269 adults and 230 additional adults for whom short-term safety data were available, 13 of 269 patients (4.8%) withdrew because of flushing (41). During the first 4 weeks about half had flushing. The mean intensity was about 4.0 on a visual analogue scale (representing "none" to "intolerable"). Patients were encouraged to use aspirin prophylactically to minimize flushing. Other nicotinic acid-related adverse effects leading to withdrawal included nausea (3.3%) sometimes with vomiting, other gastrointestinal symptoms (1.5%), and pruritus (2.6%). Once case each of gout, acanthosis nigricans, headache, palpitation, raised glucose concentrations, and shoulder pain led to patient withdrawal. Certain adverse events thought to be associated with nicotinic acid were uncommon in the study group. There was one case of peptic ulcer, amblyopia occurred in three patients, and leg aches and myalgias in one patient taking nicotinic acid with simvastatin, with a normal creatine kinase activity.

The efficacy and adverse effects of a modified-release formulation have been studied in 32 patients with type 2 diabetes (42). Of 22 patients who completed 6 months of therapy, 17 took 1000 mg/day, 3 1500 mg/day, and 2 2000 mg/day. Seven of 32 patients discontinued therapy. Of these, three withdrew after 2, 5, and 6 months because of flushing and itching. Three other patients withdrew within 2 months because of nausea, diarrhea, and dyspepsia. One patient withdrew after 7 days because of increased blood glucose concentrations. There were no significant increases in mean transaminase activities, which remained within the reference ranges in all patients.

The safety and efficacy of escalating doses of modified-release tablets of nicotinic acid (Niaspan) have been evaluated in a multicenter, placebo-controlled study in 131 patients with primary hyperlipidemia (43). The dose of nicotinic acid was initially 375 mg/day, then 500 mg/day, and then increasing in 500 mg increments at 4-week intervals to a maximum of 3000 mg/day. Changes in biochemical measurements in patients taking nicotinic acid were significant only for uric acid and phosphorus. Fasting blood glucose, bilirubin, transaminases, alkaline phosphatase, lactate dehydrogenase, and amylase were not altered. Of the 131 patients, 80 completed the study. Of the patients who withdrew, 31 did so for medical reasons (3% taking nicotinic acid and 11% placebo). Eight of the 26 patients who stopped taking nicotinic acid withdrew because of flushing (all before the 2000 mg/day dose) and 5 because of a rash. These reasons accounted for half of the dropouts with nicotinic acid. The number of patients who had episodes of flushing fell with each dose increment of nicotinic acid, suggesting tolerance. Of other adverse events, only nausea (18 and 9%), vomiting (10 and 2%), pruritus (11 and 0%), and rash (10 and 0%) were more common with nicotinic acid.

Drug–Drug Interactions

Ethanol

An apparent interaction between nicotinic acid and alcohol caused toxic delirium and lactic acidosis (44).

Nicotine

An interaction between nicotinic acid and nicotine transdermal patches has also been observed, causing flushing and dizziness (45).

Statins

Nicotinic acid increased the risk of rhabdomyolysis associated with HMG-CoA reductase inhibitors (SEDA-19, 206) (46).

References

1. Tato F, Vega GL, Grundy SM. Effects of crystalline nicotinic acid-induced hepatic dysfunction on serum low-density lipoprotein cholesterol and lecithin cholesteryl acyl transferase. Am J Cardiol 1998;81(6):805–7.
2. McKenney JM, Proctor JD, Harris S, Chinchili VM. A comparison of the efficacy and toxic effects of sustained- vs immediate-release niacin in hypercholesterolemic patients. JAMA 1994;271(9):672–7.
3. Lasagna L. Over-the-counter niacin. JAMA 1994;271(9):709–10.
4. Gibbons LW, Gonzalez V, Gordon N, Grundy S. The prevalence of side effects with regular and sustained-release nicotinic acid. Am J Med 1995;99(4):378–85.
5. Crouse JR 3rd. New developments in the use of niacin for treatment of hyperlipidemia: new considerations in the use of an old drug. Coron Artery Dis 1996;7(4):321–6.
6. Britton ML, Bradberry JC, Letassy NA, Mckenney JM, Sirmans SM. ASHP Therapeutic Position Statement on the safe use of niacin in the management of dyslipidemias. American Society of Health-System Pharmacists. Am J Health Syst Pharm 1997;54(24):2815–19.
7. Knopp RH. Clinical profiles of plain versus sustained-release niacin (Niaspan) and the physiologic rationale for nighttime dosing. Am J Cardiol 1998;82(12A):24U–8U; discussion 39U-41U.
8. Miller SM. Potential perils of niacin therapy. Clin Lab Sci 1991;4:156–8.
9. Kaanders JH, Pop LA, Marres HA, Liefers J, van den Hoogen FJ, van Daal WA, van der Kogel AJ. Accelerated radiotherapy with carbogen and nicotinamide (ARCON) for laryngeal cancer. Radiother Oncol 1998;48(2):115–22.
10. Bernier J, Stratford MR, Denekamp J, Dennis MF, Bieri S, Hagen F, Kocagoncu O, Bolla M, Rojas A. Pharmacokinetics of nicotinamide in cancer patients treated with accelerated radiotherapy: the experience of the Co-operative Group of Radiotherapy of the European Organization for Research and Treatment of Cancer. Radiother Oncol 1998;48(2):123–33.
11. Luria MH. Atherosclerosis: the importance of HDL cholesterol and prostacyclin: a role for niacin therapy. Med Hypotheses 1990;32(1):21–8.
12. Ganzer BM. Langzeitstudie zu acipimox. Pharmazie 1990;135:31.
13. Lavezzari M, Milanesi G, Oggioni E, Pamparana F. Results of a phase IV study carried out with acipimox in type II diabetic patients with concomitant hyperlipoproteinaemia. J Int Med Res 1989;17(4):373–80.

nifedipine could have posed an extra risk by causing hypotension and reflex tachycardia.

In a review of almost 800 patients randomized to beta-adrenoceptor agonists or nifedipine, the latter was associated with more frequent prolongation of pregnancy, a lower incidence of respiratory distress syndrome, and lower incidences of maternal and fetal adverse effects (44).

Fetotoxicity

The use of nifedipine during pregnancy and labor has been widely debated, although its effects on child development have not been well evaluated. In one study nifedipine did not affect the development and health of 190 children, aged 18 months, born to women with mild to moderate hypertension who had been randomized to nifedipine, given for 12–34 gestational weeks before delivery, or expectant management (45).

Susceptibility Factors

Treatment of hypertensive emergencies has been the object of a randomized comparison of isosorbide dinitrate aerosol and nifedipine in 60 adults (46). Two patients taking nifedipine had myocardial ischemia early after administration and four patients had rebound hypertension during the follow-up period. Authors who reviewed the role of nifedipine in hypertensive emergencies reached the conclusion that the use of short-acting sublingual or oral nifedipine is no longer recommended for the treatment of these urgencies because it can precipitate serious adverse reactions (47).

There has been a report of cardiovascular collapse after uncomplicated coronary artery bypass surgery in patients taking nifedipine preoperatively (48); the condition responded to intravenous calcium chloride in three patients and adrenaline in four. Nifedipine may facilitate cardiac arrest during induction of anesthesia by sensitizing the carotid sinus (49).

Drug Administration

Drug overdose

Unlike verapamil and diltiazem, overdose with nifedipine is not usually fatal. Multiple case series of pediatric nifedipine ingestion have been published, and none has reported any deaths. However, two fatal cases of ingestion of long-acting nifedipine in children have been reported: a 24-month-old girl who took 20 tablets of nifedipine 10 mg and a 14-month-old girl who took a single tablet of nifedipine 10 mg; neither responded to aggressive supportive care (50).

Drug–Drug Interactions

Alcohol

There is a substantial increase in the systemic availability of nifedipine when alcohol is taken at the same time (51).

Atenolol

The combination of nifedipine with atenolol in patients with intermittent claudication resulted in a reduction in walking distance and skin temperature, whereas either drug alone produced benefits (52).

Ciclosporin

Ciclosporin significantly inhibits the metabolism of nifedipine, leading to increased effects (53).

Fluconazole

A pharmacokinetic interaction between fluconazole and nifedipine has been reported (54).

- A 16-year-old man with neurofibromatosis type 1, a malignant pheochromocytoma with lung and bone metastases, and candidiasis of the gastrointestinal tract with fungemia was taking nifedipine for arterial hypertension. The fungal infection responded to fluconazole, but three attempts to withdraw the fluconazole resulted in recurrence of headache, palpitation, and increased blood pressure.

After careful pharmacokinetic assessment of the effects of fluconazole withdrawal on 24-hour ambulatory blood pressure and nifedipine plasma concentration, the authors concluded that fluconazole can enhance the blood-pressure lowering effects of nifedipine by increasing its plasma concentrations, most likely by inhibiting CYP3A4.

Lithium

Lithium clearance is reduced by about 30% by nifedipine (55).

Melatonin

Melatonin has a hypotensive effect in both normotensive and hypertensive subjects. In a double-blind, randomized, crossover study designed to evaluate whether evening ingestion of melatonin potentiates the antihypertensive effect of nifedipine monotherapy in 50 patients with well-controlled mild to moderate hypertension aged 38–65 years (28 men, 22 women), there was a surprising significant increase in blood pressure and heart rate throughout 24 hours (56). The authors suggested that there was competition between melatonin and nifedipine, with impairment of the antihypertensive efficacy of the calcium channel blocker.

Phenytoin

Increased serum phenytoin concentrations have been reported after the introduction of nifedipine (57,58).

Quinidine

Nifedipine may enhance the elimination of quinidine (59) and cause hypotension and a loss of antidysrhythmic effect (60).

Tacrolimus

Nifedipine can increase the blood concentration of the macrolide immunosuppressant tacrolimus (SEDA-21, 392).

Food–Drug Interactions

The effect of food on the systemic availability of two modified-release dosage forms of nifedipine for once-daily administration (Adalat OROS, a tablet with an osmotic push–pull system, and Slofedipine XL, a tablet with an acid-resistant coating) has been investigated in 24 healthy men in an open, randomized, crossover study (61). After fasted administration the systemic availability was slightly lower for Slofedipine XL than Adalat OROS, with a point estimate of 82%, mainly resulting from differences in nifedipine concentrations during the first 15 hours after administration. Maximum plasma concentrations were lower after Slofedipine XL compared with Adalat OROS (point estimate 84%). After a high-fat breakfast the differences in availability between the two products were greater than while fasting, with point estimates of 70% for AUC and 81% for C_{max}. Most striking was the lag time after food for Slofedipine XL which was more than 15 hours in 15 of 24 subjects. The availability of nifedipine from Slofedipine XL compared with Adalat OROS was only 28% over the intended dosing interval of 24 hours. The delay in nifedipine absorption when Slofedipine XL is administered may be explained by properties of the formulation, since the acid-resistant coating probably confers delayed absorption, due to prolongation of the gastric residence time, while the osmotic push–pull system is not sensitive to food. The same authors conducted a similar study in 24 healthy subjects, in which they compared Adalat OROS with Nifedicron, a product that consists of a capsule containing several mini-tablets (62). There was a higher rate of availability for Nifedicron in the fasted state, and after a high-fat breakfast the differences between the products became even more pronounced. The most important effect of concomitant food was reflected by a pronounced increase in Cmax after Nifedicron, which resulted in a more than three-fold higher mean concentration than Adalat OROS. This phenomenon may result in safety and tolerability problems.

References

1. Ricciardi MJ, Knight BP, Martinez FJ, Rubenfire M. Inhaled nitric oxide in primary pulmonary hypertension: a safe and effective agent for predicting response to nifedipine. J Am Coll Cardiol 1998;32(4):1068–73.
2. Sitbon O, Humbert M, Jagot JL, Taravella O, Fartoukh M, Parent F, Herve P, Simonneau G. Inhaled nitric oxide as a screening agent for safely identifying responders to oral calcium-channel blockers in primary pulmonary hypertension. Eur Respir J 1998;12(2):265–70.
3. Brown MJ, Palmer CR, Castaigne A, de Leeuw PW, Mancia G, Rosenthal T, Ruilope LM. Morbidity and mortality in patients randomised to double-blind treatment with a long-acting calcium-channel blocker or diuretic in the International Nifedipine GITS study: Intervention as a Goal in Hypertension Treatment (INSIGHT). Lancet 2000; 356(9227):366–72.
4. Maxwell CJ, Hogan DB, Campbell NRC, Ebly EM. Nifedipine and mortality risk in the elderly: relevance of drug formulation, dose and duration. Pharmacoepidemiol Drug Saf 2000;9:11–23.
5. Committee on Safety of Medicines. Nifedipine (Adalat) and myocardial ischaemia. Curr Probl 1979;4:1.
6. Deanfield J, Wright C, Fox K. Treatment of angina pectoris with nifedipine: importance of dose titration. BMJ (Clin Res Ed) 1983;286(6376):1467–70.
7. Yagil Y, Kobrin I, Leibel B, Ben-Ishay D. Ischemic ECG changes with initial nifedipine therapy of severe hypertension. Am Heart J 1982;103(2):310–11.
8. Stason WB, Schmid CH, Niedzwiecki D, Whiting GW, Caubet JF, Cory D, Luo D, Ross SD, Chalmers TC. Safety of nifedipine in angina pectoris: a meta-analysis. Hypertension 1999;33(1):24–31.
9. Ishibashi Y, Shimada T, Yoshitomi H, Sano K, Oyake N, Umeno T, Sakane T, Murakami Y, Morioka S. Sublingual nifedipine in elderly patients: even a low dose induces myocardial ischaemia. Clin Exp Pharmacol Physiol 1999; 26(5–6):404–10.
10. Grayson HA, Kennedy JD. Torsades de pointes and nifedipine. Ann Intern Med 1982;97(1):144.
11. Krikler DM, Rowland E. Torsade de pointes and nifedipine. Ann Intern Med 1982;97(4):618–19.
12. Nobile-Orazio E, Sterzi R. Cerebral ischaemia after nifedipine treatment. BMJ (Clin Res Ed) 1981;283(6297):948.
13. Ellrodt AG, Ault MJ, Riedinger MS, Murata GH. Efficacy and safety of sublingual nifedipine in hypertensive emergencies. Am J Med 1985;79(4A):19–25.
14. Pitlik S, Manor RS, Lipshitz I, Perry G, Rosenfeld J. Transient retinal ischaemia induced by nifedipine. BMJ (Clin Res Ed) 1983;287(6408):1845–6.
15. Bertel O, Conen LD. Treatment of hypertensive emergencies with the calcium channel blocker nifedipine. Am J Med 1985;79(4A):31–5.
16. Gill JS, Zezulka AV, Horrocks PM. Rupture of a cerebral aneurysm associated with nifedipine treatment. Postgrad Med J 1986;62(733):1029–30.
17. Murphy MB, Scriven AJ, Brown MJ, Causon R, Dollery CT. The effects of nifedipine and hydralazine induced hypotension on sympathetic activity. Eur J Clin Pharmacol 1982;23(6):479–82.
18. Struthers AD, Reid JL. Nifedipine does not influence adrenaline induced hypokalaemia in man. Br J Clin Pharmacol 1983;16(3):342–3.
19. Neaton JD, Grimm RH Jr, Prineas RJ, Stamler J, Grandits GA, Elmer PJ, Cutler JA, Flack JM, Schoenberger JA, McDonald R, et al.; Treatment of Mild Hypertension Study. Final results. Treatment of Mild Hypertension Study Research Group JAMA 1993; 270(6):713–24.
20. Tishler M, Armon S. Nifedipine-induced hypokalemia. Drug Intell Clin Pharm 1986;20(5):370–1.
21. Laporte JR, Ibanez L, Ballarin E, Perez E, Vidal X. Fatal aplastic anaemia associated with nifedipine. Lancet 1998;352(9128):619–20.
22. Pernu HE, Knuuttila ML. Macrophages and lymphocyte subpopulations in nifedipine- and cyclosporin A-associated human gingival overgrowth. J Periodontol 2001;72(2):160–6.
23. Nurmenniemi PK, Pernu HE, Knuuttila ML. Mitotic activity of keratinocytes in nifedipine- and immunosuppressive medication-induced gingival overgrowth. J Periodontol 2001;72(2):167–73.
24. Miranda J, Brunet L, Roset P, Berini L, Farre M, Mendieta C. Prevalence and risk of gingival enlargement in patients treated with nifedipine. J Periodontol 2001;72(5):605–11.
25. Goglin WK, Elliott BM, Deppe SA. Nifedipine-induced hypotension and mesenteric ischemia. South Med J 1989; 82(2):274–5.
26. Lavy A. Corrosive effect of nifedipine in the upper gastrointestinal tract. Diagn Ther Endosc 2000;6:39–41.
27. Niezabitowski LM, Nguyen BN, Gums JG. Extended-release nifedipine bezoar identified one year after discontinuation. Ann Pharmacother 2000;34(7–8):862–4.

Nimodipine

See also Calcium channel blockers

General Information

Nimodipine is a dihydropyridine calcium channel blocker.

In the absence of effective neuroprotective treatment for ischemic stroke, a double-blind, randomized, placebo-controlled trial has been performed in 454 patients in primary care (1). Nimodipine 30 mg/day or placebo was started within 6 hours after the onset of the stroke and continued for 10 days. Nimodipine had no effect on all-cause mortality or dependency in daily life. In patients with ischemic stroke documented by CT scan, nimodipine had a borderline significant adverse effect on outcome. Nimodipine was tolerated as well as placebo (7 versus 8 treatment withdrawals respectively), but the lack of benefit does not support the use of any voltage-sensitive calcium channel blocker in ischemic stroke.

It has been suggested that calcium channel blockers can be used to treat cocaine dependence, and some studies have shown reductions in cocaine-induced subjective and cardiovascular responses with nifedipine and diltiazem. The cardiovascular and subjective responses to cocaine have been evaluated in a double-blind, placebo-controlled, crossover study in five subjects pretreated with two dosages of nimodipine (2). Nimodipine 60 mg attenuated the systolic, but not the diastolic, blood pressure rise after cocaine. In three subjects, nimodipine 90 mg produced greater attenuation than 60 mg. The subjective effects of cocaine were not altered by either dosage of nimodipine.

Organs and Systems

Cardiovascular

When nimodipine was given intravenously to 87 patients with proven subarachnoid hemorrhage in a maintenance dosage of 2 mg/hour, it caused significant hypotension in one-third of cases (3). With maintenance oral administration, the incidence of hypotension was much lower. It is therefore recommended that if nimodipine is prescribed, the oral route is preferable, even in intubated patients who should receive it via a nasogastric tube.

Nervous system

Nimodipine has been routinely used to reduce cerebral vasospasm in patients with subarachnoid hemorrhage. A randomized, double-blind, placebo-controlled trial was stopped early because of excess mortality (8/75 versus 1/74 deaths with nimodipine and placebo respectively), which was attributed to an increased incidence of surgical bleeding (4). In addition, its use for cerebral protection in a cardiac valve replacement trial involving cardiopulmonary bypass was also terminated prematurely because of increased cerebrovascular complications and excessive blood loss in a small subgroup of patients (5). In traumatic subarachnoid hemorrhage, a trial in 123 patients showed a significant reduction in unfavorable outcomes (death, vegetative survival, or severe disability) at 6 months with nimodipine (25 versus 46% for placebo) (6).

References

1. Horn J, de Haan RJ, Vermeulen M, Limburg M. Very Early Nimodipine Use in Stroke (VENUS): a randomized, double-blind, placebo-controlled trial. Stroke 2001;32(2):461–5.
2. Kosten TR, Woods SW, Rosen MI, Pearsall HR. Interactions of cocaine with nimodipine: a brief report. Am J Addict 1999;8(1):77–81.
3. Porchet F, Chiolero R, de Tribolet N. Hypotensive effect of nimodipine during treatment for aneurysmal subarachnoid haemorrhage. Acta Neurochir (Wien) 1995;137(1–2):62–9.
4. Wagenknecht LE, Furberg CD, Hammon JW, Legault C, Troost BT. Surgical bleeding: unexpected effect of a calcium antagonist. BMJ 1995;310(6982):776–7.
5. Heininger K, Kuebler J. Use of nimodipine is safe. Stroke 1996;27(10):1911–13.
6. Harders A, Kakarieka A, Braakman R. Traumatic subarachnoid hemorrhage and its treatment with nimodipine. German tSAH Study Group. J Neurosurg 1996;85(1):82–9.

Niridazole

See also Benzimidazoles

General Information

Niridazole is used in the treatment of schistosomiasis and of guinea-worm (*Dracunculus medinensis*) infections; it is given in divided daily doses of 25 mg/kg for 5–10 days, depending on the infecting species. Niridazole is well tolerated in *Schistosoma hematobium* infections. It is metabolized in the liver, and its metabolites color the urine dark brown. In the treatment of schistosomiasis it has been largely superseded by newer drugs.

General adverse effects

In the treatment of schistosomiasis adverse effects were seen in 80% of inpatients and 33% of outpatients. Gastrointestinal effects were the most common, with vomiting in 50% of cases. Neurotoxic and psychiatric effects, convulsions, and cardiac effects are less common, except in patients with liver disease. Insomnia, somnolence, vertigo, nightmares, headache, weakness, jaundice, and muscle pains have all been reported (SEDA-12, 244). Toxic reactions are seen more often in *Schistosoma mansoni* infections, especially in patients with poor liver function or portocaval shunts, when neuropsychiatric complications can be expected. Some toxicity is directly related to parasite destruction and liberation of antigen rather than to the drug itself. Allergic reactions related to parasite destruction include urticaria, allergic conjunctivitis, and fever with peripheral eosinophilia. Niridazole is a potent carcinogen in mice, and tumorigenic in hamsters. It is not clear what the risks are in man, but it is of course usually given for only a brief period.

Organs and Systems

Cardiovascular

Minor electrocardiographic abnormalities, especially T wave changes, are common but are probably of no functional significance of patients (1). Dysrhythmias with prolongation of the QT interval occur in a small minority of patients (2).

Respiratory

Cough, fever, and dyspnea with pulmonary infiltration have been reported in two cases (3).

Nervous system

Headache, drowsiness, and dizziness are common with niridazole (2,4,5). More severe neuropsychiatric symptoms are more frequent in patients with liver disease, especially those with portosystemic shunts, in whom the drug bypasses the liver (6). Symptoms in these cases include insomnia, anxiety, depression, confusion, hallucinations, and convulsions; the reactions may prove fatal. The electroencephalogram can show slowed alpha rhythms, beta waves, and theta waves, as well as sharp wave and spike forms with niridazole (7). A single case of acute cortical necrosis was recorded in the much older literature, but was probably coincidental (SED-8, 691) (8). Agitation can occur in patients with abnormal liver function.

Hematologic

A peripheral eosinophilia is usual (2). Hemolysis has been reported once in glucose-6-phosphate dehydrogenase (G6PD) deficiency (SED-8, 691) (9).

Gastrointestinal

Bad taste, anorexia, nausea, vomiting, diarrhea, and abdominal pain are common with niridazole (1,2,5). Gastrointestinal bleeding has been seen (10).

Liver

Prolongation of the prothrombin time can occur (11). Niridazole is contraindicated in liver disease.

Urinary tract

Metabolites of niridazole color the urine dark brown (12,13).

Musculoskeletal

Muscle pain, joint pain, and bone pain are commonly reported but may be related to parasite destruction rather than to direct toxicity (5).

Long-Term Effects

Mutagenicity

Niridazole should not be used in pregnancy; mutagenic effects have been seen in bacteria (14).

Second-Generation Effects

Fertility

Transient reduction in spermatogenesis, apparently reversible, can occur (15).

Susceptibility Factors

Genetic factors

Caution is required when using niridazole in individuals with G6PD deficiency (16).

Hepatic disease

Niridazole should not be used in the presence of hepatic disease (17).

References

1. Abdallah A, Saif M, Abdel-Meguid M, Badran A, Abdel-Fattah F, Aly IM. Treatment of urinary and intestinal bilharziasis with Ciba 32644-Ba (Ambilhar). A preliminary report. J Egypt Med Assoc 1966;49(2):145–63.
2. Katz N, et al. Clinical trials with CIBA 32644-Ba (Ambilhar) in schistosomiasis mansoni. Folha Med 1966;53(4):561.
3. Farid Z, Bassily S, Lehman JS Jr, Ayad N, Hassan A, Sparks HA. A comparative evaluation of the treatment of *Schitosoma mansoni* with niridazole and potassium antimony tartrate. Trans R Soc Trop Med Hyg 1972;66(1):119–24.
4. Abdallah A, Saif M, el-Mawla NG, Abdel-Fattah F, Aly IM. Spaced-dosage treatment of bilharziasis with niridazole. J Egypt Med Assoc 1968;51(9):823–30.
5. Ruas A, Almeido Franco LT. The effect of CIBA 32,644-Ba in the treatment of 1,059 cases of vesical and intestinal schistosomiasis. Ann Trop Med Parasitol 1966;60(3):288–92.
6. Basmy K, Shoeb SM, Mohran Y. The role of liver dysfunction in the occurrence of the neuropsychiatric side effects of Ambilhar. J Egypt Med Assoc 1969;52(2):196–204.
7. Davidson JC. Neuropsychiatric effects and E.E.G. changes in niridazole therapy. Trans R Soc Trop Med Hyg 1969;63(5):579–81.
8. Emerit J, Saigot T, Escourolle R, Begue P. Un case de nécrose massive de la substance blanche hémisphérique au décours d'un traitement par l'Ambilhar chez une cirrhotique. [A case of massive necrosis of the hemispheric white substance during treatment with Ambilhar in a cirrhotic female patient.] Ann Med Interne (Paris) 1974;125(1):65–9.
9. McCaffrey RP, Farid Z, Kent DC. Acute haemolysis with Ambilhar treatment in glucose-6-phosphate dehydrogenase deficiency. Trans R Soc Trop Med Hyg 1972;66(5):795–7.
10. de Almeida Junior N, Penha LA, Pereira N, de Oliveira CA, de Oliveira JV, Crosara A, Habib P, Jacob M, de Oliveira S. Hemorragia digestiva no decorrer do tratamento da esquistossomose mansonica com o niridazol (pesquisas realizadas em 28 pacientes no sentido

de apurar o provavel mecanismo de sua producao). [Gastrointestinal hemorrhage during the management of schistosomiasis mansoni using niridazole (studies in 28 patients for the purpose of accelerating of proving its action mechanism).] Hospital (Rio J) 1968;74(5):1639–47.

11. Rodrigues LD, Vilela Mde P, Guimaraes RX, Jafferian PA, Miszputen SJ, Costa A. Estudo do comportamento do "tempo de protrombina" en pacientes esquisto-somoticos medicados com Ambilhar. [Study of the behavior of "prothrombin time" in schistosomatic patients using Ambilhar.] Hospital (Rio J) 1969;75(1):87–95.
12. Kelani YZ, Wilson P. Experiences with Ciba 32644 Ba (Ambilhar) in the treatment of schistosomiasis. J Kuwait Med Assoc 1969;2:151.
13. Mistry CJ, Mandanna KK. Ambilhar in amebic dysentery and hepatic amebiasis. Indian J Med Sci 1968;22(10):709–12.
14. McCalla DR, Voutsinos D, Olive PL. Mutagen screening with bacteria: niridazole and nitrofurans. Mutat Res 1975;31(1):31–7.
15. El-Beheiry AH, Kamel MN, Gad A. Niridazole and fertility in bilharzial men. Arch Androl 1982;8(4):297–300.
16. Gentillini M, Capron A, Imbert JC, Escande JP, Vernes A, Domart A. Essais thérapeutiques d'un dérivé du nitrothiazole (CIBA 32644) dans la bilharziose chronique. Etude clinique et sérologique portant sur 100 malades. [Therapeutic trials of a nitrothiazole derivative in chronic bilharziasis. Clinical and serological study of 100 patients.] Bull Mem Soc Med Hop Paris 1966; 117(4):323–41.
17. Coutinho A, Barreto FT. Treatment of hepatosplenic schistosomiasis mansoni with niridazole: relationships among liver function, effective dose, and side effects. Ann NY Acad Sci 1969;160(2):612–28.

Nitazoxanide

General Information

Nitazoxanide is a thiazolide derivative first described in 1975 and originally developed as a veterinary anti-helminthic drug. In vitro it has a documented efficacy against protozoa such as *Giardia lamblia*, *Trichomonas vaginalis*, and *Entamoeba histolytica*, and in vivo in particular against *Cryptosporidium parvum* in patients with AIDS, as well as against nematodes such as *Syphacia obvelata*, *Uncinaria stenocephala*, and *Trichuris vulpis*, and cestodes such as *Dipylidium canimum*, *Tenia pisiformis*, and *Hymenolepis nana* (1,2). Since it is also effective against *Fasciola hepatica* in vitro it has been tried in the treatment of fasciola infections in man.

Pharmacokinetics

Nitazoxanide was given to many patients, before its tolerability and pharmacokinetics were adequately assessed (1,2). In men randomly assigned to one of four treatment groups, in each of which two took a placebo and six took a single oral dose of nitazoxanide 1, 2, 3, or 4 g, first fasted and a week later with a standardized breakfast, there were no significant changes in electrocardiograms, vital signs, or laboratory tests (1). Plasma concentrations increased linearly with dose, although there was a trend to increased systemic availability at a dose of 4 g. Food approximately doubled the concentrations of the metabolites of nitazoxanide, deacetylnitazoxanide (or tizoxanide), and tizoxanide glucuronide, irrespective of dose. Tizoxanide glucuronide was eliminated more slowly than tizoxanide. Tolerability was good up to the maximum dose of 4 g. There were 89 adverse events; all were mild and none required treatment. Minor adverse events were dizziness, fatigue, discolored urine, malaise, and postural hypotension. However, the most frequent adverse events were gastrointestinal—diarrhea ($n = 13$), abdominal pain ($n = 8$), flatulence and nausea ($n = 5$), and vomiting ($n = 3$). Their frequency increased significantly with dose under fed conditions but not fasted.

Observational studies

In a village close to Alexandria in Egypt 137 patients were given nitazoxanide 500 mg bd for 6 days (3). On the 30th day 113 patients (82%) were presumed cured, with stools free of fasciola eggs. Nitazoxanide was extremely well tolerated. Only three patients reported adverse effects: abdominal pain in two and vomiting in one. The symptoms were mild and disappeared without medication or withdrawal of treatment. Together with triclabendazole, nitazoxanide can be considered for the treatment of *Fasciola hepatica* infections in man.

Placebo-controlled studies

Nitazoxanide 0.5 g bd and 1 g bd was given to 16 healthy volunteers for 7 days with food to study its pharmacokinetics and tolerability (2). The pharmacokinetics of both tizoxanide and tizoxanide glucuronide were only slightly influenced by repeated administration of nitazoxanide 0.5 g bd; the treatment group had no more adverse events than the placebo group and there was no accumulation. In contrast, repeated administration of nitazoxanide 1 g bd resulted in a significant increase in adverse events: diarrhea ($n = 9$), abdominal pain ($n = 9$), flatulence ($n = 5$), nausea ($n = 4$), and dyspepsia ($n = 1$). All reported discolored urine. Four subjects in the high-dose group reported headaches. Vital signs, electrocardiograms, and laboratory tests were normal. There was accumulation of nitazoxanide metabolites, because of solubility-limited or transport-limited elimination at the higher dose of nitazoxanide.

References

1. Stockis A, Allemon AM, De Bruyn S, Gengler C. Nitazoxanide pharmacokinetics and tolerability in man using single ascending oral doses. Int J Clin Pharmacol Ther 2002;40(5):213–20.
2. Stockis A, De Bruyn S, Gengler C, Rosillon D. Nitazoxanide pharmacokinetics and tolerability in man during 7 days dosing with 0.5 g and 1 g b.i.d. Int J Clin Pharmacol Ther 2002;40(5):221–7.
3. Rossignol JF, Abaza H, Friedman H. Successful treatment of human fascioliasis with nitazoxanide. Trans R Soc Trop Med Hyg 1998;92(1):103–4.

Nitrates, organic

See also Antianginal drugs

General Information

Organic nitrates have been in use for over 135 years, and their adverse effects are therefore well documented. The first compound of this class to be used was amyl nitrite, synthesized in 1844 by Ballard and used to treat angina pectoris by Brunton in 1869. Glyceryl trinitrate was first synthesized by Ascagne Sobrero in 1847 and was used by William Murrell to treat angina pectoris in 1879.

Nitrates have been produced in many chemical forms, but the current choice lies between the rapid-onset, short-acting glyceryl trinitrate (nitroglycerin) and the longer-acting isosorbide mononitrate and isosorbide dinitrate.

Mechanism of action

The nitrates act by releasing nitric oxide, which relaxes vascular smooth muscle. The discovery that endothelium-derived relaxing factor (EDRF) is nitric oxide (1) stimulated new interest in these drugs, as nitric oxide not only controls local vessel wall tension in response to shear stress, but also plays a role in regulating the interaction of platelets with blood vessel walls. The release of nitric oxide from the walls of atheromatous arteries is reduced, because of malfunctioning or absent endothelium. Atheromatous arteries behave differently from healthy arteries, in that these vessels vasoconstrict rather than vasodilate when stimulated by acetylcholine. This impairment of the acetylcholine vasomotor response appears to be related to serum cholesterol concentration (2).

Uses

Traditionally, nitrates have been first-line therapy in angina. They can be given to treat acute attacks, taken prophylactically before exertion or other stimuli known to provoke an attack, or used as continuous prophylaxis over 24 hours. Since angina is an episodic symptom, the first two methods are attractive, as continuous prophylaxis requires treatment over long periods when there are no symptoms. Tempering this argument is the realization that there may be silent myocardial ischemia, especially overnight, and morning angina on waking can be troublesome. In practice, a combination of continuous prophylaxis and as-required therapy is often used.

Nitrates are the drugs of choice in patients with left ventricular impairment, in whom they are of benefit when used in combination with hydralazine (3), and they should be used in preference to the calcium antagonists, which cause deterioration in myocardial function by an as yet unknown mechanism (4). In black patients with congestive heart failure taking ACE inhibitors and beta-blockers, a combination of isosorbide dinitrate plus hydralazine significantly reduced total mortality (5).

The potentially life-threatening hypotension caused by an interaction with sildenafil citrate (Viagra), a treatment for male erectile dysfunction, should be highlighted, especially in patients with coronary heart disease needing regular nitrates (6).

Observational studies

Glyceryl trinitrate can be used to treat anal fissure, as an alternative to surgery. Although glyceryl trinitrate causes resolution of symptoms in some cases, its local use as ointment is associated with frequent adverse reactions, mostly headache and anal burning (7,8). The difficulty in adjusting the dose and time of application, the high frequency of adverse reactions (up to 75% of patients), and the high rate of recurrence make the use of glyceryl trinitrate in non-surgical treatment of anal fissures questionable (9). In one case, a patient reported itching, dyspnea, and hypotension after applying glyceryl trinitrate. This unexplained systemic reaction to topical glyceryl trinitrate was reported as "anaphylactic," without a clear demonstration that it was an allergic reaction (10).

Besides its usual indications, topical glyceryl trinitrate has been used to prevent intravenous infusion failure because of phlebitis and extravasation, which occur in 30–60% of patients and can cause discomfort and harm, such as pulmonary embolism, septicemia, and increased mortality. Local application of glyceryl trinitrate patches was efficacious in several studies (11); the mechanism is probably vasodilatation and increased capillary flow. Glyceryl trinitrate is safe, since it causes only skin rashes and transient headache.

Transdermal glyceryl trinitrate is effective as an analgesic co-adjuvant for cancer pain. In combination with opiates it is well tolerated and reduces the daily consumption of morphine (12). Transdermal glyceryl trinitrate was safe in potentiating the analgesic effect of spinal sufentanil analgesia after knee surgery (13). The effects of glyceryl trinitrate include headache, a feeling of pressure in the head, nausea, vomiting, dizziness, tiredness, blackouts, and possibly penile erection and ageusia (14,15).

Placebo-controlled studies

In a multicenter, randomized, placebo-controlled, double-blind study of 0.2% glyceryl trinitrate ointment in 132 patients with anal fissures over at least 4 weeks, healing rates were similar with glyceryl trinitrate and placebo, but adverse events were more frequent in those who used glyceryl trinitrate: 34% complained of headache and 5.9% had orthostatic hypotension (16).

High-dose transdermal glyceryl trinitrate 50–100 mg given over a period of 12 hours each day for 3 months improved exercise tolerance and left ventricular systolic function in 29 patients with congestive heart failure taking a long-term ACE inhibitor (17). The most frequent adverse effects were skin irritation at the site of patch application and headache, which caused premature glyceryl trinitrate withdrawal in three patients.

Intravenous glyceryl trinitrate (starting rate 50 micrograms/minute uptitrated with blood pressure monitoring) for an average of 63 hours was very effective in preventing adverse ischemic events in 200 patients with unstable angina secondary to restenosis after coronary artery angioplasty, while heparin had no effect (18). In this acute setting, complications and adverse effects were not frequent, even if there was an excess of cases with headache or hypotension with glyceryl trinitrate, never leading to premature discontinuation. This study has shown that glyceryl trinitrate is safe and effective in

43. Packer M, Halperin JL, Brooks KM, Rothlauf EB, Lee WH. Nitroglycerin therapy in the management of pulmonary hypertensive disorders. Am J Med 1984; 76(6A):67–75.
44. Siepmann M, Kirch W. Effects of nitroglycerine on cerebral blood flow velocity, quantitative electroencephalogram and cognitive performance. Eur J Clin Invest 2000;30(9):832–7.
45. Purvin VA, Dunn DW. Nitrate-induced transient ischemic attacks. South Med J 1981;74(9):1130–1.
46. Bevan JS, Oza AM, Burke CW, Adams CB. Pituitary apoplexy following isosorbide administration. J Neurol Neurosurg Psychiatry 1987;50(5):636–7.
47. Ahmad S. Nitroglycerin and intracranial hypertension. Am Heart J 1991;121(6 Pt 1):1850–1.
48. Demey HE, Daelemans RA, Verpooten GA, De Broe ME, Van Campenhout CM, Lakiere FV, Schepens PJ, Bossaert LL. Propylene glycol-induced side effects during intravenous nitroglycerin therapy. Intensive Care Med 1988;14(3):221–6.
49. Rosenthal R. Visual hallucinations and suicidal ideation attributed to isosorbide dinitrate. Psychosomatics 1987;28(10):555–6.
50. Needleman P, Johnson EM Jr. Vasodilators in the treatment of angina. In: Gilman AG, Goodman LS, Gilman A, editors. The Pharmacological Basis of Therapeutics. 6th ed. New York: MacMillan, 1980:819.
51. Wizemann AJ, Wizemann V. Organic nitrate therapy in glaucoma. Am J Ophthalmol 1980;90(1):106–9.
52. Rodger JC. Peripheral oedema in patients treated with isosorbide dinitrate. BMJ (Clin Res Ed) 1981;283(6303): 1365–6.
53. Marshall JB, Ecklund RE. Methemoglobinemia from overdose of nitroglycerin. JAMA 1980;244(4):330.
54. Kaplan JA, Finlayson DC, Woodward S. Vasodilator therapy after cardiac surgery: a review of the efficacy and toxicity of nitroglycerin and nitroprusside. Can Anaesth Soc J 1980;27(3):254–9.
55. Kaplan KJ, Taber M, Teagarden JR, Parker M, Davison R. Association of methemoglobinemia and intravenous nitroglycerin administration. Am J Cardiol 1985;55(1):181–3.
56. Zurick AM, Wagner RH, Starr NJ, Lytle B, Estafanous FG. Intravenous nitroglycerin, methemoglobinemia, and respiratory distress in a postoperative cardiac surgical patient. Anesthesiology 1984;61(4):464–6.
57. Buenger JW, Mauro VF. Organic nitrate-induced methemoglobinemia. DICP 1989;23(4):283–8.
58. Tarburton JP, Metcalf WK. Kinetics of amyl nitrite-induced hemoglobin oxidation in cord and adult blood. Toxicology 1985;36(1):15–21.
59. Chinoy DA, Camp J, Elchahal S, Godoy C, Grossman W, Hai H, Hamilton W, Kushner M, McGreevy M, Mulvihill RJ. A multicenter comparison of adhesion, preference, tolerability, and safety characteristics of two transdermal nitroglycerin delivery systems: Transderm-Nitro and Deponit. Clin Ther 1989;11(5):678–84.
60. Hendricks AA, Dec GW Jr. Contact dermatitis due to nitroglycerin ointment. Arch Dermatol 1979;115(7):853–5.
61. Rosenfeld AS, White WB. Allergic contact dermatitis secondary to transdermal nitroglycerin. Am Heart J 1984; 108(4 Pt 1):1061–2.
62. Letendre PW, Barr C, Wilkens K. Adverse dermatologic reaction to transdermal nitroglycerin. Drug Intell Clin Pharm 1984;18(1):69–70.
63. Wilkin JK. Vasodilator rosacea. Arch Dermatol 1980;116(5):598.
64. Anonymous. Transdermal glyceryl trinitrate patches (Transiderm-Nitro). Drug Ther Bull 1986;24(2):5–6.
65. Cowan JC. Nitrate tolerance. Int J Cardiol 1986;12(1):1–19.
66. Cowan JC. Antianginal drug therapy. Curr Opin Cardiol 1990;5:453.
67. Needleman P, Johnson EM Jr. Mechanism of tolerance development to organic nitrates. J Pharmacol Exp Ther 1973;184(3):709–15.
68. Elkayam U. Tolerance to organic nitrates: evidence, mechanisms, clinical relevance, and strategies for prevention. Ann Intern Med 1991;114(8):667–77.
69. Cowan JC. Avoiding nitrate tolerance. Br J Clin Pharmacol 1992;34(2):96–101.
70. Gori T, Parker JD. Nitrate tolerance: a unifying hypothesis. Circulation 2002;106(19):2510–13.
71. Parker JO, Vankoughnett KA, Farrell B. Comparison of buccal nitroglycerin and oral isosorbide dinitrate for nitrate tolerance in stable angina pectoris. Am J Cardiol 1985;56(12):724–8.
72. Abrams J. Management of myocardial ischemia: role of intermittent nitrate therapy. Am Heart J 1990; 120(3):762–5.
73. Muiesan ML, Boni E, Castellano M, Beschi M, Cefis G, Cerri B, Verdecchia P, Porcellati C, Pollavini G, Agabiti-Rosei E. Effects of transdermal nitroglycerin in combination with an ACE inhibitor in patients with chronic stable angina pectoris. Eur Heart J 1993;14(12):1701–8.
74. Watanabe H, Kakihana M, Ohtsuka S, Sugishita Y. Randomized, double-blind, placebo-controlled study of carvedilol on the prevention of nitrate tolerance in patients with chronic heart failure. J Am Coll Cardiol 1998;32(5):1194–200.
75. Glasser SP. Prospects for therapy of nitrate tolerance. Lancet 1999;353(9164):1545–6.
76. Daniel TA, Nawarskas JJ. Vitamin C in the prevention of nitrate tolerance. Ann Pharmacother 2000;34(10):1193–7.
77. Ebright GE. The effects of nitroglycerin on those engaged in its manufacture. JAMA 1914;62:201.
78. Hogstedt C, Axelson O. Nitroglycerine–nitroglycol exposure and the mortality in cardio-cerebrovascular diseases among dynamite workers. J Occup Med 1977; 19(10):675–8.
79. RuDusky BM. Acute myocardial infarction secondary to coronary vasospasm during withdrawal from industrial nitroglycerin exposure—a case report. Angiology 2001; 52(2):143–4.
80. Lange RL, Reid MS, Tresch DD, Keelan MH, Bernhard VM, Coolidge G. Nonatheromatous ischemic heart disease following withdrawal from chronic industrial nitroglycerin exposure. Circulation 1972;46(4):666–78.
81. Danahy DT, Aronow WS. Hemodynamics and antianginal effects of high dose oral isosorbide dinitrate after chronic use. Circulation 1977;56(2):205–12.
82. Aronow WS. Nitrates as antianginal agents. Prim Cardiol 1980;6:46.
83. Andreassi MG, Picano E, Del Ry S, Botto N, Colombo MG, Giannessi D, Lubrano V, Vassalle C, Biagini A. Chronic long-term nitrate therapy: possible cytogenetic effect in humans? Mutagenesis 2001;16(6):517–21.
84. David M, Halle H, Lichtenegger W, Sinha P, Zimmermann T. Nitroglycerin to facilitate fetal extraction during cesarean delivery. Obstet Gynecol 1998;91(1):119–24.
85. Craig S, Dalton R, Tuck M, Brew F. Sublingual glyceryl trinitrate for uterine relaxation at Caeserean section—a prospective trial. Aust NZ J Obstet Gynaecol 1998; 38(1):34–9.
86. Gazzolo D, Bruschettini M, Di Iorio R, Marinoni E, Lituania M, Marras M, Sarli R, Bruschettini PL, Michetti F. Maternal nitric oxide supplementation decreases cord blood S100B in intrauterine growth-retarded fetuses. Clin Chem 2002;48(4):647–50.

87. Caponas G. Glyceryl trinitrate and acute uterine relaxation: a literature review. Anaesth Intensive Care 2001; 29(2):163–77.
88. De Caterina R. Nitrate als Thrombocytenfunktionskemmer. [Nitrates as thrombocyte function inhibitors.] Z Kardiol 1994;83(7):463–73.
89. ISIS-4 (Fourth International Study of Infarct Survival) Collaborative Group. ISIS-4: a randomised factorial trial assessing early oral captopril, oral mononitrate, and intravenous magnesium sulphate in 58,050 patients with suspected acute myocardial infarction. Lancet 1995; 345(8951):669–85.
90. Cohn JN, Johnson G, Ziesche S, Cobb F, Francis G, Tristani F, Smith R, Dunkman WB, Loeb H, Wong M, et al. A comparison of enalapril with hydralazine–isosorbide dinitrate in the treatment of chronic congestive heart failure. N Engl J Med 1991;325(5):303–10.
91. Hoit B, Gregoratos G, Shabetai R. Paradoxical pulmonary vasoconstriction induced by nitroglycerin in idiopathic pulmonary hypertension. J Am Coll Cardiol 1985; 6(2):490–2.
92. Lefebvre RA, Bogaert MG, Teirlynck O, Sioufi A, Dubois JP. Influence of exercise on nitroglycerin plasma concentrations after transdermal application. Br J Clin Pharmacol 1990;30(2):292–6.
93. Wrenn K. The hazards of defibrillation through nitroglycerin patches. Ann Emerg Med 1990;19(11):1327–8.
94. Murray KB. Hazard of microwave ovens to transdermal delivery system. N Engl J Med 1984;310(11):721.
95. Kocher HM, Steward M, Leather AJ, Cullen PT. Randomized clinical trial assessing the side-effects of glyceryl trinitrate and diltiazem hydrochloride in the treatment of chronic anal fissure. Br J Surg 2002; 89(4):413–17.
96. Lanas A, Bajador E, Serrano P, Arroyo M, Fuentes J, Santolaria S. Effects of nitrate and prophylactic aspirin on upper gastrointestinal bleeding: a retrospective case-control study. J Int Med Res 1998;26(3):120–8.
97. Tongia SK. Exaggerated tendency to postural hypotension with isosorbiddinitrate on clonidine's background activity. J Assoc Physicians India 1994;42(7):580.
98. Barletta MA, Eisen H. Isosorbide dinitrate–disopyramide phosphate interaction. Drug Intell Clin Pharm 1985; 19(10):764.
99. Abrams J, Schroeder K, Raizada V. Potentially adverse effects of sublingual nitroglycerin during consumption of alcohol. J Am Coll Cardiol 1990;15:226A.
100. Korn SH, Comer JB. Intravenous nitroglycerin and ethanol intoxication. Ann Intern Med 1985;102(2):274.
101. Shook TL, Kirshenbaum JM, Hundley RF, Shorey JM, Lamas GA. Ethanol intoxication complicating intravenous nitroglycerin therapy. Ann Intern Med 1984; 101(4):498–9.
102. Andrien P, Lemberg L. An unusual complication of intravenous nitroglycerin. Heart Lung 1986;15(5):534–6.
103. Shorey J, Bhardwaj N, Loscalzo J. Acute Wernicke's encephalopathy after intravenous infusion of high-dose nitroglycerin. Ann Intern Med 1984;101(4):500.
104. Shergy WJ, Gilkeson GS, German DC. Acute gouty arthritis and intravenous nitroglycerin. Arch Intern Med 1988;148(11):2505–6.
105. Habbab MA, Haft JI. Intravenous nitroglycerin and heparin resistance. Ann Intern Med 1986;105(2):305.
106. Pye M, Oldroyd KG, Conkie JA, Hutton I, Cobbe SM. A clinical and in vitro study on the possible interaction of intravenous nitrates with heparin anticoagulation. Clin Cardiol 1994;17(12):658–61.
107. Bechtold H, Kleist P, Landgraf K, Moser K. Einfluss einer niedrigdosierten intravenosen Nitrattherapie auf die antikoagulatorische Wirkung von Heparin. [Effect of low-dosage intravenous nitrate therapy on the anticoagulant effect of heparin.] Med Klin (Munich) 1994; 89(7):360–6.
108. Lancaster L, Fenster PE. Complete heart block after sublingual nitroglycerin. Chest 1983;84(1):111–12.
109. Antonelli D, Barzilay J. Complete atrioventricular block after sublingual isosorbide dinitrate. Int J Cardiol 1986; 10(1):71–3.
110. Hyldstrup L, Mogensen NB, Nielsen PE. Orthostatic response before and after nitroglycerin in metoprolol- and verapamil-treated angina pectoris. Acta Med Scand 1983;214(2):131–4.
111. Silfvast T, Kinnunen A, Varpula T. Laryngeal oedema after isosorbide dinitrate spray and sublingual nifedipine. BMJ 1995;311(6999):232.
112. Cheitlin MD, Hutter AM Jr, Brindis RG, Ganz P, Kaul S, Russell RO Jr, Zusman RM. Use of sildenafil (Viagra) in patients with cardiovascular disease. Technology and Practice Executive Committee. Circulation 1999; 99(1):168–77.
113. Webb DJ, Freestone S, Allen MJ, Muirhead GJ. Sildenafil citrate and blood-pressure-lowering drugs: results of drug interaction studies with an organic nitrate and a calcium antagonist. Am J Cardiol 1999; 83(5A):C21–8.
114. Bhalerao S. A new suicide. J Fam Pract 2001;50(6):551.

Nitrazepam

See also Benzodiazepines

General Information

Nitrazepam is a long-acting benzodiazepine used primarily for insomnia. However, it has a long half-life (about 24 hours) and poses a substantial risk of residual daytime effects, including sedation, psychomotor and cognitive impairment, and accidental injury (1).

Organs and Systems

Death

Between January 1983 and March 1994, 302 patients with intractable epilepsy were entered into a nitrazepam compassionate plea protocol (2). Nitrazepam increased the risk of death, especially in young patients with intractable epilepsy. The authors suggested that nitrazepam should be used with caution in young children with intractable epilepsy, especially if they have difficulties in swallowing, aspiration, pneumonia, gastroesophageal reflux, or a combination of these.

References

1. Vermeeren A. Residual effects of hypnotics: epidemiology and clinical implications. CNS Drugs 2004;18(5):297–328.
2. Rintahaka PJ, Nakagawa JA, Shewmon DA, Kyyronen P, Shields WD. Incidence of death in patients with intractable epilepsy during nitrazepam treatment. Epilepsia 1999; 40(4):492–6.

oxide in severe bronchopulmonary dysplasia. Pediatrics 1999;103(3):610–18.
27. Hermon M, Golej J, Burda G, Marx M, Trittenwein G, Pollak A. Intravenous prostacyclin mitigates inhaled nitric oxide rebound effect: a case control study. Artif Organs 1999;23(11):975–8.
28. Buratti T, Joannidis M, Pechlaner C, Wiedermann CJ. Systemic hypotension on withdrawal from inhaled nitric oxide in an adult patient with acute respiratory distress syndrome. Crit Care Med 1999;27(2):441.

Nitrofurantoin

General Information

Nitrofurantoin is a synthetic nitrofuran that belongs to a group of organic substances characterized by a heterocyclic ring consisting of four carbon atoms and one oxygen atom (1). Its mechanism of action is not understood. Nitrofurans enter bacterial cells and interact with several enzymes; thereby inhibiting bacterial growth. Nitrofurantoin is active against many Gram-positive and Gram-negative bacteria. It is particularly useful in treating urinary pathogens, including *Escherichia coli*, *Klebsiella* species, and *Proteus* species. However, *Pseudomonas aeruginosa* is almost always resistant.

After almost complete absorption from the gastrointestinal tract, nitrofurantoin produces high urinary concentrations. Blood and tissue concentrations are low. Nitrofurantoin has been used almost exclusively in the treatment and prophylaxis of urinary tract infections (1). Because of the severity of its adverse effects it should not be used as first choice.

General adverse effects

Harmless gastrointestinal adverse effects are most frequent with nitrofurantoin. Polyneuropathy occurs mainly in patients with renal insufficiency, in whom nitrofurantoin is contraindicated. Rarely, hemolytic anemia and hepatitis occur. Adverse events that are believed to be due to hypersensitivity include rashes, generalized urticaria, and acute pulmonary reactions. Although there are some in vitro data suggesting that nitrofurantoin may be a mutagen, a carcinogenic effect has not been proven in vivo. Teratogenic effects of nitrofurantoin have not been reported. High-dose oral nitrofurantoin may influence spermatogenesis and sperm motility.

Frequency

Drug-related adverse events are rare with nitrofurantoin and occur in fewer patients than with co-trimoxazole or trimethoprim, for example (1–3). The frequency of certain adverse reactions varies in different geographical areas (4,5). Lung reactions are more prevalent in Scandinavia and South Africa than in the UK, whereas polyneuropathies or gastrointestinal reactions are more frequent in the UK than in Sweden. These discrepancies are unexplained.

Organs and Systems

Cardiovascular

Except for cardiovascular collapse in anaphylactic shock, adverse cardiovascular events seem to be extremely rare with nitrofurantoin (4,5). In experimental animals, cardiotoxic effects have been described (6).

Respiratory

Acute respiratory reactions to nitrofurantoin include dyspnea, cough, interstitial pneumonitis, and pleural effusion, while interstitial pneumonitis and fibrosis are common chronic reactions (7). Nitrofurantoin causes acute lung injury more often than any other drug. Since the first well-documented case of an acute lung reaction in 1962 (8), several hundred further observations have been published (5,9). The frequency of acute severe pulmonary disease has been estimated to be one in every 5000 first administrations (10). Women aged 40–50 years are mainly affected. The acute lung reactions are not dose-related, and sensitization occurs at the earliest 1–2 weeks after the onset of exposure during the first course of therapy. Symptoms develop 2–10 hours after administration and consist of severe dyspnea, tachypnea, non-productive cough, high fever (usually with chills), cyanosis, and chest pain. Occasionally, arthralgia, backache or headache, vomiting, rash, collapse, and anaphylactic shock accompany the pulmonary symptoms (9). Lung findings include dense crackles or moist râles, predominantly at the lung bases. X-ray examination may be normal, but more often shows bilateral interstitial lower lobe infiltrates, often with pleural effusion. In one case, transient reverse ventilation-perfusion mismatch was documented by scintigraphy (11). Initially the leukocyte count is normal or raised, with neutrophilia and lymphopenia. Later, eosinophilia is common. When nitrofurantoin is withdrawn, clinical symptoms subside rapidly, usually within 1–3 days (5). However, minor X-ray changes can still be found 2 months later. Re-exposure to nitrofurantoin 50 mg re-induces the syndrome. Single cases of death due to heart failure have been reported in debilitated patients.

Acute lung reactions to nitrofurantoin are extremely rare in children (12). Lung tissue findings in acute reactions have shown minor vasculitis, granulomatous vasculitis (hypersensitivity angiitis), proliferation of endothelial cells, and empty alveoli (13). Rapidly progressing bronchiolitis obliterans with organizing pneumonia (BOOP) has been reported (14).

Chronic lung reactions are 10–20 times less frequent than acute reactions and mainly involve older patients. Reactions serious enough to require hospitalization occur in one out of 750 long-term users (15). Acute reactions do not seem to predispose to the later occurrence of chronic reactions. During long-term treatment, dyspnea and usually a non-productive cough without fever develop (15). Restrictive respiratory impairment is common. X-rays show interstitial infiltrations, often in the middle and basal lung regions. Fibrotic changes, alveolar exudates, and pleural effusions are rare. Histologically, chronic interstitial pneumonitis with varying degrees of fibrosis most often is found, and in some instances desquamative alveolitis (15–19).

Several mechanisms for the adverse lung effects of nitrofurantoin have been proposed (20–24). The pathogenesis of the acute lung reactions may be allergic (type III reactions) (18). However, there is also evidence that a cytotoxic immune mechanism (type II reactions), cell-mediated immunity (type IV reactions) (2), or direct toxic injury to lung tissue through the production of oxygen radicals (3,4) may be involved (20,21,24,25). In chronic lung reactions, the causative role of nitrofurantoin is less evident. It is supported by analogy and by the clinical course. Sometimes the skin test is positive, even in chronic lung reactions. Lymphocyte transformation tests give variable results. A polyclonal hypergammaglobulinemia is always present, with IgG predominating. Precipitating serum antibodies have not been found. Recent data have supported a toxic pathogenesis similar to that of the herbicide paraquat.

After nitrofurantoin withdrawal, the clinical symptoms regress rapidly. However, in most cases X-ray findings abate slowly and resolution is incomplete in at least 50% of patients. Occasional deaths due to cardiopulmonary failure have also been reported. The therapeutic benefit of corticosteroids is controversial, but the bulk of experience and anecdotal reports suggest that they are useful.

Atypical courses have been rarely described (5). A mixed type of reaction can occur: after an initial short fever peak, the patient becomes either afebrile or subfebrile, despite continuing to take nitrofurantoin and unabated activity of the lung process, or a typical chronic reaction converts to a typical acute reaction on re-exposure to nitrofurantoin after withdrawal. Acute reactions can occur without clinical symptoms, and can be recognized only on X-ray. Single cases of pulmonary hemorrhage, eosinophilic pneumonia, and interstitial giant cell pneumonia have also been reported (26,27).

In nitrofurantoin-induced pulmonary toxicity, in which high-resolution computed tomography initially showed a widespread reticular pattern and associated distortion of the lung parenchyma, thought to represent established and irreversible fibrosis, follow-up scans after drug withdrawal nevertheless showed resolution of pulmonary changes (28). These findings have been corroborated by a report of two middle-aged women who developed respiratory symptoms after prolonged treatment with nitrofurantoin (29). Both had impaired lung function and abnormal CT scans, and lung biopsies showed features compatible with bronchiolitis obliterans organizing pneumonia. Their condition improved when nitrofurantoin was withdrawn and glucocorticoid treatment was given.

In a patient with nitrofurantoin-induced pulmonary toxicity, in whom high resolution CT scans initially showed a widespread reticular pattern and associated distortion of the lung parenchyma, thought to represent established and irreversible fibrosis, follow-up CT scans after withdrawal of the drug showed resolution of the pulmonary changes.

- An 82-year-old woman developed a productive cough after having taken nitrofurantoin 50 mg/day for 4 years (30). She had impaired lung function and abnormal CT scans, and lung biopsies showed features compatible with bronchiolitis obliterans organizing pneumonia. The condition improved when nitrofurantoin was withdrawn and she was given a glucocorticoid.
- In a 58-year-old woman who took nitrofurantoin 100 mg/day for 11 months, pulmonary toxicity occurred, with bilateral interstitial infiltrates in the lower zones of the chest X-ray and loss of lung volume (31). High resolution CT scans showed ground-glass opacification in the mid-thoracic region, with patchy fibrosis and traction bronchiectasis. After withdrawal of nitrofurantoin and administration of prednisone, a chest X-ray 3 months later showed resolution of the pulmonary changes.

Nervous system

More than 140 cases of toxic polyneuropathy have been reported. The frequency depends on dose, tissue concentration, and renal function: in up to 90% of cases polyneuropathy occurred in patients with renal insufficiency (32). Symptoms usually start 9–45 days (at the earliest 3 days) after beginning nitrofurantoin. The neuropathy starts peripherally, predominantly affects the limbs, and remains more severe distally. Initially, there is sensory loss with paresthesia. Later, motor loss develops, often with severe muscle atrophy. As a rule, no further deterioration occurs after withdrawal of nitrofurantoin, and there may be total regression (34% of cases) or partial regression (45% of cases) (32). In some severe cases there is residual disability. The motor loss resolves more slowly and less completely than the sensory impairment. Single cases of retrobulbar optic neuritis, lateral rectus muscle palsy, and facial nerve palsy have been reported (33).

The lesions comprise degeneration of the myelin sheath of the nerves and nerve roots, with degeneration of the corresponding anterior horn cells and muscle fibers. The pathogenesis is unclear. Impairment of glutathione reductase has been considered. Even in healthy people, nitrofurantoin 400 mg/day for 2 weeks causes a significant increase in motor nerve conduction time. If strict attention is paid to the contraindication of renal insufficiency, the risk of polyneuropathy can be reduced. Careful controls for the initial symptoms of paresthesia can prevent the development of severe disablement.

While taking nitrofurantoin after urinary tract surgery, a 10-year-old girl developed diplopia and ptosis (34). A sleep test confirmed ocular myasthenia. Her signs and symptoms resolved after drug withdrawal.

Single cases of benign intracranial hypertension (pseudotumor cerebri), with and without ocular palsy, have been reported (35,36). Uncharacteristic general symptoms, with dizziness, cephalalgia, or drowsiness, are more frequent.

Trigeminal neuralgia (37) and cerebellar symptoms (38) have been attributed to nitrofurantoin.

Sensory systems

One case of crystalline retinopathy has been associated with long-term nitrofurantoin (39).

Psychological, psychiatric

Rarely, concomitant dysphoric, euphoric, or even psychotic reactions have been reported in patients taking nitrofurantoin (1).

Metabolism

One case of hyperlactatemic metabolic acidosis together with hemolytic anemia due to glucose-6-phosphate dehydrogenase deficiency has been reported (40).

Hematologic

Some cases of hemolytic anemia associated with glucose 6-phosphate dehydrogenase deficiency have been described in patients taking nitrofurantoin (41).

Single cases of nitrofurantoin-induced (or enhanced) hemolytic anemia have occurred in patients with deficiencies of other erythrocyte enzymes (enolase or glutathione peroxidase), as have isolated cases of methemoglobinemia (42).

Nitrofurantoin produces oxidant stress and cellular damage by different mechanisms (43). It can disturb folate metabolism, leading to a megaloblastic component in pre-existing (mostly hemolytic) anemia, which responds to folic acid treatment.

There have been single cases of thrombocytopenia and a severe hemorrhagic diathesis with deficiency of coagulation factors due to a nitrofurantoin-induced hepatic disorder (44). Furthermore, nitrofurantoin experimentally inhibits ADP-induced platelet aggregation (45).

Allergic agranulocytosis or neutropenia have been proven in only a few cases (46,47). Pancytopenia is also rarely seen (5).

Mouth and teeth

Some cases of parotitis, rarely proven by rechallenge, have been associated with nitrofurantoin (48). The symptoms disappear after withdrawal.

Gastrointestinal

Gastrointestinal symptoms are the most common adverse effects of nitrofurantoin. Nausea and anorexia have been most often reported (49,50), whereas abdominal pain and diarrhea are rare. These effects are dose-related and usually harmless. The manifestations occur mostly after absorption of the drug and are mediated by the central nervous system. Measures that delay absorption, such as sugar coating or the use of a macrocrystalline form of the drug, reduce these adverse effects (51).

Liver

Hepatic reactions to nitrofurantoin are rare, and different forms can be distinguished (52–54). They can be associated with fatal liver necrosis (55,56).

Data from The Netherlands suggest that acute reactions are more common than chronic ones. Acute hepatic reactions may be hepatocellular or cholestatic. In the vast majority of subjects, symptoms appear within the first 6 weeks of nitrofurantoin treatment, and in half of the patients they occur within the first week of treatment. Jaundice is most common, followed by abdominal pain, malaise, and nausea. Hepatomegaly has been reported in nearly 50% of cases, fever in 30–65%, eosinophilia in 15–50%, and a rash in 12–60%. An immunological pathogenesis has been proposed (57), but experimental data point to a toxic mechanism involving the formation of glutathione-protein mixed disulfides and/or protein alkylation (58). The prognosis after withdrawal of the drug is good, but fatal courses have been reported when the drug is continued or, rarely, even after it has been discontinued.

Chronic active hepatitis, icteric or anicteric, has been described, almost always in women taking long-term nitrofurantoin. Most patients develop symptoms after a period of about 6 months of nitrofurantoin use. Fever (0–24%), rash (0–3%), and eosinophilia (9–23%) occur rarely compared with acute cases. There is hepatomegaly in 30–60% of chronic cases (54). Sometimes a broad spectrum of autoimmune reactions, a lupus-like syndrome, or mild cholestasis can be present (59,60). Some of these cases have occurred in combination with lung reactions of the protracted acute or chronic type, or in patients with ascites and liver cirrhosis. The clinical symptoms usually improve after withdrawal, but a few cases with extensive hepatocellular necrosis have necessitated liver transplantation or ended fatally (61–64). The histological changes can persist. Re-exposure to nitrofurantoin has reproduced the pathological liver tests.

Granulomatous hepatitis, with a rash or isolated increases in serum transaminase activities, can occur in patients with lung reactions (65). In the protracted acute and in chronic lung reactions liver injury (such as chronic active hepatitis) is more frequent than in acute reactions. Such cases usually show a broad spectrum of serological autoimmune reactions (lupus-like syndrome) (66).

Pancreas

A few cases of nitrofurantoin-induced acute pancreatitis, confirmed by rechallenge, have been reported (67).

Urinary tract

Nitrofurantoin-induced crystalluria, leading to obstruction of indwelling catheters, has been described in a few patients (68).

In rare cases, interstitial nephritis has been observed (69,70).

Skin

Allergic skin reactions occur in 1–2% of patients who take nitrofurantoin and comprise about 21% of all adverse reactions to nitrofurantoin (5,71). They often occur with other reactions, such as drug fever, lung, or liver reactions. The lesions can present as pruritus, as macular, maculopapular, or vesicular rashes, urticaria, angioedema, or erythema multiforme (72). The frequency of serious cutaneous reactions (erythema multiforme, Stevens–Johnson syndrome, or toxic epidermal necrolysis) after nitrofurantoin has been estimated to be 7 cases per 100 000 exposed individuals (71).

Sweet's syndrome has been observed in association with a 7-day course of nitrofurantoin (73).

Transitory alopecia that has been reported in a few cases is dose-related (74).

Immunologic

About 20 cases of a lupus-like syndrome have been described, mostly in the Scandinavian literature. The clinical picture consisted of arthralgia or, rarely, exacerbation of a pre-existing rheumatoid arthritis and generalized lymphadenopathy, mostly associated with chronic lung and/or liver reactions, such as chronic active hepatitis (19,75,76). In patients with the lupus-like syndrome at least two immunological tests (antinuclear factor, rheumatoid factor, Coombs' test, and antibodies against smooth muscle, thyroglobulin, thyroid cell cytoplasm, or glomeruli) were positive. The lymphocyte transformation test was always positive. However, the LE cell phenomenon was always negative. As in other allergic reactions to nitrofurantoin, circulating albumin IgG complexes were found by immunoelectrophoresis, with tailing of the albumin line (77). The syndrome regresses after withdrawal.

Long-Term Effects

Drug tolerance

Nitrofurantoin is effective against Enterobacteriaceae; the rates of resistance were below 2% in a single-center study (78) and 3.5% in a multicenter study (79).

Mutagenicity

In vitro, nitrofurantoin acts as a mutagen by inhibiting DNA synthetase. In human fibroblast cultures it damages DNA (80). Treatment with nitrofurantoin for 12 months caused a significant increase in chromosome aberrations and sister chromatid exchanges in the lymphocytes of 69 children (81).

Tumorigenicity

Some studies have shown similar metabolism of nitrofurantoin and other (carcinogenic) nitrofurans. Formation of carcinogenic nitrofurantoin metabolites is therefore possible (82). However, a carcinogenic effect has not been proven for nitrofurantoin (83).

Second-Generation Effects

Fertility

High-dose oral nitrofurantoin (10 mg/kg/day) transiently reduces the sperm count in 30% of patients (84). This is due to arrest of maturation. Depression of sperm motility or ejaculate volume can also occur at lower doses (85).

Teratogenicity

Only very small amounts of nitrofurantoin cross the placenta, and teratogenic effects are not known (86). Even when it is used in the first trimester, there have been no associated fetal malformations (87). No teratogenic effects have been associated with nitrofurantoin in Denmark, Finland, Norway, and Sweden (88), or in a Hungarian case-control survey (89).

Fetotoxicity

Hemolytic anemia occurred during the first hours of life in a full-term neonate whose mother had taken nitrofurantoin during the last month of pregnancy (90). It may therefore be wise not to prescribe nitrofurantoin at the end of pregnancy.

Lactation

Nitrofurantoin is actively transported into human milk, achieving concentrations greatly exceeding those in serum. Concern is warranted for suckling infants under 1 month old or for infants with a high frequency of glucose-6-phosphate dehydrogenase deficiency or sensitivity to nitrofurantoin (91).

Susceptibility Factors

Genetic factors

Glucose-6-phosphate dehydrogenase deficiency is decisive for the development of hemolytic anemia in patients taking nitrofurantoin.

Age

Nitrofurantoin is contraindicated during the last trimester of pregnancy and in neonates, because hemolytic anemia can result from immature enzyme systems (90).

Renal disease

The main risk factor for toxic reactions to nitrofurantoin, especially polyneuropathy and gastrointestinal symptoms, is impaired renal function (32).

Drug–Drug Interactions

Estrogens

Nitrofurantoin reduces the enterohepatic circulation of estrogens (92).

Nalidixic acid

Antagonism in antibacterial efficacy between nitrofurantoin and nalidixic acid has been observed (93).

Pyridoxine

Pyridoxine accelerates the renal elimination of nitrofurantoin (94).

Interference with Diagnostic Tests

Glucose measurements

Nitrofurantoin can produce spurious positive urine glucose concentrations or raised blood glucose concentrations if reducing reagents are used (95).

References

1. D'Arcy PF. Nitrofurantoin. Drug Intell Clin Pharm 1985;19(7–8):540–7.
2. Spencer RC, Moseley DJ, Greensmith MJ. Nitrofurantoin modified release versus trimethoprim or co-trimoxazole in the treatment of uncomplicated urinary tract infection in general practice. J Antimicrob Chemother 1994;33(Suppl A):121–9.

Table 1 *Continued*

Butazone derivatives
Azapropazone
Bumadizone
Feprazone
Ketophenylbutazone
Monophenylbutazone
Oxyphenbutazone
Phenylbutazone
Pipebuzone
Pyrazine-butazone
Suxibuzone
Trimethazone
Coxibs (COX-2 inhibitors)
Celecoxib
Parecoxib
Rofecoxib
Valdecoxib
Indoleacetic acid derivatives
Acemetacin
Cinmetacin
Clometacin
Glucametacin
Indometacin
Oxametacin
Proglumetacin
Sulindac
Zidometacin

More than 100 NSAIDs are marketed or at an advanced stage of development worldwide. Their use is constantly expanding and the search for more efficacious and better-tolerated compounds is still being pursued, and has received renewed impulse with studies on selective inhibitors of cyclo-oxygenase type 2 (COX-2), nitric oxide-releasing NSAIDs, peroxidase inhibitors, enantiomers of already known NSAIDs, NSAIDs associated with zwitterionic phospholipids, and cytokine-modulating antirheumatic drugs.

Predominantly used in the management of rheumatological conditions, NSAIDs are drugs of choice in the treatment of inflammatory arthropathies. However, their use has also been extended to many non-rheumatological problems (for example dysmenorrhea, pain of different origin, neoplastic fever, migraine, thromboembolic disease, and patent ductus arteriosus; they are also used for tocolysis and in some neoplastic diseases) (1). Several clinical, epidemiological, and animal studies have suggested that NSAIDs can reduce the occurrence or progression of colorectal cancer, polyps, and perhaps other gastrointestinal tumors (2–4). Reports and epidemiological studies have shown that NSAIDs can protect against the risk of Alzheimer's disease (5,6). NSAIDs are used locally in the eye to prevent and treat postoperative cystoid macular edema, to control postoperative ocular inflammation and pain, for example after radial keratotomy or photorefractive keratectomy, and for non-surgically induced inflammatory disorders, such as allergic conjunctivitis.

The range and incidence of these conditions clearly justifies extensive use of suitable drugs, and explains the pharmaceutical industry's interest in exploiting the potential revenues of such a large market.

The effort to find new compounds is medically justified by the unsatisfactory benefit-to-harm balance of the NSAIDs that are currently available.

The adverse reactions profiles of many NSAIDs have proved to be unacceptable. Over the last 20 years, 18 NSAIDs have been withdrawn from the market or their clinical studies have been terminated because of unexpected toxicity (7). Selection of an NSAID can be difficult, since reliable information about their relative efficacy and adverse reactions is usually meager.

Although the physicochemical features, pharmacokinetics, and pharmacodynamics of individual NSAIDs differ, it is not known to what extent these differences are significant in the benefit-to-harm balance in the individual patient (8). Certainly they influence the adverse reactions and the general pattern of action of a particular subgroup of NSAIDs or a specific compound within a class, but this still provides no reliable prediction of what the individual patient will experience.

The acidic nature and lipid solubility of these compounds are important. The lipid solubility of an NSAID determines its penetration into the central nervous system and hence the incidence of nervous system-related adverse effects and perhaps adverse skin reactions (9,10). The weak acid nature affects tissue distribution, which explains why NSAIDs have actions at certain sites (for example synovial tissue of inflamed joints) and also contribute to triggering particular adverse reactions at others (for example the stomach and renal medulla) (11).

Pharmacokinetic aspects can play a critical role in the onset of certain adverse effects in some patients (12). NSAIDs are almost entirely absorbed from the gastrointestinal tract (13). The rate and the site of absorption from the gastrointestinal tract can be important; formulations designed to spare the stomach from NSAID toxicity can instead damage the intestinal wall, which seems to have been the case with Osmosin (SEDA-8, 103). There have been a few studies of the chronopharmacology of NSAIDs (SEDA-20, 90). NSAID absorption is probably better in the morning, but there are more adverse effects than when the drug is taken in the evening.

NSAIDs bind avidly to plasma proteins. High protein binding can theoretically predispose patients to drug interactions, which occur most frequently with certain NSAIDs (for example the butazones) in patients who are concomitantly taking drugs such as hypoglycemic agents or oral anticoagulants. The unbound fraction responsible for the pharmacological action of NSAIDs varies with the plasma albumin concentrations, which can be influenced by active rheumatoid arthritis, genetic factors, sex, age, pregnancy, other drugs, and diseases, particularly when the kidney and liver are involved. A correlation between anti-inflammatory action and dose or plasma concentration has been documented for only a few NSAIDs, and there is no direct evidence that an increase in unbound drug concentration is associated with greater toxicity. However, there is convincing evidence that the dose contributes to certain adverse effects (for example gastrointestinal and renal). A record-linkage study has shown an association between NSAID dosage and upper gastrointestinal bleeding (14).

NSAIDs can be roughly divided into those with short and long half-lives. Although the difference in clinical effects between these two categories is poorly understood, half-lives have served as a rough guide for NSAID dosage regimens, compounds with long half-lives being administered only once a day. These NSAIDs also have a greater potential to cause adverse effects, at least in some patients. As the half-lives of this type of NSAID vary widely in different patients, drug accumulation can occur in some individuals. When using an NSAID with a long half-life, loading doses can be given to achieve high drug concentrations quickly, but can be associated with increased adverse effects, particularly gastrointestinal intolerance.

NSAIDs are mainly cleared by the liver, and their clearances would be expected to fall with age (13). Their metabolites are generally inactive and excreted in the urine, which as a rule contains very little unchanged drug. Conversely, several NSAIDs that are themselves inactive can be used as prodrugs, since they have active metabolites; some of these compounds, such as sulindac, undergo enterohepatic recycling. Claims that these prodrugs are less toxic than other compounds are not supported by any firm evidence. Some NSAIDs, including carprofen, fenoprofen, indometacin, ketoprofen, and naproxen are metabolized to acylglucuronides; the metabolites are retained and hydrolysed to re-form the parent compound. This is probably one of the mechanisms of toxicity in patients with renal insufficiency.

Pharmacodynamic mechanisms can also be crucial. The main mechanism of action is inhibition of cyclo-oxygenase (COX) activity and consequently of prostaglandin synthesis (15–17). Two forms of COX have been identified: COX-1, which is constitutively expressed in many cells and tissues, and COX-2, which is selectively induced by proinflammatory cytokines at the site of inflammation. The discovery of a second COX enzyme has led to the hypothesis that the toxicity associated with the clinically useful NSAIDs is caused by inhibition of COX-1, whereas the anti-inflammatory properties are caused by the inhibition of COX-2 (18). A selective COX-2 inhibitor may therefore have better anti-inflammatory activity with greater safety than existing NSAIDs. The in vitro potency of NSAIDs as inhibitors of prostaglandin synthesis, which tends to match their anti-inflammatory potency in vivo, varies from one anti-inflammatory agent to the next (19,20). Other mechanisms that are poorly understood may be implicated in determining both a drug's activity and its adverse effects.

These data provide a basis for the practical use of NSAIDs. There can be no doubt that some NSAIDs are more toxic than others, notably those that have the greatest inhibitory effect on cyclo-oxygenase. NSAIDs that inhibit both cyclo-oxygenase and lipoxygenase are particularly toxic. The fact that some NSAIDs are more toxic to single organs than others seems to depend on the physicochemical and metabolic characteristics of single drugs or groups of similar drugs. Despite numerous studies, reliable comparisons of the adverse effects of the different drugs are scanty. However, some data have been produced from the data bank centers of the Arthritis Rheumatism and Aging Medical Information System (ARAMIS) and have been reviewed (SEDA-17, 102). If selective COX-2 inhibitors are confirmed to have less gastrointestinal toxicity than the old NSAIDs, we should have new drugs with fewer risks. However, doubts are emerging about whether COX-1 inhibition makes a contribution to the anti-inflammatory activity of NSAIDs and whether COX-2 activity is implicated in mucosal healing and protective processes (SEDA-22, 109).

The categories of patients who are at higher risk of adverse reactions when treated with NSAIDs are well known and can largely be deduced from what has been said above. They include the elderly (especially women), pregnant women (and their fetuses), neonates, patients with liver, kidney, or cardiac disorders, and those with hypertension, multiple myeloma, peptic disorders, or active rheumatoid arthritis. Greater awareness of these risk factors among medical practitioners, limiting the use of NSAIDs to cases in which there is a precise indication, informing patients, developing systems for monitoring unwanted adverse effects, and carrying out adequate well-designed experimental studies would do much to ensure better use of these drugs. Many of the adverse effects of NSAIDs are, with negligible differences, common to all of them.

Organs and Systems

Cardiovascular

Hypertension

NSAIDs can cause or aggravate hypertension and interact negatively with the effects of antihypertensive drugs, including diuretics, although contrasting data from experimental and clinical studies have been published (21).

The mechanisms by which NSAIDs affect cardiovascular function are complex and controversial. They may include reduced blood flow, a reduction in the filtered load of sodium, an increase in tubular reabsorption of sodium, and a reduction in the synthesis of PGE-1, which may be associated with raised blood viscosity and increased peripheral vascular resistance. This is perhaps the primary mechanism, which is due to increased renal synthesis of endothelin-1.

Meta-analyses

In a meta-analysis of the hypertensive effects of NSAIDs or aspirin (1.5 g/day or greater) in short-term intervention studies; 54 studies and 123 NSAID treatment arms were included (22). Of the 1324 participating subjects, 92% were hypertensive; they had a mean age of 46 years and none was over 65 years. The major outcome studied was the change in mean arterial pressure. The effects of NSAIDs on blood pressure were found solely in hypertensive subjects; among these, the increase in mean arterial pressure, after adjusting for possible confounders (for example dietary salt intake) was different among different NSAIDs. The increase in mean arterial pressure was 3.59 mmHg for indometacin (57 treatment arms), 3.74 mmHg for naproxen (4 arms), and 0.45 mmHg for piroxicam (4 arms). However, mean arterial pressure fell by 2.59 mmHg with placebo (10 arms), by 0.83 mmHg with ibuprofen (6 arms), 1.76 mmHg with aspirin (4 arms), and 0.16 mmHg with sulindac (23 arms).

Overall, only the effects of indometacin on mean arterial pressure were statistically significantly different from those found with placebo, showing that in this population the effects of NSAIDs on blood pressure were modest and varied considerably among different drugs. However, one must take into account the important limitations of the analysis: the patients were mostly young, the studies included in the meta-analysis were small and short-term, and information on possible confounders was incomplete. The significance of the results of this study is therefore doubtful.

Another meta-analysis provided more complete and useful results (23). Its primary aim was to produce an estimate of the overall effect of NSAIDs on blood pressure, and its secondary aims were to evaluate the mechanisms by which NSAIDs alter blood pressure and to determine susceptibility factors. Moreover, as NSAIDs have been associated with raised blood pressure in normotensive individuals and in both treated and untreated hypertensive subjects, the authors tried to discover different effects in these subgroups. Finally, they studied whether different NSAIDs alter blood pressure to the same degree.

In all, 50 randomized placebo-controlled trials and 16 randomized comparisons of two or more NSAIDs met the selection criteria. These studies included 771 young volunteers or patients aged 47 years or younger. The studies were small (the mean sample size per trial was 16); many different NSAIDs and antihypertensive drugs were used, but indometacin was used in more than half of all the trials; the duration of therapy with NSAIDs or antihypertensive drugs was 1 week or longer, but in most studies it was less than 3 months. NSAIDs raised supine mean blood pressure by 5.0 mmHg (95% CI = 1.2, 8.7), but had no significant effect on variables measured to assess possible mechanisms (such as body weight, daily urinary sodium output, creatinine clearance, or urinary prostaglandin excretion). Overall, the data suggested that NSAIDs do not appear to increase blood pressure primarily by increasing salt and water retention, because weight and urinary sodium were not altered by NSAIDs and inhibition of blood pressure control was not more marked in patients taking diuretics compared with other antihypertensive drugs. In addition NSAIDs did not significantly alter plasma renin activity or 24-hour urinary excretion of prostaglandin E_2 and 6-ketoprostaglandin $F_{1\alpha}$. Other factors may therefore contribute to the increase in blood pressure caused by NSAIDs. In particular, a potential effect of NSAIDs on peripheral vascular resistance should be considered (24,25). There is good evidence to suggest an important role for prostaglandins in the modulation of two major determinants of blood pressure, vasoconstriction of arteriolar smooth muscle and control of extracellular volume.

NSAIDs inhibited the effects of all antihypertensive drug categories. However, in patients taking beta-blockers and vasodilators, NSAIDs produced a greater increase in supine mean blood pressure than in patients taking diuretics, but only the pooled inhibitory effect of NSAIDs on the effects of beta-blockers achieved statistical significance. When the data were analysed by type of NSAID the meta-analysis showed that all NSAIDs increased supine blood pressure, and that piroxicam, indometacin, and ibuprofen produced the most marked increases. However, only piroxicam had a statistically significant effect with respect to placebo. Aspirin, sulindac, and flurbiprofen caused the smallest increases in blood pressure.

In conclusion this meta-analysis has provided more clear evidence that, as a group, NSAIDs significantly increase arterial pressure and can antagonize the blood pressure-lowering effect of some antihypertensive drugs, by mechanisms that are still unclear. Although the hypertensive effect of NSAIDs was more marked in hypertensive subjects taking antihypertensive drugs than in normotensive subjects not taking antihypertensive drugs, the difference was not statistically significant and its clinical relevance is unclear. It is worth noting that the effects of NSAIDs on blood pressure were similar in patients taking antihypertensive drugs for months or only a few days.

This study also had two main limitations: first, most of the trials were small, which precluded definitive conclusions about the effects of individual NSAIDs or individual antihypertensive drug classes; secondly, in most studies, therapy was short term and the patients were relatively young, making generalization of the results difficult, as NSAIDs are most often prescribed long term and for elderly people.

Prospective studies

A case-control study of the effects of NSAID therapy on arterial pressure has been performed in subjects aged 65 years and over, drawn from a large database (the State of New England Medicaid Program) to determine whether NSAIDs affect blood pressure (26). The investigators calculated the odds ratio (OR) for the initiation of antihypertensive therapy in patients taking NSAIDs relative to non-users after adjusting for possible confounding factors. The 9411 patients had started taking antihypertensive drugs between 1981 and 1990, and a similar number of controls were randomly selected. The date of the first prescription for an antihypertensive drug was defined as the index date. Of those who took antihypertensive drugs, 41% had taken an NSAID during the year before the index date, compared with 26% of the control subjects. This risk increased with the recency of NSAID therapy, and was greatest among recent users (those with a supply of NSAIDs ending more than 60 days before the index date) (OR = 2.10; 95% CI = 1.95, 2.26). For former users (those with a supply of NSAIDs ending more than 60 days before the index date) the adjusted OR compared with non-users was 1.66 (CI = 1.54, 1.80). There was a dose-response relation, with adjusted ORs of 1.55 (CI = 1.38, 1.74), 1.64 (CI = 1.44, 1.87), and 1.82 (CI = 1.62, 2.05) for low, medium, and high daily doses of NSAIDs respectively. The unadjusted ORs for ibuprofen, piroxicam, meclofenamate, and indometacin, were separately calculable, and for each of these drugs the OR increased with increasing dose. The relation between cumulative duration of NSAID use and the initiation of antihypertensive therapy was also examined in recent users. The risk was greatest in those who had used an NSAID for 30–90 days and was less for those who had used an NSAID for less than 30 days or for more than 90 days.

The results of this study suggest that the effects of NSAIDs on blood pressure in older patients taking NSAIDs may be clinically important. Given that 15% of the control group were recent users of NSAIDs, and assuming that the adjusted OR of 1.66 represents a causal association of these drugs with the initiation of antihypertensive therapy, the proportion of cases attributable to the use of these drugs in this sample of elderly population was nearly one in ten.

Despite the high prevalence of the use of minor analgesics (aspirin and paracetamol) there is little information available on the association between the use of these analgesics and the risk of hypertension. A prospective cohort study in 80 020 women aged 31–50 years has provided some useful information (27). The women had participated in the Nurses' Health Study II and had no previous history of hypertension. The frequency of use of paracetamol, aspirin, and NSAIDs was collected by mailed questionnaires and cases of physician-diagnosed hypertension were identified by self-report. During 164 000 person-years of follow-up, 1650 incident cases of hypertension were identified. Overall 73% of the cohort had used paracetamol at least 1–4 days/month, 51% had used aspirin, and 77% had used an NSAID. Compared with non-users of paracetamol the age-adjusted relative risk (RR) of hypertension was significantly increased even in women who had used paracetamol for only 1–4 days/month (RR = 1.22; CI = 1.07, 1.39). There seemed to be a dose-response relation, as the RR of hypertension compared with non-users was 2.00 (CI = 1.52, 2.62) in women who had taken paracetamol for 29 days/month or more. For women using aspirin or NSAIDs at a frequency of 1–4 days/month the RRs were 1.18 (CI = 1.02, 1.35) and 1.17 (CI = 1.02, 1.36) respectively. However, after adjusting for age and other potential risk factors, only paracetamol and NSAIDs, but not aspirin, remained significantly associated with a risk of hypertension. In summary, the data from this study support the view that paracetamol and NSAIDs are strongly associated with an increased risk of hypertension in women, the risk increasing with increasing frequency of use. Aspirin did not seem to be associated with an increased risk. This conclusion contrasts with the results of some short-term studies that have shown no effect of paracetamol on blood pressure (28,29).

However, the results from this study must be interpreted with caution, as there were some limitations: the assessments of analgesic use and hypertension were made using a self-reported questionnaire; relative risk can be influenced by many potentially confounding variables; the results are relevant only for young women and cannot be extrapolated to the general population.

The impact of NSAIDs on blood pressure in elderly people has been evaluated in three epidemiological studies, with similar findings (SEDA-19, 92). The use of NSAIDs was significantly associated with hypertension or the use of antihypertensive drugs. Reliable data are available for hypertension in the elderly. Recent users of NSAIDs have a 1.7-fold increase in the risk of initiating antihypertensive therapy compared with non-users, and the use of NSAIDs significantly predicts the presence of hypertension (OR = 1.4; 95% CI = 1.1, 1.7) (21).

Conclusions

The overall results of these studies have provided convincing evidence that NSAIDs and paracetamol can raise arterial blood pressure in a dose-related fashion, interfere with the actions of antihypertensive drugs, and prompt the need for new antihypertensive therapy.

Even if the increase in mean blood pressure is probably modest (less than 5.0 mmHg) the clinical relevance of such an increase can be large, especially in elderly people. In fact, an overview of randomized clinical trials of antihypertensive treatment has shown that a 5–6 mmHg increase in diastolic blood pressure over a few years can be associated with a 67% increase in the incidence of strokes and a 15% increase in coronary heart disease (30). These effects are apparent in both normotensive and hypertensive patients.

Whether these results apply with certainty to patients taking NSAIDs is not known, because these studies included patients not taking NSAIDs, but it is wise to consider this probability. The type and dose of NSAID may be important, but more studies are needed to document this. Hypertensive and elderly patients seem to be particularly at risk. In patients taking long-term NSAIDs, or even paracetamol, periodic monitoring of blood pressure appears to be warranted.

Congestive heart failure

Much less is known about the risk of congestive heart failure with NSAIDs. The rate of hospitalization for congestive heart failure in more than 10 000 patients over 55 years of age during exposure to both diuretics and NSAIDs was compared with the rate in those exposed to diuretics alone (31). At mean follow up of 4.7 years, there was an increased risk of hospitalization when diuretics and NSAIDs were used concomitantly (RR = 1.8; 95% CI = 1.4, 2.4).

In 600 elderly patients with documented congestive cardiac failure there was a possible or probable link between NSAIDs and heart failure in 27 cases (32). In some, the mechanism was apparently a reduction in the effect of furosemide. In others the NSAID may have caused an imbalance in circulatory homeostasis. Pre-existing renal impairment was not observed in any of the 27 cases. This study suggests that in elderly people congestive heart failure may be a complication of NSAIDs.

In a matched case-control study the relation between the recent use of NSAIDs and hospitalization with congestive heart failure in elderly patients has been analysed (33). Cases (n = 365) were patients admitted to hospital with a primary diagnosis of congestive heart failure; controls (n = 658) were patients without congestive heart failure. Structured interviews were used to obtain information on several possible risk factors, such as a history of heart disease and the type and dosage of NSAIDs used. The use of NSAIDs (other than low-dose aspirin) in the previous week was associated with a doubling of the chance of a hospital admission with congestive heart failure (adjusted OR = 2.5, CI = 1.2, 3.3). The risk was even higher in patients with a history of heart disease, in whom the use of NSAIDs was associated with an increased risk of a first admission with congestive heart failure (OR = 11; CI = 0.7, 45), but not in those without a history of heart disease (OR = 1.6; CI = 0.7, 3.7). In contrast to the results of a previous study (31), the risk of admission to hospital with congestive heart failure was positively related to the dose of NSAID consumed in the previous week and was higher with long half-life NSAIDs than with short half-life NSAIDs. The authors estimated that, assuming that these relations were causal, NSAIDs might be responsible for about 19% of hospital admissions with congestive heart failure. If confirmed, this burden of illness resulting from NSAID-related congestive heart failure may rival that resulting from damage to the gastrointestinal tract and would represent an under-recognized public health problem. In any case, this study reinforces the timely suggestion that NSAIDs should be used with great caution in patients with a history of cardiovascular disease. This recommendation must also include the use of the selective COX-2 inhibitors, until more information is available.

Respiratory

As 2–20% of adult asthmatics have aspirin hypersensitivity (34), they must be considered at risk from NSAIDs. The mechanism is related to a deficiency in bronchodilator prostaglandins; prostaglandin inhibition may make arachidonic acid produce more leukotrienes with bronchoconstrictor activity. Oral challenge in asthmatic patients is an effective but potentially dangerous method for establishing the presence of aspirin hypersensitivity (35). Occasionally, bronchospasm may be part of an anaphylactoid reaction to NSAIDs; zomepirac was withdrawn for this reason. Intriguingly bee-keepers may be at increased risk for severe reactions from bee stings if they are taking NSAIDs, and it has been suggested that NSAIDs should be prescribed with particular caution for them (36).

Nervous system

NSAIDs cause headaches and confusion in a relatively small number of patients. Headache and dizziness are common with indometacin, and it has been suggested that its chemical similarity to serotonin, which can cause severe headaches, may be responsible (37). Headache due to long-term use of ibuprofen has been reported in children (38,39).

The Australian Drug Reaction Advisory Committee has reported paresthesia as a class effect of NSAIDs, although it is rare and reversible (40).

Studies on the link between falls in elderly people and NSAIDs have yielded conflicting and inconsistent data (41,42), and an increased risk of falls with NSAIDs is difficult to explain.

Some rarer adverse effects, such as aseptic meningitis, have been reported with ibuprofen, sulindac, and tolmetin (37) in patients with systemic lupus erythematosus. A case-control study showed no increased risk of intracerebral hemorrhage in patients using aspirin or other NSAIDs in low dosages as prophylaxis against thrombosis (43).

Sensory systems

Eye disorders, such as blurred vision, ocular discomfort, irritation, and more severe problems, such as optic or retrobulbar neuritis and papilledema, have been described (SEDA-19, 96).

Psychological, psychiatric

Behavioral changes have been reported with indometacin (44).

- A 92-year-old man with a history of senile dementia of the Alzheimer type, glaucoma, and constipation took indometacin 25 mg for pseudogout. After six doses he became very agitated and confused and was physically and verbally aggressive. Indometacin was withdrawn and he recovered over 10 days with the help of haloperidol 0.5 mg/day (45).

NSAIDs should probably be included as one of the many groups of drugs that can cause confusion in the elderly.

Cognitive function in elderly out-patients was assessed in a large retrospective study by a questionnaire; there were no significant differences in the total scores of users and non-users of NSAIDs (SEDA-17, 106). Another study showed that performance in sensorimotor coordination and short-term memory tests can improve in healthy elderly volunteers who take indometacin (46). NSAIDs have also been associated with a reduced risk of Alzheimer's disease (47).

Electrolyte balance

NSAIDs can interfere with fluid and electrolyte homeostasis, thereby causing edema, hyponatremia, hyperkalemia, and blunting of the natriuretic effects of diuretics (48,49).

Hematologic

NSAIDs have been reported to cause potentially severe hematological disorders: thrombocytopenia, agranulocytosis, aplastic anemia, and hemolytic anemia (50). Thrombocytopenia is generally mild and reversible and has a low case-fatality rate, but deaths from bleeding have been reported, particularly with indometacin, oxyphenbutazone, and phenylbutazone (50).

Pyrazolone derivatives and butazones are most frequently blamed for causing agranulocytosis and aplastic anemia (SEDA-9, 85) (SEDA-11, 89). Unfortunately, no reasonably accurate estimate of the overall incidence of either disease or of the risk associated with the use of any particular NSAID is available. The results of the International Agranulocytosis and Aplastic Anemia study (51) have been reviewed in detail (SEDA-11, 89) (SED-11, 171). This epidemiological study was organized by the manufacturer (Hoechst) of the widely incriminated drug dipyrone. The overall annual community agranulocytosis incidence was 4.4 per million (6.2 including hospital cases), with a fatality rate of 10% and an annual mortality rate of 0.4 per million. Analgesics significantly associated with agranulocytosis were dipyrone, indometacin, and two butazones (oxyphenbutazone and phenylbutazone). Other pyrazolones, such as amidopyrine (which is an acknowledged cause of agranulocytosis), or other NSAIDs could not be evaluated because of the small number of cases.

A population-based, case-control study in patients hospitalized with neutropenia has confirmed both the association between NSAIDs and neutropenia and the differences between different classes of NSAID (52). The data on aplastic anemia are also of interest, since this was the first study to provide excess risk estimates of this adverse effect in NSAID users. The overall annual incidence was 2.2 per million, with a 2-year fatality rate of 40%. A significantly increased risk for aplastic anemia was associated with any exposure to three drugs: indometacin (multivariate rate ratio 13), butazones (8.7), and, unexpectedly, diclofenac (8.8). Whatever the interpretations by different manufacturers, the study confirmed that dipyrone can cause agranulocytosis and that indometacin can cause aplastic anemia (53). The high relative risk of diclofenac for aplastic anemia is unexpected and requires confirmation.

Hemolytic anemia has occasionally been associated with NSAIDs; many reports involved mefenamic acid, ibuprofen and sulindac (54). No evidence has been found that any NSAID, except aspirin, constitutes a particular risk for subjects with glucose-6-phosphate dehydrogenase deficiency.

A prospective study on bleeding complications in 23 patients undergoing dermatological surgery has shown that NSAIDs and aspirin need not be withdrawn routinely preoperatively, unless the bleeding time is prolonged (55). Relatively few patients developed a prolonged bleeding time while taking aspirin or other NSAIDs and only few had significant intraoperative blood loss. There is variation in the response of patients for unknown reasons and so the recommendation that NSAIDs should be withdrawn before elective surgery awaits confirmation (SEDA-19, 96).

Gastrointestinal

Peptic ulceration

Prostaglandins have a protective effect on the gastrointestinal mucosa. All NSAIDs that non-selectively inhibit prostaglandin synthesis cause gastrointestinal mucosal damage. Direct NSAID-mediated acid damage has been identified as a mechanism of gastrointestinal toxicity (56). Several in vitro and animal studies have provided evidence of early vascular changes and have highlighted the role of leukocyte adhesion to the endothelium in NSAID-induced gastropathy. The pathogenesis of NSAID-associated gastrointestinal damage has been reviewed (SEDA-17, 104).

Clinical presentation

Features of upper gastrointestinal toxicity during NSAID therapy range from relatively mild symptoms (such as heartburn, dyspepsia, and stomach discomfort) to more severe and potentially life-threatening states (for example gastrointestinal erosion or ulceration, bleeding, or perforation). Although dyspepsia is one of the major factors that limit the use of NSAIDs in patients with rheumatic diseases, it does not necessarily predict mucosal damage. There is no close correlation between objective gastroscopy findings and subjective intolerance of medications, or between acute or chronic damage and complications. Epigastric pain was the most common symptom in patients admitted to hospital with hematemesis and/or melena, whether treated or not with NSAIDs in the 14 days before admission (SEDA-17, 103).

"NSAID gastropathy" is the term proposed by Roth and Bennett to describe upper gastrointestinal lesions associated with NSAID therapy. It has its own specific features (primarily antral and prepyloric localization, especially in elderly women), which differentiate it from classic peptic ulcer disease (57). Damage to the upper gastrointestinal tract can also involve the duodenum and, albeit infrequently, the esophagus.

Frequency

Gastrointestinal damage by NSAIDs is a major health problem. Estimates of the absolute risk vary from about two cases of serious upper gastrointestinal adverse effects per 10 000 person-months (58) to a seven-fold increase in the risk of hospitalization in patients with rheumatoid arthritis (59). Estimates of hospitalization for ulcer complications and the excess of gastrointestinal deaths in the UK have shown that 20–30% of all cases of ulcer complications in subjects aged over 60 which result in hospitalization are directly attributable to the use of NSAIDs, and that some 10% culminate in death (60). For the UK, this means that at least 2000 cases of bleeding are caused every year with about 200 deaths (61), in association with about 11 million prescriptions. The relative risk reported in different studies has generally been in the range of 3:1 to 5:1 (62).

In 2747 patients with rheumatoid arthritis, those taking NSAIDs were five times more likely (hazard ratio of 5.2) to be hospitalized for an upper gastrointestinal event (63). The risk of hospitalization for a gastrointestinal event was 15.8 per 1000 person-years in individuals taking NSAIDs, compared with 3.2 per 1000 person-years for controls. Such figures mean that on average one to two out of every 100 patients taking NSAIDs for 1 year are hospitalized for a gastrointestinal event (most commonly an ulcer).

The conclusion of a meta-analysis of 16 studies was that NSAID users have an approximately three-fold greater relative risk of developing serious adverse gastrointestinal events than non-users (64). This has been confirmed by a review (65).

Several authors have suggested that the upper gastrointestinal toxicity shortly after exposure does not persist (SEDA-22, 108), either because there is adaptation to NSAID-induced mucosal damage or because in these studies susceptible patients were selected. However, a population-based, cohort study has provided evidence that upper gastrointestinal toxicity is constant during exposure to NSAIDs and continues for some time after treatment stops (66).

Susceptibility factors

Case-control and surveillance studies have confirmed that the susceptibility factors for peptic ulcer disease are age, a history of ulcers and/or gastric bleeding, combination with corticosteroids, combination with other NSAIDs, and possibly smoking (SEDA-14, 84). The combination of NSAIDs, smoking, and alcohol increased the risk of gastrointestinal perforation nearly 11 times (OR = 10.7; CI = 3.8, 30) (SEDA-21, 97). Data on patients with rheumatoid arthritis taking NSAIDs show that the predisposition to gastrointestinal events is related to the severity of the disease (63). Other potential risk factors are sex (female), the musculoskeletal diseases for which NSAIDs are used, the NSAID taken, and dosage. The presence of gastric mucosal erosions at endoscopy was associated with an increased risk of a gastric ulcer, irrespective of prophylactic treatment (misoprostol versus sucralfate) in chronic NSAID users with osteoarthritis evaluated in a large randomized controlled trial (67). This was confirmed in other studies (SEDA-20, 86) (68,69), suggesting that the presence or absence of erosions is a better predictor of the risk of ulceration than the number of erosions.

The role of *Helicobacter pylori* *Helicobacter pylori* and non-steroidal anti-inflammatory drugs (NSAIDs) account for nearly all gastroduodenal ulcers and serious ulcer complications, but the interaction between infection with *H. pylori* and the use of NSAIDs in the pathogenesis of NSAID-induced gastropathy is controversial. In fact, studies that have examined these two susceptibility factors have yielded conflicting results about whether *H. pylori* infection increases the risk of toxicity in NSAID users, has no effect, or may even be protective (70–72).

Since we reviewed this topic 10 years ago (SEDA-16, 103) (SEDA-17, 105) a large amount of information has accumulated and merits further attention.

The pathophysiological mechanisms Among possible common pathophysiological mechanisms of importance are those that compromise the effectiveness of the gastroduodenal mucus–bicarbonate barrier, those that cause recruitment and activation of neutrophils, and those that can interfere with the process of mucosal adaptation (70). Both NSAIDs and aspirin can reduce the effectiveness of mucosal defences, by inhibiting gastroduodenal prostaglandin synthesis and by reducing mucosal blood flow (73). On the other hand *H. pylori* infection can damage the mucus–bicarbonate barrier, by increasing gastric acid secretion and reducing the viscosity of gastric mucus (74). Contrasting data have been reported on the effect of *H. pylori* on mucosal blood flow (75,76) and on mucosal prostaglandin production. However, although *H. pylori* increases mucosal prostaglandin synthesis, the combination of *H. pylori* with NSAIDs or aspirin causes a marked fall in mucosal prostaglandin synthesis, showing that the stimulatory effect of prostaglandin production by *H. pylori* is insignificant in the presence of NSAIDs or aspirin (76,77).

Gastric ulceration induced by NSAIDs is a neutrophil-dependent process (78) and the association of *H. pylori* infection with neutrophil infiltration has also been well documented. Gastric injury by NSAIDs is minimal in neutropenic animals, and the cumulative incidence of peptic ulcers in long-term NSAID users is increased in the presence of neutrophil infiltration in the mucosa of patients who are *H. pylori*-positive, suggesting a possible link between NSAIDs and *H. pylori* in the pathogenesis of peptic ulcers (79,80).

The ability of the gastroduodenal mucosa to adapt to repeated exposure to NSAIDs and aspirin is well documented, and some reports have shown the possible involvement of *H. pylori* in this process (76,81). In one endoscopic study in volunteers, mucosal adaptation to naproxen after 4 weeks of treatment occurred in 53% of *H. pylori*-positive subjects and in 81% in *H. pylori*-negative subjects (82). Similar results were found in another study in volunteers who took aspirin for 2 weeks; mucosal adaptation to the injury caused by aspirin was clearly impaired in the presence of *H. pylori* and was restored after *H. pylori* eradication (83).

In summary, NSAIDs and *H. pylori* can cause adverse effects on gastroduodenal mucosal protective mechanisms in different ways, and so the interaction between these two susceptibility factors might allow damage to occur more readily when NSAIDs are taken in the presence of *H. pylori* infection. However, despite this experimental evidence, the interaction between *H. pylori* infection and use of NSAIDs in the pathogenesis of peptic ulcers and their complications is still unclear from clinical studies.

Clinical studies Most of the early studies of the interaction between *H. pylori* infection and the use of NSAIDs were based on observational studies in long-term NSAID users and gave conflicting results (79, 84–91). In some studies there were significantly more ulcers in NSAID users who were *H. pylori*-positive then in users who were not infected (79,84,85). However, these findings were not confirmed by other investigators (86–89), and they probably reflect a complex relation between *H. pylori* infection and NSAID-associated gastropathy, as well as heterogeneity of methods across studies. For example, differences in population studied (for example the type of NSAID exposure, the age of the patient) and even in the definition of ulcer at endoscopy make direct comparison of results difficult. Most of the few published prospective trials did not show that *H. pylori* is a susceptibility factor for NSAID-induced gastroduodenal damage (77,92–94), and two long-term longitudinal studies (69,95) gave conflicting results, although the data have mostly been derived from studies in small numbers of young healthy volunteers at very low risk of gastropathy, and the results must therefore be treated with great caution. Thus, despite numerous studies we do not have convincing evidence for or against a link between *H. pylori* and NSAIDs in the development of peptic ulcers.

A meta-analysis has helped to clarify this issue (96). The aim was to assess the presence and magnitude of any possible interaction in peptic ulcer disease between these two susceptibility factors, with particular attention to bleeding peptic ulcer disease, the sites of ulceration, and the effect of *H. pylori* eradication. In all, 61 relevant studies were identified, 36 of which were excluded for various reasons. Thus, 25 studies were left for analysis, of which 16 observational studies (eight cross-sectional studies, seven case-control studies, and one cohort study) provided data on the prevalence of peptic ulcer disease in 1633 NSAID users, with data on *H. pylori* status for 1625 patients. The pooled frequency of peptic ulcer disease in NSAID users was 42% in those who were *H. pylori*-positive and 25% in those who were *H. pylori*-negative (OR = 2.12; 95% CI = 1.68, 2.67).

The frequencies of uncomplicated peptic ulcer disease in NSAID users and non-users were compared in eight case-control studies; however, the NSAID users and controls were not matched by age in three studies and so, because *H. pylori* infection is age-dependent, the prevalence of infection was analysed in only five studies.

Overall, *H. pylori* infection was diagnosed in 47% of the NSAID users and 46% of the controls, but peptic ulcer disease was significantly more common in the NSAID users (36% versus 8.3%; OR = 5.14; CI = 1.35, 20). Compared with patients who were *H. pylori*-negative and were not taking NSAIDs, the risk of ulcer in *H. pylori*-infected NSAID users was very high (OR = 61; CI = 10, 373). *H. pylori* infection increased the risk of peptic ulcer disease in NSAID users 3.53 times in addition to the risk associated with NSAID use (OR = 19). Similarly, in the presence of a risk of peptic ulcer disease associated with *H. pylori* infection (OR = 18) the use of NSAIDs increased the risk of peptic ulcer disease 3.55 times. *H. pylori* infection and NSAID use, respectively, increased the risk of ulcer bleeding 1.79 times and 4.85 times; the risk of ulcer bleeding increased to 6.13 when both factors were present.

From these data we can conclude that both *H. pylori* infection and NSAID use independently and significantly increase the risk of peptic ulcer and ulcer bleeding and that there is synergism in the development of peptic ulcer and ulcer bleeding between *H. pylori* infection and NSAID use.

The meta-analysis also showed that one-third of patients taking long-term NSAIDs have gastric or duodenal ulcers, irrespective of *H. pylori* status and study design. However, peptic ulcer disease was significantly more common in *H. pylori*-infected NSAID users than in non-infected users, suggesting a possible interaction between NSAID use and *H. pylori* infection for the development of peptic ulcers.

Moreover, the meta-analysis clarified another uncertainty: whether in NSAID takers *H. pylori* infection is as important a risk factor for gastric ulcer as it is for duodenal ulcer. A pooled analysis of four studies (75,97–99) showed that *H. pylori* infection is less closely associated with gastric ulcer than with duodenal ulcer in both NSAID users and non-users, and that while NSAID use has a major role in the development of gastric ulcer, duodenal ulcer is more closely related to *H. pylori* infection.

Further convincing evidence for the existence of a possible interaction between *H. pylori* and NSAIDs in the pathogenesis of ulcer has been obtained by investigating the effects of *H. pylori* eradication on the occurrence of NSAID-related ulcers and their complications (for example bleeding), although some divergent findings have been reported from these studies (100,101).

In a prospective, randomized trial of the effect of eradication of *H. pylori* before the start of NSAID therapy on the subsequent risk of ulcer occurrence, patients who required new NSAID treatment and who had *H. pylori* infection but no pre-existing ulcers on baseline endoscopy were recruited (100). Of these patients, 100 were randomly allocated to naproxen for 8 weeks, either alone or preceded by a 1-week course of *H. pylori* eradication. Endoscopy was repeated after 8 weeks or if naproxen was withdrawn early because of adverse effects. The primary end-point of the study was the cumulative rate of gastric and duodenal endoscopic ulcers. At 8 weeks *H. pylori* was eradicated in 40 patients (89%) who took eradication therapy and in none of those who had no pretreatment. Twelve (26%) of those who had no eradication therapy developed ulcers compared with three (7%) who had eradication therapy, two of whom had failure of eradication. Thus, only one patient with successful eradication developed ulcers with naproxen. These data suggest that NSAID-induced ulceration can be reduced by eradication of *H. pylori* before naproxen administration and suggest that *H. pylori* infection is a susceptibility factor for NSAID-induced ulcer disease. Some therefore believe that determination of *H. pylori* infection and eradication in infected patients should be recommended before starting NSAID therapy.

However, the data from this study contrasted with those from another randomized, controlled trial, the HELP study, in which the effect of *H. pylori* eradication was investigated in a different population of 285 patients who had used long-term NSAID therapy, those with current or previous peptic ulcers, or dyspepsia, or both (101). The patients were randomly assigned to omeprazole plus 1 week of eradication therapy ($n = 142$) or to omeprazole plus placebo for 1 week ($n = 143$). They took omeprazole until their ulcer healed or dyspepsia resolved, after which they continued taking the NSAID, with follow-up assessment of ulcer and dyspepsia at 1, 3, and 6 months. The estimated probabilities of being ulcer-free at 6 months were similar in the two groups: 0.56% (95% CI = 0.47, 0.65) with eradication treatment and 0.53 (0.44, 0.62) with control treatment. Moreover, fewer gastric ulcers healed in those who had taken eradication therapy than in the controls (7% versus 100% at 8 weeks). These data suggest that *H. pylori* eradication therapy not only did not reduce the rate of development of peptic ulcer or dyspepsia at 6 months, but actually led to impaired healing of gastric ulcers. On the basis of these results *H. pylori* eradication seems not to be justified.

These conflicting results can probably be explained by important differences in the characteristics of the patients and the study methods. The inclusion criteria in the two studies were mutually exclusive: patients with long-term NSAID use and a history of ulceration were excluded in the first study and included in the second. Furthermore, there were differences in the definition of endoscopic ulcers, the eradication regimen, the definition of *H. pylori* infection, and the length of follow-up.

Data from a later eradication study helped to clarify these uncertainties. The aim of the study was to determine whether among NSAID-naive patients positive for *H. pylori* who have dyspepsia or a history of ulcer and who are about to start long-term NSAID treatment, eradication of *H. pylori* infection reduces the risk of ulcers (102). Bismuth was replaced by omeprazole in the eradication regimen, the observation period was increased to 6 months, and the frequencies of both complicated and symptomless ulcers were assessed. Patients were randomly assigned to omeprazole triple therapy (eradication group, $n = 51$) or omeprazole with placebo antibiotics (control group, $n = 51$) for 1 week. All took diclofenac 100 mg/day for 6 months. The 6-month probability of having ulcers was 12% (95% CI = 3.1, 21) in the eradication group and 34% (21, 48) in the placebo group. The 6-month probability of complicated ulcers was 4.2% (1.3, 9.7) in the eradication group and 27% (15, 40) in the placebo group. These statistically significant differences suggested that screening and treatment for *H. pylori* depletion or hypoalbuminemia and those in which there is pre-existing renal impairment due to age, atherosclerosis, hypertensive renal disease, or other intrinsic renal disease. Although the functional renal insufficiency is usually mild and reversible within a few days of withdrawing NSAIDs, it can also be severe and irreversible, so early recognition is essential. All NSAIDs can cause this complication.

A case-control study on recent use of NSAIDs and functional renal impairment at the time of hospitalization showed that there was a weak association between the use of NSAIDs and renal dysfunction. Patients at higher risk had a history of renal disease or of gout and hyperuricemia. While NSAID dosages were only weakly related to renal impairment, there was a statistically significant difference between compounds with half-lives under or over 4 hours: the OR increased from 1.2 (95% CI = 0.6, 2.4) to 4.8 (CI = 1.5, 16) for compounds with half-lives over 12 hours (156). Therefore, long half-life drugs should be avoided in subjects at risk of renal impairment.

A case-control study provided convincing epidemiological evidence that the use of NSAIDs was associated with the risk of hospitalization for acute renal insufficiency (relative risk about 2.0) (SEDA-19, 95) (157).

Acute interstitial nephritis, which is distinct from the methicillin-like form, is the most important type of organic renal damage caused by NSAIDs. Distinguished by a nephrotic syndrome, often with renal insufficiency, the histological picture is an acute interstitial nephritis combined plus a glomerular lesion with fusion of the epithelial foot process. Patients had usually been taking NSAIDs over a long period of time. Acute interstitial nephritis has been reported relatively often in patients taking fenoprofen.

The acute flank pain syndrome associated with reversible renal insufficiency is very rare. It has usually been reported with suprofen (SEDA-12, 89), but flurbiprofen and ibuprofen have also been implicated (SEDA-18, 100).

Membranous nephropathy is rare and causes the nephrotic syndrome, usually with minimal-change glomerulopathy, with or without interstitial nephritis (SEDA-11, 85). A retrospective study provided more data on the frequency and clinical characteristics of membranous nephropathy associated with NSAIDs (158). It confirmed that it is rare (13 of 125 patients diagnosed during the last 20 years met the strict criteria for NSAID-associated membranous nephropathy), and the nephrotic syndrome is reversible after prompt withdrawal. The pathogenesis is unknown but seems to be immune-mediated, given the characteristic deposition of IgG and C3.

Renal papillary necrosis has been reported after long-term intake or abuse of aspirin and other NSAIDs (SEDA-11, 85) (SEDA-12, 79).

Chronic renal disease

The relation between long-term heavy exposure to analgesics and the risk of chronic renal disease has been the object of intensive toxicological and epidemiological research for many years (SEDA-24, 120) (159). Most of the earlier reports suggested that phenacetin-containing analgesics probably cause renal papillary necrosis and interstitial nephritis. In contrast, there is no convincing epidemiological evidence that non-phenacetin-containing analgesics (including paracetamol, aspirin, mixtures of the two, and NSAIDs) cause chronic renal disease. Moreover, findings from epidemiological studies should be interpreted with caution, because of a number of inherent limitations and potential biases in study design (160). Two methodologically sound studies have provided information on this topic.

The first was the largest cohort study conducted thus far to assess the risk of renal dysfunction associated with analgesic use (161). Details of analgesic use were obtained from 11 032 men without previous renal dysfunction participating in the Physicians' Health Study (PHS), which lasted 14 years. The main outcome measure was a raised creatinine concentration defined as 1.5 mg/dl (133 μmol/l) or higher, and a reduced creatinine clearance of 55 ml/minute or less. In all, 460 men (4.2%) had a raised creatinine concentration and 1258 (11%) had a reduced creatinine clearance. Mean creatinine concentrations and creatinine clearances were similar among men who did not use analgesics and those who did. This was true for all categories of analgesics (paracetamol and paracetamol-containing mixtures, aspirin and aspirin-containing mixtures, and other NSAIDs) and for higher risk groups, such as those aged 60 years or over or those with hypertension or diabetes.

These data are convincing, as the large size of the PHS cohort should make it possible to examine and detect even modest associations between analgesic use and a risk of renal disease. Furthermore, this study included more individuals who reported extensive use of analgesics than any prior case-control study. However, the study had some limitations, the most important being the fact that the cohort was composed of relatively healthy men, most of whom were white. These results cannot therefore be generalized to the entire population. However, the study clearly showed that there is not a strong association between chronic analgesic use and chronic renal dysfunction among a large cohort of men without a history of renal impairment.

The second study was a Swedish nationwide, population-based, case-control study of early-stage chronic renal insufficiency in men whose serum creatinine concentration exceeded 3.4 mg/dl (300 μmol/l) or women whose serum creatinine exceeded 2.8 mg/dl (250 μmol/l) (162). In all, 918 patients with newly diagnosed renal insufficiency and 980 controls were interviewed and completed questionnaires about their lifetime consumption of analgesics. Compared with controls, more patients with chronic renal insufficiency were regular users of aspirin (37% versus 19%) or paracetamol (25% versus 12%). Among subjects who did not use aspirin regularly, the regular use of paracetamol was associated with a risk of chronic renal insufficiency that was 2.5 times as high as that for non-users of paracetamol. The risk increased with increasing cumulative lifetime dose. Patients who took 500 g or more over a year (1.4 g/day) during periods of regular use had an increased odds ratio for chronic renal insufficiency (OR = 5.3; 95% CI = 1.8, 15). Among subjects who did not use paracetamol regularly, the regular use of aspirin was associated with a risk of chronic renal insufficiency that was 2.5 times as high as that for non-users of aspirin. The risk increased significantly with an increasing cumulative lifetime dose of aspirin. Among the patients with an average intake of 500 g or more of aspirin per year during periods of regular use, the risk of chronic renal insufficiency was increased about three-fold (OR = 3.3; CI = 1.4, 8.0). Among patients who used paracetamol in addition to aspirin, the risk of chronic renal insufficiency was increased about two-fold when regular aspirin users served as the reference group, (OR = 2.2; CI = 1.4, 3.5) and non-significantly when regular paracetamol users were used as controls (OR = 1.6; CI = 0.9, 2.7). There was no relation between the use of other analgesics (propoxyphene, NSAIDs, codeine, and pyrazolones) and the risk of chronic renal insufficiency. Thus, the regular use of paracetamol, or aspirin, or both was associated dose-dependently with an increased risk of chronic renal insufficiency. The OR among regular users exceeded 1.0 for all types of chronic renal insufficiency, albeit not always significantly. These results are consistent with exacerbating effects of paracetamol and aspirin on chronic renal insufficiency, regardless of accompanying disease.

How can we explain the contrasting results of these two studies? A possible explanation lies in the different populations studied. In PHS, relatively healthy individuals were enrolled while in the Swedish study all the patients had pre-existing severe renal or systemic disease, suggesting that such disease has an important role in causing analgesic-associated chronic renal insufficiency. People without pre-existing disease who use analgesics may have only a small risk of end-stage renal disease.

Prevention

While misoprostol has been shown to limit NSAID-induced gastric damage, three studies failed to show that misoprostol prevents NSAID-induced impairment of renal function. However, another showed that it prevents ciclosporin-induced renal damage in renal transplant patients (163). Further studies are therefore required to assess the protective effect of misoprostol on renal function (SEDA-16, 106).

Skin

Skin reactions are often reported with NSAIDs, but the true incidences with individual NSAIDs are unknown. There are very few specific epidemiological studies, and most information comes from single case reports and data from national spontaneous reporting systems. A major study on nearly 20 000 patients showed that 0.3% of 9118 patients taking analgesics and NSAIDs developed skin reactions that could be attributed to these drugs (164).

Although usually mild, skin reactions very often require withdrawal of treatment. At times they can be severe, and isoxicam was withdrawn from the market because of the high frequency of severe adverse skin reactions (SEDA-10, 88).

There are various types of NSAID-induced rashes. The main morphological patterns are urticarial, maculopapular, vesicular, and exfoliative. Skin reactions to NSAIDs are probably of phototoxic origin and can be associated with systemic hypersensitivity or other allergic reactions. More rarely, NSAIDs can exacerbate pre-existing skin disease (for example psoriasis, acne). Phototoxic reactions were very common with benoxaprofen (30–50% of patients treated in the UK), and were one reason why it did not receive licensing approval in Australia or the Benelux countries. Other NSAIDs, such as azapropazone, piroxicam, and fenbufen, have been reported to cause higher than average rates of photosensitivity (165). NSAIDs were among the causal agents of phototoxic reactions most commonly reported to the Australian Adverse Drug Reactions Advisory Committee (166,167).

Widespread use of naproxen, sulindac, diclofenac, and diflunisal probably explains why they were the most frequently implicated, rather than because they have a greater tendency to cause these adverse effects. NSAIDs differ in their ability to cause adverse skin reactions in terms of both frequency and severity: pyrazolones, butazones, and oxicams are most often blamed, and among the arylalkanoic acid derivatives fenbufen and carprofen are most often incriminated.

The types of skin adverse effect also vary with different compounds. The most serious life-threatening reactions, such as erythema multiforme and its variants (Stevens–Johnson syndrome, toxic epidermal necrolysis, exfoliative erythroderma) are uncommon and occur mainly with the butazone derivatives and to a lesser extent with piroxicam, sulindac, and possibly fenbufen. In large series reported in France, Germany, and the USA, NSAIDs are most often implicated: 12 (44%) of the most commonly implicated 29 drugs (168).

Although all NSAIDs can cause urticaria, particularly in aspirin-sensitive patients, it is more common with pyrazolone derivatives. Photosensitivity is principally a problem with azapropazone, carprofen, tiaprofenic acid, and piroxicam (SEDA-9, 84).

The reasons for these different effects of different NSAIDs are poorly understood. The only physicochemical characteristic that seems to be important in determining a particular propensity for adverse skin reactions is lipophilicity (10), which probably affects NSAID distribution to the skin. The longer half-lives of lipophilic compounds may concomitantly facilitate the persistence of skin reactions. Although there are no clear relations between the other pharmacological and kinetic characteristics of NSAIDs and effects on the skin, less lipophilic drugs with short half-lives might be preferable.

There are no clearly identifiable predisposing factors for most adverse skin reactions. Urticaria and photosensitivity are exceptions. Many NSAIDs can cause urticaria (sometimes associated with angioedema) in aspirin-sensitive patients. Probably not immunological in origin, the reaction may be related to prostaglandin inhibition in a patient whose cutaneous mastocytes are more susceptible to the stabilizing effect of prostaglandins. Skin testing in patients with a history of urticarial and/or anaphylactic reactions to analgesics is of little value in identifying patients at risk and can be dangerous (169,170). Skin pigmentation and environmental factors that influence the radiant exposure dose are clearly very important in determining the risk of a phototoxic reaction.

Since the extreme rarity of life-threatening reactions, such as erythema multiforme and toxic epidermal adaptation to continued administration of aspirin in humans. Gastroenterology 1998;114(2):245–55.

84. Martin DF, Montgomery E, Dobek AS, Patrissi GA, Peura DA. *Campylobacter pylori*, NSAIDS, and smoking: risk factors for peptic ulcer disease. Am J Gastroenterol 1989;84(10):1268–72.
85. Li EK, Sung JJ, Suen R, Ling TK, Leung VK, Hui E, Cheng AF, Chung S, Woo J. *Helicobacter pylori* infection increases the risk of peptic ulcers in chronic users of non-steroidal anti-inflammatory drugs. Scand J Rheumatol 1996;25(1):42–6.
86. Heresbach D, Raoul JL, Bretagne JF, Minet J, Donnio PY, Ramee MP, Siproudhis L, Gosselin M. *Helicobacter pylori*: a risk and severity factor of non-steroidal anti-inflammatory drug induced gastropathy. Gut 1992;33(12):1608–11.
87. Loeb DS, Talley NJ, Ahlquist DA, Carpenter HA, Zinsmeister AR. Long-term nonsteroidal anti-inflammatory drug use and gastroduodenal injury: the role of *Helicobacter pylori*. Gastroenterology 1992;102(6):1899–905.
88. Graham DY, Lidsky MD, Cox AM, Evans DJ Jr, Evans DG, Alpert L, Klein PD, Sessoms SL, Michaletz PA, Saeed ZA. Long-term nonsteroidal antiinflammatory drug use and *Helicobacter pylori* infection. Gastroenterology 1991;100(6):1653–7.
89. Shallcross TM, Rathbone BJ, Wyatt JI, Heatley RV. *Helicobacter pylori* associated chronic gastritis and peptic ulceration in patients taking non-steroidal anti-inflammatory drugs. Aliment Pharmacol Ther 1990;4(5):515–22.
90. Upadhyay R, Howatson A, McKinlay A, Danesh BJ, Sturrock RD, Russell RI. *Campylobacter pylori* associated gastritis in patients with rheumatoid arthritis taking non-steroidal anti-inflammatory drugs. Br J Rheumatol 1988;27(2):113–16.
91. Publig W, Wustinger C, Zandl C. Non-steroidal anti-inflammatory drugs (NSAID) cause gastrointestinal ulcers mainly in *Helicobacter pylori* carriers. Wien Klin Wochenschr 1994;106(9):276–9.
92. Lanza FL, Evans DG, Graham DY. Effect of *Helicobacter pylori* infection on the severity of gastroduodenal mucosal injury after the acute administration of naproxen or aspirin to normal volunteers. Am J Gastroenterol 1991;86(6):735–7.
93. Thillainayagam AV, Tabaqchali S, Warrington SJ, Farthing MJ. Interrelationships between *Helicobacter pylori* infection, nonsteroidal antiinflammatory drugs and gastroduodenal disease. A prospective study in healthy volunteers. Dig Dis Sci 1994;39(5):1085–9.
94. Goggin PM, Collins DA, Jazrawi RP, Jackson PA, Corbishley CM, Bourke BE, Northfield TC. Prevalence of *Helicobacter pylori* infection and its effect on symptoms and non-steroidal anti-inflammatory drug induced gastrointestinal damage in patients with rheumatoid arthritis. Gut 1993;34(12):1677–80.
95. Kim JG, Graham DY. *Helicobacter pylori* infection and development of gastric or duodenal ulcer in arthritic patients receiving chronic NSAID therapy. The Misoprostol Study Group. Am J Gastroenterol 1994;89(2):203–7.
96. Huang JQ, Sridhar S, Hunt RH. Role of *Helicobacter pylori* infection and non-steroidal anti-inflammatory drugs in peptic-ulcer disease: a meta-analysis. Lancet 2002;359(9300):14–22.
97. Voutilainen M, Sokka T, Juhola M, Farkkila M, Hannonen P. Nonsteroidal anti-inflammatory drug-associated upper gastrointestinal lesions in rheumatoid arthritis patients. Relationships to gastric histology, *Helicobacter pylori* infection, and other risk factors for peptic ulcer. Scand J Gastroenterol 1998;33(8):811–16.
98. Santucci L, Fiorucci S, Patoia L, Di Matteo FM, Brunori PM, Morelli A. Severe gastric mucosal damage induced by NSAIDs in healthy subjects is associated with *Helicobacter pylori* infection and high levels of serum pepsinogens. Dig Dis Sci 1995;40(9):2074–80.
99. Caselli M, Pazzi P, LaCorte R, Aleotti A, Trevisani L, Stabellini G. *Campylobacter*-like organisms, nonsteroidal anti-inflammatory drugs and gastric lesions in patients with rheumatoid arthritis. Digestion 1989;44(2):101–4.
100. Chan FK, Sung JJ, Chung SC, To KF, Yung MY, Leung VK, Lee YT, Chan CS, Li EK, Woo J. Randomised trial of eradication of *Helicobacter pylori* before non-steroidal anti-inflammatory drug therapy to prevent peptic ulcers. Lancet 1997;350(9083):975–9.
101. Hawkey CJ, Tulassay Z, Szczepanski L, van Rensburg CJ, Filipowicz-Sosnowska A, Lanas A, Wason CM, Peacock RA, Gillon KR. Randomised controlled trial of *Helicobacter pylori* eradication in patients on non-steroidal anti-inflammatory drugs: HELP NSAIDs study. Helicobacter Eradication for Lesion Prevention. Lancet 1998;352(9133):1016–21.
102. Chan FK, To KF, Wu JC, Yung MY, Leung WK, Kwok T, Hui Y, Chan HL, Chan CS, Hui E, Woo J, Sung JJ. Eradication of *Helicobacter pylori* and risk of peptic ulcers in patients starting long-term treatment with non-steroidal anti-inflammatory drugs: a randomised trial. Lancet 2002;359(9300):9–13.
103. Aalykke C, Lauritsen JM, Hallas J, Reinholdt S, Krogfelt K, Lauritsen K. *Helicobacter pylori* and risk of ulcer bleeding among users of nonsteroidal anti-inflammatory drugs: a case-control study. Gastroenterology 1999;116(6):1305–9.
104. Labenz J, Peitz U, Kohl H, Kaiser J, Malfertheiner P, Hackelsberger A, Borsch G. *Helicobacter pylori* increases the risk of peptic ulcer bleeding: a case-control study. Ital J Gastroenterol Hepatol 1999;31(2):110–15.
105. Cullen DJ, Hawkey GM, Greenwood DC, Humphreys H, Shepherd V, Logan RF, Hawkey CJ. Peptic ulcer bleeding in the elderly: relative roles of *Helicobacter pylori* and non-steroidal anti-inflammatory drugs. Gut 1997;41(4):459–62.
106. Santolaria S, Lanas A, Benito R, Perez-Aisa M, Montoro M, Sainz R. *Helicobacter pylori* infection is a protective factor for bleeding gastric ulcers but not for bleeding duodenal ulcers in NSAID users. Aliment Pharmacol Ther 1999;13(11):1511–18.
107. Chan FK, Chung SC, Suen BY, Lee YT, Leung WK, Leung VK, Wu JC, Lau JY, Hui Y, Lai MS, Chan HL, Sung JJ. Preventing recurrent upper gastrointestinal bleeding in patients with *Helicobacter pylori* infection who are taking low-dose aspirin or naproxen. N Engl J Med 2001;344(13):967–73.
108. Hawkey CJ, Karrasch JA, Szczepanski L, Walker DG, Barkun A, Swannell AJ, Yeomans ND. Omeprazole compared with misoprostol for ulcers associated with non-steroidal antiinflammatory drugs. Omeprazole versus Misoprostol for NSAID-induced Ulcer Management (OMNIUM) Study Group. N Engl J Med 1998; 338(11):727–34.
109. Yeomans ND, Tulassay Z, Juhasz L, Racz I, Howard JM, van Rensburg CJ, Swannell AJ, Hawkey CJ. A comparison of omeprazole with ranitidine for ulcers associated with nonsteroidal antiinflammatory drugs. Acid Suppression Trial: Ranitidine versus Omeprazole for NSAID-associated Ulcer Treatment (ASTRONAUT) Study Group. N Engl J Med 1998;338(11):719–26.
110. Silverstein FE, Graham DY, Senior JR, Davies HW, Struthers BJ, Bittman RM, Geis GS. Misoprostol reduces serious gastrointestinal complications in patients with rheumatoid arthritis receiving nonsteroidal anti-inflammatory drugs. A randomized, double-blind, placebo-controlled trial. Ann Intern Med 1995;123(4):241–9.

111. Graham DY. Critical effect of *Helicobacter pylori* infection on the effectiveness of omeprazole for prevention of gastric or duodenal ulcers among chronic NSAID users. Helicobacter 2002;7(1):1–8.
112. Hawkey CJ, Langman MJ. Non-steroidal anti-inflammatory drugs: overall risks and management. Complementary roles for COX-2 inhibitors and proton pump inhibitors. Gut 2003;52(4):600–8.
113. Garcia Rodriguez LA, Jick H. Risk of upper gastrointestinal bleeding and perforation associated with individual non-steroidal anti-inflammatory drugs. Lancet 1994;343(8900):769–72.
114. Langman MJ, Weil J, Wainwright P, Lawson DH, Rawlins MD, Logan RF, Murphy M, Vessey MP, Colin-Jones DG. Risks of bleeding peptic ulcer associated with individual non-steroidal anti-inflammatory drugs. Lancet 1994;343(8905):1075–8.
115. Koch M, Capurso L, Dezi A, Ferrario F, Scarpignato C. Prevention of NSAID-induced gastroduodenal mucosal injury: meta-analysis of clinical trials with misoprostol and H2-receptor antagonists. Dig Dis 1995;13(Suppl 1): 62–74.
116. Simon TJ, Berger ML, Hoover ME, Stauffer LA, Berline RG. A dose ranging study of famotidine in prevention of gastroduodenal lesions associated with non-steroidal anti-inflammatory drugs (NSAIDs): results of a US multicenter trial. Am J Gastroenterol 1994;89:1644.
117. Singh G, Ramey DR, Morfeld D, Shi H, Hatoum HT, Fries JF. Gastrointestinal tract complications of nonsteroidal anti-inflammatory drug treatment in rheumatoid arthritis. A prospective observational cohort study. Arch Intern Med 1996;156(14):1530–6.
118. Graham DY, Agrawal NM, Roth SH. Prevention of NSAID-induced gastric ulcer with misoprostol: multicentre, double-blind, placebo-controlled trial. Lancet 1988;2(8623):1277–80.
119. Levine JS. Misoprostol and nonsteroidal anti-inflammatory drugs: a tale of effects, outcomes, and costs. Ann Intern Med 1995;123(4):309–10.
120. Ekstrom P, Carling L, Wetterhus S, Wingren PE, Anker-Hansen O, Lundegardh G, Thorhallsson E, Unge P. Prevention of peptic ulcer and dyspeptic symptoms with omeprazole in patients receiving continuous non-steroidal anti-inflammatory drug therapy. A Nordic multicentre study. Scand J Gastroenterol 1996;31(8):753–8.
121. Cullen D, Bardhan KD, Eisner M, Kogut DG, Peacock RA, Thomson JM, Hawkey CJ. Primary gastroduodenal prophylaxis with omeprazole for non-steroidal anti-inflammatory drug users. Aliment Pharmacol Ther 1998;12(2):135–40.
122. Wynne HA, Long A. Patient awareness of the adverse effects of non-steroidal anti-inflammatory drugs (NSAIDs). Br J Clin Pharmacol 1996;42(2):253–6.
123. Herxheimer A. Many NSAID users who bleed don't know when to stop. BMJ 1998;316(7130):492.
124. Semble EL, Wu WC, Castell DO. Nonsteroidal antiinflammatory drugs and esophageal injury. Semin Arthritis Rheum 1989;19(2):99–109.
125. Taha AS, Dahill S, Nakshabendi I, Lee FD, Sturrock RD, Russell RI. Oesophageal histology in long term users of non-steroidal anti-inflammatory drugs. J Clin Pathol 1994;47(8):705–8.
126. Scheiman JM, Patel PM, Henson EK, Nostrant TT. Effect of naproxen on gastroesophageal reflux and esophageal function: a randomized, double-blind, placebo-controlled study. Am J Gastroenterol 1995;90(5):754–7.
127. Langman MJ, Morgan L, Worrall A. Use of anti-inflammatory drugs by patients admitted with small or large bowel perforations and haemorrhage. BMJ (Clin Res Ed) 1985;290(6465):347–9.
128. Bjarnason I, Macpherson A. The changing gastrointestinal side effect profile of non-steroidal anti-inflammatory drugs. A new approach for the prevention of a new problem. Scand J Gastroenterol Suppl 1989;163:56–64.
129. Bjarnason I, Hayllar J, MacPherson AJ, Russell AS. Side effects of nonsteroidal anti-inflammatory drugs on the small and large intestine in humans. Gastroenterology 1993;104(6):1832–47.
130. Allison MC, Howatson AG, Torrance CJ, Lee FD, Russell RI. Gastrointestinal damage associated with the use of nonsteroidal antiinflammatory drugs. N Engl J Med 1992;327(11):749–54.
131. Lang J, Price AB, Levi AJ, Burke M, Gumpel JM, Bjarnason I. Diaphragm disease: pathology of disease of the small intestine induced by non-steroidal anti-inflammatory drugs. J Clin Pathol 1988;41(5):516–26.
132. Kwo PY, Tremaine WJ. Nonsteroidal anti-inflammatory drug-induced enteropathy: case discussion and review of the literature. Mayo Clin Proc 1995;70(1):55–61.
133. Speed CA, Bramble MG, Corbett WA, Haslock I. Nonsteroidal anti-inflammatory induced diaphragm disease of the small intestine: complexities of diagnosis and management. Br J Rheumatol 1994;33(8):778–80.
134. Gargot D, Chaussade S, d'Alteroche L, Desbazeille F, Grandjouan S, Louvel A, Douvin J, Causse X, Festin D, Chapuis Y, et al. Nonsteroidal anti-inflammatory drug-induced colonic strictures: two cases and literature review. Am J Gastroenterol 1995;90(11):2035–8.
135. Giardiello FM, Hansen FC 3rd, Lazenby AJ, Hellman DB, Milligan FD, Bayless TM, Yardley JH. Collagenous colitis in setting of nonsteroidal antiinflammatory drugs and antibiotics. Dig Dis Sci 1990;35(2):257–60.
136. Rampton DS, McNeil NI, Sarner M. Analgesic ingestion and other factors preceding relapse in ulcerative colitis. Gut 1983;24(3):187–9.
137. Rampton DS, Sladen GE. Relapse of ulcerative proctocolitis during treatment with non-steroidal anti-inflammatory drugs. Postgrad Med J 1981;57(667):297–9.
138. Kaufmann HJ, Taubin HL. Nonsteroidal anti-inflammatory drugs activate quiescent inflammatory bowel disease. Ann Intern Med 1987;107(4):513–16.
139. Felder JB, Korelitz BI, Rajapakse R, Schwarz S, Horatagis AP, Gleim G. Effects of nonsteroidal antiinflammatory drugs on inflammatory bowel disease: a case-control study. Am J Gastroenterol 2000; 95(8):1949–54.
140. Bonner GF, Walczak M, Kitchen L, Bayona M. Tolerance of nonsteroidal antiinflammatory drugs in patients with inflammatory bowel disease. Am J Gastroenterol 2000;95(8):1946–8.
141. Garcia Rodriguez LA, Williams R, Derby LE, Dean AD, Jick H. Acute liver injury associated with nonsteroidal anti-inflammatory drugs and the role of risk factors. Arch Intern Med 1994;154(3):311–16.
142. Fry SW, Seeff LB. Hepatotoxicity of analgesics and anti-inflammatory agents. Gastroenterol Clin North Am 1995;24(4):875–905.
143. Benjamin SB, Ishak KG, Zimmerman HJ, Grushka A. Phenylbutazone liver injury: a clinical-pathologic survey of 23 cases and review of the literature. Hepatology 1981;1(3):255–63.
144. ADRAC. Diclofenac sodium and hepatic injury. Aust Adv Drug React Bull 1986;June.
145. Wilholm BE, Myrhed M, Ekman E. Trends and patterns in adverse drug reactions to non-steroidal anti-inflammatory drugs reported in Sweden. In: Rainsford KD, Velo GP, editors. Side-effects of Anti-inflammatory Drugs, Part I. Clinical and Epidemiological Aspects. Lancaster: MTP Press, 1987:55.

146. Brooks PM. Side-effects of non-steroidal anti-inflammatory drugs. Med J Aust 1988;148(5):248–51.
147. De Ledinghen V, Heresbach D, Fourdan O, Bernard P, Liebaert-Bories MP, Nousbaum JB, Gourlaouen A, Becker MC, Ribard D, Ingrand P, Silvain C, Beauchant M. Anti-inflammatory drugs and variceal bleeding: a case-control study. Gut 1999;44(2):270–3.
148. Richards IM, Fraser SM, Capell HA, Fox JG, Boulton-Jones JM. A survey of renal function in outpatients with rheumatoid arthritis. Clin Rheumatol 1988;7(2):267–71.
149. Allred J, Wong W, Kafetz K. Elderly people taking non-steroidal anti-inflammatory drugs are unlikely to have excess renal impairment. Postgrad Med J 1989; 65(768):735–7.
150. Dunn MJ, Simonson M, Davidson EW, Scharschmidt LA, Sedor JR. Nonsteroidal anti-inflammatory drugs and renal function. J Clin Pharmacol 1988;28(6):524–9.
151. Stillman MT, Schlesinger PA. Nonsteroidal anti-inflammatory drug nephrotoxicity. Should we be concerned? Arch Intern Med 1990;150(2):268–70.
152. Whelton A, Stout RL, Spilman PS, Klassen DK. Renal effects of ibuprofen, piroxicam, and sulindac in patients with asymptomatic renal failure. A prospective, randomized, crossover comparison. Ann Intern Med 1990;112(8):568–76.
153. Murray MD, Brater DC. Adverse effects of nonsteroidal anti-inflammatory drugs on renal function. Ann Intern Med 1990;112(8):559–60.
154. Eriksson LO, Sturfelt G, Thysell H, Wollheim FA. Effects of sulindac and naproxen on prostaglandin excretion in patients with impaired renal function and rheumatoid arthritis. Am J Med 1990;89(3):313–21.
155. Sandler DP, Burr FR, Weinberg CR. Nonsteroidal anti-inflammatory drugs and the risk for chronic renal disease. Ann Intern Med 1991;115(3):165–72.
156. Henry D, Page J, Whyte I, Nanra R, Hall C. Consumption of non-steroidal anti-inflammatory drugs and the development of functional renal impairment in elderly subjects. Results of a case-control study. Br J Clin Pharmacol 1997;44(1):85–90.
157. Evans JM, McGregor E, McMahon AD, McGilchrist MM, Jones MC, White G, McDevitt DG, MacDonald TM. Non-steroidal anti-inflammatory drugs and hospitalization for acute renal failure. QJM 1995;88(8):551–7.
158. Radford MG Jr, Holley KE, Grande JP, Larson TS, Wagoner RD, Donadio JV, McCarthy JT. Reversible membranous nephropathy associated with the use of nonsteroidal anti-inflammatory drugs. JAMA 1996;276(6):466–9.
159. Delzell E, Shapiro S. A review of epidemiologic studies of nonnarcotic analgesics and chronic renal disease. Medicine (Baltimore) 1998;77(2):102–21.
160. McLaughlin JK, Lipworth L, Chow WH, Blot WJ. Analgesic use and chronic renal failure: a critical review of the epidemiologic literature. Kidney Int 1998;54(3):679–86.
161. Rexrode KM, Buring JE, Glynn RJ, Stampfer MJ, Youngman LD, Gaziano JM. Analgesic use and renal function in men. JAMA 2001;286(3):315–21.
162. Fored CM, Ejerblad E, Lindblad P, Fryzek JP, Dickman PW, Signorello LB, Lipworth L, Elinder CG, Blot WJ, McLaughlin JK, Zack MM, Nyren O. Acetaminophen, aspirin, and chronic renal failure. N Engl J Med 2001;345(25):1801–8.
163. Moran M, Mozes MF, Maddux MS, Veremis S, Bartkus C, Ketel B, Pollak R, Wallemark C, Jonasson O. Prevention of acute graft rejection by the prostaglandin E1 analogue misoprostol in renal-transplant recipients treated with cyclosporine and prednisone. N Engl J Med 1990;322(17):1183–8.
164. Kaiser U, Sollberger J, Hoigné R, Wymann R, Fritschy D, Maibach R. Haut-Nebenwirkungen unter richt-Steroidalen Analgetika-Entzundungshemmexn und sogenannten leichten Analgetika. Mitteilung aus dem komprehensiven Spital Drug Monitorin Bern (CHDMB). [Skin side effects of non-steroidal anti-inflammatory analgesics and so-called minor analgesics. Report from the Berne Comprehensive Hospital Monitor.] Schweiz Med Wochenschr 1987; 117(49):1966–70.
165. Fowler PD. Aspirin, paracetamol and non-steroidal anti-inflammatory drugs. A comparative review of side effects. Med Toxicol Adverse Drug Exp 1987;2(5):338–66.
166. ADRAC. Photosensitivity reactions: a sunburnt country. Aust Adv Drug React Bull 1983;March.
167. ADRAC. A sunburnt country revisited. Aust Adv Drug React Bull 1987;February.
168. Roujeau JC, Stern RS. Severe adverse cutaneous reactions to drugs. N Engl J Med 1994;331(19):1272–85.
169. Paul E, Hellwich M. Die Wertigkeit des intracutanen Hauttestes bei Analgetika-Unverträglichkeit im Vergleich zur oralen Provokation. [Value of the intracutaneous skin test in analgesic intolerance in comparison with oral provocation.] Z Hautkr 1987;62(9):705–14.
170. Maucher OM, Fuchs A. Kontakturtikaria im Epikutantest bei Pyrazolonallergie. [Contact urticaria caused by skin test in pyrazolone allergy.] Hautarzt 1983;34(8):383–6.
171. Roujeau JC, Bracq C, Huyn NT, Chaussalet E, Raffin C, Duedari N. HLA phenotypes and bullous cutaneous reactions to drugs. Tissue Antigens 1986;28(4):251–4.
172. Powles AV, Griffiths CE, Seifert MH, Fry L. Exacerbation of psoriasis by indomethacin. Br J Dermatol 1987;117(6):799–800.
173. Sendagorta E, Allegue F, Rocamora A, Ledo A. Generalized pustular psoriasis precipitated by diclofenac and indomethacin. Dermatologica 1987;175(6):300–1.
174. Berger TG, Dhar A. Lichenoid photoeruptions in human immunodeficiency virus infection. Arch Dermatol 1994;130(5):609–13.
175. Wallace CA, Farrow D, Sherry DD. Increased risk of facial scars in children taking nonsteroidal antiinflammatory drugs. J Pediatr 1994;125(5 Pt 1):819–22.
176. Adamski H, Benkalfate L, Delaval Y, Ollivier I, le Jean S, Toubel G, le Hir-Garreau I, Chevrant-Breton J. Photodermatitis from non-steroidal anti-inflammatory drugs. Contact Dermatitis 1998;38(3):171–4.
177. Le Coz CJ, Bottlaender A, Scrivener JN, Santinelli F, Cribier BJ, Heid E, Grosshans EM. Photocontact dermatitis from ketoprofen and tiaprofenic acid: cross-reactivity study in 12 consecutive patients. Contact Dermatitis 1998;38(5):245–52.
178. Kranke B, Szolar-Platzer C, Komericki P, Derhaschnig J, Aberer W. Epidemiological significance of bufexamac as a frequent and relevant contact sensitizer. Contact Dermatitis 1997;36(4):212–15.
179. Ophaswongse S, Maibach H. Topical nonsteroidal anti-inflammatory drugs: allergic and photoallergic contact dermatitis and phototoxicity. Contact Dermatitis 1993;29(2):57–64.
180. Gniazdowska B, Rueff F, Przybilla B. Delayed contact hypersensitivity to non-steroidal anti-inflammatory drugs. Contact Dermatitis 1999;40(2):63–5.
181. Iwakiri K, Hata M, Miura Y, Numano K, Yuge M, Sasaki E. Allergic contact dermatitis due to bendazac and alclometasone dipropionate. Contact Dermatitis 1999;41(4):218–39.
182. Beller U, Kaufmann R. Contact dermatitis to indomethacin. Contact Dermatitis 1987;17(2):121.
183. Pulido Z, Gonzalez E, Alfaya T, Alvarez JA, Cena M, de la Hoz B. Allergic contact dermatitis from indomethacin. Contact Dermatitis 1999;41(2):112.

184. Bujan JJ, Morante JM, Guemes MG, Del Pozo Losada J, Capdevila EF. Photoallergic contact dermatitis from piketoprofen. Contact Dermatitis 2000;43(5):315.
185. Albes B, Marguery MC, Schwarze HP, Journe F, Loche F, Bazex J. Prolonged photosensitivity following contact photoallergy to ketoprofen. Dermatology 2000;201(2):171–4.
186. Offidani A, Cellini A, Amerio P, Simonetti O, Bossi G. A case of persistent light reaction phenomenon to ketoprofen? Eur J Dermatol 2000;10(2):153–4.
187. Kanitakis J, Souillet AL, Faure M, Claudy A. Ketoprofen-induced pemphigus-like dermatosis: localized contact pemphigus? Acta Derm Venereol 2001;81(4):304–5.
188. Kawada A, Aragane Y, Asai M, Tezuka T. Simultaneous photocontact sensitivity to ketoprofen and oxybenzone. Contact Dermatitis 2001;44(6):370.
189. Goday Bujan JJ, Garcia Alvarez-Eire GM, Martinez W, del Pozo J, Fonseca E. Photoallergic contact dermatitis from aceclofenac. Contact Dermatitis 2001;45(3):170.
190. Valenzuela N, Puig L, Barnadas MA, Alomar A. Photocontact dermatitis due to dexketoprofen. Contact Dermatitis 2002;47(4):237.
191. Henschel R, Agathos M, Breit R. Photocontact dermatitis after gargling with a solution containing benzydamine. Contact Dermatitis 2002;47(1):53.
192. Sugiura M, Hayakawa R, Xie Z, Sugiura K, Hiramoto K, Shamoto M. Experimental study on phototoxicity and the photosensitization potential of ketoprofen, suprofen, tiaprofenic acid and benzophenone and the photocross-reactivity in guinea pigs. Photodermatol Photoimmunol Photomed 2002;18(2):82–9.
193. Green JJ, Manders SM. Pseudoporphyria. J Am Acad Dermatol 2001;44(1):100–8.
194. Maerker JM, Harm A, Foeldvari I, Hoger PH. Naproxeninduzierte pseudoporphyrie. [Naproxen-induced pseudoporphyria.] Hautarzt 2001;52(11):1026–9.
195. Rashad S, Revell P, Hemingway A, Low F, Rainsford K, Walker F. Effect of non-steroidal anti-inflammatory drugs on the course of osteoarthritis. Lancet 1989; 2(8662):519–22.
196. Huskisson EC, Berry H, Gishen P, Jubb RW, Whitehead J. Effects of antiinflammatory drugs on the progression of osteoarthritis of the knee. LINK Study Group. Longitudinal Investigation of Nonsteroidal Antiinflammatory Drugs in Knee Osteoarthritis. J Rheumatol 1995;22(10):1941–6.
197. al Arfag A, Davis P. Osteoarthritis 1991. Current drug treatment regimens. Drugs 1991;41(2):193–201.
198. Schnitzer TJ, Popovich JM, Andersson GB, Andriacchi TP. Effect of piroxicam on gait in patients with osteoarthritis of the knee. Arthritis Rheum 1993;36(9):1207–13.
199. Varghese D, Kodakat S, Patel H. Non-steroidal anti-inflammatories should not be used after orthopaedic surgery. BMJ 1998;316(7141):1390–1.
200. Stone PG, Richards E. NSAIDs need not usually be withheld after orthopaedic surgery. BMJ 1998;317(7165):1079.
201. Godden D. Effects of NSAIDs on bone healing have been widely reported in maxillofacial journals. BMJ 1999;318(7191):1141.
202. Dimar JR 2nd, Ante WA, Zhang YP, Glassman SD. The effects of nonsteroidal anti-inflammatory drugs on posterior spinal fusions in the rat. Spine 1996;21(16):1870–6.
203. Altman RD, Latta LL, Keer R, Renfree K, Hornicek FJ, Banovac K. Effect of nonsteroidal antiinflammatory drugs on fracture healing: a laboratory study in rats. J Orthop Trauma 1995;9(5):392–400.
204. Smith G, Roberts R, Hall C, Nuki G. Reversible ovulatory failure associated with the development of luteinized unruptured follicles in women with inflammatory arthritis taking non-steroidal anti-inflammatory drugs. Br J Rheumatol 1996;35(5):458–62.
205. Akil M, Amos RS, Stewart P. Infertility may sometimes be associated with NSAID consumption. Br J Rheumatol 1996;35(1):76–8.
206. Mendonca LL, Khamashta MA, Nelson-Piercy C, Hunt BJ, Hughes GR. Non-steroidal anti-inflammatory drugs as a possible cause for reversible infertility. Rheumatology (Oxford) 2000;39(8):880–2.
207. Stevenson DD, Sanchez-Borges M, Szczeklik A. Classification of allergic and pseudoallergic reactions to drugs that inhibit cyclooxygenase enzymes. Ann Allergy Asthma Immunol 2001;87(3):177–80.
208. Eaton RA. A comparison of anaphylactoid reactions associated with non-steroidal anti-inflammatory drugs. ADR Highlights 1981;8116.
209. Strom BL, Carson JL, Schinnar R, Sim E, Morse ML. The effect of indication on the risk of hypersensitivity reactions associated with tolmetin sodium vs other nonsteroidal anti-inflammatory drugs. J Rheumatol 1988;15(4):695–9.
210. Czerniawska-Mysik G, Szczeklik A. Idiosyncrasy to pyrazolone drugs. Allergy 1981;36(6):381–4.
211. Anonymous. Sensitisation to bee and wasp stings with NSAIDs/ACE inhibition. Reactions 1999;3:747.
212. Stevens DL. Could nonsteroidal antiinflammatory drugs (NSAIDs) enhance the progression of bacterial infections to toxic shock syndrome? Clin Infect Dis 1995; 21(4):977–80.
213. Barnham M, Anderson AW. Non-steroidal anti-inflammatory drugs (NSAIDs). A predisposing factor for streptococcal bacteraemia? Adv Exp Med Biol 1997;418:145–7.
214. Rivey MP, Allington DR, Henry Dunham AL. Necrotising fasciitis in an elderly patient: case report. Pharm Technol 1998;14:58–62.
215. Kahn LH, Styrt BA. Necrotizing soft tissue infections reported with nonsteroidal antiinflammatory drugs. Ann Pharmacother 1997;31(9):1034–9.
216. Dubach UC, Rosner B, Pfister E. Epidemiologic study of abuse of analgesics containing phenacetin. Renal morbidity and mortality (1968–1979). N Engl J Med 1983;308(7):357–62.
217. Dubach UC, Rosner B, Sturmer T. An epidemiologic study of abuse of analgesic drugs. Effects of phenacetin and salicylate on mortality and cardiovascular morbidity (1968 to 1987). N Engl J Med 1991;324(3):155–60.
218. Gago-Dominguez M, Yuan JM, Castelao JE, Ross RK, Yu MC. Regular use of analgesics is a risk factor for renal cell carcinoma. Br J Cancer 1999;81(3):542–8.
219. Bonati M, Bortolus R, Marchetti F, Romero M, Tognoni G. Drug use in pregnancy: an overview of epidemiological (drug utilization) studies. Eur J Clin Pharmacol 1990;38(4):325–8.
220. Ostensen M, Ostensen H. Safety of nonsteroidal anti-inflammatory drugs in pregnant patients with rheumatic disease. J Rheumatol 1996;23(6):1045–9.
221. Nielsen GL, Sorensen HT, Larsen H, Pedersen L. Risk of adverse birth outcome and miscarriage in pregnant users of non-steroidal anti-inflammatory drugs: population based observational study and case-control study. BMJ 2001;322(7281):266–70.
222. Chan LY, Yuen PM, Kristensen P. Risk of miscarriage in pregnant users of NSAIDs. BMJ 2001;322(7298):1365–6.
223. Kristensen P. Risk of miscarriage in pregnant users of NSAIDs. Miscarriages also occur in women intending to have induced abortions. BMJ 2001;322(7298):1366.
224. Anonymous. Pregnant woman should avoid NSAIDs, says RCOG. Pharm J 2001;266:178.
225. Keirse MJNC. Indomethacin tocolysis in preterm labour. In: Cochrane Library. CDROM and online versions.

Oak moss resin

General Information

Oak moss resin is an extract of *Evernia prunasti* found in many after-shave lotions and some perfumes (1).

Organs and Systems

Immunologic

Oak moss resin is usually reported as a contact allergen in those who use perfumed products, but is also reported in rural and forestry workers (2). Perfumes are recognized as being potential sensitizers in soluble oils (3), but oak moss as a specific sensitizer within a coolant has not previously been reported.

- A 47-year-old atopic man gave a 3-year history of dermatitis of his hands, forearms, and face (4). He had worked for 24 years as an engineer, grinding components for printing presses. During an enforced absence from work, he noticed that his rash had resolved, but it relapsed within 2 days of his return. Further remissions were noted during his annual holidays, but the rash would always recur within 2 days of returning to work. His skin eruption continued to deteriorate until the coolant used during the grinding process was withdrawn. His rash subsequently resolved and did not recur. Patch testing with standard series, oils and coolants, the constituents of fragrance mix, and his own coolant gave strong positive reactions to fragrance mix, balsam of Peru (*Myroxylon pereirae*), sodium metabisulfite, diethanolamine, and oak moss, and a smaller reaction to his own coolant. The manufacturer of the coolant was contacted for information on the individual constituents of the oil. Further patch tests were then carried out with these components plus the individual components of the fragrance used within it. There were strong positive reactions to oak moss resin and monoethanolamine.

This case highlights the importance of patch testing with individual components of a suspected product in occupational dermatitis. This reduces the chance of false positive reactions and of missing a relevant allergen.

References

1. Held JL, Ruszkowski AM, Deleo VA. Consort contact dermatitis due to oak moss. Arch Dermatol 1988;124(2):261–2.
2. Goncalo S, Cabral F, Goncalo M. Contact sensitivity to oak moss. Contact Dermatitis 1988;19(5):355–7.
3. Hodgson G. Eczemas associated with lubricants and metalworking fluids. Dermatol Dig 1976;Oct:11–15.
4. Owen CM, August PJ, Beck MH. Contact allergy to oak moss resin in a soluble oil. Contact Dermatitis 2000;43(2):112.

Ocular dyes

General Information

Fluorescein

Topical fluorescein dye is often used during slit lamp examination, because it helps in identifying corneal epithelial defects (1). Fluorescein retinal angiography was first described in 1961 (2); rapid intravenous injection of fluorescein displays retinal circulation velocity and the fine architecture and integrity of the blood retinal barrier. This is associated with minor adverse events in 21% of cases and potential life-threatening adverse events in 0.5% (3).

Fluorescein angiography using oral sodium fluorescein involves the use of 10 ml of a 10% solution of sodium fluorescein, the same material that is generally used for intravenous injection in conventional fluorescein angiography. Retinal photography starts 15 minutes after ingestion and continues for 1 hour. The camera, the photography, and film processing techniques are the same as those used for conventional fluorescein angiography. In 97% of 2625 eyes, adequate photographs for clinical use were obtained after oral fluorescein (4). Only 1.7% of the patients had minimal itching, discomfort, or nausea after oral sodium fluorescein. There were no anaphylactic or other severe adverse effects.

Complications of the use of fluorescein, all of which were reversible in a few hours or days, have been reported (5,6). Most of the complications were associated with the use of a larger quantity of fluorescein than recommended. The most frequent adverse effect of intravenous fluorescein is nausea; urticaria, hypersalivation, rhinorrhea, and chills have been seen in a few cases.

Serious or fatal accidents during fluorescein angiography have been assessed in an international survey involving 594 687 angiographies. The incidence of fatal accidents was one case per 49 557 angiographies, and of non-fatal but serious accidents one case per 18 020 angiographies. The total number of accidents reported was 45 cases, equal to one per 13 215 angiographies.

Indocyanine green

Indocyanine green, used for infrared angiography of the choroidal vessels, is well tolerated intravenously and its adverse effects are less pronounced than those of intravenous fluorescein (7).

Methylthioninium chloride (methylene blue)

Methylthioninium chloride is somewhat irritating, and topical anesthesia is recommended before its use; prolonged systemic exposure can cause the fundus to turn visibly blue (8).

Rose bengal

Discomfort and irritation are more pronounced with rose bengal than with fluorescein. Discoloration of the skin of the patient's eyelids and the examiner's fingers as well as ocular staining are more persistent than when fluorescein is used (9).

102. Morrison D, Clark D, Goldfarb E, McCoy L. Worsening of obsessive-compulsive symptoms following treatment with olanzapine. Am J Psychiatry 1998;155(6):855.
103. al-Mulhim A, Atwal S, Coupland NJ. Provocation of obsessive-compulsive behaviour and tremor by olanzapine. Can J Psychiatry 1998;43(6):645.
104. Jonkers F, De Haan L. Olanzapine-induced obsessive-compulsive symptoms in a patient with bipolar II disorder. Psychopharmacology (Berl) 2002;162(1):87–8.
105. Lykouras L, Zervas IM, Gournellis R, Malliori M, Rabavilas A. Olanzapine and obsessive-compulsive symptoms. Eur Neuropsychopharmacol 2000;10(5):385–7.
106. de Haan L, Beuk N, Hoogenboom B, Dingemans P, Linszen D. Obsessive-compulsive symptoms during treatment with olanzapine and risperidone: a prospective study of 113 patients with recent-onset schizophrenia or related disorders. J Clin Psychiatry 2002;63(2):104–7.
107. al Jeshi A. Paranoia and agitation associated with olanzapine treatment. Can J Psychiatry 1998;43(2):195.
108. Licht RW, Arngrim T, Cristensen H. Olanzapine-induced galactorrhea. Psychopharmacology (Berl) 2002;162(1):94–5.
109. Kingsbury SJ, Castelo C, Abulseoud O. Quetiapine for olanzapine-induced galactorrhea. Am J Psychiatry 2002;159(6):1061.
110. Canuso CM, Hanau M, Jhamb KK, Green AI. Olanzapine use in women with antipsychotic-induced hyperprolactinemia. Am J Psychiatry 1998;155(10):1458.
111. Gazzola LR, Opler LA. Return of menstruation after switching from risperidone to olanzapine. J Clin Psychopharmacol 1998;18(6):486–7.
112. Potenza MN, Wasylink S, Epperson CN, McDougle CJ. Olanzapine augmentation of fluoxetine in the treatment of trichotillomania. Am J Psychiatry 1998;155(9):1299–300.
113. Popli AP, Konicki PE, Jurjus GJ, Fuller MA, Jaskiw GE. Clozapine and associated diabetes mellitus. J Clin Psychiatry 1997;58(3):108–11.
114. Wirshing DA, Spellberg BJ, Erhart SM, Marder SR, Wirshing WC. Novel antipsychotics and new onset diabetes. Biol Psychiatry 1998;44(8):778–83.
115. Ober SK, Hudak R, Rusterholtz A. Hyperglycemia and olanzapine. Am J Psychiatry 1999;156(6):970.
116. Ramankutty G. Olanzapine-induced destabilization of diabetes in the absence of weight gain. Acta Psychiatr Scand 2002;105(3):235–6.
117. Fertig MK, Brooks VG, Shelton PS, English CW. Hyperglycemia associated with olanzapine. J Clin Psychiatry 1998;59(12):687–9.
118. Lindenmayer JP, Patel R. Olanzapine-induced ketoacidosis with diabetes mellitus. Am J Psychiatry 1999;156(9):1471.
119. Gatta B, Rigalleau V, Gin H. Diabetic ketoacidosis with olanzapine treatment. Diabetes Care 1999;22(6):1002–3.
120. Bettinger TL, Mendelson SC, Dorson PG, Crismon ML. Olanzapine-induced glucose dysregulation. Ann Pharmacother 2000;34(7–8):865–7.
121. Melkersson KI, Hulting AL, Brismar KE. Elevated levels of insulin, leptin, and blood lipids in olanzapine-treated patients with schizophrenia or related psychoses. J Clin Psychiatry 2000;61(10):742–9.
122. Cohn TA, Remington G, Kameh H. Hyperinsulinemia in psychiatric patients treated with olanzapine. J Clin Psychiatry 2002;63(1):75–6.
123. Bonanno DG, Davydov L, Botts SR. Olanzapine-induced diabetes mellitus. Ann Pharmacother 2001;35(5):563–5.
124. Roefaro J, Mukherjee SM. Olanzapine-induced hyperglycemic nonketonic coma. Ann Pharmacother 2001; 35(3):300–2.
125. Lindenmayer JP, Smith RC, Singh A, Parker B, Chou E, Kotsaftis A. Hyperglycemia in patients with schizophrenia who are treated with olanzapine. J Clin Psychopharmacol 2001;21(3):351–3.
126. Meatherall R, Younes J. Fatality from olanzapine induced hyperglycemia. J Forensic Sci 2002;47(4):893–6.
127. Budman CL, Gayer AI. Low blood glucose and olanzapine. Am J Psychiatry 2001;158(3):500–1.
128. Bryden KE, Kopala LC. Body mass index increase of 58% associated with olanzapine. Am J Psychiatry 1999;156(11):1835–6.
129. Zullino DF, Quinche P, Hafliger T, Stigler M. Olanzapine improves social dysfunction in cluster B personality disorder. Hum Psychopharmacol 2002;17(5):247–51.
130. Gupta S, Droney T, Al-Samarrai S, Keller P, Frank B. Olanzapine-induced weight gain. Ann Clin Psychiatry 1998;10(1):39.
131. Gupta S, Droney T, Al-Samarrai S, Keller P, Frank B. Olanzapine: weight gain and therapeutic efficacy. J Clin Psychopharmacol 1999;19(3):273–5.
132. Sheitman BB, Bird PM, Binz W, Akinli L, Sanchez C. Olanzapine-induced elevation of plasma triglyceride levels. Am J Psychiatry 1999;156(9):1471–2.
133. Bronson BD, Lindenmayer JP. Adverse effects of high-dose olanzapine in treatment-refractory schizophrenia. J Clin Psychopharmacol 2000;20(3):382–4.
134. Littrell KH, Petty RG, Hilligoss NM, Peabody CD, Johnson CG. Weight loss associated with olanzapine treatment. J Clin Psychopharmacol 2002;22(4):436–7.
135. Powers PS, Santana CA, Bannon YS. Olanzapine in the treatment of anorexia nervosa: an open label trial. Int J Eat Disord 2002;32(2):146–54.
136. Ellingrod VL, Miller D, Schultz SK, Wehring H, Arndt S. CYP2D6 polymorphisms and atypical antipsychotic weight gain. Psychiatr Genet 2002;12(1):55–8.
137. Sacchetti E, Guarneri L, Bravi D. H(2) antagonist nizatidine may control olanzapine-associated weight gain in schizophrenic patients. Biol Psychiatry 2000;48(2):167–8.
138. Littrell KH, Johnson CG, Littrell SH, Peabody CD. Effects of olanzapine on polydipsia and intermittent hyponatremia. J Clin Psychiatry 1997;58(12):549.
139. Beasley CM Jr, Tollefson GD, Tran PV. Safety of olanzapine. J Clin Psychiatry 1997;58(Suppl 10):13–17.
140. Steinwachs A, Grohmann R, Pedrosa F, Ruther E, Schwerdtner I. Two cases of olanzapine-induced reversible neutropenia. Pharmacopsychiatry 1999;32(4):154–6.
141. Naumann R, Felber W, Heilemann H, Reuster T. Olanzapine-induced agranulocytosis. Lancet 1999;354(9178):566–7.
142. Anonymous. Olanzapine: hematological reactions. CMAJ 1998;159(1):81–2, 85–6.
143. Gajwani P, Tesar GE. Olanzapine-induced neutropenia. Psychosomatics 2000;41(2):150–1.
144. Gardner I, Zahid N, MacCrimmon D, Uetrecht JP. A comparison of the oxidation of clozapine and olanzapine to reactive metabolites and the toxicity of these metabolites to human leukocytes. Mol Pharmacol 1998;53(6):991–8.
145. Kodesh A, Finkel B, Lerner AG, Kretzmer G, Sigal M. Dose-dependent olanzapine-associated leukopenia: three case reports. Int Clin Psychopharmacol 2001;16(2):117–19.
146. Meissner W, Schmidt T, Kupsch A, Trottenberg T, Lempert T. Reversible leucopenia related to olanzapine. Mov Disord 1999;14(5):872–3.
147. Dettling M, Cascorbi I, Hellweg R, Deicke U, Weise L, Muller-Oerlinghausen B. Genetic determinants of drug-induced agranulocytosis: potential risk of olanzapine? Pharmacopsychiatry 1999;32(3):110–12.
148. Buchman N, Strous RD, Ulman AM, Lerner M, Kotler M. Olanzapine-induced leukopenia with human leukocyte antigen profiling. Int Clin Psychopharmacol 2001;16(1):55–7.

149. Felber W, Naumann R, Schuler U, Fulle M, Reuster T, Garcia K, Heilemann H. Are there genetic determinants of olanzapine-induced agranulocytosis? Pharmacopsychiatry 2000;33(5):197–9.
150. Swartz JR, Ananth J, Smith MW, Burgoyne KS, Gadasally R, Arai Y. Olanzapine treatment after clozapine-induced granulocytopenia in 3 patients. J Clin Psychiatry 1999;60(2):119–21.
151. Benedetti F, Cavallaro R, Smeraldi E. Olanzapine-induced neutropenia after clozapine-induced neutropenia. Lancet 1999;354(9178):567.
152. Konakanchi R, Grace JJ, Szarowicz R, Pato MT. Olanzapine prolongation of granulocytopenia after clozapine discontinuation. J Clin Psychopharmacol 2000;20(6):703–4.
153. Oyewumi LK, Al-Semaan Y. Olanzapine: safe during clozapine-induced agranulocytosis. J Clin Psychopharmacol 2000;20(2):279–81.
154. Dernovsek MZ, Tavcar R. Olanzapine appears haematologically safe in patients who developed blood dyscrasia on clozapine and risperidone. Int Clin Psychopharmacol 2000;15(4):237–8.
155. Chatterton R. Experiences with clozapine and olanzapine. Aust NZ J Psychiatry 1998;32(3):463.
156. Finkel B, Lerner A, Oyffe I, Rudinski D, Sigal M, Weizman A. Olanzapine treatment in patients with typical and atypical neuroleptic-associated agranulocytosis. Int Clin Psychopharmacol 1998;13(3):133–5.
157. Lambert T. Olanzapine after clozapine: the rare case of prolongation of granulocytopaenia. Aust NZ J Psychiatry 1998;32(4):591–2.
158. Bogunovic O, Viswanathan R. Thrombocytopenia possibly associated with olanzapine and subsequently with benztropine mesylate. Psychosomatics 2000;41(3):277–8.
159. Onofrj M, Thomas A. One further case of pancytopenia induced by olanzapine in a Parkinson's disease patient. Eur Neurol 2001;45(1):56–7.
160. Mathias S, Schaaf LW, Sonntag A. Eosinophilia associated with olanzapine. J Clin Psychiatry 2002;63(3):246–7.
161. Perkins DO, McClure RK. Hypersalivation coincident with olanzapine treatment. Am J Psychiatry 1998;155(7):993–4.
162. Doucette DE, Grenier JP, Robertson PS. Olanzapine-induced acute pancreatitis. Ann Pharmacother 2000;34(10):1128–31.
163. Woodall BS, DiGregorio RV. Comment: olanzapine-induced acute pancreatitis. Ann Pharmacother 2001;35(4):506–8.
164. Doucette DE, Robertson PS. Comment: olanzapine-induced acute pancreatitis. Ann Pharmacother 2001;35:508.
165. Vernon LT, Fuller MA, Hattab H, Varnes KM. Olanzapine-induced urinary incontinence: treatment with ephedrine. J Clin Psychiatry 2000;61(8):601–2.
166. Heckers S, Anick D, Boverman JF, Stern TA. Priapism following olanzapine administration in a patient with multiple sclerosis. Psychosomatics 1998;39(3):288–90.
167. Deirmenjian JM, Erhart SM, Wirshing DA, Spellberg BJ, Wirshing WC. Olanzapine-induced reversible priaprism: a case report. J Clin Psychopharmacol 1998;18(4):351–3.
168. Gordon M, de Groot CM. Olanzapine-associated priapism. J Clin Psychopharmacol 1999;19(2):192.
169. Compton MT, Saldivia A, Berry SA. Recurrent priapism during treatment with clozapine and olanzapine. Am J Psychiatry 2000;157(4):659.
170. Kuperman JR, Asher I, Modai I. Olanzapine-associated priapism. J Clin Psychopharmacol 2001;21(2):247.
171. Matthews SC, Dimsdale JE. Priapism after a suicide attempt by ingestion of olanzapine and gabapentin. Psychosomatics 2001;42(3):280–1.
172. Raz A, Bergman R, Eilam O, Yungerman T, Hayek T. A case report of olanzapine-induced hypersensitivity syndrome. Am J Med Sci 2001;321(2):156–8.
173. Elian AA. Fatal overdose of olanzepine. Forensic Sci Int 1998;91(3):231–5.
174. Gerber JE, Cawthon B. Overdose and death with olanzapine: two case reports. Am J Forensic Med Pathol 2000;21(3):249–51.
175. Stephens BG, Coleman DE, Baselt RC. Olanzapine-related fatality. J Forensic Sci 1998;43(6):1252–3.
176. Favier JC, Da Conceicao M, Peyrefitte C, Aussedat M, Pitti R. Intoxication mortelle à l'olanzapine. [Fatal intoxication with olanzapine.] Cah Anesthesiol 2002; 50:29–31.
177. Cohen LG, Fatalo A, Thompson BT, Di Centes Bergeron G, Flood JG, Poupolo PR. Olanzapine overdose with serum concentrations. Ann Emerg Med 1999;34(2):275–8.
178. Gardner DM, Milliken J, Dursun SM. Olanzapine overdose. Am J Psychiatry 1999;156(7):1118–19.
179. Dobrusin M, Lokshin P, Belmaker RH. Acute olanzapine overdose. Hum Psychopharmacol 1999;14:355–6.
180. Bosch RF, Baumbach A, Bitzer M, Erley CM. Intoxication with olanzapine. Am J Psychiatry 2000;157(2):304–5.
181. O'Malley GF, Seifert S, Heard K, Daly F, Dart RC. Olanzapine overdose mimicking opioid intoxication. Ann Emerg Med 1999;34(2):279–81.
182. Bonin MM, Burkhart KK. Olanzapine overdose in a 1-year-old male. Pediatr Emerg Care 1999;15(4):266–7.
183. Catalano G, Cooper DS, Catalano MC, Butera AS. Olanzapine overdose in an 18-month-old child. J Child Adolesc Psychopharmacol 1999;9(4):267–71.
184. Bond GR, Thompson JD. Olanzapine pediatric overdose. Ann Emerg Med 1999;34(2):292–3.
185. Heimann SW. High-dose olanzapine in an adolescent. J Am Acad Child Adolesc Psychiatry 1999;38(5):496–8.
186. Yip L, Dart RC, Graham K. Olanzapine toxicity in a toddler. Pediatrics 1998;102(6):1494.
187. Malek-Ahmadi P, Simonds JF. Olanzapine for autistic disorder with hyperactivity. J Am Acad Child Adolesc Psychiatry 1998;37(9):902.
188. Callaghan JT, Bergstrom RF, Ptak LR, Beasley CM. Olanzapine. Pharmacokinetic and pharmacodynamic profile. Clin Pharmacokinet 1999;37(3):177–93.
189. Olesen OV, Linnet K. Olanzapine serum concentrations in psychiatric patients given standard doses: the influence of comedication. Ther Drug Monit 1999;21(1):87–90.
190. Lucas RA, Gilfillan DJ, Bergstrom RF. A pharmacokinetic interaction between carbamazepine and olanzapine: observations on possible mechanism. Eur J Clin Pharmacol 1998;54(8):639–43.
191. Linnet K, Olesen OV. Free and glucuronidated olanzapine serum concentrations in psychiatric patients: influence of carbamazepine comedication. Ther Drug Monit 2002;24(4):512–17.
192. Markowitz JS, DeVane CL. Suspected ciprofloxacin inhibition of olanzapine resulting in increased plasma concentration. J Clin Psychopharmacol 1999;19(3):289–91.
193. de Jong J, Hoogenboom B, van Troostwijk LD, de Haan L. Interaction of olanzapine with fluvoxamine. Psychopharmacology (Berl) 2001;155(2):219–20.
194. Zullino DF, Delessert D, Eap CB, Preisig M, Baumann P. Tobacco and cannabis smoking cessation can lead to intoxication with clozapine or olanzapine. Int Clin Psychopharmacol 2002;17(3):141–3.
195. Deshauer D, Albuquerque J, Alda M, Grof P. Seizures caused by possible interaction between olanzapine and clomipramine. J Clin Psychopharmacol 2000;20(2):283–4.

Opioids and hypnotic drugs are often used to prevent increased intracranial pressure and the subsequent reduction in cerebral perfusion pressure. However, it is still uncertain whether opioids can cause increased intracranial pressure. The effects of a bolus injection and infusion of sufentanil, alfentanil, and fentanyl on cerebral hemodynamics and electroencephalographic activity have been studied in a randomized crossover study in six patients with increased intracranial pressure after severe head trauma (34). All three infusions were associated with a significant increase in intracranial pressure (9, 8, and 5.5 mmHg respectively) 3–5 minutes after the bolus opioid injection. Intracranial pressure gradually fell and returned to baseline after 15 minutes. This increase was associated with significant falls in mean arterial pressure and cerebral perfusion pressure throughout the study period. The electroencephalogram changed from a fast to a reduced activity pattern, with an improvement in background activity. It is therefore advisable to avoid using bolus injections of opioids in patients with head injury and to use continuous infusion for sedation.

Endocrine

Morphine reduces the response of the hypothalamus to afferent stimulation (35). In many species, opioids alter the equilibrium point of the hypothalamic heat-regulatory mechanisms.

In patients undergoing surgery, opioids inhibit the stress-induced release of ACTH (36).

Secretion of luteinizing hormone (LH) and thyrotropin is suppressed by opioids, whereas the release of prolactin and, in some cases, growth hormone is enhanced (37).

Gastrointestinal

Opioids reduce the secretion of hydrochloric acid and have a marked effect on gastrointestinal motility. Gastric emptying is prolonged and the likelihood of esophageal reflux is increased (38). Tone in the antral part of the stomach and first part of the duodenum is increased. The passage of gastric contents through the duodenum can be delayed by as much as 12 hours, retarding the absorption of orally administered drugs (39). In 260 patients with malignant disease, 23–40% vomited and 8–10% felt nauseated (SEDA-17, 79). Transdermal hyoscine (scopolamine) can reduce these problems (SEDA-17, 79).

Biliary and pancreatic and intestinal secretions are reduced by morphine, and digestion in the small intestine is delayed.

Constipation is usual (SEDA-17, 79). The tone of the anal sphincter is increased and the usual reflex relaxation response to rectal distension is reduced.

Biliary tract

Therapeutic doses of opioids constrict the sphincter of Oddi, and biliary tract pressure rises ten-fold. Patients with biliary colic can have exacerbation of pain after morphine. Likewise, opioids such as fentanyl, morphine, and dextropropoxyphene can cause bile duct spasm (SEDA-21, 85).

"It is standard teaching that morphine should not be used to treat patients with pancreatitis because it causes a rise in biliary and pancreatic pressure" (40). From this starting point, this comprehensive review discusses current approaches to opioid analgesia in pancreatitis, pointing out that morphine has been reported to cause biliary colic in individuals without biliary tract disease and that pethidine (meperidine) has become the analgesic of choice. Constriction of the sphincter of Oddi and the basal tone of the sphincter and the frequency of phasic contractions have been measured using endoscopic retrograde cholangiopancreatography (ERCP); an increase in basal tone is believed to be the best indication of sphincter dysfunction. Morphine sulfate in intravenous doses of 2.5–5 micrograms/kg caused increased contractions but no change in basal pressure, while doses of 10 micrograms/kg and over caused a rise in basal pressure. Pethidine increased contractions but not basal tone, while tramadol had no effect on basal pressure in a small study. Among mixed opiate agonist/antagonists, pentazocine increased basal pressure. Buprenorphine, a partial opiate agonist, resulted in no pressure changes, while the antagonist naloxone 0.4 mg intravenously had no effect alone on the sphincter basal pressure and did not stop the increase in pressure caused by morphine. However, case reports have suggested that naloxone reduces sphincter spasm in clinical situations.

Urinary tract

The urinary voiding reflex is inhibited by opioids, and both the tone of the external sphincter and the volume of the bladder increase; urinary retention is therefore common.

Skin

Flushing of the face, neck, and upper thorax can follow therapeutic doses of opioids. These effects may be partly due to release of histamine, which is also implicated in the sweating and pruritus seen after opioid administration. Opioid effects on neurons may partly be involved in the pruritus, as pruritus is provoked by opioids that do not release histamine and is abolished by small doses of naloxone.

Urticaria at the site of injection is due to histamine release. It is seen with pethidine and morphine, but not with oxymorphone, methadone, fentanyl, or sufentanil. Wheal and flare responses to various opioids differ (41).

Sexual function

Although long-term administration of low-dose opioids, especially intrathecally, improves quality of life through improved pain control, it can compromise it by causing impaired sexual function. Low testosterone concentrations have been reported in heroin addicts (42) and subjects in a methadone maintenance program (43).

In prospective non-randomized non-blinded evaluation of the effects of a 12-week course of intrathecal opioids for the control of chronic non-cancer pain on the hypothalamic–pituitary–gonadal axis in 12 men, it was suppressed and serum testosterone concentrations fell (44). This effect not only reduces quality of life through sexual dysfunction but can also increase the risk of spinal osteoporosis in men, with an increased risk of vertebral and hip fractures. Patients receiving long-term intrathecal opioid therapy need to be informed of potential hypothalamic–pituitary–gonadal axis suppression as a result of the treatment, and testosterone replacement after hypothalamic–pituitary–gonadal axis surveillance during treatment should be considered if indicated.

Death

Opiates are widely used all over the world, but recently concerns about opiate use (and deaths from such use) have increased in Australia and the UK (45). The rate of opiate overdose deaths in these countries increased dramatically between 1985 and 1995. Throughout that period, it was four to ten times higher in Australia than the UK, but the rate of increase may have been greater in the UK in the latter half of the period, since the difference in rate narrowed substantially during that time. Methadone maintenance treatment, established in Australia in 1969 and in the UK in 1970, has become the main treatment for opiate dependence in both countries. About half of the opiate deaths in the UK were attributed at least in part to methadone. By contrast, considerably fewer (18%) opiate overdose deaths in Australia were attributed to methadone. The authors suggested that the discrepancy in the rates between the two countries could be artefacts of the differences in (a) the documentation of these deaths, (b) the rate of opiate dependence, (c) the route of opiate administration, (d) opiate purity, and, most importantly, (e) the method of delivery of methadone maintenance treatment.

Methadone-related fatalities have been reported from all countries in which methadone has been used for either detoxification or maintenance treatment of opiate users. These fatalities are often defined as cases of poisoning due to methadone or as polydrug intoxication with methadone as the leading cause of death. Methadone maintenance treatment was introduced in Germany in 1989, and 1396 drug-related deaths were reported from 1990 to 1999 in Hamburg (46). While the absolute numbers of drug-related deaths by poisoning did not change over this period, the rise in methadone-associated deaths paralleled a fall in the number of heroin-associated deaths. From 1990 to 1998, the rate of monovalent heroin intoxication in cases of poisoning fell from 60% to 11%, while the rate of polydrug intoxication increased. Poisoning caused by methadone combined with other substances first gained significance 4 years after methadone maintenance treatment was introduced in Hamburg. Since 1994, methadone-related deaths have increased steadily, and by 1997–1998 the numbers had increased exponentially. In the first 6 months of 1999, 60% of all cases of poisoning among drug addicts showed the presence of methadone. When strict guidelines for describing such poisonings were used, 39 poisonings in 1998 (40%) were predominantly caused by methadone, six of them being monovalent methadone intoxication. About two-thirds of all methadone-related poisonings concerned drug addicts who never stayed in methadone maintenance treatment, implying that they obtained methadone from outside of regular treatment. Almost 10 years after the introduction of methadone maintenance treatment in Hamburg, methadone replaced heroin as the leading cause of death due to poisoning. At the same time, however, the absolute number of drug-related deaths and poisonings fell slightly. While methadone maintenance treatment has clearly reduced overall morbidity and mortality in addicts globally, some issues remain unresolved. There are significant differences in the delivery of methadone maintenance treatment from one country to another. The authors reported that in some patients the starting doses of methadone are quite high and potentially lethal. This is especially so when the patients are also using other drugs and attempting to wean off them. Thus, continued polydrug use in treatment is an important risk factor for mortality. Many patients receive take-home doses for a week at a time. While this is useful in a select group of patients, it is not useful in those who sell methadone to buy heroin and combine the two drugs without knowledge of their half-lives and potential complications. The authors suggested changes in methadone maintenance treatment policy, in order to reduce the chances of accidental overdose/poisoning. Specifically, they recommended: a substantial improvement in quality assurance; a more restrictive methadone take-home policy (at least for patients with evidence for concomitant opiate use); and evaluating heroin or long-acting acetylmethadol as alternatives.

Another report from Australia reviewed all the accidental illicit drug deaths that occurred in the Sydney area in 1995–1997 (47). There were 3559 autopsies, of which 4% were considered accidental illicit drug deaths; of these deaths, 121 were men and 22 were women. While the highest number of male deaths occurred in the 25–35 year age group, female deaths were evenly spread from ages 20–35. Almost half (49%) of the deaths occurred from morphine poisoning, 27% from multiple drug toxicity, and 21% from heroin toxicity combined with alcohol. Methadone was detected in 19 cases (13%); 12 of these people were enrolled in a methadone maintenance program. Methadone intoxication alone was responsible for two deaths (1%) only. Methadone was present in the blood in a potentially fatal concentration in 13 cases, while 113 people (80%) had a heroin concentration in the fatal range and 91% had detectable concentrations of heroin. There were no significant neurological findings in the 143 cases studied. More than 50% of those with methadone detected also had heroin in their blood. Unfortunately, this appears to show that some people who participate in a methadone program may still die from accidental heroin overdose. Thus, the authors emphasized the importance of education of heroin users about the risk of accidental overdose.

There is excess mortality in heroin users compared with the general population. The prevalence and experience of heroin overdose in drug users in a general practice in Ireland were examined during 5 months (48). Of the 33 patients identified, 24 agreed to participate. They had had their first overdose on average 5 years after starting to use heroin. Ten had taken an overdose themselves, 23 had witnessed an overdose, 22 knew a victim of fatal overdose, and 4 had been present at a fatal overdose. However, they reported poor understanding of how to deal with an overdose. Despite maintenance treatment mean follow-up of 68 days (maximum 13 months) there was an incidence of less than 10% (105).

Intrathecal opioids used in obstetrics are well tolerated by mother and child (SED-11, 139, 140) (106–108).

Morphine is the opioid most often chosen for intrathecal administration.

Respiratory

Respiratory depression occurs more often after intrathecal than after epidural opioid administration and can be more of a problem in old age or when there is pre-existing respiratory disease (SED-11, 139) (109,110). The time of onset is variable but usually occurs within 6–10 hours of the opioid injection, although delays of up to 11 hours have been reported (111). There have been two cases of prolonged respiratory depression lasting 18 hours after single doses of 3 and 5 mg (111). Repeated doses of naloxone were required, but each incremental dose did not alter the level of analgesia.

It has been suggested that opioid-naive patients may be more susceptible to respiratory depression and that posture may also be important (SED-11, 139) (112).

Return of normal respiration can take up to 23 hours. Peak expiratory flow rate (PEFR) was significantly better in patients who had received intrathecal rather than intravenous morphine after cardiac surgery, but mean $PaCO_2$ was significantly higher in patients given intrathecal morphine 2 mg, rather than intrathecal or intravenous morphine 1 mg (113). The effect was dose-dependent (114).

Nervous system

Central adverse effects are as expected; with the exception of constipation, urinary retention, and respiratory depression, these effects tend to be transient and disappear within a few days of starting therapy.

Drowsiness, miosis, and respiratory depression have been reported after intracerebroventricular administration of morphine in two of 55 patients who received morphine 1–1.5 mg (115). A third patient developed visual hallucinations and behavioral disorders after 1 mg. All effects were rapidly reversed by naloxone.

Myoclonic spasms of the legs have been described after intrathecal morphine, and were abolished by intrathecal bupivacaine (116).

Hyperalgesia and myoclonus were reported after high-dose intrathecal morphine (SEDA-17, 87).

Temporary, totally reversible motor and sensory paralysis has been reported after intrathecal morphine 1.6 mg and was attributed not to a direct spinal action of morphine but to cardiovascular changes occurring as a result of pain relief (117).

Gastrointestinal

There is a high incidence of nausea and vomiting with intrathecal diamorphine, which may not be dose-related (118). Two studies have suggested that the incidence of nausea and vomiting in labor is higher with intrathecal than with epidural opioids (119,120).

Urinary tract

Urinary retention has been described in one of a series of patients who had been given pentazocine 5 mg intrathecally (121); others have since reported similar findings.

Skin

Pruritus is a frequent adverse effect after intrathecal administration, with an incidence of one-third with buprenorphine (122) and diamorphine (123) and over 70% for both diamorphine and morphine (124,125). In one study the incidence of pruritus was higher with morphine than with methadone; analgesia was also superior (124). Pruritus has also been reported with intrathecal pethidine (meperidine). Treatment was not reported to be necessary. This effect is not reported to occur after intrathecal beta-endorphin (126,127). The mechanism of pruritus is not well understood and has been attributed to a disturbance of thiamine metabolism (128) and to a disturbance of afferent input at supraspinal as well as at spinal receptor sites (129).

Infection risk

Reactivation of *Herpes simplex* infection after epidural administration of opioids is well known. However, there have been reports of reactivation of *Herpes simplex* after intrathecal morphine for cesarean section (SEDA-17, 87) (SEDA-18, 84).

Susceptibility factors

Knowledge of the use of spinal opioids in children is limited, but adverse effects are similar to those reported in adults (SEDA-18, 85) (130–132). Dysphoria has also been reported, but attributed to systemic absorption (132).

Epidural route

The adverse effects reported with epidural administration are similar to those reported with the intrathecal route. Again, old age and respiratory disease probably dispose to respiratory depression (133). As can be predicted from pharmacokinetic considerations, delayed respiratory depression is more common with epidural morphine than with fentanyl (134).

Epidural administration of opioids has been reviewed (SEDA-21, 92). Morphine causes less respiratory depression and provides better analgesia when it is given by continuous infusion than by intermittent bolus. The authors concluded that epidural fentanyl offers no advantage over the intravenous route and that the mechanism of analgesia is by a systemic effect due to the vascular absorption of this lipophilic drug. However, the administration of lipophilic opioids together with a local anesthetic offers the advantage of using lower doses of both drugs, giving comparable analgesia with a reduction in adverse effects.

Patient-controlled epidural analgesia (PCEA) with fentanyl gives superior analgesia and reduces opioid doses, but without a reduction in adverse effects. However, PCEA with sufentanil offers no advantage (SEDA-19, 87).

Studies of the use of the partial opioid agonist butorphanol to reduce the adverse effects of epidural morphine have not provided evidence of benefit (SEDA-19, 86). Epidural meptazinol has been described as being well tolerated (135).

Respiratory
Respiratory depression occurs less often after epidural than intrathecal opioid administration (109,110). It has been suggested that older patients and those with increased intrathoracic or intra-abdominal pressure are particularly at risk and require reduced dosages (133). In a retrospective study, in which over 6000 patients received epidural morphine, 220 epidural pethidine, and 90 intrathecal morphine, respiratory depression requiring naloxone occurred in about 0.33% after epidural morphine and 5.5% after intrathecal morphine (110). Only two of the patients who received epidural morphine had respiratory depression later than 6 hours after the last dose of opioid. Only three of the 22 patients who had respiratory depression after epidural morphine had not received opioids in addition to epidural morphine during or after the operation. Ten were over 70 years old and 10 had thoracic injections. In another study of 2000 women who received 9000 doses of epidural pethidine 50 mg there was only one case of respiratory depression; this was due to migration of the catheter into the subarachnoid space (136).

The time taken for diffusion of poorly lipid-soluble opioids, such as morphine, from the lumbar subarachnoid space to the fourth ventricle is the most likely explanation for the delayed onset of respiratory depression. It has been suggested that the frequency of respiratory depression can be influenced by the position of the patient and the form of administration, as well as by the dosage of the opioid and the volume of the solution (112).

Doxapram has been used to treat respiratory depression after epidural morphine (137). However, the patient still required endotracheal intubation and mechanical ventilation to correct severe hypercapnia.

Markedly lipid-soluble opioids have also been reported to cause respiratory depression. There was profound respiratory depression 100 minutes after the administration of fentanyl 100 micrograms epidurally (138), whilst epidural sufentanil caused apnea within a couple of minutes, reversed by nalbuphine (139). Epidural buprenorphine 150 micrograms produced prolonged time-dependent biphasic depression of carbon dioxide response in six healthy volunteers. The second maximum occurred at 8–10 hours after injection (140). Similar cases have been reported by others.

Respiratory depression occurred 3.5 hours after a 2.5-year-old child had been given a caudal epidural of 100 micrograms/kg of morphine (141). The effects were successfully reversed by intravenous naloxone.

The efficacy of up to two doses of epidural hydromorphine 1.5 mg has been evaluated in 10 women after cesarean section (142). The mean duration of analgesia was 19.3 hours. Adverse effects were pruritus (56–70%), nausea (11–20%), and vomiting (less than 10%). There was a significant increase in venous PCO_2 3 hours after the second dose of hydromorphine. There was no delayed respiratory depression.

Extradural diamorphine 5 mg, extradural phenoperidine 2 mg, and intramuscular diamorphine 5 mg have been compared (143). Extradural diamorphine produced more prolonged and intense analgesia and there were no serious adverse effects.

Epidural opioids have a much better safety margin in patients who are already tolerant to such drugs (144). Tolerance has also not proven to be a problem (145).

Cardiovascular
Both severe hypotension and severe hypertension have occurred after epidural pethidine (146,147).

There were symptoms of shock lasting 2–3 hours in two women with advanced cancer who were given epidural buprenorphine 300 micrograms after becoming tolerant to epidural morphine (148). The buprenorphine was given 12 hours after the last dose of morphine. Symptoms started within 2 hours of administration and remitted spontaneously.

Nervous system
Myoclonic seizures after epidural morphine 25 mg/hour and after intrathecal hydromorphone have been reported (149).

- A 30-year-old known epileptic woman who had undergone cesarean section developed a tonic-clonic seizure 6 hours after epidural morphine (150).

Two cases of Menière-like syndrome (SEDA-16, 83) (151), and vertical nystagmus and blurred vision (SEDA-16, 83) (SEDA-17, 86), have been reported after epidural morphine.

Catatonia has been reported after a continuous infusion of epidural morphine (152). Hallucinations were thought to be an important sign of impending intoxication.

Mechanical difficulties, in the form of backflow of solution from epidural catheters, occurred in 31 of 32 patients and there were neurological complications in a further two of eight patients in whom the catheter had been tunnelled and connected to a subcutaneous access port; epidural fibrosis with compression of the spinal cord was presumed to be the cause (144).

Epidural fibrosis is a reported complication after long-term epidural morphine administration (SEDA-17, 85).

Psychological, psychiatric
Psychomotor symptoms have been noted subsequent to epidural buprenorphine (153).

Gastrointestinal
Whereas a high incidence (50%) of delayed (6 hours) nausea and vomiting has been reported in volunteers who received epidural morphine (154), there is a low incidence postoperatively (155). In another series the incidence of nausea (12%) and vomiting (24%) was similar whether morphine was used intramuscularly or epidurally or saline was injected epidurally (156). In labor the incidence of this adverse effect is low with epidural opioids (136,157) compared with intrathecal opioids (119,120). The incidence appears to fall with repeated dosing and is very low in patients with cancer who require long-term opioids (111,158). Nausea and vomiting have also been reported after fentanyl (159,160) and pethidine (161). The effects are abolished by intravenous naloxone without loss of analgesia (162).

Urinary tract
Current evidence suggests that the urodynamic effects of epidural morphine are not dose-related, and the incidence is similar to that reported after intramuscular injections. Urinary retention is more frequent after the use of epidural opioids in volunteers compared with patients

41. Levy JH, Brister NW, Shearin A, Ziegler J, Hug CC Jr, Adelson DM, Walker BF. Wheal and flare responses to opioids in humans. Anesthesiology 1989;70(5):756–60.
42. Mendelson JH, Mello NK. Plasma testosterone levels during chronic heroin use and protracted abstinence. A study of Hong Kong addicts. Clin Pharmacol Ther 1975;17(5):529–33.
43. Spring WD Jr, Willenbring ML, Maddux TL. Sexual dysfunction and psychological distress in methadone maintenance. Int J Addict 1992;27(11):1325–34.
44. Roberts LJ, Finch PM, Pullan PT, Bhagat CI, Price LM. Sex hormone suppression by intrathecal opioids: a prospective study. Clin J Pain 2002;18(3):144–8.
45. Hall W, Lynskey M, Degenhardt L. Trends in opiate-related deaths in the United Kingdom and Australia, 1985–1995. Drug Alcohol Depend 2000;57(3):247–54.
46. Heinemann A, Iwersen-Bergmann S, Stein S, Schmoldt A, Puschel K. Methadone-related fatalities in Hamburg 1990–1999: implications for quality standards in maintenance treatment? Forensic Sci Int 2000;113(1–3):449–55.
47. Garrick TM, Sheedy D, Abernethy J, Hodda AE, Harper CG. Heroin-related deaths in Sydney, Australia. How common are they? Am J Addict 2000;9(2):172–8.
48. Cullen W, Bury G, Langton D. Experience of heroin overdose among drug users attending general practice. Br J Gen Pract 2000;50(456):546–9.
49. Christie B. Gangrene bug killed 35 heroin users. West J Med 2000;173(2):82–3.
50. Gill JR, Graham SM. Ten years of "body packers" in New York City: 50 deaths. J Forensic Sci 2002;47(4):843–6.
51. Koch A, Reiter A, Meissner C, Oehmichen M. Ursache des Todes von Heroinkonsumenten mit niedrigen Morphin-Konzentrationen im Blut. [Cause of death in heroin users with low blood morphine concentration.] Arch Kriminol 2002;209(3–4):76–87.
52. Suresh S, Anand KJ. Opioid tolerance in neonates: mechanisms, diagnosis, assessment, and management. Semin Perinatol 1998;22(5):425–33.
53. Eddy NB, Halbach H, Isbell H, Seevers MH. Drug dependence: its significance and characteristics. Bull World Health Organ 1965;32(5):721–33.
54. Kleber HD, Riordan CE. The treatment of narcotic withdrawal: a historical review. J Clin Psychiatry 1982;43(6 Pt 2):30–4.
55. Kolb L, Himmelsbach CK. Clinical studies of drug addiction. III. A clinical review of withdrawal treatment with a method of evaluating abstinence syndromes. Am J Psychiatry 1938;94:759.
56. Isbell H, Vogel VH, Chapman KW. Present status of narcotic addiction with particular reference to medical indications and comparative addiction liability of the newer and older analgesic drugs. JAMA 1948;138:1019.
57. Glossop M, Johns A, Green L. Opiate withdrawal: in-patient vs out-patient programmes and preferred vs random assignment to treatment. BMJ (Clin Res Ed) 1986;293:103.
58. Gossop M, Green L, Phillips G, Bradley B. What happens to opiate addicts immediately after treatment: a prospective follow up study. BMJ (Clin Res Ed) 1987;294(6584):1377–80.
59. Kleber HD. Detoxification from narcotics. In: Lowinson L, Ruiz P, editors. Substance Abuse. Baltimore: Williams and Wilkins, 1981:317.
60. Phillips GT, Gossop M, Bradley B. The influence of psychological factors on the opiate withdrawal syndrome. Br J Psychiatry 1986;149:235–8.
61. Gossop M, Bradley B, Phillips GT. An investigation of withdrawal symptoms shown by opiate addicts during and subsequent to a 21-day in-patient methadone detoxification procedure. Addict Behav 1987;12(1):1–6.
62. Gossop M, Griffiths P, Bradley B, Strang J. Opiate withdrawal symptoms in response to 10-day and 21-day methadone withdrawal programmes Br J Psychiatry 1989;154:360–3.
63. Newman RG, Whitehill WB. Double-blind comparison of methadone and placebo maintenance treatments of narcotic addicts in Hong Kong. Lancet 1979;2(8141):485–8.
64. Lowinson JH, Marion IJ, Joseph H, Dole VP. Methadone maintenance. In: Lowinson JH, Ruiz P, Millman RB, editors. Substance Abuse: A Comprehensive Textbook. 2nd ed. Baltimore: Williams and Wilkins, 1992:550.
65. Ball JC, Ross A. The Effectiveness of Methadone Maintenance Treatment. New York: Springer-Verlag, 1991.
66. Gold MS, Redmond DE Jr, Kleber HD. Noradrenergic hyperactivity in opiate withdrawal supported by clonidine reversal of opiate withdrawal. Am J Psychiatry 1979;136(1):100–2.
67. Gold MS, Byck R, Sweeney DR, Kleber HD. Endorphin–locus coeruleus connection mediates opiate action and withdrawal. Biomedicine 1979;30(1):1–4.
68. Anonymous. Clonidine treatment for acute opiate withdrawal. Med Lett 1979;21:100.
69. Charney DS, Kleber HD. Iatrogenic opiate addiction: successful detoxification with clonidine. Am J Psychiatry 1980;137(8):989–90.
70. Charney DS, Sternberg DE, Kleber HD, Heninger GR, Redmond DE Jr. The clinical use of clonidine in abrupt withdrawal from methadone. Effects on blood pressure and specific signs and symptoms. Arch Gen Psychiatry 1981;38(11):1273–7.
71. Rounsaville BJ, Kosten T, Kleber H. Success and failure at outpatient opioid detoxification. Evaluating the process of clonidine- and methadone-assisted withdrawal. J Nerv Ment Dis 1985;173(2):103–10.
72. Kleber HD, Riordan CE, Rounsaville B, Kosten T, Charney D, Gaspari J, Hogan I, O'Connor C. Clonidine in outpatient detoxification from methadone maintenance. Arch Gen Psychiatry 1985;42(4):391–4.
73. Ghodse H, Myles J, Smith SE. Clonidine is not a useful adjunct to methadone gradual detoxification in opioid addiction. Br J Psychiatry 1994;165(3):370–4.
74. Charney DS, Heninger GR, Kleber HD. The combined use of clonidine and naltrexone as a rapid, safe, and effective treatment of abrupt withdrawal from methadone. Am J Psychiatry 1986;143(7):831–7.
75. National Institute on Drug Abuse. Drug Dependence in Pregnancy: Clinical Management of Mother and Child. Services Research Monograph Series. NIDA, DHEW Publication, No. ADM 79-678.
76. National Institute on Drug Abuse. Drug Dependence in Pregnancy: Clinical Management of Mother and Child. Services Research Monograph Series. NIDA, DHEW Publication, No. ADM, 79-678. Rockville, MD, 1979.
77. Finnegan LP. Pulmonary problems encountered by the infant of the drug-dependent mother. Clin Chest Med 1980;1(3):311–25.
78. Ghodse AH, Reed JL, Mack JW. The effect of maternal narcotic addiction on the newborn infant. Psychol Med 1977;7(4):667–75.
79. Olofsson M, Buckley W, Andersen GE, Friis-Hansen B. Investigation of 89 children born by drug-dependent mothers. I. Neonatal course. Acta Paediatr Scand 1983;72(3):403–6.
80. Rosen TS, Johnson HL. Children of methadone-maintained mothers: follow-up to 18 months of age. J Pediatr 1982;101(2):192–6.
81. Johnson HL, Rosen TS. Prenatal methadone exposure: effects on behavior in early infancy. Pediatr Pharmacol (New York) 1982;2(2):113–20.
82. Herman NL, Calicott R, Van Decar TK, Conlin G, Tilton J. Determination of the dose–response relationship

for intrathecal sufentanil in laboring patients. Anesth Analg 1997;84(6):1256–61.
83. Arkoosh VA, Cooper M, Norris MC, Boxer L, Ferouz F, Silverman NS, Huffnagle HJ, Huffnagle S, Leighton BL. Intrathecal sufentanil dose response in nulliparous patients. Anesthesiology 1998;89(2):364–70.
84. Herman NL, Choi KC, Affleck PJ, Calicott R, Brackin R, Singhal A, Andreasen A, Gadalla F, Fong J, Gomillion MC, Hartman JK, Koff HD, Lee SH, Van Decar TK. Analgesia, pruritus, and ventilation exhibit a dose–response relationship in parturients receiving intrathecal fentanyl during labor. Anesth Analg 1999;89(2):378–83.
85. Lo WK, Chong JL, Chen LH. Combined spinal epidural for labour analgesia—duration, efficacy and side effects of adding sufentanil or fentanyl to bupivacaine intrathecally vs plain bupivacaine. Singapore Med J 1999;40(10):639–43.
86. Mardirosoff C, Dumont L. Two doses of intrathecal sufentanil (2.5 and 5 microgram) combined with bupivacaine and epinephrine for labor analgesia Anesth Analg 1999;89(5):1263–6.
87. D'Angelo R, Evans E, Dean LA, Gaver R, Eisenach JC. Spinal clonidine prolongs labor analgesia from spinal sufentanil and bupivacaine. Anesth Analg 1999;88(3):573–6.
88. Lardizabal JL, Belizan JM, Carroli G, Gonzalez L, Campodonico L, Aguillaume CJ. A randomized trial of nalbuphine vs meperidine for analgesia during labor. Ref Gynecol Obstet 1999;6:245–8.
89. Hallworth SP, Fernando R, Bell R, Parry MG, Lim GH. Comparison of intrathecal and epidural diamorphine for elective caesarean section using a combined spinal-epidural technique. Br J Anaesth 1999;82(2):228–32.
90. Caranza R, Jeyapalan I, Buggy DJ. Central neuraxial opioid analgesia after caesarean section: comparison of epidural diamorphine and intrathecal morphine. Int J Obstet Anesth 1999;8(2):90–3.
91. Fanshawe MP. A comparison of patient controlled epidural pethidine versus single dose epidural morphine for analgesia after caesarean section. Anaesth Intensive Care 1999;27(6):610–14.
92. Vercauteren MP, Mertens E, Schols G, Mol IV IV, Adriaensen HA. Patient-controlled extradural analgesia after caesarean section: a comparison between tramadol, sufentanil and a mixture of both. Eur J Pain 1999;3(3): 205–10.
93. Cooper DW, Saleh U, Taylor M, Whyte S, Ryall D, Kokri MS, Desira WR, Day H, McArthur E. Patient-controlled analgesia: epidural fentanyl and i.v. morphine compared after caesarean section. Br J Anaesth 1999;82(3):366–70.
94. Siddik-Sayyid S, Aouad-Maroun M, Sleiman D, Sfeir M, Baraka A. Epidural tramadol for postoperative pain after Cesarean section. Can J Anaesth 1999;46(8):731–5.
95. Ron M, Menashe M, Scherer D, Palti Z. Fetal heart rate decelerations following the administration of meperidine-promethazine during labor. Int J Gynaecol Obstet 1982;20(4):301–5.
96. Tejavej A, Siripoonya P, Saungsomboon A, Chiewsilp D. Morphine and birth asphyxia. J Med Assoc Thai 1984;67(Suppl 2):73–9.
97. Belsey EM, Rosenblatt DB, Lieberman BA, Redshaw M, Caldwell J, Notarianni L, Smith RL, Beard RW. The influence of maternal analgesia on neonatal behaviour: I. Pethidine Br J Obstet Gynaecol 1981;88(4):398–406.
98. McQuay H, Moore A. Be aware of renal function when prescribing morphine. Lancet 1984;2(8397):284–5.
99. Sear JW, Hand CW, Moore RA, McQuay HJ. Studies on morphine disposition: influence of renal failure on the kinetics of morphine and its metabolites. Br J Anaesth 1989;62(1):28–32.
100. Bogod D. Advances in epidural analgesia for labour: progress versus prudence. Lancet 1995;345(8958):1129–30.
101. Collis RE, Davies DW, Aveling W. Randomised comparison of combined spinal-epidural and standard epidural analgesia in labour. Lancet 1995;345(8962):1413–16.
102. Cousins MJ, Mather LE. Intrathecal and epidural administration of opioids. Anesthesiology 1984;61(3):276–310.
103. Madrid JL, Fatela LV, Alcorta J, Guillen F, Lobato RD. Intermittent intrathecal morphine by means of an implantable reservoir: a survey of 100 cases. J Pain Symptom Manage 1988;3(2):67–71.
104. Dautheribes M, Guerin J. Analgesie par voie intrathécal Aproposde 50 cas. [Intrathecal analgesia. Apropos of 50 cases.] Neurochirurgie 1988;34(3):194–7.
105. Gestin Y, Pere N, Solassol C. Morphinothérapie isobare intrathécale au long cours. [Long-term intrathecal isobaric morphine therapy.] Ann Fr Anesth Reanim 1986;5(4): 346–50.
106. Blain PG, Lane RJ, Bateman DN, Rawlins MD. Opiate-induced rhabdomyolysis. Hum Toxicol 1985;4(1):71–4.
107. Bonnardot JP, Colau JC, Maillet M, Millot F, Salat-Baroux J. Analgesïe morphinique par voie intrathécalean cours de L'accouchement. [Morphine analgesia by the intrathecal route.] J Gynecol Obstet Biol Reprod (Paris) 1982;11(5):619–23.
108. Schmidt WK, Tam SW, Shotzberger GS, Smith DH Jr, Clark R, Vernier VG. Nalbuphine. Drug Alcohol Depend 1985;14(3–4):339–62.
109. Kossmann B, Dick W, Bowdler I, et al. The analgesic action and respiratory side effects of epidural morphine. A double-blind trial on patients undergoing vaginal hysterectomy. Reg Anaesth 1984;9:55.
110. Gustafsson LL, Schildt B, Jacobsen K. Adverse effects of extradural and intrathecal opiates: report of a nationwide survey in Sweden. Br J Anaesth 1982;54(5):479–86.
111. Glynn CJ, Mather LE, Cousins MJ, Wilson PR, Graham JR. Spinal narcotics and respiratory depression. Lancet 1979;2(8138):356–7.
112. Eriksen HO, Jensen FM. Bivirkninger ved anvendelse af opiater epidwalt og opinalt. [Adverse effects of epidural and spinal opiates.] Ugeskr Laeger 1982;144(36):2627–30.
113. Fitzpatrick GJ, Moriarty DC. Intrathecal morphine in the management of pain following cardiac surgery. A comparison with morphine i.v. Br J Anaesth 1988;60(6):639–44.
114. Yamaguchi H, Watanabe S, Motokawa K, Ishizawa Y. Intrathecal morphine dose–response data for pain relief after cholecystectomy. Anesth Analg 1990;70(2):168–71.
115. Lazorthes Y. Intracerebroventricular administration of morphine for control of irreducible cancer pain. Ann NY Acad Sci 1988;531:123–32.
116. Glavina MJ, Robertshaw R. Myoclonic spasms following intrathecal morphine. Anaesthesia 1988;43(5):389–90.
117. Kleiner LI, Krzeminski J, Rosenwasser RH. Temporary motor and sensory paralysis associated with intrathecal administration of morphine. Neurosurgery 1989; 24(5):756–8.
118. Barron DW, Strong JE. The safety and efficacy of intrathecal diamorphine. Pain 1984;18(3):279–85.
119. Baraka A, Noueihid R, Hajj S. Intrathecal injection of morphine for obstetric analgesia. Anesthesiology 1981;54(2):136–40.
120. Scott PV, Bowen FE, Cartwright P, Rao BC, Deeley D, Wotherspoon HG, Sumrein IM. Intrathecal morphine as sole analgesic during labour. BMJ 1980;281(6236):351–5.
121. Swaraj, Saxena R, Sabzposh SW, Shakoor A. Effect on intrathecal pentazocine on postoperative pain relief. J Indian Med Assoc 1988;86(4):93–6.

Severe fluid retention resistant to furosemide and fluid restriction was observed in 10 patients randomized to receive subcutaneous oprelvekin 50 μg/kg/day to prevent mucositis and acute graft-versus-host disease after allogeneic stem cell transplantation (2). One patient also had a large but reversible increase in serum transaminases.

A preliminary study of the thrombopoietic effect of oprelvekin (50 μg/kg/day for 21 days) in patients with refractory immune thrombocytopenic purpura was halted, since all of the first seven patients had adverse effects without significant changes in the platelet count (3). Adverse effects consisted of conjunctival injection, diffuse aches and joint pains, marked pedal edema, petechiae, and mild anemia. In addition, one patient had a neuropathy, which resolved more than 1 month after oprelvekin withdrawal.

References

1. Dorner AJ, Goldman SJ, Keith JC. Interleukin-11. Biological activity and clinical studies. BioDrugs 1997; 8:418–29.
2. Antin JH, Lee SJ, Neuberg D, Alyea E, Soiffer RJ, Sonis S, Ferrara JL. A phase I/II double-blind, placebo-controlled study of recombinant human interleukin-11 for mucositis and acute GVHD prevention in allogeneic stem cell transplantation. Bone Marrow Transplant 2002;29(5):373–7.
3. Bussel JB, Mukherjee R, Stone AJ. A pilot study of rhuIL-11 treatment of refractory ITP. Am J Hematol 2001; 66(3):172–7.

Orciprenaline

See also Adrenoceptor agonists

General Information

Orciprenaline is somewhat beta$_2$-selective compared with isoprenaline, but is by no means free of cardiac effects (1). Individual susceptibility to these varies, but it would seem that about one individual in 10 will experience tachycardia after usual therapeutic doses. At normal doses (for example 20 mg qds) "jitteriness" and nervousness are not uncommon, and about one patient in 12 suffers from cramps or numbness in the extremities. Lactic acidosis has been described in one patient as a result of concomitant use of orciprenaline, theophylline, and glucocorticoids. Other susceptibility factors and interactions are as for isoprenaline.

Reference

1. Sasaki T, Takishima T, Sugiura R. Comparison of fenoterol and orciprenaline with regard to broncho-dilating action and beta$_2$-selectivity. J Int Med Res 1980;8(3):205–16.

Organic solvents

General Information

Lighter fuels, benzene, toluene, cleaning fluids (carbon tetrachloride), petrol, paraffin, and even the fluorocarbon propellants found in various household sprays and medications have all been used, particularly by children, to produce changes in consciousness. They are all inhaled, often with the aid of a plastic bag, and, since they are lipid-soluble, they are readily concentrated in brain tissue. As with many anesthetics there is an early period of hyperactivity, excitement, and intoxication, followed by sedation and confusion. Prolonged or regular use can cause serious toxicity with bone-marrow depression, cardiac dysrhythmias, peripheral neuropathy, cerebral damage, and liver and kidney disorders (SEDA-12, 37) (1).

Reference

1. Carlan SJ, Stromquist C, Angel JL, Harris M, O'Brien WF. Cocaine and indomethacin: fetal anuria, neonatal edema, and gastrointestinal bleeding. Obstet Gynecol 1991;78(3 Part 2):501–3.

Orgotein

General Information

Orgotein, an enzyme (CuZn superoxide dismutase) that is present in all mammalian cells, is obtained from bovine liver by several steps, including chromatography. It can be given parenterally or topically. Reliable published clinical experience of its properties is limited. In Germany, marketing approval for orgotein was suspended because of severe reactions and deaths, mostly due to hypersensitivity (SEDA-18, 107).

Organs and Systems

Immunologic

Two anaphylactic reactions have been reported, one after intra-articular injection, the other after submucosal bladder injection of orgotein. An IgE-mediated mechanism was demonstrated in the first case (SEDA-12, 94) (SEDA-14, 96).

Drug Administration

Drug administration route

Painful local subcutaneous reactions, erythema, urticaria, and pruritus have been observed after topical administration (1), as have fever and swelling, redness, heat, and pain at the injection site after intravenous administration (2).

References

1. Huber W, Menander-Huber KB. Orgotein. Clin Rheum Dis 1980;6:465.
2. Lund-Olesen K, Menander-Huber KB. Intra-articular orgotein therapy in osteoarthritis of the knee. A double-blind, placebo-controlled trial. Arzneimittelforschung 1983;33(8):1199–203.

Ornidazole

General Information

Used in single large doses for the treatment of *Trichomonas urogenitalis* or *Giardia* infections, ornidazole can cause gastrointestinal symptoms (SEDA-11, 597) (1).

Organs and Systems

Nervous system

- A meningeal syndrome with fever has been reported in a 65-year-old man on the fourth day of administration of ornidazole (500 mg tds) (2). Spontaneous recovery occurred within a few days and without sequelae.

Liver

Ornidazole can cause hepatotoxic damage resembling acute cholestatic hepatitis (3).

References

1. Chaisilwattana P, Bhiraleus P, Patanaparnich P, Bhadrakom C. Double blind comparative study of tinidazole and ornidazole as a single dose treatment of vaginal trichomoniasis. J Med Assoc Thai 1980;63(8):448–53.
2. Mondon M, Ollivier L, Daumont A. Méningite aseptique rapportée a l'ornidazole au cours d'une endocardite infectieuse. [Aseptic meningitis ornidazole-induced in the course of infectious endocarditis.] Rev Med Interne 2002;23(9):784–7.
3. Tabak F, Ozaras R, Erzin Y, Celik AF, Ozbay G, Senturk H. Ornidazole-induced liver damage: report of three cases and review of the literature. Liver Int 2003;23(5):351–4.

Orphenadrine

See also Adrenoceptor agonists

General Information

Orphenadrine is related to an antihistamine (diphenhydramine), and appears to have been developed in the hope of producing a greater effect in Parkinson's disease by combining both anticholinergic and antihistaminic effects in a single molecule.

In the doses commonly used, any of the well-recognized anticholinergic effects can occur. Some patients become drowsy, whilst others are stimulated. With increasing dosages, some patients go into coma; others have agitation, convulsions, and marked euphoria, perhaps with hallucinations and disorientation.

Organs and Systems

Cardiovascular

Non-sustained ventricular tachycardia has been attributed to orphenadrine (1).

- A 57-year-old woman had been taking a formulation containing orphenadrine 15 mg and paracetamol 450 mg bd for musculoskeletal pain. She was also taking propafenone 600 mg/day for paroxysmal atrial fibrillation. After 5 days she developed severe palpitation. Holter monitoring showed frequent brief episodes not only of atrial fibrillation but also of non-sustained ventricular tachycardia. After the orphenadrine was withdrawn the palpitation ceased.

The authors pointed out the potential problems of anticholinergic drugs like orphenadrine in patients taking antidysrhythmic drugs.

Long-Term Effects

Drug abuse

Orphenadrine abuse has been described (SEDA-14, 122).

Drug Administration

Drug overdose

In overdosage, orphenadrine has been stated to be relatively toxic (SEDA-3, 124). Although some patients have survived doses grossly in excess of the usual maximum of 400 mg/day, the therapeutic margin can vary. On occasion doses of as little as 2–3 g have produced a fatal outcome within 6–12 hours. The clinical picture of intoxication tends to be characterized by coma with seizures, apnea, disturbances of cardiac rhythm, and shock; physostigmine should only be used cautiously and preferably after the most severe toxic phase has been overcome (2).

References

1. Dilaveris P, Pantazis A, Vlasseros J, Gialafos J. Non-sustained ventricular tachycardia due to low-dose orphenadrine. Am J Med 2001;111(5):418–19.
2. Sangster B, van Heijst AN, Zimmerman AN. Treatment of orphenadrine overdose. N Engl J Med 1977;296(17):1006.

rheumatoid arthritis: a comparison with aspirin. Semin Arthritis Rheum 1986;15:90.
5. Purdum PP 3rd, Shelden SL, Boyd JW, Shiffman ML. Oxaprozin-induced fulminant hepatitis. Ann Pharmacother 1994;28(10):1159–61.
6. Carucci JA, Cohen DE. Toxic epidermal necrolysis following treatment with oxaprozin. Int J Dermatol 1999;38(3):233–4.
6. Suyama T, Fujiwara H, Takenouchi K, Ito M. Drug eruption and liver injury caused by terfenadine and oxatomide. Eur J Dermatol 2002;12(4):385–6.
7. Origoni M, Ferrari D, Rossi M, Gandini F, Sideri M, Ferrari A. Topical oxatomide: an alternative approach for the treatment of vulvar lichen sclerosus. Int J Gynaecol Obstet 1996;55(3):259–64.

Oxatomide

See also Antihistamines

General Information

Oxatomide is a second-generation antihistamine (SED-12, 371) (SEDA-18, 185) (SEDA-21, 176).

Organs and Systems

Respiratory

In some cases of asthma exacerbation of bronchospasm has occurred when patients have taken oxatomide (1,2).

Nervous system

Oxatomide caused drowsiness in 37–56% of treated patients (3,4).

Liver

Acute cytolytic hepatitis has been attributed to oxatomide (5). An eruption and liver damage has been described in an elderly woman taking several different antihistamines; oral rechallenge with both terfenadine and oxatomide caused erythema, and there was mild liver dysfunction after oxatomide (6).

Skin

When oxatomide was used topically in a gel in 22 patients with vulvar lichen sclerosus, in a concentration sufficient to relieve pruritus, some patients withdrew from treatment because of a burning sensation (7).

References

1. Banham SW, Moran F. A clinical trial of oxatomide in asthma. Br J Clin Pract 1980;34(11–12):323–6.
2. Castaner J. Oxatomide. Drugs Future 1978;3:465.
3. Barlow JL, Beitman RE, Tsai TH. Terfenadine, safety and tolerance in controlled clinical trials. Arzneimittelforschung 1982;32(9a):1215–17.
4. Brompton Hospital/Medical Research Council Collaborative Trial. A controlled trial of oxatomide in the treatment of asthma with or without perennial rhinitis. Clin Allergy 1981;11(5):483–90.
5. De Parades V, Roulot D, Neyrolles N, Rautureau J, Coste T. Hepatite cytolotique au cours de l'administration d'oxatomide. [Acute cytolytic hepatitis during administration of oxatomide.] Gastroenterol Clin Biol 1994;18(3):294.

Oxazepam

See also Benzodiazepines

General Information

Oxazepam is a relatively short-acting benzodiazepine with a half-life of about 9 hours. As well as being used as a drug in its own right, it is a metabolite of temazepam and desmethyldiazepam.

Passiflora incarnata extract has been compared with oxazepam in a double-blind, randomized trial in 26 outpatients with DSM-IV generalized anxiety disorder (1). Both were effective, but oxazepam had a more rapid onset of action and caused significantly more problems relating to work performance.

Organs and Systems

Psychological, psychiatric

An important behavioral adverse effect of benzodiazepines, hostility and aggression in response to provocation, is less common with oxazepam than with its closely related analogue lorazepam (2). In a study of the effects of oxazepam on implicit versus explicit memory processes, as a function of time-course the effects of oxazepam (30 mg) or placebo on directly comparable tests of implicit memory and explicit memory were examined at three times in 60 healthy volunteers. Before the plasma concentration had peaked, oxazepam impaired cued recall performance relative to placebo but did not impair priming. At the time of the peak, oxazepam impaired performance in both memory tasks. After the peak, cued recall performance in the oxazepam group remained significantly impaired relative to placebo. However, oxazepam-induced impairments in priming were only marginal, suggesting that oxazepam-induced impairments in implicit memory processes begin to wane after theoretical peak drug concentrations. The results support the hypothesis that benzodiazepines cause impaired implicit memory processes time-dependently (3).

In 30 subjects who were given an acute dose of oxazepam 30 mg, lorazepam 2 mg, or placebo, both drugs impaired explicit memory relative to placebo. Also, both oxazepam and lorazepam impaired priming performance. The results suggested that episodic memory is time-dependently impaired by both benzodiazepines (4).

References

1. Akhondzadeh S, Naghavi HR, Vazirian M, Shayeganpour A, Rashidi H, Khani M. Passionflower in the treatment of

generalized anxiety: a pilot double-blind randomized controlled trial with oxazepam. J Clin Pharm Ther 2001;26(5):363–7.
2. Bond A. Drug induced behavioural disinhibition. CNS Drugs 1998;9:41–57.
3. Buffett-Jerrott SE, Stewart SH, Bird S, Teehan MD. An examination of differences in the time course of oxazepam's effects on implicit vs explicit memory. J Psychopharmacol 1998;12(4):338–47.
4. Buffett-Jerrott SE, Stewart SH, Teehan MD. A further examination of the time-dependent effects of oxazepam and lorazepam on implicit and explicit memory. Psychopharmacology (Berl) 1998;138(3–4):344–53.

Oxazolidinones

General Information

The oxazolidinones have a unique mechanism of action, involving inhibition of the first step in protein synthesis. The first marketed member of the class, linezolid, has inhibitory activity against a broad range of Gram-positive bacteria, including methicillin-resistant *Staphylococcus aureus* (MRSA), glycopeptide-intermediate *Staphylococcus aureus* (GISA), vancomycin-resistant enterococci (VRE), and penicillin-resistant *Streptococcus pneumoniae*. It also has activity against certain anerobes, including *Clostridium perfringens*, *Clostridium difficile*, *Peptostreptococcus* species, and *Bacteroides fragilis*. The most frequently reported adverse effects are diarrhea, headache, nausea and vomiting, insomnia, constipation, rash, and dizziness; thrombocytopenia has also been documented in a few patients (about 2%) (1,2).

In controlled phase III studies, linezolid was as effective as vancomycin in patients with infections caused by MRSA and VRE. It is effective both intravenously and orally. Although technically classified as bacteriostatic against a number of pathogens in vitro, linezolid behaves in vivo like a bactericidal antibiotic.

The pharmacokinetics of linezolid in adults are not altered by hepatic or renal function, age, or sex to an extent that requires dose adjustment. Linezolid is metabolized via morpholine ring oxidation, which is independent of CYP450; linezolid is therefore unlikely to interact with medications that induce or inhibit CYP450 enzymes. Plasma linezolid trough concentrations after a 1-hour infusion of 600 mg bd were 0.54–5.3 μg/ml and CSF linezolid trough concentrations were 1.46–7.0 μg/ml; the ratio between CSF and plasma linezolid trough concentrations always exceeded 1 (mean, 1.6; range 1.2–2.3) (3). There was good rapid penetration of linezolid into bone, fat, and muscle (4,5). The mean peak plasma concentration of linezolid was 18.3 μg/ml in six healthy men who took 600 mg orally every 12 hours for five doses. There was good penetration into inflammatory fluid (6,7).

General adverse effects

Linezolid is generally well tolerated (8–10). The most frequently reported adverse events were diarrhea, headache, nausea and vomiting, insomnia, constipation, rash, and dizziness. Thrombocytopenia was also documented in few patients (about 2%). In a phase II, open, multicenter study of intravenous linezolid followed by oral linezolid suspension, both in a dose of 10 mg/kg every 12 hours in 66 children, the most common adverse effects were diarrhea (10%), neutropenia (6.4%), and raised alanine transaminase activity (6.4%) (11).

In children the common adverse events have been similar to those found in adults, although thrombocytopenia has not been as common (12).

Organs and Systems

Nervous system

Peripheral and optic neuropathy occurred in a 76-year-old man after he had taken linezolid for about 6 months (13).

Hematologic

Linezolid has been associated with reversible myelosuppression (14), which appears to be related to the duration of therapy, with a higher risk after more than 2 consecutive weeks of treatment (15). Myelosuppression with red cell hypoplasia has been reported in three patients taking linezolid 600 mg bd. The bone marrow changes were similar to those seen in reversible chloramphenicol toxicity. Another patient had sideroblastic anemia after taking linezolid for 2 months (16,17).

- Red cell hypoplasia and thrombocytopenia occurred in a 66-year old man who took linezolid 600 mg bd (18).
- Reversible pure red blood cell aplasia occurred in a 52-year-old black man who had taken linezolid for 8 weeks (19).

Pancytopenia in two cases was reported with linezolid 600 mg bd (20).

In 19 patients there was thrombocytopenia in six of those who had taken it for more than 10 days; gastrointestinal bleeding was observed in one patient and four required platelet transfusions (21). Of 71 patients who took linezolid for 1–44 days, 48 took it for more than 5 days; among those 48, thrombocytopenia, with a 32–89% reduction in platelet count, occurred in 23; the platelet count fell to below 100×10^9/l in nine (22).

Susceptibility Factors

Age

In single-dose pharmacokinetic studies children had a greater plasma clearance (0.34 l/hour/kg for children aged 3 months to 16 years) than adults (0.10 l/hour/kg) (12).

Drug–Drug Interactions

Selective serotonin re-uptake inhibitors (SSRIs)

Serotonin syndrome was reported in a 56-year-old white woman who received intravenous linezolid shortly after withdrawal of a selective serotonin reuptake inhibitor, paroxetine (23).

Phenytoin

In human liver microsomes with cDNA-expressed CYP2C19, oxcarbazepine and its 10-monohydroxy metabolite inhibited CYP2C19-mediated phenytoin metabolism at therapeutic concentrations (22). Thus, co-administration of oxcarbazepine with phenytoin could significantly increase serum phenytoin concentrations.

Steroid oral contraceptives

In a placebo-controlled study in healthy women, oxcarbazepine 900 mg/day reduced the serum concentrations of ethinylestradiol and levonorgestrel by about 50% (23). This confirms that oxcarbazepine may reduce the efficacy of the contraceptive pill, as does carbamazepine. Women taking oxcarbazepine should be given a contraceptive that contains 50 μg of ethinylestradiol and they should be monitored for signs of insufficient contraceptive cover, such as breakthrough bleeding.

Warfarin

Oxcarbazepine does not modify the anticoagulant activity of warfarin (17).

References

1. Perucca E. The new generation of antiepileptic drugs: advantages and disadvantages. Br J Clin Pharmacol 1996;42(5):531–43.
2. Schachter SC. The next wave of anticonvulsants: focus on levetiracetam, oxcarbazepine and zonisamide. CNS Drugs 2000;14:229–49.
3. Anonymous. Two new drugs for epilepsy. Med Lett Drugs Ther 2000;42(1076):33–5.
4. Lott RS, Helmboldt K. A carbamazepine analogue for partial seizures in adults and children with epilepsy Formulary 2000;35:219–33.
5. Shorvon S. Oxcarbazepine: a review. Seizure 2000; 9(2):75–9.
6. Kramer G. Oxcarbazepine (Trileptal): a new antiepileptic drug for mono- and add-on-therapy. Aktuel Neurol 2000;27:59–71.
7. Barcs G, Walker EB, Elger CE, Scaramelli A, Stefan H, Sturm Y, Moore A, Flesch G, Kramer L, D'Souza J. Oxcarbazepine placebo-controlled, dose-ranging trial in refractory partial epilepsy. Epilepsia 2000;41(12):1597–607.
8. Beydoun A, Sachdeo RC, Rosenfeld WE, Krauss GL, Sessler N, Mesenbrink P, Kramer L, D'Souza J. Oxcarbazepine monotherapy for partial-onset seizures: a multicenter, double-blind, clinical trial. Neurology 2000;54(12):2245–51.
9. Glauser TA, Nigro M, Sachdeo R, Pasteris LA, Weinstein S, Abou-Khalil B, Frank LM, Grinspan A, Guarino T, Bettis D, Kerrigan J, Geoffroy G, Mandelbaum D, Jacobs T, Mesenbrink P, Kramer L, D'Souza J. Adjunctive therapy with oxcarbazepine in children with partial seizures. The Oxcarbazepine Pediatric Study Group. Neurology 2000;54(12):2237–44.
10. Sachdeo R, Beydoun A, Schachter S, Vazquez B, Schaul N, Mesenbrink P, Kramer L, D'Souza J. Oxcarbazepine (Trileptal) as monotherapy in patients with partial seizures. Neurology 2001;57(5):864–71.
11. Gatzonis SD, Georgaculias N, Singounas E, Jenkins A, Stamboulis E, Siafakas A. Elimination of oxcarbazepine-induced oculogyric crisis following vagus nerve stimulation. Neurology 1999;52(9):1918–19.
12. Schmidt D, Arroyo S, Baulac M, Dam M, Dulac O, Friis ML, Kalviainen R, Kramer G, van Parys J, Pedersen B, Sachdeo R. Recommendations on the clinical use of oxcarbazepine in the treatment of epilepsy: a consensus view. Acta Neurol Scand 2001;104(3):167–70.
13. Sachdeo RC, Wassertein AG, D'Souza J. Oxcarbazepine (Trileptal) effect on serum sodium. Epilepsia 1999;40(Suppl 7):103.
14. Isojarvi JI, Huuskonen UE, Pakarinen AJ, Vuolteenaho O, Myllyla VV. The regulation of serum sodium after replacing carbamazepine with oxcarbazepine. Epilepsia 2001; 42(6):741–5.
15. Sachdeo RC, Wasserstein A, Mesenbrink PJ, D'Souza J. Effects of oxcarbazepine on sodium concentration and water handling. Ann Neurol 2002;51(5):613–20.
16. Pierach CA. Oxcarbazepine and hepatic porphyria. Epilepsia 2002;43(4):455.
17. Baruzzi A, Albani F, Riva R. Oxcarbazepine: pharmacokinetic interactions and their clinical relevance. Epilepsia 1994;35(Suppl 3):S14–19.
18. Raitasuo V, Lehtovaara R, Huttunen MO. Effect of switching carbamazepine to oxcarbazepine on the plasma levels of neuroleptics. A case report. Psychopharmacology (Berl) 1994;116(1):115–16.
19. Rosche J, Froscher W, Abendroth D, Liebel J. Possible oxcarbazepine interaction with cyclosporine serum levels: a single case study. Clin Neuropharmacol 2001;24(2):113–16.
20. Zaccara G, Gangemi PF, Bendoni L, Menge GP, Schwabe S, Monza GC. Influence of single and repeated doses of oxcarbazepine on the pharmacokinetic profile of felodipine. Ther Drug Monit 1993;15(1):39–42.
21. May TW, Rambeck B, Jurgens U. Influence of oxcarbazepine and methsuximide on lamotrigine concentrations in epileptic patients with and without valproic acid comedication: results of a retrospective study. Ther Drug Monit 1999;21(2):175–81.
22. Lakehal F, Wurden CJ, Kalhorn TF, Levy RH. Carbamazepine and oxcarbazepine decrease phenytoin metabolism through inhibition of CYP2C19. Epilepsy Res 2002;52(2):79–83.
23. Fattore C, Cipolla G, Gatti G, Limido GL, Sturm Y, Bernasconi C, Perucca E. Induction of ethinylestradiol and levonorgestrel metabolism by oxcarbazepine in healthy women. Epilepsia 1999;40(6):783–7.

Oxitropium

See also Anticholinergic drugs

General Information

Oxitropium is an anticholinergic drug that is used in the treatment of asthma.

In a single blind, randomized, crossover study, in 12 patients the bronchodilator effects of salmeterol 50 micrograms and oxitropium 200 and 400 micrograms were compared with placebo. All treatments were taken from a metered dose inhaler. The peak effect of salmeterol was delayed but the effect was more prolonged than the effect of oxitropium. The response to salmeterol 50 micrograms exceeded the response to oxitropium 200 micrograms over 12 hours. Between 3 and 12 hours the response to salmeterol was greater than the response to oxitropium 400 micrograms, but the difference was not significant. There were no significant changes in pulse rate, blood pressure, or the electrocardiogram with any of the four treatments. No patients complained of adverse symptoms and none noticed any difference in the taste of the different inhalers (1).

Organs and Systems

Immunologic

Total serum IgE has been measured in 36 patients with allergic rhinitis and 11 healthy subjects given a submaximal dose of oxitropium bromide 600 micrograms by inhalation (2). FEV_1 was greater than 80% of predicted in all subjects. Baseline FEV_1 correlated negatively with serum IgE concentration. Oxitropium bromide inhalation produced an increase in FEV_1 (mean 155 ml) that was significantly greater in allergic patients with high serum IgE than in healthy subjects (64 ml) or in those with allergic rhinitis and low serum IgE (82 ml). The effect of an inhaled $beta_2$-adrenoceptor agonist (orciprenaline) was similar in all three groups. These findings may explain some of the variation in response to inhaled antimuscarinic drugs in patients with asthma. The data also suggested that IgE may itself modify airway tone by an increase in cholinergic responsiveness.

References

1. Cazzola M, Matera MG, Di Perna F, Calderaro F, Califano C, Vinciguerra A. A comparison of bronchodilating effects of salmeterol and oxitropium bromide in stable chronic obstructive pulmonary disease. Respir Med 1998;92(2):354–7.
2. Endoh N, Ichinose M, Takahashi T, Miura M, Kageyama N, Mashito Y, Sugiura H, Ikeda K, Takasaka T, Shirato K. Relationship between cholinergic airway tone and serum immunoglobulin E in human subjects. Eur Respir J 1998;12(1):71–4.

Oxolamine

General Information

Oxolamine citrate is a synthetic derivative of 3,5-disubstituted 1,2,4-oxodiazole. It has been used to treat cough in some European countries for more than two decades.

Organs and Systems

Psychological, psychiatric

Evidence has accumulated that oxolamine can cause hallucinations in children, especially those under 10 years of age (1,2); some cases have been confirmed by re-exposure to the drug.

References

1. Anonymous. Hallucinaties door oxolamine (Bredon). Bull Bijwerk Geneesmd 1986;2:10–11.
2. McEwen J, Meyboom RH, Thijs I. Hallucinations in children caused by oxolamine citrate. Med J Aust 1989;150(8):449–50.

Oxybuprocaine

See also Local anesthetics

General Information

Oxybuprocaine is an ester of para-aminobenzoic acid. It is a popular local anesthetic for use in ophthalmology.

Organs and Systems

Cardiovascular

An episode of severe bradycardia, with no perceptible cardiac output, was reported in a previously healthy patient after one drop of 0.4% oxybuprocaine was applied to each eye (1).

Sensory systems

When used in the eye, oxybuprocaine can enter the anterior chamber, and fibrinous iritis and moderate corneal swelling have been described (SED-12, 257) (2). Abuse has often been reported and can lead to keratopathy, severe visual impairment, and even enucleation (3).

Skin

There have been two reports of patients scheduled for tonometry who developed periorbital dermatitis following the topical instillation of local anesthetic eye drops (4). The first patient reacted strongly positive on patch testing to Thilorbin AT (oxybuprocaine, fluorescein, phenylmercuric borate, polysorbate 20, mannitol) and also to oxybuprocaine alone. The second reacted to Conjucain EDO (oxybuprocaine, sorbitol, sodium hydroxide) and to oxybuprocaine alone. The authors believed these to be the only described cases of a delayed hypersensitivity reaction to oxybuprocaine, an ester local anesthetic commonly used for topical anesthesia in the eye.

References

1. Christensen C. Bradycardia as a side-effect to oxybuprocaine. Acta Anaesthesiol Scand 1990;34(2):165–6.
2. Haddad R. Fibrinous iritis due to oxybuprocaine. Br J Ophthalmol 1989;73(1):76–7.
3. Rosenwasser GO, Holland S, Pflugfelder SC, Lugo M, Heidemann DG, Culbertson WW, Kattan H. Topical anesthetic abuse. Ophthalmology 1990;97(8):967–72.
4. Blaschke V, Fuchs T. Periorbital allergic contact dermatitis from oxybuprocaine. Contact Dermatitis 2001;44(3):198.

Hepatic disease

In end-stage cirrhosis, reduced clearance and prolonged half-life of oxycodone may necessitate dosage reduction (SEDA-22, 101).

Drug Administration

Drug formulations

A double-blind, randomized, crossover comparison of modified-release or immediate-release oxycodone has been carried out in 30 patients with cancer pain (8). There were no significant differences between the two groups with respect to pain intensity or acceptability of therapy. More than 80% of the patients did not require rescue medication. Adverse effects were similar with the two formulations and occurred in relatively low numbers compared with previous morphine studies. The greatest difference in adverse effects was in the incidence of vomiting, which occurred in 6% of those given immediate-release morphine, and none of those given modified-release morphine. The modified-release formulation provided equal analgesia with the benefit of less frequent dosing.

In a systematic review of the safety and efficacy of modified-release oxycodone 16 trials were identified; 7 addressed the safety and efficacy of oxycodone for the treatment of non-cancer pain (9). In these studies, modified-release oxycodone offered no significant advantage over immediate-release oxycodone. There was no consistent beneficial effect on quality of life, despite adequate analgesia. Opioid adverse effects, such as constipation, nausea, vomiting, and drowsiness, were more frequent and severe with oxycodone than with placebo. In six studies, modified-release oxycodone was compared with immediate-release oxycodone in cancer and non-cancer pain. In only one study was modified-release oxycodone superior; in the other five there were no significant differences in analgesic effect. In five randomized, double-blind comparisons there was no advantage in analgesic efficacy nor a consistent reduction in adverse effects with modified-release oxycodone compared with modified-release morphine, hydromorphone, or methadone.

Drug administration route

Oxycodone has been available in oral form for at least 70 years and is rarely given by other routes. In a study of subcutaneous oxycodone hydrochloride 100 mg/ml for opioid rotation in 63 patients with cancer pain (maximum dose 4.5–660 mg in 24 hours for 1–49 days) there was local toxicity in only two cases, and this included central pallor of the skin at the needle site with surrounding erythema and bruising; there was no necrosis (10). The design of the study made it difficult to compare the adverse effects profile of subcutaneous oxycodone with oral oxycodone or other opioids. Randomized controlled trials are needed to support the conclusions that subcutaneous oxycodone is free from adverse effects and is a better vehicle for analgesia in terminal cancer.

References

1. Levanen J. Ketamine and oxycodone in the management of postoperative pain. Mil Med 2000;165(6):450–5.
2. Roth SH, Fleischmann RM, Burch FX, Dietz F, Bockow B, Rapoport RJ, Rutstein J, Lacouture PG. Around-the-clock, controlled-release oxycodone therapy for osteoarthritis-related pain: placebo-controlled trial and long-term evaluation. Arch Intern Med 2000;160(6):853–60.
3. Hale ME, Fleischmann R, Salzman R, Wild J, Iwan T, Swanton RE, Kaiko RF, Lacouture PG. Efficacy and safety of controlled-release versus immediate-release oxycodone: randomized, double-blind evaluation in patients with chronic back pain. Clin J Pain 1999;15(3):179–83.
4. Watson CP, Babul N. Efficacy of oxycodone in neuropathic pain: a randomized trial in postherpetic neuralgia. Neurology 1998;50(6):1837–41.
5. Kaplan R, Parris WC, Citron ML, Zhukovsky D, Reder RF, Buckley BJ, Kaiko RF. Comparison of controlled-release and immediate-release oxycodone tablets in patients with cancer pain. J Clin Oncol 1998;16(10):3230–7.
6. Bruera E, Belzile M, Pituskin E, Fainsinger R, Darke A, Harsanyi Z, Babul N, Ford I. Randomized, double-blind, cross-over trial comparing safety and efficacy of oral controlled-release oxycodone with controlled-release morphine in patients with cancer pain. J Clin Oncol 1998; 16(10):3222–9.
7. Fishbain DA, Goldberg M, Rosomoff RS, Rosomoff H. Atypical oxycodone withdrawal syndrome. Pain Management 1989;Mar/Apr:76.
8. Stambaugh JE, Reder RF, Stambaugh MD, Stambaugh H, Davis M. Double-blind, randomized comparison of the analgesic and pharmacokinetic profiles of controlled- and immediate-release oral oxycodone in cancer pain patients. J Clin Pharmacol 2001;41(5):500–6.
9. Rischitelli DG, Karbowicz SH. Safety and efficacy of controlled-release oxycodone: a systematic literature review. Pharmacotherapy 2002;22(7):898–904.
10. Gagnon B, Bielech M, Watanabe S, Walker P, Hanson J, Bruera E. The use of intermittent subcutaneous injections of oxycodone for opioid rotation in patients with cancer pain. Support Care Cancer 1999;7(4):265–70.

Oxyfedrine

See also Adrenoceptor agonists

General Information

Oxyfedrine is a vasodilator and has been used in angina pectoris and myocardial infarction.

Organs and Systems

Sensory systems

Impairment of the sense of taste is a particular complication of oxyfedrine therapy; 21 such cases have been reviewed since 1985 (1) and they continue to be reported to national monitoring centers. This adverse effect usually occurs within 4 weeks after the start of therapy and is slowly reversible after the drug is withdrawn.

Reference

1. von Rudiger F, Lantzsch W. Schmeckstörungen als Nebenwirkung des Myofedrin. HNO Praxis 1985;10:201.

Oxygen

General Information

The duration and extent of hyperoxygenation during anesthesia are generally limited. However, in intensive care, a patient's exposure to oxygen can become prolonged and dangerous. Oxygen toxicity can cause adverse effects in numerous tissues, including the lungs, nervous system, eyes, red blood cells, and liver, because of their susceptibility to chemical toxicity by mechanisms such as lipid peroxidation (SED-12, 242) (1).

Organs and Systems

Respiratory

The adverse effects of high-dose oxygen on the lungs take the form of an initial exudation of blood and fibrinous fluid into the alveoli followed by proliferation of fibroblasts and alveolar cells (2). The proliferative phase can be permanent (3). It is reflected in a reduced vital capacity and a reduced diffusion capacity (4) and appears to be proportional to the units of pulmonary toxic dose (UPTD) administered; 1 UPTD is equivalent to 1 absolute atmosphere × 1 minute of exposure. If exposure exceeds 1000 UPTD it can be difficult to predict the outcome (5), owing to inter-patient differences in susceptibility.

Nervous system

High doses of oxygen can cause convulsant activity resembling tonic-clonic seizures (6) and is associated with reduced concentrations of GABA in the brain. Such fits may not be apparent in sedated patients.

Sensory systems

Oxygen toxicity in the eye can cause tunnel vision by an effect on the retina (7) and, in neonates, retrolental fibroplasia (8) (SED-12, 242).

Hematologic

Oxygen toxicity in red blood cells can cause hemolysis (SED-12, 242) (9).

References

1. Kovachich GB, Haugaard N. Biochemical aspects of oxygen toxicity in the metazoa. In: Gilbert DL, editor. Oxygen and the Living Processes: An Inter-Disciplinary Approach. New York: Springer Verlag, 1981:210.
2. Nash G, Blennerhassett JB, Pontoppidan H. Pulmonary lesions associated with oxygen therapy and artifical ventilation. N Engl J Med 1967;276(7):368–74.

3. Kapanci Y, Tosco R, Eggermann J, Gould VE. Oxygen pneumonitis in man. Light- and electron-microscopic morphometric studies. Chest 1972;62(2):162–9.
4. Clark JM, Lambertsen CJ. Pulmonary oxygen toxicity: a review. Pharmacol Rev 1971;23(2):37–133.
5. Wright WB. Use of the University of Pennsylvania Institute for Environmental Medicine procedure for calculation of pulmonary oxygen toxicity. US Navy Exp Diving Unit Rep 1972;2:72.
6. Donald KW. Oxygen poisoning in man. I and II. BMJ 1947;1:667, 712.
7. Behnke AR, Forbes HS, Motley EP. Circulatory and visual effects of oxygen at 3 atmosphere pressure. Am J Physiol 1935;114:436.
8. Nichols CW, Lambertsen C. Effects of high oxygen pressures on the eye. N Engl J Med 1969;281(1):25–30.
9. Larkin EC, Adams JD, Williams WT, Duncan DM. Hematologic responses to hypobaric hyperoxia. Am J Physiol 1972;223(2):431–7.

Oxygen-carrying blood substitutes

General Information

The development of oxygen-carrying blood substitutes, which can act as alternatives for allogenic erythrocyte transfusions, has progressed significantly in the last decade. It is important for the laboratory medicine community to be aware of their effects on routine laboratory testing and the settings in which they might be used (1).

The characteristics of an ideal emulsion for use as a blood substitute are absence of red cell incompatibility, absence of a risk of transmission of infectious diseases, a long duration of conservation, easy access, and rheological parameters similar to those of blood (2).

Oxygen carriers can be divided into two classes: hemoglobin-based oxygen carriers, prepared from hemoglobin of human or bovine origin, and synthetic perfluorocarbons.

Hemoglobin-based oxygen carriers

There are three sources of hemoglobin from which oxygen carriers have been developed: human, bovine, and recombinant. Hemoglobin-based oxygen carriers have benefits, such as the lack of pathogen transmission, no need for cross-matching, and increased stability and storage time; however, compared with erythrocyte transfusions, they have a short half-life. Of various hemoglobin-based oxygen carriers under development, two (Polyheme and Hemopure) have been tested in phase III studies. One product, Hemopure—polymerized hemoglobin of bovine origin—has been licensed for human use in South Africa. The tetrameric hemoglobin easily dissociates in vivo into dimers and monomers that are quickly eliminated by the kidneys. As the administration of tetrameric hemoglobin is associated with renal insufficiency, intermolecular cross-linking of hemoglobin has been performed using different agents to polymerize hemoglobin. Newly developed hemoglobin-based oxygen carriers are conjugated hemoglobin or packed hemoglobin in nanocapsules or lipid vesicles (3–6).

Perfluorocarbons

Perfluorocarbons are synthetic, fluorinated hydrocarbons that increase the amount of oxygen dissolved in the fluid phase of the blood. Perfluorocarbon emulsions are heavy, low-viscosity liquids, inert, and optically clear, with a high specific gravity and good surface tension. Their chemical and physical properties make them a suitable temporary intraoperative tool to flatten the retina during surgery, and they have gained wide acceptance in the surgical management of complicated retinal detachment (7). Perfluorocarbons have a transport capacity that is greater than that of blood under hyperoxic conditions (2).

The available formulations include perfluoro-octyl bromide, perfluoro-octylethane, perfluorodichloro-octane, Fluosol-DA (70% perfluorodecalin plus 30% perfluorotripropylamine), Oxygent™ (perflubron, perfluoro-octyl bromide) (5), and LiquiVent (perflubron). Second-generation perfluorocarbons are now used in anemia, trauma, high blood loss surgery, perioperative hemodilution, ischemia, and organ conservation for transplantation. Phase III studies of one of the perfluorocarbons, Oxygent™, are proceeding in cases in which tissue oxygenation is required and when it is desirable to avoid allogeneic blood transfusion.

General adverse effects

Hemoglobin-based oxygen carriers

Hemoglobin-based oxygen carriers bind endogenous nitric oxide, thereby causing transient hypertension, esophageal dysfunction, and abdominal discomfort. In a phase II study using *O*-raffinose cross-linked hemoglobin (Hemolink™) in patients undergoing coronary artery bypass grafting surgery raised blood pressure, probably caused by binding of *O*-raffinose cross-linked hemoglobin to nitric oxide, and jaundice were observed (8). Jaundice was expected, owing to metabolism of cell-free hemoglobin.

Perfluorocarbons

Perfluorocarbon blood substitutes are reported to have several adverse effects, the clinical significance of which is not currently fully understood. They include a dose-related, flu-like illness 4–6 hours after infusion (2,9). Symptoms included back pain, malaise, flushing, and transient fever (10); arterial hypotension, tachycardia, a high leukocyte count, and thrombocytopenia can also occur. These symptoms are most likely cytokine-mediated, as the perfluorocarbon particles are cleared by cells of the reticuloendothelial system (11). The most important adverse effect of LiquiVent is the risk of intravascular passage of the perfluorocarbon. Phagocytosis by alveolar macrophages has been demonstrated by cytology. Larger doses of emulsion particles can lead to hepatic engorgement and temporary impairment of immune defences (2).

Third-generation emulsions are currently in early preclinical development (2). The absence of toxicity of these new emulsions has been demonstrated in endothelial cell cultures and in animal organ preservation studies.

In a phase II study in 25 patients undergoing ardiac surgery a perflubron emulsion (AF0144) was well tolerated (12).

Organs and Systems

Cardiovascular

A modified hemoglobin solution, DCLHb, has been associated with an increase in mean arterial pressure. This has been proposed to be due to binding to nitric oxide, stimulation of the production of endothelin, and sensitization and/or potentiation of beta-1 and beta-2 adrenoceptor responses to catecholamines (2).

It has been suggested that cell-free hemoglobin, particularly low molecular weight hemoglobin, such as tetrameric hemoglobin, has the ability to come more closely to the endothelial cell lining of blood vessels than erythrocytes and to extravasate into the subendothelial space. There, hemoglobin might scavenge nitrous oxide and so induce vasoconstriction and hypertension (3,5,9). A randomized, controlled phase II study has suggested that hemoglobin raffimer (Hemolink) is safe and effective in patients undergoing coronary artery bypass surgery. The incidence of hypertension was higher in the treated group, but blood pressure management prevented serious hypertension-related events (13).

Another hemoglobin substitution product, liposome-encapsulated tetrameric hemoglobin, can exacerbate the manifestations of septic shock (2).

Respiratory

In premature neonates and children with respiratory distress syndrome treated with a perfluorocarbon, pneumothorax has been observed (2).

Sensory systems

Corneal epithelial damage has been attributed to a perfluorocarbon (14).

- An elderly man underwent vitreoretinal surgery for retinal detachment. Perfluorodecalin was used to repair the retina and was left in situ for 8 weeks and removed via the pars plana. One month later he developed a non-healing corneal epithelial defect associated with limbitis. Perfluorodecalin was found under the superior conjunctiva. A biopsy showed vacuoles in the conjunctival stroma surrounded by inflammatory cells. On surgical removal of the perfluorodecalin from the subconjunctival space, the epithelial defect healed.

Although the high surface tension of perfluorocarbons allows closure of retinal breaks and prevents them from flowing into the subretinal space, particularly during intraocular manipulation, they can gain entry into the subretinal space, resulting in residues in the eye (15,16). The removal of perfluorocarbons is recommended at the end of surgery, but they can be left in the eye for limited periods of time (17).

- A 29-year-old man with a high degree of myopia developed a rhegmatogenous retinal detachment due to a giant retinal tear following blunt trauma (18). After surgical treatment perfluorodecalin was left in the eye as a tamponade; 2 weeks later it was removed and 20% sulfahexafluoride was injected. On the following day the retina was flat and residual perfluorodecalin was not detected in the vitreous cavity. A week later he developed severe pain in the operated eye and his vision worsened. There was a marked cellular response in the vitreous cavity and total retinal detachment. Examination with retroillumination showed that there was residual perfluorocarbon trapped in the retrolental space. There also appeared to be a precipitate of pigmented cells adherent to the vitreous surface of the posterior lens capsule, as seen on slit lamp biomicroscopy. Posterior capsulotomy removed the obstruction caused by the deposits, confirming the suspicion of the site of the pigmentary infiltration. A small amount of heavy liquid was found subretinally and removed. Although retinal reattachment was not possible due to very severe proliferative vitreoretinopathy, the intravitreal inflammation resolved.

Hematologic

Administration of erythrocytes can cause neutrophil priming, which leads to a dysfunctional inflammatory response. This neutrophil priming, which has been associated with the occurrence of multiple organ failure after trauma, was not observed after administration of Polyheme, a glutaraldehyde-cross-linked hemoglobin product (3).

In a randomized, double-blind, placebo-controlled study in healthy volunteers coagulation responses (using bleeding time) and hemostasis were examined for 14 days after dosing with either saline or perfluorocarbon emulsion (1.2 or 1.8 g/kg) (19). There were no postinfusion changes in bleeding time or differences in in vivo agonist-induced platelet aggregation. There was a fall in platelet count, but this recovered to baseline within 7 days. The intravascular half-life of perfluorocarbon for the first 24 hours was dose-dependent (9.4 hours and 6.1 hours with 1.8 and 1.2 g/kg respectively). The authors concluded that perfluorocarbon does not affect coagulation, at least in healthy volunteers.

Transient thrombocytopenia can occur 3–4 days after perfluorocarbon (10). In several studies the fall in platelet count was 30–40%, and platelet counts returned to normal in 7–10 days. The use of radioactively labelled platelets showed increased platelet clearance, thought to be due to alteration of the platelet surface by the perfluorocarbon emulsion.

Gastrointestinal

Occasionally, gastrointestinal disorders have been related to the use of hemoglobin-based oxygen carriers, possibly through binding of nitrous oxide, causing gastrointestinal smooth muscle spasm (9,20).

Liver

In a single-blind, randomized study, four of 55 surgical patients who were treated with Hemopure developed jaundice without an increase in serum bilirubin (21). Similarly, in a double-blind, randomized study of 98 patients undergoing cardiac surgery, Hemopure was related to some cases of jaundice (22).

Urinary tract

Purification of haemoglobin avoids free hemoglobin, which can cause nephrotoxicity (2).

Skin

In a single-blind, randomized study, two of 55 surgical patients who were treated with Hemopure had ecchymotic rashes (21).

Immunologic

Hemoglobin solutions do not have the antigenic properties of the blood groups.

Drug Administration

Drug contamination

The main limitation of bovine hemoglobin is the risk of transmission of bovine spongiform encephalopathy and the development of antibodies to bovine proteins (2).

References

1. Scott MG, Kucik DF, Goodnough LT, Monk TG. Blood substitutes: evolution and future applications. Clin Chem 1997;43(9):1724–31.
2. Remy B, Deby-Dupont G, Lamy M. Red blood cell substitutes: fluorocarbon emulsions and haemoglobin solutions. Br Med Bull 1999;55(1):277–98.
3. Stowell CP. Hemoglobin-based oxygen carriers. Curr Opin Hematol 2002;9(6):537–43.
4. Squires JE. Artificial blood. Science 2002;295(5557):1002–5.
5. Chang TM. Oxygen carriers. Curr Opin Investig Drugs 2002;3(8):1187–90.
6. Winslow RM. Blood substitutes. Curr Opin Hematol 2002;9(2):146–51.
7. Blinder KJ, Peyman GA, Desai UR, Nelson NC Jr, Alturki W, Paris CL. Vitreon, a short-term vitreoretinal tamponade. Br J Ophthalmol 1992;76(9):525–8.
8. Cheng DC. Safety and efficacy of O-raffinose cross-linked human hemoglobin (Hemolink) in cardiac surgery. Can J Anaesth 2001;48(Suppl 4):S41–8.
9. Jahr JS, Nesargi SB, Lewis K, Johnson C. Blood substitutes and oxygen therapeutics: an overview and current status. Am J Ther 2002;9(5):437–43.
10. Spence RK. Perfluorocarbons in the twenty-first century: clinical applications as transfusion alternatives. Artif Cells Blood Substit Immobil Biotechnol 1995;23(3):367–80.
11. Flaim SF, Hazard DR, Hogan J, Peters RM. Characterization and mechanism of side-effects of Oxygent HT in swine. Biomater Artif Cells Immobilization Biotechnol 1991;19:383–5.
12. Hill SE, Leone BJ, Faithfull NS, Flaim KE, Keipert PE, Newman MF. Perflubron emulsion (AF0144) augments harvesting of autologous blood: a phase II study in cardiac surgery. J Cardiothorac Vasc Anesth 2002;16(5):555–60.
13. Hill SE, Gottschalk LI, Grichnik K. Safety and preliminary efficacy of hemoglobin raffimer for patients undergoing coronary artery bypass surgery. J Cardiothorac Vasc Anesth 2002;16(6):695–702.
14. Ramaesh K, Bhagat S, Wharton SB, Singh J. Corneal epithelial toxic effects and inflammatory response to

perfluorocarbon liquid. Arch Ophthalmol 1999;117(10): 1411–13.
15. Chang S, Ozmert E, Zimmerman NJ. Intraoperative perfluorocarbon liquids in the management of proliferative vitreoretinopathy. Am J Ophthalmol 1988;106(6):668–74.
16. Chang S, Reppucci V, Zimmerman NJ, Heinemann MH, Coleman DJ. Perfluorocarbon liquids in the management of traumatic retinal detachments. Ophthalmology 1989; 96(6):785–91.
17. Kertes PJ, Wafapoor H, Peyman GA, Calixto N Jr, Thompson H. The management of giant retinal tears using perfluoroperhydrophenanthrene. A multicenter case series. Vitreon Collaborative Study Group. Ophthalmology 1997;104(7):1159–65.
18. Singh J, Ramaesh K, Wharton SB, Cormack G, Chawla HB. Perfluorodecalin-induced intravitreal inflammation. Retina 2001;21(3):247–51.
19. Leese PT, Noveck RJ, Shorr JS, Woods CM, Flaim KE, Keipert PE. Randomized safety studies of intravenous perflubron emulsion. I. Effects on coagulation function in healthy volunteers. Anesth Analg 2000;91(4):804–11.
20. Anonymous. Human haemoglobin—Hemosol: Hemolink. BioDrugs 2002;16(3):223–5.
21. Sprung J, Kindscher JD, Wahr JA, Levy JH, Monk TG, Moritz MW, O'Hara PJ. The use of bovine hemoglobin glutamer-250 (Hemopure) in surgical patients: results of a multicenter, randomized, single-blinded trial. Anesth Analg 2002;94(4):799–808.
22. Levy JH, Goodnough LT, Greilich PE, Parr GV, Stewart RW, Gratz I, Wahr J, Williams J, Comunale ME, Doblar D, Silvay G, Cohen M, Jahr JS, Vlahakes GJ. Polymerized bovine hemoglobin solution as a replacement for allogeneic red blood cell transfusion after cardiac surgery: results of a randomized, double-blind trial. J Thorac Cardiovasc Surg 2002;124(1):35–42.

Oxymetazoline and xylometazoline

General Information

Oxymetazoline and xylometazoline are alpha-adrenoceptor agonists, which seem to be better tolerated than other topically used drugs of this sort.

Organs and Systems

Ear, nose, throat

Nasal irritation, with dryness of the mouth and throat, can occur; a rebound effect on the nasal mucosa was found in some 5% of cases studied (1).

Sensory systems

The development of an acute retinal artery obstruction in a young, otherwise healthy man was associated with excessive use of an oxymetazoline nasal spray. Platelet coagulation studies indicated a platelet aggregation hypersensitivity to adenosine diphosphate and adrenaline. Predisposition to sympathomimetic drug-induced platelet fibrin embolus formation may have played a role in this case (2).

Oxymetazoline has a vasoconstrictor effect and this has been reported to have caused an ischemic retinopathy (3).

- A 43-year-old woman with hypertension and diabetes mellitus used 2–3 puffs of oxymetazoline nasal spray and experienced painless blurring of vision in the right eye, with a corrected acuity of 20/400 (20/50 on the left). Apart from background diabetic retinopathy she had edema of the optic disk. Several weeks later she used the spray again and this time developed blurred vision in the left eye. There was disk pallor on both sides and acuities were 20/400 on the right and 20/70 on the left. There were also segmental inferior field defects in both eyes. After 6 weeks both eyes had recovered somewhat, but only to 20/200 and 20/50 respectively: there was no further improvement after a year.

The authors concluded that this was sequential bilateral ischemic retinopathy due to oxymetazoline.

Long-Term Effects

Drug withdrawal

The interruption of a high dose nasal spray therapy precipitated a prolonged panic disorder in a healthy man (SEDA-13, 109).

Second-Generation Effects

Fetotoxicity

Repeated use of an oxymetazoline nasal spray has been associated with changes in fetal heart rate demonstrated as a non-reactive, non-stress test and late decelerations in a patient at 41 weeks of gestation; 6 hours after the last dose these changes gradually disappeared (4).

Susceptibility Factors

Age

Systemic adverse reactions of ocular administration have been reported in young children (5).

Drug Administration

Drug overdose

An unusual response to an overdose of oxymetazoline (0.05% nasal spray) occurred in an elderly patient who used the product several times daily; the patient, who had pre-existing cerebellar degeneration and peripheral neuropathy, developed severe bradycardia and oscillations in systolic pressure between 236 and 60 mmHg. Withdrawal of the spray resulted in complete recovery (6).

References

1. Feinberg AR, Feinberg SM. The "nose drop nose" due to oxymetazoline (Afrin) and other topical vasoconstrictors. IMJ Ill Med J 1971;140(1):50–2.

2. Magargal LE, Sanborn GE, Donoso LA, Gonder JR. Branch retinal artery occlusion after excessive use of nasal spray. Ann Ophthalmol 1985;17(8):500–1.
3. Fivgas GD, Newman NJ. Anterior ischemic optic neuropathy following the use of a nasal decongestant. Am J Ophthalmol 1999;127(1):104–6.
4. Baxi LV, Gindoff PR, Pregenzer GJ, Parras MK. Fetal heart rate changes following maternal administration of a nasal decongestant. Am J Obstet Gynecol 1985;153(7):799–800.
5. Higgins GL 3rd, Campbell B, Wallace K, Talbot S. Pediatric poisoning from over-the-counter imidazoline-containing products. Ann Emerg Med 1991;20(6):655–8.
6. Glazener F, Blake K, Gradman M. Bradycardia, hypotension, and near-syncope associated with Afrin (oxymetazoline) nasal spray. N Engl J Med 1983;309(12):731.

Oxyphenbutazone

See also Non-steroidal anti-inflammatory drugs

General Information

Oxyphenbutazone is a parahydroxylated analogue of phenylbutazone, and is one of its active metabolites. It has the same spectrum of activity, therapeutic uses, interactions, dangers, and contraindications. In April 1985, Ciba-Geigy decided to stop sales of systemic dosage forms of oxyphenbutazone worldwide. They stated that they had reached this decision because a survey had shown that although the recommended limitations on the use of phenylbutazone had been widely respected, the same could not be said of oxyphenbutazone. Evidence that oxyphenbutazone was more likely to cause death due to bone marrow failure than phenylbutazone (1) was provided by data from the UK's Committee on Safety of Medicines. Furthermore, according to Ciba-Geigy's re-assessment in January 1984, deaths per million prescriptions of oxyphenbutazone were 5.5 (USA) to 12.8 (UK) compared with phenylbutazone (3.8–7.6 deaths per million prescriptions) (SEDA-9, 87).

Reference

1. Anonymous. Phenylbutazone and oxyphenbutazone: time to call a halt. Drug Ther Bull 1984;22(2):5–6.

Oxyphencyclamine

General Information

Oxyphencyclamine is an anticholinergic drug, which is claimed to act for some 12 hours. However, the wide range of oral doses used (10–50 mg/day) indicate doubt about its potency.

Oxyphenonium

See also Anticholinergic drugs

General Information

Like methanthelinium, oxyphenonium is an anticholinergic drug with relatively marked ganglion-blocking effects, but it seems to have little effect on the central nervous system; an oral dose of 5–10 mg given several times a day produces typical anticholinergic effects. Its efficacy is rather poor (1).

Reference

1. Martan A, Voigt R, Halaska M. Untersuchungen zur medikamentosen Behandlung der Urge-Inkontinenz der Frau. [Drug therapy of urge incontinence in the female.] Zentralbl Gynakol 1993;115(5):205–9.

Oxytocin and analogues

General Information

Oxytocin is a hypothalamic nonapeptide that selectively stimulates the smooth muscle of the uterus and mammary glands. It is used in the induction or augmentation of labor and to prevent postpartum hemorrhage, and is well tolerated and effective in a wide range of infusion rates and concentrations. Contraindications to its use include placenta previa or vasa previa, a previous classical uterine incision, pelvic structural deformities, and an abnormal fetal presentation. Large fetal size and high maternal parity are relative contraindications. Prior non-classical cesarean delivery should not preclude oxytocin therapy.

Uterine contractions and fetal heart rate should be monitored during oxytocin administration (SEDA-13, 1310) (1,2). There is no significant increase in uterine complications or in fetal morbidity or mortality in women with a previous cesarean section, although oxytocin-treated patients had a higher rate of failed trial of labor for reasons that are unclear (3). Oxytocin is structurally similar to vasopressin, and like the latter has water-retaining properties when used in pharmacological doses.

Oxytocin is in common use during induction of labor and in the third stage of labor to prevent uterine atony and postpartum hemorrhage. Carbetocin, a synthetic analogue with a half-life 4–10 times longer than the native hormone, has been studied in trials; both agents cause a small transient fall in blood pressure (less than 4 mmHg) (4). Common mild adverse effects of both drugs include headache, flushing, a feeling of warmth, a metallic taste, and abdominal pain.

Organs and Systems

Cardiovascular

Tachycardia and a fall in blood pressure are common and usually short-lived after oxytocin administration during labor. There has been one reported maternal death after a hypovolemic woman was given a bolus dose of oxytocin 10 units (5).

In 34 women undergoing cesarean section at full term under spinal anesthesia, heart rate and cardiac output increased significantly within 2 minutes of the rapid administration of either 5 or 10 units of oxytocin, with an associated 10 mmHg fall in mean arterial pressure in those who received 10 units (6). There were significant ST segment changes in 11 of 26 women undergoing cesarean section, with raised concentrations of troponin I in two; however, the relationship to oxytocin administration was not clear in this report (7).

- A previously fit 19-year-old woman had severe ST segment depression and increased troponin concentrations after a bolus dose of oxytocin 5 units (8).

Ventricular tachycardia has been reported in two patients with pre-existing prolongation of the QT interval, immediately after oxytocin was begun (9).

Fluid balance

Fluid retention causing severe hyponatremia and convulsions has been observed in neonates after administration of oxytocin and salt-poor fluids to the mother during labor.

Acute water intoxication has produced maternal cerebral edema and convulsions in under 50 reported cases, both with intravenous and intranasal administration (10). The risk is higher in women given high doses of the drug in combination with salt-poor intravenous fluids. In rare cases this has been fatal.

Hematologic

Maternal oxytocin administration increases the rate of neonatal physiological jaundice in a dose-dependent manner (SEDA-13, 1310) (11). This effect may be due to hemodilution and an increased rate of hemolysis.

Second-Generation Effects

Pregnancy

In a retrospective analysis of 2774 women who had had one prior cesarean delivery, there was a 1% incidence of uterine rupture in women who were given oxytocin, compared with 0.4% in non-augmented controls with spontaneous labor (12). Six women needed emergency hysterectomy. The odds ratio for uterine rupture in the oxytocin-treated women was 4.6 by logistic regression analysis (CI = 1.5,14). The small number of events limited the study: it had only 30% power to detect changes of that magnitude. However, it is reasonable to proceed cautiously, with close clinical observation, given the potentially severe outcome.

- Uterine rupture occurred when oxytocin was started 5 hours after the administration of a second misoprostol tablet for induction of labor, although the usual recommendation is to wait at least 12 hours (13).
- A 36-year-old multiparous woman had a ruptured uterus after labor was induced at 24 weeks with misoprostol 200 μg and augmented with oxytocin (14).

The risk of uterine rupture is increased by previous cesarean section, fetal weight over 4 kg, and the use of oxytocin (SEDA-24, 506) (15,16). In 24 women with uterine rupture after oxytocin, the dose and duration of use of oxytocin were 10% higher than in controls; this difference was not statistically significant, but the power of the study was limited by the small sample size (17).

References

1. Owen J, Hauth JC. Oxytocin for the induction or augmentation of labor. Clin Obstet Gynecol 1992;35(3): 464–75.
2. ACOG. Technical Bulletin Number 157. Int J Obstet 1991;39:139.
3. Chelmow D, Laros RK Jr. Maternal and neonatal outcomes after oxytocin augmentation in patients undergoing a trial of labor after prior cesarean delivery. Obstet Gynecol 1992: 80(6):966–71.
4. Dansereau J, Joshi AK, Helewa ME, Doran TA, Lange IR, Farine D, Schulz ML, Horbay GL, Griffin P, Wassenaar W. Double-blind comparison of carbetocin versus oxytocin in prevention of uterine atony after cesarean section. Am J Obstet Gynecol 1999;180(3 Pt 1): 670–6.
5. Why mothers die 1997–1999. The confidential enquiries into maternal deaths in the United Kingdom. London: RCOG Press, 2001.
6. Pinder AJ, Dresner M, Calow C, Shorten GD, O'Riordan J, Johnson R. Haemodynamic changes caused by oxytocin during caesarean section under spinal anaesthesia. Int J Obstet Anesth 2002;11(3):156–9.
7. Moran C, Ni Bhuinneain M, Geary M, Cunningham S, McKenna P, Gardiner J. Myocardial ischaemia in normal patients undergoing elective Caesarean section: a peripartum assessment. Anaesthesia 2001;56(11):1051–8.
8. Spence A. Oxytocin during Caesarean section. Anaesthesia 2002;57:710–11.
9. Liou SC, Chen C, Wong SY, Wong KM. Ventricular tachycardia after oxytocin injection in patients with prolonged Q-T interval syndrome—report of two cases. Acta Anaesthesiol Sin 1998;36(1):49–52.
10. Mayer-Hubner B. Pseudotumour cerebri from intranasal oxytocin and excessive fluid intake. Lancet 1996; 347(9001):623.
11. Sakala EP, Kaye S, Murray RD, Munson LJ. Oxytocin use after previous cesarean: why a higher rate of failed labor trial? Obstet Gynecol 1990;75(3 Pt 1):356–9.
12. Zelop CM, Shipp TD, Repke JT, Cohen A, Caughey AB, Lieberman E. Uterine rupture during induced or augmented labor in gravid women with one prior cesarean delivery. Am J Obstet Gynecol 1999;181(4):882–6.
13. Fletcher H, McCaw-Binns A. Rupture of the uterus with misoprostol (prostaglandin El) used for induction of labour. J Obstet Gynaecol 1998;18(2):184–5.

14. Al-Hussaini TK. Uterine rupture in second trimester abortion in a grand multiparous woman. A complication of misoprostol and oxytocin. Eur J Obstet Gynecol Reprod Biol 2001;96(2):218–19.
15. Aboyeji AP, Ijaiya MD, Yahaya UR. Ruptured uterus: a study of 100 consecutive cases in Ilorin, Nigeria. J Obstet Gynaecol Res 2001;27(6):341–8.
16. Diaz SD, Jones JE, Seryakov M, Mann WJ. Uterine rupture and dehiscence: ten-year review and case-control study. South Med J 2002;95(4):431–5.
17. Goetzl L, Shipp TD, Cohen A, Zelop CM, Repke JT, Lieberman E. Oxytocin dose and the risk of uterine rupture in trial of labor after cesarean. Obstet Gynecol 2001;97(3):381–4.